Clinical
Medicine
Selected Problems With
Pathophysiologic Correlations

CLINICAL MEDICINE

Selected Problems With Pathophysiologic Correlations

Edited and with contributions by

H. VERDAIN BARNES, M.D.

Professor and Chairman
Department of Medicine
Wright State University School of Medicine
Dayton, Ohio

Associate editors

JAMES W. AGNA, M.D.
BARRETT H. BOLTON, M.D.
KIM GOLDENBERG, M.D.
H. BRADFORD HAWLEY, M.D.
CHARLES B. PAYNE, JR., M.D.

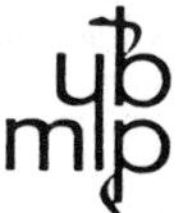

YEAR BOOK MEDICAL PUBLISHERS, INC.
Chicago • London • Boca Raton

1 2 3 4 5 6 7 8 9 0 ME 91 90 89 88 87

Library of Congress Cataloging-in-Publication Data

Barnes, H. Verdain (Herman Verdain), 1935–
    Clinical medicine.

    Includes bibliographies and index.
    1. Internal medicine. I. Title. [DNLM: 1. Diagnosis,
Differential—problems. 2. Internal Medicine—problems.
3. Pathology—problems. WB 18 B261c]
RC46.B26 1988   616   87-16052
ISBN 0-8151-0489-8

Sponsoring Editor: Richard H. Lampert
Assistant Director, Manuscript Services: Frances M. Perveiler
Production Manager, Text and Reference/Periodicals: Etta Worthington

DEDICATION

We wish to dedicate this volume to our parents, wives,
and children who have supported us in our profession.

CONTRIBUTORS

A. K. AGARWAL, M.D.
Clinical Instructor of Medicine
Wright State University
School of Medicine
Dayton, Ohio

JAMES W. AGNA, M.D.
Professor of Medicine
Wright State University
School of Medicine
Dayton, Ohio

ARNOLD ALLEN, M.D.
Professor of Psychiatry
Wright State University
School of Medicine
Dayton, Ohio

SHERMAN J. ALTER, M.D.
Assistant Professor of Pediatrics
Wright State University
School of Medicine
Dayton, Ohio

JOSEPH ASKENAZI, M.D.
Clinical Associate Professor of Medicine
Wright State University
School of Medicine
Dayton, Ohio

DENNIS D. BARBER, M.D.
Associate Professor of Obstetrics and Gynecology
Wright State University
School of Medicine
Dayton, Ohio

CHRISTOPHER J. BARDE, M.D.
Assistant Professor of Medicine
Wright State University
School of Medicine
Dayton, Ohio

H. VERDAIN BARNES, M.D.
Professor and Chairman
Department of Medicine
Wright State University
School of Medicine
Dayton, Ohio

MICHAEL A. BAUMANN, M.D.
Assistant Professor of Medicine
Wright State University
School of Medicine
Dayton, Ohio

JACK M. BERNSTEIN, M.D.
Associate Professor of Medicine and Microbiology and
   Immunology
Wright State University
School of Medicine
Dayton, Ohio

BLAINE BLOCK, M.D.
Clinical Associate Professor of Otolaryngology
Wright State University
School of Medicine
Dayton, Ohio

BARRETT H. BOLTON, M.D.
Professor of Medicine and Pharmacology
Wright State University
School of Medicine
Dayton, Ohio

JOHN D. BULLOCK, M.D., M.S.
Professor of Ophthalmology
Wright State University
School of Medicine
Dayton, Ohio

JAE C. CHANG, M.D.
Clinical Professor of Medicine
Wright State University
School of Medicine
Dayton, Ohio

NICHOLAS P. CHRISTOFF, M.D.
Clinical Instructor in Medicine
Wright State University
School of Medicine
Dayton, Ohio

MAX A. CLARK, D.O.
Assistant Professor of Obstetrics and Gynecology
Wright State University
School of Medicine
Dayton, Ohio

STEVEN M. COHEN, M.D.
Assistant Professor of Medicine
Wright State University
School of Medicine
Dayton, Ohio

MICHAEL P. COYLE, M.D.
Resident Instructor of Medicine
Wright State University
School of Medicine
Dayton, Ohio

PHIL D. CRAFT, M.D.
Clinical Associate Professor of Plastic and Reconstructive
  Surgery
University of Tennessee
College of Medicine
Chattanooga, Tennessee

JORGE CRESPO, M.D.
Associate Professor of Medicine
Wright State University
School of Medicine
Dayton, Ohio

JOHN S. CZACHOR, M.D.
Resident Instructor of Medicine
Wright State University
School of Medicine
Dayton, Ohio

MARGARET M. DUNN, M.D.
Assistant Professor of Surgery
Wright State University
School of Medicine
Dayton, Ohio

DANIEL W. ELLIOT, M.D.
Professor and Chair of Surgery
Wright State University
School of Medicine
Dayton, Ohio

TONI I. EVANS, M.D.
Assistant Professor of Medicine
Wright State University
School of Medicine
Dayton, Ohio

ALICE FARYNA, M.D.
Associate Professor of Medicine
Wright State University
School of Medicine
Dayton, Ohio

EDWARD B. FEINBERG, M.D.
Clinical Assistant Professor of Ophthalmology
University of Tennessee
College of Medicine
Chattanooga, Tennessee

H. ALLAN FELLER, M.D.
Clinical Associate Professor of Medicine
Wright State University
School of Medicine
Dayton, Ohio

JOHN A. FLEISHMAN, M.D.
Fellow of Ophthalmology
Wright State University
School of Medicine
Dayton, Ohio

RONALD D. FOSTER, M.D.
Clinical Assistant Professor of Medicine
Wright State University
School of Medicine
Dayton, Ohio

KIM GOLDENBERG, M.D.
Associate Professor of Medicine
Wright State University
School of Medicine
Dayton, Ohio

ROBERT A. GOLDENBERG, M.D.
Associate Professor and Chair of Otolaryngology
Wright State University
School of Medicine
Dayton, Ohio

N. GOPALSWAMY, M.D.
Associate Professor of Medicine
Wright State University
School of Medicine
Dayton, Ohio

JACK S. GRUBER, M.D.
Assistant Professor of Obstetrics and Gynecology
Wright State University
School of Medicine
Dayton, Ohio

SATYENDRA C. GUPTA, M.D.
Associate Professor of Medicine
Wright State University
School of Medicine
Dayton, Ohio

JOHN J. HALKI, M.D., Ph.D.
Associate Professor and Chair of Obstetrics and
  Gynecology and Pharmacology and Toxicology
Wright State University
School of Medicine
Dayton, Ohio

GLENN C. HAMILTON, M.D.
Professor and Chair of Emergency Medicine and Associate
  Professor of Medicine
Wright State University
School of Medicine
Dayton, Ohio

ROBERT A. HAWKINS, M.D.
Clinical Assistant Professor of Medicine
Wright State University
School of Medicine
Dayton, Ohio

H. BRADFORD HAWLEY, M.D.
Professor of Medicine and Associate Professor of
    Postgraduate Medicine and Continuing Education
Wright State University
School of Medicine
Dayton, Ohio

ABRAHAM HELLER, M.D.
Professor of Psychiatry
Wright State University
School of Medicine
Dayton, Ohio

JAMES V. HENNESSEY, M.D.
Clinical Assistant Professor of Medicine
Wright State University
School of Medicine
Dayton, Ohio

RICHARD J. HILDEBRANDT, M.D.
Professor of Obstetrics and Gynecology
Wright State University
School of Medicine
Dayton, Ohio

TIMOTHY G. JANZ, M.D.
Assistant Professor of Medicine and Emergency Medicine
Wright State University
School of Medicine
Dayton, Ohio

SMITH L. JOHNSTON, III, M.D.
Resident Instructor of Medicine and Aerospace Medicine
Wright State University
School of Medicine
Dayton, Ohio

LARRY M. JONES, M.D.
Clinical Assistant Professor in Surgery
Wright State University
School of Medicine
Dayton, Ohio

RUSSELL A. JONES, M.D.
Clinical Assistant Professor of Medicine
University of Tennessee
College of Medicine
Chattanooga, Tennessee

HYTHAM A. KADRIE, M.D.
Clinical Assistant Professor of Medicine
University of Tennessee
College of Medicine
Chattanooga, Tennessee

PATRICK A. KELLEY, M.D.
Clinical Assistant Professor of Medicine
University of Tennessee
College of Medicine
Chattanooga, Tennessee

PAUL KEZDI, M.D.
Professor Emeritus of Medicine
Wright State University
School of Medicine
Dayton, Ohio

HOBART E. KLAAREN, M.D.
Professor and Chair of Orthopedic Surgery
Wright State University
School of Medicine
Dayton, Ohio

JAMES T. LEHNER, M.D.
Associate Professor of Orthopedic Surgery
Wright State University
School of Medicine
Dayton, Ohio

HOWARD P. LISS, M.D.
Assistant Professor of Medicine
Wright State University
School of Medicine
Dayton, Ohio

MICHAEL J. MARKUS, M.D.
Clinical Instructor of Medicine
Wright State University
School of Medicine
Dayton, Ohio

THOMAS MATHEWS, M.D.
Associate Professor of Neurology and Pathology
Wright State University
School of Medicine
Dayton, Ohio

STEPHEN D. McDONALD, M.D.
Associate Professor of Medicine
Wright State University
School of Medicine
Dayton, Ohio

SIDNEY F. MILLER, M.D.
Clinical Professor of Surgery
Wright State University
School of Medicine
Dayton, Ohio

CHETNA MITAL, M.D.
Resident Instructor of Medicine
Wright State University
School of Medicine
Dayton, Ohio

CLYDE T. MIYAKI, M.D.
Clinical Instructor of Medicine
Wright State University
School of Medicine
Dayton, Ohio

VENKATACHALAM MUTHIAH, M.D.
Clinical Assistant Professor of Medicine
Wright State University
School of Medicine
Dayton, Ohio

WILLIAM A. NAHHAS, M.D.
Professor of Obstetrics and Gynecology
Wright State University
School of Medicine
Dayton, Ohio

JAIME PACHECO, M.D.
Associate Professor of Medicine
Wright State University
School of Medicine
Dayton, Ohio

JOHN G. PATY, JR., M.D.
Clinical Associate Professor of Medicine
University of Tennessee
College of Medicine
Chattanooga, Tennessee

CHARLES B. PAYNE, JR., M.D.
Associate Professor of Medicine
Wright State University
School of Medicine
Dayton, Ohio

JAMES B. PEOPLES, M.D.
Associate Professor of Surgery
Wright State University
School of Medicine
Dayton, Ohio

SAMUEL E. PITNER, M.D.
Professor and Chair of Neurology
Wright State University
School of Medicine
Dayton, Ohio

JOSEPH PREMANANDAN, M.D.
Clinical Assistant Professor of Medicine
Wright State University
School of Medicine
Dayton, Ohio

ANDREW RITTENBERRY, M.D.
Clinical Associate Professor of Surgery
University of Tennessee
College of Medicine
Chattanooga, Tennessee

MEINHARD ROBINOW, M.D.
Professor of Pediatrics
Wright State University
School of Medicine
Dayton, Ohio

MOSHEN SAKHAII, M.D.
Clinical Associate Professor of Medicine
Wright State University
School of Medicine
Dayton, Ohio

MOHAMMAD G. SAKLAYEN, M.D.
Assistant Professor of Medicine
Wright State University
School of Medicine
Dayton, Ohio

HOWARD J. SCHWARTZ, M.D.
Professor of Medicine
Case Western Reserve University
School of Medicine
Cleveland, Ohio

RICHARD A. SERBIN, M.D.
Clinical Professor of Medicine
Wright State University
School of Medicine
Dayton, Ohio

ADEL N. SHENOUDA, M.D.
Clinical Associate Professor of Medicine
University of Tennessee
College of Medicine
Chattanooga, Tennessee

DANIEL SIMON, M.D.
Clinical Assistant Professor of Medicine
Wright State University
School of Medicine
Dayton, Ohio

TIMOTHY B. SORG, M.D.
Assistant Professor of Medicine
Wright State University
School of Medicine
Dayton, Ohio

ALVIN L. STEIN, M.D.
Clinical Assistant Professor of Medicine
Wright State University
School of Medicine
Dayton, Ohio

JOSEPH STEMPLE, Ph.D.
Professor of Otolaryngology
Wright State University
School of Medicine
Dayton, Ohio

A. G. SURYAPRASAD, M.D.
Associate Professor of Medicine
Wright State University
School of Medicine
Dayton, Ohio

DIETMAR V. TRULZSCH, M.D.
Assistant Professor of Medicine
Wright State University
School of Medicine
Dayton, Ohio

MARGARET A. TURK, M.D.
Assistant Professor of Physical Medicine and Rehabilitation
    and Pediatrics
Wright State University
School of Medicine
Dayton, Ohio

ROBERT P. TURK, M.D.
Clinical Associate Professor of Surgery
Wright State University
School of Medicine
Dayton, Ohio

BARRY A. WARNER, D.O.
Assistant Professor of Medicine
Wright State University
School of Medicine
Dayton, Ohio

SYLVAN L. WEINBERG, M.D.
Clinical Professor of Medicine
Wright State University
School of Medicine
Dayton, Ohio

LARRY W. WEPRIN, M.D.
Clinical Assistant Professor of Medicine
Wright State University
School of Medicine
Dayton, Ohio

GILBERT L. WERGOWSKE, M.D.
Assistant Professor of Medicine
Wright State University
School of Medicine
Dayton, Ohio

J. H. WITTOESCH, M.S., M.D.
Clinical Associate Professor of Surgery
Wright State University
School of Medicine
Dayton, Ohio

ROBERT T. WITTY, M.D., Ph.D.
Clinical Associate Professor of Medicine
Wright State University
School of Medicine
Dayton, Ohio

HOWARD F. WUNDERLICH, M.D.
Assistant Professor of Medicine
Wright State University
School of Medicine
Dayton, Ohio

JACKSON JOE YIUM, M.D.
Clinical Professor of Medicine
University of Tennessee
College of Medicine
Chattanooga, Tennessee

PREFACE

The ability to relate underlying pathophysiology to the clinical manifestations of a patient's illness is critical to the understanding and practice of clinical medicine. This book:

1. Emphasizes the clinical–pathologic correlations of a broad spectrum of disorders, typically with a table depicting the relationships.

2. Provides a discussion of the major features of the clinical presentation, clinical course, differential diagnosis, diagnostic criteria, and basic concepts of therapy for over 135 common or catastrophic disorders.

3. Is concise, with chapters ranging from two to five pages and containing an average of three useful tables or figures and six key annotated references.

This book was conceived and designed for the medical student who is making the transition into the world of clinical medicine. This major milestone in medical education is often difficult and there is a need for a concise presentation of the subject matter, which can provide a general overview and stimulate the student to seek additional depth from a standard comprehensive specialty text.

The methods used by medical schools to facilitate this transition are varied, but the goal is to reorient the student's focus toward integrating basic science and basic knowledge of pathophysiology into the clinical practice of medicine. Although there are outstanding encyclopedic pathophysiology and clinical medicine texts available to the student, "user friendliness" (to borrow from the language of computer technology) regarding focused, easily readable information is hard to find. For example, in the 1980s, the time required for the student beginning clinical medicine to read a typical pathophysiology textbook of over 1,000 pages and a clinical medicine textbook of 1,500 to 2,200 pages is substantial; for most students, amounting to in excess of 250 hours of concentrated reading time. Furthermore, there may not be a standard format for correlating the pathophysiologic findings of a disorder with its clinical manifestations.

Over the years many of our students have asked about a concise, carefully formatted, readable text with a focus on clinical-pathologic correlations. This book attempts to meet these needs with a relatively short, easily readable text with a standard format. To accomplish these goals, only selected topics could be included and each would need to be brief and accurate rather than fully comprehensive. The topics included were selected on the basis of their relative frequency of occurrence or potential catastrophic outcome when viewed from the perspective of clinical practice. They were identified from a review of the introduction to clinical medicine and the third-year core clerkship content of several medical schools, plus a review of the available literature defining the most common problems encountered in the clinical practice of medicine.

The authors were recruited from the faculty of the Wright State University School of Medicine and, to a lesser extent, the University of Tennessee College of Medicine in Chattanooga. Each chapter was edited by a professional medical editor, followed by author confirmation and an external peer review.

This text can be used as a basic or supplemental text for students in their introduction to medicine and core clinical clerkships. In addition, it may be used by residents in training and perhaps busy practitioners as a quick, up-to-date review of selected topics. We hope it is user friendly and will serve as a practical guide to a better understanding of clinical medicine while stimulating the desire to attain a greater depth of knowledge from the more detailed and comprehensive pathophysiology and clinical medicine texts as well as the current medical literature.

H. VERDAIN BARNES, M.D.

JAMES W. AGNA, M.D.

BARRETT H. BOLTON, M.D.

KIM GOLDENBERG, M.D.

H. BRADFORD HAWLEY, M.D.

CHARLES B. PAYNE, JR, M.D.

ACKNOWLEDGMENTS

A significant component in the preparation of this text was the review and critique of the chapters by an outstanding group of peer reviewers who graciously provided their expertise to specific chapters. We wish to express our deep appreciation to:

MURRY D. ALTOSE, M.D.
Case Western Reserve University
School of Medicine
Cleveland, Ohio

JOHN AMATRUDA, M.D.
University of Rochester
School of Medicine and Dentistry
Rochester, New York

DOUGLAS L. BECHARD, M.D.
University of Tennessee
College of Medicine
Chattanooga, Tennessee

FRANK H. BOEHM, M.D.
Vanderbilt University
School of Medicine
Nashville, Tennessee

ROBERT C. CODDINGTON, M.D.
University of Tennessee
College of Medicine
Chattanooga, Tennessee

DONALD D. BROWN, M.D.
University of Iowa
College of Medicine
Iowa City, Iowa

ANNE DAVIDSON, M.D.
Wright State University
School of Medicine
Dayton, Ohio

PETER DENSON, M.D.
University of Iowa
College of Medicine
Iowa City, Iowa

JOHN FLAHERTY, M.D.
The Johns Hopkins
School of Medicine
Baltimore, Maryland

HERBERT FLESSA, M.D.
University of Cincinnati
College of Medicine
Cincinnati, Ohio

THOMAS E. HOBBINS, M.D.
University of Maryland
School of Medicine
Baltimore, Maryland

RICHARD J. KOZERA, M.D.
University of Cincinnati
College of Medicine
Cincinnati, Ohio

WILLIAM LAWTON, M.D.
University of Iowa
College of Medicine
Iowa City, Iowa

DENNIS E. NIEWOEHNER, M.D.
University of Minnesota
Medical School
Minneapolis, Minnesota

GEORGE PAULSON, M.D.
Ohio State University
College of Medicine
Columbus, Ohio

KENNETH SCHER, M.D.
Wright State University
School of Medicine
Dayton, Ohio

CHARLES STRATTON, M.D.
Vanderbilt University
School of Medicine
Nashville, Tennessee

KENNETH WALKER, M.D.
Emory University
School of Medicine
Atlanta, Georgia

ROBERT W. SUMMERS, M.D.
University of Iowa
College of Medicine
Iowa City, Iowa

ANDREW WELTON, M.D.
The Johns Hopkins University
School of Medicine
Baltimore, Maryland

ALEXANDER S. TOWNES, M.D.
University of Tennessee
College of Medicine
Memphis, Tennessee

Our professional medical editor, Martha Tacker, Ph.D., of Richmond, Indiana, provided us with invaluable editing.

We also express our appreciation to William D. Sawyer, M.D., Dean of the Wright State University School of Medicine, for his encouragement and support, to the Wright State University School of Medicine Word Processing Center for the preparation of the final manuscript, and to Joyce G. Barnes, the coordinating secretary for the book.

THE EDITORS

CONTENTS

PREFACE   xii

ACKNOWLEDGMENTS   xiv

Part I
GENERAL CLINICAL PROBLEMS

1. USE AND LIMITATIONS OF DIAGNOSTIC TESTS   3

    Kim Goldenberg

2. ACID-BASE DISORDERS   8

    Jackson Joe Yium

3. FEVER OF UNKNOWN ORIGIN   16

    Howard F. Wunderlich

4. JAUNDICE   23

    Dietmar V. Trulzsch

5. HYPERTENSION   28

    Kim Goldenberg

6. HEADACHE   37

    Samuel E. Pitner

7. COMA AND STATES OF DIMINISHED CONSCIOUSNESS   44

    Samuel E. Pitner

8.   DEMENTIA   50

     Thomas Mathews

9.   DYSPNEA   57

     Charles B. Payne, Jr.

10. HEMOPTYSIS   61

     Timothy G. Janz

11. GASTROINTESTINAL BLEEDING   65

     Christopher J. Barde

12. BOWEL OBSTRUCTION   70

     Dan W. Elliot

13. ABDOMINAL TRAUMA   77

     Larry M. Jones

14. STINGING INSECT VENOM ALLERGY   82

     Howard J. Schwartz

15. GENETIC DISEASES APPEARING AS CATASTROPHIC ILLNESSES: APPROACHES
     TO DIAGNOSIS   85

     Meinhard Robinow

16. MALNUTRITION   87

     Smith L. Johnston, III and Kim Goldenberg

17. THERMAL INJURIES   95

     Sidney F. Miller

18. WOUND HEALING   101

     Phil D. Craft

Part II
CIRCULATORY DISORDERS

19. ANGINA PECTORIS   109

A. G. Suryaprasad

20. ACUTE MYOCARDIAL INFARCTION   117

Moshen Sakhaii and Sylvan L. Weinberg

21. CONGESTIVE HEART FAILURE   126

Satyendra C. Gupta

22. CARDIOMYOPATHY   134

A. G. Suryaprasad

23. VENTRICULAR ARRHYTHMIAS   144

Joseph Askenazi and A. K. Agarwal

24. ATRIAL ARRHYTHMIAS   152

Satyendra C. Gupta

25. MITRAL VALVE DISEASE   159

Paul Kezdi

26. AORTIC VALVE DISEASE   165

Satyendra C. Gupta

27. TRAUMATIC HEART DISEASE   175

Moshen Sakhaii and Sylvan L. Weinberg

28. PERIPHERAL ARTERY DISEASE   180

Margaret M. Dunn

29. VENOUS INSUFFICIENCY   187

James B. Peoples

30. DEEP VEIN THROMBOSIS   **190**

Steven M. Cohen

Part III
RESPIRATORY DISORDERS

31. CHRONIC AIRFLOW OBSTRUCTION   **199**

Charles B. Payne, Jr.

32. LUNG CANCER   **204**

Charles B. Payne, Jr.

33. ACUTE BACTERIAL PNEUMONIA   **210**

Jorge Crespo

34. ATYPICAL PNEUMONIA   **218**

Charles B. Payne, Jr.

35. LUNG ABSCESS   **223**

Timothy B. Sorg

36. ASTHMA   **227**

Glenn C. Hamilton

37. ADULT RESPIRATORY DISTRESS SYNDROME   **235**

Jorge Crespo

38. INTERSTITIAL LUNG DISEASE   **241**

Charles B. Payne, Jr.

39. SARCOIDOSIS   **246**

Alvin L. Stein

40. CYSTIC FIBROSIS   **250**

Howard P. Liss

41.   PNEUMOTHORAX   254

Howard P. Liss

42.   PLEURAL EFFUSION   258

Howard P. Liss

Part IV
INFECTIOUS DISEASES

43.   UPPER RESPIRATORY INFECTION: STREPTOCOCCAL PHARYNGITIS AND THE
      COMMON COLD   265

Toni I. Evans and Kim Goldenberg

44.   INFECTIOUS MONONUCLEOSIS   269

Jack M. Bernstein

45.   INFLUENZA   273

Jack M. Bernstein

46.   ACUTE SINUSITIS   277

Steven M. Cohen

47.   URINARY TRACT INFECTION   280

Adel N. Shenouda

48.   BACTEREMIA AND SEPTIC SHOCK   284

Jorge Crespo

49.   INFECTIVE ENDOCARDITIS   289

H. Bradford Hawley

50.   CLOSTRIDIAL INFECTIONS   295

Michael J. Markus and H. Bradford Hawley

51.   INFECTION IN THE IMMUNOCOMPROMISED HOST   302

Howard F. Wunderlich

52. SEXUALLY TRANSMITTED DISEASES   309

Dennis D. Barber

53. ACQUIRED IMMUNODEFICIENCY SYNDROME (AIDS)   317

Timothy B. Sorg

54. PARASITIC DISEASES   324

Barrett H. Bolton

55. TUBERCULOSIS   331

Howard P. Liss

56. HISTOPLASMOSIS   338

H. Bradford Hawley

Part V
GASTROINTESTINAL DISORDERS

57. ESOPHAGEAL REFLUX   345

Christopher J. Barde

58. PEPTIC ULCER DISEASE   349

N. Gopalswamy

59. GASTRIC CARCINOMA   354

N. Gopalswamy and Christopher J. Barde

60. GALLBLADDER DISEASE   358

James B. Peoples

61. VIRAL HEPATITIS   361

Dietmar V. Trulzsch

62. ALCOHOLIC CIRRHOSIS   368

Christopher J. Barde

63.   HEPATOCELLULAR CARCINOMA   373

Larry W. Weprin

64.   PANCREATITIS   377

Christopher J. Barde

65.   ADULT DIARRHEAL ILLNESSES   381

Clyde T. Miyaki and Christopher J. Barde

66.   INFLAMMATORY BOWEL DISEASE   387

N. Gopalswamy

67.   ACUTE APPENDICITIS   394

Dan W. Elliot

68.   DIVERTICULOSIS COLI   400

Dan W. Elliot

69.   PERIANAL DISEASES   406

J. H. Wittoesch

70.   COLORECTAL CARCINOMA   411

Robert P. Turk

71.   COMMON HERNIAS   416

Margaret M. Dunn

Part VI
HEMATOLOGIC DISORDERS

72.   COAGULATION DISORDERS   423

Barrett H. Bolton

73.   IRON DEFICIENCY ANEMIA   429

Jaime Pacheco and Michael A. Baumann

74.   HEMOLYTIC ANEMIAS   433

Jaime Pacheco and Michael A. Baumann

75.   MEGALOBLASTIC ANEMIA   440

Jaime Pacheco and Michael A. Baumann

76.   MYELOPROLIFERATIVE DISEASES   445

Michael A. Baumann and Jaime Pacheco

77.   ACUTE NONLYMPHOCYTIC LEUKEMIA   450

Michael A. Baumann and Jaime Pacheco

78.   CHRONIC LYMPHOCYTIC LEUKEMIA   455

Russell A. Jones

79.   NON-HODGKIN'S LYMPHOMA   461

Michael A. Baumann and Jaime Pacheco

80.   HODGKIN'S DISEASE   466

Russell A. Jones

81.   MULTIPLE MYELOMA   472

Jae C. Chang

Part VII
ENDOCRINE AND METABOLIC DISORDERS

82.   DIABETES INSIPIDUS   481

Barry A. Warner and James V. Hennessey

83.   HYPERTHYROIDISM   487

H. Verdain Barnes

84.   HYPOTHYROIDISM   494

Richard A. Serbin

85. THYROIDITIS   499

James V. Hennessey and Barry A. Warner

86. ADRENAL CRISIS   505

James W. Agna

87. DIABETES MELLITUS   510

Stephen D. McDonald

88. FASTING HYPOGLYCEMIA   516

Barry A. Warner and James V. Hennessey

89. HYPERNATREMIA   521

Joseph Premanandan

90. HYPONATREMIA   524

Joseph Premanandan

91. HYPERKALEMIA AND HYPOKALEMIA   529

Daniel Simon

92. HYPERMAGNESEMIA AND HYPOMAGNESEMIA   541

James W. Agna

93. HYPERCALCEMIA AND HYPOCALCEMIA   546

James W. Agna

94. HYPOPHOSPHATEMIA   553

Mohammad G. Saklayen

Part VIII
RENAL AND REPRODUCTIVE DISORDERS

95. NEPHROLITHIASIS   561

Mohammad G. Saklayen and Chetna Mital

96. GLOMERULONEPHRITIS   567

Nicholas P. Christoff

97. NEPHROTIC SYNDROME   577

Robert T. Witty

98. ACUTE RENAL FAILURE   583

Venkatachalam Muthiah

99. CHRONIC RENAL FAILURE   590

H. Allan Feller

100. HYPERNEPHROMA   596

Gilbert L. Wergowske

101. PROSTATE CANCER   600

Barrett H. Bolton

102. BENIGN BREAST DISEASE   606

Margaret M. Dunn

103. BREAST CANCER   610

Andrew B. Rittenberry

104. DYSMENORRHEA   617

Dennis D. Barber

105. AMENORRHEA   620

Jack S. Gruber

106. PREGNANCY COMPLICATIONS   628

Richard J. Hildebrandt

107. MENOPAUSE AND CLIMACTERIC   633

John J. Halki

108. UTERINE CARCINOMA   639

Max A. Clark

109. OVARIAN CARCINOMA   644

William A. Nahhas

Part IX
EYE AND EAR DISORDERS

110. COMMON SYMPTOMS OF OTOLOGIC DISEASE   651

Robert A. Goldenberg

111. OTITIS MEDIA   657

Sherman J. Alter

112. HOARSENESS   661

Blaine Block and Joseph Stemple

113. COMMON OCULAR DISORDERS   668

John A. Fleishman and John D. Bullock

114. REFRACTIVE ERRORS   675

John A. Fleishman and John D. Bullock

115. STRABISMUS AND AMBLYOPIA   678

John A. Fleishman and John D. Bullock

116. GLAUCOMA   683

John A. Fleishman and John D. Bullock

117. EYELID AND CONJUNCTIVAL DISEASES   688

Edward B. Feinberg

118. RETINAL DISEASES   691

John A. Fleishman and John D. Bullock

119. OCULAR MALIGNANCY   698

John A. Fleishman and John D. Bullock

Part X
NERVOUS SYSTEM AND PSYCHIATRIC DISORDERS

120. STROKE: OCCLUSIVE CEREBRAL VASCULAR DISEASE   707

Samuel E. Pitner

121. INTRACRANIAL HEMORRHAGE   714

Samuel E. Pitner

122. SEIZURE DISORDERS   719

Thomas Mathews

123. INTRACRANIAL TUMORS   725

Thomas Mathews

124. MENINGITIS   733

John S. Czachor and H. Bradford Hawley

125. BRAIN ABCESS   740

Michael P. Coyle and Timothy B. Sorg

126. PARKINSON'S DISEASE   745

Patrick A. Kelley

127. MYASTHENIA GRAVIS   749

Hytham A. Kadrie

128. MULTIPLE SCLEROSIS   753

Thomas Mathews

129. NEUROMUSCULAR DISORDERS   757

Samuel E. Pitner and Margaret A. Turk

130. CEREBRAL PALSY   764

Margaret A. Turk and Samuel E. Pitner

131. ANXIETY DISORDERS   771

Abraham Heller and Arnold Allen

132. DEPRESSION   774

Arnold Allen and Abraham Heller

133. SCHIZOPHRENIA   780

Abraham Heller and Arnold Allen

134. SUBSTANCE ABUSE   785

Abraham Heller and Arnold Allen

Part XI
JOINT, CONNECTIVE TISSUE AND SKELETAL DISORDERS

135. RHEUMATOID ARTHRITIS   793

Alice Faryna

136. SYSTEMIC LUPUS ERYTHEMATOSUS   799

Robert A. Hawkins

137. SYSTEMIC VASCULITIS   807

Alice Faryna

138. RAYNAUD'S PHENOMENON   816

Alice Faryna and Kim Goldenberg

139. PROGRESSIVE SYSTEMIC SCLEROSIS   821

John G. Paty, Jr.

140. POLYMYALGIA RHEUMATICA AND GIANT CELL ARTERITIS   824

John G. Paty, Jr.

141. OSTEOPOROSIS   828

Gilbert L. Wergowske

142. OSTEOARTHRITIS   833

Ronald D. Foster and Robert A. Hawkins

143. GOUT AND PSEUDOGOUT   838

Toni I. Evans

144. SEPTIC ARTHRITIS   844

Alice Faryna and Kim Goldenberg

145. OSTEOMYELITIS   850

John S. Czachor and H. Bradford Hawley

146. COMMON FRACTURES   858

Hobart E. Klaaren

147. SCOLIOSIS AND SPINAL DEFORMITIES   860

James T. Lehner

148. BURSITIS AND TENDONITIS   867

John G. Paty, Jr.

149. INTERVERTEBRAL DISC DISEASE   873

Samuel E. Pitner

INDEX   881

Clinical Medicine

Selected Problems With Pathophysiologic Correlations

part I

General Clinical Problems

USE AND LIMITATIONS OF DIAGNOSTIC TESTS

Kim Goldenberg, M.D.

The contribution of the history, physical examination, and laboratory studies to the formulation of a differential diagnosis is traditionally considered to be about 75%, 20%, and 5%, respectively. The exponential growth of laboratory tests in the past 30 years, however, including noninvasive measurements of most body secretions in picomolar quantities and invasive measurements of most body tissues by radiography or biopsy, requires the modern physician to have a comprehensive understanding of the use and limits of these tests. Because over 50 billion dollars per year are spent on hospital laboratory tests, it is not surprising that cost containment is an increasing problem along with scrutiny of medical bills by third-party payers. The appropriate use of tests requires some familiarity with testing characteristics (sensitivity and specificity) and, more importantly, with the clinical basis for ordering a particular test, including the physician's estimate of the likelihood that the patient has the disease and of the prevalence of the disease. Some factors to be considered before ordering a test include whether (1) the test is intended to exclude or confirm a diagnosis, (2) the test results will significantly change the probability of a disease, (3) further action is needed if results are abnormal or false positive, (4) the mean value for normal and diseased persons are known, and (5) the test is invasive or noninvasive.

TO EXCLUDE A POTENTIAL DIAGNOSIS

A 30-year-old black woman complains of photosensitivity of one year's duration. If no other clinical findings are present, the differential diagnosis should initially include potentially common and catastrophic diseases. One such disease is systemic lupus erythematosis (SLE). The likelihood of this disease is very low given that only one of eleven criteria is evident in this patient. A very sensitive test to detect the disease is required because if the test result is negative, the disease would be virtually excluded. For example, if the antinuclear antibody (ANA) test had a sensitivity of 99% (99 positive tests in 100 patients with the disease), then only 1 out of 100 persons with SLE would have a negative test result.

Most very sensitive tests are usually not very specific and vice versa. If the ANA test had a specificity of 80% (80 negative results in 100 normal people), then 20 out of 100 normal persons would have a positive test. This high false-positive rate is the price paid when a test is not very specific for a disease. An advantage to tests such as the ANA, in which there is a range of abnormal values represented by a titer rather than a distinct cutoff level, is that the specificity for the disease increases the higher the titer. For example, a 1:80 titer for the ANA test is fairly nonspecific, whereas a 1:640 titer makes SLE more likely.

The need for a very sensitive test to help exclude a disease can be applied to symptoms and signs as well as to laboratory tests. For example, a 30-year-old woman complains of three episodes of palpitations per month and has a family history of Graves' disease. The most common physical finding, (i.e., the finding with the highest sensitivity) in Graves' disease is a goiter (found in 97 of 100 patients). The presence of a goiter, however, is not specific for Graves' disease and may be found in other thyroid diseases. In contrast, the absence of a goiter would almost certainly exclude Graves' disease because only 3 of 100 patients with that disease do not have a goiter.

TO CONFIRM A DIAGNOSIS

If a test with a high sensitivity and low specificity is used to exclude a disease, but the test result is unexpectedly positive, another test becomes necessary to confirm the diagnosis. For example, if the 30-year-old black woman with photosensitivity has a positive ANA test (a test with high sensitivity and low specificity), another test is required. A test for SLE with a high specificity might include an antinuclear double-stranded DNA test (anti-DNA test). If the specificity is 98% (98 negative tests in 100 normal persons), then only 2 of 100 normal persons would have a positive test. Thus a positive test result is highly specific for SLE and would strongly support the presence of the disease. A negative test result, however, would not exclude the disease; this is because the anti-DNA test may have a relatively poor sensitivity of 73% (i.e., only 73 of 100 patients with SLE will have a positive test).

The trade-off between high sensitivity and low specificity can be applied to symptoms and signs as well as laboratory tests. For example, a 70-year-old patient with dyspnea on exertion, while performing routine activities of daily living, might have disease involving the pulmonary or cardiac system. Dyspnea is a sensitive indicator of heart failure, but is not specific for heart failure. In contrast, the physical finding of an S_3 ventricular gallop would be specific for heart failure in this patient (i.e., elderly without other diseases) and would strongly support its presence. The poor sensitivity of an S_3 gallop for detecting heart failure, however, would mean that its absence would not exclude the disease. Few tests have both a high sensitivity and specificity, and there are no tests that are 100% accurate given observer, laboratory, and subject variability.

PROBABILITY OF DISEASE: BEFORE AND AFTER A TEST

"Medicine is a science of uncertainty and an art of probability."[1] Given a test result, the probability of a patient having a disease (posttest probability) depends to a greater extent on the probability of his or her having the disease before ordering the test (pretest probability) than on the test characteristics of sensitivity and specificity (Bayes' theorem). Pretest proba-

bility is based on clinical judgment or disease prevalence or both. Perhaps one of the best tested applications of Bayes' theorem is in cardiac stress testing. If a stress test has a sensitivity of 70% and specificity of 80% (for > 1-mm ST depression) the probability of having significant coronary artery disease can be predicted, if a patient's age, sex, and chest pain description are given. These predictions of having coronary artery disease depend on the extent of ST depression and have been substantiated by both coronary arteriograms and autopsy studies. Formulations of posttest probabilities are shown in Table 1–1.

For example, if a 30-year-old man complains of several minutes of sharp chest pain which is unrelated to activity, studies show that he has less than a 5% chance of having coronary artery disease before ordering any test. A positive stress test (> 1-mm ST depression) increases the likelihood of disease from 5% to 16% and is, therefore, not helpful in confirming the disease. A negative stress test, however, decreases the likelihood of disease from 5% to 2%, and thus, would virtually exclude coronary artery disease. In this setting either test result hardly changes the likelihood of the disease.

Similar limitations on the outcome of testing are found when the likelihood of disease is very high or very low. For example, a 65-year-old man with the tight chest pain characteristic of angina pectoris has about a 95% probability of having significant coronary artery disease. A positive stress test increases the likelihood of disease from 95% to 99%. A negative stress test decreases the likelihood of disease from 95% to 88% and, therefore, is not particularly helpful in excluding the disease. In this setting, too, the likelihood of the disease is not much affected by either test result.

The optimal benefit of a test occurs when the uncertainty of whether a patient has or does not have disease is greatest. For example, a 45-year-old man who complains of burning chest pain, which is worse with activity, has about a 50% probability of having coronary artery disease. A positive stress test in this setting would increase the likelihood of coronary ar-

---

[1]Sir William Osler, quoted by William B. Bean in *Sir William Osler: Aphorisms*. Springfield, Ill. Charles C. Thomas, 1961.

TABLE 1–1.
Formulation of Posttest Probability Based on Bayes' Theorem

POSTTEST PROBABILITY GIVEN A POSITIVE TEST

$$= \frac{\text{pretest probability} \times \text{sensitivity}}{\text{pretest probability} \times \text{sensitivity} + (1 - \text{pretest probability}) \times (1 - \text{specificity})}$$

POSTTEST PROBABILITY GIVEN A NEGATIVE TEST

$$= \frac{\text{pretest probability} \times (1 - \text{sensitivity})}{\text{pretest probability} \times (1 - \text{sensitivity}) + (1 - \text{pretest probability}) \times \text{specificity}}$$

tery disease from 50% to 78%, and a negative test would decrease the likelihood from 50% to 27%. Although the test in this setting does not confirm or exclude the disease, a significant change in probability occurs. The importance of pretest probability as illustrated by this example is general and, therefore, widely applicable in the evaluation of clinical problems on the interpretation of test outcome.

THE UNEXPECTED ABNORMAL RESULT

Physicians deal with an unexpected abnormal test result in a variety of ways, including observation, repetition of the test, ordering other tests, and immediate treatment based on the results. An example is a 45-year-old asymptomatic man with an elevated aspartate transcarbamoylase (AST) level on a routine screening panel. The decision strategy depends on the extent of deviation from normal. Most laboratories define the normal boundaries for upper and lower limits as contained within two standard deviations (i.e., to include 95% of the normal population). Therefore, 2.5% of the normal population will be below the lower limit, and 2.5% will be above the upper limit of normal. Most borderline values or values just outside the limits defined by the laboratory are from normal individuals. The differential diagnosis, therefore, depends in part on the extent of enzyme elevation. After requestioning the patient for obvious causes of an elevated AST level, such as infection, drug or ethanol use, and not receiving an answer to pinpoint a cause, several possible strategies are available.

For a minimally elevated AST, observation of the patient with reassessment at a future date

or an immediate repeat of the test would not likely affect the outcome of the disease. The first strategy is possible in a compliant patient who could be reassured and the second in a noncompliant patient who could not be effectively reassured. Moderate-to-severe elevations of the AST level would suggest a pathologic condition requiring additional testing. Treatment with a medication or hospitalization would not be warranted in this patient, but there are circumstances in which the unexpected abnormal result could lead to this strategy.

For example, in a 45-year-old asymptomatic man, a history of diabetes and an unexpected elevation of the MB isoenzyme of creatine kinase (CK) suggests the possibility of a "silent" myocardial infarction. Further testing with an ECG would be helpful but would not influence the decision to hospitalize this patient for observation because a normal ECG would not exclude the diagnosis of coronary artery disease. Fortunately, on a statistical basis this scenario is uncommon. The unexpected abnormal test result is usually minimally elevated, which often represents a false-positive result, or it is moderately-to-severely elevated with the cause usually revealed during the comprehensive history and physical examination or unmasked by further specific questioning and examination of the patient.

EXPECTATIONS FROM A TEST PANEL OR BATTERY

A test panel or battery of tests is frequently ordered to screen for disease and contain costs; multiple tests are usually less expensive than ordering fewer individual tests. Most laboratory tests have a 95% confidence interval, or a 5% false-positive rate. When ordering multiple tests, therefore, the false-positive rate increases in proportion to the number of tests ordered. For example, the 12 tests in a routine chemistry panel together will have a 46% false-positive rate assuming that each test is independent regarding the information it provides. We know, however, that in a typical chemistry panel the elevation of the alkaline phosphatase and aspartate transcarbamoylase levels may reflect the same or different pathophysiologic changes. Similarly, the serum creatinine and blood urea nitrogen levels, are, in part, interdependent. For any disease process it is unlikely that more than half of the tests are interdependent; if 6 out of the 12 tests are interdependent, a high false-positive rate of 26% occurs. The routine ordering of a test panel or battery of 12 chemistries can, therefore, be expected to result in an overall false-positive result 26% to 46% of the time, when no underlying pathologic change is present. These routinely encountered false-positive tests can be effectively analyzed with the strategies discussed in the previous section.

TENDENCY OF REPEATED TESTS TO MOVE TOWARD THE MEAN VALUE

A test value, in a normal person, that is minimally elevated or depressed just outside the normal range will often, on repeat testing, revert to a value within the normal range. This fundamental law of nature is statistically called regression to the mean; for example, if the mean potassium level of the normal population is 4.0 mEq/L and the standard deviation is 0.25 mEq/L, the normal range (which includes two standard deviations above and below the mean) is then defined as a potassium value between 3.5 and 4.5 mEq/L. If the potassium value is 3.4 mEq/L in a patient, then repeating the test will produce a number closer to 4.0 mEq/L if no pathologic condition is affecting the potassium level. In contrast, if the potassium value outside the normal range is the result of a disease in the patient, then repeat testing will usually give a result closer to the mean value of that measurement for the associated disease. For example, if the mean value of potassium in a group of patients with primary aldosteronism

is 3.1 mEq/L, then repeating the measurement for a patient with an original value of 2.5 mEq/L would tend to move the value closer to 3.1 mEq/L.

This same principle applies to physical signs such as blood pressure. For example, an initial blood pressure of 144/94 mm Hg in a 30-year-old person has on repeated measurement about a 25% chance of reverting toward the population mean, which is less than 140/90 mm Hg. Multiple measurements of blood pressure over several weeks will, therefore, often bring perceived mild elevations back toward normal. This occurs in part because the patient is less anxious when having the pressure measured in a familiar environment and in part due to a regression toward the mean. This concept is also helpful in understanding why patients with severe elevations of blood pressure may have lower values on repeated measurement but rarely low enough to be considered normal. For example, a 50-year-old patient with an initial blood pressure of 190/120 mm Hg may revert on repetition to a more moderately elevated blood pressure reading (e.g., 170/110), but even the mean blood pressure readings for this person will still be in the high range and will require urgent treatment. The chance of this patient's blood pressure reverting to normal on subsequent readings without treatment is remote.

INVASIVE VERSUS NONINVASIVE TESTS

"The appearance of the bull changes as one leaves the grandstand and enters the ring."[2] In choosing between invasive and noninvasive tests whose sensitivities and specificities are similar, the noninvasive test is usually preferred by the patient. Invasive tests are, however, usually much more sensitive and specific than their noninvasive counterparts. The choice of the appropriate test involves a comparison of the potential risks and benefits of the procedure and a consideration of the patient's perception and wishes. Invasive procedures are often ordered when clinical uncertainty exists. Unless the outcome is significantly affected by the result, however, the risk of morbidity and

---

[2] Old Spanish proverb.

mortality often exceeds the benefit. For example, a 50-year-old patient with a five-year history of chronic renal disease of undetermined cause and no recent change in renal status would not benefit from a renal biopsy. The minimal gain of information regarding the prognosis would generally not outweigh the risk of the procedure. In contrast, a patient with an acute onset of renal failure of undetermined cause and rapid progression might benefit from a renal biopsy if treatment and outcome could be affected by the result.

The rapid evolution of tests and increasing public awareness have created a modern agenda regarding the patient's desire to know everything about his or her care and a desire to preserve autonomy in decisions concerning that care. Morris Abrams, the previous chairperson of the President's Commission on Bioethics and Medicine which evaluated the use of technology, recently published their findings in over 16,000 pages of manuscript. The fundamental and unanimous finding of this committee was that 95% of the public considered their autonomy to be paramount regarding medical decisions about their care. In general, the greater the risk of the procedure or treatment, the more involved the person wished to be in the decision-making process. The ultimate choice of invasive versus noninvasive tests, therefore, often rests as much with the patient as it does on the clinical judgment of the caring physician.

In summary, the flourishing of laboratory tests has caused a number of common problems to develop for the modern, discerning physician. Because symptoms are not pathognomonic for a disease and clinical findings are only suggestive, a very sensitive test is indicated to exclude common and catastrophic diseases. In contrast, when a disease is strongly suspected because of a previous test or from clinical examination, a specific test is indicated to confirm the diagnosis. In considering the probability of a disease, although the test characteristics (sensitivity and specificity) are important, the pretest probability has the greatest influence on posttest probability; this concept of Bayes' theorem emphasizes clinical judgment over any test result. Given the large array of available tests, abnormal findings with potential false-positive results are common. Strategies for dealing with abnormal results include further observation, repeat testing, other testing, and treatment. Multiple test panels or batteries regularly produce abnormal test results. These abnormalities are often false-positive results when the test value is only minimally elevated or depressed from the normal range. Repeating, these will often result in normal values as the previous borderline or minimally abnormal values regress toward the normal mean value. Finally, invasive tests are best ordered when the disease outcome is affected by the results and when the patient's sense of autonomy is preserved.

REFERENCES

Bradwell AR, Carmalt MHB, Whitehead TP: Explaining the unexpected abnormal results of biochemical profile investigations. *Lancet* 1974; II:1071–1074. *A succinct discussion helpful in understanding abnormal tests from a panel or battery.*

Cutler P: *Problem Solving in Clinical Medicine: From Data to Diagnosis,* ed 2. Baltimore, Williams & Wilkins, Co, 1985. *A comprehensive review of problem solving and data management, with numerous examples for each organ system.*

Goldenberg K, Snyder DK: Screening for primary aldosteronism: Hypokalemia and hypertension. *J Gen Intern Med* 1986; 1:368–372. *How to determine a test cutoff level when using a common test to detect a rare disease.*

Griner PF, Mayewski RJ, Mushlin AI, Greenland P: Selection and interpretation of diagnostic tests and procedures: Principles and applications. *Ann Intern Med* 1981; 94(part 2):553–600. *The best presentation of the principles that are used in understanding, choosing, and interpreting diagnostic tests.*

Griner PF, Panzer RJ, Greenland P: *Clinical Diagnosis and the Laboratory: Logical Strategies for Common Medical Problems.* Chicago, Year Book Medical Publishers, 1986. *Principles of test selection and interpretation, with numerous clinical examples, which emphasize a systematic approach to the integration of clinical information.*

Knotman DD, Curada N, Tan EN: Profiles of antinuclear antibodies in systemic rheumatic diseases. *Ann Intern Med* 1975; 83:464–469. *A concise review of laboratory tests in rheumatic disease.*

McNeil BJ, Keeler E, Adelstein SJ: Primer on certain elements of decision making. *N Engl J Med* 1975; 293:211–215. *A pithy review of fundamental con-*

cepts regarding testing and decision making, with some examples.

Weiner DA, Ryan TJ, McCabe CH: Exercise stress testing. Correlations among history of angina, ST-segment response and prevalence of coronary-artery disease in the coronary artery surgery study (CASS). *N Engl J Med* 1979; 301:230–235. *A comprehensive presentation of how the exercise stress test is interpreted as a function of the pretest clinical findings.*

Weinstein MC, Fineberg HV: *Clinical Decision Analysis.* Philadelphia, WB Saunders Co, 1980. *An in-depth analysis of the decision-making process including the advantages and disadvantages of a variety of test strategies.*

Wong ET, McCarron MM, Shaw ST Jr: Ordering of laboratory tests in a teaching hospital: Can it be improved? *JAMA* 1983; 249:3076–3080. *A review of the pros and cons of hospital testing and a presentation of a potential strategy for modifying it.*

2 ACID–BASE DISORDERS

Jackson Joe Yium, M.D.

The pH of normal blood ranges from 7.36 to 7.44 with an average of 7.40. The pH can also be expressed as the hydrogen-ion concentration, which is 40 mEq/L for an average pH. Although the hydrogen-ion concentration appears to be more precise in asssessing acid–base disturbances, clinicians use the pH because it is easy to measure and is a widely available clinical test. Blood pH is maintained by an effective interaction of the carbonic acid-bicarbonate buffer system and the lung and kidney functions. The body's buffers include carbonic acid/bicarbonate, phosphates, and protein buffers which respond to the need to buffer H^+ or to form an acid. Daily activities, such as eating, sleeping, and exercising, generate an enormous quantity of H^+ ion (approximately 12,000 mEq/day), which is virtually all channeled into the formation of carbonic acid (H_2CO_3) so that is can be eliminated by the lungs as the carbonic acid is broken down to CO_2 and H_2O (i.e., $H_2CO_3 \rightarrow CO_2 + H_2O$). A small amount of H^+ ion (75–100 mEq/day) is not converted into carbonic acid and other acids (sulfuric and phosphoric acid and other organic acids) and must be eliminated by the kidney. There is a complex interdependency of these body systems to maintain a normal pH (Table 2–1).

The Henderson-Hasselbach equation characterizes the pH of the blood. This equation is

$$pH = 6.1 \log \frac{[HCO_3]}{H_2CO_3}$$

The bicarbonate concentration is determined by metabolic and renal factors. The carbonic acid concentration is related to ventilatory changes by the lung. For clinical purposes the carbonic acid concentration is derived from measurement of the arterial partial pressure of carbon dioxide (Pa_{CO_2}) multiplied by 0.03 (the solubility coefficient for CO_2 at 37°C). The modified Henderson-Hasselbach equation is

$$pH + \log \frac{[HCO_3]}{0.03 \times Pa_{CO_2}}$$

The normal values for the critical acid–base factors are given in Table 2–1, and a classification of the simple acid–base disturbances is given in Table 2–2. A decrease in pH by an increasing hydrogen-ion concentration (pH < 7.36) is acidosis or acidemia. An increase of the pH (pH > 7.44) by a decrease in hydrogen-ion concentration is alkalosis or al-

TABLE 2–1.

Regulation of Blood ph and Normal Values of Acid–Base Serum Factors

BODY COMPONENTS

1. *Body buffer systems*—participate in immediate and long-term response to acid or alkaline challenges
Extracellular buffers—Carbonic acid/bicarbonate, phosphates, proteins
Intracellular buffers—Hemoglobin, proteins, organic phosphate complexes in bone
Maintains body pH = 7.36 to 7.44; H+ = 39 to 42 mEq/L
2. *Lungs*—ventilation of carbon dioxide = 10 to 12 moles/day; maintains Pa_{CO_2} = 37 to 45 mm Hg. Compensates for metabolic acidosis by increasing ventilation, compensates for metabolic alkalosis by decreasing ventilation.
3. *Kidneys*—Reclamation by the renal tubules of bicarbonate filtered from the blood by the glomeruli. Approximately 4500 mEq/day. Excretion as titratable acids and ammonium of 50 to 100 mEq hydrogen/day generated by breakdown of food stuffs. Compensates for respiratory alkalosis by decreasing $[H^+]$ excretion, compensates for respiratory acidosis by increasing $[HCO_3]$ absorption.
Maintains serum bicarbonate = 24 to 26 mEq/L

TABLE 2–2.

Classification of Some Common Causes of Simple Acid–Base Disorders

RESPIRATORY ACIDOSIS: PRIMARY DECREASE IN CO_2 RELEASED BY THE LUNGS.
Pa_{CO_2} is increased.
Acute—Sudden changes in Pa_{CO_2} without renal compensation—serum bicarbonate normal or slightly increased.
Example: Sedative or illicit drug (heroin, cocaine) overdose. Attempt at weaning from mechanical ventilator.
Chronic—Accompanied by renal compensation—serum bicarbonate is high.
Example: Chronic obstructive lung disease; neurological disease with respiratory paralysis—Guillain-Barré syndrome; spinal cord injury.
RESPIRATORY ALKALOSIS: PRIMARY INCREASE IN CO_2 RELEASED BY THE LUNGS.
Pa_{CO_2} is low. Example: Anxiety, hyperventilation syndrome, pneumonia, pregnancy, hepatic coma, CNS injury.
METABOLIC ACIDOSIS: PRIMARY DECREASE IN SERUM BICARBONATE LEVEL RESULTING FROM AN ACCUMULATION OF STRONG ACIDS OR LOSS OF BICARBONATE FROM EXTRACELLULAR FLUID.
Normal anion gap—Serum chloride increased. Example: Renal tubular acidosis, tubule-interstitial renal disease.
Increased anion gap—Increase in unmeasured anions. Example: Diabetic ketoacidosis, lactic acidosis, chronic renal insufficiency (uremic acidosis), alcohol intoxication.
METABOLIC ALKALOSIS: PRIMARY INCREASE IN SERUM BICARBONATE.
Sodium chloride-responsive—Due to volume contraction with secondary mineralocorticoid excess usually accompanied by hypokalemia. Example: Non-potassium-sparing diuretic use, gastrointestinal losses due to vomiting or suctioning.
Sodium chloride-resistant—Primary mineralocorticoid excess with volume expansion. Usually have hypertension and hypokalemia. Example: Cushing's syndrome, primary aldosteronism.
Increased bicarbonate loads—Increased oral or intravenous intake of bicarbonate or alkalizing salts. Example: Infusions of acetate with total parental alimentation.

kalemia. When the major initiating process is related to respiration and ventilation produces an increase or decrease in Pa_{CO_2}, it is a *respiratory* acidosis or alkalosis, respectively. A primary increase or decrease in the serum bicarbonate results in a *metabolic* alkalosis or acidosis, respectively. For each initiating process, there is a normal physiologic response to compensate for the change. Respiratory acidosis will be compensated for by an increase in bicarbonate reabsorption by the kidney causing a rise in serum bicarbonate. Acute metabolic acidosis will be compensated by hyperventilation and a concomitant fall in Pa_{CO_2}.

An acid–base disturbance in which the initiating abnormality is counteracted by an appropriate physiologic response is termed a *simple* acid–base disorder. The compensatory process is not always complete and may be limited by other physiologic responses or underlying pathology. In a *mixed* acid–base disorder, two or more concurrent processes may effectively nullify any major effect on the pH, such as respiratory acidosis and metabolic alkalosis, or may markedly worsen the abnormality, such as respiratory and metabolic acidosis.

DIAGNOSIS OF ACID–BASE DISORDERS

Accurate and reliable laboratory data are critical in the diagnosis and management of acid–base disorders. In the clinical assessment of an acid–base disorder it is *always* necessary to know the values of any *two* of the following three parameters (1) arterial pH, (2) arterial P_{CO_2}, and (3) serum bicarbonate concentration. Additionally, it is important to evaluate the full serum electrolyte pattern to determine the chloride, potassium, and bicarbonate concentrations. Measurement of serum urea nitrogen (SUN) and serum creatinine provide important information about the patient's renal function and volume status. In many instances, an acid–base disturbance can be determined by correlating the physical examination, clinical setting, and electrolyte pattern. For example, a patient with protracted nausea and vomiting, low blood pressure of 90/60 mm Hg, respirations of 12, tachycardia of 130 with a low normal serum sodium of 135 mEq/L, low potassium 2.5 mEq/L, low normal chloride 95 mEq/L, and elevated bicarbonate 35 mEq/L would be expected to have a metabolic alkalosis.

An acid–base disturbance should be considered in patients with unexplained changes in their clinical condition, such as confusion, seizures, hypotension, tachypnea, or cardiac arrhythmias. Acute respiratory acidosis and alkalosis may be detected by a sudden development of respiratory distress accompanied by a change in respiratory rate. Severe alkalosis may cause tetany and seizures. In patients with a chronic illness, acid–base changes may be subtle, asymptomatic, or lead to relatively nonspecific symptoms, such as weakness or anorexia. In these cases, the monitoring of serum electrolytes and arterial pH and/or P_{CO_2} will be necessary to detect and characterize acid–base changes. Examples include patients treated with diuretics and patients with chronic obstructive pulmonary disease, liver disease, or renal insufficiency. Tables 2–3 through 2–6 list the expected range of compensatory response for the Pa_{CO_2} or serum bicarbonate and some of the signs and symptoms that may be associated with common acid–base disturbances.

METABOLIC ACIDOSIS AND ALKALOSIS

Metabolic acidosis and alkalosis result from alterations in the serum bicarbonate concentration. Metabolic acidosis, as a pathophysiologic state, is characterized by a gain in strong acids or loss of bicarbonate from the extracellular fluid (Table 2–3). The serum bicarbonate will be decreased. It can be classified on the basis of changes in the unmeasured anions, *the anion gap* (AG), into an increased or normal AG acidosis. The anion gap is calculated by subtracting the sum of the serum chloride and bicarbonate concentrations from the serum sodium concentration (i.e., $AG = [Na^+] - ([Cl^-] + [HCO_3^-])$; normal 12–14 mEq/L). This estimates the quantity of anions not routinely measured, such as negatively charged proteins, the anions of organic acids, sulfates, and phosphates. Acidosis due to an increase in organic acids, such as keto or lactic acidosis or the acidosis of chronic renal insufficiency, in which the organic acids, sulfates, and phosphates accumulate, is characterized by an increased anion gap (> 14 mEq/L) and decrease in serum chloride. If a base accumulates, the anion gap will remain normal, as in renal tubular acidosis which produces a hyperchloremic acidosis in which serum bicarbonate reduction is offset by the renal retention of chloride.

Severe acidosis (pH ≤ 7.0) may cause profound physiologic disturbances including severe hypotension and heart failure. At the cellular level, changes in pH affect both O_2 saturation (Bohr effect) and the release of O_2 at the tissue level by the red blood cells through the oxygen-binding enzyme—2,3-diphosphoglycerate (2,3 DPG). The Bohr effect produces an increase in O_2 saturation by acidosis and a decrease in saturation by alkalosis. This is an immediate effect. Chronic changes alter the concentration of 2,3 DPG. Acidosis decreases red blood cell binding of O_2 with an increased release of O_2 to the tissue. Acidosis may be accompanied by hyperkalemia due primarily to shifts of potassium from intracellular sites to the extracellular fluid compartments as in the case of the acidosis of chronic renal failure. Re-

TABLE 2–3.
Metabolic Acidosis
Signs and symptoms: Tachypnea, confusion, hypotension, anorexia.
Findings related to cause of acidosis (i.e., sepsis, shock, renal failure)

	SERUM ACID–BASE FACTORS					
NORMAL VALUES	pH 7.36–7.44	Pa_{CO_2} 37–45 mm Hg	HCO_3 24–26 mEq/L	Na^+ 135–145 mEq/L	K^+ 3.5–4.5 mEq/L	Cl 95–105 mEq/L
DIRECTION OF CHANGE IN METABOLIC ACIDOSIS	↓	↓ Compensatory response*	↓ Primary abnormality	⇔ No change	↑ ↑ (usually)[†]	↑ or ↓
TYPICAL VALUES: NORMAL ANION GAP‡ < 14 mEq/L	7.20	25	10	140	6.5[†]	115
ELEVATED ANION GAP > 14 mEq/L§	7.20	25	10	140	5.5	100

* Expected range of compensation: Pa_{CO_2} decrease of 1.5 mm Hg [HCO_3^-] + 8 ± 2 mEq/L. ‖
† Low potassium occurs with renal tubular acidosis (Types I and II, see text).
‡ As occurs with mild renal failure due to interstitial nephritis.
§ As occurs with diabetic ketoacidosis and lactic acidosis.
‖ Data from Narins and Emmett, 1980.

TABLE 2–4.
Metabolic Alkalosis
Signs and symptoms: Confusion, rhythm disturbances, weakness, paresthesia, tetany.

	SERUM ACID–BASE FACTORS					
NORMAL VALUES	pH 7.36–7.44	Pa_{CO_2} 37–45 mm Hg	HCO_3^- 24–26 mEq/L	Na^+ 135–145 mEq/L	K^+ 3.5–4.5 mEq/L	Cl^- 95–105 mEq/L
DIRECTION OF CHANGE IN METABOLIC ALKALOSIS	↑	↑ Compensatory response*	↑ Primary abnormality	⇔ No change	↓ Usually	↓
TYPICAL VALUES[†]	7.50	48	40	138	2.5	85

* Expected range of compensation: Pa_{CO_2} increases 0.6 mm Hg for each mEq/L increase in [HCO_3^-].‡
† As occurs with severe vomiting, diuretics, primary aldosteronism.
‡ Data from Narins and Emmett, 1980.

nal tubular acidosis (RTA) is a group of disorders related to abnormal tubular transport of hydrogen or bicarbonate ions. Two types of RTA involving abnormalities of the "distal" and "proximal" tubules (Types I and II) are associated with hypokalemia due to renal potassium wasting. Another type (Type IV) may cause hyperkalemia due to renal potassium retention and low aldosterone secretion.

Metabolic alkalosis is characterized by a gain in bicarbonate or a loss of nonvolatile acids from the extracellular fluid (Table 2–4) and results in an increase in the serum bicarbonate concentration. It is probably the most common acid–base disturbance encountered in clinical practice. It can be classified into two main groups, based on the patient's volume status— *sodium chloride responsive* or *sodium chloride resistant.* These terms are used to characterize the volume state and should not be taken to mean that saline infusion be used to distinguish the two processes. Sodium chloride-responsive alkalosis is the most common, resulting from a loss of sodium, hydrogen, potassium, and chloride ions resulting in volume depletion. Common causes are the loss of hydrogen and chloride ions from the gastrointestinal tract by vomiting or nasogastric suction, or loss of sodium and potassium chloride through the kidney from the use of non–potassium-sparing diuretics. Chloride lost through the gastrointestinal tract or kidneys leads to volume depletion which is a stimulus for enhanced sodium absorption by the kidney which is accompanied by increased bicarbonate absorption. Volume depletion states, besides causing enhanced bicarbonate and sodium absorption, lead secondarily to an increased secretion of aldosterone from the adrenal glands which enhances potassium and hydrogen excretion by the kidneys. Hypokalemia with a body deficit in potassium results in a cellular loss of potassium and enhanced bicarbonate and sodium reabsorption by the kidney. In the absence of diuretic administration, measurement of urine chloride levels will be low (< 20 mEq/L).

Sodium chloride-resistant alkalosis is less common. In this setting hormones with mineralocorticoidlike action initiate sodium retention by the kidney which leads to a concomitant loss of hydrogen and potassium ions. Examples are Cushing's syndrome (an excess of corticosteroid hormones) and primary aldosteronism. These patients are volume expanded, hypokalemic, and may be hypertensive. Urine chloride levels will be elevated (> 20 mEq/L).

An increase in body buffers through the infusion or increased oral intake of bicarbonate, lactate, or acetate may also cause metabolic alkalosis.

The assessment of metabolic alkalosis requires an evaluation of the patient's volume status to establish whether there has been a volume loss (chloride ion loss) as an initiating factor (sodium chloride-responsive alkalosis), or if the potassium and hydrogen ion loss is due to an initiating mineralocorticoid effect (sodium chloride-resistant alkalosis). Measurement of urine chloride may be helpful in making the distinction.

RESPIRATORY ACIDOSIS AND ALKALOSIS

Respiratory acidosis and respiratory alkalosis are ventilation-induced acid–base abnormalities. Respiratory alkalosis occurs when CO_2 excretion exceeds production (Table 2–5). Factors that stimulate alveolar hyperventilation cause respiratory alkalosis, except in the case of a primary metabolic acidosis in which case the response is secondary. In an acute disturbance, patients are tachypnic and may be in respiratory distress. Examples are anxiety, hysteria with hyperventilation syndrome, seizures, and pneumonia. Chronic respiratory alkalosis occurs in pregnancy, hepatic coma, and certain central nervous system disorders. In some cases, such as hepatic coma and salicylate overdose, respiratory alkalosis may be accompanied by the development of lactic acidosis.

Respiratory acidosis results from a primary decrease in alveolar ventilation relative to the rate of CO_2 production (Table 2–6). In acute respiratory acidosis, the rise in serum bicarbonate is typically less than in chronic states in which the kidney has compensated by increasing bicarbonate reabsorption. Acute respiratory acidosis occurs when there is a relatively sudden depression in ventilation, such as in a sedative overdose. Evidence of respiratory distress is apparent, and there may be apnea and cyanosis. Chronic respiratory acidosis is common in patients with chronic obstructive pulmonary disease (COPD).

MIXED ACID–BASE DISORDERS

Mixed acid–base disorders are common in hospitalized and critically ill patients. These disturbances result from multiple organ failure including the lung and usually require mechanical ventilation. Mixed disorders should be suspected when the initiating abnormality in ventilation or hydrogen-ion concentration does not produce the expected pH change or the change is more profound than expected. Unexplained changes in the anion gap or inappropriate compensatory responses in Pa_{CO_2} or serum bicarbonate may also indicate a mixed acid–base disorder. Assessment of these patients includes an evaluation of their volume status; knowledge of the type of fluids admin-

TABLE 2–5.
Respiratory Alkalosis
Signs and symptoms: Paresthesia, weakness, convulsions, tetany, tachypnea.

			SERUM ACID–BASE FACTORS			
	pH	Pa_{CO_2}	HCO_3^-	Na^+	K^+	Cl^-
NORMAL VALUES	7.36–7.44	37–45 mm Hg	24–26 mEq/L	135–145 mEq/L	3.5–4.5 mEq/L	95–105 mEq/L
DIRECTION OF CHANGE IN ACUTE RESPIRATORY ALKALOSIS	↑	↓ Primary abnormality	↓ Compensatory response*	———	No change ———	———
TYPICAL VALUES†	7.60	20	20	140	4	95

* Expected range of compensation:
    Acute: [HCO_3^-] falls 2 mEq/L per 10-mm Hg fall in Pa_{CO_2}.
    Chronic: [HCO_3^-] falls 5 mEq/L per 10-mm Hg fall in Pa_{CO_2}.‡
† Acute anxiety, hepatic coma, central nervous system injury.
‡ Data from Narins and Emmett, 1980.

TABLE 2–6.
Respiratory Acidosis
Signs and symptoms: Acute and chronic confusion, cyanosis, wheezes, coma, apnea.

			SERUM ACID–BASE FACTORS			
	pH	Pa_{CO_2}	HCO_3^-	Na^+	K^+	Cl^-
NORMAL VALUES	7.36–7.44	37–45 mm Hg	24–26 mEq/L	135–145 mEq/L	3.5–4.5 mEq/L	95–105 mEq/L
DIRECTION OF CHANGE IN RESPIRATORY ACIDOSIS	↓	↑ Primary abnormality	↑ Compensatory response*	⇔	⇔	↓ or minor change
TYPICAL VALUES: CHRONIC†	7.30	55	33	140	5	99
ACUTE‡	7.20	55	27	140	5	105

* Expected range of compensation:
    Acute: [HCO_3^-] increase of 1 mEq/L per 10-mm Hg increase in Pa_{CO_2}.
    Chronic: [HCO_3^-] increase of 3.5 mEq/L per 10-mm Hg increase of Pa_{CO_2}.§
† Chronic obstructive lung disease.
‡ Acute respiratory failure due to drug overdose.
§ Data from Narins and Emmett, 1980.

istered intravenously; medications; sites and types of fluid losses (diarrhea, nasogastric suction); and mechanical ventilator settings. In some cases of multiple organ failure coupled with mechanical ventilation, the dominant acid–base abnormality may not be clear. Examples of mixed acid–base disturbances are provided in Table 2–7.

The mixed acid–base disturbance of *respiratory acidosis* and *metabolic alkalosis* is usually a consequence of chronic or acute respiratory failure. Metabolic alkalosis may ensue because of volume depletion due to a diuretic or gastrointestinal losses of hydrogen and chloride ions. This leads to an exaggerated bicarbonate reabsorption by a kidney, which is already attempting to compensate for a respiratory acidosis. The serum bicarbonate level and Pa_{CO_2} will be elevated while the pH will be normal or only slightly increased.

TABLE 2–7.
Mixed Acid–Base Disturbances

1. RESPIRATORY ACIDOSIS AND METABOLIC ALKALOSIS

pH: Normal or increased $\dfrac{[HCO_3^-] \uparrow \uparrow *}{Pa_{CO_2} \uparrow}$

Serum: $[K^+] \downarrow$; $[Cl^-] \downarrow$; $[HCO_3^-] \uparrow$
Example: Chronic obstructive lung disease causing respiratory acidosis; diuretic-induced metabolic alkalosis

2. RESPIRATORY ACIDOSIS AND METABOLIC ACIDOSIS

pH: Decreased $\dfrac{[HCO_3^-] \downarrow}{Pa_{CO_2} \uparrow}$

Serum: $[K^+] \uparrow$; $[HCO_3^-] \downarrow$ or normal
Example: Cardiopulmonary arrest causing respiratory acidosis and cardiac arrest with shock and acidosis

3. RESPIRATORY ALKALOSIS AND METABOLIC ALKALOSIS

pH: Increased $\dfrac{[HCO_3^-] \uparrow}{Pa_{CO_2} \downarrow}$

Serum: $[K^+] \downarrow$; $[Cl^-] \downarrow$; $[HCO_3^-] \uparrow$
Example: Postoperative patient with hyperventilation causing respiratory alkalosis and volume depletion due to nasogastric suction and metabolic alkalosis

4. RESPIRATORY ALKALOSIS AND METABOLIC ACIDOSIS

pH: Normal or increased $\dfrac{[HCO_3^-] \downarrow}{Pa_{CO_2} \downarrow \downarrow}$

Serum: $[K^+] \downarrow$; $[HCO_3^-] \downarrow$
Example: Liver disease with hyperventilation causing respiratory alkalosis, and a development of lactic acidosis

5. METABOLIC ACIDOSIS AND METABOLIC ALKALOSIS

pH: Variable—acidotic or alkalotic $\dfrac{[HCO_3^-]}{Pa_{CO_2}}$ variable

Serum: $[K^+] \downarrow$; $[Cl^-] \downarrow$; anion gap $\uparrow \uparrow$ (see text)
Example: Metabolic alkalosis from nausea and vomiting, plus acidosis (lactic acidosis or ketoacidosis)

* Arrows indicate expected direction of change; severity of underlying process will determine exact magnitude.

The mixed disturbance of *respiratory acidosis* and *metabolic acidosis* is characterized by profound acidosis, a low serum bicarbonate level, and a high Pa_{CO_2}. This disturbance may be encountered in patients with acute cardiorespiratory failure.

Respiratory alkalosis and *metabolic alkalosis* occur with hyperventilation in patients with a metabolic alkalosis. Such hyperventilation can be due to central nervous system trauma, liver disease, or a high mechanical ventilation rate. The serum bicarbonate level is high, and Pa_{CO_2} is low. These patients may be significantly alkalotic (pH > 7.5).

Metabolic acidosis is normally compensated by hyperventilation. However, sustained overventilation can lead to a normal pH or mild alkalosis producing a mixed disorder of *respiratory alkalosis* and *metabolic acidosis*. The serum bicarbonate level and the Pa_{CO_2} will be low, but the pH will be inappropriately near normal or slightly alkalotic.

The pH, Pa_{CO_2}, and bicarbonate levels in a mixed disorder depend on the severity of the two processes and the degree to which each counteracts the effects of the other. The diagnosis should be suspected when there is an unusual electrolyte pattern (e.g., a patient with a metabolic alkalosis from severe nausea and vomiting who then develops a lactic acidosis). The patient may have a normal pH, or be only mildly acidotic. The serum bicarbonate level would then be normal or slightly low, the chloride level very low, potassium concentration normal or low, and the anion gap very high. The high anion gap suggests a significant unmeasured amount of hydrogen ions, with only minimal acidosis or a less-than-expected degree of acidosis (i.e., a mixed *metabolic acidosis-alkalosis*). Such a patient could have the following laboratory values: pH = 7.30; Pa_{CO_2} = 30 mm Hg; HCO_3^- = 20 mEg/L; Na_+ = 135 mEq/L; K^+ = 3.5 mEq/L; Cl^- = 85 mEq/L; AG = 30.

PRINCIPLES OF THERAPY

A main principle of therapy in all acid–base disturbances is correction of the initiating process. This is especially true for metabolic acidosis and alkalosis. For example, the treatment of diabetic ketoacidosis is directed at lowering of the hyperglycemia with insulin, which also decreases the liver's production of acetoacitic and beta-hydroxybutyric acid. Only when the acidosis is severe (pH < 7.0), and there may be compromise of the cardiovascular system, is cautious bicarbonate infusion therapy recommended to raise the pH to around 7.20.

In other acidoses in which there has been an accumulation of lactic acid or a loss of body buffers (renal failure, RTA), bicarbonate is used. In lactic acidosis, bicarbonate is given while treatment is directed at correcting the initiating process (shock, sepsis, or others).

Treatment of metabolic alkalosis depends on the type. In saline-responsive alkalosis, volume depletion should be corrected with sodium chloride infusion, diuretics should be discontinued, and potassium losses should be replaced. Rarely is the alkalosis so severe and resistant to treatment that acidifying agents such as dilute hydrochloric acid or ammonium chloride are necessary. These agents must be used cautiously because they may have serious side-effects. Treatment for the saline-resistant metabolic alkalosis consists of a replacement of potassium loss and efforts to remove the cause of the mineralocorticoid steroid excess. Because these patients may be volume expanded, hypokalemic, and hypertensive, treatment with a potassium-sparing diuretic such as spironolactone may be indicated.

Most cases of acute respiratory alkalosis are short-lived, and treatment is directed at the underlying cause such as anxiety, pneumonia, or seizures. In chronic cases, in which alkalosis is not severe and pH is not over 7.5, no treatment is usually needed. In the more severe cases, if the sustained hyperventilation is tiring, then control of respiration by mechanical ventilation may be necessary.

Treatment of acute respiratory acidosis is primarily directed at measures to improve ventilation, which may include clearing of the upper airway by suction, assisted or mechanical ventilation, and intubation or tracheostomy. In chronic respiratory acidosis due to chronic obstructive pulmonary disease, pharmacologic agents such as bronchodilators are used.

As with the other acid–base disorders, the treatment of mixed abnormalities depends on correcting the initiating factor. For example, a patient with respiratory failure from circulatory collapse will need assisted ventilation and supported circulation. Manipulation of the ventilation may be necessary in patients on mechanical ventilators. In the case of hypoventilation and CO_2 retention the ventilatory rate can be increased. In a patient on a mechanical ventilator with anxiety and hyperventilation, sedation or voluntary respiration paralysis can be utilized to decrease the ventilatory rate.

REFERENCES

Barrett EJ, DeFronzo RA: Diabetic ketoacidosis: Diagnosis and treatment. *Hosp Pract* 1984; 19:89–104. *A practical overview of a common acid–base disturbance.*

Mitchell JH, Wildenthal K, Johnson RL Jr: The effects of acid–base disturbances on cardiovascular and pulmonary function. *Kidney Int* 1972; 1:375–389. *A good review of pathophysiological effects of acid–base disturbances on the cardiovascular system.*

Narins RG, Emmett M: Simple and mixed acid–base disorders: A practical approach. *Medicine* 1980; 59:161–187. *A comprehensive view of a complex subject.*

Narins RG, Jones ER, Stom MC, Rudnich MR, Baste CP: Diagnostic strategies in disorders of fluid, electrolyte and acid–base homeostasis. *Am J Med* 1982; 72:496–519. *A thorough explanation of the relationships between acid–base and electrolyte changes.*

Schrier RW (ed): Renal and Electrolyte Disorders, 3. Boston, Little, Brown & Co, 1986. *An affordable, up-to-date text which will be a suitable reference for most clinicians and medical students.*

Seldin DW, Rector FC Jr: The generation and maintenance of metabolic alkalosis. *Kidney Int* 1972; 1:306–321. *A classic. Metabolic alkalosis has never been explained so well.*

FEVER OF UNKNOWN ORIGIN

Howard F. Wunderlich, M.D.

There is a tendency to label an undiagnosed febrile illness that has not responded to a few days of antibiotic therapy as a fever of undetermined origin. However, the term *fever of unknown origin* should be reserved for the fever in those patients with *documented* daily temperature elevations above 101°F and for which 1 week of routine laboratory tests have failed to elucidate the cause. The addition of the criterion that the fever has lasted at least 2 or 3 weeks helps eliminate a protracted viral illness as a cause (Petersdorf and Beeson, 1961). Further clinical and laboratory study identifies the etiology in all but 5% to 10% of cases.

CLINICAL SIGNS AND SYMPTOMS

Three features of the patient's history help to determine the cause and source of a fever of unknown origin: general systemic symptoms that give credence to a serious disorder causing the fever, clues to an anatomic source, and environmental exposure to a potential cause of fever.

Among the general systemic symptoms are the pattern of fever and association of the fever with administration of antibiotics or other drugs such as antineoplastic or anti-inflammatory agents. Other symptoms are the night sweats, chills or rigors, and weight loss with or without changes in appetite. Patients who have factitious fever or drug fever rarely have any of these. Although these symptoms are nonspecific, they are a measure of how seriously one should pursue identifying a cause.

A relapsing pattern of fever is the most significant. In a clinical study by Sheon and Van Ommen (1963), it was the most common pattern, and progression from a relapsing to daily pattern portended a poorer prognosis. A relapsing fever is found in all diagnostic groups, but tends to occur most often in neoplastic diseases and noninfectious inflammatory conditions. Diseases such as Hodgkin's and non-Hodgkin's lymphomas, leukemia, metastatic carcinoma, Crohn's disease, and ulcerative colitis, as well as systemic lupus erythematosis, are diagnoses associated with a relapsing pattern. In addition, such infections as tuberculosis, brucellosis, malaria, Colorado tick fever, Charcot's biliary fever, and infectious mononucleosis have been reported to have a relapsing fever.

In eliciting an anatomic source of the fever, abdominal, chest, or musculoskeletal pain may be clues to the presence of abdominal abscesses, osteomyelitis, pericarditis, pleuritis, or connective tissue disease. Abdominal pain is the most helpful in localizing the source. Surprisingly, cough and urinary symptoms are not as likely to assist in localization, but should be sought in the history. Mental changes may be a helpful clue in a diagnosis of central nervous system disease, but are not specific regarding a cause.

Environmental and epidemiologic data may help in interpreting the clinical clues. Exposure in the workplace to people, animal products, chemicals, solvents, and aerosols may stimulate a hypersensitivity reaction or may lead to an infection such as brucellosis or a neoplasm involving the liver or bone marrow. A history of travel and exposure to animals is also important. A lack of sanitary conditions in the workplace or home may lead to hepatitis, typhoid fever, or tuberculosis. Queries regarding avocations may reveal such unusual exposures as spelunking (histoplasmosis), hunting (tularemia), or pigeon breeding (ornithosis). Of importance in the social history are habits (e.g., intravenous drug abuse and sexual preference) which may be very important in suggesting the possibility of endocarditis or the acquired immunodeficiency syndrome. The family history may also be relevant. Tuberculosis exposure, a history of familial fever suggesting familial Mediterranean fever, or family background of inflammatory bowel disease can be pertinent in identifying an occult source of fever.

In addition to fever, there may be important and rather obscure physical findings. Examination of the integument, mucous membranes, and nailbeds may reveal a macular or vesicular rash, petechiae, purpura, nodules, or plaques; samples of these may be taken for culture or histologic study. Lymphadenopathy should be sought and, if present, categorized as either localized or diffuse. Biopsy may be fruitful. Lymphoma, infectious mononucleosis, sarcoidosis, and hypersensitivity angiitis may appear with a diffuse lymphadenopathy. Chest findings such as crackles, rubs, or signs of pleural effusion may pinpoint a location for culture or biopsy. Often, however, the culture and biopsy findings do not correlate with the chest x-ray findings or they are helpful only in more advanced states of the disease than associated with fever of unknown origin. Heart murmurs are the hallmark of endocarditis, but may occur in atrial myxomas, marantic endocarditis, and connective tissue disease. A systolic ejection murmur is common in febrile patients with or without anemia and is often of no diagnostic significance, whereas a changing or new regurgitant murmur may be helpful. Abdominal tenderness may help localize disease, and the presence of ascites may lead to a diagnostic paracentesis. Hepatomegaly with or without splenomegaly may be nonspecific, but granulomatous diseases or neoplastic diseases may later be found with needle biopsy or exploration. Acute joint swelling with inflammatory signs is helpful in leading the examiner to consider a connective tissue disease. Although it is important to document and pursue abnormal physical findings, they are often nondiagnostic and need to be placed in perspective with the entire spectrum of the clinical findings.

PATHOPHYSIOLOGY

No one particular organ system can be singled out as an especially common source of the fever, although the lymphoreticular and hema-topoietic systems seem to be frequently involved. Because of its role in filtration and the immunologic response to foreign antigens, the reticuloendothelial system may develop a response to disease that both produces many of the signs and symptoms discussed previously, but it may also serve as a check point to systemic invasion and may contain, therefore, storehouses of information.

Microscopic sections of lymph nodes may yield both histopathologic information and specimens for culturing. The sections may show benign hyperplasia, granulomatous disease, lymphadenitis with or without necrosis, or nests of tumor cells. With these techniques, one may diagnose lymphomatous conditions, identify tubercle bacilli, or, with special stains, make the diagnosis of cat-scratch disease or Whipple's disease.

Moreover, the liver or bone marrow may produce granulomatous or neoplastic changes in response to systemic disease or disease localized in the liver or bone. Sarcoidosis, brucellosis, histoplasmosis, miliary tuberculosis, or any of a variety of hemic or neoplastic conditions may evolve in these tissues and be recognized by their characteristic histopathologic changes or with special stains and cultures.

Fever is a nonspecific but highly sensitive response to a leukocyte pyrogen released by polymorphonuclear leukocytes, monocytes, or macrophages. The height of the fever does not allow one to differentiate among the different causes of fever of unknown origin, but the biochemical consequences or derangements in metabolism can be used to localize and characterize disease. The catabolism that often causes weight loss and cachexia is a result of tissue breakdown stimulated by an overzealous immune system, unchecked neoplasms, widespread infection, or hormonal imbalance. This tissue breakdown may lead to the escape of increased amounts of antibodies or leukocytes into the circulation which can be measured as gamma globulin or specific antibodies to autoantigens or foreign antigens. It also may cause the escape of increased amounts of tissue enzymes from muscle, heart, liver, pancreas, or a variety of other organs as well as measurable dysfunction of these organs. Abnormal levels of hormone from the pituitary, thyroid, or adrenal glands may also be primarily or secondarily associated with the cause of the fever.

DIFFERENTIAL DIAGNOSIS

Although a myriad of conditions may be initially seen because of a fever of unknown origin, it is useful to group these conditions into four categories: infections, neoplasms, connective tissue diseases, and miscellaneous causes. As seen in Table 3–1, infections account for 30% to 40% of cases, neoplasia 20% to 30%, connective tissue diseases 10% to 15%, and miscellaneous 15% to 25%. There are some instances in which no diagnosis can be elucidated. A recent study by Larson, Featherstone, and Petersdorf (1982) (see Column 1 of Table 3–1) reports that the incidence of neoplastic and noninfectious granulomatous diseases has increased, particularly the incidences of the lymphoma/leukemia group of illnesses and granulomatous hepatitis group have increased.

The most common infections are abdominal abscesses, tuberculosis, cytomegalovirus, urinary tract infections, sinusitis, osteomyelitis, and catheter-related infections. In Larson et al.'s (1982) study of fever of undetermined origin (see Column 1 of Table 3–1) endocarditis, brucellosis, typhoid fever, and malaria are strikingly absent. However, in earlier reviews both Petersdorf and Beeson (1961) (see Column 2 of Table 3–1) and Sheon and Van Ommen (1963) (see Column 3 of Table 3–1) had a much higher incidence of endocarditis, 14% and 46%, respectively. Infections still cause 30% of fevers of unknown origin.

Neoplastic diseases account for 31% of cases in Larson et al.'s (1982) series, the most frequent being non-Hodgkin's lymphoma and leukemia, followed by Hodgkin's disease and other lymphoreticular malignancies. In one-third of the neoplastic disease, solid tumors, frequently in the abdomen, are present. These are hypernephroma and hepatoma, two each, and a variety of malignancies including cervical, gastric, and pancreatic tumors and several, obscure sarcomas (mesothelioma, leiomyosarcoma, and spindle cell).

Collagen diseases have been found to be decreased in Larson et al.'s (1982) review (see Column 1 of Table 3–1) primarily as a result of the declining incidences of rheumatic fever and systemic lupus erythematosis. However, the incidence of Still's disease has increased over that found in Sheon and Van Ommen's (1963) series (Column 3 of Table 3–1) as did

that of polyarteritis nodosa. Other causes are giant cell arteritis, panarteritis, and rheumatic fever, all one case each. Notably absent are polymyalgia rheumatica or temporal arteritis. The connective tissue diseases account for 9% of cases.

The miscellaneous group consists of granulomatous diseases (i.e., granulomatous hepatitis, Crohn's disease, sarcoidosis, and erythema nodosum). The incidence of this group has increased in recent years. Granulomatous hepatitis was the subject of a study published in 1973 by Simon and Wolff who looked at all of the most important causes of granulomata in the liver. Tuberculosis and sarcoidosis were the most common causes, accounting for 50% to 65% of cases, but 20% of cases could not be categorized and the causes remained obscure. Fever was present in all cases, but hepatomegaly was found in only seven of thirteen cases and jaundice in only three. Liver biopsy was the most helpful diagnostic procedure. Patients were given a trial of antituberculosis therapy first, and if that was unsuccessful, corticosteroids were given with successful results in nine of ten cases, but there were two relapses. Additionally, the miscellaneous group in Larson et al.'s (1982) review (see Column 1 of Table 3–1) contains three cases each of hematoma and factitious fever and one case each of pulmonary embolism, familial Mediterranean fever, myxoma, and nonspecific pericarditis. The miscellaneous group totals 18% of all fever of unknown origin cases. Such obscure causes of fever as drug fever, Fabry's disease, hyperlipidemia, cyclic neutropenia, or central/hypothalamic disorders are absent. These can produce an obscure fever requiring a thorough neuroendocrine and metabolic evaluation. Etiocholanolone is no longer considered a cause of fever of unknown origin. There are 13 (12%) undiagnosed cases representing an increase over the original series by Petersdorf and Beeson (1961) (see Column 2 of Table 3–1).

DIAGNOSIS

The diagnostic studies begin with further study of abnormal results from the routine tests. If there are abnormalities on urinalysis, an intravenous pyelogram (IVP) or renal scan may be performed. Appropriate sputum studies for

TABLE 3–1.
Comparative Cause of Fever of Undetermined Origin in 242 Cases*

CAUSE OF FEVER	FREQUENCY OF CAUSE IN THREE CLINICAL STUDIES (NUMBER OF CASES)		
	LARSON, FEATHERSTONE, PETERSDORF (1982)	PETERSDORF AND BEESON (1961)	SHEON AND VAN OMMEN (1963)
Infection	(32)	(36)	(13)
Abdominal abscess	11	11	2
Subphrenic	3	2	1
Splenic	2	0	0
Diverticular	2	0	0
Liver and biliary	3	7	1
Pelvic	1	2	0
Mycobacterial	5	11	3
Cytomegalovirus	4	0	0
Infectious mononucleosis	0	0	1
Urinary tract	3	3	0
Sinusitis	2	0	0
Osteomyelitis	2	0	0
Catheter infection	2	0	0
Candidiasis	1	0	0
Amoebiasis	1	0	1
Endocarditis	0	5	5
Wound infection	1	0	0
Psittacosis	0	2	0
Brucellosis	0	1	0
Malaria	0	1	0
G. C. arthritis	0	1	0
Cirrhosis with *Escherichia coli* infection	0	1	0
Streptococcal sepsis	0	0	1
Neoplasia	(33)	(19)	(10)
Lymphoproliferative	17	6	5
Leukemia	5	2	1
Solid tumors	11	9	4
No diagnosis	0	2	
Collagen disease	(9)	(15)	(8)
Still's disease	4	2	1
Vasculitis	4	2	4
Rheumatic fever	1	6	0
Systemic lupus erythematosis	0	5	3
Miscellaneous	(18)	(23)	(6)
Granulomatous hepatitis	4	2	
Crohn's disease	2	0	1
Sarcoidosis	2	2	
Hematoma	3	0	
Pulmonary embolism	1	3	
Familial Mediterranean fever	1	0	
Factitious fever	3	3	
Periodic fever	0	5	
Other	2	8	5
Undiagnosed	(13)	(7)	(0)
TOTAL	105	100	37

* Based on data from the series found in respective review articles.

cytology, routine culture, acid-fast staining, and fungal smears and cultures should be done for patients with abnormal chest x-ray films. Likewise, if a lymph node or skin lesion exists, it may be necessary to take a biopsy specimen for culture.

Often, however, there is no obvious specific place to begin other than with evidence of anemia or an increased erythrocyte sedimentation rate by the Westergren method. An algorithm for the diagnosis of fever of unknown origin is shown in Figure 3–1. This begins after routine blood and urine cultures and normal chest x-ray films and urinalyses have provided no evidence supporting a specific cause. Skin tests for anergy using *Candida*, mumps, or trichophytin antigens as well as a 5TU Mantoux test for a tuberculin reaction are placed, and liver function studies are ordered to assess disease in this organ. If the skin tests reveal anergy, one must look at the patient's state of nutrition and the lymphocyte count. If the lymphocyte count is abnormally low ($< 1500/$ mL), one should consider the patient's lifestyle and evaluate the patient for the acquired immunodeficiency syndrome. If the lymphocyte count is elevated, a mononucleosis-like syndrome may be present, and appropriate serologic studies should be ordered for the Epstein-Barr virus, cytomegalovirus, or toxoplasmosis. If the lymphocyte counts are normal, observation of the fever pattern and further diagnostic tests or trials are appropriate as indicated. A positive tuberculin test indicates the need to consider active tuberculosis, and cultures of urine and nasogastric secretions would be indicated even if the chest x-ray films were normal.

Biliary liver enzyme determinations can be used to screen for infiltrative or inflammatory liver disease, and the liver can be evaluated with radionuclide scanning or ultrasonagraphy. The carcinoembryonic antigen (CEA) or alphafetoprotein levels can be determined if there is an obvious mass on scanning. If they are elevated a computed tomography (CT) scan may be used to delineate a hepatoma or abdominal mass. The serum protein electrophoresis provides a useful screen for increased gamma globulin levels and any abnormal paraprotein patterns (i.e., monoclonal spike). This screen can point toward the connective tissue diseases or multiple myeloma as a cause. The determi-

nation of the levels of antibodies to nucleoprotein or rheumatoid factor or a VDRL can also be used to screen for these diseases. The gallium citrate scan can be used to screen for abdominal and other diseases. Radiocontrast barium studies of the gastrointestinal tract can be helpful if symptoms or signs point toward inflammatory bowel disease or an extrinsic bowel mass (i.e., a hepatic, pancreatic, or colonic mass). Measurement of the levels of agglutinins which normally cause fever, screening echocardiograms, or fungal serologic tests are not helpful unless clinically indicated or if special circumstances of exposure exist.

Generally, the diagnostic study of a case of fever of unknown origin is performed in three steps. The noninvasive laboratory and nucleoradiographic tests are performed first; the bone marrow, liver biopsy, or lymph node biopsy is next, especially if earlier studies suggest that abnormalities exist in these areas; an exploratory laparotomy or therapeutic trial is the final step.

Exploratory laparotomies can be helpful after unrewarding diagnostic procedures from steps one or two have been tried and if symptoms or signs suggest an intra-abdominal process. A positive gallium scan or CT scan of the abdomen showing a mass or organ enlargement may help substantiate the usefulness of an exploratory procedure. The laparotomy is nothing but a very invasive, investigative foray into the abdomen for purposes of liver biopsy, splenectomy, lymph node or kidney biopsy, and inspection. Laparoscopy or percutaneous organ or mass aspiration may be substituted for a laparotomy in some instances. Although a laparotomy will provide diagnostically useful information in most cases, CT scanning and subcutaneous biopsy techniques may have supplanted exploratory laparotomy in some cases. In the situations outlined above, however, laparotomy may still prove fruitful.

The therapeutic trial consists of using empirical antibiotic or corticosteroid therapies to treat clinically suspected but unproven causes. This often involves isoniazid and rifampin for suspected tuberculosis, streptomycin for suspected brucellosis, or chloroquine for suspected malaria. The therapy should be specific with certain goals and limits. Corticosteroids may be used if temporal arteritis or a vasculitis is suspected.

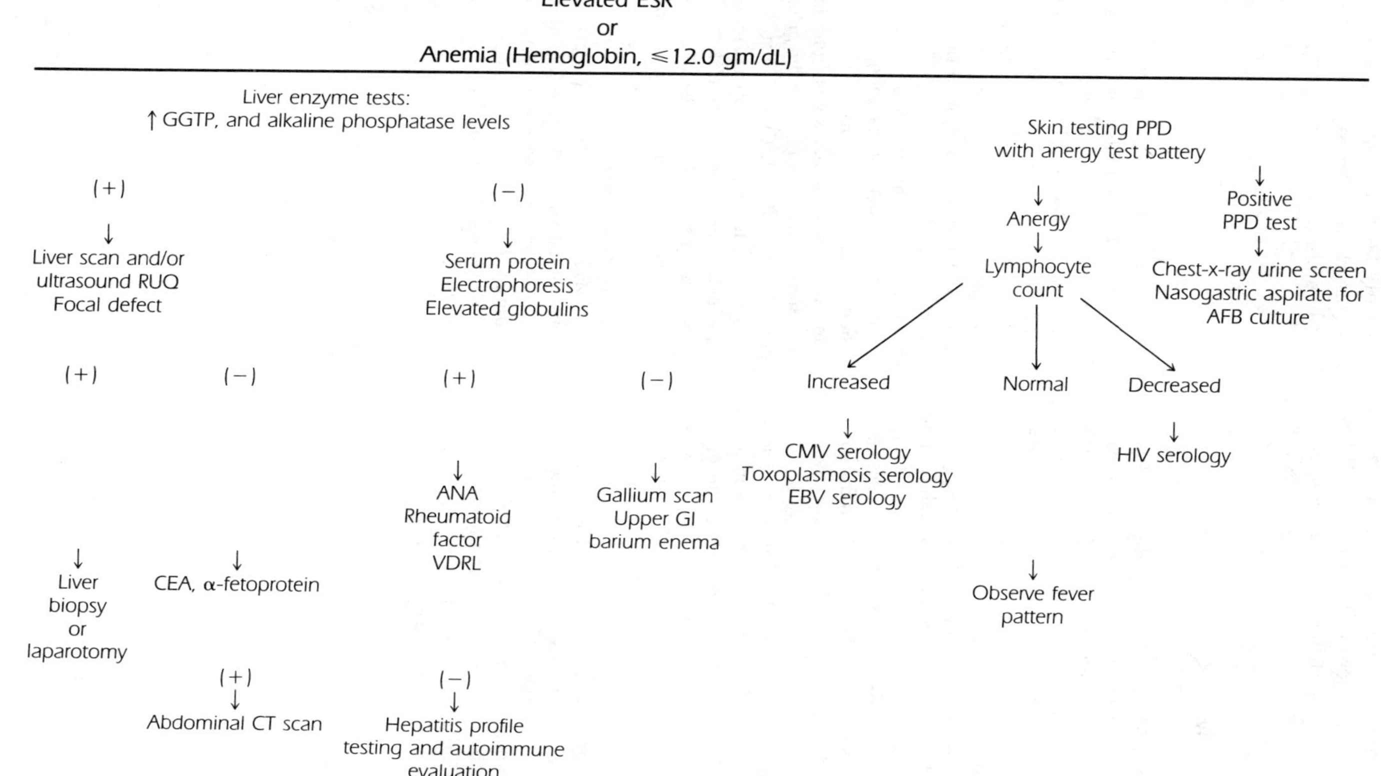

FIG 3–1.
Algorithm for the diagnosis of fever of unknown origin.

Prior to specific trials of drugs, nonsteroidal anti-inflammatory drugs (such as naproxen) or salicylates can be used generally either to control or help differentiate from other causes fever secondary to neoplastic disease. Whatever the response to either general or specific treatments, the patient will need complete and regular reevaluation.

In some instances, the diagnostic dilemma may only become apparent after a great deal of time, effort, and forbearance on the part of both the physician and the patient.

REFERENCES

Chang JC, Gross HM: Utility of naproxen in the differential diagnosis of fever of undetermined origin in patients with cancer. *Am J Med* 1984; 76:597–603. *A discussion of an innovative concept that naproxen effectively reduces fever in cases of tumor but not infection, presenting evidence from a clinical study.*

Dinarello CA, Wolff SM: Approach to the patient with fever of unknown origin, in Mandell GL (ed): *The Principles and Practice of Infectious Diseases* New York, John Wiley & Sons, 1985, pp 347–351. *A recent textbook chapter on a practical approach to and treatment of a patient with fever of unidentified origin.*

Geraci JE, Weed LA, Nichols DR: Fever of obscure origin—The value of abdominal exploration in diagnosis. *JAMA* 1959; 169:1306–1315. *One of the early articles supporting the value of exploratory laparotomy in cases of fever of unknown origin and showing a rewarding yield of diagnostic information.*

Larson EB, Featherstone HJ, Petersdorf RG: Fever of undetermined origin: Diagnosis and follow-up of 105 cases, 1970–1980. *Medicine* 1982; 61:269–291. *A more recent sequel to the 1961 version updating the causes of fever of undetermined origin.*

Molavi A, Weinstein L: Persistent perplexing pyrexia: Some comments on etiology and diagnosis. *Med Clin North Am* 1970; 54:379–396. *An insightful review of the common and uncommon causes of fever of unknown origin with six case examples.*

Petersdorf RG, Beeson PB: Fever of unexplained origin. Report on 100 cases. *Medicine* 1961; 40:1–30. *The classic description of 100 cases of fever of unknown origin describing the causes classified into the traditional diagnostic categories of the 1950s.*

Sheon RP, Van Ommen RA: Fever of obscure origin. *Am J Med* 1963; 34:486–499. *A review of 60 patients with fever of unknown origin which correlates the symptoms, signs, and laboratory data with the cause and reviews the prior literature.*

Simon HB, Wolff SM: Granulomatous hepatitis and prolonged fever of unknown origin: A study of 13 patients. *Medicine* 1973; 52:1–21. *A report on a particularly nebulous area of hepatology involving fever of unknown origin cases with liver granulomas; an approach to diagnosis and therapy is discussed.*

Wolff SM, Fauci AS, Dale DC: Unusual etiologies of fever and their evaluation. *Annu Rev Med* 1975; 26:277–281. *A discussion of the unusual spectrum of illness found in a small group of patients with persistent fever defying clinical and laboratory diagnosis.*

4　JAUNDICE

Dietmar V. Trulzsch, M.D.

Jaundice is caused by an increased serum level of bilirubin (normal range 0.2 to 1.0 mg/dL). Patients with bilirubin levels higher than 2 mg/dL appear visibly jaundiced.

Bilirubin is formed as a metabolic end product from the heme moiety of hemoglobin, and to a lesser extent, of cytochromes. Cells of the reticuloendothelial system, particularly in the spleen, break down the ring structure of the heme, probably with the microsomal enzyme heme oxygenase, releasing carbon monoxide. The biliverdin formed is reduced to bilirubin (specifically the isomer designated bilirubin IXα), which in the blood is bound to albumin (some covalently) and is taken up by the liver, which extracts it efficiently.

In the liver cells, the free bilirubin binds to cytoplasmic proteins such as ligandin (MW 46,000) and is transported to the endoplasmic reticulum when conjugation with two molecules of glucuronic acid takes place. The bilirubin diglucuronide is now more water-soluble and can be excreted into the biliary system at the canalicular plasma membrane. Excretion is the rate-limiting step in the liver cell's overall handling of bilirubin.

Gut bacteria deconjugate and reduce bilirubin to urobilinogen, which is reabsorbed and reexcreted by the liver, thus undergoing an enterohepatic circulation. Complete obstruction of the bile duct abolishes urobilinogen production. On the other hand, if the capacity of the liver to extract urobilinogen is overwhelmed, urobilinogen appears in the urine and can be detected with Ehrlich's diazo reaction.

Four types of bilirubin are found: α bilirubin—unconjugated, β bilirubin—monoglucuronide, γ bilirubin—diglucuronide, δ bilirubin—covalently bound to albumin. Except for the unconjugated or indirect bilirubin, all other (conjugated) fractions are more water-soluble and react directly in the van den Bergh reaction (i.e., without the solubilizing methanol). Despite the two carboxyl groups, unconjugated bilirubin appears apolar, because the molecule is folded on itself in the "ZZ" configuration. It is not excreted in urine.

CLINICAL SIGNS AND SYMPTOMS

The patient with a history of fever may have jaundice resulting from leptospirosis, Q fever, mononucleosis, cytomegaly, hepatitis B (fever only in the prodromal stage), miliary tuberculosis, liver abscess, cholangitis (Charcot's triad: pain, shaking chills, and jaundice), and occasionally drugs (halothane, isoniazid, hydantoin, methyldopa, rifampicin). A history of alcohol or intravenous drug abuse, blood transfusions, and recent travel which may lead to the cause for jaundice should be documented. Right upper quadrant or epigastric pain is common in biliary tract disease, frequently in conjunction with a long history of colic and fatty-food intolerance. Very deep-seated upper abdominal pain and mental depression are reported in cancer of the pancreas. A dull ache in the right upper quadrant is common in the acute phase of viral hepatitis, in acute right heart failure, and other conditions in which the capsule of the liver is under tension from sudden expansion. Pruritus suggests cholestasis, particularly in primary biliary cirrhosis.

The physical examination of jaundiced patients should focus on the cutaneous manifestations of chronic liver disease (spider nevi, palmar erythema). Jaundice is noted first in the conjunctivae, where subtle changes are better seen under natural light. Inspection of the eye in Wilson's disease may reveal a brownish Kayser-Fleischer corneal ring. Hepatic fetor appears in hepatic coma. Lymphadenopathy in conjunction with pharyngitis may indicate mononucleosis. Occasionally patients with massive portal hypertension manifest a caput medusae with venous blood flow centrifugal from the umbilicus. A venous hum may then be audible over the recanalized umbilical vein (Cruveilhier-Baumgarten syndrome). Venous hums over the liver are found in hepatoma. Malignant implants at the liver capsule may cause a friction rub.

The size of the liver should be determined by careful palpation. Most diseases of the liver (including fatty liver, cirrhosis, extrahepatic biliary obstruction, and hepatitis) result in hepatomegaly. The liver can then be appreciated either as a fullness in the right upper quadrant or by palpation of the edge on deep inspiration. If the liver is nonpalpable in a jaundiced patient, percussion of the upper and lower border is useful to estimate the size. Disappearance of liver dullness can be detected in fulminant hepatitis and is an ominous sign. Very large livers more than five finger breadths below the right costal margin are seen in tumorous infiltration or amyloidosis. A palpable gallbladder may indicate malignant obstruction, but is also found in inflammatory conditions. A palpable spleen may indicate portal hypertension in chronic liver disease or infiltration in the course of viral infections such as hepatitis and mononucleosis, of bacterial infection such as sepsis, or of neoplasm.

Ascites is often present. Usually over 75% of the cells in ascitic fluid are lymphocytes. A polymorphonuclear leukocyte count over 500/mm^3, a pH less than 7.35, and an elevated level of lactate and lactate dehydrogenase (LDH) suggest spontaneous bacterial peritonitis. Bloody ascites is frequently seen in cases of malignancy like hepatoma or of other peritoneal implants. The ascitic fluid should be cultured for aerobic and anaerobic bacteria and for tubercle bacilli. High concentrations of protein are found in hepatic vein obstruction (Budd-Chiari syndrome). High concentrations of amylase indicate pancreatic ascites. Chylous ascites is caused by leakage from the lymphatic system, as with malignant erosion of the thoracic duct.

PATHOPHYSIOLOGY

The various types of jaundice and some of their causes are listed in Table 4–1. Every step in the handling of bilirubin can be a cause of hyperbilirubinemia. Excess production of bilirubin may be a consequence of increased red cell destruction, as in spherocytosis, sickle cell anemia, or immune hemolytic anemia. Intramedullary hemolysis, seen in pernicious anemia, can be another cause of mild jaundice. The increased supply of bilirubin leads to higher blood levels of unconjugated bilirubin, which is eventually completely excreted via bile because no urinary losses take place.

The albumin binding of bilirubin is considered an enhancing factor in its uptake by the sinusoidal cell membrane. It is not surprising, therefore, that drugs such as the sulfonamides, which compete for this binding site, can cause hyperbilirubinemia.

Glucuronidation of bilirubin is accomplished by the microsomal enzyme bilirubin UDP-glucuronyl transferase. This enzyme develops late in fetal life, explaining why neonates may have difficulty handling an increased bilirubin load. The enzyme is completely absent in patients with Crigler-Najjar syndrome Type I. Babies born with this enzyme defect usually die from kernicterus. A marked reduction of glucuronidation, as in Crigler-Najjar syndrome Type II, results in conspicuous jaundice in otherwise healthy individuals. Gilbert's disease has an even milder unconjugated hyperbilirubinemia, which manifests mainly in fasting or stressful situations.

Excretion of bilirubin diglucuronide is impaired in the familial Dubin-Johnson or Rotor's syndromes. This step becomes rate limiting also in many common hepatocellular diseases such as viral hepatitis, drug reactions, and alcoholic hepatitis in which uptake and conjugation are still preserved, but excretion of the bilirubin glucuronide is inhibited, resulting in a predominantly conjugated hyperbilirubinemia.

CLINICAL–PATHOLOGIC CORRELATIONS

Excess production of bilirubin, leading to increased levels of free bilirubin in the blood (unconjugated hyperbilirubinemia), is not ac-

TABLE 4–1.
Pathophysiologic Mechanisms of Jaundice

TYPE OF JAUNDICE	CAUSES
HEPATOCELLULAR JAUNDICE	
Hereditary Disorders of Bilirubin Metabolism	
A. Unconjugated hyperbilirubinemias	
1. Gilbert's disease	Decreased UDP-glucuronyl transferase activity (enzyme inducible by phenobarbital); impaired uptake of bilirubin; mild hemolysis in 50% of patients
2. Crigler-Najjar syndrome (Type I)	Absent UDP-glucuronyl transferase activity
3. Crigler-Najjar syndrome (Type II)	Markedly decreased UDP-glucuronyl transferase activity (enzyme inducible by phenobarbital)
B. Conjugated hyperbilirubinemias	
1. Dubin-Johnson syndrome	Impaired biliary excretion of conjugated bilirubin; black liver
2. Rotor's syndrome	Impaired biliary excretion of conjugated bilirubin; liver not pigmented
Hepatitis	Dropout of liver cells leads to impaired excretion of conjugated bilirubin
A. Infectious *acute*	Viral hepatitis A and B, non-A non-B, delta, mononucleosis, cytomegalic virus, herpes, leptospirosis
B. Infectious *chronic*	Viral hepatitis B, non-A non-B, delta
C. "Lupoid hepatitis"	Autoimmune mechanisms
D. Toxic	Alcohol, amanita, carbon tetrachloride
E. Drug-induced	Halothane, isoniazid, alpha-methyldopa, quinidine
Circulatory Failure	Centrizonal necrosis of liver cells
A. Acute heart failure and shock	
B. Congestive heart failure	
Cirrhosis of the Liver	
A. Micronodular	Alcohol, malnutrition
B. Macronodular	Postnecrotic after viral hepatitis, Wilson's disease, hemochromatosis
CHOLESTATIC JAUNDICE	
Intrahepatic	
A. Hepatocellular	Alcoholic hepatitis, viral hepatitis
B. Drug-induced	Chlorpromazine, oral contraceptives, methyl testosterone
C. Benign recurrent cholestasis	Familial (Tygstrup, Kühn)
D. Cholestasis of pregnancy	Familial in Scandinavia and Chile
E. Sclerosing cholangitis	Inflammatory bowel disease, usually ulcerative colitis
Extrahepatic (Surgical Jaundice)	Common-duct stone, tumor stricture, carcinoma of head of pancreas, pancreatitis
HEMOLYTIC JAUNDICE	
Hemolytic anemias	Liver's capacity to conjugate bilirubin is overwhelmed by excess amounts of unconjugated bilirubin
Large hematoma	
Lung infarction	

companied by bilirubinuria. The stool color also remains normal. Although the liver is not primarily involved in hemolytic jaundice, multiple transfusions required to treat the anemia may lead to iron overload and subsequent hepatocellular damage with fibrosis. Iron is stored predominantly in Kupffer's cells.

Hepatocellular jaundice is clinically characterized by cola-colored urine due to the bilirubinuria. Because there is bile flow, the stool color is only somewhat lighter than normal.

Swelling of the liver may lead to a dull ache in the right upper quadrant. In severe disease, the death of many liver cells decreases the vital metabolic functions of the liver. Protein synthesis may be compromised, leading to decreased albumin levels in the blood, which then may be followed by edema. If portal hypertension is also present, ascites may ensue. Decreased synthesis of coagulation factors, which is not correctable by vitamin K, results in a bleeding tendency. Detoxification of nitrogenous compounds (ammonia, mercaptans, aromatic amino acids, gamma-aminobutyric acid (GABA), octopamine) is impaired when liver damage is severe, explaining hepatic encephalopathy or coma.

The clinical signs and symptoms in cholestasis are determined by the degree of obstruction. Complete obstruction of the common bile duct leads to progressively increasing jaundice, dark urine, and clay-colored stools. Patients frequently suffer from severe pruritus, even before jaundice appears (as in primary biliary cirrhosis), possibly due to increased bile acid concentration.

Increased hepatic synthesis of cholesterol leads to hypercholesterolemia, manifested by xanthomas, which are deposits of cholesterol in the skin. Longstanding cholestasis creates a malabsorption syndrome due to the diminished bile acid concentration in the gut. Vitamins A, D, E, and K are normally absorbed with other lipids and the bile acids in mixed micelles. In chronic cholestasis, vitamin K deficiency is noted first and explains the bleeding tendency, which is easily corrected with parenteral vitamin K. Vitamin D deficiency decreases calcium absorption and accounts for the bone demineralization. Vitamin A malabsorption causes night blindness.

The liver tends to respond uniformly to any injury. It is virtually impossible to discriminate between the various forms of viral hepatitis, halothane, or isoniazid-induced hepatitis. Conditions as different as Wilson's disease or chronic active hepatitis can have an identical histologic picture. Nevertheless, various symptoms and signs frequently correlate with certain pathologic changes.

Jaundice with clay-colored stools for more than 1 week suggests complete obstruction of the common bile duct. Totally acholic stools are very rarely seen in nonmechanical cholestasis. Pruritus occurs in chronic cholestasis, sometimes even before jaundice becomes visible. Fluctuating jaundice may be caused by floating common bile duct stones, whereas malignant obstruction of the bile ducts is characterized by relentlessly increasing jaundice. If such painless jaundice is accompanied by an enlarged, palpable gallbladder (Courvoisier's gallbladder), malignancy is very likely.

In the jaundiced patient, right upper quadrant pain is typical of gallstone disease, congestive heart failure, liver abscess, cholangitis, or even metastasis to the liver. Splenomegaly may indicate portal hypertension, hemolysis, or infections like mononucleosis. It is not found in extrahepatic biliary obstruction.

DIFFERENTIAL DIAGNOSIS

The differential diagnosis of jaundice is listed in Table 4–2.

In Gilbert's disease, Crigler-Najjar syndrome, Dubin-Johnson syndrome, or Rotor's syndrome, there is frequently a family history of jaundice. Familial cholestasis has also been reported. In persons up to age 35 years, Wilson's disease is a consideration. Hepatitis A is common in children, while hepatitis B is seen most frequently in the sexually active age group. Of the liver diseases with a sex predominance, chronic active autoimmune hepatitis is observed mainly in young girls. Primary biliary cirrhosis occurs in women about 50 years old. In contrast, primary sclerosing cholangitis is more a disease of men about 35 years old (M:F = 2:1).

DIAGNOSIS

Laboratory studies help classify icteric patients as having hemolytic, hepatocellular, or cholestatic jaundice. A mildly elevated serum level of unconjugated bilirubin and no bilirubin in the urine is typical of hemolytic jaundice. Because most coagulation factors are synthesized in the liver, a prolonged prothrombin time that cannot be corrected by vitamin K is a sensitive indicator of liver damage. Correction of the prothrombin time with vitamin K is seen in longstanding cholestasis and is due to fat malabsorption (no bile salts for micelle formation!). High serum levels of cholesterol occur in cholestasis, particularly in primary biliary cirrhosis. However, in fulminant hepatitis, a fall in cholesterol levels is ominous. Triglyceride levels are frequently high in alcoholic hepatitis and are sometimes accompanied by hemolysis (Zieve syndrome).

Regarding changes in levels of the serum proteins, an increase of polyclonal gamma globulins with a concomitant decrease of albumin is

TABLE 4–2.
Differential Diagnosis of Common Causes of Jaundice

	ACUTE VIRAL HEPATITIS	DRUG-INDUCED CHOLESTASIS	EXTRAHEPATIC OBSTRUCTION	
			STONE	TUMOR
HISTORY	Contact	Drug exposure	Cholelithiasis	-
Onset	Sudden	Sudden	Slow (sometimes fast)	Slow
Pruritus	Transient or absent	Variable	+	+ +
Pain	Mild ache	-	+/-	-/+
Type of jaundice	Rapid onset, slow recovery	Variable; occasional rash	Moderate (fluctuates)	Progressive, deep
Fever	At onset	At onset	-	-
Palpable gallbladder	-	-	-	+
LABORATORY FINDINGS				
Stool color	Light	Light	Light (fluctuates)	Acholic
Urine urobilinogen	+ (early -)	+ (early -)	+/-	-
Serum transaminases	+ + + +	+ +	+	+
Serum alkaline phosphatase	+	+ + + +	+ + +	+ + + +
Serum bilirubin	+ to + + +	+	+ + +	+ + + +
RADIOLOGIC FINDINGS				
Plain abdominal film	-	-	Gallstones in 10% of patients	-
Ultrasound, CT	-	-	Dilated ducts, gallstones	Dilated ducts, enlarged pancreas
ERCP, PTC	-	-	Common-duct stones. Level of obstruction defined	Rat-tailing of bile duct

typical of chronic liver disease. Reduced levels of alpha$_1$-antitrypsin may indicate an inborn metabolic error as a cause of cirrhosis and emphysema. Decreased ceruloplasmin is characteristic of Wilson's disease. The presence of α_1-fetoprotein supports the diagnosis of hepatoma.

Of the serum enzymes, alkaline phosphatase, leucine aminopeptidase, and 5'-nucleotidase levels are augmented in cholestasis. On the other hand, the levels of aspartate aminotransferase (AST, GOT) and alanine aminotransferase (ALT, GPT) are elevated in hepatocellular jaundice, as in viral hepatitis and, to a lesser degree, in alcoholic hepatitis, cirrhosis, or drug-induced hepatitis. An increased level of lactate dehydrogenase alone is a useful indicator of hemolysis or occasionally of malignancy. High serum iron and ferritin levels are conspicuous signs of hemochromatosis.

Further differentiation of the various forms of jaundice requires more invasive testing. Distinguishing medical from surgical cholestasis is particularly important and requires radiologic examination. If ultrasonography detects dilated bile ducts, endoscopic retrograde cholangiopancreatography or percutaneous "skinny" needle cholangiography will define the nature and level of obstruction. Supplementary to ultrasonography, either a computed tomography (CT) or nuclear magnetic resonance scan can be used to detect dilated bile ducts, hepatic metastasis, abscesses, or an enlarged head of the pancreas. If metastatic or other focal involvement of the liver is initially suspected, a ^{99m}Tc sulfur colloid scan will be most useful, and a biopsy guided through a laparoscope usually leads to a histologic diagnosis. A "blind" liver biopsy is an excellent and relatively safe method, in the absence of ascites and coagulopathies, of obtaining tissue in situations such as chronic active hepatitis and micronodular cirrhosis, which involve the liver homogenously.

PRINCIPLES OF PREVENTION AND THERAPY

The treatment of jaundiced patients depends on the underlying pathologic changes. Notably, the induction of glucuronyl transferase by phenobarbital can be used to clear the jaundice in patients with Crigler-Najjar Type II syndrome who are otherwise healthy. Sufferers from Gilbert's disease need reassurance about the benign nature of their condition. Patients with Wilson's disease *must be recognized early* so that penicillamine can be started. Patients with hemochromatosis may benefit greatly from repeated phlebotomy, particularly if cirrhosis is not yet present. Alcohol and noxious drugs causing jaundice must be discontinued. Unfortunately for the vast majority of patients with hepatocellular disorders, no rational treatment is available. The physician must protect patients from unnecessary or even harmful therapy in such cases.

Harmful drugs must also be stopped in cases of cholestasis. If an obstruction of the extrahepatic biliary system is present, surgery is needed to decompress the bile ducts and to avoid the development of cholangitis. In longstanding unrelieved cholestasis, fat-soluble vitamins A, D, and K must be provided. In advanced biliary cirrhosis, liver transplantation may eventually be required to avert impending liver failure.

REFERENCES

Gollan JL, Schmid R: Bilirubin update: Formation, transport and metabolism. *Prog Liver Dis* 1982;7:261–283. *Biochemical aspects of jaundice. See also Volume 8 of the same series (1986), Chapters 7–9.*

Popper H, Schaffner F: Cholestasis, in Berk JE (ed): *Bockus Gastroenterology,* ed 4, vol 5. Philadelphia, WB Saunders, 1985; 2697–2731. *Up-to-date monograph on cholestasis.*

Schaffner F (ed): The management of chronic liver disease. *Semin Liver Dis* 1985;5:209–307. *Authoritative evaluation of treatment modalities in jaundiced patients.*

Sherlock S: *Disease of the Liver and Biliary System* ed 7. Oxford, Blackwell, 1985. *Comprehensive text of liver disease. The important aspects of jaundice and cholestasis are discussed in Chapters 13 and 14.*

Wolkoff AW (ed): Bilirubin metabolism and hyperbilirubinemia. *Semin Liver Dis* 1983;3:1–86. *Pathophysiology and metabolic abnormalities of jaundice.*

5   HYPERTENSION

Kim Goldenberg, M.D.

High blood pressure is a hemodynamic abnormality which is epidemiologically defined by an increased morbidity and mortality from vascular changes in the cardiac, cerebral, and renal systems. Elevation of systolic blood pressure is more important than elevation of diastolic as a predictor of vascular disease, but diastolic blood pressure is referred to more often because of extensive clinical study of this measurement. An abnormal blood pressure in adults (18 years and older) is defined as a pressure of 140/90 mm Hg or more. Based on this criterion there is a hypertension prevalence in this country of up to sixty million people with the rate for black Americans greater than for white Americans. The definitions, however, are different for pediatric, adolescent, pregnant, and geriatric patients (Table 5–1). In adults, 95% of hypertensive patients have no known underlying disease. This group with primary (also called idiopathic or essential) hypertension probably contains multiple subsets or patients with varying causes related to genetic predisposition and environmental influence. In the remaining 5% of hypertensive patients with secondary causes, at least seven diseases are identified. The most common causes of secondary hypertension are renal parenchymal and vascular disease (3%) followed by endocrine disorders (1%), coarctation of the aorta, and drugs (1%) (Table 5–2). In children and adolescents and those with accelerated or malignant hypertension, however, there is a relatively higher percentage of secondary causes.

CLINICAL SIGNS AND SYMPTOMS

Early in the disease process of mild, primary hypertension, there are usually no symptoms. As the disease progresses, nonspecific symptoms are often reported such as fatigue, dizziness, tinnitus, nose bleed, and irritability. These symptoms are not, however, always related to blood pressure. Hypertension is usually insidious and develops over months or years; it may appear abruptly with end-organ damage (Table 5–3), but does so only rarely in primary hypertension or more commonly with a secondary disease.

Early primary hypertension shows no characteristic signs. As the disease progresses, a gallop rhythm (S_4 heart sound) and venticular heave may develop, and with advancing disease, end-organ damage may predominate, with specific signs of one or more organs (Table 5–3). Of the end-organ systems (retinal, neurologic, cardiac, and renal) that are commonly effected by hypertension, however, the renal and neurologic systems characteristically do not produce any abnormal physical signs until very late in the disease process. The retina, long considered a window to the microvascular changes in hypertension, produces physical signs that are more characteristic with advanced (grade 3 and 4 retinopathy) than with early disease (grades 1 and 2). This is because grades 1 and 2 retinopathy are also seen in arteriolosclerosis of aging. Grades 3 and 4 retinopathy in hypertension may also be difficult

TABLE 5–1.
Definitions of High Blood Pressure

AGE (YEARS)	BLOOD PRESSURE (MM HG)
3–5*	≥ 116/76
6–9*	≥ 122/78
10–12*	≥ 126/82
13–15*	≥ 136/86
16–18*	≥ 142/92
≥ 18	≥ 140/90
Diastolic: mild†	90–104
moderate	105–114
severe‡	≥ 115
Systolic: isolated§	≥160

* Childhood and adolescent hypertension cutoff levels are not known. Levels shown are averages of the 95th to 99th percentile (National Heart, Lung and Blood Institute).

† Hypertension in the third-trimester of pregnancy is defined as a diastolic pressure ≥85 mm Hg or a mean blood pressure ≥ 95 mm Hg. *Preeclampsia* is hypertension plus edema, proteinuria with or without coagulation, and/or liver function abnormalities. *Eclampsia* is hypertension, proteinuria and edema, plus convulsions with or without premonitory headache, severe epigastric pain, hyperreflexia, and decreased intravascular volume.

‡ Severe (and less often mild or moderate) hypertension may include the following: Accelerated hypertension is rapidly increasing hypertension (diastolic BP > 120) associated with grade 3 retinopathy (i.e., hemorrhages/exudates). Malignant hypertension is accelerated hypertension associated with grade 4 retinopathy (i.e., papilledema).

§ Isolated systolic hypertension, most often in patients >55 years old is usually associated with a pulse pressure >80 mm Hg.

to distinguish from that resulting from coexisting diabetes or glaucoma.

In untreated patients with mild, essential hypertension, end-organ damage may not fully develop for 10 to 20 years or more. With persistently higher blood pressure, the likelihood of developing end-organ damage sooner in the course of the disease is increased. Untreated patients with severe hypertension and grade 4 retinopathy (i.e., papilledema) are at the greatest risk; the mortality rate of these patients if left untreated is 50% at 2 months and 90% at 1 year. Even with effective treatment, the mortality rate may still be as high as 50% at 4 years in this small group of patients with severe hypertension and retinopathy. Hypertension that is secondary to renal or endocrine disease may appear insidiously or abruptly, with increased risks directly proportional to the increased blood pressure levels.

TABLE 5–2.
Types of Hypertension, Associated Pathophysiologic Mechanisms, and Clinical Features

TYPE	MECHANISMS	SYMPTOMS/SIGNS
Primary hypertension	Increased sensitivity or reactivity of arteriolar smooth muscle wall in the presence of increased adenosine	Early manifestations include dizziness, headache, paresthesias, irritability, gallop rhythm (S_4), ventricular heave, polyuria, and nocturia (none of these are proven to be caused by small vessel changes). All manifestations are shown in Table 5–3. Severe hypertension is rare.
Secondary hypertension Chronic renal disease	Infarction, inflammation (immunologically mediated), infection, obstructive uropathy, or rarely neoplasia with secondary ischemia. Volume overload is a major contributor to hypertension. Much less frequently, increased release of renin and angiotensin occurs.	Hematuria, polyuria, nocturia, flank pain. Hypertension severity usually, but not always, parallels the extent of renal failure.
Renal vascular disease	Renal artery obstruction, with secondary ischemia and secretion of renin and angiotensin	Abdominal bruit with a systolic or systolic-diastolic murmur heard lateral to the umbilical area, sudden onset of flank pain, nocturia. Moderate-to-severe hypertension is common.
Oral contraceptive use	Increased estrogen secretion, causing increased renin and aldosteronism, with sodium retention; increased progesterone, causing decreased aldosterone excretion	Headache, edema. Hypertension, when present, is commonly mild, but may be severe or even accelerated.
Coarctation of the aorta	Mechanical obstruction of cardiac output by increased proximal arterial resistance. Secondary increase in renin-angiotensin levels and stiumulation of adrenergic nervous system	Radial-femoral delay, right arm pressure greater than left arm if coarctation before the left subclavian artery; should be weak pulse at or below femoral artery, and blood pressures in the leg 10 mm Hg below arm, intercostal pulsations, precordial murmur
Pheochromocytoma	Adenoma producing catecholamines such as norepinephrine, epinephrine, and dopamine with pressor effects. High circulating levels of catecholamines producing decreased postural reflex sensitivity and plasma volume in some patients	Headache, perspiration, palpitations, pallor, tremor, nausea, weakness, anxiety, chest or epigastric pain, flushing, dyspnea, tachycardia, orthostatic hypotension, and moderate-to-severe hypertension
Cushing's syndrome	Adenoma or hyperplasia, producing cortisol, which causes sodium and extracellular fluid retention and increased vascular reactivity to vasoconstrictor factors and angiotensin	Truncal obesity, plethoric facies, hypertension, hirsutism, muscle weakness, menstrual disorders, acne, bruising, mental disorders, and backache
Primary aldosteronism	Adenoma or hyperplasia, producing aldosterone, which results in sodium or extracellular fluid retention and increased tissue sodium in susceptible individuals	Muscle weakness, polyuria and/or arrhythmias secondary to hypokalemia; hypertension usually, but not always, moderate to severe

The long-term prognosis of patients with primary or secondary hypertension who are treated early in their disease and are well controlled is excellent. If antihypertensive medication is removed at a later time, the blood pressure commonly either immediately elevates or returns more slowly to previous abnormal levels in no more than 6 to 18 months. Control of blood pressure, therefore, requires lifelong maintenance with diet or medication or both. Untreated hypertension results in high mortality rates for coronary artery disease (50%), cerebral vascular accidents (33%), and chronic renal failure (15%) and in morbidity due to visual deficits with retinopathy. Control of high blood pressure is, therefore, paramount because hypertension and cardiovascular diseases are the leading causes of death in nonprimitive societies.

PATHOPHYSIOLOGY

The mean blood pressure is determined by the product of cardiac output and total peripheral resistance, albeit an abnormality of the latter factor is considered the hallmark of primary hypertension. Cardiac output is, in turn, determined by the product of stroke volume and heart rate, where the stroke volume is predominantly influenced by the preload, afterload, and cardiac contractility. Total peripheral resistance is inversely related to the fourth power of the vessel radius, which is primarily determined by smooth muscle contractility.

Blood pressure is influenced, therefore, by organ systems that control these hemodynamic factors, usually acting in concert rather than alone. For example, the adrenal medulla secretes norepinephrine which can augment both cardiac output and total peripheral resistance. The adrenal cortex produces both aldosterone and cortisol, which can lead to sodium and volume retention with a concomitant initial increase in cardiac output. Stimulation of receptors found in the peripheral sympathetic nervous system can produce constriction (alpha receptors) or dilatation (beta receptors) or both, leading to changes in total peripheral resistance. Local neurohumoral control of peripheral resistance is influenced by enkephalins, kallikreinkinins, endorphins, prostaglandins,

TABLE 5–3.
Hypertension with Dominant Symptoms and Signs of a Single Organ System

ORGAN SYSTEMS	CLINICAL MANIFESTATIONS
Retina	Visual changes
	Arteriolar narrowing
	Arteriolar-vein nicking
	Hemorrhages
	Exudates
	Papilledema
Neurologic	Occipital headaches
	Visual changes
	Paresthesias
	Nervousness
	Dizziness
	Vertigo
	Tinnitus
	Sensory deficit
	Motor deficit
	Mental changes
Cardiac	Angina pectoris
	Dyspnea
	Orthopnea
	Palpitations
	Ventricular heave
	S_4 heart sound
	S_3 heart sound
	Edema
Renal	Polyuria
	Nocturia
	Fatigue
	Anorexia
	Edema

vasopressin, and other vasoactive substances. Total peripheral resistance can also be increased locally by the potent vasoconstrictor angiotensin, whose production in the renal juxtaglomerular apparatus is stimulated by renin. Perhaps the predominant modulator of smooth muscle contraction at the local level comes from adenosine, a necessary precursor for most energy-dependent mechanisms. Each of these factors may contribute singularly or in combination to the development of primary or secondary hypertension because each neurohumoral agent can produce specific types of secondary hypertension (Table 5–2). The major macroscopic and microscopic findings seen in primary and secondary hypertension are shown in Table 5–4.

The biochemical basis for hypertension is unknown, but one logical and common hypothesis involves an augmented dietary salt intake with an abnormal ability to handle that salt at the membrane transport level, either in

TABLE 5–4.
Typical Macroscopic and Microscopic Features of Diseases Causing Hypertension

TYPE OF HYPERTENSION	MACROSCOPIC FEATURES	MICROSCOPIC FEATURES
Primary hypertension	Macroangiopathy with hypertrophy and fibrosis of the aorta	Microangiopathy with hyalinosis (or hyalinization) and fibrinoid necrosis of renal, cerebral, cardiac, and retinal vessels
Secondary hypertension Chronic renal disease	Usually small kidneys depending on disease	Variable with disease, but often ischemic changes
Renal vascular disease	Kidneys often small and firm Arteries stenosed	Kidneys show diffuse ischemic atrophy, often with crowded glomeruli, and atrophic tubules with interstitial fibrosis. Arteries show atheromatous plaques or fibromuscular dysplasia.
Coarctation	Aorta shows sharp membranelike constrictions.	Constrictions may show hypertrophy and plaquelike formation.
Pheochromocytoma	Adrenal medulla is pale gray or light brown with areas of hemorrhage/necrosis. Extra-adrenal disease (~10%) usually in and around sympathetic ganglia.	Adrenal tumor (5%–10% malignant) composed of mature pheochromyocytes with variable cytologic features. Cells are arranged in large trabeculae or small alveoli. Extra-adrenal disease occurs in chromaffin tissue.
Cushing's syndrome Pituitary Cushing's	Adrenal cortical hyperplasia. Glands are usually bilaterally enlarged, yellow and have an uneven surface due to the increased bulk of the cortex but unaltered medulla.	Bilateral adrenal hyperplasia with occasional nodules (tiny adenomas) Wide inner zone of compact cells is lipid-depleted, whereas the remaining zona reticularis and fasciculata are lipid-laden and thickened.
Adrenal Cushing's	Adrenal cortical macroadenomas are usually unilateral, encapsulated firm, yellow, and fleshy. Carcinomas may look like adenomas or be grossly enlarged with capsular invasion.	Adrenal adenomas consist of zona fasciculata-like cells which are usually well encapsulated; necrosis and calcification may be seen. Carcinoma generally shows large vesicular nuclei and cellular pleomorphism, but the distinction between adenoma and carcinoma is sometimes difficult.
Ectopic Cushing's	Adrenal glands are similar to pituitary Cushing's except they are heavier with a more thickened cortex; hypertrophied cells often extend to the medulla.	Bilateral adrenal cortical hyperplasia is similar to pituitary Cushing's except for a distinctive lack of dense lipid-laden cells.
Iatrogenic Cushing's	Adrenal cortex, firm and small	Adrenal cortical atrophy
Primary aldosteronism	Adrenal glands have similar gross features of hyperplasia as seen in pituitary Cushing's and macroadenoma as seen in adrenal Cushing's.	Adenoma with lipid-laden clear cells are similar to those of the zona fasciculata, and compact cells are similar to those of the zona glomerulosa with hybrid forms. Bilateral adrenal hyperplasia of the zona glomerulosa cells is diffuse or nodular.

the renal tubule or at the vascular smooth muscle site or both. Because membrane transport proteins are genetically determined, any defect in these proteins could make a patient more susceptible to environmental influence. For example, a membrane transport defect that results in increased intracellular sodium may increase calcium transport by a sodium-dependent pump mechanism. Calcium, in turn, causes increased vascular tone, which, if persistent, would eventually lead to functional and then structural changes in the arteriolar wall. Thickening of the arteriolar wall with a decrease in lumen radius increases total peripheral resistance, the pathologic hallmark of primary hypertension. Defects in the membrane transport systems of hypertensive patients and their progeny have included active (Na-K-ATPase) sodium pump and passive (Na-Na countertransport and Na-K-cotransport) systems. For example, a decreased Na-K-cotransport system has been found in up to 80% of patients with primary hypertension. No consistently abnormal genetic pattern or marker, however, has emerged. Because no consistent defects in membrane transport have emerged, a natriuretic hormone has been postulated to inhibit sodium transport. Recently, a newly discovered "atrial" natriuretic peptide has been described which plays a role in blood pressure homeostasis without inhibiting sodium transport. Its role in hypertension has not been defined. In addition, a high-salt diet has also been shown to augment neurogenic vasoconstriction. For example, a high-salt diet in salt-sensitive individuals will augment the vasoconstriction associated with certain reflexes, such as changing position from supine to standing.

Thus, a number of possible abnormalities are being actively studied which will increase our understanding of essential hypertension.

CLINICAL–PATHOLOGIC CORRELATIONS

The clinical features of hypertension are dependent, in part, on whether it is primary or secondary in origin because secondary causes have associated features related to the particular pathologic changes in the disease. The effects of primary and secondary hypertension produce the same symptoms related to end-organ damage (Table 5–5).

DIFFERENTIAL DIAGNOSIS

The differential diagnoses of various types of hypertension are shown in Table 5–2. A complete history, a physical examination, and baseline laboratory tests (see diagnostic section) are sufficient to screen for end-organ damage in primary and secondary hypertension and for the causes of secondary hypertension as well. Features of the history and physical examination that suggest secondary causes include a history of drug use such as alcohol, birth control pills, or sympathomimetic agents; accelerated hypertension with grade 3 or 4 retinopathy; onset of hypertension when less than 20 years old or over 55 years old; severe hypertension; unexpected end-organ damage; and unresponsiveness to adequate medications especially if previously well-controlled. Certain diseases have distinguishing features that might help in the differential diagnosis. For example, renal artery stenosis should be suspected if an abdominal bruit is heard lateral from the midline and has a diastolic component (50% of patients), if the patient is a white woman less than 30 years old or a white man more than 50 years old both with a sudden onset of hypertension, if the hypertension is difficult to control with medication, or if the patients' renal function suddenly deteriorates. A significant difference in the appearance of a palpable pulse felt simultaneously in the radial and femoral arteries suggests coarctation of the aorta.

Detection of pheochromocytoma, like renal vascular disease, requires a high index of suspicion because the blood pressure elevations may be unusually labile. Paroxysms of certain adrenergic manifestations (Table 5–2) occur in about half the patients. Rare associated diseases that might aid in the differential diagnosis include the multiple endocrine neoplastic syndromes (MEN, types II and III). The MEN II, Sipple's syndrome, consists of pheochromocytoma, medullary carcinoma of the thyroid, and hyperparathyroidism. MEN III, mucosal neuroma syndrome, consists of pheochromocytoma, medullary carcinoma of the thyroid, and multiple mucosal neuromas often

TABLE 5–5.
Clinical–Pathologic Correlations for Hypertension

CLINICAL FINDINGS	PATHOLOGIC/PHYSIOLOGIC FINDINGS
RETINA	
Grades 1 and 2	Arteriolar hypertrophy/fibrosis
Light reflex broadening	Hyaline deposition (collagen deposition in
Arteriole-venous crossing changes	arteriosclerosis of aging)
Arteriole narrowing	
Grade 3	Capillary endothelial breaks in the radial peripapillary
Linear hemorrhages (flame/boat-shaped)	vessels
Cotton wool spots	Axonal mitochondrial swelling
Hard exudates	Fatty aggregations with fibrin
Grade 4	Vessel-wall leakage of plasma and obstruction to
Papilledema	axoplasmic flow
CARDIAC SYSTEM	
Ventricular gallop rhythm	Ventricular hypertrophy and/or dilatation
Ventricular heave	Increased cardiac output
Congestive heart failure	Increased adrenergic stimulation
Arrhythmias	Increased total peripheral resistance
RENAL SYSTEM	
Polyuria	Small-vessel hyaline changes
Proteinuria	Fibrinoid degeneration and atrophy
Hematuria	
NERVOUS SYSTEM	
Cerebral or subarachnoid bleeding	Small-vessel fibrinoid necrosis
Cerebral or lacunar infarction	Large-vessel atherosclerosis
Hypertensive encephalopathy	Genetic aneurysmal dilatations near the circle of Willis

in association with a marfinoid habitus. At least 5% of patients with pheochromocytoma have neurofibromatosis, often incomplete, consisting of five or more café au lait spots, vertebral deformities, and kyphoscoliosis.

A high index of suspicion is also needed to diagnose primary aldosteronism; although most patients present with unexpected hypokalemia when no renal, gastrointestinal, or cellular losses are apparent, some of the patients may present with normokalemia. Also, salt intake dramatically affects the serum potassium level. For example, a severely restricted salt diet can correct hypokalemia, and a high-salt diet can produce significant hypokalemia. Although these three diseases (renovascular disease, pheochromocytoma, and primary aldosteronism) are often difficult to diagnose, most causes of secondary hypertension are usually more apparent from the history and physical examination. Table 5–2 lists the most common types of hypertension (selected differential diagnoses) consistent with the estimates of prevalence in several large, primary-care surveys. An exhaustive list of all causes of secondary hypertension

can be found in standard textbooks of medicine.

DIAGNOSIS

Because the diagnosis of primary and secondary hypertension is predominantly based on a comprehensive history and physical examination, screening tests are mainly helpful in assessing end-organ damage, risk factors, and secondary causes not apparent in a routine comprehensive evaluation. Routine laboratory tests usually include a hematocrit to detect anemia or polycythemia, a blood glucose level in a fasting patient to detect diabetes mellitus, a creatinine measurement and urine analysis to detect renal parenchymal or renal vascular disease, and a plasma potassium level to detect primary aldosteronism and to use as a baseline for future antihypertensive therapy. An ECG is obtained to determine ventricular hypertrophy, and plasma cholesterol and uric acid levels are measured for potential risk-factor reduction.

Rarely a patient may have features of second-

TABLE 5–6.
Laboratory Evaluation in Selected Cases of Secondary Hypertension

DIAGNOSIS	SCREENING TESTS	ADDITIONAL TESTS
Chronic renal disease	Serum creatinine Blood urea nitrogen Urine analysis Hematocrit	Renal isotope scan Renal ultrasound (See Chapter 99, Chronic Renal Failure)
Renal vascular disease	Serum creatinine Blood urea nitrogen Urine analysis	Renal isotope scan Intravenous pyelogram (rapid sequence) Digital subtraction angiography Renal arteriography, Renal vein renins
Coarctation of the aorta	Chest x-ray film	Aortography

Pheochromocytoma	Spot urine metanephrine
	> 1 μg/mg of creatinine
	24-hr urine for metanephrine,
	   vanillylmandelic acid, and
	   catecholamines
		Plasma catecholamine levels before and
		   after inhibition of the sympathetic
		   nervous system (0.3 mg clonidine)
		Abdominal computed tomography (CT
		   scan)
		Magnetic resonance imaging

Cushing's syndrome	Morning cortisol level (> 5 mg/dl) after
	   dexamethasone (1 mg) given at
	   bedtime
		Plasma cortisol/urinary 17-hydroxy-
		   corticoid levels in response to low or
		   high dose of dexamethasone; pituitary
		   CT scan, metyrapone test, plasma
		   ACTH, adrenal CT scan.

Primary aldosteronism	Serum potassium level (unprovoked)
	< 3.5 mEq/L) or rapidly developing
	   hypokalemia with diuretics
		Urine potassium >30 mEq/24 hr when
		   patient is hypokalemic and not taking
		   diuretics
		Plasma renin activity after stimulation
		   (low-salt diet)
		Plasma/urine aldosterone after suppression
		   (high-salt diet)
		Abdominal CT scan
		Magnetic resonance imaging
		Iodocholesterol nuclear medicine adrenal
		   scan

ary hypertension without any abnormality in baseline history, physical examination, and laboratory tests. Additional laboratory screening tests that might be obtained in these patients are shown in Table 5–6. In general, for each diagnosis the related screening and additional tests are listed in Table 5–6 in increasing order of cost or risk of invasive procedures or both. These laboratory tests, therefore, should not be routinely obtained on all patients because of the cost and the risk of a false-positive result. According to Bayes' theorem, when the prevalence or pretest likelihood of the disease being present is low, as found with most cases of hypertension, the posttest likelihood is also low irrespective of the sensitivity and specificity of the test (see Table 1–1). Because coarctation of the aorta, renal vascular disease, pheochromocytoma, and primary aldosteronism can each require expensive and invasive

testing for their definitive diagnosis, it is wise not to order specific screening tests for these diseases unless there is clinical suspicion of their presence.

PRINCIPLES OF PREVENTION AND THERAPY

Control of hypertension clearly and markedly reduces the risk of end-organ damage in the cardiac, cerebral, and renal systems and in the retina. Risk reduction by antihypertensive medication increases with increasing blood pressure levels from mild to severe. The value of pharmacologic intervention for diastolic pressures between 90 and 95 mm Hg has yet to be proven. Hypertension is best treated with a weight-reducing diet (if appropriate), sodium restriction, or medications that interfere with a myriad of mechanisms that are potentially responsible for hypertension. For example, diuretics can increase sodium excretion, while alpha-, beta-, and ganglionic-receptor blocking agents can decrease stimulation of the sympathetic nervous system at the receptor site; vasodilators and angiotensin-converting enzyme inhibitors can directly reduce smooth muscle-wall constriction, and calcium channel-blocking agents can locally prevent calcium-related smooth muscle contraction. The benefits of treatment in elderly patients with isolated systolic hypertension have yet to be proven, but limited trials suggest risk is reduced. Caution, therefore, must be exercised in reducing the blood pressure of elderly patients so the treatment does not become more of a problem than the disease. In pediatric and adolescent patients, in whom the long-term effects of mild hypertension are unknown, close follow-up and treatment are needed if the hypertension persists (National Heart, Lung and Blood Institute). In contrast, hypertensive pregnant patients have immediate risks of fetal morbidity and mortality, which are dramatically reduced by control of blood pressure.

Overall, adult patients have an excellent prognosis with adequate treatment, whether it be diet, salt restriction, medications, or a combination of the three. Although secondary hypertension is usually treated by eliminating the underlying disease, treatment does not automatically eliminate the hypertension, and therefore the risks and benefits for each patient must be carefully assessed. In primary and secondary hypertension, evaluation should include the patients' risk factor profile of cigarette usage, hyperlipidemia, and history of diabetic, renal, cardiac, and neurologic problems; these risk factors must enter into the decision of when and how to treat mild elevations of systolic and diastolic blood pressure. For example, preexisting cardiac disease requires more urgency in treating mild blood pressure elevations; and diabetes mellitus, which develops with diuretic therapy, requires changing of antihypertensive medications. In the elderly a rapid lowering of blood pressure can induce a stroke, the very problem treatment is trying to prevent.

REFERENCES

Ferguson RK, Vlasses PH: Hypertensive emergencies and urgencies. *JAMA* 1986; 255:1607–1613. *A review of the classification and treatment for acute hypertensive episodes.*

Follow B: Physiological aspects of primary hypertension. *Physiol Rev* 1982; 62:347–504. *A comprehensive review of hypertension physiology.*

Genest J, Kuchel O, Hammet P, Cantin M (eds): *Hypertension,* ed 2. New York, McGraw-Hill, 1984. *The best, detailed presentation of the pathophysiology and clinical features of essential and secondary hypertension with an international perspective.*

The Joint National Committee on Detection, Evaluation and Treatment of High Blood Pressure: The 1984 report of the Joint National Committee on Detection, Evaluation and Treatment of High Blood Pressure. *Arch Intern Med* 1984; 144:1045–1057. *A unified approach to screening, classifying, and treating high blood pressure; supported by the majority of national medical organizations in the United States.*

Kaplan NM: *Clinical Hypertension,* ed 4. Baltimore, Williams & Wilkins Co, 1986. *A detailed review of primary and secondary causes of hypertension with emphasis on clinical applicability.*

Koch-Weser J: Management of hypertension in the elderly. *N Engl J Med* 1980; 302:1397–1401. *A concise discussion of systolic hypertension in the elderly.*

Laragh JH: Atrial natriuretic hormone, the renin-aldosterone axis, and blood-pressure-electrolyte homeostasis. *N Engl J Med* 1985; 313:1330–1340. *A review of atrial natriuretic hormone physiology.*

Lindheimer MD, Katz AI: Current concepts: Hypertension and pregnancy. *N Engl J Med* 1985; 313:675–680. *A concise review of the classification, pathophysiology, and management of preeclampsia and eclampsia.*

Loggie JMH, Horan MJ, Gruskin AB, Hohn AR, Dunbar JB, Havlik RJ (eds): *NHLBI Workshop on Juvenile Hypertension.* New York, Biomedical Information Corp, 1984. *A comprehensive review of current issues in juvenile hypertension.*

National Heart, Lung, and Blood Institute's Task Force on Blood Pressure Control in Children: Report of the second task force on blood pressure control in children. *Pediatrics* 1987; 79:1–25. *Recommendations for the evaluation and treatment of childhood hypertension.*

HEADACHE

Samuel E. Pitner, M.D.

Chronic recurrent headache has been estimated to be the third most frequent complaint of patients seeing a primary care physician; 9% of the population is thought to miss at least one day of work each year because of it. In these patients, headache is a disease in itself; however, it also can be a symptom of serious disease, and it is important to make a precise diagnosis regarding the cause of a patient's headaches.

In order to produce headache, there must be some noxious stimulation of the pain-sensitive structures about the head or neck. The structures and stimuli are listed in Table 6–1. Note that only a small number of intracranial structures are pain sensitive. Pain can be produced by recurrent pathophysiologic stimulation of a pain-sensitive structure as well as by anatomical pathologic changes such as invasion by tumor.

There is no universally accepted classification of headache. However, 20 years ago a committee of the National Institutes of Health attempted to develop a standard classification of headache. This is now the most commonly used classification, and a slight modification is shown in Table 6–2. This classification is based both on the anatomical structure giving rise to the pain and the responsible pathophysiologic stimulus.

The first five types of headache listed in Table 6–2 account for the vast majority of chronic and recurrent headaches and represent headache as a "disease" itself, as opposed to headache as a symptom. The last four types of headache are much less frequent and even may occur only once, at the most, in a lifetime. These represent headache as a symptom of a specific disease.

The remainder of this chapter will be devoted to considering the various types of headaches individually and considering their clinical aspects in depth.

TYPES OF HEADACHES

VASCULAR HEADACHE OF THE MIGRAINE TYPE

The pain in vascular headaches of the migraine type is due to recurrent arterial dilation. The term "migraine" itself is a corruption of the Greek *hemicrania*, meaning pain in half of the head. The name is aptly taken because this tendency to involve only one side of the head—at least at the onset of pain—can be said to be the hallmark of migraine headaches. The pathophysiologic changes in an artery during the course of a vascular headache occur in a definite sequence. Except in the case of classic migraine (in which cerebral or retinal vessels are affected), only branches of the external carotid artery are involved. The first phase of the headache is *vasoconstriction*, which generally is asymptomatic. In the case of classic migraine, this vasoconstriction also involves intracranial arteries and gives rise to some of the fleeting neurologic symptoms that are often seen as an "aura." The next phase is *vasodilation*. Here the pain, which is nearly always unilateral, begins. Arising as it does from an artery, it usually is throbbing in character, at least at the onset. Finally, once the headache has been underway for a number of minutes or hours, sustained dilation of the vessel is believed to result in *edema of the vessel wall*. In this situation, the vessel is unable to respond

TABLE 6–1.

Production of Headache by Stimulation of Pain-Sensitive Structures

PAIN-SENSITIVE STRUCTURE	USUAL TYPE OF STIMULUS	TYPE OF HEADACHE PRODUCED*
COVERINGS OF CRANIUM		
Arteries	Sustained dilation	Vascular (I, III, IV, and VI)
Muscles	Sustained contraction	Muscle contraction or tension (II, III, and some IX)
Other soft tissues	Variable	Variable (IV, VIII, and IX)
INTRACRANIAL STRUCTURES		
Venous sinuses, large veins, dural and large cerebral arteries, basal dura mater, cranial nerves V, IX, and X, spinal nerves C-1, C-2, and C-3	Distortion, traction, and/or inflammation	Traction headache (VII) Some inflammatory headaches (VIII)

* Roman numerals in this column refer to the specific headache types shown in Table 6–2.

TABLE 6–2.

Classification of Headache

    I. Vascular headache of the migraine type
       A. "Classic" migraine
       B. "Common" migraine
       C. "Cluster" headache
       D. "Complicated" migraine
   II. Muscle contraction ("tension") headache
  III. Combined headache: Vascular and muscle contraction
  IV. Headache of nasal vasomotor reaction ("sinus headache")
   V. Headache of delusional, conversion, or hypochondriacal states ("psychogenic headache")
  VI. Nonmigrainous vascular headache
 VII. Traction headache (headache of intracranial origin)
VIII. Headache due to overt cranial inflammation
       A. Intracranial
       B. Extracranial
  IX. Headache due to disease of ocular, aural, nasal and sinus, dental, or other cranial or neck structures.

well to vasoconstrictor medication. Hence, the pathophysiologic changes lead to one of the primary principles of treatment of the migraine syndrome—if treating with vasoconstrictor medication, give it early in the course of the headache.

Within the migraine syndrome, various subtypes are recognized: classic migraine, common migraine, cluster headache, and complicated migraine. The first three are by far the most common, and their features are shown in Table 6–3. In complicated migraine, neurologic symptoms are prominent, which is of primary importance in the neurologic differential diagnoses distinguishing complicated headache from more serious diseases such as intracranial aneurysms.

The importance of the location and type of pain has already been mentioned. Classic and common migraine tend to remit during pregnancy and are exacerbated by oral contraceptives. The most common immediate prodromal symptom or aura is a scintillating scotoma, followed in frequency by hypesthesia, both of which occur only in patients with classic migraine. Patients with both common and classic migraine may experience a vague feeling of malaise or bloating for up to 24 hours before an attack. In addition to nausea and vomiting (and not noted in Table 6–3), patients with classic migraine and common migraine usually are photophobic during migraine attacks and generally find some relief from an ice cap or a cold cloth as opposed to heat. A family history of

TABLE 6–3.
Features of the Major Types of Migraine Headache

TYPE OF HEADACHE	AGE AND SEX CHARACTERISTICS	LATERALITY	PRODROMA	FREQUENCY AND DURATION	AUTONOMIC DISTURBANCES	FAMILY HISTORY	PERSONALITY PROFILE	ASSOCIATED FEATURES
Classic migraine	Onset during teenage years Ends with menopause Female:male, 2.5:1	Alternating hemicrania is usual	Both long-term and immediate	Variable frequency; lasts few hours	Nausea and vomiting	Nearly always	Very constant, precise, and perfectionist	Abnormal EEG and allergy are common
Common migraine	Onset during teenage years Ends with menopause Female:male, 2.5:1	Unilateral only at onset	Long-term only	Variable frequency; lasts many hours	Nausea and vomiting frequent	Usually	Similar to but less constant than classic migraine patient	
Cluster headache	Onset between ages 20 and 30 years Male:female, 5:1	Always unilateral	None	Occurs in clusters; usually nocturnal; lasts many minutes	Ipsilateral tearing and rhinorrhea constant	None	Inconstant	Histamine sensitivity

migraine is so frequent in both classic and common migraine that many have postulated that an autosomal recessive gene is involved. A personality profile also has been developed for patients with migraine. EEG abnormalities are not uncommon in these patients, particularly during an attack. Anyone given an injection of histamine will have a vascular headache; however, patients with cluster headache are said to be unusually sensitive to histamine. At one time this syndrome was known as histamine headache or histamine cephalgia.

Historical points are all important in establishing the diagnosis of migraine. A physical examination and laboratory studies both usually provide no diagnostic help.

MUSCLE CONTRACTION HEADACHE

Muscle contraction (tension) headache is thought to be the most common type of headache. The mechanism producing this type of headache is sustained contraction of the posterior neck muscles. Experimentally, it has been shown in electromyographic studies in volunteers that when a susceptible individual is presented with psychologically stressful material, there is increasing sustained contraction of the posterior neck muscles, building up until a tension headache begins. There is an interesting—although unproven—evolutionary theory as to why stress selectively should affect these muscles. This theory holds that, in quadripeds, the posterior neck muscles are in a state of readiness to contract for the startled animal to look around and get set for either "fight or flight." Thus, selective contraction of posterior nuchal muscles under stress may be a vestigial "startle" reflex which has been handed down from our grazing ancestors.

In any event, the muscle contraction, or tension, headache is the most common of all chronic recurrent headaches. It is usually bilateral from onset. Most patients do not experience it as throbbing in character, but steady and continuous. These two points help in differentiating muscle contraction headache from vascular headaches. The muscle contraction headache tends to be sustained, often lasting for days or even weeks. Often, its onset is late in the day. The patient may complain of a feeling of "too tight a cap" or a constricting band around the head.

Here, too, the diagnosis is based largely on history. However, many of these patients have tenderness of the scalp and neck muscles to palpation during a headache. No laboratory studies are particularly helpful in diagnosing this condition.

In a patient with chronic recurrent headache, the differential diagnosis usually is between vascular (migrainous) headache and muscle contraction (tension) headache. The differential diagnosis of these two conditions is shown in Table 6–4.

COMBINED HEADACHE

Combined headache, the third major category of chronic recurrent headache, is a mixture of common migraine and muscle contraction headache. It can be very difficult to treat.

HEADACHE OF NASAL VASOMOTOR REACTION

The pathophysiologic basis of the headache of nasal vasomotor reaction ("sinus" headache) is intranasal vasodilation. Thus, it essentially is a vascular headache occurring within the nose. It may coexist with structural nasal or sinus disease, but more often it does not. The condition with which it most frequently is associated is vasomotor rhinitis, not chronic sinusitis.

The pain-sensitive intranasal structures include the nasal mucosa about the sinus ostia and the turbinates. Most of the rest of the nasal and sinus mucosa is not particularly pain sensitive. Generally, pain in the sensitive structures is experienced locally before it becomes generalized. One exception to this is pain from the sphenoid ostia, which is referred to the vertex of the head.

Some of the clinical characteristics of this type of headache are that it usually tends to be diurnal and relatively mild. It often comes on in the midmorning and spontaneously remits by midafternoon. The upright position tends to worsen this headache. Head jolt or sudden turning of the head or coughing will exacerbate any headache; however, these events occasionally can precipitate the sinus headache. The diagnosis of this type of headache can be confirmed by the cessation of pain after a local anesthetic is applied to the mucosa of the turbinates and ostia of the sinuses.

TABLE 6–4.
Differential Diagnosis of Migraine and Muscle Contraction (Tension) Headaches

FINDING	MIGRAINE (CLASSIC AND COMMON)	MUSCLE CONTRACTION HEADACHE
Location at onset		
Unilateral	+ + + +*	+
Bilateral	+	+ + + +
Throbbing character of pain	+ + + +	+ +
Neurologic prodromata	+ + + +	+
Duration		
Continuous	0	+
Less than 1 day	+ + +	+ +
Frequency		
Constant or daily	0	+ +
Less than 1 per week	+ + +	+
Family history of headache	+ + +	+ +
Age of onset		
Before age 20 years	+ + +	+
After age 20 years	+ +	+ + +
Vomiting with attack	+ + +	+

* Scale (0 to + + + +) shows relative frequency of finding, with + + + + being most frequent.

HEADACHE OF DELUSIONAL, CONVERSION OR HYPOCHONDRIACAL STATES

Headache of delusional, conversion, or hypochrondriacal states (headache of psychogenic origin) is relatively unusual and has no known pathophysiology. Its clinical features are extremely variable. The only effective therapy is treatment of the underlying psychiatric disorder.

As previously noted, these first five types of headache are important because: (1) they account for the majority of chronic recurrent headaches seen in a primary care practice, and (2) they represent headache as a disease as opposed to headache as a symptom. The last group of headaches we will consider, although numerically quite infrequent, is more important because they may be symptoms of serious underlying disease.

NONMIGRAINOUS VASCULAR HEADACHES

Nonmigrainous vascular headaches are similar to migraine headaches in that arterial dilation causes the pain. They differ from migraine headaches in that they are not chronic and recurrent, but are precipitated by specific agents or illness. The most common of these is the headache of influenza or other systemic viral infections, which usually is vascular in origin.

Other types include arterial dilation associated with early carbon monoxide poisoning, intake of nitrites and nitrates (whether in medication or through industrial exposure), withdrawal of caffeine (a mild vasoconstrictor) in the person who drinks a lot of coffee, and ergot withdrawal in the patient who has taken too much ergotrate over too long a time for migraine headaches. A postconvulsive headache, usually a feature of a postictal state (see Chapter 122, Seizure Disorders), also is a vascular headache. An episode of loss of consciousness *followed* by a severe headache on recovery always suggests a seizure rather than syncope. Acute pressor reactions, as seen in pheochromocytoma, some hypertensive headaches, and (although this may be recurrent in some cases) the "hangover" headache complete this group of headaches.

TRACTION HEADACHE

Traction headache is caused by traction on or distortion of the relatively few pain-sensitive intracranial structures. Noxious stimulation of each of the intracranial structures listed in Table 6–1 can produce referred pain in certain areas. The pain of aneurysmal distention (like that of many migraine attacks) is felt behind the eye. (Only 10% of intracranial aneurysms give rise to pain prior to rupture, however.)

Stretching of the upper cervical nerve roots, as may occur in herniating posterior fossa tumors in children, produces a suboccipital headache. Frequently traction headache occurs in the morning and may be associated with nausea and projectile vomiting. Headache only rarely is the first symptom of brain tumor. Headache usually is a symptom at some point in the course of most intracranial hemorrhages (see Chapter 121, Intracranial Hemorrhage).

A thorough neurologic examination is the best way to exclude this cause of headache. Only rarely is headache present in a patient who has an intracranial mass without some abnormality on the neurologic examination. The laboratory study of the greatest value in the diagnosis of this type of headache is computed tomography (CT scan); a second choice is a combination of an EEG and radioisotope brain scan if CT scanning is not available. Computed tomography of all patients complaining of headache is not cost-effective and cannot be recommended.

HEADACHE DUE TO OVERT CRANIAL INFLAMMATION

Intracranial inflammation, as exemplified by bacterial meningitis, produces a very severe headache because of the inflammation of the pain-sensitive intracranial structures. Extracranial inflammation is the mechanism producing headache in temporal arteritis. This collagen disorder occurs almost exclusively in patients over 60 years of age and usually produces a unilateral headache, often with edema and tenderness about the involved superficial temporal artery. These patients most frequently have an elevated erythrocyte sedimentation rate. Diagnosis can be made with certainty only by biopsy of the superficial temporal artery. Recognition of this type of headache is particularly important because many of these patients will become blind from the arteritic involvement of the retinal arteries if the disorder is not diagnosed and corticosteroid treatment is not instituted.

HEADACHE DUE TO DISEASE OF CRANIAL AND NECK STRUCTURES

Noxious stimulation of any of these structures can produce headache. Fortunately, if one takes a thorough history, there nearly always has been some discomfort in the involved structure before a generalized headache ensues.

Disease of the temporomandibular joint occasionally can produce a unilateral headache similar to common migraine. Although most laymen believe the eyes are a common cause of headache, this is not true; less than 5% of chronic recurrent headaches can be traced to ocular disease. Although individuals with presbyopia and astigmatism may develop headache, myopia, the most common refractive error, only rarely causes it. Relatively mild heterophorias can cause an ocular headache, but severe heterotropias cannot. Only if the refractive error or extraocular muscle imbalance can be corrected by muscle contraction will these conditions cause headache.

OTHER

Two types of headache that are difficult to classify are the hypertensive headache and the posttraumatic headache. The hypertensive headache is predominantly a nonmigrainous vascular headache, although other factors may be present. Multiple factors play a role in posttraumatic headaches.

DIAGNOSIS

The diagnosis of headache type is predominantly made by the history. Whereas some types of headache may have significant physical findings or laboratory data, these have been discussed under the type of headache. It is not cost-effective to do a cerebral CT scan of every headache patient; nonetheless, one should use this procedure liberally if the initial clinical manifestation is not typical of one of the other syndromes described above.

THERAPY

Therapy of headache is shown in Table 6–5. Note that therapy for some headaches is quite specific, whereas for others treatment is quite general. Use of any of the agents listed in the table requires complete familiarity with the given drug and often requires laboratory tests during the treatment.

TABLE 6–5.
Treatment of Headache

TYPE OF HEADACHE	TREATMENT OF ACUTE EPISODE	PROPHYLAXIS*
I. Migraine	Ergotamine derivatives	Propranolol (Methysergide) (Biofeedback)
II. Muscle contraction headache	Nonnarcotic analgesics	Mild sedatives (Relaxation training) (Muscle relaxants)
III. Combined headache	As for types I and II	Amitriptyline (Others as noted above)
IV. Nasal vasomotor headache	Nonnarcotic analgesics	Oral decongestants No smoking
V. Psychogenic headache	None	Treatment of underlying psychiatric problem
VI. Nonmigrainous vascular headache	Variable	Remove cause
VII. Traction headache	Nonnarcotic analgesics	Treat intracranial cause
VIII. Inflammatory headache	Nonnarcotic analgesics	Treat cause
IX. Miscellaneous headache	Nonnarcotic analgesics	Treat cause

* Main method of treatment is listed first, other frequently used treatments are shown in parentheses.

REFERENCES

American Association for the Study of Headache: *Headache. This monthly journal, published under the auspices of the Association, emphasizes therapeutic trials of new drugs.*

Appenzeller O (ed): *Pathogenesis and Treatment of Headache.* New York, Spectrum, 1976. *An excellent short monograph on the topic by leading experts in the field.*

Dalessio, DJ (ed): *Wolff's Headache and Other Head Pain.* ed 4. New York, Oxford University Press, 1980. *The standard reference work on the subject.*

Raskin NH, Appenzeller O: Headache in Smith JK (ed): *Major Problems in Internal Medicine, Vol 19.* Philadelphia, WB Saunders Co. 1980. *Scholarly, well-referenced monograph by two outstanding authorities in the field.*

7 COMA AND STATES OF DIMINISHED CONSCIOUSNESS

Samuel E. Pitner, M.D.

An all too common problem in most emergency rooms is the patient who has been brought in and is unable to give any history because of diminished consciousness. Most conditions that produce coma or diminished consciousness are life threatening and represent true medical emergencies.

Coma is defined as a state of unresponsiveness from which the patient cannot be aroused; even painful stimuli produce either no response or, at the most, a reflex response. Normalcy is a state of alert awareness; there are many gradations of diminished responsiveness between this and frank coma. Unfortunately, there is no general agreement about the meaning of related terms such as *stupor, lethargy,* and *semicoma.* For the purposes of this discussion, we will use the term *obtundation* to refer to any degree of diminished consciousness.

CLINICAL SIGNS AND SYMPTOMS

The histories of obtunded patients must be obtained from others such as relatives, friends,

police, or ambulance drivers. Important points are the mode of onset (abrupt or gradual and if preceded by a period of confusion), recent complaints (focal neurologic episodes, headache, behavioral changes), previous medical history (including diabetes and alcoholism), and access to drugs.

The first things to be assessed in the physical examination are the state of the airway, respiration, and circulation; support of vital functions is all important, and this takes precedence over history taking and further examination. A general physical examination may show evidence of systemic illness, needle marks, trauma, or signs of meningeal irritation. As much of a standard neurologic examination as possible should be performed; most obtunded patients are unable to cooperate for even such basic parts as manual muscle testing, however. Because of this, those portions of the examination discussed here are those that are practical even in truly comatose patients and that ultimately lead to the correct diagnosis and therapy by categorizing patients into one of the three groups of major pathophysiologic causes of coma or obtundation: (1) intracranial mass lesions, (2) primary brainstem lesions, and (3) toxic, metabolic, or diffuse lesions. These key parts of the examination are shown in Table 7–1, together with additional observations to be made in patients who are obtunded but not truly comatose.

Asymmetric cheek movements on respiration or decreased muscle tone on one side of the body may be the only lateralizing signs in true coma. In less severely obtunded patients, spontaneous movement of only one side of the body or withdrawal of only one arm and leg to pain should be sought. Presence of lateralized or other focal abnormalities almost invariably means a patient has a mass or primary brainstem lesion.

TABLE 7–1.
Key Observations In Diminished Consciousness

COMATOSE AND OBTUNDED PATIENTS
Lateralizing signs
Pupillary responses
Reflex eye movements
Respiratory pattern
Posture and tone
ADDITIONAL OBSERVATIONS FOR OBTUNDED PATIENTS
Response to pain
Motor responses
Eye opening
Corneal reflexes
Spontaneous eye movement
Verbal responses
Deep tendon reflexes

Pupillary responses have the greatest variety in primary brainstem lesions; small and reactive pupils are seen with upper midbrain lesions, midpoint and fixed pupils with upper pons lesions, pinpoint pupils with central pontine lesions, and small but reactive pupils with medullary lesions. A supratentorial mass located laterally in the anterior or middle fossa may produce herniation of the uncus of the hippocampus through the tentorium cerebelli with compression of the third cranial nerve, producing at first a dilated and then a dilated and fixed pupil ipsilateral to the mass. As rostro-caudal deterioration of brainstem function continues, one or both pupils then become midpoint and fixed and continue so until death. In cases of supratentorial masses that are near the midline in the saggital plane, the direction of brain herniation is more nearly directly downward, and unilateral pupil dilation does not occur. In this sequence of events ("central herniation"), after rostro-caudal deterioration of function has reached the pontine level, both pupils remain midpoint and fixed until death. With notable exceptions such as narcotic overdoses and glutethimide poisoning, coma of toxic, metabolic, or diffuse origin tends to spare the pupillary responses.

Reflex eye movements that are tested in the obtunded or comatose patient usually either cannot be tested or else produce quite different responses in alert and awake individuals. Nevertheless, the expected if not totally normal responses to these tests indicate that the vestibular apparatus, cranial nerve VIII and its brainstem connections, and the nuclei of the cranial nerves III, IV, and VI and their interconnections via the medial longitudinal fasciculus (all of which spread out over a vertical distance of about 5 cm in the brainstem) are functioning. These tests are the oculocephalic ("doll's eye") and oculovestibular (caloric) responses. These are illustrated in Fig. 7–1; full technical details of these tests are beyond the scope of this discussion. Generally, these responses are preserved in patients with toxic, metabolic, or diffuse lesions until quite late in the course of the illness. Patients with primary brainstem lesions show the greatest variety of abnormal reflex eye movements, and these movements are lost relatively early in the course of the rostro-caudal progression of mass lesions.

Of the various respiratory patterns, Cheyne-Stokes respiration occurs in patients with cardiac and pulmonary disorders, as well as in some normal people during sleep. In a patient with altered consciousness, its presence implies either bilateral hemispheric or midbrain disease, as does posthyperventilation apnea. Midbrain to upper pontine lesions have been described as producing central neurogenic hyperventilation; usually these are primary lesions rather than secondary effects of mass lesions. Atactic and apneustic breathing usually indicate a primary brainstem lesion. Progressively slower respirations culminating in respiratory arrest are commonly seen in patients with a herniating mass. The related phenomena of yawning or hiccupping in patients with a mass lesion and a clear sensorium often are thought to be very early signs of herniation.

Posture and tone often can be checked by the reflex response to painful stimuli even in a comatose patient. Supraorbital notch pressure or vigorous rubbing of the sternum with the knuckles usually are quite effective stimuli. Differences in responses on the two sides of the body usually indicate a structural lesion. In upper midbrain dysfunction, regardless of cause, decorticate posturing may occur; with upper pontine dysfunction, decerebrate rigidity may be induced by stimulation. In the final stages of rostro-caudal deterioration in cases of mass lesions and of primary medullary lesions, flaccidity may be prominent. Paradoxically, metabolic lesions often show very striking decerebrate posturing to stimulation, but in association with preservation of most of the other brainstem reflexes.

The physical examination, as modified for the poorly responsive patient, will allow this initial determination of the general type of lesion present in most instances.

PATHOPHYSIOLOGY AND CLASSIFICATION

Cognition and orientation are functions of the cerebral hemispheres; wakefulness itself is a function of the upper brainstem in general and the ascending reticular activating system (RAS) in particular. An infant with hydranencephaly (a severe variant of hydrocephalus in which there are no functioning cerebral hemispheres) has an intact RAS and thus has normal

A. Oculovestibular Reflex (Caloric Test)

Supine; head up 35° to stimulate horizontal canal

Conjugate deviation of eyes to right

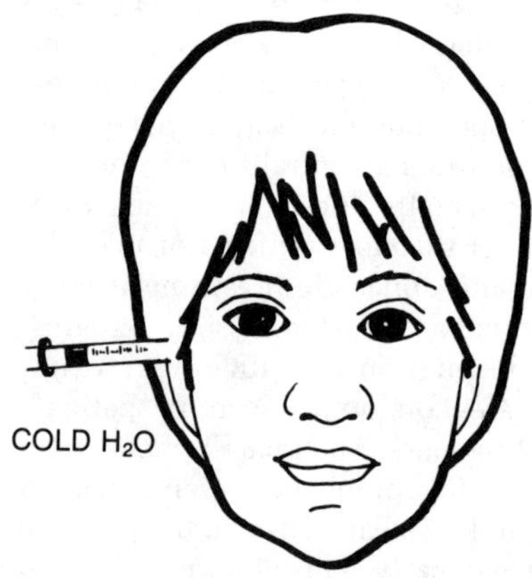

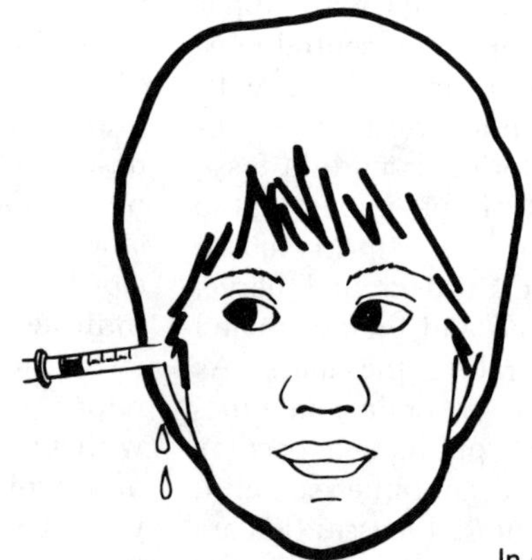

In conscious patient, would expect nystagmus with quick component to the left

B. Oculocephalic Reflex (''Doll's Eye Test'')

Patient supine; examiner at head

Rotation of head

Head position after rotation

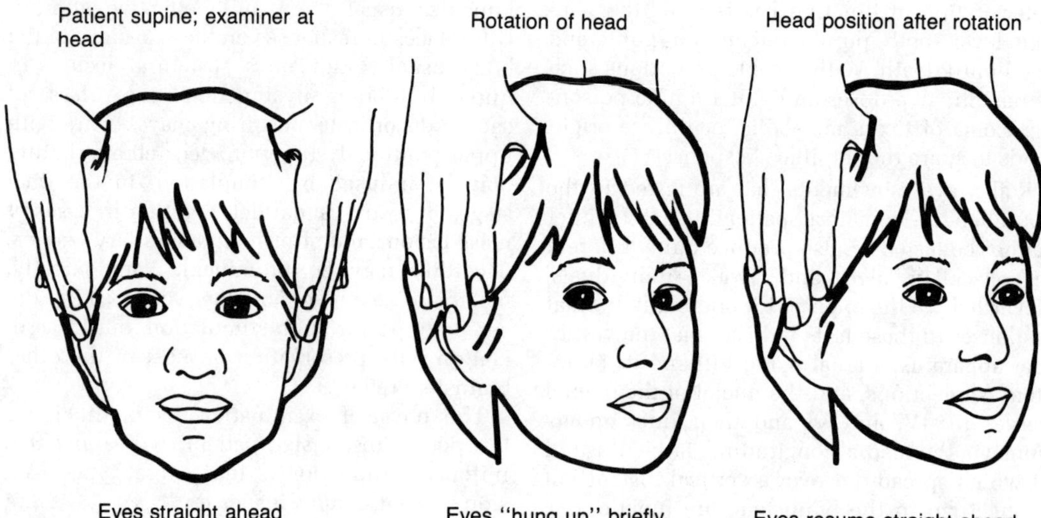

FIG 7–1.

Reflex eye movement tests. In **A,** only the right horizontal semicircular canal is stimulated. In **B,** the entire vestibular apparatus and (probably) the proprioceptive fibers in the neck muscles are stimulated. In both tests, the afferent fibers, vestibular brain stem connections, median longitudinal fasciculus, and the right sixth nucleus and cranial nerve (which innervates the lateral rectus muscle) together with left third nucleus and cranial nerve (which innervates medial rectus muscles) are shown to be functional.

sleep–wake cycles and is clearly conscious. Only lesions involving the RAS produce obtundation. Primary brainstem lesions, such as infarctions in the territory of the basilar artery or its branches, affect the RAS from their onset. Only one type of hemisphere lesion, a mass lesion, can produce *secondary* anatomical changes in the RAS and thus produce obtundation. Mass lesions of the hemispheres produce brain shifts and herniations of brain tissue through dural structures and result in secondary brainstem distortion or actual hemorrhage into the brainstem. Diseases that produce both primary and secondary anatomic lesions in the brainstem also occur in specific areas of the brain and thus usually produce focal (localized) lesions in addition. Thus, such findings as hemiparesis on examination of an obtunded patient strongly suggest a structural brain lesion. Primary brainstem lesions and hemispheric mass lesions with secondary effects on the brainstem each account for just under one of every five patients presenting to an emergency room with obtundation.

Somewhat over three of every five obtunded patients presenting to an emergency room will not have a localized anatomic lesion of the RAS, but will have a pathophysiologic lesion of either a toxic or metabolic origin. Even in these cases, there may be anatomic changes. For example, in cerebral hypoxia there are both metabolic defects and, if the condition is severe and protracted, diffuse necrosis of certain cortical layers (laminar necrosis). This large group of patients can best be considered to have toxic, metabolic, or diffuse (as opposed to focal) neurologic lesions. As a group, and in contrast to those patients with either a mass or primary brainstem lesion, these patients do not show focal neurologic signs on examination. Much of the physical examination in obtunded patients is directed toward separating the patients with focal neurologic signs (and anatomic lesions) from patients with metabolic or diffuse lesions. One percent of patients presenting in "coma" have psychogenic unresponsiveness; these will not be considered further in this discussion.

TABLE 7–2.
Characteristics, Common Causes, and Useful Diagnostic Studies In Coma

LESION TYPE	COMMON CAUSES (% OF PATIENTS IN LESION CATEGORY)	DIAGNOSTIC STUDIES
SUPRATENTORIAL MASS LESIONS		
Focal signs early	Hematomas (75%); tumors (7%); infarcts (9%); abscess (6%); other (3%)	CT scan, if available; if not, skull X-ray films; echoencephalogram; electroencephalogram
Rostro-caudal progression Signs point to one anatomical area Asymmetric motor signs are usual; pupil and reflex eye problems late		(If mass is suspected, do not do a lumbar puncture!)
PRIMARY BRAINSTEM LESIONS		
History suggests stem lesion *or* sudden onset of coma	Subtentorial masses; cerebellar hematoma, abscess, infarct or tumor (18%); Non-mass lesions (82%); stem infarcts, pons hemorrhage, other	CT scan, if available; if not, skull X-ray films; echoencephalogram; electroencephalogram
Brainstem signs from onset Cranial nerve involvement, pupil and reflex eye movement involvement from onset Wide range of respiratory patterns		
TOXIC, METABOLIC, OR DIFFUSE LESIONS		
Confusion precedes coma Eye reflexes preserved Focal signs rare	Extrinsic toxins (45%); metabolic (22%); diffuse and mixed (33%)	Venous blood studies: (levels of: glucose, BUN, electrolytes; osmolality); arterial blood studies: (pH, P_{O_2} P_{CO_2}); ECG; CSF studies; later, detailed studies of blood and urine for toxins, etc.

DIFFERENTIAL DIAGNOSIS

The major specific lesions causing coma or obtundation and the diagnostic studies most useful in further delineating the cause are shown in Table 7–2.

COURSE AND PROGNOSIS

It is very important to monitor the course of the poorly responsive patient. The best way to do this is to avoid terms such as *stupor*, which have no generally accepted meaning, and to describe the exact response of the patient (e.g., "arouses when name is called but drifts back to sleep when not stimulated"). One way to follow changes in a patient's condition is the use of various scoring systems to keep track of the state of consciousness. One widely accepted system, the Glasgow Coma Scale, is shown in Table 7–3.

By the time any disease process has produced a loss of consciousness, the outlook for survival, in general, is not good. Even with prompt and proper diagnosis, the outcome leaves much to be desired. Specific prognostic indicators in situations such as persistent coma following resuscitation from cardiac arrest are important, but are beyond the scope of this discussion.

BRAIN DEATH

Brain death occurs when the organ is so extensively damaged that there is not only no potential for recovery of consciousness, but there is no longer even brain stem function to sustain vital functions such as pulse, blood pressure, and respiration, one or more of which, usually respiration, is being maintained by external means. In contrast, irreversible coma and "persistent vegetative state" are situations in which most or all vital functions of the brainstem are intact, but no cognition or other functions of higher centers are present. In these conditions, unfortunate but protracted survival can occur. In true brain death, cessation of all vital function is inevitable in at the most several days, and the cessation of cerebral circulation as well as electrical function is attested to by the massive necrosis of the brain ("respirator brain") found at autopsy.

The legal status of brain death varies from state to state, and various criteria have been proposed. The criteria of the Ad Hoc Committee of the Harvard Medical School (Table 7–4) are the most widely accepted criteria for this diagnosis. These have been criticized as too conservative because of the requirement of persistence for 24 hours, which is much longer than in other proposed criteria and perhaps is an impediment to obtaining donor organs fit for

TABLE 7–3.
The Glasgow Coma Scale*

RESPONSE	STIMULUS	SCORE
Eye opening (E)	Spontaneous	4
	To speech	3
	To pain	2
	Nil	1
Best motor response (M)	Obeys	6
	Localizes	5
	Withdraws	4
	Abnormal flexion	3
	Extension	2
	Nil	1
Verbal response (V)	Oriented	5
	Confused	4
	Words	3
	Sounds	2
	Nil	1
Coma score (E + M + V) = 15 (normal) to 3 (coma)		

* Derived from Jennett B, Bond M: Assessment of outcome after severe brain damage. A practical scale. *Lancet* 1975; 1: 480–484.

transplantation. Review of alternative proposals is beyond the scope of this discussion. Documented recoveries of patients meeting these criteria for brain death have been seen in patients with massive sedative drug overdoses and those with hypothermia, so the presence of these two conditions must be excluded before the patient is declared dead.

TABLE 7–4.
The Harvard Brain-Death Criteria*

Unresponsive coma
Apnea
Absence of cephalic reflexes
Absence of spinal reflexes
Absence of drug intoxication or hypothermia
Isoelectric electroencephalogram (EEG)†
Persistence of condition for 24 hours

* Derived from Report of the Ad Hoc Committee of the Harvard Medical School to Examine the Definition of Brain Death: A definition of irreversible coma. *JAMA* 1968; 205: 85–88.

† An isoelectric EEG is one showing no evidence of brain electrical activity ("cerebral electrical silence"); the EEG must be performed under the detailed technical requirements for such recordings as outlined by the American EEG Society. Liberalized criteria have been proposed which allow spinal reflexes to be present and which, with arteriographic evidence of the absence of cerebral circulation, allow death to be declared after periods as short as 30 minutes.

REFERENCES

Fisher CM: The neurological examination of the comatose patient. *Acta Neurolog Scand* 1969;45 (suppl 36): 1–56. *A scholarly and lucid discussion of the subject, written before computed tomography was in use.*

Jennett B, Bond M: Assessment of outcome after severe brain damage: A practical scale. *Lancet* 1975;1:480–484. *The first appearance of the Glasgow scale. Designed for a neurosurgical unit to follow head injuries, it has found much wider application.*

Plum F, Posner JD: *The Diagnosis of Stupor and Coma.* ed 3, Vol 19 of Contemporary Neurology Series. Philadelphia, FA Davis, 1980. *The major reference work devoted strictly to this topic. The chapters entitled "Prognosis in Coma" and "Brain Death" are complete and authoritative summaries of these subjects not available elsewhere. If the full book tells you more about coma than you really want to know, the final, summary chapter, "Approach to the Unconscious Patient," wraps it all up in 20 pages.*

Tindall RSA: Evaluation and treatment of the comatose patient, in Rosenberg R (ed): *The Treatment of Neurological Disease.* New York, Spectrum, 1979, pp 1–15. *A short and concise approach to the subject with plenty of tables and algorithms.*

8 DEMENTIA

Thomas Mathews, M.D.

Dementing illnesses have become a major health care problem in the developed nations. The prevalence of dementia increases dramatically with chronologic age. An estimated 5% of the population over 65 years of age will develop severe dementia, and another 5% to 10% will show mild cognitive dysfunction. In the group over 80 years of age, the prevalence of dementia may exceed 20%. More than 50% of nursing home patients have dementing disorders. The most common cause of dementia, Alzheimer's disease, is an age-related disorder. Demographic studies show that the population of the United States is aging rapidly (Table 8–1) and that the fastest growing segment of the population is the "very old" (over 80 years), in which Alzheimer's disease is most prevalent.

Dementia or decreased mentation is a symptom complex characterized by impairment of cognitive function. Many cortical functions are affected, although some may be more involved than others. Dementia is usually insidious and progressive, although it can occasionally be acute or static (as with cerebral anoxia or trauma). Most dementias are irreversible, but some may be arrested or even reversed. Dementias are due to pathologic derangements in the brain. They must not be equated with the mild decrements in memory common in normal aging.

The general features of dementia are discussed here first, followed by the specific details of various dementing disorders.

CLINICAL SIGNS AND SYMPTOMS

The ABCs of dementia are changes in affect, behavior, and cognition. The cardinal feature of dementia is cognitive impairment. Memory, abstract thinking, judgment, problem solving, language, and visual-spatial skills are involved. Behavioral symptoms may consist of personality changes, apathy and lack of drive, paranoid ideation, delusions, impulsiveness, dysinhibition, loss of social graces, and poor personal hygiene. Affective changes include depression, irritability, labile mood, anxiety, and somatization.

In many dementias there is a paucity of neurologic abnormalities, in contrast to the striking cognitive derangement. The motor, sensory, cerebellar, and visual systems are usually normal. Frontal lobe "release" signs such as grasp and palmomental or snout reflexes are com-

TABLE 8–1.
The Number of Elderly Persons in the United States*

PERSONS	1985	1990	2000
Ages 65–74	16.9 million	18.0 million	18.0 million
Ages 75–84	9.0 million	10.0 million	12.0 million
Age 85 and older	2.7 million	3.5 million	5.0 million
Total 65 and older	28.6 million	31.5 million	35.0 million
Total elderly as % of total population	11.8%	12.7%	13.0%

* Projections from U.S. Census Bureau. Table from Appel (1986), Courtesy Year Book Medical Publishers.[2]

mon; and aphasias and apraxias may be present. Neurologic signs such as myoclonus or chorea may be seen in specific dementing neurologic syndromes (see under Clinical-Pathologic Correlations).

DIFFERENTIAL DIAGNOSIS

Several conditions can mimic dementia. Normal aging is commonly associated with forgetfulness and mild memory loss and can be mistaken for early dementia. Senescent forgetfulness is not progressive and does not impair independent living.

Delirium or acute confusional states cause global cognitive impairment. They affect attention, memory, thinking, and judgment. Illusions, hallucinations, and agitation are common. Delirium is distinguished from dementia by the impairment of arousal and consciousness in delirious states. Delirium is usually acute in onset and brief in duration. Delirium can be caused by a wide variety of systemic illnesses, infections, metabolic and electrolyte derangements. Prescription and over-the-counter drugs are an important cause of delirium. Acute CNS lesions (e.g., hypoxia, stroke, and meningitis) can also cause delirium.

Depression is common in the aged. Depressed elderly patients may show cognitive impairment which ranges from mild memory impairment to severe confusion, mutism, and incontinence. This may be indistinguishable from an organic dementia. The dementia associated with depression (pseudodementia) is reversible with antidepressant therapy. Other disorders occasionally mistaken for dementia include mental retardation, schizophrenia, malingering, and aphasia.

DIAGNOSIS

The diagnosis involves resolving two issues: (1) Recognition of dementia, which is a clinical determination based on a careful history and a mental status examination. Psychometric tests may be of value. (2) Identifying the cause of the dementia. Dementia is a symptom complex and can be caused by many different diseases. It is imperative to determine the cause of the dementia by clinical examination and laboratory investigation. Table 8–2 lists routine and

TABLE 8–2.
Diagnostic Tests for Dementia

ROUTINE TESTS
Complete blood count
Urinalysis
ECG
Blood chemistry studies
Vitamin B_{12} and folate levels
Thyroid profile
Serologic studies for syphilis
CT scan of head
X-ray film of chest
FOR SELECTED CASES
Cerebrospinal fluid studies
Drug screening tests
Isotope cisternogram
Electroencephalogram
Brain biopsy

selected tests in the diagnostic approach to dementia.

Dementia is a manifestation of chronic brain failure. Like liver or renal failure, dementia has many different causes (Fig. 8–1). Identification of the specific cause by appropriate laboratory tests is essential because 10% to 20% of dementia cases have underlying causes that can be arrested or reversed. This group of "treatable" dementias include the toxic-metabolic encephalopathies, depression, cerebral masses, infections, and hydrocephalus. The 80% of patients with irreversible dementias are those with Alzheimer's disease, multi-infarct dementia, and degenerative neurologic disorders (Fig. 8–1).

CLINICAL–PATHOLOGIC CORRELATIONS

Selected dementing disorders are described below in greater detail. Their clinical-pathologic correlations are summarized in Table 8–3.

ALZHEIMER'S DISEASE

Alzheimer's disease, a devastating disorder, is the fourth leading cause of death in the United States. The etiology is unknown, and there is no specific treatment. The emotional impact on the families, the socioeconomic consequences, and the utilization of health resources are enormous. Alzheimer's disease includes both presenile dementia and senile dementia depending

ETIOLOGY OF DEMENTIA

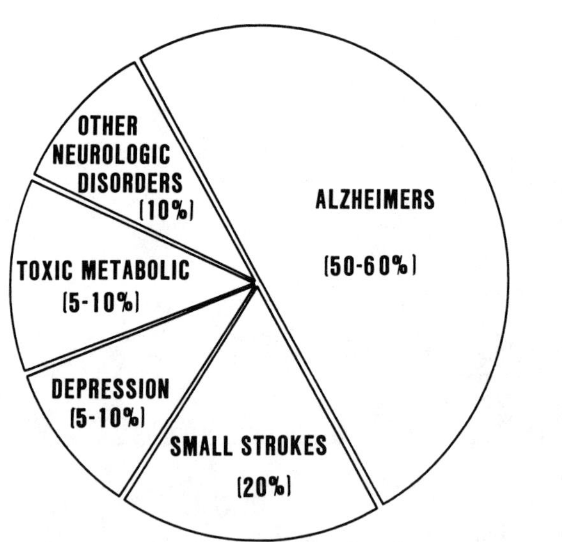

FIG 8–1.
Percentages of major causes of dementia and a differential of the other neurologic and toxic-metabolic etiologies.

on whether its onset is before or after a person is 65 years old. Alzheimer's disease accounts for 50% to 60% of all dementias. It is most common in persons older than 60 years, and the prevalence increases with age, exceeding 20% in those over 80 years of age.

Clinical Features

The intellectual deterioration is insidious but steadily progressive. The initial forgetfulness progresses to confusion and disorientation and impairment of language and gait. By this time the patient needs much assistance in activities of daily living. In the late stages the patient is bedridden and survives in a vegetative state. Death is usually from aspiration or intercurrent infection and may occur from 2 to 20 years after onset.

Diagnosis

There is no specific diagnostic test for Alzheimer's disease. It remains a clinical-pathologic diagnosis by brain biopsy or at autopsy. Computed tomography (CT scanning) and autopsy frequently show cortical atrophy and ventricular dilatation (Fig. 8–2). However, cerebral atrophy is frequent in normal aging and is often indistinguishable from the atrophy of Alzheimer's disease. There is often no correlation between severity of dementia and the degree of atrophy seen in CT scan.

Pathologic Changes

Microscopic abnormalities characteristically seen in Alzheimer's disease consist of neuronal loss, senile (neuritic) plaques, and neurofibrillary tangles. These changes are scattered throughout the cerebral cortex, but are particularly abundant in the hippocampus and amygdala. They are not unique to Alzheimer's disease and may be found in smaller numbers in the normal aging brain. Senile plaques are spherical aggregates of degenerating dendrites, axon terminals, and glial cells and processes in the neuropil. The central core of the plaque contains amyloid. Neurofibrillary tangles are thickened twisted neurofibrils located in the neuronal perikariyon. Ultrastructurally, tangles are paired filaments twisted around each other in a helical fashion (paired helical filaments). Tangles may be seen in other neurologic disorders (e.g., parkinsonism and pugilistic dementia). Hippocampal neurons may show

TABLE 8–3.
Dementia: Clinical–Pathologic Correlations

DEMENTING DISORDER	MAJOR CLINICAL FEATURES	AREAS OF MAXIMAL INVOLVEMENT	HISTOLOGY/IOCHEMISTRY/ PATHOPHYSIOLOGY
Alzheimer's disease	Dementia	Cerebral cortex Hippocampus Amygdala Nucleus basalis	Neuronal loss Senile plaques Neurofibrillary tangles ↓ Acetylcholine
Huntington's disease	Dementia Chorea Autosomal dominant history	Caudate and putamen Cerebral cortex	Neuronal loss in caudate ↓ Acetylcholine and GABA
Multi-infarct dementia	Dementia Gait disorder Pseudobulbar palsy Corticospinal signs Hypertension Diabetes	Cerebral cortex Central white matter Basal ganglia Internal capsule	Multiple small infarcts Small vessel occlusions Arteriolar necrosis
Normal pressure hydrocephalus	Gait disorder Incontinence Dementia	Dilated ventricles without cortical atrophy	↓ CSF circulation Meningeal fibrosis
Creutzfeldt-Jakob disease	Dementia Myoclonus Extrapyramidal Cerebellar	Cerebral cortex Basal ganglia Cerebellum	Spongiform changes Neuronal loss Astrocytosis "Slow virus" infection
Parkinson's disease	Akinesia Tremor Rigidity Gait disorder	Substantia nigra Locus ceruleus	Depigmentation Lewy inclusion bodies Neuronal loss ↓ Nigrostriatal dopamine
Wilson's disease	Dementia Extrapyramidal Kaiser-Fleischer ring Liver involvement Autosomal recessive history	Basal ganglia Liver Cornea Kidney	↓ Ceruloplasmin Copper deposition in tissues

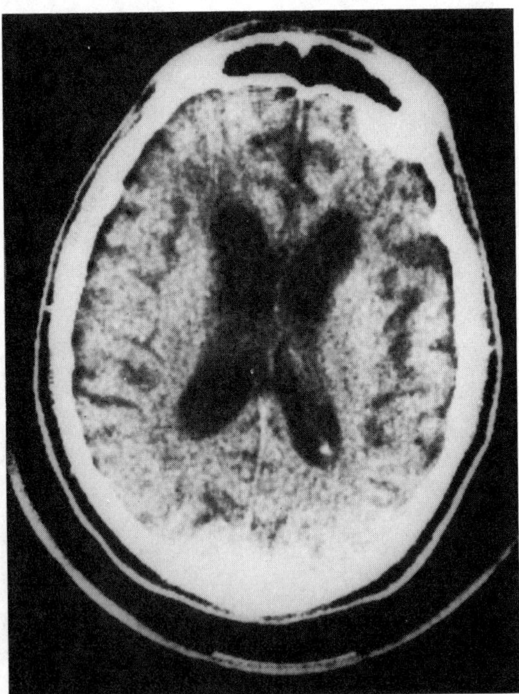

FIG 8–2.
CT scan in Alzheimer's disease showing cortical atrophy and ventricular dilatation. Similar degrees of atrophy are common in normal aging.

granulovacuolar degeneration. The cytoplasm shows vacuolation with a central granular particle. There is neuronal loss and shrinkage of dendritic arborizations in the cortex which is greater than that seen in normal aging.

In Alzheimer's disease the brain shows a consistent decrease of the neurotransmitter acetylcholine and the enzyme necessary for its synthesis, choline acetyl transferase. Acetylcholine-producing neurons are concentrated in a small area in the basal forebrain nuclei (nucleus basalis of Meynert). Their axons transport the neurotransmitter widely throughout the cortex. In Alzheimer's disease this cholinergic neuronal system is selectively damaged. Less consistent decreases of norepinephrine, serotonin, and somatostatin have also been noted in some cases of Alzheimer's disease.

Etiology

The etiology of Alzheimer's disease is unknown, but several hypotheses are under study. Genetics may play a role in programming cer-

tain neuronal systems for premature death. The vast majority of Alzheimer's disease is sporadic, but in a few families there is an autosomal dominant transmission. In identical twins there is an increased concordance of Alzheimer's disease. Population studies of Alzheimer's disease show a higher risk for Alzheimer's disease in first-degree relatives of probands. Alzheimer's disease has a close relationship with Down's syndrome (trisomy 21). Virtually all patients with Down's syndrome who live past 35 years will show the clinical, pathologic, and biochemical findings of Alzheimer's disease. An increased frequency of Down's syndrome has been noted in the families of Alzheimer's disease. This suggests that abnormalities in chromosomes may have a role in the development of Alzheimer's disease. A viral cause has been suggested. Slowly progressive dementing disorders (e.g., Creutzfeldt-Jakob disease and kuru) have been shown to be due to transmissible agents, presumably unconventional or "slow" viruses. However, Alzheimer's disease has not been transmitted to animals, and no infectious agent has been identified. Environmental toxins have been suggested as a cause of Alzheimer's disease. Aluminum levels in the brain are increased in Alzheimer's disease, but elevated levels are also seen in dialysis dementia and other encephalopathies. Increased aluminum may be a consequence of neuronal injury rather than its cause. Memory loss is postulated to be due to a selective loss of cholinergic neurons in the basal forebrain nuclei. The selective vulnerability of this neuronal system may be due to a toxic or infectious agent or to the lack of a trophic hormone. Other hypotheses under scrutiny include immune system abnormalities, disordered cerebral blood flow, and multifactorial causes (e.g., a toxic or infectious insult in a genetically predisposed individual).

Principles of Treatment

The course of Alzheimer's disease cannot be arrested or reversed. Many different pharmacologic modes of treatment to improve memory have met with little or no success. Strategies to increase acetylcholine levels in the brain using its precursors lecithin and choline, cholinomimetic drugs, or choline esterase inhibitors (physostigmine) have resulted in little or no significant benefit. Symptomatic and supportive treatments of the depression, agitation, psychosis, wandering, and sleep disturbances are provided with antidepressants, neuroleptics, or sedative drugs. Nonpharmacologic strategies such as a structured environment and structured activities, group therapy, reality orientation, and behavioral modification are useful. The primary caregivers must be assisted through day care, social services, and self-help support groups.

MULTIPLE INFARCT DEMENTIA

Multiple strokes account for 20% of all dementias. Dementia is associated with corticobulbar and pyramidal dysfunction resulting in pseudobulbar palsy, a shuffling gait, hyperreflexia, and Babinski's signs. There are multiple strokes in the cortex, central white matter, and basal ganglia due to occlusion of small or penetrating blood vessels. Small-vessel disease is usually due to hypertension or diabetes mellitus. This syndrome can also be caused by multiple strokes of any etiology (e.g., emboli, vasculitis, and so forth). The clinical course is punctuated by repeated acute episodes and stepwise deterioration. Progression may be arrested by vigorous treatment of the hypertension.

NORMAL PRESSURE HYDROCEPHALUS

Normal pressure hydrocephalus consists of a triad of dementia, gait impairment, and urinary incontinence. In normal pressure hydrocephalus there is no ventricular obstruction, but there is a delay in the circulation of cerebrospinal fluid (CSF) in the subarachnoid space or in its absorption by the arachnoid villi. Delayed CSF flow is often due to meningeal fibrosis secondary to previous meningitis, subarachnoid hemorrhage, head trauma, or surgery. In many cases the predisposing cause is unknown. A lumbar puncture shows normal pressure and may be followed by transient clinical improvement. It is unclear why CSF pressure is normal despite a blockage of CSF circulation. A CT scan typically shows marked ventricular enlargement without cortical atrophy (Fig. 8–3). Delayed circulation and absorption of CSF can be demonstrated by radionuclide cisternography in which a radioisotope is

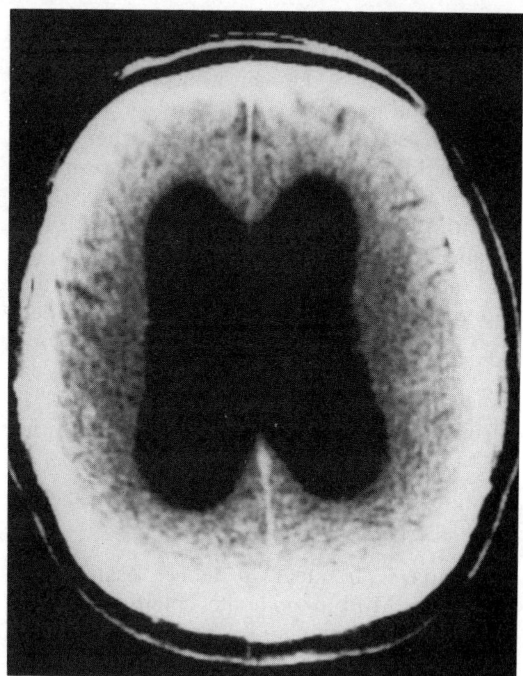

FIG 8–3.
CT scan in normal pressure hydrocephalus. Marked ventricular dilatation in a 60-year-old man with gait impairment, urinary incontinence, and mild dementia. He had bacterial meningitis in childhood.

injected into the CSF by lumbar puncture. Patients with the classic triad and the typical radiologic findings may show dramatic reversal of their neurologic abnormalities after operative shunting of CSF into the peritoneum or the vascular system.

HUNTINGTON'S DISEASE

Dementia is associated with choreiform or athetoid movements. Huntington's disease is an autosomal dominant disorder which usually begins between ages 20 and 40 years. Huntington's disease may begin with abnormal movements or with dementia. Psychiatric symptoms such as depression, personality changes, or psychosis are common early features of dementia. Chorea consists of quick involuntary nonpurposeful movements of the extremities. Gait, speech, and swallowing may be affected. The course of the disease is usually 20 to 30 years. Marked atrophy of the caudate nucleus and putamen may be detected by a CT scan. There is a lesser degree of neuronal loss in the cerebral cortex and other subcortical nuclei. The levels of the neurotransmitters acetylcholine and gamma-aminobutyric acid (GABA) are decreased in the basal ganglia whereas the level of dopamine is unchanged. This results in a dopaminergic-cholinergic imbalance. Neuroleptic drugs such as haloperidol restore the balance by blocking dopamine transmission and may ameliorate the movement disorder. Molecular genetic studies have helped to identify the probable locus of the Huntington's disease gene in chromosome 4. Future advances based on these studies may assist in early diagnosis and identification of high-risk patients.

PARKINSONISM

Dementia is frequent in other basal ganglia disorders. Mild-to-moderate cognitive impairment often accompanies the tremor, rigidity, akinesia, and gait disorder of parkinsonism.

WILSON'S DISEASE

Wilson's disease is an autosomal recessive disorder of copper metabolism. There is a deficiency of the copper-binding globulin ceruloplasmin, and copper is deposited in the brain (lenticular nuclei), liver, and kidneys. Mental, cognitive, and extrapyramidal symptoms are common. Copper deposits in the cornea result in the Kayser-Fleischer ring. Because of frequent liver involvement, the disorder is referred to as hepatolenticular degeneration. Penicillamine therapy may arrest or reverse the neurologic symptoms.

CREUTZFELDT-JAKOB DISEASE

Creutzfeldt-Jakob Disease is a rare disorder in which rapidly progressive dementia is associated with myoclonus, rigidity, and ataxia. This disease is an example of a degenerative dementing disorder which has been proven to be due to a filtrable agent, probably a "slow" or unconventional virus. Creuetzfeldt-Jakob disease can be transmitted to animals by inoculation of infected human brain tissue. There have also been well-documented studies of man-to-man transmission through contaminated neurosurgical instruments and corneal transplants, as well as from the use of infected pituitary growth hormone extract.

TOXIC-METABOLIC DEMENTIAS

Toxic-metabolic dementias are important because they include many of the treatable dementias. Drugs, chronic alcoholism, deficiency of vitamin B_{12} and folate, and hypothyroidism may result in progressive intellectual deterioration.

CHRONIC INFECTIONS

Chronic infections of the CNS are uncommon, but potentially treatable causes of dementia. Patients with tertiary syphilis, fungal and tuberculous meningitis, sarcoidosis, Whipple's disease, and viral encephalitides can present with dementia. Dementia is a frequent complication of AIDS, resulting from an opportunistic viral fungal or parasitic infection of the CNS, or due to a chronic encephalitis from the AIDS virus itself.

REFERENCES

Appel SH: Alzheimer's disease, in Appel SH (ed): *Current Neurology*, Vol 6. Chicago, Year Book Medical Publishers, 1986, pp 289–324. *An excellent review of current developments in Alzheimer's disease.*

Hutton JT (ed): Dementia. *Neurologic Clin North Am* 1986; 4(2). *This multiauthored monograph is recommended as the best reference text on dementia.*

Katzman R: Dementia, in Appel SH (ed): *Current Neurology*, Vol 5. New York, John Wiley & Sons, 1984, pp 91–116. *A comprehensive account of the clinical and pathologic features of the dementias.*

Khachaturian ZS: Diagnosis of Alzheimer's disease. *Arch Neurol* 1985; 42:1097–1105. *A research workshop report summarizing current knowledge and future directions of research.*

NIA Task Force: Senility reconsidered. Treatment possibilities for mental impairment in the elderly. *JAMA* 1980; 244:259–263. *A brief but well-written overview of normal aging, delirium, and dementia.*

Reisberg B: *Alzheimer's Disease.* New York, Free Press, 1983. *The psychosocial aspects of Alzheimer's disease are well described.*

9 DYSPNEA

Charles B. Payne, Jr., M.D.

Dyspnea (shortness of breath) is defined as a sensation of labored or difficult breathing. Physiologic breathlessness occurs appropriately after exertion and increases in intensity proportionally to the magnitude of the workload. This chapter will discuss pathologic dyspnea, which, in the opinion of the patient, occurs inappropriately. Dyspnea is a symptom and may cause a great deal of suffering, anxiety, and impairment of functional ability. Because dyspnea is subjective, it is imprecisely measured. Sensations felt to be of no consequence to a stoic person may produce severe complaints in an anxious patient. When the patient and the physician disagree on the appropriateness of breathlessness, medical intervention and physiologic testing, which may be extensive, are often necessary to resolve the difference of opinion.

Although no theory explains dyspnea fully, one hypothesis is that the sensation may occur when external respiration (breathing) is inadequate to keep pace with cellular respiration. If the output of the respiratory system is inappropriate for the "drive" to breathe, this disparity is interpreted as dyspnea. Dyspnea may occur as a symptom of pulmonary disease or of diseases not primarily involving the respiratory system, and it may occur in the absence of significant disease of any organ system.

CLINICAL SIGNS AND SYMPTOMS

A detailed medical history must be obtained with particular emphasis on the patient's use of tobacco. Smoking should be recorded in pack-years or bowls of pipe tobacco consumed per unit time. Smoking is intimately involved in the pathogenesis not only of parenchymal lung diseases, but also in cardiac and peripheral vascular diseases associated with shortness of breath or exercise limitation. The history must elicit exactly what the patient means by shortness of breath. This may vary from accurate estimates of the number of stairs climbed to produce breathlessness to being unable to "fill the lungs" on deep breathing or sighing. Some complaints actually refer to "choking" or "tightness" of the chest. Several methods of rating dyspnea are described in Table 9–1.

Specific inquiries must be made regarding where, when, and under what circumstances dyspnea arises and whether or not there are other associated symptoms. Postural changes that elicit or decrease dyspnea must be recorded. Dyspnea that occurs when the patient lies flat is called orthopnea. In patients with lung disease, breathing discomfort is immediate or immediately worsened upon lying down. Dyspnea beginning 1 or 2 hours after lying down at night is called paroxysmal nocturnal dyspnea and strongly suggests congestive heart failure or mitral stenosis. The acute onset of dyspnea suggests an acute process such as pulmonary emboli, pneumothorax, cardiac or noncardiac pulmonary edema, or aspiration of a foreign body. A subacute or chronic onset suggests more indolent disease. Shortness of breath at rest but not during exertion is usually psychogenic.

A complete physical examination must be performed with particular emphasis on the cardiovascular and pulmonary systems. The respiratory rate should be measured unobtrusively when the patient's attention is diverted. The normal resting respiratory rate is 14 to 20 breaths per minute in adults. Although physical findings will suggest specific laboratory tests, determination of the hemoglobin level or hematocrit, the leukocyte count, and blood glucose and urea nitrogen levels should

---

TABLE 9–1.
Methods for Rating Dyspnea

I. Dyspnea Graded on a 0-to-4 Scale
   Grade 0—No dyspnea with normal activity
   Grade 1—More dyspnea than for a person of the same age on level walking, climbing two flights of stairs, or going up an incline
   Grade 2—More dyspnea than and an inability to keep pace with a person of the same sex/age on level walking
   Grade 3—Dyspnea on level walking and while performing everyday chores
   Grade 4—Dyspnea during personal activities such as dressing, talking, and so forth
II. Linear Estimation of Dyspnea (Visual Analogue Scale of Stark and Gamble)

(15 to 20 cm)

Not at all breathless   Very breathless

III. Magnitude Scaling of Loads to Breathing
   Based on Steven's psychophysical law, $\psi = K\Theta^n$, where K is a constant, n = increase in sensation (ψ) for an increase in physical stimulus (Θ). The subject is instructed to assign an open-ended number to the perceived magnitude of an added load to breathing (either elastic or resistive).
   If the natural log of the estimated number is plotted against the increasing loads, an exponential relationship is seen. The exponent for elastic loads appears to be about 1, while for resistive loads, values of 0.75 to 0.80 are reported.

---

be routine. An electrocardiogram and a standard chest x-ray film are needed. Tests of pulmonary function such as simple spirometry to detect restriction or obstruction are quite useful. More detailed testing may be required.

PATHOPHYSIOLOGY

Stimulation of irritant receptors in the nose, pharynx, and airways signals the effector organs to initiate protective behavior such as breathholding, coughing, sneezing, and avoidance. Chemical pollution, extremes of temperature, or antigenic materials, when inhaled, may initiate diffuse bronchospasm with wheezing and dyspnea.

Chemoreceptors in the blood, brain, and elsewhere respond to changes in blood pH and carbon dioxide and oxygen tensions by varying the respiratory rate and depth to maintain homeostasis. Mechanoreceptors in the lung, chest-wall musculature, and diaphragm detect changes in length–tension relationships such as alterations in lung or chest-wall compliance or in the resistance to airflow. The output of these receptors is fed into the central nervous system. Thermoreceptors, mechanoreceptors, and vasomotor neuron impulses from the whole body provide stimuli that modify the central control of ventilation.

Cortical control of ventilation enables us to suspend breathing, sigh voluntarily, speak, and carry out other essential body functions for which a Valsalva or Mueller maneuver is required. The integration of stimuli from peripheral receptors enables us to suspend cortical control during sleep and most activities without conscious awareness of breathing. Experiments have shown that awareness may be quickly recruited by techniques that focus concentration on the act of breathing.

There is a complex hierarchy of stimuli and responses. The central pontine respiratory center (controller) initiates inspiratory and expiratory signals to the respiratory musculature (effectors), which result in the minute ventilation (V_{min}). Disorders of the integrative brainstem centers are known to produce markedly dysrhythmic breathing, apnea, and disorders of sleep. The various receptors provide the input signals to the central controller as well as necessary feedback loops that tune respiratory output to the environment. Cheyne-Stokes respiration is the classic example of abnormal timing of the feedback circuit. In this condition, delays in the stimuli resulting from altered partial pressures of carbon dioxide or oxygen result in periodic apnea and hyperpnea as the controller "hunts" for the optimal level of V_{min}. Because of the altered timing of the feedback circuit, the arterial oxygen tension (Pa_{O_2}) is actually highest during the periods of apnea.

In general, chemoreceptor responses that are evolutionarily "old" appear to be less impor-

TABLE 9–2.
Pulmonary Diseases and Probable Mechanisms of Dyspnea Production

PULMONARY DISEASE	PROBABLE MECHANISMS OF DYSPNEA
Chronic airflow obstruction	Alterations in lung and chest-wall compliance.
Emphysema	Ventilation/perfusion mismatch with hypercapnia and
Chronic bronchitis	hypoxemia.
Interstitial lung diseases	Compliance may be altered by increased lung water or
Adult respiratory distress	inflammatory or fibrotic or neoplastic infiltrates.
syndrome	Hypoxemia drives breathing as disease progresses.
Pneumoconioses	
Lymphangitic carcinomatosis	
Sarcoidosis	
Infectious diseases	Increased airway resistive loads.
Viral and bacterial bronchitis	Alterations in compliance and ventilation/perfusion
Bronchiolitis	mismatching.
Asthma	Increased resistive loads to airflow with changes in lung
	compliance and chest-wall compliance.
Pulmonary hypertension	Stimulation of cardiac and pulmonary stretch receptors and
	baroreceptors with hypoxemia.

tant than other input signals in the fine tuning of ventilation in normal humans. In disease states with the anesthetic effects of increased levels of carbon dioxide and the depressant effects of drugs and trauma, the hierarchy may be rearranged. Substantial hypoxemia is normally well tolerated before dyspnea is produced. In some patients with neuromuscular paralysis who are mechanically ventilated producing chronic hypocapnea and alkalosis, attempts to normalize the pH and Pa_{CO_2} by reducing V_{min} result in dyspnea. Oxygen therapy is frequently prescribed for patients with dyspnea resulting from mechanical abnormalities of the lung or chest wall such as infiltrating neoplasms. If these patients are hypoxemic because of intrapulmonary shunts, neither the hypoxemia nor the dyspnea is corrected with oxygen, which is both expensive and illogical therapy.

The difficulties of carrying out invasive experiments in primates and humans and the problems in extrapolating findings in lower mammals to humans make studies of the pathogenesis, mechanisms, and treatment of dyspnea difficult to design and to interpret. This is currently an active and fruitful area of research.

PULMONARY CONDITIONS ASSOCIATED WITH DYSPNEA

Dyspnea may be produced by alterations of the environment such as extremes of temperature and humidity, alterations of lung and chest-wall compliance, and changes in airway tone and caliber. Pulmonary diseases that alter gas tensions of carbon dioxide and oxygen from ventilation/perfusion ratio changes may cause breathlessness. A listing of some of these diseases and the probable mechanisms of dyspnea production is shown in Table 9–2. The detection of these pulmonary conditions is based on the historical and objective findings discussed under each disease.

NONPULMONARY CONDITIONS ASSOCIATED WITH DYSPNEA

In many nonpulmonary diseases the actual mechanism of dyspnea production is poorly understood. Early in most of these diseases, there may be few symptoms. At which level of disease dyspnea becomes an initial complaint is not recorded for most. Table 9–3 lists major nonpulmonary illnesses and the presumed mechanisms of dyspnea production. Psychogenic dyspnea is a diagnosis of exclusion. The diagnosis may be made only after organic causes are eliminated by careful and thorough examination. In addition, there should be a history and positive findings consistent with a psychiatric disorder.

LABORATORY INVESTIGATIONS IN DYSPNEA

Diagnostic studies for the underlying disease processes will usually be rewarded with a sat-

TABLE 9–3.
Nonpulmonary Diseases and Presumed Mechanisms of Dyspnea Production

NONPULMONARY DISEASE	PRESUMED MECHANISM OF DYSPNEA
Heart failure	Altered lung compliance from increased lung water. Inadequate cardiac output and oxygen transport during exertion, especially in pulmonic stenosis. Activation of vascular stretch receptors in mitral stenosis.
Anemia	Tachypnea occurs without dyspnea early. Orthopnea and exertional dyspnea occur late. Hypoxemia in respiratory center stimulates breathing. Diminished oxygen delivery to respiratory muscles.
Hyperthyroidism	Cause is not well understood. Common symptom unrelated to heart failure.
Obesity	Altered chest-wall compliance requiring increased work to breathe. Increased blood volume prior to heart failure with lung compliance change because of increased lung water.

Mechanical disorders of the spine
  Scoliosis
  Kyphosis
	Degree of dyspnea usually proportional to degree of deformity. Abnormal stretch receptors and compliance change. Hypoxemia and hypercapnea with increased lung water when heart failure occurs late.

Neuromuscular diseases
  Amyotrophic lateral sclerosis
  Guillain-Barré syndrome
  Myasthenia gravis
	Apparently little reflex stimulation. Dyspnea occurs late with vital capacity severely reduced to about 1 L. Ventilation must be carefully monitored.

Pulmonary embolic disease	Obstruction of pulmonary vasculature by embolized material alters compliance, ventilation perfusion relationships with reduced arterial oxygenation or a widened arterial-alveolar oxygen gradient and causes pulmonary hypertension together with remodeling of pulmonary vessels.

isfactory explanation of the symptom of dyspnea. The most common requirement for more complex testing occurs in the fields of sports medicine and in disability evaluations. In these areas, exercise testing with determination of blood oxygen tensions or saturation, oxygen consumption, and carbon dioxide production under exercise conditions on an ergometer or treadmill may be required. On occasion catheterization of the pulmonary artery may be used to measure intravascular pressures and to obtain a sample of mixed venous blood to measure oxygen content. Cardiac output measurements by a variety of methods may be added.

Additional pulmonary laboratory studies may include determination of the lung volumes, maximum voluntary ventilation, airway resistance, diffusing capacity for carbon monoxide, compliance, and frequency dependency of compliance. Methacholine studies or other challenge tests may be required to detect hyperactive airways. These studies are not routine and should be based on a real need to know after most other diagnostic tests have been performed.

PRINCIPLES OF TREATMENT

Dyspnea should never be treated without a diagnosis of the underlying condition that produces it. In most clinical situations, management of the underlying disease is the preferred method of therapy. In some patients with proven lung disease, in whom dyspnea is the cause of great discomfort and suffering, efforts to reduce the symptom of dyspnea without compromising the respiratory drive to breathe may be useful. The use of diazepam, dihydrocodeine, and promethazine for this condition has been studied. Promethazine currently appears to be the most promising agent because it reduces the level of breathlessness for a constant V_{min} in normal subjects. The effectiveness of drug therapy in patients with chronic lung disease has not yet been proven. A variety of meditation and biofeedback techniques are currently under investigation.

REFERENCES

Altose MD: Assessment and management of breathlessness. *Chest* 1985; 88(2):77s–83s. *A good description of the physiologic mechanisms of dyspnea together with an introduction to direct magnitude scaling measurements and current therapy.*

Burki NK: Dyspnea. *Clin Chest Med* 1980; 1:47–55. *An excellent and brief review of the theories of dyspnea production and their experimental basis with a bibliography citing early work.*

Killian KJ, Mahutte CK, Campbell EJM: Magnitude scaling of externally added loads to breathing. *Am Rev Respir Dis* 1981; 123:12–15. *A description of the complexities of measuring the output variables of the respiratory control system and the difficulty of drawing conclusions.*

Sivaprasad R, Payne CB Jr: Nonpulmonary causes of dyspnea. *Radiol Clin North Am* 1984; 22:463–465. *A brief review paper with references to the scanty literature on nonpulmonary dyspnea.*

Stark RD, Gambles SA, Lewis JA: Methods to assess breathlessness in healthy subjects: A critical evaluation and application to analyse the acute effects of diazepam and promethazine on breathlessness induced by exercise or by exposure to raised levels of carbon dioxide. *Clin Science* 1981; 61:429–439. *A description of the visual analogue scale method of Aitken in the clinical measurement of dyspnea.*

10   HEMOPTYSIS

Timothy G. Janz, M.D.

Hemoptysis is defined as the expectoration of blood or blood-stained sputum from the lower respiratory tract. It typically occurs after cough and frequently recurs over several hours or days. Fortunately most episodes of hemoptysis are mild; however, serious underlying disease accounts for approximately 80% of the cases.

The amount of hemoptysis correlates with the urgency of evaluation. Massive hemoptysis is defined as greater than 200 ml of blood in one episode or greater than 600 ml of blood in 24 hours. Massive hemoptysis is life threatening, not because of exsanguinating hemorrhage, but because of asphyxiation, which is the leading cause of death. As little as 150 ml of blood can result in suffocation.

CLINICAL SIGNS AND SYMPTOMS

Clinically, hemoptysis must be differentiated from hematemesis (Table 10–1) and from bleeding from the upper respiratory tract (i.e., epistaxis). The differentiation can usually be made with a careful history and physical exam-

TABLE 10–1.
Differentiation of Hemoptysis and Hematemesis

FEATURES	HEMOPTYSIS	HEMATEMESIS
Blood Characteristics		
Character	Frothy	Smooth nonfrothy
Color	Bright red	Dark red
pH	Alkaline	Acidic
History	Coughing	GI symptoms

ination. Once hemoptysis is established, the history should include the amount, character, and duration of bleeding. Some patients are able to localize the site of bleeding by an ill-defined, vague, pulling-type sensation in the chest. The patient should be questioned about past medical history, current medications, exposure to tuberculosis, thrombophlebitis, trauma, and history of preexisting lung disease, rheumatic fever, and smoking.

A thorough physical examination is essential. There may be signs of pulmonary consolidation accompanied by rhonchi or rales. Wheezing suggests airway obstruction; however, a pulmonary friction rub suggests pulmonary infarction. A diastolic murmur of mitral stenosis or a third heart sound may indicate a cardiovascular cause. Cutaneous ecchymosis or purpura points toward a bleeding dyscrasia. Clubbing of the digits suggests lung neoplasm or lung abscess. Deep venous thrombophlebitis may indicate pulmonary embolism as a cause of hemoptysis. The absence of the gag reflex may be associated with aspiration and lung abscess.

PATHOPHYSIOLOGY

The pathophysiology of bleeding into the respiratory tract can be accounted for by two basic mechanisms: (1) disruption of the integrity of the pulmonary vascular walls, and (2) disorders in coagulation or hemostasis. Distur-

TABLE 10–2.
Clinical–Pathologic Correlations for Hemoptysis

DISEASE PROCESS	CLINICAL FINDINGS — CLINICAL PRESENTATION	PATHOLOGIC FINDINGS
CARDIOVASCULAR		
Pulmonary infarction	Tachypnea, tachycardia, pleuritic chest pain friction rub, signs of thrombophlebitis	Vessel necrosis
Mitral stenosis	Diastolic heart murmur, right ventricular thrust, opening mitral snap, loud first heart sound	Pulmonary hypertension
Pulmonary edema	Pink frothy sputum, bilateral pulmonary rales, distended neck veins, S_3, pedal edema	Pulmonary hypertension
MISCELLANEOUS		
Bleeding dyscrasias	Cutaneous ecchymosis or purpura, bleeding gingiva, epistaxis, hematuria	Abnormal blood coagulation or hemostasis
Pulmonary arteriovenous malformations	Pulmonary bruits, telangiectasia	Ruptured bronchial artery
INFECTIOUS		
Chronic bronchitis	Smoking history, chronic cough and sputum production, rhonchi/wheezing	Mucosal ulceration
Bronchiectasis	Digital clubbing, with or without cough and copious sputum production, coarse rales	Mucosal ulceration, ruptured bronchial artery
Lung abscess	Cough, foul-smelling sputum, fever, localized lung dullness with bronchial or absent breath sounds, digital clubbing	Vessel necrosis
Tuberculosis and fungal diseases	Cough, with or without sputum production, weight loss, cachexia, anorexia, fever, night sweats	Vessel necrosis, ruptured bronchial artery or aneurysm
NEOPLASTIC		
Carcinoma of the lung	Smoking history, chronic cough, weight loss, cachexia, anorexia	Mucosal ulceration, vessel necrosis
TRAUMATIC		
Blunt or penetrating chest trauma	Puncture wounds, localized chest ecchymosis or contusion, localized chest pain or tenderness, subcutaneous emphysema, signs of hemothorax or pneumothorax	Mucosal ulceration or laceration, rupture or laceration of pulmonary vascular structures
Foreign body aspiration	Localized wheezing, possible rales, signs of consolidation or hyperinflation	Mucosal ulceration or laceration

TABLE 10–3.
"Chocolate MINT" (Mnemonic for remembering categories of hemoptysis)

CATEGORY OF HEMOPTYSIS	CAUSES
Cardiovascular	Pulmonary infarction, mitral stenosis, pulmonary edema, pulmonary hypertension, congenital heart disease
Miscellaneous	Idiopathic, iatrogenic, bleeding diathesis, pulmonary arteriovenous malformations, emphysematous bullae or cysts, broncholithiasis
Infectious	Chronic bronchitis, bronchiectasis, lung abscess, tuberculosis, fungal or bacterial pneumonias
Inflammatory	SLE, Goodpasture's syndrome, Wegener's granulomatosis, polyarteritis nodosa
Neoplasms	Bronchogenic carcinoma, bronchial adenoma, hemangiomas, disease metastatic to the lung
Trauma	Penetrating or blunt chest trauma, foreign-body aspiration, noxious gas inhalation, protracted coughing

bances in the pulmonary vasculature can be caused by mucosal ulceration or laceration, direct necrosis of vascular walls, pulmonary hypertension, or rupture of a dilated bronchial artery or an aneurysm. The correlations of the clinical features with the pathophysiologic findings for the various disease processes are listed in Table 10–2.

DIFFERENTIAL DIAGNOSIS

Causes of hemoptysis can usually be classified into one of the following categories: infectious or inflammatory, neoplastic, cardiovascular, traumatic, and miscellaneous (Table 10–3).

The most common cause of hemoptysis is infection. Chronic bronchitis and bronchiectasis can account for up to 50% to 60% of all cases. Chronic bronchitis is one of the most common causes of mild hemoptysis and is associated with ulceration of the airway mucosa. Approximately 50% of bronchiectasis cases are associated with hemoptysis; in some instances massive bleeding occurs. Like bronchitis, bronchiectasis causes bleeding by ulceration of the airway mucosa. Lung abscesses are usually caused by anaerobic organisms after aspiration of oropharyngeal secretions. In 10% to 15% of these patients, hemoptysis will develop, and, in half of the patients, it will be massive. In the past, tuberculosis was the most common cause of hemoptysis; however, its occurrence has declined in recent years. While mild bleeding in tuberculosis is due to necrosis of the vessel walls, massive hemorrhage is secondary to rup-

ture of bronchial arteries or aneurysms. Because it can lead to massive, life-threatening hemorrhage, tuberculosis must always be considered in the evaluation of hemoptysis. Virtually any bacterial or fungal pneumonia can be associated with hemoptysis, although the hemoptysis is usually mild.

Other inflammatory disorders can also be associated with hemoptysis. It may occur secondary to a necrotizing vasculitis in diseases such as systemic lupus erythematosis (SLE), Goodpasture's syndrome, polyarteritis nodosa, and Wegener's granulomatosis.

Neoplasm has become a common cause of hemoptysis, especially if the patient is older than 45 years. Bronchogenic carcinoma accounts for 20% to 40% of all hemoptysis. Bleeding is usually mild and appears late in the course of lung cancer. Bronchial adenoma is an uncommon vascular tumor primarily involving the large airways. It is accompanied by hemoptysis in half the cases, and at times the bleeding is massive. Other pulmonary tumors, including carcinoma metastatic to the lungs, are rare causes of hemoptysis. Because of the high association between lung neoplasms and hemoptysis, this symptom in a smoker warrants a thorough evaluation with fiberoptic bronchoscopy and sputum cytology.

Among the cardiovascular causes of hemoptysis, pulmonary infarction is the most important because diagnosis and treatment must be instituted promptly. Although hemoptysis is part of the classic triad for pulmonary infarction (i.e., hemoptysis, dyspnea, and pleuritic chest pain), it occurs in only 35% of cases. Less common cardiovascular causes of mild pulmonary bleeding include pulmonary edema, mitral stenosis, and other causes of pulmonary hypertension.

Penetrating and blunt chest trauma may result in pulmonary bleeding. Penetrating wounds result in direct injury to lung parenchyma. Blunt trauma is associated with pulmonary contusion or rupture of bronchi from rapid deceleration. Foreign body aspiration, especially in the pediatric age group, can result in local laceration and ulceration of the airway mucosa. Noxious gas inhalation and severe, protracted coughing may also be associated with mild airway bleeding.

Miscellaneous causes of hemoptysis include pulmonary arteriovenous malformations, bleeding diathesis, and iatrogenic or idiopathic causes. Idiopathic hemoptysis, which accounts for 10% to 20% of all cases, is a diagnosis of exclusion and requires the following: (1) a normal chest x-ray film, (2) normal findings with fiberoptic bronchoscopy, (3) a normal bronchogram, and (4) a sputum examination negative for pathogenic organisms and malignant cytology.

DIAGNOSIS

A thorough evaluation will lead to a diagnosis of hemoptysis in 80% to 90% of actual cases. In addition to a thorough history and physical examination, the initial evaluation should include measurement of the arterial blood gases, a complete blood count, a coagulation profile that includes a platelet count, and sputum for Gram's stain, for acid-fast stain, for cytologic studies, and for various cultures. Although normal in half the cases, the chest x-ray film is an essential part of the evaluation. Other radiologic studies may include chest tomography, chest computed tomography (CT scan), a ventilation-perfusion lung scan, and, if bronchiectasis is suspected, bronchography.

Fiberoptic bronchoscopy is an integral part of the work-up. It allows direct visualization of the tracheobronchial tree, as well as acquisition of quality sputum samples. In addition to the specific diagnostic utility of fiberoptic bronchoscopy, it can localize the site of active bleeding in almost 90% of cases.

PRINCIPLES OF THERAPY

The definitive therapy of hemoptysis is treating the underlying disease process. The management of pulmonary hemorrhage depends on its severity. Mild hemoptysis may only require rest and cough suppression with an antitussive agent such as low doses of codeine. Treatment of moderate-to-severe hemoptysis may also include rest and cough suppression and, in addition, keeping the involved lung (if known or suspected) in a dependent position, administering supplemental oxygen, and assuring a patent airway.

Massive hemoptysis requires emergency intubation for adequate airway control. Life-threatening hemorrhage usually requires surgical resection of the involved area of the lung. Several procedures may be attempted to keep the airway open and to control the hemorrhage prior to surgery; these include rigid-tube bronchoscopy with packing the site of bleeding, placement of a Fogarty catheter to balloon tamponade the involved bronchus, insertion of a double-lumen endotracheal tube (Carlens tube) to pack the involved mainstem bronchus while maintaining a patent airway in the noninvolved bronchus, and selective endotracheal intubation of the nonbleeding mainstem bronchus. Major contraindications to surgical therapy include advanced bilateral pulmonary disease, inability to localize the site of bleeding, widespread metastatic disease, and severe pulmonary function impairment. Medical management of nonsurgical candidates consists of selective pulmonary angiography with embolization of the bleeding bronchial artery. Surgical therapy is associated with approximately 18% mortality versus 32% for medical therapy; thus, surgical management remains the treatment of choice for massive hemoptysis.

The overall prognosis in patients with hemoptysis depends on the underlying disease process causing the bleeding. Generally speaking, the prognosis of patients with idiopathic hemoptysis is good-to-excellent.

REFERENCES

Athanasoulis CA: Therapeutic applications of angiography. *N Engl J Med* 1980; 302(20):1117–1125. *A relatively recent article describing selective angiography and its application to hemoptysis.*

Conlan AA, Hurwitz SS, Krige L, Nicolaou N, Pool R: Massive hemoptysis: Review of 123 cases. *J Thorac Cardiovasc Surg* 1983; 85:120–124. *A recent review of medical versus surgical management of hemoptysis.*

Orban DJ: Hemoptysis in the emergency setting. *Top Emerg Med* 1980; 2(1):67–77. *A concise, easily read review with emphasis on acute care.*

Parsons GH: Hemoptysis. *J Fam Pract* 1978; 7(2): 353–359. *A good review with emphasis on differential diagnosis and clinical evaluation.*

Pierce JA: Hemoptysis, in Blacklow RS (ed): *Signs and Symptoms,* ed 6. Philadelphia, JB Lippincott, Co, 1977, pp 337–340. *A review of hemoptysis emphasizing the clinical assessment.*

Putman JS, Tellis CJ: Hemoptysis. *Primary Care* 1978; 5(1):67–80. *A detailed discussion with illustrative case presentations.*

11 GASTROINTESTINAL BLEEDING

Christopher J. Barde, M.D.

Patients with gastrointestinal bleeding present in one of three ways. Those with acute hemorrhage have hematemesis, melena, or hematochezia (bright red blood from the rectum). Those with occult bleeding, in which the rate of bleeding is slower, have blood in the stools which is not visible but may be detected with chemical testing. Those with no visual or chemical evidence of blood in the stools may have symptoms or signs of a recent blood loss, such as lethargy, worsening of heart failure, or tachycardia. Gastro-intestinal bleeding is also identified by the site of bleeding, upper and lower gastrointestinal bleeding divided arbitrarily by the ligament of Treitz.

CLINICAL SIGNS AND SYMPTOMS

The history should concentrate on the hemodynamic status of the patient. The symptoms of orthostasis, dizziness, syncope, and rapid heartbeat suggest a volume loss of 20% or more. Precipitating factors are vomiting (Mal-lory-Weiss tear), use of ulcerogenic medications or anticoagulants, and recurrence of ulcer symptoms. A thorough history is also necessary to rule out concomitant disease that may be causing the bleeding (cirrhosis or peptic ulcer) or may be complicated by the bleeding (atherosclerotic heart disease or chronic pulmonary disease).

Finally, attempts are made to localize the source of bleeding through the patient's descriptions of blood loss or pain. Hematemesis points to an upper gastrointestinal lesion, though at least 20% of duodenal ulcers will have an unremarkable history. Melena suggests an upper gastrointestinal source, though small bowel and right colonic lesions may produce melena. Small amounts (5 to 30 ml) of bright red blood lost through the rectum are most frequently from hemorrhoids, though the possibility of polyps, cancer, and colitis should always be considered and evaluated.

The physical examination may give an estimate of the amount of blood lost in acute gastrointestinal bleeding. Orthostasis is the change in blood pressure when going from a supine to a sitting position. A drop of 20 mm Hg systolically, of 10 mm Hg diastolically, or an increase in the pulse rate by 20 beats per minute represents a possible volume loss of 20%. The presence of hypotension and tachycardia represents a possible volume loss of 40%.

An examination of the skin is made for the stigmata of liver disease (jaundice, spider angiomas, palmar erythema), purpura, telangiectasis, or dermal fibromas. Lymphadenopathy may suggest a malignancy. The nares and pharynx should be inspected so that posterior epistaxis is not confused with upper gastrointestinal bleeding. The abdomen is inspected for surgical scars suggesting prior gastric or colonic surgery. With an upper gastrointestinal hemorrhage, the bowel sounds are usually hyperactive. Pain in the epigastrium may be a sign of ulcer, though 15% to 20% of patients will have no pain. Colonic bleeding is usually painless, but when pain occurs, it is usually in the right or left lower quadrant. The presence of hepatomegaly or ascites suggests esophageal varices as a possible source. The rectum is examined for hemorrhoids or low-lying tumors and may reveal melena or hematochezia. A nasogastric aspirate should be collected in all cases of acute hemorrhage, though it will be negative in 20% of patients who have bled from duodenal ulcers. It is important to identify patients at high risk for a complication from gastrointestinal bleeding, such as patients with chronic pulmonary, cardiac, and neurovascular disease.

The natural history of gastrointestinal bleeding is known because of the paucity of medical modalities to arrest hemorrhage. The bleeding in about 80% of patients with upper gastrointestinal bleeding and in 75% of patients with lower gastrointestinal bleeding stops without treatment. The average mortality rate is 8% to 10%, but this may vary from 0% to 100% depending on the source of bleeding, the incidence of rebleeding, and the type of patient. Those with massive bleeding have a higher mortality rate regardless of the source of hemorrhage. The mortality rate is increased by 2 to 8 times if 6 units of packed red blood cells (RBCs) are infused before an operation and by 6 to 24 times if over 10 units are infused. The presence of cirrhosis decreases the survival rate regardless of the patient's age. Patients with lower plasma levels of albumin have a higher

mortality rate should they go to surgery. Finally, the older patient with a coexistent disease has a greater mortality rate.

The relationship between the source of bleeding and mortality varies from 0% for hemorrhoids to 100% for untreated aortoenteric fistulas. The mortality rate for bleeding esophageal varices is 50%, but approaches 95% if the hematocrit is less than 20%. Finally, mortality rates increase for patients who have recurrent bleeding in the hospital. The mortality rate for duodenal ulcer increases from between 1% and 7% to between 12% and 30% with rebleeding. For gastric ulcer, the rate increases from between 7% and 16% to between 25% and 48% and for varices from between 22% and 63% to between 56% and 70% with rebleeding. The risk of a first recurrent hemorrhage in diverticulosis is 20% to 25%, but the risk of a second recurrence is over 50%.

PATHOPHYSIOLOGY

The numerous causes of upper and lower gastrointestinal bleeding can be divided into several categories on the basis of the pathologic features. These are inflammation of the mucosa, physical tearing, varices, diverticula, tumor, and vascular malformations. Any gastrointestinal organ can develop mucosal inflammation that may progress to ulceration. The inflamed areas show erythema that may progress to petechial hemorrhage, exudation, and then ulceration with a visible depression. The mucosa will show an inflammatory response in the lamina propria, but with progression the inflammation will go beyond the muscularis mucosa, and ulceration may ensue.

A Mallory-Weiss tear from vomiting is a linear mucosal tear at the esophagogastric junction. While usually minor, the depth of the tear determines the clinical and pathologic findings. Varices may arise throughout the abdomen but are most critical in the esophagus where they lie close to the surface and may rupture. These large blue serpiginous vessels protrude into the lumen.

Diverticular bleeding comes from a minute rupture in one of the intramural arteries where it passes adjacent to the diverticulum. The rupture is associated with a focus of medial thinning in the artery.

Tumors (polyps or cancers) protrude into the lumen and have a hyperemic appearance from

TABLE 11–1.
Clinical–Pathologic Correlations for Gastrointestinal Bleeding

| | | PATHOLOGIC FINDINGS | |
CLINICAL FINDINGS	CAUSE	PATHOLOGIC FEATURES	TYPE OF BLEEDING
Dyspepsia, variable	Esophagitis, gastritis, duodenitis	Erosion of small vessels	Hematemesis, heme-positive stool
Dyspepsia, variable	Ulcer	Small vessels to medium arteries	Hematemesis, melena, or heme-positive stool
Change in bowel movement	Colitis	Superficial vessels, may be diffuse	Heme-positive stools, rectal bleeding
Without symptoms	Varices	Submucosal or sub-epithelial veins	Hematemesis, melena, or heme-positive stool
History of vomiting	Mallory-Weiss tear	Mucosal or submucosal tear	Hematemesis
Change in bowel movement	Tumor or polyp	Neovascularization	Intermittent or continuous, slow bleeding
Without symptoms	Angiodysplasia or arteriovenous malformation	Smaller vessels	Melena, heme-positive stool
Without symptoms	Aortoenteric fistula	Fistula from an infected graft to bowel	Intermittent melena but eventual exsanguination

neovascularization. They will usually have extreme friability or an ulceration that causes the bleeding.

Four other types of vascular lesions can be seen throughout the bowel and appear as bright red mucosal lesions against a paler mucosa. Angiodysplasia is a flat lesion, often less than 5 mm in diameter and has dilated, tortuous, thin-walled veins and venules. Telangiectases are histologically similar but may be larger and have a clinically distinct pattern. Hemangiomas are nodular and represent clusters of enlarged nonectatic, nontortuous mucosal capillaries. Arteriovenous malformations are over 5 mm in diameter and composed of thickened arteries and veins without the normal capillary connection.

CLINICAL–PATHOLOGIC CORRELATIONS

In gastrointestinal bleeding the correlation between the clinical findings and the pathologic lesion is poor (Table 11–1). This may be related to differences in pain perception, vascular lesions that bleed without pain, different rates of bleeding, and gastrointestinal motility.

DIFFERENTIAL DIAGNOSIS

The history and physical examination may help distinguish between an upper and a lower gastrointestinal source of bleeding but may not help identify the cause. In patients with dyspepsia and bleeding, 75% have an ulcer causing the blood loss. In patients with no dyspepsia, 35% have ulcers as the source of bleeding. Nor does the patient's use of aspirin or alcohol help predict the cause of bleeding. In patients with significant liver disease, only 20% have varices as the source of hemorrhage. Physicians predict the correct source of bleeding less than 40% of the time, and their success rates are independent of their amount of experience. The clinical history and the relative frequencies of various lesions help to arrive at a differential diagnosis (Table 11–2).

TABLE 11–2.
Etiology of Gastrointestinal Bleeding

CAUSE	FREQUENCY (% OF PATIENTS)
CAUSE OF UPPER GI BLEEDING	
Duodenal ulcer	22–39
Gastric ulcer	12–22
Varices	10–20
Erosive gastritis	12–30
Esophagitis	8–12
Duodenitis	9
Mallory-Weiss tear	8
Cancer	3–7
CAUSE OF RECTAL BLEEDING	
Upper gastrointestinal	10
Small intestine	5
Colonic	
Diverticulosis	25
Vascular dysplasia	10
Neoplasm	15
Colitis	5
Ischemia	2
Miscellaneous	8
Undiagnosed	20

DIAGNOSIS

The history and physical examination help localize the source of bleeding. A history of hematemesis or blood on nasogastric aspiration correlates with an upper gastrointestinal lesion. Unfortunately, 20% of bleeding duodenal lesions will have no blood in the nasogastric aspirate. A history of melena suggests an upper gastrointestinal lesion.

The complete blood cell count (CBC) helps to gauge the magnitude of bleeding, though with a massive hemorrhage the intravascular volume may take 6 hours to equilibrate so the true hemoglobin value can be determined. The PT/PTT and platelet count will identify coagulation defects. Other routine tests help assess metabolic and liver function.

Contrast radiographs in the evaluation of bleeding have been largely replaced by endoscopy, radionuclide scans, and angiography. The source of upper gastrointestinal bleeding is identified 90% to 95% of the time by endoscopy and only 80% to 85% by double-contrast x-ray films (with a lower percentage with single contrast films). Because 15% of patients have more than one site of bleeding, radiologic techniques are unable to differentiate the active site. Table 11–3 shows the error rates in patients with rectal bleeding in whom a barium enema showed a normal intestine or only diverticula.

The ability to identify the bleeding site decreases with time. A specific bleeding lesion can be diagnosed 65% to 80% of the time when endoscopy is done in the first 24 hours, but only 20% to 30% of the time after 48 hours. When the site of bleeding is not known, radionuclide scanning using technetium (Tc)-labeled RBCs should be performed. This technique can detect rates of bleeding as low as 0.1 ml/minute, and because the agent stays in the vascular system for 24 hours, intermittent bleeding can be detected thus increasing the test sensitivity to 45% with a 91% specificity. Angiography may be used after a positive radionuclide scan to better identify the lesion, to carry out therapeutic embolization, or to detect vascular lesions like arteriovenous malformations and leiomyomas.

PRINCIPLES OF THERAPY

The initial step in managing gastrointestinal hemorrhage is to stabilize the patient's hemodynamic status. Intravenous fluids can correct

TABLE 11–3.
Barium Enema in Detecting Rectal Bleeding

CLINICAL SIGN	RESULTS OF BARIUM ENEMA	FREQUENCY OF RESULT (% OF PATIENTS)
Acute bleeding	Negative	53
	Diverticula only	44
Heme-positive stool	Negative	19
	Diverticula only	32

intravascular volume depletion, but transfusions are often needed to improve the oxygen-carrying capacity. This improvement may be critical in patients with ischemic heart disease or chronic pulmonary disease. When to transfuse depends on the patient's age, the severity of bleeding, and the associated medical problems. In general, younger patients can tolerate lower hemoglobin values. Patients who have chronic blood loss with microcytic indices may not need transfusions unless angina or neurologic complaints are evident. In older patients, correction of the hematocrit to between 30% and 36% is usually adequate, though volume overload or hepatitis may result. Coagulation defects in patients with active bleeding must be corrected.

Noninvasive medical therapy has been limited to gastric lavage and cimetidine and vasopressin administration, but none of these has proven to be effective. A nasogastric tube is useful to localize the bleeding, monitor its recurrence, and to empty the stomach prior to endoscopy. Neither lavage with ice, an ice-saline, or epinephrine solution will stop active bleeding. Cimetidine is frequently given for hemorrhage. It does not alter the patient's requirement for transfusions or decrease the number of rebleeding episodes, but should still be used in patients with peptic ulcer disease or to prevent stress ulcerations. Vasopressin as a treatment of esophageal varices, is probably not of benefit and can cause hyponatremia and ischemia of small vessels. Balloon tamponade (Sengstaken-Blakemore tube) for esophageal varices is effective in' temporarily arresting variceal bleeding, but subsequent definitive therapy is usually needed.

To date there are no convincing data that early endoscopy alters the morbidity or mortality of bleeding patients. The recent advent of therapeutic endoscopy (injection of varices with sclerosing agents, bicap electrocoagulation, or laser coagulation) is promising. Angiographic embolization of selected bleeders has also been of benefit. The indications for surgical treatment are massive bleeding, perforation, significant rebleeding within 48 hours, and a requirement of 8 or more units of blood. These indications must be tempered by the patient's general condition. The management of gastrointestinal bleeding should involve the gastrointestinal endoscopist and surgeon early in the patient's presentation to help in the decision-making process.

REFERENCES

Bernan J, Rueff B: Treatment of acute variceal bleeding. *Clin Gastroenterol* 1985; 14:185–207. *Excellent, well-referenced review of medical treatments for variceal bleeding.*

Bunker SR, Brown JM, McAuley RJ, et al.: Detection of gastrointestinal bleeding sites. *JAMA* 1982; 247:789–792. *A good discussion of the use and limitation of radionuclide scanning in detecting the source of bleeding.*

Forde KA: Colonoscopy in acute rectal bleeding. *Gastrointest Endosc* 1981; 27:219–220. A report that colonoscopy can be performed acutely and that diverticular bleeding is not as frequent a cause as previously claimed.*

LaBrooy ST, Misiewicz JJ, Edwards J, et al.: Controlled trial of cimetidine in upper gastrointestinal hemorrhage. *Gut* 1979; 20:892–895. *One of several studies showing that cimetidine does not control acute gastrointestinal bleeding or alter transfusion requirements.*

Meyer CT, Troucale FJ, Galloway S, et al.: Arteriovenous malformations of the bowel: An analysis of 22 cases and a review of the literature. *Medicine* 1981; 60:36–48. *An extensive review of arteriovenous malformations.*

Morrissey JF: Clinical approach to diagnostic endoscopy in patients with upper gastrointestinal bleeding. *Dig Dis Sci* 1981; 26:6s–11s. *An excellent discussion of the timing and findings of endoscopy in acute gastrointestinal bleeding.*

Peterson WL: Gastrointestinal bleeding, in Sleisinger MH, Fordtran JS (eds): *Gastrointestinal Disease.* Philadelphia, WB Saunders Co, 1983, pp 177–207. *An extensive discussion and general review of gastrointestinal bleeding, with over 100 references.*

12   BOWEL OBSTRUCTION

Dan W. Elliott, M.D.

The term *bowel obstruction* implies a mechanical barrier preventing the progress of the normal bowel content through the lumen toward the anus. An obstruction that is partial or incomplete may produce only some unpleasant symptoms. An obstruction that stops the flow of all liquid and gas is complete and not compatible with life. Very profound pathologic changes follow within a few hours and demand relief, usually by a surgical operation.

CLINICAL SIGNS AND SYMPTOMS

Regardless of the underlying cause, the symptoms of bowel obstruction depend very much on the level in the bowel at which obstruction occurs (Table 12–1). When the obstruction is sufficiently high, at the pylorus, for instance, vomiting completely decompresses the stomach. This also occurs if the obstruction is in the duodenum or in the first 30 to 60 cm of the jejunum.

In obstruction below the ampulla of Vater, the vomitus is dark green due to a high bile content. Mechanical obstruction may be suspected, but the bowel sounds are not characteristic of obstruction, the abdomen shows no distention, and plain x-ray films of the abdomen are normal. When barium contrast is given, the point of obstruction is revealed. Because the fluid losses from this vomiting are voluminous and high in sodium content, tachycardia and serious dehydration follow very quickly.

Generally, the lower the point of obstruction, the later vomiting appears and the less voluminous it becomes. In the mid-small bowel the onset of obstruction is heralded by severe crampy pain rising to a crescendo, with relief of pain between peristaltic rushes. Abdominal distention is moderate. The bowel sounds are initially hyperactive, but after a few hours grow silent. There is usually generalized abdominal tenderness. The diagnosis can be confirmed by plain x-ray films of the abdomen without contrast, but these must always be taken with the patient in two positions. The film with the patient lying supine will reveal a few loops of distended gas-filled small bowel. With the patient in the upright or lateral decubitus position, characteristic air–fluid levels will be seen. These air–fluid levels indicate the absence of effective peristalsis, which normally mixes air and gas together. The bowel distal to the obstruction is empty and collapsed. The colon normally contains gas and should be visible in plain films. When all gas disappears from the colon, the presence of complete bowel obstruction is confirmed (Figs. 12–1 and 12–2).

When the lower small bowel is involved, the abdominal pain is characteristically more steady, diffuse, and periumbilical. Vomiting occurs later and is feculent. The abdominal distention is marked. Tachycardia and dehy-

TABLE 12–1.
Clinical–Pathologic Correlations for Bowel Obstruction in Adults

| CLINICAL FINDINGS | | PATHOLOGIC FINDINGS | MECHANICAL OBSTRUCTION |
SYMPTOMS AND SIGNS	PHYSICAL SIGNS	RADIOGRAPHIC	SITE
Frequent vomiting, bilious if below pylorus; pain relieved by vomiting; no abdominal distention	Rapid dehydration; tachycardia; abdomen normal, no bowel sounds between vomiting	Plain normal (contrast agent reveals obstruction)	Duodenum, first foot of jejunum
Cramps with crescendo, then relief; moderate vomiting; bile-stained	Moderate abdominal distention; tachycardia; bowel sounds hyperactive early, silent late	A few gas-filled loops of small bowel; air–fluid levels; no gas in colon	Low jejunum Ileum
Generalized steady periumbilical pain; some cramps; vomiting late and feculent	Marked abdominal distention; tachycardia; bowel sounds early rushes, silent late	Many stepladder loops of gas-filled small bowel; air–fluid levels, no gas in colon	Low ileum
Midline lower abdominal cramps, then steady pain; bloating; vomiting very late and feculent	Marked abdominal distention; visible peristalsis; bowel sounds tinkling; tachycardia; dehydration	Enormous gas-filled colon loops with or without a less distended gas-filled small bowel	Distal colon

dration are out of proportion to the external fluid losses. They are due to the marked shifts of fluid into the obstructed loops and within the abdomen. The x-ray films show a large number of gas-filled loops of small bowel above the point of obstruction, but no gas in the colon.

Most colonic obstructions occur distally, in the descending, sigmoid, or upper rectum. These characteristically produce midline lower abdominal pain well below the umbilicus. The pain may be crampy at the onset, but quickly becomes steady with a sensation of bloating. Vomiting appears very late, if at all, and will be feculent. The abdominal distention is the most marked seen with obstruction and may be accompanied by visible peristalsis. The bowel sounds do not reflect hyperactive peristalsis, but only the tinkling of gas bubbles. Tachycardia and dehydration are just as marked as in higher levels of obstruction. The x-ray films of the abdomen show enormously dilated loops of colon filled with gas down to the point of obstruction. If the ileocecal valve is incompetent (as it usually is against high pressure), the small bowel may also be filled with gas, but is less distended. If the valve is competent, the cecum may be enormously dilated. The cecal wall is relatively thin and is usually the first point involved with patchy gangrene, followed by perforation.

The physical examination is significant and should always include a careful appraisal of the degree of dehydration and hypovolemia present. Tachycardia is an important clue. Fever is usually absent or low grade until very late in the course. The degree of abdominal distention will provide a significant guide to the level of obstruction. It is particularly important to search for small hernias of which the patient may have been unaware. These can occur at the umbilicus, in healed incisions, and in the groins of both male and female patients. Tenderness over the femoral triangle may be the only definite clue to a femoral or obturator hernia. These are notoriously prone to incarcerate and strangulate the bowel. A rectal examination should always be done, searching for a tumor in the pelvic cul-de-sac and looking at the character of the stool. Evidence of peritoneal irritation with rigidity and rebound tenderness is an ominous sign of advanced changes in the bowel. Continuous severe pain felt in either the abdomen or the back requires

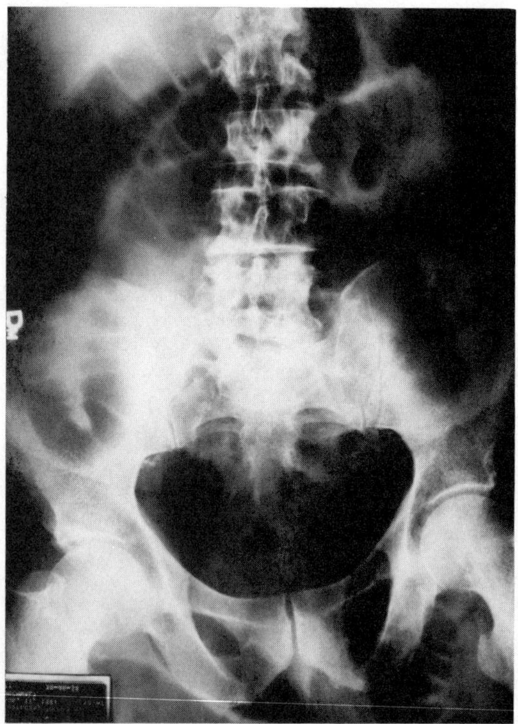

FIG 12–1.
Plain x-ray film of the abdomen with the patient supine. The patient is an adult with complete small-bowel obstruction due to incarceration in a left inguinal hernia. The small bowel is dilated and filled with gas and can be seen in the hernia; no gas at all can be seen in the colon.

urgent attention. Nothing is more painful than ischemic tissue. This sign may herald a strangulated obstruction.

PATHOPHYSIOLOGY

Obstruction usually becomes complete quite suddenly. Regardless of the cause, the pathologic changes secondary to obstruction follow a reasonably constant pattern. The bowel proximal to the point of obstruction distends with liquid and gas whether anything is taken by mouth or not. Gas in the lumen of the bowel builds up quickly. This is mostly swallowed air in the early stages of obstruction.

Fluid also enters the obstructed segment because normal reabsorption of water from the gut lumen is prevented. Distended bowel increases the normal bowel process of secreting fluid into the lumen. Pressure within the lumen of the distended bowel rises. If the obstruction

is very high in the small bowel, vomiting may relieve this pressure both early and late. When the obstruction is more distal, vomiting appears but much later. It is probably reflex in origin and will not evacuate sufficient fluid to reduce the pressure. As the pressure mounts, lymph and venous drainage are impaired, causing the bowel wall to become enormously edematous. Huge quantities of interstitial fluid are also lost because these tissues weep ascitic fluid. This results in rapid development of dehydration, tachycardia, and eventually hypovolemia sufficient to cause shock and death.

The initial response of the bowel wall is to increase the vigor and frequency of peristalsis. Bowel sounds are hyperactive and may be audible without a stethoscope. In thin persons, peristaltic motion of the bowel can be seen through the abdominal wall. As edema of the bowel wall progresses, the smooth muscle eventually becomes fatigued. In late stages of obstruction, the bowel sounds disappear except for the high-pitched tinkling of ineffective peristalsis, and the abdomen grows silent.

Eventually pressures grow sufficient to impede arterial circulation to the mucosa, which will become necrotic and bleed into the lumen. As bacteria proliferate, the vomiting, which started as bilious, becomes feculent in odor and appearance. Patches of gangrene in the intestinal wall coalesce and penetrate to the serosa, eventually causing gross perforation. This releases a lethal mixture of bacteria, necrotic tissue, and blood into the peritoneal cavity which, upon absorption, causes septic shock.

Below the point of obstruction, gas and luminal fluid are normally absorbed and the bowel becomes collapsed and empty. There may be a bowel movement or two immediately after the onset of obstruction in response to the intense initial peristalsis. Within a few hours of obstruction, obstipation is complete. No matter at what level the obstruction develops, no further passage through the anus will occur.

The obstruction is called *simple* if it occurs at only one point in the bowel. Vomiting may partially decompress the bowel above a simple obstruction if it is not too far distal. The introduction of a suction tube may also lower pressures and reverse this progressive cascade of events. However, a volvulus of small or large bowel around a fixed adhesive band, for instance, can produce a "closed loop." This loop of bowel is caught between two points of obstruction, one proximal and one distal. It cannot be decompressed by vomiting or proximal suction. The closed loop may proceed to gangrene and perforation even though the obstructed bowel proximal to this loop is decompressed. Surgical relief is required for closed-loop obstruction.

Both external and internal hernias can "incarcerate" bowel with or without obstruction. However, incarcerated tissues may twist in such a way as to shut off the arterial blood supply. This becomes a "strangulated" obstruction and requires prompt surgical intervention.

DIFFERENTIAL DIAGNOSIS

The causes for bowel obstruction are numerous and depend very much on whether small or large bowel is involved (Table 12–2). In adults by far the most frequent cause for small-bowel obstruction is a single adhesive band, usually the result of a prior abdominal or pelvic operation. Congenital bands also occur, and the absence of prior surgery does not rule out an adhesive band as the cause of obstruction. The band may have been present for months or years, but what has now caused the obstruction is the volvulus of a loop of bowel around it. The possibility of a closed-loop obstruction must be kept in mind. The second most frequent cause is an external hernia, most frequently in the groin. Other less frequent causes include primary tumors of the small bowel. Although rare, these may progress to complete obstruction or may be the lead point in intussusception. More frequently, the neoplasms causing obstruction are metastatic, recurrent, or generalized carcinomatosis. Other causes include primary volvulus which can occur without a postoperative band. Granulomatous enteritis and radiation injury can progress to complete obstruction. In the elderly, vascular occlusion may paralyze a segment of bowel and produce a typical small-bowel obstruction.

In the large bowel, by contrast, the causes for obstruction are much more likely to be neoplastic. The most frequent is adenocarcinoma of the sigmoid colon. Acute diverticulitis is a much less frequent cause for complete obstruction, but it may result in fibrotic stenosis similar to that in ischemic and granulomatous colitis. Volvulus of the sigmoid colon is a distinctive form of acute complete colonic obstruction

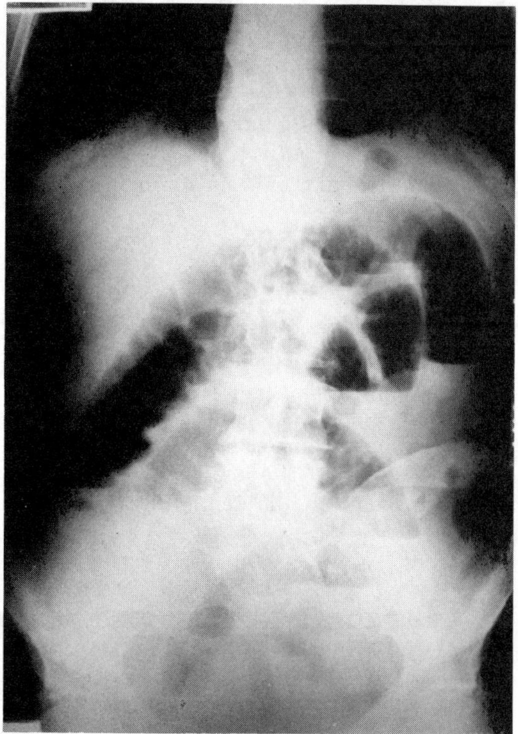

FIG 12–2.
Plain x-ray film of the abdomen with the patient upright. This is the same patient as shown in Fig 12–1. Air-fluid levels are seen in multiple loops of small bowel, while no gas can be seen in the colon.

occurring usually in the elderly with a history of constipation. It invariably produces a two-point obstruction with a completely closed loop. It is usually possible to recognize volvulus on plain films of the abdomen and very important to do so. Decompression through the rectum may be possible by introducing a tube into the closed loop with the aid of a sigmoidoscope. When successful, this decompression leads to complete detorsion and provides relief of obstruction.

The age of the patient is a guide to the likely causes for obstruction. In infancy and early childhood, external hernias predominate. Ileocolonic intussusception has its peak incidence at the age of 2 years and is rare in later childhood. In adults a careful history can provide important clues. Of particular importance is the history of prior operations, hernias, regional enteritis, or radiation. With adhesive bands or incarcerated hernias, the onset is sudden and unexpected. With tumors there may be long history of partial obstructive symptoms, crampy pain, change in bowel habits, or bleeding in the stool. The incidence of tumors among all causes for bowel obstruction rises steadily as age advances (Table 12–3), but even in the elderly, adhesive bands remain the most common cause.

DIAGNOSIS

X-ray films of the abdomen with the patient flat and also upright are the most definitive aids in diagnosis. A chest film is helpful in ruling out air free in the abdomen, suggesting a perforated bowel or stomach. The x-ray films are particularly important in differentiating obstruction from paralytic ileus, its most frequent mimic. In paralytic ileus the obstruction is partial, localized, and due to paralysis of peristalsis near an extrinsic inflammatory process such as appendicitis or pancreatitis. The principal x-ray finding of ileus is distention in both small and large bowel of roughly equal degree (Figure 12–3).

Laboratory investigations include a CBC, urinalysis, and measurement of values for amylase, electrolytes, blood urea nitrogen, and creatinine as a minimum. Leukocytosis is usually absent in early obstruction and then progresses in proportion to the degree of dehydration. Modest elevations of amylase are seen in bowel obstructions of all causes, but high levels are more suggestive of pancreatitis. Electrolyte abnormalities are of particular importance be-

TABLE 12–2.
Causes of Mechanical Obstruction of the Small and Large Bowel in Adults*

SMALL BOWEL (N = 349)		LARGE BOWEL (N = 70)	
CAUSE	INCIDENCE (% OF CASES)	CAUSE	INCIDENCE (% OF CASES)
Adhesive bands	60	Cancer	63
External hernia	15	Diverticulitis	13
Neoplasms		Volvulus	7
Extrinsic	10	Hernia	5
Intrinsic	3	Other causes	12
Other causes	12	Stenosis	
Volvulus		Bands	
Vascular occlusion		Ischemic colitis	
Regional enteritis		Radiation	
Intussusception			
Radiation			

* Data compiled by author in unpublished studies.

TABLE 12–3.
Causes of Mechanical Obstruction of the Bowel in Patients of Various Ages (N = 303)*

	PERCENT OF CASES IN VARIOUS PATIENT AGE RANGES (YEARS)				
CAUSE	0–10	11–20	21–40	41–60	61–90
Hernias	57	30	23	25	43
Adhesive bands	2	51	59	51	27
Tumors	1	0	5	9	17
Intussusception	32	4	0	0	2
Others	8	15	13	15	11

* Data compiled by author in unpublished studies.

cause they require correction for safe operation. Arterial blood gas values can be helpful because profound metabolic acidosis may be the earliest clue to an ischemic bowel. Unfortunately, no laboratory or x-ray finding provides a reliable guide to the progress of obstruction or the presence of impending or actual gangrene, and none should be relied on for this purpose.

PRINCIPLES OF THERAPY

Partial bowel obstruction and paralytic ileus can be effectively treated with nasogastric suction and decompression. In a few instances decompression from above may sufficiently unload a twisted or incarcerated loop to allow release of obstruction. However, this is a risky venture in complete obstruction. Undue delay in operation may lead to progressive necrosis. Nevertheless, nasogastric suction should always be instituted in the presence of bowel obstruction. The stomach is very likely to be loaded with regurgitated small bowel contents. Serious aspiration of vomitus can occur prior to operation or at the induction of anesthesia. Short tubes decompressing only the stomach are probably as effective as the specialized long tubes devised to pass distally into the small bowel. There are, however, cases in which nonoperative therapy is best, such as in abdominal carcinomatosis, radiation injury, inflammatory bowel disease, and when there have been numerous previous operations for obstruction. In such cases, specialized long tubes can be helpful.

Recognition of complete bowel obstruction should not be the occasion for rushing the patient to surgery before there has been a serious effort made to correct dehydration and hypovolemia. Large volumes of intravenous fluids containing balanced electrolytes, such as Ringer's lactate solution, are almost always needed. Debilitated, anemic, or badly depleted patients may need albumin, plasma, or blood as well. Metabolic acidosis must be corrected. Potassium losses are serious in bowel obstruction, but potassium must not be given until a good flow of urine is assured. Once the operation has been scheduled, a combination of antibiotics should be administered intravenously before operation to minimize postoperative

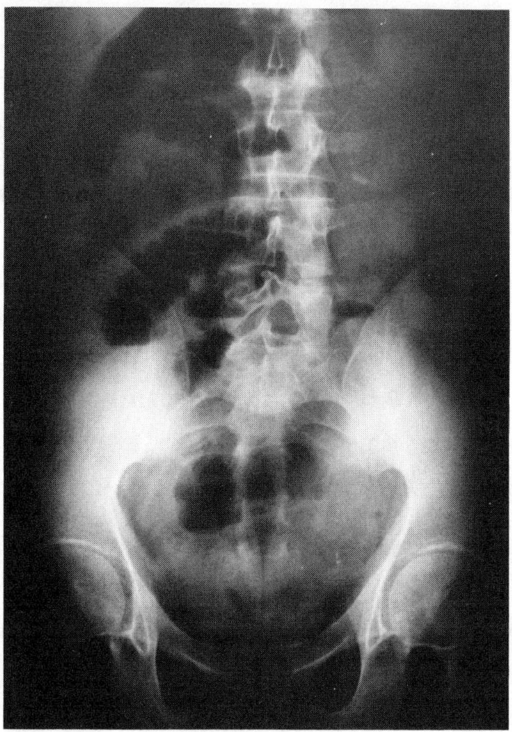

FIG 12–3.
Plain x-ray film of the abdomen with the patient supine. The patient is a 12-year-old child with acute appendicitis. There are a few loops of dilated gas-filled small bowel on the right side near the appendix. Some gas is also visible in the transverse colon at the top of the film. These are the signs of a partially obstructing paralytic ileus.

sepsis. Drugs are selected to oppose as broad a spectrum of colon organisms as possible and should include an agent active against the anaerobes. Cultures taken from peritoneal fluid are often positive for multiple organisms when the bowel is compromised, even though no gross necrosis or perforation is apparent.

The more severely ill the patient, the longer the period of preparation needed. Careful monitoring of the pulse rate, temperature, blood pressure, and urine flow through an indwelling catheter is important to assure optimum preparation. Occasionally the pain of ischemia or developing peritonitis must shorten preparation, but 3 to 6 hours of fluid therapy are almost always essential.

The results of surgery for bowel obstruction depend to a great extent on what must be done to relieve the obstruction. Results are better for small-bowel obstruction than for large. In adult patients of all ages simple obstruction without strangulation has a mortality rate of less than 5% with most of the deaths occurring in the elderly. Strangulated obstruction raises the death rate to 8% if the operation is performed within 36 hours of the onset of symptoms and to more than 25% in those cases delayed beyond 36 hours. In contrast, the results of treatment of large-bowel obstruction are not nearly so good as the overall results with small-bowel obstruction probably because so many cases occur in older patients with advanced cancer. Mortality rates as high as 22% have been reported.

Bowel obstruction is a disorder in which early diagnosis, prompt and adequate preparation with intravenous fluids and antibiotics, and well-timed surgical intervention can minimize necrosis, gangrene, and perforation. The quality of the care given these patients is critical in determining their outcome.

REFERENCES

Barnett WO, Petro AB, Williamson JW: A Current appraisal of problems with gangrenous bowel. *Ann Surg* 1976; 183(6):653–659. *A comprehensive review of problems in managing gangrenous bowel shows how delay increases morbidity and mortality and emphasizes the value of preoperative preparation.*

Brolin RE: Partial small bowel obstruction. *Surgery* 1984; 95(2):145–149. *A careful review of experience with partial bowel obstruction shows frequent resolution in response to nasogastric tube suction.*

Jones RS: Intestinal obstruction, in Sabiston DC, Jr (ed): *Textbook of Surgery*, ed 13. Philadelphia, WB Saunders Co, 1986, pp 905–914. *A comprehensive discussion of small bowel obstruction with interesting illustrations and selected pertinent references; includes principles of preparation and operative treatment.*

Kerry RL, Ransom HK: Volvulus of the colon: Etiology, diagnosis, and treatment. *Arch Surg* 1969; 99:215–222. *This comprehensive review of experience with volvulus of the colon shows results of both nonsurgical and surgical methods of treatment.*

Sarr MG, Bulkley GB, Zuidema GD: Preoperative recognition of intestinal strangulation obstruction. Prospective evaluation of diagnostic capability. *Am J Surg* 1983; 145:176–182. *A well-documented account of a prospective effort made to determine the presence or absence of necrotic bowel preoperatively, showing how unreliable most signs are.*

Schrock TR: Large intestine, in Way LW (ed): *Current Surgical Diagnosis and Treatment*, ed 7. Los Altos, Lange Medical Publishers, 1985, pp 592–601, 613–615. *A relatively concise discussion of obstruction of the colon by tumors and volvulus; includes principles and results of treatment.*

Shatila AH, Chamberlain BE, Webb WR: Current status of diagnosis and management of strangulation obstruction of the small bowel. *Surgery* 1976; 132:299–303. *The clinical findings and causes in simple and strangulation obstruction are compared, and early operation is shown to lower the mortality rate.*

Umpleby HC, Williamson RCN: Survival in acute obstructing colorectal carcinoma. *Dis Colon Rectum* 1984; 27:299–304. *This objective review of colon obstruction due to carcinoma shows the many reasons for a very high rate of complications and mortality during treatment.*

13 ABDOMINAL TRAUMA

Larry M. Jones, M.D.

Injury to the abdominal organs may be the result of a penetrating object, such as a knife or bullet, or of a blunt force applied to the abdomen, such as a seat belt injury. Although the operative treatment may be the same for any injury regardless of its cause, the method of diagnosing injuries associated with the two basic types of trauma differs. It is generally well accepted that injuries that penetrate into the peritoneal space require surgical exploration. Blunt trauma, on the other hand, may often be treated nonoperatively. The decision to explore or not explore the abdomen of a victim of blunt trauma can be one of the most difficult to make. A good history of how the injury was received along with the results of the physical examination of the patient may lead the physician to suspect injuries of specific intra-abdominal organs. This index of suspicion will suggest to the physician the use of x-ray films and other diagnostic tests. These results will either confirm or deny the need for laparotomy.

All trauma patients, regardless of the type of trauma and organ injury, must be approached initially in the same manner. The ABCs (airway, breathing, cardiac) of resuscitation must be strictly followed. Securing a patent airway is always the first priority. Second, full expansion of the lungs with respiratory exchange of gases must be assured, such as by decompression of a tension pneumothorax. Third, cardiovascular function must be assessed and appropriate treatment carried out, such as drainage of pericardial tamponade or control of hemorrhage.

Any discussion of the fundamentals of abdominal trauma must include a definition of the abdomen. Because the confines of the abdominal cavity change with the diaphragm during respiration, most surgeons recognize the nipple line of the chest as the external landmark for the upper limit of the abdomen. The lower limit is a line drawn across at the inferior level of the public rings anteriorly and at the level of the skin fold between the buttocks and thighs posteriorly. When evaluating abdominal trauma, remember that the patient has a posterior surface as well as an anterior one. Both must be examined. The intra-abdominal organs must also be thought of as occupying intraperitoneal or extraperitoneal positions.

Abrasions and contusions over the lower ribs should point out the possibility of an underlying liver laceration or splenic rupture. Lacerations of the liver or spleen frequently produce pain over the involved organ. Bleeding from these injuries may cause diaphragmatic irritation with pain referred to the shoulder and neck area. There may be guarding of the abdominal wall musculature. The entire abdomen may be distended, especially if there has been significant hemorrhage. Some patients will present with signs of hypovolemic shock.

Injuries to the gallbladder and common bile duct are usually found incidentally at laparotomy. Their presence is suggested preoperatively by peritoneal lavage, outlined below.

The pancreas may be injured as a result of gunshot or knife wounds or as a result of compression against the vertebral column by blunt force. Pancreatic injury is usually found at laparotomy during exploration of the lesser sac. Preoperatively, the physician may suspect pancreatic injury by the presence of Turner's sign (ecchymosis of the flanks), Cullen's sign (periumbilical ecchymosis secondary to retroperitoneal blood dissecting around the abdomen anteriorly), or vertebral fractures in the T10 to L2 area. The patient may complain of upper abdominal pain and show signs of guarding. The serum amylase level may be elevated.

The stomach is less frequently injured as a result of blunt trauma than of penetrating trauma. Regardless of the cause, the patient will complain of abdominal pain and display guarding and rebound tenderness. A nasogastric tube passed into the stomach may return blood. An upright chest x-ray film or left lateral decubitus x-ray film of the abdomen may show free intraperitoneal air.

Duodenal disruption initially appears as pain in the right upper quadrant. Signs of peritoneal irritation and pneumoperitoneum in x-ray films will be present if there is laceration with spillage of the intestinal contents into the peritoneal space. Because part of the duodenum is retroperitoneal, spillage into this area may cause right flank pain. In this case free intraperitoneal air will not be seen on x-ray film. However, a retroperitoneal air pattern may be seen just below the liver and may extend down to outline the right kidney.

Small-bowel injuries are usually due to penetrating trauma. Blunt force, however, can produce small bowel injuries, particularly near the ligament of Treitz and the terminal ileum. The patient will complain of generalized abdominal pain. Spillage of intestinal contents will produce rebound tenderness and guarding. Pneumoperitoneum may be seen on the x-ray film.

The colon may sustain penetrating traumatic injury anywhere along its course. Blunt trauma may also cause injury anywhere along the colon, but most commonly this type of force causes injury to the cecum. Perforation and spillage of large-intestine contents into the peritoneal space will result in generalized abdominal pain with guarding and rebound tenderness. Pneumoperitoneum may be present.

The rectum is an extraperitoneal organ. Injuries to this part of the bowel are easily overlooked and can be life threatening. Most rectal injuries are penetrating injuries. Many result from gunshot or shotgun wounds or foreign bodies inserted into the rectum. Blunt trauma to the pelvis may also result in penetration of the rectal wall by sharp pieces of fractured bone. When this occurs, the pelvic fracture is considered an open fracture. Suspicion of rectal injury should be raised by the history. Digital rectal exam may reveal gross blood. Proctosigmoidoscopy should always be performed on patients with this finding.

Patient with injuries to the back and flank should be suspected of having renal trauma as well. In fact, back and flank pain may be the only symptom of a kidney injury. Hematuria, an inconsistent finding, is absent in 20% of renal injuries. Injury to the ureter is extremely rare; the diagnosis is made based on a clinical suspicion that renal injury may have occurred and subsequent confirmation by intravenous pyelogram.

Injuries to the urinary bladder are commonly the result of trauma to the bony pelvis. These patients usually have hematuria. The diagnosis is made by cystogram. This x-ray study must include oblique or lateral views of the bladder to rule out perforations of this organ's posterior wall.

Urethral injuries are more common in men than in women and are associated with pelvic trauma. Blood at the external urethral meatus or a freely movable or displaced ("high-riding") prostate on digital rectal examination should alert the physician to the possibility of urethral disruption. Perineal ecchymosis and scrotal hematoma may also be present. The diagnosis is made by a retrograde urethrogram. Foley catheters should not be placed in these patients until the urethrogram rules out such an injury.

Information about injuries of the major abdominal vessels is mainly academic, because over half of these patients will die before resuscitation efforts can begin. Clinically these patients present in profound shock. Triage and transport to the operating suite must be rapid. The only hope for survival rests in surgical control of the hemorrhage.

Peritoneal lavage is a procedure often used to determine the presence of intra-abdominal injury. It may be performed by a "semi-open" method, but the "open" technique, described below, is becoming more popular and is the one endorsed by the American College of Surgeons in their Advanced Trauma Life Support Course.

First, the stomach and urinary bladder are decompressed by passing a nasogastric tube and Foley catheter. Pneumoperitoneum is ruled out by appropriate x-ray studies. The periumbilical area and lower abdomen are prepared and draped. Local anesthesia with 1% lidocaine is achieved for a distance of 3 to 5 cm one-third of the way from the umbilicus to the

TABLE 13–1.
Indications for Peritoneal Lavage

1. Equivocal results of physical examination
2. Unexplained hypovolemia
3. Altered pain response, perhaps associated with head or spinal cord
4. Injury with questionable penetration of the peritoneum
5. Patients unavailable for immediate follow-up physical examinations, such as those receiving a general anesthetic for nonabdominal surgery

pubis. An incision is made down to the peritoneum. The peritoneum is then opened under direct vision, and a peritoneal dialysis catheter is inserted toward the hollow of the pelvis. Aspiration through an attached syringe is performed, and if 5 ml or more of gross blood is returned, laparotomy is indicated. If gross blood is not obtained, the dialysis catheter is connected to a 1-liter bottle containing normal saline, which is infused into the abdominal cavity. After infusion is complete, the bottle is placed on the floor, and the fluid is siphoned out of the abdomen. Red and white blood cell counts, amylase and bilirubin levels, and Gram's-stain reactions are determined for the fluid collected. Values indicating the need for laparotomy are a RBC count $> 100,000/\text{mm}^3$, WBC count $> 500/\text{mm}^3$, amylase level > 100 U/liter, the presence of bile, or Gram's stain reactions showing enteric organisms or food fibers.

Certain patients undergoing peritoneal lavage will require a slight change in the technique. Patients who have suffered pelvic fractures should have the peritoneum approached from a supraumbilical incision. Patients with abdominal scars from previous surgery may require peritoneal exposure in either of the lower abdominal quadrants rather than the midline.

Peritoneal lavage is indicated in a number of clinical situations (Table 13–1). The most common indication is the patient with an equivocal physical examination. However, because peritoneal lavage is an invasive procedure with possible complications, it should not be a substitute for thorough, repeated physical examinations. The procedure is absolutely contraindicated for those patients who have obvious indications for laparotomy.

It must be remembered that peritoneal lavage is useful in the diagnosis of intraperitoneal injury only. Retroperitoneal injuries will not be diagnosed with this procedure. In cases of suspected retroperitoneal injury computed tomography (CT scan) of the abdomen may be helpful if time and the condition of the patient permits.

The clincal-pathologic correlations for abdominal trauma are summarized in Table 13–2 (see pp. 80–81).

REFERENCES

Blaisdell FW, Trunkey DD (eds): *Trauma Management, Vol I: Abdominal Trauma.* New York, Thieme-Stratton, 1982. *Discusses all aspects of abdominal trauma, including surgical treatment, in a concise manner.*

Committee on Trauma, American College of Surgeons: *Advanced Trauma Life Support Course for Physicians.* Chicago, American College of Surgeons, 1984. *Aspects of initial diagnosis, resuscitation, and treatment of immediate life-threatening injuries are discussed.*

Committee on Trauma, American College of Surgeons: *Early Care of the Injured Patient,* ed 2. Philadelphia, WB Saunders Co, 1982. *Standard guidelines for the care of trauma patients.*

Root HD, Hauser CW, McKinley CR, et al.: Diagnostic peritoneal lavage. Surgery 1965; 57:633–637. *The original article describing catheter paracentesis and diagnostic peritoneal lavage.*

TABLE 13–2.
Clinical–Pathologic Correlations

ORGAN INJURED	ASSOCIATED PHYSICAL FINDINGS	X-RAY FINDINGS	PERITONEAL LAVAGE RESULTS	OTHER TESTS
Liver	Contusions, abrasions of lower right chest; fractures of lower right ribs; tenderness in right upper quadrant; may have referred pain in right shoulder-neck area; abdominal guarding; severe hemorrhage associated with abdominal distention and signs of shock	Chest and abdominal x-ray films often normal	Gross blood	Liver scan or CT scan may be helpful, particularly in diagnosing and following subcapsular hematomas of the liver without free rupture into the peritoneal space
Gallbladder	Pain in right upper quadrant	May show other injuries; no specific findings for isolated gallbladder injury	Bile on lavage	
Spleen	Contusions, abrasions of lower left chest; fractures of lower left rib cage; tenderness in left upper quadrant; may have referred pain in left shoulder-neck area; abdominal guarding and rebound; signs of hypovolemic shock may be present	Chest and abdominal x-ray films often normal; may see displacement of gastric bubble due to blood	Gross blood	Spleen scan or CT scan may be helpful, particularly in diagnosing and following subcapsular hematomas of spleen
Stomach	Upper abdominal pain; guarding and rebound tenderness; nasogastric tube drainage may be bloody	Upright chest x-ray film shows pneumoperitoneum	Blood, food fibers, possibly *Candida* with Gram's stain	
Duodenum	Pain in right upper quadrant or right flank	Pneumoperitoneum, if ruptured free into abdominal cavity; retroperitoneal rupture may have air collection below the liver shadow or air outlining the right kidney shadow	Perforation into the abdominal cavity may show food fibers, bile, and amylase in fluid with lavage; retroperitoneal rupture has no abnormal findings with lavage	CT scan of upper abdomen may be helpful with retroperitoneal injury
Small intestines	Generalized abdominal pain with signs of peritoneal irritation	Pneumoperitoneum may be present but not always seen	Amylase may be elevated; bile and food fibers may be present	

Colon	Generalized abdominal pain with guarding and rebound	Pneumoperitoneum may be present	Food fibers and enteric bacteria seen with Gram's stain	
Pancreas	Upper abdominal pain; guarding; Turner's sign; Cullen's sign	Not diagnostic; suspect this injury with fractures of the T11–L2 vertebral bodies seen on abdominal x-ray films	No abnormal findings	Serum amylase may be elevated; CT scan of the abdomen may be helpful
Rectum	External evidence of perineal trauma including contusions and ecchymosis; blood on the examining finger following digital rectal examination	Suspect in patients with severe pelvic fractures, gunshot or shotgun pellet fragments within the pelvic hollow on x-ray films; foreign body inserted into the rectum may also be seen on x-ray films	No abnormal findings	Proctosigmoidoscopy
Kidney/ureter	Pain in the upper abdomen and flank	Intravenous pyelogram is indicated: may show extravasation or no or poor visualization of the nephrogram	No abnormal findings	Hematuria, including microscopic hematuria, may be absent in up to 20% of kidney injuries
Urinary bladder	Suspect in patients with severe, unstable pelvic fractures	Pelvic fractures; cystogram diagnostic, include oblique or lateral views	No abnormal findings with extra-peritoneal bladder rupture; may see increase in bladder catheter drainage with infusion of lavage fluid, with intraperitoneal rupture	
Urethra	Blood at external urethral meatus; hematoma of scrotum. Ecchymosis of perineal region mobile or "high-riding" prostate	Suspect with pelvic fractures (pubic ring); retrograde urethrogram is diagnostic	Not indicated	Foley catheter should not be placed

14 STINGING INSECT VENOM ALLERGY

Howard J. Schwartz, M.D.

Anaphylactic, Type I, or IgE-mediated hypersensitivity to the venoms of stinging hymenoptera insects is the source of significant morbidity in the United States and may account for 35 or more deaths each year. It is an allergic syndrome due to the presence of specific antivenom IgE antibodies. Its occurrence is not limited to persons with other types of allergic diseases so the risk of developing stinging insect allergy extends beyond atopic people. All members of the general population are at risk of developing this type of allergy.

CLINICAL SIGNS AND SYMPTOMS

Typically, the patient presents to an emergency room as a person who was stung once, on an extremity, while involved in some sort of outdoor activity during the warm weather months. The patient will first experience some local pain, but will continue his or her activity and, within several minutes, will suddenly not feel well. He or she may become apprehensive, may feel warm, flushed, or hot all over, may become lightheaded or dizzy and go inside to "rest." The patient may then decide he or she is "ill" and note diffuse erythema, hives, and swelling of the face or lips. The condition may then progress to include other symptoms such as palpitations and dyspnea.

The past history usually indicates the patient has had "many" previous "bee" stings without incident, and there will usually be no history or other allergies.

The anaphylactic syndromes due to insect sting allergy are no different than anaphylaxis from other causes. The manifestations may be cutaneous, respiratory, cardiovascular, gas-trointestinal, or a combination. Most reactions begin within 10 to 15 minutes of the sting, but may not reach peak intensity for a somewhat longer period. Specific symptoms vary from flushing, hives, and angioedema to nausea, abdominal cramps, symptoms of upper airway edema, chest tightness, lightheadedness, hypotension, collapse, and shock. Most fatalities occur in older adults.

PATHOPHYSIOLOGY

The major stinging insects—honeybee, yellow jacket, hornet, and wasp—belong to the Hymenoptera order of the class Insecta. The honeybee is a member of the Apoidea family, and the yellow jacket, hornet, and wasp are members of the Vespoidea family. Allergic individuals may be sensitive to one, several, or all of these stinging insects. In many areas of the United States, the yellow jacket is the most common cause of acute stinging insect allergic reactions, perhaps because it is the most likely insect to be disturbed during outdoor activities. These epidemiologic "facts" vary considerably from case to case. Patient identification of the causative insect is usually difficult and often unreliable, unless the patient can state that the insect died after the sting leaving the venom sac *in situ*. This is characteristic only of the honeybee. Other insects do not die after a single sting.

Normally some degree of local swelling, redness, heat, and itching occur at the site of the insect sting because insect venom contains a variety of enzymes and toxins capable of causing substantial local inflammation. While such reactions can be the cause of considerable patient distress, they are not harbingers of severe allergic reactions.

Anaphylactic reactions involve the reaction of specific IgE antibodies present on mast cells with allergen and the subsequent release of the mediators of immediate hypersensitivity.

Unusual reactions have been reported including vasculitis, neuritis, encephalitis, and renal disease. The pathophysiologic mechanisms in these unusual reactions to insect sting are not well understood.

It has been speculated that, on occasion, a person may experience a toxic reaction following multiple insect stings ("envenomation"). The symptoms may resemble those of anaphylaxis, but the history will characteristically feature a large number of stings being suffered at one time. On later testing of the patient, IgE antivenom antibodies are absent.

DIFFERENTIAL DIAGNOSIS

A specific sensitivity to insect venoms should be documented after the patient has recovered and is several weeks past the acute event. Current recommendations are to test with each of the five available venom preparations all patients who have a history suggesting systemic insect allergy. Skin testing is begun at very dilute concentrations and continued, if negative, up to a concentration of 1 μg/ml. Mixtures should not be used. A positive skin test in this setting is interpreted as evidence of an immunologically specific reaction. Use of venom concentrations above 1 μg/ml can be irritating to the skin and lead to nonspecific skin responses. In the past, whole-body insect preparations were used for the diagnosis and therapy of stinging insect allergy. These materials lack potency, are unreliable, and should no longer be used for these purposes.

On occasion, it may be helpful to obtain serologic evidence of stinging insect allergy. The *in vitro* radioallergosorbent test (RAST) can be used because it can detect venom-specific circulating IgE. The RAST is not as sensitive as the skin test but is useful for quantitating antibody titers. However, it should be recognized that perhaps 15% to 20% of the patients with positive venom skin tests do not react to the RAST.

DIAGNOSIS

The diagnosis of an acute allergic event following an insect sting is usually obvious. Stings will not go unrecognized; the pain of the sting will usually call attention to it having happened. The symptoms that then develop are typical of allergy. Identification of the specific causative insect is usually unreliable.

PRINCIPLES OF PREVENTION AND THERAPY

The management of persons with a good history of allergic reactions to an insect sting and who have evidence of specific antivenom IgE by skin or serologic testing is based on the substantial increased risk these persons have of a severe reaction to a subsequent sting, especially if the patient is an adult. Therapeutic considerations include (1) measures to reduce exposure (avoidance); (2) making certain the patient always possesses, and knows how to use, emergency medications in the event of a subsequent sting reaction; and (3) specific venom immunotherapy.

Avoidance involves the use of proper clothing, including shoes, long-sleeve shirts, long-leg pants, and gloves when working outdoors and avoiding the use of scented perfumes, deodorants, and cosmetics. Smooth-textured, snug-fitting, subdued-colored clothing is preferred for outdoor activity. Food and strong odors attract insects, so great care should be taken when picnicking outdoors.

For patients with known stinging insect allergy, epinephrine in prefilled syringes (Epi-Pen, ANA-kit) should always be available, and the patient must be instructed in its use.

Venom immunotherapy has been documented to be highly effective in preventing subsequent anaphylactic sting reactions in sensitive persons. Fifty to sixty percent of allergic persons not given immunotherapy react following a subsequent sting whereas less than 5% of venom-treated persons react. Venom immunotherapy is associated with a reduction in titers of venom-specific IgE, and the stimulation of venom-specific IgG. Selecting patients appropriate for immunotherapy and selecting the venoms to be used in immunotherapy are components with which the allergist is best equipped to deal, and patients should be referred to a subspecialist for these considerations.

At present it is unclear whether venom immunotherapy must be lifelong or whether criteria can be developed for the safe cessation of venom immunotherapy. While current recommendations call for treatment lasting indefinitely, several studies in progress suggest that criteria for cessation are likely within the next several years.

Medical therapy of sting anaphylaxis involves the same principles as treating an acute allergic reaction from any cause. Subcutaneous epinephrine is the treatment of choice with the dosage depending on the circumstances. It can be repeated at 20- to 30-minute intervals, if necessary. Antihistamines may help flushing, pruritis, and urticaria and can be given orally or parenterally, but are not very helpful in severe anaphylaxis. Oxygen, intravenous fluids, pressors, and theophylline may be helpful, depending on the symptoms. Upper airway patency must be maintained. Upper airway edema is the most common pathologic finding in fatal insect sting anaphylaxis, and signs for its possible presence or development must be monitored. Corticosteroids have no place in the primary treatment of anaphylaxis and should not be used except to deal with symptoms such as pruritis and urticaria, which may linger from hours to days.

REFERENCES

Golden DBK, Johnson K, Addison BI, Valentine MD, Kagey-Sobotka A, Lichtenstein LM: Clinical and immunologic observations in patients who stop venom immunotherapy. *J Allergy Clin Immunol* 1986; 77:435–442. *Current important research findings dealing with the need for long-term treatment.*

Levine MI, Lockey RF (eds): *Monograph on Insect Allergy*. Milwaukee, American Academy of Allergy and Immunology, 1986. *Excellent review of the field in a very readable format.*

Mauriello PM, Barde SH, Georgitis JW, Reisman RE: Natural history of large local reactions from stinging insects. *J Allergy Clin Immunol* 1984; 74:494–498. *Important paper in its negative findings.*

Reisman RE, Dvorin DJ, Randolph CC, Georgitis JW: Stinging insect allergy: Natural history and modification with venom immunotherapy. *J Allergy Clin Immunol* 1985; 75:735–740. *A series of significant observations in a long-term study.*

Schwartz HJ: Appropriate evaluation and therapy of stinging insect hypersensitivity. *Arch Intern Med* 1984; 144:1560–1561. *Brief discussion of consensus position of how to deal with patients with this disease.*

Schwartz HJ, Squillace DL, Sher Th, et al.: Studies in stinging insect hypersensitivity: Postmortem demonstration of antivenom IgE antibody in possible sting-related death. *Am J Clin Pathol* 1986; 85:607–610. *Extends the potential relevance of stinging insect allergy and application of in vitro tests.*

Valentine MD: Insect venom allergy: Diagnosis and treatment. *J Allergy Clin Immunol* 1984; 73:299–304. *Important review of the work in the field by a leading researcher in this subject.*

15 GENETIC DISEASES APPEARING AS CATASTROPHIC ILLNESSES: APPROACHES TO DIAGNOSIS

Meinhard Robinow, M.D.

All genetic disorders are uncommon and many are quite rare, but all of them combined account for a substantial part of serious human illness. While many genetic diseases manifest themselves as slow deterioration of an organ system, a few can appear as acute catastrophic illnesses. Table 15–1 lists some of the most important of these genetic disorders. It is evident that they can mimic some of the common illnesses caused by extrinsic factors.

Because the number of genetic disorders is huge and still rapidly growing, it is a hopeless task to keep abreast of the field by memorization. How then can a physician suspect a genetic disorder and eventually arrive at the correct diagnosis? I believe a systematic, stepwise approach can be helpful.

The initial step should be to take a brief and targeted personal and family history. The important questions to ask are:

1. Has the patient ever had an episode similar to the present one?
2. Have any other family members ever suffered from a similar problem?
3. Is there a history of *any* genetic disease in the family? This is a necessary question due to the variable expressivity of many autosomal dominant disorders (e.g., neurofibromatosis or myotonic dystrophy). The patient may not be aware that a genetic disorder in a relative may be the same as his or her own.
4. Were the patient's parents blood relatives? This question is important if the patient is a member of a religious isolate (e.g., Amish or Hutterite) or if he or she comes from a part of the world where consanguineous marriages are prevalent (most Arab countries).

Parental consanguinity increases the likelihood of recessive disorders.

Two considerations can be clues to a genetic cause. First, a genetic disorder should be considered if, in any given case, the combination of signs and symptoms does not seem to make sense, if it does not fit into the physician's past medical experience. For instance, a patient may present with abdominal pain so severe as to suggest a surgical emergency, but the simultaneous presence of a psychiatric disturbance and an acute neuropathy fits no common surgical emergency. A genetic disorder should be considered as an alternative. The correct diagnosis in this case is acute intermittent porphyria, not an extremely rare disease, but sufficiently uncommon so that few physicians will have seen it in their own practice. The correct diagnosis may be life saving.

The second clue to genetic causation is the occurrence of a serious or catastrophic illness at an unexpectedly young age. An example would be the discovery of an aortic aneurysm in a teenager or young adult. The patient's youth rules against such common causes of aneurysms as atherosclerosis or syphilis and suggests a possible genetic cause. A search for associated signs such as tall stature, scoliosis, and lens dislocation, points to the correct diagnosis, namely Marfan's syndrome.

Once the suspicion of genetic disease has been raised, how can one arrive at a specific diagnosis? If attention has been paid to the personal history, family history, and the above mentioned clues, the diagnosis may become obvious, provided the condition is fairly common. If the condition is rare and one's personal

TABLE 15–1.
Genetic Disorders that May Appear as Catastrophic Illnesses

INITIAL SYMPTOMS	GENETIC DISORDER	MODE OF INHERITANCE*	ASSOCIATED FINDINGS	USUAL AGE AT APPEARANCE
Paroxysmal abdominal pain	Intermittent porphyria	AD	Bizarre neurologic and psychiatric symptoms; red urine	Usually young women
Paroxysmal abdominal pain	Fabry's disease	XL	Angiokeratoma; chronic renal disease	Young adults
Paroxysmal abdominal pain	Familial Mediterranean fever	AR	Fever; amyloidosis	Any age
Paroxysmal abdominal pain	Hereditary pancreatitis	AD	Elevated serum and urine amylase levels	Adolescents or young adults
Spontaneous rupture of bowel or large artery	Ehlers-Danlos syndrome, type IV	AD or AR	Excessive bruising; lax finger joints	Children or young adults
Colon cancer	Gardner's syndrome	AD	Intestinal polyps; multiple osseous and soft tissue tumors; sebaceous cysts	Young adults
Reye's syndrome-like episodes	Carnitine deficiency	AR	Muscle cramps	Young adults
Severe nose bleeds and hemoptyses	Hereditary teleangiectasia	AD	Teleangiectasias of lips; pulmonary AV fistulas	Any age
Acute, profound muscle paralysis	Periodic paralysis	AD	Hypokalemia (rarely hyperkalemia) during attacks	Any time after puberty
Ruptured berry aneurysms	Adult polycystic kidneys	AD	Renal and hepatic cysts	Young adults
Thromboembolic disease	Homocystinemia	AR	Marfanoid habitus; osteoporosis; dislocated lenses	Usually young adults
Esophageal stricture	Epidermolysis bullosa dystrophica	AR	Blisters; abrasions; milia; loss of nails	Usually teenager or young adults
Renal calculi	Lesch-Nyhan syndrome	XL	Athetoid cerebral palsy	Children or young adults

* AD = autosomal dominant; AR = autosomal recessive; XL = X-linked.

knowledge insufficient, a consultant with special competence in genetic diseases may help solve the diagnostic puzzle. Another aid that is gradually becoming available is the computer. A diagnostic computer-based system for congenital anomalies and genetic diseases is now available on floppy disk.[1] Once the computer has identified a group of potential diagnoses, a literature search for references can be initiated by consulting appropriate textbooks or McKusick's catalog of *Mendelian Inheritance in Man* (McKusick, 1986).

REFERENCES

McKusick VA: *Mendelian Inheritance in Man,* ed 7. Baltimore, Johns Hopkins University Press, 1986. *A comprehensive, brief classification of genetic disorders.*

[1]For information, contact the Center for Birth Defects Information Services, 171 Harrison Avenue, Boston, MA 02111.

16 MALNUTRITION

Smith L. Johnston, III, M.D.
Kim Goldenberg, M.D.

Malnutrition occurs when there is an inadequate supply of proteins, calories, or micronutrients (vitamins, minerals, and trace elements). It predisposes to, initiates, or is caused by a disease process. Malnutrition can affect every organ system of the body and usually involves multiple systems.

The classic syndromes of infantile marasmus (deficiency of proteins and calories with stunted growth, loss of adipose tissue, and generalized wasting of lean body mass) and kwashiorkor (deficiency of protein with growth failure, hypoalbuminemia, edema, fatty liver, and preservation of adipose tissue) are common in the greater than one billion humans suffering from hunger and malnutrition in Third World countries. Combinations of these syndromes are also common in the geriatric, poor, and hospitalized populations of developed nations. Clinical manifestations of vitamin deficiency have been reported in approximately 10% of Americans over the age of 60 years with deficiencies of folic acid, thiamine, riboflavin, nicotinic acid, pyridoxine, ascorbic acid, and vitamin A being the most common. The most likely predisposing factors leading to malnutrition in the United States are low socioeconomic status, drug and alcohol abuse, depression and isolation in the aged, anorexia nervosa, malabsorption, and inadequate intake by hospitalized patients.

CLINICAL SIGNS AND SYMPTOMS

The patient with malnutrition usually has a gradual onset of the following signs and symptoms: generalized weakness, weight loss, decreased exercise tolerance, cold intolerance, generalized aches (thorax, pelvis, lower extremities), anxiety, amenorrhea, impotence, and increased frequency and duration of minor infections. A careful diet history to ascertain the quantity of food intake and its biologic quality over a specific period of time along with a thorough medical history should be the first step in the evaluation of every medical patient suspected of being malnourished. The signs and symptoms of an underlying disease process may mask or exacerbate those of malnutrition. This is especially true in the hospitalized patient requiring parenteral nutrition and multiple medications with a sustained stress such as major surgery, burns, or respirator.

The patient with malnutrition usually has early physical signs in the visible organs (hair, eyes, skin, oral mucosa, and teeth) such as cheilosis, paleness, dry flaking skin, glossitis, loss of subcutaneous fat, temporal muscle wasting, and dental caries. In infants and children, the syndromes of marasmus and kwashiorkor may be present. In the advanced stages of malnutrition, diffuse muscle wasting, brittle hair and nails, perifollicular petechiae, marked weakness, and a progressive decrease in all vital signs are common.

An evaluation of weight may be misleading because an obese person could lose a large amount of weight and present with a normal weight for height. Therefore, a quantification of weight loss for one- and six-month time intervals is important when possible. Also, with primary protein deficiency, the total body weight may even be increased due to edema and a maintenance of adipose tissue. A list of clinical signs and symptoms with possible correlating nutrition deficiency is presented in Table 16–1.

The classic syndromes of marasmus and kwashiorkor are well defined. If a person is chronically malnourished from birth, retarded brain and somatic growth may develop along with poor dentition and atrophy of the gastrointestinal, pancreatic, and biliary systems, which further intensifies the malnutrition.

If primary starvation or nosocomial malnutrition persists, with critical protein depletion, the following can occur: anemia with pallor and fatigue, hypoalbuminemia with decreased amounts of transport proteins and clotting factors, decreased cell-mediated immunity with associated bronchopneumonia or urinary tract infection or both, decreased structural and visceral protein integrity with associated decubitus ulcers, acceleration of cachexia by the hypermetabolism and anorexia associated with infectious and malignant processes, and overwhelming infection and sepsis with total body failure.

PATHOPHYSIOLOGY

Total body homeostasis requires an adequate intake of nutrients to provide fuel for immediate metabolic requirements, to expand glycogen reserves in liver and muscle, to maintain protein for structural integrity and function of visceral organs, and to store calories as triglycerides in adipose tissue (14 kg of triglycerides equals approximately 125,000 calories, or over a month of basal survival fuel). In malnutrition, this sequence is in part reversed with hormone and metabolic adaptations directed toward the preservation of vital proteins and the central nervous system.

The central physiologic adaptive roles of simple starvation are initiated by glucose maintenance. Whenever there is a significant decrease in the amount of glucose absorbed from the gut (8 to 10 hours of starvation), insulin secretion decreases and glucagon, growth hormone, and cortisol secretion increase resulting in a mobilization of free fatty acids from adipose tissue and amino acids from muscle for oxidative metabolism and gluconeogenesis. Glucose is required for optimal function of the brain, fibroblasts, and polymorphonuclear leukocytes.

The progression of starvation appears to lead to an adaptive decrease in the body's basal metabolic rate by the following mechanisms: a decrease in extrathyroidal conversion of thyroxine (T_4) to triiodothyronine (T_3) and an increase in the conversion of T_4 to reverse T_3 (inactive form), a decrease in T_3-receptor synthesis, a decrease in the production and turnover of catecholamines, a decrease in the levels of cofactors (micronutrients) due to the decrease in dietary intake, and a decrease in neurotransmitter synthesis due to a decrease in the intake of tryptophan and phenylalinine.

The brain with continued starvation begins to use progressively more ketoacids for fuel. At 2 weeks, ketoacid production is usually maximal. Ketoacids increase acidity thus necessitating an increase in ammonia production by the kidney to prevent the loss of cations in the urine and to preserve fluid volume. At this point the brain begins to use ketoacids preferentially as fuel. Gluconeogenesis from proteins also decreases thus sparing the visceral loss of critical proteins. If starvation continues, free fatty acids are depleted and a critical level of protein for life cannot be maintained.

TABLE 16–1.
Clinical–Pathologic Correlations for Vitamin Deficiencies

DEFICIENCY	CLINICAL FINDINGS	PATHOLOGIC FINDINGS
FAT-SOLUBLE VITAMINS		
Vitamin A	Retinal degeneration Skin and eye dryness Delayed wound healing Increased susceptibility to infection	Visual pigment (rhodopsin) synthesis decrease Mucopolysaccharides synthesis decrease Possible steroid activity Decreased cellular growth and membrane stabilization
Vitamin D_3 (cholecalciferol)	Retarded bone growth, abnormal bone formation (osteomalacia)	Low levels of activated vitamin D, which decreases maintainence of calcium and phosphate concentrations in plasma and extracellular fluid and therefore inhibits bone matrix calcification
Vitamin E (tocopherol)	Erythrocyte hemolysis in infants nutritional muscular dystrophy	Decreased antioxidant activity which stabilizes lysosomes, lipid membranes, and other cell structures
Vitamin K (phylloquinone)	Bleeding abnormalities Hemolytic disease of newborn	Decreased carboxylation of glutamic acid residues which alters binding of calcium required for synthesis of clotting factors II, VII, IX, X
WATER-SOLUBLE VITAMINS		
Vitamin C (L-ascorbic acid)	Poor wound healing, ecchymosis Scurvy	Decreased hydroxylation of proline and lysine used in the biosynthesis of collagen and basement membrane microvasculature endothelium
	Weakness, irritability Hypochromic macrocytic anemia	Decreased synthesis of noradrenaline and steroids Decreased incorporation of iron into ferritin, altered folate metabolism
Vitamin B_1 (thiamine)	Beriberi (wet) Cardiac failure Muscular weakness	Decreased α-ketoglutaric, pyruvic acid metabolism, co-carboxylase activity, and nicotinamide-adenine dinucleotide phosphate (NADP) energy metabolism
	Beriberi (dry) Neurologic deficits	Decreased acetylcholine synthesis
Vitamin B_2 (riboflavin)	Oral mucosal, skin, and corneal derangements	Decreased amounts of coenzyme in flavoprotein enzyme system [flavin adenine dinucleotide (FAD), flavin mononucleotide (FMN)] which catalyze oxidation in electron transport system essential for cellular growth
Niacin (nicotinic acid)	Dementia, weakness, dermatitis, diarrhea (pellagra)	Decreased amounts of nicotinamide adenine dinucleotide (NAD) and NADP required in intracellular respiratory mechanisms of all cells (mitochondrial electron transport) Decreased oxidation of glucose-6-phosphate Degeneration of axis cylinders of the pyramidal cells of the cortex and myelin degeneration
Vitamin B_6 (pyridoxine)	Oral mucosal and skin lesions, neurologic deficits, red cell microcytosis	Abnormal synthesis and catabolism of all amino acids More than 60 pyridoxal phosphate-dependent enzyme systems are associated with nitrogen metabolism
Vitamin B_{12}* (cyanocobalamin)	Ataxia, paresthesias, depression, memory abnormalities	Decreased synthesis of methionine, succinyl-coenzyme A, DNA, and myelin with subacute combined degeneration of the spinal cord
	Megaloblastic anemia	Decreased activation of folic acid coenzymes
Folate*	Megaloblastic anemia	Decreased amounts of coenzyme purine and pyrimidine synthesis, and for conversion of deoxyuridylic acid to thymidylic acid for DNA synthesis and cellular replication
Biotin	Oral mucosal and skin lesions, alopecia	Decreased co-carboxylation reactions for intermediate metabolism of carbohydrates, proteins, and fats
	Fatigue, depression	Decreased gluconeogenesis, RNA metabolisms and altered cholesterol
Pantothenic acid	Breakdown of skin and gut epithelium Neurologic abnormalities	Decreased conversion to Coenzyme A, which catalyzes acyl transfers in the synthesis of free fatty acids, cholesterol, and citric acid

* Both vitamin B_{12} and Folate are metabolically interrelated for DNA synthesis and, therefore, for growth.

TABLE 16–2.
Clinical–Pathologic Correlations for Trace Elements and Minerals

DEFICIENCY	CLINICAL FINDINGS	PATHOLOGIC FINDINGS
TRACE ELEMENTS		
Iron	Weakness, pallor, angular stomatitis, anemia	Decreased hemoglobin synthesis, oxygen, electron transport
Zinc	Skin rashes, alopecia, growth retardation	Decreased activity of the more than 70 metalloenzymatic reactions essential for synthesis of protein, DNA, and RNA
Iodine	Hypothyroidism, goiter, delayed growth	Decreased thyroid function
Chromium	Glucose intolerance, impaired release of free fatty acids	Potentiation of insulin Impaired release of free fatty acids
Selenium	Cardiomyopathy, muscle pain	Decreased activity of glutathione peroxidase; heavy metal interactions
Copper	Anemia, disturbance of ossification	Decreased elastin cross-linking, oxidative enzyme activity, iron interaction
Fluorine	Caries, possibly osteoporosis	Structure of teeth and possibly of bones
MINERALS		
Calcium	Tetany, convulsions	Decreased nerve and muscle conduction
	Bone abnormalities	Decreased bone matrix formation
Phosphorus	Muscular and neurologic abnormalities	Decreased ATP energy metabolism
	Bone abnormalities	Bone formation
Magnesium	Neurologic, cardiac, and skeletal muscle abnormalities	Decreased neuromuscular transmission
	Growth failure	Decreased amount of cofactor for oxidative phosphorylation
		Decreased nucleic acid synthesis
Sodium	Hypotension, muscular weakness	Disrupted body fluid homeostasis
Potassium	Muscular weakness, polyuria	Decreased cell-membrane transport
		Decreased neurotransmitter propagation

The above scenario of total starvation is rare in the United States. More frequently there is a partial or total lack of high biologic protein or micronutrient ingestion, with adequate or increased carbohydrate ingestion (alcohol, refined sugars). This state is similar to kwashiorkor in children, with insulin playing the central role. Insulin increases, thus decreasing lipolysis, and increasing lipogenesis with a subsequent loss of free fatty acids for oxidation. Concurrently the increased insulin level decreases the mobilization and redistribution of essential muscle amino acids for use by the liver. This explains how an obese, hospitalized person on intravenous 5% dextrose and 0.9% normal saline infusion can develop a severe protein deficiency, become edematous and immunocompromised, and develop an overwhelming infection.

Another physiologic variation occurs with malnutrition caused by hypermetabolism as with trauma, burns, infections, and major surgery. These conditions can produce an increased demand for protein synthesis and energy. The basal intake of proteins, calories, and micronutrients must be increased accordingly or malnutrition will result.

CLINICAL–PATHOLOGIC CORRELATIONS

Table 16–1 correlates the pathologic processes and clinical findings of specific vitamin deficiency, and Table 16–2 correlates those features of specific mineral and trace element deficiency. The correlation of the clinical effects of protein or calorie deficiency is discussed above.

DIFFERENTIAL DIAGNOSIS

Table 16–3 presents the many causes of malnutrition divided into five basic categories: (1) inadequate intake, (2) increased metabolism, (3) malabsorption, (4) impaired utilization, and (5) increased excretion.

TABLE 16–3.
Differential Diagnosis of Malnutrition

INADEQUATE OR UNBALANCED INTAKE

1. Low socioeconomic status
2. Indigent/geriatric populations
3. Alcohol and/or drug abuse
4. Dental pathologic changes (edentulous)
5. Food faddism
6. Iatrogenic
7. Psychiatric (anorexia nervosa, depression)

EXCESSIVE INTAKE

1. Megavitamin therapy (especially fat-soluble vitamins A and D)
2. Caloric imbalance/obesity
3. Medications, mineral excesses [antacids (magnesium, aluminum)]

INCREASED METABOLISM (REQUIREMENTS)

1. Major surgery, severe trauma, burns
2. Chronic illness (cancer, infections, fever)
3. Pregnancy, lactation, menstruation
4. Infancy, adolescence
5. Endocrine abnormality (hyperthyroidism, pheochromocytoma)
6. Psychiatric/psychologic abnormalities (mania, stress)

MALABSORPTION

1. Pancreatic, cholestatic, small-bowel diseases
2. After GI surgery (gastrectomy, small-bowel resection)
3. Inflammatory bowel disease
4. Parasitic infections
5. Blind-loop syndrome
6. Sprue, celiac disease, gluten-sensitive enteropathy
7. Malignancy of GI tract
8. Zollinger-Ellison disease

IMPAIRED UTILIZATION OR METABOLISM

1. Antagonist drugs (chemotherapeutics–amino acids, antacids–phosphorus, diuretics–K^+ and Mg^+, oral contraceptives–folic acid, antituberculin–B_6, anticonvulsants–vitamin D, tetracycline–calcium)
2. Genetic deficiencies [lactase deficiency (maple-syrup urine), homocystinuria, Hartnup disease]
3. Endocrinologic abnormalities (diabetes mellitus, hyperlipidemias, thyroid disease, hypothalamic abnormalities, Cushing's disease, Addison's disease)
4. Food allergies (dairy products, xanthines, tartrazines)

INCREASED EXCRETION

1. Nephrotic syndrome, protein-losing enteropathy
2. Burns
3. Dialysis
4. Fistulas, catheter drainage

DIAGNOSIS

Assessment of a patient's nutrition status for diagnostic and therapeutic purposes requires refined medical acumen. A careful history and physical examination for clinical signs and symptoms are the first priority. In the early stages of a malnutrition state, clinical manifestations may not be evident. In advanced disease, these manifestations may be masked by an underlying disease. A nutrition profile or index is required, with dietary, anthropometric, biochemical, and immunologic testing. The minimal data obtained should include height and weight and levels of albumin, transferrin, electrolytes, blood urea nitrogen, creatinine, glucose, cholesterol, and lymphocytes. The anthropometric measurements help to quantitate the physiochemical composition of the lost weight, taken at 6-month intervals (> 10% body weight loss is significant) and 1-month intervals (> 5% body weight loss is significant),

TABLE 16–4.
Nutritional Deficiencies: Laboratory Procedures for Diagnosis and Therapy*

NUTRIENT	LABORATORY MEASUREMENTS	VALUE SHOWING DEFICIENCIES
Protein		
	Serum albumin	< 3.3 gm/dL
	Serum transferrin	< 200 mg/dL
	Urine nitrogen (24 hr)	< 12 gm/24 hr
	Blood urea nitrogen	< 10 mg/dL
	Creatinine-Height Index (CHI)	
Protein-Calories	$= \dfrac{\text{actual 24hr creatinine excretion}}{\text{ideal 24hr creatinine excretion}} \times 100\%$	< 80%
	Total lymphocyte count	
	$= \text{WBC (cells/mm}^3) \times \dfrac{\%\ \text{lymphocytes}}{100}$	< 200/mm^3
	Delayed cutaneous hypersensitivity (skin tests)	≤ 1 of 3
	Hemoglobin	< 12 mg/dL
	Complete blood count	Anemia normocytic microcytic macrocytic
VITAMINS		
Vitamin D	Serum 25-OH vitamin D	< 8 ng/mL
	Serum calcium × phosphorus product	< 40 mg/dL
	Alkaline phosphatase (King-Armstrong)	> 40 unit/dL
Vitamin A	Serum Vitamin A (fasting patient)	< 10 μg/dL
Vitamin C	Leukocyte ascorbate concentration	< 7 mg/dL
	Serum ascorbic acid	< 0.2 mg/dL
Vitamin B$_1$	Erythrocyte transketolase activity after thiamine diphosphate challenge	> 15% increase
Vitamin B$_2$	Erythrocyte glutathione reductase activity	> 1.2
	Urine B$_2$ (24 hr)	50 μg/24 hr
Niacin	Urine N-methyl-2-pyridine	
	5-Carboxamine: N-methylnicotinamide	< 1
Vitamin B$_6$	Serum transaminase erythrocyte (tryptophan load test)	> 1.5 > 50 mg/24 hr
Folate	Erythrocyte folate	< 150 ng/mL
	Serum folate	< 3 ng/mL

Vitamin B_{12}	Serum B_{12} + therapeutic trial	< 140 pg/mL
	Shilling test	
Biotin	Whole blood biotin	< 0.82 mg/mL
	Urine biotin (24 hr)	< 24g/24 hr
Vitamin K	K challenge	(5–10 mg) with decreased pro-thrombin time
MINERALS		
Calcium	Serum calcium	< 8.5 mg/dL
Phosphorus	Serum phosphorus	< 2.5 mg/dL
Magnesium	Serum magnesium	< 1.8 mg/dL
Sodium	Serum sodium	< 135 mEq/L
Potassium	Serum potassium	< 3.5 mEq/L
Chloride	Serum chloride	< 95 mEq/L
TRACE ELEMENTS		
Iron	Plasma iron	< 40 μg/dL
	Hemoglobin, mean corpuscular volume	Decreased
Iodine	Radioactive-iodine uptake	10%–50%/24 hr
	Protein-bound iodine (PBI)	< 3.6 μg/dL
	T_3, T_4	Decreased
	Thyroid-stimulating hormone	Increased
Copper	Serum copper	< 70 μg/dL
Fluoride	None	———

* Laboratory values may vary depending on the laboratory used.

TABLE 16–5.
Nutritional Assessment Checklist

1. Daily body weight
2. Weekly anthropometric measurements, albumin level, renal studies (blood urea nitrogen, creatinine, electrolyte levels)
3. Calorie count (food diary)
4. Medication and possible adverse nutrition interactions
5. Basal metabolic rate calculation
6. Depression or other psychiatric disorders
7. Ability to swallow and chew food (dentures)
8. Prompt recognition of need for nasogastric, peripheral, or central intravenous feeding
9. Unnecessarily prolonged withholding of nutrition for diagnostic testing (colonoscopy) or therapy (pancreatitis)
10. Use of nutrition-support team members
11. Past and most recent alcohol and/or drug use
12. Fluid intake and output

and should include a measurement of triceps skin-fold thickness, mid-arm muscle circumference, and creatinine height index. In children a decrease of 20% or greater in growth height and weight over a 6-month period is significant. Table 16–4 lists the most commonly used laboratory procedures for assessing patients with a suspected nutrition abnormality. It must be emphasized that these tests, with wide confidence limits, provide only estimations, especially in the elderly. They may convey misleading information in hepatic disease, nephrosis, protein-losing enteropathy, dehydration, infection, and certain drug interactions.

PRINCIPLES OF PREVENTION AND THERAPY

According to Butterworth and Weinsier in Goodhart and Shils (1980): "To a considerable extent, physician-induced malnutrition is the result of inappropriate emphasis on a complex modern treatment program while fundamental principles of nutrition remain in the background." Current reports state that the incidence of malnutrition in seriously ill medical/surgical patients is 25% to 70% after 2 weeks of hospitalization. Hospital-organized nutrition-support teams (physicians, nurses, nutritionists, and pharmacists) can contribute significantly to the prevention of malnutrition.

Table 16–5 lists the parameters to be followed in the therapy and prevention of malnutrition. A discussion of the individual therapeutic dosages of specific micronutrients is beyond the scope of this chapter and the Manual of Nutritional Therapeutics (Kilpers, Clouse, and Stenson, 1984) is recommended.

REFERENCES

Blackburn GL, Thornton PA: Nutritional assessment of the hospitalized patient. *Med Clin North Am* 1979; 63(5):1103–1114. *A complete article on nutritional assessment with excellent bibliography.*

Cahill GF Jr: Starvation in man. *Clin Endocrinol Metab* 1979; 5(2):397–415. *Classic comprehensive work on the physiology, biochemistry, and endocrinology of starvation.*

Goodhart RS, Shils ME: *Modern Nutrition in Health and Disease,* ed 6. Philadelphia, Lea & Febiger, 1980, pp 1–1220. *Most comprehensive textbook on nutrition.*

Heymsfield SB, Andrews JS, Horowitz J, Galloway JR, Shronts EP: Nutritional disorders, in Hurst JW: *Medicine for the Practicing Physician.* Boston, Butterworth, 1983, pp 155–183. *Excellent overview of most common nutritional disorders with therapeutic, preventive, and cost containment information.*

Kilpers DN, Clouse RE, Stenson WF: *Manual of Nutritional Therapeutics.* ed 1. Boston, Little, Brown & Co, 1984, pp 1–161. *Extensive data on micronutrients with emphasis on therapeutic modalities.*

Mertz W: The essential trace elements. *Science* 1981;

213:1332–1338. *Concise review of trace elements and their clinical signs and symptoms in deficient states.*

Rudman D: Biological considerations in the approach to clinical medicine, Section 5: Nutrition, in Braunwald E, Isselbacher KJ, Petersdorf RG, Wilson JD, Martin JB, Fauci AS (eds): *Harrison's Principles of Internal Medicine*, ed 11. New York, McGraw-Hill Book Co, 1987, pp 383–397. *Best overall section on nutrition in major textbook of internal medicine.*

Russell RM, Marliss EB, Rivlin RS, Tasman-Jones C: Nutritional diseases, in Wyngaarden JB, Smith LH (eds): *Cecil Textbook of Medicine*, ed 17. Philadelphia, WB Saunders Co, 1985, pp 1174–1209. *Thorough presentations of clinical signs and symptoms and metabolism of vitamins and trace minerals.*

Weinsier RL, Hunker EM, Krumdieck CL, Butterworth CE Jr: A prospective evaluation of general medical patients during the course of hospitalization. *Am J Clin Nutr* 1979; 32:418–426. *Excellent guidelines for nutritional assessment and monitoring.*

17 THERMAL INJURIES

Sidney F. Miller, M.D.

The skin is the largest single organ in the human body and serves several important functions. Three of the most important are (1) heat regulation, (2) preventing loss of extracellular fluid, and (3) preventing invasion of surface bacteria into the body. All of these functions are lost when the protective barrier of the skin is lost. A variety of injuries to the skin may produce this unwanted result, but the most common is thermal injury due to burns. An estimated 2 million people suffer burn injuries yearly, and, of these, 106,000 require hospitalization and 6,000 die (Pruitt, 1985) Chemical burns, electrocution, and certain bacterial infections that produce widespread skin injury (toxic epidermal necrolysis) produce similar injuries to the skin, however, each has unique features which can be reviewed in standard reference texts.

CLINICAL SIGNS AND SYMPTOMS

The magnitude of the injury to the skin is related to the depth of the injury and the extent of the body surface involved (Figure 17–1). Additional factors having an adverse effect on the patient's outcome include age, associated injuries, and preexisting illnesses.

The skin heals as the epidermis is regenerated by migration of epithelial cells from the hair follicles and sweat and sebaceous glands in the dermis.

Burn injuries are defined as superficial (first degree), partial-thickness (second degree), and full-thickness (third degree).

Superficial burns involve only the epidermis, which is readily regenerated. The most common examples of superficial burns are sunburns and mild flash or steam burns. These burns are red, painful, and occasionally form blisters, but heal rapidly because the underlying dermis is intact.

Partial- and full-thickness burns are so named because either part or all of the dermis is involved. Partial-thickness burns might heal if enough of the dermal hair follicles and sweat and sebaceous glands survive the injury. Full-thickness burns by definition will not heal because all of the dermis is destroyed, and the skin must be replaced, usually by grafting.

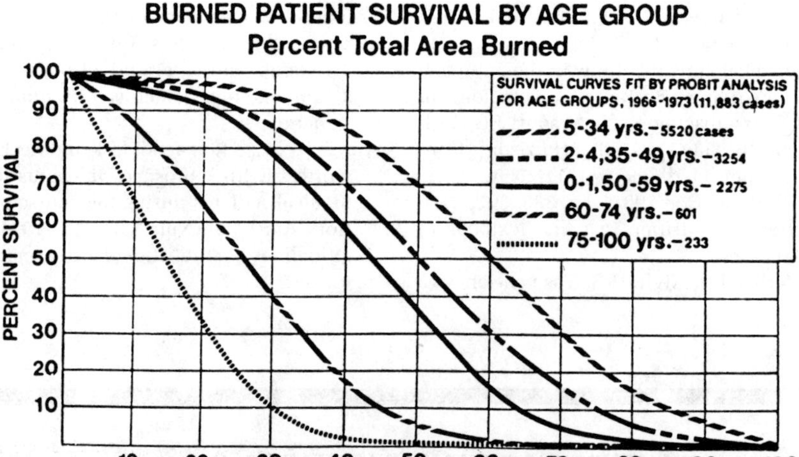

FIG 17–1.
Burn patient survival by age group (percent total body surface burned). Survival of the burn patient varies with not only size of the burn injury but also age. The 5 to 34-year age group has the best survival for all burn sizes, while the 75 to 100-year age group has the worst. [From National Burn Information Exchange (2, p. 10)]

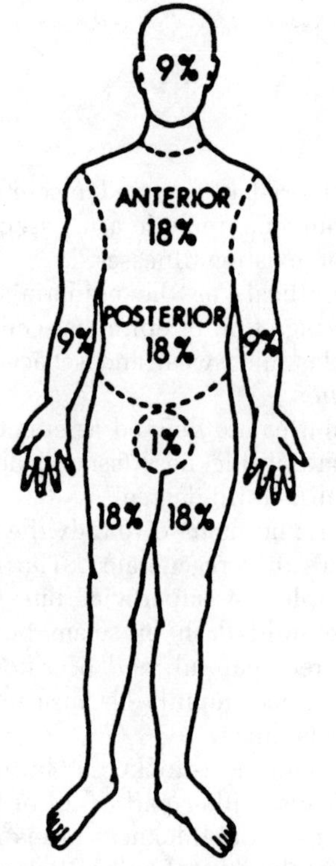

FIG 17–2.
The Rule of Nines is used to quickly estimate the total body surface involved with burns in adults. The head and each arm are considered 9% of the body surface. The anterior trunk, posterior trunk, and each leg each represent 18% of the body surface.

Partial-thickness burns are red, wet, and painful. Hyperemia occurs, rapidly producing the red appearance. Cell damage produces leakage of intracellular and intravascular fluid into the extracellular space producing edema and bullae (blisters), which frequently break producing the wet surface. The dermal nerves are intact and irritated by loss of the overlying epidermis and by edema, both of which produce pain. The sensation to touch, pressure, and pin prick is present.

Full-thickness burns may be red, brown-black, or pale pearly white and are dry and painless. The appearance of these burns depends on the burning agent, but the skin may actually become transparent with thrombosed subdermal veins visible. The skin has a dry leathery feel because most of the water in the skin has been "boiled" out. Because all the dermal elements are destroyed including the dermal nerves, full-thickness burns are painless.

The severity of the burn injury is also a function of the amount (percentage) of the body surface burned. The rule of nines (Fig 17–2) is commonly used to estimate burn size. A good reference for smaller burn is the patient's palm, which represents 1% of the body surface. Special tables are available for estimating burn size in children (Lund and Browder charts).

CLINICAL–PATHOLOGIC CORRELATIONS

The major burn affects almost all body systems (Table 17–1). Many of these are a direct effect of the burn injury and occur early in the course of treatment. Some result from loss of the skin, complications of various therapies, infections, or malnutrition. The primary pathophysiology of burn injuries is related to the following:

1. Loss of skin function
2. Associated injuries (inhalation and others)
3. Nutritional needs
4. Stress-related changes (in the gastrointestinal, cardiac, and renal systems)
5. Psychosocial efforts

LOSS OF SKIN FUNCTION

Early in the course of the burn injury massive amounts of water are lost into and out of the burn area. Depending on the size of the burn injury and the patient's state of health prior to the injury, various degrees of shock occur. Because the skin plays a major role in heat regulation, patients with large partial- and full-thickness burns lose their ability to regulate their body temperature and the temperature drops toward the ambient temperature.

Later, because the protective barrier function of the skin is lost and as the patient's wounds rapidly become colonized with bacteria, usually from the patient's own respiratory and gastroinestinal tract, bacteria readily gain access to the blood leading to sepsis. Seeding of the lungs (pneumonia or abscess), brain (abscess), or other sites may occur.

Additionally because the healed partial-thickness and grafted full-thickness burns contain large amounts of scar (fibroblast) tissue, the normal elasticity of the skin is lost. The grafted skin does not have sweat and sebaceous glands and, therefore, some or most of the body's ability to regulate its temperature by sweat glands and the lubricating function of the sebaceous glands are permanently lost.

ASSOCIATED INJURIES (INHALATION AND OTHERS)

A variety of associated injuries may occur with the burn injury. These are related to the injury mechanism and will have various effects on the outcome. Falls or automobile accidents may produce fractures and internal injuries as well as burns.

The most commonly occurring associated injury is an inhalation injury. Although frequently referred to as an "inhalation burn," heat has essentially no role in producing these injuries. The moisture content of the upper airways cools hot gases to body temperature before these gases reach the lungs. Damage is caused by the production of noxious gases during combustion of plastics, vinyls, and synthetic materials made from petroleum products. These noxious gases include hydrogen cyanide, hydrogen sulfide, hydrochloric acid, and carbon monoxide. These gases produce varying degrees of damage to the tracheobronchial tree, cause direct cellular damage, or produce systemic effects by destroying erythrocytes or by binding oxygen (carbon monoxide) and making it unavailable to the tissue for normal cellular functions.

Damage to the tracheobronchial tree produces varying degrees of airway obstruction and alveolar collapse. This damaged tracheobronchial epithelium is also more susceptible to colonization by blood-borne bacteria from the damaged skin.

NUTRITIONAL EFFECTS AND NEEDS

The basic energy expenditure (BEE) of the resting person is defined by the Harris-Benedict equations (formulas).[1] This requirement is increased markedly with any type of stress. With burn patients, the BEE may be increased by as much as 100%. The burn patients may require 4000 to 6000 kcal daily for the several weeks of their hospitalization. Failure to meet these energy requirements in the form of both calorie and protein intake has far-reaching clinical effects. These clinical effects can be seen not only in poor wound healing, but also in an increased risk of sepsis and nutrition-related complications such as bleeding gastric (stress) ulcers, loss of muscle strength, poor neutrophil function, and an increased mortality rate. The

---

[1] Male BEE = 66.47 + 13.75(W) + 5.00(H) − 6.75(A)
Female BEE = 655.10 + 9.56(W) + 1.85(H) − 4.68(A)
where W = weight in kg.
     H = height in cm.
     A = age in years.

TABLE 17–1.
Burn Injury: Clinical-Pathologic Correlations

ORGAN SYSTEM	CLINICAL FINDING	CAUSES	DIAGNOSIS	TREATMENT
CNS	Confusion (early)	Hypoxia	Arterial blood gas	Oxygen
	Confusion (late)	Sepsis	Wound cultures, brain scan	Antibiotics
		Brain abscess	Brain scan	Antibiotics, possible drainage
		Metabolic disorders	Trace metal analysis	Treat deficiencies
		Depression	Psychological tests	Psychological support
	Seizures	Hypoxia	Arterial blood gas	Oxygen
		Electrical injury	Electroencephalogram	Dilantin
		Sepsis/abscess	Wound cultures, brain scan	Antibiotics
Eye	Conjunctivitis	Transmitted infection	Conjunctival culture	Ophthalmic antibiotics
	Cataracts	High-voltage electrical arc	Ophthalmologic examination	Surgery
Ear	Hearing loss	Aminoglycosides	Auditometry	Limit use, monitor blood levels of drug
Larynx	Trachial stenosis	Prolonged intubation	Laryngoscopy	Tracheostomy
		Direct chemical injury	Laryngoscopy	Direct reconstructive surgery
Lung	Adult respiratory distress syndrome	Inhalation injury or fluid overload	Bronchoscopy or chest x-ray	Resiratory support
	Pneumonia/abscess	Sepsis or airway contamination	Bronchoscopy or chest x-ray	Antibiotics and pulmonary toilet
Stomach	Stress ulcers	Malnutrition	Gastroscopy	Antacids, nutritional support, surgery
Liver	Hepatitis	Blood transfusions	Laboratory diagnosis	General supportive care
	Hepatic failure	Sepsis/malnutrition	Laboratory diagnosis	Antibiotics, nutritional support
Kidney	Renal failure (early)	Shock	Laboratory diagnosis	Fluid restitution
	Tubular necrosis (acute)	Myoglobinuria in electrical injury	Inspection of urine	Fluids, diuretics, alkalinization of urine
	Renal failure (late)	Sepsis	Wound and blood cultures	Infection control, possible dialysis
Urinary bladder	Cystitis	Prolonged catheterization	Urine analysis	Catheter removal, antibiotics

key factors to monitor in these patients are their weight, serum albumin levels, the total lymphocyte count, and their ability to respond to a battery of skin tests. Patients whose weight drops to below 80% of their admission weight or who do not respond to skin tests are estimated to have a three to five times higher risk of dying from their burn injury than patients who maintain their nutritional state.

STRESS-RELATED CHANGES

The burn injury places great stress on the whole body. Early in the course of the injury, large amounts of fluids are required to treat the burn shock caused by massive fluid losses. These large fluid changes put a great amount of stress on the heart, particularly in patients with preexisting heart disease. Adequate fluid volumes are also required to maintain renal blood flow. Toxic chemicals (myoglobin, in electrical injuries) and drugs (aminoglycoside antibiotics) may damage the kidneys. Any preexisting renal problems will only complicate the patient's renal problems. Bacteremia or frank sepsis can initiate or magnify these renal problems.

Either because of increased gastric acid production or because of loss of the protective gastric mucus barrier, burn patients have a high risk of developing "stress" ulcers. These "stress" ulcers can be a single duodenal ulcer (Curling's ulcer), which can bleed or perforate, or, more commonly, can appear as diffuse bleeding gastritis with multiple small punctate ulcers.

PSYCHOSOCIAL EFFECTS

The burn patient is faced with a myriad of psychosocial problems from the moment he or she is hospitalized until, frequently, months after discharge. Loss of home or other family members in the fire will lead to depression or guilt or both during the early stages when the patient's energies and own medical needs are equally or more important. As healing occurs, concerns arise about the appearance of the healing or grafted area. Questions about acceptance by family, spouse, and others plague the patient. Leaving the sheltered environment of the burn unit at discharge brings the specter of facing friends and strangers with an altered appearance resulting from the burn injury. Even-

tually the patient must return to work or become permanently dependent on societal welfare, with the patient facing another set of psychosocial concerns.

PRINCIPLES OF THERAPY

The initial evaluation of the burn patient must address all the factors discussed under "Clinical-Pathologic Correlations." Burn injuries are classified as minor, moderate, and major burns. Most minor burns (burns that cover less than 10% of the surface area and have no injury to the dermis) can be managed through outpatient services or in any hospital. Moderate burns (burns that cover more than 10% but less than 25% of the surface area and have less than 10% of body surface full-thickness burn) unless they involve the face, hands, feet, perineum or have associated inhalation injury, can be managed at most larger hospitals. Major burns (those that cover more than 25% of the body, have more than 10% of body surface full-thickness burn, have associated injuries or medical conditions, or are chemical or electrical injuries) should be treated in burn treatment centers.

The burn injury is one that still has an associated risk of tetanus, and tetanus immunization guidelines established by the Committee on Trauma of the American College of Surgeons (1984) should be followed in all burn cases.

A variety of formulas have been advanced as guides to the management of shock in burn patients. The variety of these formulas suggests that a range of fluid requirements be obtained during the initial 48 hours of therapy. The most commonly used of these guides today is the Parkland formula which recommends giving 4 ml of lactate-Ringer's solution/kg body weight/% of body surface burned during the first 24 hours of hospitalization. One half of this fluid is given during the first 8 hours and the other half during the next 16 hours. Example: for a 70-kg patient with 40% of the body burned

$$4 \text{ ml lactate-Ringer's solution} \times 70 \text{ kg} \times 40\%$$
$$= 11,200 \text{ ml}$$

During first 8 hours: 5600 ml total given; 700 ml/hour

The adequacy of fluid replacement in adults is monitored by:

1. Urine output (at least 1 ml/kg/hour)
2. Serum hematocrit (less than 55%)
3. Serum osmolality (less than 350 mOsm/kg serum water)

Fluid overload, equally harmful, must be avoided by monitoring the central venous pressure and/or pulmonary artery wedge pressure measurements. Patients with preexisting heart disease should receive digitalis.

The skin is the primary organ of injury, and therapy is directed to protecting the skin in all areas of partial-thickness burns and replacing the skin with autografts in all areas of full-thickness burns. Initially, the damaged skin is sterile, but colonization of the damaged or dead skin by bacteria/microorganisms rapidly occurs. The wounds are gently washed and debrided twice daily in a sterile environment to limit colonization of the wounds. Topical antibiotics and bulky dressings are applied. The sooner the dead (full-thickness burn) areas are removed and covered with autologous skin grafts, the better is the patient's chance for survival. Skin grafting is, however, limited by the availability of donor sites and frequently must be performed in a stepwise fashion. Cadaver skin and artificial skin substitutes afford only temporary help because they are rapidly rejected by the patient.

Physical therapy is started early in the course of the hospitalization. This therapy is directed at maintaining a full range of motion of the uninvolved extremities and maximizing the function of the involved body parts.

Topical antibiotics, care in as sterile an environment as possible, and removal and replacement of dead skin as rapidly as possible are the hallmarks of infection control. Colonization of the burn wound occurs from the patient's own respiratory and gastrointestinal tract. Aggressive treatment of pulmonary and urinary tract infections is important. Liberal use of systemic broad-spectrum antibiotics is to be avoided because their use leads to overgrowth of the burn wounds with resistant organisms or fungi and yeast, which are extremely difficult to treat. Systemic antibiotics, when used, are used only to treat specific organisms in the blood that are identified by growing in cultures, and then the narrowest-spectrum antibiotic possible should be used.

Wound samples are routinely cultured twice weekly, and blood samples are cultured whenever the patient's temperature goes above 102° F. This routine monitoring is necessary to allow changes or additions to the antibiotic therapy to be made as promptly as possible.

Assessment of the patient's calorie and protein needs is made at the time of admission, using standard formulas. These nutritional needs can be met by supplements given with and between meals, by special tube feedings, or by intravenous hyperalimentation. Monitoring of the patient's nutritional status is performed daily by the burn unit's dietitian.

Laboratory assessment of the patient's nutritional status is also performed on a regular basis and includes weight of the patient, calorie intake, urine urea and creatinine output, serum albumin and transferrin levels, lymphocyte counts, and skin tests.

A variety of psychosocial services, including occupational therapy, psychology, and social work, are available to burn patients from the moment of admission. These services provide support to the patient and his or her family during the lengthy period of hospitalization and recovery. How well each patient does, however, is most dependent on the patient's preexisting support systems. Patients with a strong family and religious and employer support are better able to withstand the onslaught of psychosocial problems encountered during and after hospitalization.

REFERENCES

American College of Surgeons, Committee on Trauma: *Bulletin of the American College of Surgeons* 1984; 69:22–23. *Describing tetanus immunization guidelines.*

Baxter CR, Shires T: Physiological response to crystalloid resuscitation of severe burns. *Ann NY Acad Sci* 1968; 150:874–894. *Classic article on crystalloid resuscitation of severe burn injury and third space affect.*

Curreri PW, Richmond D, Marvin JA, et al.: Dietary

requirements of patients with major burns. *J Am Diet Assoc* 1974; 65:415–417. *Further delineation of dietary and nutritional requirements of major burn patients.*

Feller I, Jones CA: *Nursing the Burned Patient.* Ann Arbor, Mich, The Institute for Burn Medicine, 1974. *Compiled statistics and patient care information from the National Burn Information Exchange. The NBIE represents a large pooled database of national burn patient data.*

Hummel R (ed): *Clinical Burn Therapy.* Boston, John Wright- PSG, 1982, p. 17. *Best general text.*

Miller SF: The outpatient management of minor burns. *Am Fam Physician* 1977; 16:167–172. *Identifies principles and management of outpatient minor burns.*

Miller SF, Finley RK, Alkire S: Intervertebral disc space infection: Late sequelae of burn wound sepsis. *Bulletin and Clinical Review of Burn Injuries* 1984; Oct/Nov/Dec 1:41. *Unusual late complication of burn wound sepsis.*

Morath MA, Miller SF, Finley RK: Nutritional indicators of postburn bacteremic sepsis. *JPEN* 1981; 5:488–491. *Classic article relating sepsis with malnutrition in burn patients.*

Pruitt B, Jr: The universal trauma model. *Bulletin of the American College of Surgeons* 1985; 70:2–13. *Best text for MD, RN, PT, OT dietary.*

Rutten P, Blackburn GL, Flatt JP, Hallowell E, Cochran D: Determination of optimal hyperalimentation infusion rate. *J Surg Res* 1977; 18:477–483. *Article defining the nutritional needs of burn patients.*

18   WOUND HEALING

Phil D. Craft, M.D.

Wound healing is a fascinating series of events which will ordinarily restore the integrity and structural strength of damaged tissues. Though some of these events may occur within hours or days, the less dramatic aspects, such as scar maturation, may require years. Wound healing and a cosmetically satisfactory scar are not inevitable. The physician must understand healing and in particular those aspects that can be manipulated to provide the most satisfactory results for the patient.

The initial evaluation of a wound must not overshadow the importance of thoroughly assessing the general condition of the patient. After it is determined that the patient is not in a potentially life-threatening situation, those aspects of a patient's medical history that might interfere with the normal healing of a wound can be evaluated. For example, a patient may have had a previous injury or illness or may be taking a medication that may compromise healing.

The physician should estimate the extent of the local injury. Although the injection of a local anesthetic will make wound inspection more comfortable for the patient, it should be used with caution until potential nerve damage in the wound area has been determined. After the wound has been thoroughly explored and its extent identified, the physician can begin treatment.

EPIDERMAL WOUNDS

Epithelial integrity is important in the regulation of temperature and water metabolism and as a barrier against bacterial invasion. Small wounds are ordinarily of little consequence. For wounds that involve large surface areas, the restoration of epithelial integrity through healing is critically important.

Basic epidermal wounds include abrasions and first- and second-degree burns. In these

TABLE 18–1.
Compound Wounds

TYPE	CAUSE	CHARACTERISTICS
Contusion	Blunt force	Skin intact Subcutaneous tissue crushed Bleeding, which may be profuse Ecchymosis or localized hematoma
Puncture	Stab	Small wound at entry of stab with deeper wounds possibly extensive
Laceration	Cut	No uniformity at edges of cut May be contaminated
Incision	Cut	Uniform and clean
Avulsion	Crush or tear	Irregular margins Possibly contaminated Possibly loss of tissue
Burn	Heat	Depth variable Skin and possibly deeper tissue are part of coagulum

wounds the injury is usually deeper in the central part of the wound and more superficial in the periphery.

The wound defect fills with a mixture of blood, or blood components, and necrotic debris which forms a coagulum. If allowed to dehydrate, this coagulum will form a scab. The scab will temporarily provide a barrier to the loss of heat and fluid and to the invasion by bacteria.

Within hours after a wound is sustained, epithelialization begins from the intact periphery and from surviving skin appendages. The basilar epithelial cells dedifferentiate, their desmosomal attachments to the basement membrane and protoplasmic bridges to adjacent cells break up, and the cells migrate as a sheet into the wound. This migration continues by an ameboidlike movement until there is contact with other epithelial cells, producing "contact inhibition." The fixed basal cells adjacent to the wound then begin to proliferate by mitosis to replace the migrating cells, and eventually to add the stratification characteristic of normal skin.

TREATMENT OF EPIDERMAL WOUNDS

An epidermal wound must be cleaned. If the wound becomes contaminated with foreign matter/material, an appropriate anesthetic and judicious debridement may be required. In contamination with a pigmented material, aggressive removal using a dry sponge, scrub brush, or even a mechanical dermabrader may be

necessary to prevent a "traumatic tattoo." The tatto is actually entrapped pigment which, because of its superficial location in the dermis, may remain visible and appear as a "dirty" scar.

After the wound has been cleaned (debrided), a dry crust should be allowed to form. Fine-mesh gauze may be used as a substitute for crust formation. The crust will ordinarily separate from the epithelized wound in 7 to 10 days. The patient should be advised to avoid severe sunlight for several months to prevent possible hyperpigmentation.

COMPOUND WOUNDS

Compound wounds involve an injury of the structures deep to the dermis and add a series of complex features that normally progress to restore wound strength. Although physicians see a tremendous variety of deep wounds, most can be categorized into one or more of the types listed in Table 18–1. In large part, the type and extent of a wound dictate the care necessary for the best results, although many general (Table 18–2) and local (Table 18–3) factors will influence the outcome of treatment.

STAGES OF WOUND HEALING

Compound wounds add to the process of epithelialization: the dynamic phases of inflammation, fibroplasia, contraction, and scar maturation.

TABLE 18–2.
General Factors That Delay Wound Healing

Age
Nutrition status
   Vitamin deficiencies—particularly of A, D, C, K, thiamine, riboflavin, and pantothenic acid
   Protein depletion
Fluid–electrolyte balance
   Dehydration, edematous conditions, or both
Medication, such as immunosuppresives, glucocorticoids, and anticoagulants
Diseases, such as diabetes mellitus, hemophilia, and other disease states in which nutrition, fluid–electrolyte imbalance, or methods of treatment compromise the normal progression of wound healing

TABLE 18–3.
Local Factors That Delay Wound Healing

Devitalized tissue
   Tissue damage at time of injury
   Tissue destruction by dessication before closure
   Cellular injury from use of excessively strong antiseptics
   Compromised tissue converted to an avascular state, such as by excessively restrictive dressings or an underlying expanding hematoma
Seroma or hematoma, which provide excellent conditions for bacterial growth
Bacterial infection
Retained foreign body, including buried suture material
Failure to close a dead space
Closure under tension
Improper approximation of wound edges

Inflammatory phase

The traumatic event with its attendant tissue destruction, hemorrhage, and perhaps contamination initiates an inflammatory response. Initially, this response is characterized by transient vasoconstriction and a propensity for certain blood elements to stick to the endothelium of the small vessels in the injured area. Concurrently, serum, fibrin, and platelets collect and plug many of the small venules and lymphatic channels. When histamine is released from mast cells, and perhaps other cell types, the vasoconstriction is replaced by vasodilation with an attendant increase in blood flow. Histamine also causes the small venule walls to become more permeable, thus allowing plasma and blood elements to escape into the zone of injury. Lymphatic obstruction by fibrin and the escape of plasma into the extravascular spaces cause the wound to become edematous. This isolates the wound from the surrounding normal tissue.

In the inflammatory phase of wound healing, polymorphonuclear leukocytes and monocytes leave the small venules in the same proportions as they exist in the blood. If the wound is clean or minimally contaminated, both types of cells will, through active phagocytosis, rapidly clear the wound of cellular and foreign debris, and thus end the inflammatory phase. When the inflammatory process is prolonged (Tables 18–2 and 18–3), monocytic infiltration becomes, in part, more pronounced as a result of the relatively shorter life span of polymorphonuclear leukocytes. In either case, successful macrophage function marks the end of the inflammatory phase, which, in most "clean" wounds, lasts only a few days.

Fibroplastic phase

During epithelialization and throughout the inflammatory phase, the wound depths will have been primed with a luxurious ingrowth of endothelial buds. These give the wound the typical beefy red color of granulation tissue. From tissues nearby, undifferentiated mesenchymal cells rapidly evolve into migratory fibroblasts. These migratory fibroblasts, as well as those produced through "simple" mitosis, travel to the wound presumably along a fibrin network deposited early after the traumatic event.

With arrival in the damaged zone, the fibroblasts produce an amorphous mixture of fluids, electrolytes, mucopolysaccharides, and glycoproteins, which together are referred to as *ground substance*. Although the ground substance is the basic medium through which metabolites diffuse, its most important function may be its participation in determining the ultimate configuration of the collagen fibrils.

Once the environment in the damaged area is satisfactory, collagen is synthesized by mechanisms not yet fully understood. In the simple clean wound, biochemical evidence of hydroxyproline, a measure of collagen concentration, is noted by the third day. From the fourth day on, the amount of hydroxyproline in the wound increases rapidly with the height of activity occurring from days 5 through 12 with a continuing increase until about day 21. Thereafter, the increase is minimal and beyond the day 42 no increase is measurable.

During the early days after injury, the wound surfaces are held together not with collagen but by the protein coagulum, neovascular channels, and epithelial cohesion. With the appearance of collagen, the tensile strength parallels the content of collagen for about 28 days. Thereafter, the tensile strength slowly increases, even though the collagen content begins to decrease. The nearly imperceptible increase in tensile strength is probably related to more cross-linking within and between tropocollagen molecules and to a physical change in the organizational weave of the fiber mesh. This may be regulated by a factor in the ground substance.

Contraction phase

Wound contraction is the mechanical push–pull at the margin of a wound which progressively decreases the denuded surface area. Grillo and others (1958) have shown that the prime force in a contracting wound is located just beneath the advancing dermal edge. Although many of the active forces are yet to be identified, striated fibroblasts—myofibro-

blasts—have been identified in this zone. When a wound in the contraction phase is exposed to smooth-muscle stimulants such as prostaglandin E, a contractile force can be observed.

A regrettable feature of wound healing is that the forces associated with contraction do not subside when wound coverage has been achieved. The continuation of these significant contraction forces may cause a hypertrophic scar, keloid scar, and wound contraction. These deformities can be minimized by the use of splinting, which is appropriate in the treatment of a burn involving a flexion crease, or by the use of pressure or corticosteroid injections, which are appropriate in the treatment of a localized but unsightly hypertrophic scar.

Scar maturation phase

The maturation that occurs during the months or years after a wound has occurred is a manifestation of the improving structural quality of the collagen and the reorganization of the hyperplastic vascular channels into more efficient conduits. In adults, these changes may occur during a period of a few months, especially in wounds on or near the face. In children, the reconstructive process may require years.

TREATMENT OF COMPOUND WOUNDS

Before beginning the treatment of a wound, the physician should obtain a complete medical history from the patient. He or she should know whether the patient has allergies, diseases, takes medications, engages in strenuous activities, or is exposed to factors that might compromise care. Details about how the injury was sustained are helpful in predicting the magnitude of the general and local trauma to the patient. Information must also be obtained about previous tetanus immunizations.

The physician should not only examine the obvious wound, but should also assess the possibility of more serious injury. At that time, the wound can be clinically classified as clean, contaminated, or infected. A *clean wound* is one made under aseptic, primarily surgical, conditions and will not be considered further. A *contaminated wound* is any wound less than 6 to 8 hours old or a wound made through tis-

TABLE 18–4.
Clinical Types of Wound Healing

First intention:	Healing of a clean wound closed with sutures
Second intention:	Healing without closure by sutures or taping
Third intention:	Late approximation of a granulating wound by suturing (secondary suturing usually after failure of initial closure)
Delayed primary suture:	The contaminated wound is electively left open for a few days and then closed by suturing

sues that contain pathogenic organisms, such as a facial wound extending into the mouth. An *infected wound* is one in which bacterial growth is probable. The features used to determine if a wound is infected include local changes, such as suppuration and cellulitis, and systemic changes, such as an increase in body temperature and leukocytosis. A wound is presumed to be infected if it occurred longer than 8 hours before treatment or if the wound extends into a zone of infection. The examination should also determine whether a local or a general anesthetic is needed.

After an infection has been drained or rendered clean by local wound-care techniques, small wounds may simply be allowed to heal. Larger wounds may require further debridement and subsequent coverage by various grafts or flap techniques. The prime purpose of treatment is always early coverage of the wound and a rapid restoration of integrity and function.

REFERENCES

Bryant WM: Wound healing. In *Ciba Clinical Symposia*, 29(3). Summit, NJ, Ciba Pharmaceutical Co, 1977. *A brief, fairly comprehensive, well-illustrated review of wound healing in skin, bone, tendon, and nerve.*

Grillo HC, Watts GT, and Gross J: Studies in wound healing. I. Contraction and wound contents. *Ann Surg J* 1958; 148:145.

Ketchum LD, Cohen IK, Masters FW: Hypertrophic scars and keloids. *Plast Reconstr Surg* 1974; 53:140–154. *An excellent review of treatment modalities for hypertrophic scars and keloids.*

Klein L: Collagen structure and metabolism, in Krizek, TJ, Hoopes JE (eds): *Symposium on Basic Science in Plastic Surgery*, Vol 15. St Louis, CV Mosby Co, 1976, pp 80–86. *A good, short review on collagen.*

Longacre JJ: *The Ultrastructure of Collagen.* Springfield, Ill, Charles C Thomas, 1976. *A book for the student of collagen.*

Madden JW, Arem AJ: Wound healing: Biologic and clinical features, in Sabiston DC, Jr (ed): *Textbook of Surgery.* Philadelphia: WB Saunders Co, 1981, pp 265–286. *An abbreviated and concise review of pertinent aspects of wound repair.*

Moutandon D: Wound healing, in *Clinics in Plastic Surgery*, Vol 4(3). Philadelphia, WB Saunders Co, 1977. *An in-depth look at wound healing with good practical application.*

Peacock EE, Jr.: Wound healing and wound care, in Schwartz SI (ed): *Principles of Surgery.* New York, McGraw-Hill Book Co, 1983, pp 289–312. *An abbreviated but concise review of wound healing.*

Peacock EE, Jr, Van Winkle W, Jr: *Surgery and Biology of Wound Repair.* Philadelphia, WB Saunders Co, 1970. *An extensive, well-done, in-depth book on wound healing.*

Rohrich RJ, and Spicer TE: Wound healing/hypertrophic scars and keloids, in Barton FE, Jr (ed). *Selected Readings in Plastic Surgery*, Vol 4(1). Dallas, Baylor University Medical Center, 1986. *An overview of the more discrete problems of wound healing/care.*

part II

Circulatory Disorders

19 ANGINA PECTORIS

A. G. Suryaprasad, M.D.

Angina pectoris is a common clinical syndrome which signals a transient deficit in myocardial perfusion (ischemia). It may best be defined as discomfort in the chest or adjacent areas, with evidence of myocardial dysfunction, but without necrosis. The phrase literally means "strangling in the chest" and was coined in 1768 by William Heberden. Myocardial ischemia is an absolute or relative lack of blood supply to the myocardium, most commonly as a result of a 50% or more proximal luminal compromise of a major epicardial coronary artery.

CLINICAL SIGNS AND SYMPTOMS

The typical angina pectoris patient is an obese man, aged 50 to early 60 years. The cardinal features of typical, classic, or Heberden's angina include "visceral" or poorly localized discomfort or pain described as viselike, constricting, crushing, squeezing, or heaviness. The patient may use gestures such as a clenched fist placed over the center of the chest to indicate the nature of the discomfort. The pain may radiate either to the left shoulder, elbow, neck, or jaw, or to both arms, is predictably brought on by exercise or emotion, lasts 5 to 15 minutes, and is usually relieved within 3 minutes by rest or by sublingual nitroglycerin. The pain, almost always retrosternal and rarely strictly submammary, commonly presents as shoulder, arm, or jaw pain with or without associated substernal discomfort.

Diaphoresis, nausea, vomiting, or a sense of impending doom (angor animi) is commonly associated with the pain. Risk factors such as heavy cigarette smoking, hypertension, hypercholesterolemia, a family history of premature heart disease, or diabetes mellitus may be present (see Table 19–1 for the variability in clinical features).

In atypical angina pectoris, one or two features such as the quality of chest pain, the location, or the precipitating cause do not fit the classical description; however, the relationship of the pain to exertion is the most constant and helpful identifying feature.

Stable angina pectoris is angina that has a predictable pattern (i.e., is brought on by a constant amount of exertion or emotional stress), and may remain stable over weeks or months. However, there is practically always a recognizable precipitating cause which increases the myocardial oxygen demand.

Unstable angina pectoris is broadly of three types: (1) effort angina of recent onset, (2) "crescendo angina" with a recent change in pattern, and (3) rest angina which sometimes lasts as long as 30 minutes with or without electrocardiographic (ECG) changes and is not relieved by nitroglycerin. In variant or Prinzmetal's angina, typical but often more prolonged episodes of anginal pain occur cyclically at rest, the ST segment in the ECG is most often elevated, there is a high incidence of arrhythmias, but exercise tolerance is usually good. Angina decubitus is defined as angina during recumbency.

Although seldom crucial to the diagnosis, the physical examination may provide many helpful clues. During an anginal attack, blood pressure and heart rate often rise, and a transient holosystolic murmur, or an atrial gallop sound may be heard. Rarely, paradoxical splitting of the second heart sound may occur transiently. Aortic stenosis or hypertrophic cardiomyopathy may aggravate angina, while mitral valve prolapse may be an alternate cause for an exertional but often atypical chest pain syndrome, especially in a young female (see Table 19–2 for a summary of the important signs).

TABLE 19–1.
Historical Features of Angina Pectoris

PRIMARY SITE	REFERRAL SITE	QUALITY OF PAIN	PROVOKING FACTORS
Sternum or adjacent areas (96%)*	Jaw (9%)	Pressure, heavy weight, tightness, or choking sensation (60%–70%)	Exercise in general
Localized to chest only (34%)	Right arm (10%)	Burning, sharp, etc. (30%–40%)	Arm exercise, especially above head
	Right wrist (13%)	Gradual increase in intensity which then declines	Cold weather, walking against wind
Left shoulder, arm, and wrist (30%)			Coitus
Right arm, lower jaw (10%)	Neck (22%)		
Back or interscapular area (5%)			Fright, anger

* Percentages are percent of cases with this feature. Derived from Julian, 1985; Cohn and Braunwald, 1984; and from personal experience.

TABLE 19–2.
Physical Signs in Angina Pectoris

GENERAL EXAMINATION	CARDIAC EXAMINATION	NEGATIVE CLUES
Elevated blood pressure	Precordial systolic bulge	Precordial tenderness
Elevated pulse rate	Fourth heart sound	Midsystolic click and/or late systolic murmur (suggestive of mitral valve prolapse)
Sweating, pallor	Transient systolic murmur of papillary muscle dysfunction	
Xanthalasma	Paradoxical splitting of S_2 (rare)	
Retinal arteriolar changes	Third heart sound (rare)	
Vertical or diagonal ear lobe crease	Systolic murmur of aortic stenosis or idiopathic hypertrophic subaortic stenosis	

Because angina is a highly variable syndrome, validation of its occurrence is imprecise. Nonetheless, the annual incidence in the United States has been estimated as 0.5% for men and 0.1% for women aged 50 years and more. The factors that determine prognosis are largely based on the underlying cause of the angina, which in 85% to 90% of the cases is obstructive coronary artery disease (CAD). Prognosis is determined to a greater extent by the underlying left ventricular function, and to a lesser extent by the initial clinical presentation.

In patients with relatively stable angina, the mortality rate is about 4% per year, with 44% of the deaths being very sudden. One in four male patients with relatively stable angina can expect an acute coronary event within 5 years. Acute coronary events are more common as initial symptoms in women. The in-hospital mortality from unstable angina pectoris is around 3%. Nonfatal myocardial infarction (MI) rates in patients with unstable angina are 8% to 17%. The long-term outlook is poor, with 39% dying within 5 years and 52% within 10 years. A high-risk subset with 20% mortality and a 28% MI rate has been delineated and is characterized by continued episodes of chest pain despite aggressive medical therapy. The 5-year mortality rate for this subset is 73%. With improvements in coronary bypass surgery and the advent of new techniques such as percutaneous transluminal coronary angioplasty (PTCA), the prognosis of unstable angina pectoris has no doubt improved considerably.

Left ventricular (LV) function and the extent and location of coronary obstructions primarily determine prognosis. Left main coronary artery (LMCA) and three-vessel disease with poor LV function have the worst prognosis. The approximate annual mortality rates vary with the extent of coronary artery disease as follows: one-vessel disease 2.2%, two-vessel disease 7%, three-vessel disease 11%, and LMCA obstruction 20%. Among the nonarteriographic factors that indicate poor outlook are resting ECG changes such as left ventricular hypertrophy (LVH), ST–T segment changes, conduction defects, ventricular arrhythmias, and cardiomegaly. Administering beta-blockers immediately after MI seems to reduce the risk of MI and death for 1 or 2 years. Surgical treatment of LMCA or advanced three-vessel disease with poor LV function favorably influences the outcome.

PATHOPHYSIOLOGY

Myocardial ischemia stems from inadequate oxygen supply by coronary blood flow to a region of myocardium. The myocardial cells function essentially aerobically as attested to by the profusion of mitochondria and oxidative enzymes present. Oxygen is nearly 75% extracted from the blood even under resting conditions, and any need for increased oxygen must be met for the most part by increased coronary blood flow (autoregulation). Ischemia results in biochemical disruption, leading to anaerobic glycolysis and the production of lactate and kinins (bradykinin or kallikrein), which may mediate the sensation of pain by stimulating local nerve endings. From these endings, nerve impulses are carried to the cardiac sympathetic plexus, the spinal cord, and higher levels of the brain. This "visceral" pain is referred to the somatic structures innervated by the same spinal segments. The same location and paths of reference may be shared by the esophagus, stomach, and pulmonary vasculature. Figure 19–1 lists the factors that determine myocardial ischemia and their consequences.

Two mechanisms of ischemia have been recognized. The first, in which the pattern of angina is fixed ("fixed angina"), occurs with increased myocardial oxygen demand where supply is limited because of obstructive coronary disease. The mechanism usually present in rest or variant angina is related predominantly to diminished supply, which occurs during coronary spasm with no evidence of increased demand manifested by antecedent alteration in heart rate or blood pressure. Both mechanisms may be operative in patients with "mixed angina pectoris" in whom varying degrees of spasm are superimposed on fixed disease, resulting in a dynamic coronary obstruction.

CLINICAL–PATHOLOGIC CORRELATIONS

The major clinical-pathologic correlations of angina are listed in Table 19–3. In clinically significant angina pectoris, a 70% or more obstruction of one or more epicardial coronary arteries is present with transient ST segment changes in the ECG and LV function changes in the form of transient wall motion abnormali-

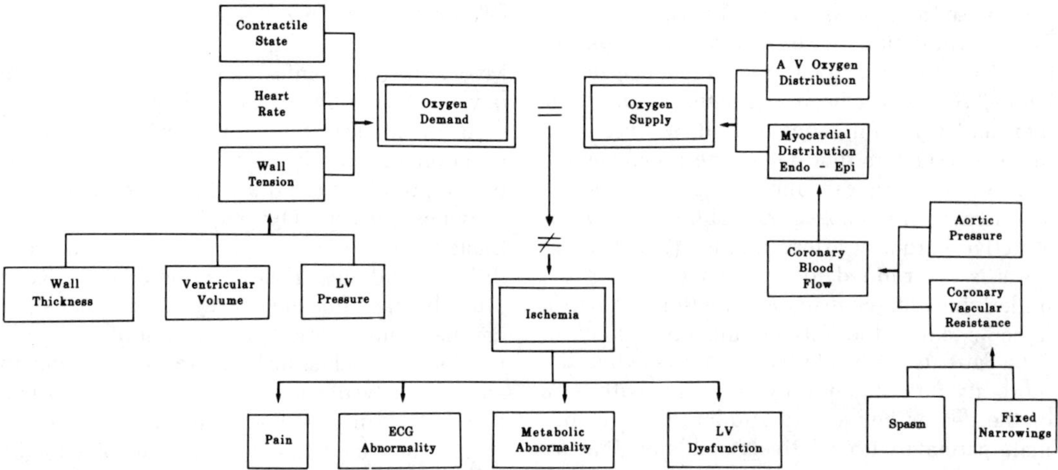

FIG 19–1.
The pathophysiology of myocardial ischemia. The factors contributing to myocardial oxygen requirement are listed at the left. The factors regulating myocardial blood flow are listed at the right, and the consequences of myocardial ischemia are listed at the bottom of the figure.

TABLE 19–3.
Clinical-Pathologic Correlations of Angina Pectoris

CLINICAL FINDINGS	PATHOLOGIC FINDINGS
Typical angina pectoris	Coronary artery disease (CAD)* (90% prevalence)
Atypical angina pectoris	CAD (50% prevalence)
Nonanginal chest pain	CAD (16% prevalence)
Angina with "normal" coronary arteries (10%–20%)	Aortic valve disease, hypertrophic cardiomyopathy, mitral stenosis, pulmonary hypertension
	Small-vessel disease
	Dilated cardiomyopathy
	Oxy-hemoglobin dissociation defects
Prinzmetal's (variant) angina	Coronary spasm superimposed on normal coronary arteries (21%) or atheromatous lesion (79%)
Unstable angina pectoris	Multivessel CAD
	Low incidence of occlusive thrombi
	Coronary vasospasm
	Platelet aggregation (transient)
Cardiac arrhythmias (ventricular ectopic rhythms, or conduction defects)	Extensive (2V or 3V) CAD
	Severe LV dysfunction (EF < 40%)
Congestive heart failure	LV aneurysm
	Mitral regurgitation due to papillary muscle dysfunction
	Global dysfunction: "ischemic cardiomyopathy"
"Silent" myocardial ischemia (Abnormal ECG: ST–T changes) (Ventricular arrhythmias or MI patterns in ECG)	CAD
	Diminished pain threshold
	Autonomic neuropathy in diabetes
(4%–5% of the population)	Psychological denial of pain

* Seventy percent or more narrowing of a major epicardial coronary artery.

ties. Signs and symptoms of heart failure or arrhythmias may also be present in cases of extensive obstructive disease. The characteristic lesion is an "atherosclerotic plaque" comprising arterial smooth muscle cells and lipids with various degrees of fibrosis.

DIFFERENTIAL DIAGNOSIS

Meticulous analysis of the history is crucial in the differential diagnosis of angina. Table 19–4 lists disorders that produce episodic chest pain, along with key differentiating features. Table 19–5 presents information about the differentiation of anginal pain from musculoskeletal chest pain and chest pain of gastrointestinal origin. Pericarditis, esophageal spasm, and exercise-induced asthma mimic angina of effort. Spontaneous attacks of angina pectoris are hard to differentiate from esophageal, gastric, or skeletal pain. Careful attention to the history and judicious use of laboratory studies are important in making this differentiation. The pain of reflux esophagitis may be mistaken for decubitus angina. Objective reproduction of the pain by acid perfusion (Bernstein's test) and esophageal manometry are helpful in making the diagnosis.

DIAGNOSIS

Because angina is a symptom, diagnosis depends primarily on correct interpretation of the patient's complaints. Laboratory studies are important in documenting ischemia objectively and in delineating the pathophysiologic mechanisms. The resting ECG during a pain-free period may be normal in more than half the patients, but during pain, ECG changes such as ST depression or T-wave changes occur in 80% to 90% of patients. The ambulatory ECG provides an elegant way of correlating ECG changes with the patient's symptoms over a period of 24 to 48 hours.

Exercise stress tests are designed to provoke myocardial ischemia by graded dynamic exercise on a treadmill or bicycle ergometer with continuous ECG and blood pressure monitoring. The primary criterion for a diagnosis of ischemia is a horizontal or downsloping ST depression of at least 1 mm at 0.08 seconds after the J point. The tests also help measure exercise capacity, assess prognosis, and suggest an approach to therapy. Maximal benefit from noninvasive stress test is obtained in patients with atypical anginal pain with a pretest likelihood of 50% coronary disease. In them a positive test raises the likelihood of CAD to 85%, and a negative test reduces it to 15%.

Thallium 201 myocardial perfusion imaging enhances the sensitivity and specificity of exercise stress testing. Thallium 201 is injected intravenously at the peak of exercise and is distributed in the myocardium proportionately to perfusion. Areas of hypoperfusion show up as filling defects. These areas show uptake of isotope in the scans obtained during the washout period 4 hours after exercise, indicating reversible myocardial ischemia.

Radionuclide ventriculography provides an estimate of global and regional LV function by blood pool imaging (multiple-gated acquisition scan, MUGA), with ECG gating using technetium-tagged red cells. It gives clues to myocardial ischemia in the form of wall motion abnormalities which may be studied at rest and during exercise.

Coronary angiography is an invasive procedure which is most precise in documenting coronary anatomy and LV function. Coronary arteries are imaged in various oblique projections after selective injection of contrast agents. The mortality rate is about 0.1% with potential morbidity from infection, vascular occlusion, MI, arrhythmias, or stroke. Indications for this procedure include preoperative assessment, diagnosis of obscure chest pain syndromes, assessing results of surgical or medical therapy.

Pacing stress studies and ergonovine induction of coronary spasm are other valuable approaches to provoking myocardial ischemia. These invasive procedures are low in sensitivity and specificity compared to stress testing.

Esophageal function tests such as acid perfusion, esophageal manometry, or 24-hour ambulatory monitoring of pH in the esophagus may be valuable in suggesting or excluding reflux esophagitis or esophageal motility disorders as underlying causes for anginalike chest pain when the coronary angiogram is normal.

PRINCIPLES OF THERAPY

Management of angina pectoris begins with the precise recognition and substantiation of the cause and clinical prognosis. All current ther-

TABLE 19–4.
Differential Diagnosis of Episodic Chest Pain

TYPE OR CAUSE OF PAIN	SITE	DURATION	SENSATION	PROVOCATION	RELIEF	COMMENT
Effort angina	Substernal	5–15 min	Deep (visceral) pressure	Exercise Emotion	Rest (in < 3 min) Nitroglycerin (in < 3 min)	Gradual onset and ending
Rest angina	Substernal, radiates to arms, jaw, neck	5–30 min	Visceral pressure	Spontaneous recumbency Smoking	Nitroglycerin	Often nocturnal or at same time of day
Mitral prolapse	Left anterior	Minutes to hours	Superficial stabbing	No pattern Question posture	Time	Associated with panic attack, skeletal abnormalities, wide changes in heart rate, and arrhythmias
Esophageal spasm	Substernal with radiation to elbow, fingers, or neck	5–60 min	Pressure or burning	Spontaneous Cold liquids Exercise (question)	Nitroglycerin	Mimics angina
Reflux esophagitis	Substernal Epigastric	5–60 min	Burning or visceral	Recumbency Lack of food	Food Antacids	Rarely radiates Nocturnal
Peptic ulcer	Epigastric	Hours	Burning	Nocturnal Lack of food "Acid" food	Milk Antacids	Generally not aggravated by exercise
Biliary	Epigastric, radiates to right scapular area and shoulder	Hour	Visceral waxes and wanes	Fatty foods Spontaneous	Time Analgesics	Colic
Pleurisy and lung disease	Left/right side of chest Substernal	30 or more minutes	Sharp Visceral	Deep breathing Coughing Spontaneous	Rest Time Bronchodilators	Dyspnea, wheezing, pleural rub, x-ray evidence of pleurisy or lung disease
Chest wall (musculoskeletal)	Many areas	Variable (Seconds to hours to days)	Superficial Sharp or dull aching	Deep breathing Twisting Bending	Local heat Analgesics	Tenderness sharply localized and reproduced by manipulation Pain lingers long after exertion
Hyperventilation	Substernal	2–3 min	Deep pressure (visceral)	Emotion Tachycardia	Stop deep breathing Remove stimulus	Circumoral tingling Numbness Tingling in fingers Dizziness
Psychoneurosis	Inframammary	Seconds to hours	Poorly described Highly variable	Severe anxiety	Reassurance Sedative	Might be associated with mitral valve prolapse

TABLE 19–5.
Differential Diagnosis of Common Disorders Mimicking Angina Pectoris

FEATURES	ANGINA PECTORIS	GI DISORDER	SKELETAL DISORDER
Onset of illness	First episode generally vivid Gradual onset	Not specific	Not specific
Duration of illness	Usually less than 5 years without objective findings on ECG	Highly variable Usually years Seasonal exacerbation	Highly variable
Pertinent history	Risk factors: Cigarette smoking Diabetes Premature death in family Hypertension Cholesterol	Dyspepsia (indigestion)	History of trauma
Duration (each attack)	5–15 min or until patient cannot continue and must stop effort. Relief in 1–3 min.	Variable. Usually 30 min to hours. Pain of esophageal spasm closely mimics angina.	Minutes to hours after rest. Patient can continue effort.
Precipitation	Effort Emotion	Nervous tension. Food may relieve pain. Cold or hot liquids may aggravate esophageal pain. Recumbency might aggravate.	Movement may cause pain that lasts long after exertion ceases
Relief	Cessation of effort Nitroglycerin	Eructation Milk, antacids Change in position Nltroglycerin (in > 3 min)	Change in position Local heat Analgesics
Time of day	May be nocturnal Usually associated with roughly constant degree of effort May occur soon after arising	Early morning, related to food Nervous tension relieved by antacids	Worse in evening after a day of physical exertion Relieved by local heat, analgesics
Seasonal/weather	Easily precipitated in cold weather with less exertion	May have periodicity in duodenal ulcer Otherwise no relationship	May be worse in winter and damp weather

apy is essentially palliative because no definitive cure for the atherosclerotic process exists. All patients require medical management. If medical measures fail, coronary bypass surgery or angioplasty are valuable options for control of symptoms. These procedures may prevent MI or sudden death when used early in cases of unstable angina or in certain high-risk subsets of patients such as in those with LMCA disease.

General therapeutic measures such as smoking cessation and weight reduction, a diet low in saturated fat, and control of diabetes, hypertension, and hyperlipidemia should be vigorously pursued as there is evidence (although not conclusive) of their efficacy in retarding progression of atherosclerosis. A regular exercise program, although not proven to delay the atherosclerotic process, is valuable in improving the patient's exercise tolerance and his or her physical and mental state. Walking and swimming are recommended.

Specific measures are recommended on the basis of clinical evaluation, ECG, and chest x-ray studies. Patients may be categorized as having angina pectoris, noncardiac chest pain, or pain related to other cardiac disorders such as mitral valve prolapse, or chest pain of uncertain origin. Stress testing helps identify high-risk patients in urgent need of angiography. Patients with LMCA stenosis narrowed (more than 50%) or three-vessel disease, with objec-

tively documented ischemia provoked within 3 minutes of exercise, are best treated surgically. All other patients should initially be treated medically.

Drug therapy is aimed at reducing factors that increase myocardial oxygen demand (preload, afterload, an increased heart rate, or increased myocardial contractility), or improving perfusion by coronary vasodilation. Nitrates, beta-blockers, and calcium-channel blockers are used. Sublingual nitroglycerin is most valuable in mild episodic angina. In moderate angina, combining nitrates with beta-blockers or calcium-channel blockers is effective.

Coronary bypass surgery is primarily indicated for angina that remains disabling despite aggressive medical treatment, for LMCA disease, or for three-vessel CAD with poor LV function. Percutaneous transluminal coronary angioplasty has emerged as a viable therapeutic option predominantly in single proximal CAD or in multivessel CAD. It is contraindicated in LMCA disease.

Therapy of unstable angina pectoris is initially medical with rest, rhythm monitoring, and administration of nitrates, beta-blockers, and calcium-channel blockers. If symptoms do not subside, intra-aortic balloon counterpulsation may help stabilize the patient's condition before urgent angiography and angioplasty, or surgical treatment.

REFERENCES

Achuff SC, Ross RS: Thoracic pain and angina pectoris, in Harvey AM, Johns RJ, McKusick VA, Owens AH, Ross RS (eds): *The Principles and Practice of Medicine*, ed 21. Norwalk, Conn, Appleton-Century-Crofts, 1984, pp 246–257. *Good coverage of differential diagnosis.*

Christie LG, Conti CR: Systematic approach to evaluation of angina-like chest pain: Pathophysiology and clinical testing with emphasis on objective documentation of myocardial ischemia. *Am Heart J* 1981; 102(5):897–912. *Excellent presentation of diagnosis and pathophysiology.*

Cohn PF, Braunwald E: Chronic ischemic heart disease, in Braunwald E (ed): *Heart Disease: A Textbook of Cardiovascular Medicine*, ed 2. Philadelphia, WB Saunders Co, 1984, pp 1334–1383. *Thorough coverage of all aspects of chronic ischemic heart disease.*

Heberden W: Some account of a disorder of the breast. *Med Trans Royal College Physicians (London)* 1772; 2:59 (See Braunwald: *Heart Disease*, ed 2, p 1374). *Classic reference on the history of angina pectoris. Best clinical description.*

Julian DG (ed): *Angina Pectoris*, ed 2. London, Churchill Livingston, 1985. *Most current and exhaustive text on the subject.*

Kannel WB, Feinleib M: Natural history of angina pectoris in the Framingham study. *Am J Cardiol* 1972; 29:154–163. *Classic reference on epidemiology.*

Mulcahy R, Daly L, Graham I, et al.: Unstable angina: Natural history and determinants of prognosis. *Am J Cardiol* 1981; 48:525–528. *The results of conservative treatment in 101 patients compare favorably to the results of intensive medical or surgical treatment. Postadmission persistence of pain indicates an adverse prognosis; the 1-year cardiac mortality rate was 10%.*

Russell RO Jr, Kouchoukos NT, Rogers WJ, et al.: Unstable angina pectoris; National cooperative study group to compare medical and surgical therapy. IV. Results in patients with left anterior descending coronary artery disease. *Am J Cardiol* 1981; 48:517–524. *An excellent comparison of treatment in unstable angina.*

Weinblatt E, Frank CW, Shapiro S, Sager RV: Prognostic factors in angina pectoris—a prospective study. *J Chron Dis* 1968; 21:231–245. *Good coverage of prognosis.*

20 ACUTE MYOCARDIAL INFARCTION

Moshen Sakhaii, M.D.
Sylvan L. Weinberg, M.D.

Myocardial infarction is a complex phenomenon which can be defined as necrosis or death of a segment of the myocardium caused by acute occlusion of a coronary artery. In the vast majority of patients with this disease there is significant atherosclerotic occlusion of one or more coronary arteries. Subsequent thrombus formation leads to complete occlusion of the lumen in most instances of acute myocardial infarction.

CLINICAL SIGNS AND SYMPTOMS

The most common clinical manifestation is a very disagreeable sensation usually in the substernal or left precordial region, radiating to the shoulders, neck, jaws, arms, and especially the left arm. There are, however, cases in which the pain is manifested primarily in the upper part of the abdomen, or even in such unusual locations as the interscapular region, teeth, and ears. The duration and intensity of discomfort varies considerably, being described as severe tightness, constricting, explosive, or boring which frequently gives rise to angor animi, a feeling of impending doom. Rarely, the chest pain is characterized as sharp, stabbing, or crushing. The pain of myocardial infarction is felt for at least 30 minutes in most cases and may last for several hours.

Heberden's description of angina pectoris also applies to the pain of acute myocardial infarction except that in the presence of myocardial infarction, unlike angina, the pain does not abate when the patient stands still. Those patients who have preexisting angina may be aware of a difference in the character, severity, and duration of the pain of myocardial infarction. A recent change in the character of previous angina in some patients may be a prodrome to myocardial infarction. This is the so-called syndrome of crescendo or unstable angina pectoris.

Disorders of cardiac rhythm range from ventricular fibrillation and ventricular tachycardia (which is usually fatal if not treated), to sinus bradycardia and complete heart block. The so-called sudden cardiac death usually occurs in the first few hours after the onset of myocardial infarction and is almost always due to ventricular fibrillation. Supra-ventricular arrhythmias are not uncommon, especially in the presence of right ventricular infarction or, less frequently, atrial infarction or acute atrial dilation. When the damage to the heart is extensive, there are progressive signs and symptoms of left ventricular pump failure and eventual cardiogenic shock. Heart block varies from first and second degree AV block to complete heart block. The latter may be related to AV nodal conduction abnormalities or to subnodal heart block, which carries a much greater risk, usually due to extensive infarction, eventual left ventricular failure, and arrhythmias.

Another common symptom is dyspnea, which is usually related to acute left ventricular failure. Profuse perspiration is common. Gastrointestinal symptoms such as nausea and vomiting are also common, especially when the infarction is in the inferoposterior region of the left heart. Light-headedness, fainting, and syncope may also occur.

The clinical signs of myocardial infarction are primarily those of a sudden impairment in left ventricular mechanical function and a subsequent surge of the sympathetic discharges. These include the aforementioned profuse perspiration, as well as peripheral vasoconstriction, pulmonary rales, and a fourth and occasionally a third heart sound, especially when the damage is substantial. A systolic murmur of mitral regurgitation secondary to the papillary muscle dysfunction is also common in the early stages of myocardial infarction. Other auscultative findings include paradoxic split of the second heart sound and attenuation of first and second heart sounds.

The jugular venous pressure may be elevated, especially if there is right ventricular involvement. Arterial hypotension is also common, whether it be due to an enhanced vagal tone, hypovolemia, or actual acute left ventricular pump failure. Arterial hypertension may be seen in cases of a small myocardial infarction in younger patients with hyperdynamic and hyperkinetic (hyperbeta) cardiovascular states.

Signs of cardiac dysrhythmia, when present, can also be detected. A precordial bulge is occasionally palpated (or seen), especially when there is massive anterior infarction. Pulmonary rales may be present, depending on the size of the myocardial infarction and the subsequent rise in pulmonary capillary wedge pressure.

Fever is not unusual after the first day of myocardial infarction and is due to the inflammatory process and, if present, fibrinous pericarditis. The symptom should not be interpreted as a sign of infection elsewhere. Routine culture of the blood, urine, and sputum should be avoided. Oliguria is also possible. Acute

pulmonary edema and left ventricular pump failure are usually directly related to the size of myocardial infarction.

Because of significant improvement in the treatment of myocardial infarction, the natural history of this disease process is difficult to describe; however, silent myocardial infarction may follow the path of natural history.

The modern era of the treatment of myocardial infarction began in the late 1950s with the introduction of electrical defibrillation and external cardiac massage. The advent of cardiac monitoring facilities and the explosion in electronic technical advances, coupled with defibrillators and cardiac massage led to the introduction of the coronary care unit in 1962 by Dr. Hughes Day at Bethany Hospital in Kansas City. Within a decade these units had proliferated throughout the world.

The coronary care unit is generally credited with reducing mortality in acute myocardial infarction from between 30% to 40% to about 15%. In the 1970s there was a movement toward reducing the myocardial oxygen demand using multiple pharmacologic interventions. In the 1980s there is a strong temptation to increase myocardial oxygen supply by various forms of early reperfusion and even coronary revascularization. It is hoped that these forms of treatment will further reduce the short- and long-term mortality of myocardial infarction. The rapid spread and popularity of coronary care units contributed significantly to the modern management of acute myocardial infarction. There is, however, the potential for excessive and occasionally unnecessary treatment, which may become harmful.

Major complications may occur in each of the three phases of the natural history of acute myocardial infarction. The first phase is the initial 24 to 48 hours after the acute coronary occlusion and the onset of symptoms. The most common complications are atrial and most importantly ventricular arrhythmias, disturbances of intraventricular conduction, hypovolemia, and cardiogenic shock.

The second phase is from day three to the end of the first week of myocardial infarction. During this phase, the aforementioned complications may occur, but not as commonly as in the first phase. Specific complications during this period include rupture of the left ventricle in the area of the interventricular septum, rupture of the free wall of the left ventricle, or rupture of the papillary musculature. Fibrinous pericarditis, expansion of myocardial infarction, and subsequent shock may also occur. In the case of a large anteroseptal myocardial infarction, it is not unusual to have an intramural thrombus, usually within the apex of the left ventricle (Fig 20–1). Subsequent cerebrovascular accidents or peripheral arterial embolization of the thrombus are not very common, but can occur. Other complications include deep venous thrombophlebitis and pulmonary embolism. Formation of a false aneurysm always precedes external rupture of the left ventricle. These patients are rather fortunate, because the ruptured area is sealed off by the pericardium, which progressively bulges out, producing a thin-walled aneurysmal sac. There is, however, a chance of rupture of the false aneurysm, which results in immediate death due to tamponade. Postinfarction angina, especially if it becomes difficult to control, usually signifies significant underlying disease and a poor prognosis. Psychological disturbances, including anxiety, phobia, depression, reduction of the libido, and diminished self-esteem, are not uncommon. We can also add the side-effects of medications as iatrogenic complications.

The third phase is from the time of discharge to the end of the second year after the onset of infarction. The mortality rate for patients who survive acute myocardial infarction depends on the size and location of the myocardial infarction. Major complications during this phase are the occurrence of sudden cardiac death syndrome, reinfarction, and postinfarction angina pectoris. Pharmacologic as well as interventional treatment and psychological support may significantly reduce the mortality and reinfarction rate during this stage.

PATHOPHYSIOLOGY AND CLINICAL-PATHOLOGIC CORRELATIONS

Acute occlusion of a major coronary branch by a thrombus is usually the immediate cause of myocardial infarction. Coronary vasospasm, especially when protracted, may play a role in the genesis of thrombosis and subsequent myocardial necrosis. In a vast majority of the cases (more than 85%), the thrombosis is superimposed on the preexisting atherosclerotic

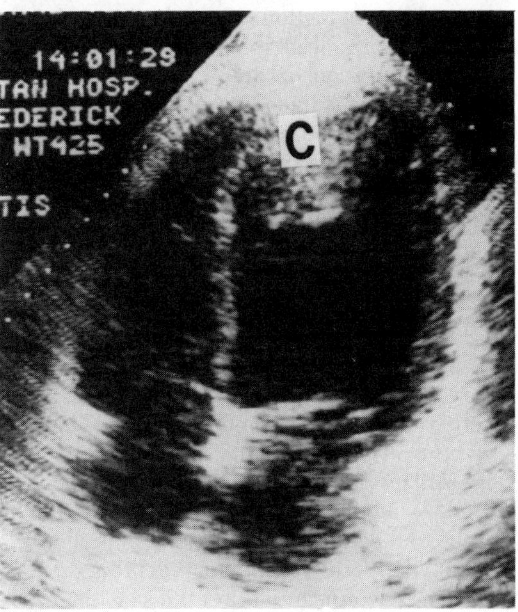

FIG 20–1.
2D echocardiogram, taken a week after an anteroseptal myocardial infarction in a 42-year-old white male. Letter C represents a large blood clot within an apical segment of the heart. Also there is bulging and thinning of the IV septum and enlargement of the L.V.

plaque. Why a stable plaque becomes unstable and initiates a thrombosis is the dilemma. At the present time, suspected factors include ulceration of the plaque, subintimal hemorrhage, inability of the disturbed endothelium to produce prostacyclin, and a hypercoagulable state along with a high level of catecholamines. In very rare cases coronary arteritis, metabolic alterations, pheochromocytoma, anomalous origin of the coronary arteries, abnormal hemoglobin dissociation curve, or possibly small-vessel disease and CNS disorders may contribute to the genesis of a myocardial infarction. A sudden increase in myocardial oxygen demand could theoretically lead to myocardial infarction, but is not considered a significant cause in pathogenesis of this disease.

Myocardial infarction triggers a chain of events that leads to disturbed pumping function of the heart and disorders of heart rhythm. Acute myocardial ischemia quickly leads to stiffness and loss of contractility of the affected segment of the left ventricle. In most cases, excessive catecholamine release occurs, especially if there is an element of pump failure and sudden reduction of the cardiac output. These, in turn, lead to manifestations of peripheral vasoconstriction including pallor, coolness of the skin, and sweating. Stimulation of vagal reflexes particularly from damage to infero-posterior segments of the left ventricle commonly lead to bradycardia, peripheral vasodilation, and hypotension. Hypotension is an inevitable manifestation of a severe drop in cardiac output and poor tissue oxygenation. Physiologically, as well as prognostically, this is in sharp contrast to hypotension that is secondary to massive damage to the left ventricle (usually anteroseptal) peripheral vasoconstriction. Reduction of the mean coronary arterial pressure and rise in left ventricular end diastolic pressure initiates a vicious cycle with more damage to the segments of myocardium that are in jeopardy. Activation of collateral circulation, which is usually related to the pressure gradient, may significantly limit the size of a myocardial infarction and its eventual outlook.

Right ventricular infarction is thought to occur in up to 25% of the cases of inferoposterior myocardial injury. This may lead to symptoms that can be confused with those of cardiogenic shock. In predominantly right ventricular infarction, pulmonary congestion and pulmonary edema are usually absent. The neck veins are usually distended, and atrial arrhythmias are common. Because of the rise in the right ventricular end diastolic pressure and the subsequent rise in right atrial pressure, there have been a few reports of opening of the foramen ovale with a right-to-left shunt, leading to profound hypoxemia. Infarctions of the atria have been reported.

Pathologically, myocardial infarction may be divided into two major types:

1. A transmural infarct, which leads to necrosis of the entire thickness of the ventricular wall (Q infarct).
2. A nontransmural infarction, which leads to a patchy necrosis of the subendocardium or focal areas within the intramural myocardium, without extending all the way to the ventricular wall (non-Q infarct).

Although gross changes may not appear in the myocardium for several hours, the paleness of the heart followed by cyanosis is seen rather early. About 20 hours after infarction the afflicted myocardium will appear tan or reddish-purple, and, in the case of a transmural infarct, with serofibrinous exudate may be evident on the epicardium. These changes can persist for 48 hours. The infiltration of neutrophils will then cause some gray or yellow lines within the damaged segment. This zone gradually widens, and after 8 to 10 days the thickness of the myocardial wall is reduced as necrotic muscles are replaced by monocellular cells. At this time the appearance of the infarcted zone is yellowish with a reddish-purple band of granulation tissue in its periphery. Yet there is another area, in the so-called twilight or border zone. This segment might improve with time or, if the necrosis continues, can lead to further deterioration of the left ventricular function. After a few weeks, the afflicted segment becomes thin and progressively whitens, leading to a firm scar. The scarring process begins at the periphery of the infarct and gradually moves inward. The endocardium of the infarcted area is usually thickened and grayish in color.

Damage to the conduction system is usually a sign of extensive myocardial infarction and carries a grave prognosis.

DIFFERENTIAL DIAGNOSIS

A careful clinical history and the electrocardiogram (ECG) will usually establish the proper diagnosis. In rare occasions, dissection of the thoracic aorta could become a major differential diagnosis. The pain of aortic dissection is commonly referred to as sharp; stabbing, crushing, or tearing. Its common location is retrosternal, interscapular; and if dissection progresses, the pain may follow the path of dissection. It is important to bear in mind that dissection of the ascending aorta may be associated with a myocardial infarction. A careful history, alteration of peripheral pulses, chest x-ray, 2D echo, CAT scan of the aorta, and ultimately an aortogram will establish the proper diagnosis. Among others, motility disorders of the esophagus, diseases of the upper gastrointestinal tract, and gallbladder diseases can cause confusing pictures. However, the ECG signs, if present, are extremely helpful. The alteration in serum enzymes almost always complements the ECG signs. At times, significant changes in the repolarization segment of the ECG can become confusing when there is CNS disease such as intracerebral bleeding. Early repolarization, local irritation of the chest wall, or nonspecific chest pain, pain of pericarditis, or pleuritis usually should not cause problems with the diagnosis. Location of the pain, however, can be misleading. Again, changes on the ECG and serum enzymes will always be helpful. Pulmonary embolus can occasionally be confused with myocardial infarction. Fractured ribs and myocardial contusion, the so-called learned pain syndrome, hyperventilation, conversion reactions, valvular diseases, cardiomyopathy, and congenital heart diseases may sometimes mimic some of the symptoms and signs of myocardial infarction. In a minority of cases the attack of myocardial infarction could be called "silent." However, a careful clinical history may reveal symptoms and signs of myocardial infarction that are either denied or were so trivial they went unrecognized.

DIAGNOSIS

Aside from ECG changes and the clinical history, the serum level of creatinine kinase and its MB band will reach its peak within 6 to 18 hours. This is followed by a rise in the transaminase level within 24 hours and subsequent elevation of the lactic dehydrogenase concentration. Other laboratory findings include an elevated erythrocyte sedimentation rate and occasionally leukocytosis. The chest x-ray film may be normal or it may reveal signs of early pulmonary edema. Atrial gallop and to a lesser degree third heart sound may be present.

Although ECG findings and enzyme elevations may contribute to a diagnosis of myocardial infarction, the essence of the diagnosis is clinical. Like all the clinical entities in medicine, the history is of prime importance. Clinical suspicion of myocardial infarction or acute coronary disease always takes precedence over laboratory findings. Where clinical suspicion is strong, based on history and physical findings, a normal ECG and cardiac enzymes should not deter the diagnosis or the patient's admission to a coronary care unit.

A two-dimensional echocardiogram and radionuclide studies are complementary, but are usually unnecessary to establish the initial diagnosis.

The ECG findings in a transmural infarction are usually straightforward. However, in the presence of complete left bundle branch block, preexisting myocardial infarction, Wolff-Parkinson-White syndrome, left ventricular hypertrophy, pacemaker rhythm, and cardiomyopathies, the initial alterations in the ECG may be difficult to interpret. A previous ECG could be potentially useful. A variety of conduction anomalies and arrhythmias may be present.

PRINCIPLES OF PREVENTION AND THERAPY

Management of myocardial infarction includes supportive treatment, treatment of cardiac arrhythmias, hemodynamic interventions, limitation of the infarct size, and ultimately, efforts at revascularization that may include use of thrombolytic therapy, transluminal angioplasty, or even surgical revascularization.

SUPPORTIVE TREATMENT

Symptomatic relief is indispensable. It not only supresses the agonizing discomfort, but it may also reduce the associated hemodymic burden. Narcotics continue to be the treatment of choice. Although the response to narcotics varies from one patient to another, from our experience we have found morphine or its analogues in doses of 3 to 15 mg to usually be effective. If there is no response within 2 to 3 minutes, repeated doses can be given until the pain subsides. Nitroglycerin, given sublingually or IV, occasionally rather rapidly relieves the chest pain. Sublingual nifedipine is effective at times. After the disappearance of the chest pain or at least reduction of its intensity, the patient usually requires a great deal of reassurance. Suppression of anxiety, as with benzodiazepines and other similar agents is imperative. Nasal oxygen in low doses, usually 2 to 4 L per minute, is recommended for the great majority of patients with myocardial infarction. Delay in treatment of the chest discomfort and its associated anxiety is not justified because one contemplates the interventional treatment available. Observation in the coronary care unit and bedrest for the first 24 hours are generally the rule. Of course, the duration of bedrest will vary from one patient to another based on several factors, most importantly, the size of myocardial infarction and its associated complications. We do recommend administration of heparin, especially in the presence of acute anterior myocardial infarction. The partial thromboplastin time does not necessarily need to be lengthened more than one and a half to twice the baseline value. This treatment should, at least to some degree, prevent the formation of an intramural thrombus and deep venous thrombophlebitis.

TREATMENT OF CARDIAC ARRHYTHMIAS

Early administration of intravenous lidocaine is being cited by some as a way to reduce the incidence of ventricular fibrillation. The treatment of ventricular fibrillation is immediate cardioversion. Similar treatment is needed for sustained ventricular tachycardia. Long-term

antiarrhythmic drug therapy may be needed. Beta-adrenergic-receptor blocking agents may diminish the size of the myocardial infarction in selected cases if administered early. Furthermore, these agents may reduce the incidence of ventricular fibrillation and postinfarction angina. The treatment of bradyarrhythmias varies from administration of atropine and isoproterenol to insertion of a temporary cardiac pacemaker.

TREATMENT OF POTENTIAL COMPLICATIONS AND HEMODYNAMIC DISTURBANCES

Despite general measures, if the patient continues to have signs of left ventricular failure, we recommend insertion of a Swan-Ganz catheter, an arterial line, and continuous monitoring of pulmonary as well as arterial pressure. The main treatment for this situation, aside from ef-

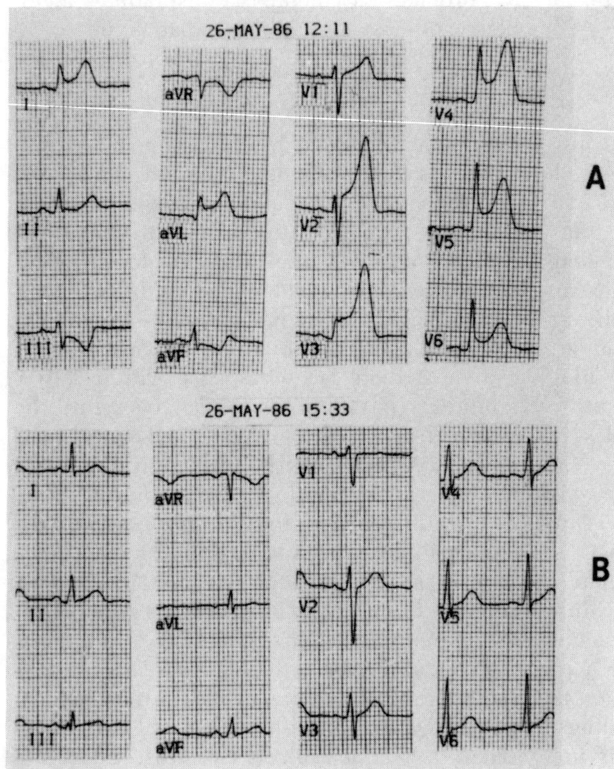

FIG 20–2.
A 41 year old white male presents to the ER + − 1.5 hr. after the onset of severe chest discomfort. **A**, 12 lead ECG showing acute anterolateral myocardial infarction. **B**, resolution of ST elevation after successful reperfusion.

forts to reperfuse when possible, includes vaso-dilator therapy, administration of a positive inotropic agent such as dopamine in a dose of 3 to 10 μg/kg minute or dobutamine infusion. Administration of digitalis is not routinely recommended. In the presence of atrial arrhythmias, especially atrial fibrillation, administration of low doses of digitalis is strongly recommended.

If the symptoms of left ventricular failure continue, or if the patient continues to have recurrent angina, intra-aortic balloon counterpulsation (IABCP) is recommended. Occurrence of major complications, such as rupture of the left ventricle, is usually catastrophic. Rupture of the left ventricular free wall leads to immediate tamponade and electromechanical dissociation and is usually fatal. Treatment of the rupture of the interventricular septum is stabilization of the patient's blood pressure and efforts to relieve pulmonary congestion; however, if the patient continues to be hypotensive, surgical repair may become necessary. Rupture of the posterior papillary muscle, which usually occurs with a limited infero-posterior myocardial infarction, requires immediate surgical repair and replacement of the mitral valve. In these circumstances, however, one ideally should have the details of the coronary artery disease by cardiac catheterization in order to perform a complete coronary revascularization.

LIMITATION OF THE INFARCT SIZE AND INTERVENTIONAL THERAPY

Every effort should be made to reduce myocardial oxygen demand and increase myocardial oxygen supply. The methods to reduce myocardial oxygen demand are limited. Agents such as beta-adrenergic receptor blockers, preload and afterload reducers, and antiinflamatory agents such as ibuprofen and possibly polarizing solution could prove to be useful. An important point, however, is to maintain an adequate mean arterial pressure and tissue oxygenation. The diastolic pressure especially should not be significantly reduced because the coronary perfusion is primarily in diastole. Experimentation with other agents such as hyaluronidase, corticosteroids, and indomethacin has proved not to be useful and possibly harmful. IABCP when indicated may be useful.

THROMBOLYTIC THERAPY

Thrombolytic therapy is becoming increasingly popular. Significant deterioration of the wall motions begins within minutes after acute coronary artery occlusion. Myocardial necrosis follows progressively within the first several hours. It is generally believed that reperfusion within the first few hours after the onset of chest pain could prove to be useful in selected cases, especially in those with anterior myocardial infarction. Rapid intravenous administration of up to 1.5 million units of streptokinase in 1 hour is currently the accepted dosage. Before initiating this treatment, establish two reliable IV lines. An arterial line will be ideal. Be prepared for treatment of possible reperfusion arrhythmias. Avoid IM injection. Intracoronary streptokinase instillation remains experimental; it should be administered only in laboratories with sufficient personnel, a rigid protocol, and an experienced interventional cardiologist.

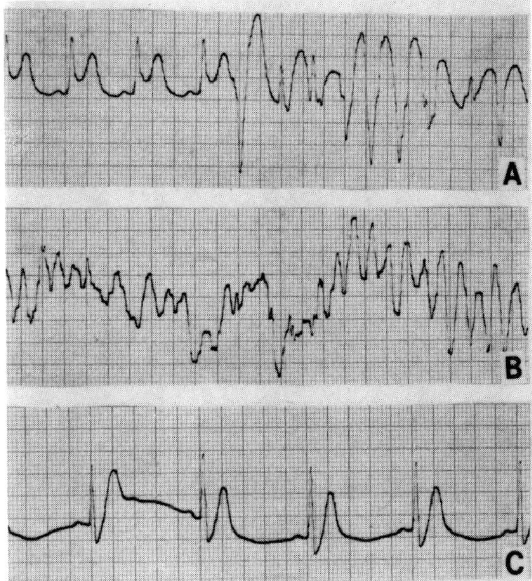

FIG 20–3.
Continuous ECG on same patient (Fig 20–2). **A,** approximately 40 minutes after infusion of 1.5 mil. u. IV, SK chest pain begins to subside, frequent ventricular arrhythmias appear. **B,** within a minute, pt. goes into ventricular fibrillation requiring several D/C cardioversions. **C,** less than one minute later, sinus rhythm is restored, ST segment normalizes, and chest pain vanishes.

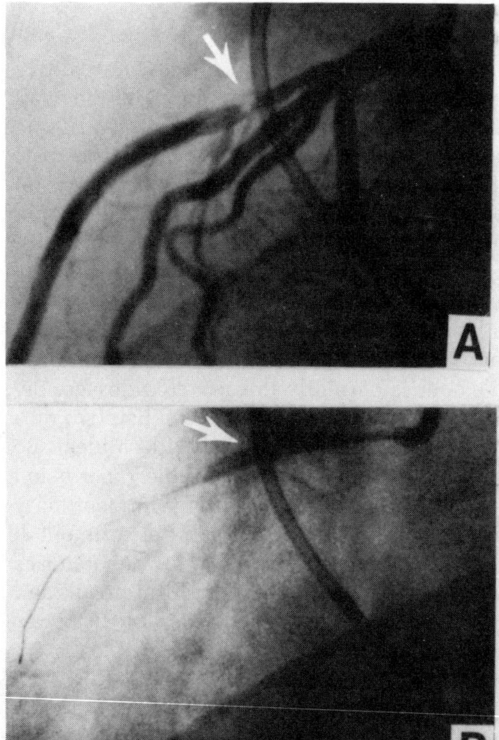

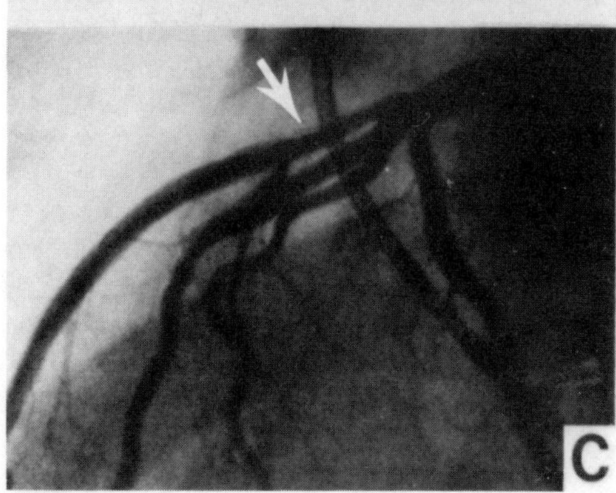

FIG 20–4.
Coronary arteriogram in same patient (Figs. 20–2 and 20–3). **A**, critical stenosis of the left anterior descending coronary artery RAO view (reversed). **B**, coronary angioplasty balloon in position, inflated. **C**, after dilation, the pressure gradient normalizes and the stenotic lesion normalizes.

Complications of thrombolytic therapy include bleeding, allergic reaction, cardiac arrhythmias, and hypotension. Furthermore, hemorrhage within the infarcted or inflamed myocardium may also occur, further depressing the myocardial function. Bleeding complications, thus far, are the major limitation, precluding its use in those who are recovering from a surgical procedure done within the past several weeks, who have had a cerebrovascular accident in the past several months, who have an active gastrointestinal ulcer, who have an allergy to the drug, and, finally, some who are over the age of 75 years.

Clot-specific agents such as tissue plasminogen activators (tPA) may be preferred; however, this agent is very expensive and has similar bleeding complications. It is twice as effective as streptokinase (IV streptokinase is effective in 35-40%, of cases, whereas IV tPA is effective in 60-70% of cases). Successful recanalization with a thrombolytic agent is signified by the disappearance of the chest pain, resolution of the ST segment elevation (Fig 20–2), early and rapid rise in creatinine kinase isoenzyme levels, a variety of cardiac arrhythmias (Fig 20–3), and hypotension. Because the reperfusion syndrome, especially the presence of arrhythmia, can become difficult to control, a trained physician should be present or immediately available when this treatment is initiated.

Administration of heparin according to a strict schedule is mandatory after successful thrombolysis (e.g., a PTT of 70-80 seconds). It is generally felt that in those who have successful reperfusion, early cardiac catheterization followed by percutaneous transluminal coronary angioplasty or complete coronary revascularization may be needed to prevent recurrent myocardial infarction, reduce the mortality rate, and improve the left ventricular function (Fig 20–4). There is a school of thought, which is gaining popularity, that advocates percutaneous transluminal coronary angioplasty as the initial interventional approach without waiting for the result of thrombolytic agents.

PROGNOSIS

The physician at the bedside using clinical observation and limited laboratory data can make a reasonably accurate appraisal of the patient's prognosis. Inferior myocardial infarction has a much lower mortality than anterior infarction. Bundle branch block, particularly one developing acutely, indicates an extremely poor prognosis, a mortality rate perhaps approaching 45% to 50%. Patients in cardiogenic shock have an acute mortality rate between 70% and 80%. Cardiogenic shock associated with myocardial infarction is to be distinguished from hypotension related to hypovolemia and/or a vasodepressor response. The distinction can be made clinically or with the use of a Swan-Ganz catheter. Patients in congestive failure, especially those who have ventricular tachycardia or atrial fibrillation, have unfavorable short-term prognosis. The presence of atrial fibrillation or supraventricular tachyarrhythmias increases the mortality rate in the acute phase. The ventricular arrhythmias occurring during reperfusion, even spontaneous or after thrombolytic therapy, do not indicate an unfavorable prognosis; quite the opposite. The overall prognosis, however, decreases with each decade of life and is worst for the oldest age group.

An understanding of prognosis is vital in selecting therapy. For example, the use of interventional therapy with cardiac catheterization and percutaneous transluminal coronary angioplasty (PTCA) or thrombolytic techniques may be appropriate in a patient with a massive anterior infarction with hypotension for which the mortality rate is in between 40% and 60%. This approach, however, may be contraindicated in a patient with an uncomplicated inferior wall myocardial infarction for which the acute mortality rate may be as low as 5% and where the area of the myocardial damage is likely to be small.

PREVENTION

Efforts to prevent myocardial infarction are primarily related to a modification of the risk factors for coronary atherosclerosis. In survivors of an acute myocardial infarction, it is prudent to determine the status of the coronary arteries. Some investigators recommend performing a cardiac catheterization in most patients with acute myocardial infarction, Others recommend an early (predischarge) stress test, and if it proves to be abnormal at 75% of the predicted heart rate, they then recommend a cardiac catheterization study. We favor the former approach; the stress test complements the anatomical data. Furthermore, pharmacologic as well as reperfusion procedures may favorably alter the prognosis. Beta-adrenergic receptor blocking agents studied in the United States and in several European countries may prove to be beneficial. It appears that administration of these agents in sufficient dose (e.g., propranolol at 60 to 80 mg tid) starting early after myocardial infarction may be especially beneficial in the first 12 to 48 months after the onset of the infarction.

In view of the threat of superimposed thrombosis, therapy to suppress platelets and blood coagulation is ideal. Although multiple risk factors are being described in the genesis of coronary artery disease, the family history appears to be the most important variable. Modification of the risk factors, especially cigarette smoking, hyperlipidemia, and modification of life-style, may have a significant effect.

REFERENCES

Erbel RA, Pop T, Henrick K-J, et al.: Percutaneous transluminal coronary angioplasty after thrombolytic therapy, a perspective controlled randomized trial. *JACE* 1986; 8:485–495. *Hospital mortality rate was 14% for thrombolysis alone and 8% for thrombolysis and angioplasty.*

Feldman RL: Coronary thrombosis, coronary spasm and coronary atherosclerosis, speculations on the link between unstable angina and acute myocardial infarction *AJC* 1987; 59:1187–1190.

Fine DG, Weiss AT, Sapoznikov D, et al.: Importance of early initiation of intravenous streptokinase therapy for acute myocardial infarction. *AJC* 1986; 58:411–417. *A timing of therapy in relation to the onset of pain is critical.*

Gillespie JA, Moss AJ: Post-infarction risk profiling: Past, present and future considerations. *JACE* 1986; 8:50–51. *A concise review.*

Kelly DT: Clinical decisions in patients following myocardial infarction. *Current Probl Cardiol* 1985; 10:485–497. *A well-referenced review.*

Mitchell JRA: Back to the future: So what will fibrinolytic therapy offer your patient with myocardial infarction? *Brit Med J* 1986; 292:915–917. *A historical perspective.*

Proudfit WL: Origin of concept of ischemic heart

disease. *Br Heart J* 1983; 4:5209–5212. *A historical review.*

Proudfit WL: Variations on a theme from Heberden: Symptoms in angina pectoris. *Cleve Clin Q* 1984; 51:1–5. *A clinical review of the symptoms of angina.*

Ross R: Factors influencing athrogenesis, in Hurst JW (ed): *The Heart.* New York, McGraw-Hill Book Co, 1986, pp 801–1009. *An in-depth discussion of pathophysiology.*

Schroder R, Neuhause K-L, Leizorovicz A, et al.: A prospective placebo-controlled double-blind multicenter trial of intravenous streptokinase in acute myocardial infarction (ISAM): Long term mortality and morbidity. *JACE* 1987; 9:197–203. *Steptokinase alone is not impressive with respect to mortality and reinfarction.*

Sobel BE: Coronary thrombolysis: Progress and promise. *J Cardiovasc Pharm,* 1984; 6:s910–s913. *A concise review and a historical perspective.*

Wissler RW: Principles of the pathogenesis of atherosclerosis; in Braunwald E (ed): *Heart Disease.* Philadelphia, WB Saunders Co, 1984, pp 1183–1334. *A comprehensive discussion of pathogenesis.*

<h1>21   CONGESTIVE HEART FAILURE</h1>

Satyendra C. Gupta, M.D.

Congestive heart failure (CHF) is not a specific disease; it is a clinical syndrome in which the heart fails to meet the metabolic and oxygen needs of the body under varying circumstances. It may occur as a manifestation or complication of many types of heart disease and is brought about by conditions causing an increase in preload (volume) or afterload (pressure), a decrease in myocardial contractility, or by impaired ventricular filling (Table 21–1). A diagnosis of CHF is not complete until the underlying cardiac disorder has been identified.

The clinical manifestation of CHF result from (1) reduced cardiac output either at rest or in response to stress, (2) fluid retention, and (3) increased pressure in the pulmonary and systemic venous systems. The term "forward failure" means that most of the patient's symptoms result from a low cardiac output. "Backward failure" implies that the patient's symptoms result from elevated venous pressure behind the failing ventricle.

While "left-sided heart failure" refers to symptoms and signs of elevated pressure and congestion in the pulmonary veins and capillaries, "right-sided heart failure" relates to the symptoms and signs of elevated pressures and congestion in the systemic veins and capillaries.

CLINICAL SIGNS AND SYMPTOMS

The main symptoms of left-sided heart failure are dyspnea, paroxysmal nocturnal dyspnea, orthopnea, cough, hemoptysis, fatigue, and insomnia. Cardiac dyspnea usually begins as shortness of breath after strenuous exertion, and eventually the patient is dyspneic at rest. Occasionally the patient complains of a dry, nonproductive cough at night when recumbent. Insomnia associated with heart failure is often due to Cheyne-Stokes respiration, which can occur because of decreased cerebral blood flow to the respiratory center. Many patients with left-sided heart failure present with acute pulmonary edema, which develops suddenly with extreme shortness of breath and frothy, blood-tinged sputum.

The usual symptoms of right-sided heart failure are swelling of the ankles, right-quadrant abdominal pain, and, occasionally,

TABLE 21–1.
Etiology of CHF*

| INCREASED WORKLOAD | | DECREASED MYOCARDIAL CONTRACTILITY | RESTRICTED FILLING |
INCREASED VOLUME (PRELOAD)	INCREASED PRESSURE (AFTERLOAD)		
Valvular insufficiency	Hypertension	Cardiomyopathy	Constrictive pericarditis
Left-to-right shunts	Aortic and pulmonic stenosis	Coronary artery disease	Cardiac tamponade
Chronic severe increase in cardiac		Acute myocarditis	Restrictive cardiomyopathy
output (high output failure)			Mitral stenosis
Anemia			
Arteriovenous fistula			
Thyrotoxicosis			
Paget's disease			
Pregnancy			
Beriberi			
Fever and infection			

* A patient may have more than one cause of CHF.

abdominal swelling, weakness, and unexplained weight gain. At night with rest, decreased metabolic demands, and redistribution of edema, diuresis occurs and the patient may complain of nocturia.

Physical findings vary widely with the extent and duration of cardiac failure and with the involvement of one or both ventricles. While the diagnosis may be difficult in mild heart failure, severe failure is often apparent at a glance. Although cardiomegaly is usually present, it is absent in patients with constrictive pericarditis, restrictive cardiomyopathy, and in CHF resulting from acute insults (e.g., acute myocardial infarction, rupture of heart valves or chordae tendinae, or interventricular septum, and secondary to sudden arrhythmias). A gallop rhythm (third heart sound) and functional mitral, or tricuspid insufficiency murmurs (systolic murmurs) may be noted on auscultation secondary to ventricular dilatation.

The pulmonic component of the second heart sound is accentuated when pulmonary hypertension occurs. Tachycardia, decreased amplitude of peripheral pulses, and pulses alternans (variation in an every-other-beat systolic pressure despite a regular sinus rhythm) may be present. Bilateral basilar rales are present.

As failure worsens, pulmonary edema develops and wheezing may be noted. Patients with acute pulmonary edema are dyspneic and anxious. They expectorate frothy pink sputum and sometimes show Cheyne-Stokes respiration.

The physical findings of right-sided heart failure include neck vein distention, hepatomegaly, and peripheral edema. Hepatojugular reflux (a rise in jugular venous pressure when pressure is exerted on the abdomen) may be an early sign of right-sided heart failure. Bilateral or unilateral pleural effusion is sometimes detected. Unilateral effusions are usually located on the right side. Ascites is seen in constrictive pericarditis and sometimes in chronic heart failure.

Valvular heart disease, congenital heart disease, or hypertensive or ischemic heart disease may be the basis for cardiac failure and should be sought.

About 3 million adults in the United States suffer from CHF. An annual mortality rate of 10% to 12% is described among the 250,000 patients newly diagnosed as having heart failure each year. This number is expected to increase in the next few decades, both because the prevalence of CHF increases with age and because patients with various cardiac diseases are living longer owing to advances in medical and surgical management. The incidence of cardiac failure more than doubles for each decade of life from 45 to 75 years. The Framingham study (Kannel et al., 1982) found that the probability of death within four years of the onset of overt cardiac failure is 52% for men and 34% for women. Although patients usually respond well to initial treatment, their conditions often deteriorate and reach a point of refractoriness to therapy.

PATHOPHYSIOLOGY

Under conditions of increased workload, cardiac output may be augmented in three ways. Healthy humans and those with acute CHF use all three major physiologic mechanisms during exercise. A more rapid heartbeat is the simplest way to increase cardiac output. Second, the Frank-Starling mechanism states that, within limits, heart performance is a function of the length of myocardial fibers at the onset of contraction. A longer initial fiber length or a larger diastolic ventricular volume results in improved performance.

The third means of increasing left ventricular output is increased sympathetic stimulation. With increased sympathetic stimulation, normal or abnormal ventricles are capable of performing more work at any given level of fiber length or diastolic volume. However, increased sympathetic activity also increases the peripheral vascular resistance, which in turn increases the impedance to left ventricular ejection, resulting in further aggravation of ventricular dysfunction. In chronic CHF, myocardial hypertrophy with or without cardiac chamber dilatation increases the mass of contractile tissue and allows the heart to maintain a normal cardiac output in spite of the increased demand for work.

Impaired systolic function is most often accentuated in heart failure, but signs and symptoms of congestion can also occur from incomplete myocardial relaxation, which impairs filling and results in abnormal diastolic function. The venous pressure is increased, and, in-

TABLE 21–2.
Macroscopic and Microscopic Features of CHF

ORGAN	MACROSCOPIC FEATURES	MICROSCOPIC FEATURES
Heart	Enlarged with dilated chambers	Underlying condition determines features
	Normal size in pericardial disease and restrictive cardiomyopathy	
Lungs	Enlarged, firm, dark, and filled with bloody fluid	Engorged capillaries
		Thickened alveolar septa
	Brown hemosiderin deposits present in chronic CHF	Extravasation of large mononuclear cells containing RBCs, hemosiderin granules, or both
		Medial hypertrophy and intimal hyperplasia of pulmonary vessels
Liver	Enlarged, firm, and filled with fluid (acute heart failure)	Dilated central hepatic veins and sinusoids
	Atrophic, nutmeg appearance from the dark red areas of central	RBCs replace hepatocytes
	venous congestion and the lighter, fatty areas in the periphery of the lobules	Central lobular necrosis and atrophy
		Sclerosis of hepatic veins
Spleen	Enlarged	Fibrosis and dilated sinusoids
		Small infarcts
Pancreas, kidney, brain, and gastrointestinal tract	Engorged	Chronic venous congestion
		Engorged and dilated capillaries
		Occasional small infarcts, especially if atrial fibrillation is present

directly, the end-diastolic volume and cardiac output are decreased.

The three compensatory mechanisms mentioned above may be adequate to maintain the pumping performance of the heart at a relatively normal level for some time; nonetheless, the potential of each of these mechanisms is limited and will not be adequate if the increased work demand of the heart increases progressively with time, or if other diseases, such as coronary artery disease, affect the heart, resulting in ultimate heart failure. The major gross and microscopic findings in CHF are shown in Table 21–2.

CLINICAL–PATHOLOGIC CORRELATIONS

The clinical features of CHF are the result of (1) left ventricular dysfunction, (2) low cardiac output, (3) increased back pressures in the cardiac chambers, and (4) sympathetic stimulation with vasoconstriction and its effect on the renin-angiotension-aldosterone system. A summary of the major clinical-pathologic correlations is shown in Table 21–3.

DIFFERENTIAL DIAGNOSIS

The conditions that mimic CHF are shown in Table 21–4. The initial manifestations of acute pulmonary embolism are a sudden onset of chest pain and dyspnea in bedridden patients, in patients who have recently undergone surgery, and in patients with a leg injury or thrombophlebitis. The diagnosis of pulmonary embolism is best established by a ventilation-perfusion scan and pulmonary angiography. Hyperventilation is suspected in patients with an onset of severe dyspnea in association with severe anxiety. The chest x-ray film should show a heart of normal size and normal pulmonary vascular markings, unless there is associated lung disease.

TABLE 21–3.
Clinical–Pathologic Correlations of CHF

CLINICAL FINDINGS	HEMODYNAMIC CHANGES	PATHOPHYSIOLOGY
Dyspnea on exertion	Left ventricular dysfunction	Transportation of fluids into interstitial lung space
Dyspnea at rest	Increased left ventricular filling pressure	
Nocturnal cough	Increased left atrial pressure	Decreased lung compliance
Tachypnea	Increased pulmonary venous pressure	Noncompliance of left ventricle
S_3 heart sound	Increased pulmonary capillary wedge pressure	
Orthopnea		Recumbent Position
Orthopnea		Augmentation of intrathoracic blood volume
		Elevation of diaphragm
Paroxysmal nocturnal dyspnea		
Pulmonary edema		Transudation of fluids into alveoli
Frothy, blood-tinged sputum		Bronchospasms
Coarse, bubbling rales		Excessive bronchial secretions
Wheezing		Congestion of bronchial mucosa
Central cyanosis		Impaired pulmonary oxygen exchange
Malor flush (common in mitral stenosis and pulmonary hypertension)		Low arterial oxygen saturation
P_2 heart sound accentuated	Increased pulmonary artery pressure	Decreased thoracic duct drainage
Hepatomegaly	Increased right ventricular filling pressure	Decreased lymphatic drainage
Edema	Increased right atrial pressure	Decreased comparative plasma oncotic pressure
Ascites	Increased venous pressure	
Jugular venous distention		
Hydrothorax		
Peripheral cyanosis	Low cardiac output	Sympathetic stimulation with vasoconstriction
Fatigue		
Oliguria, azotemia		Decreased renal perfusion
Mental confusion		Increased renin release
Insomnia		Increased angiotensin formation
Anxiety		Increased aldosterone release
Edema		Increased sodium retention

TABLE 21–4.
Conditions Mimicking CHF

ACUTE HEART FAILURE	CHRONIC HEART FAILURE
Acute pulmonary embolism	Chronic lung disease
Acute hyperventilation	Chronic obstructive pulmonary disease
Viral pneumonia	Pulmonary emphysema
Acute asthma	Alveolar-capillary diffusion defects
Acute intoxication with smoke or kerosene	Cirrhosis of the liver with ascites
	Nephrotic syndrome
	Chronic venous insufficiency

Viral pneumonia that occurs suddenly may mimic acute heart failure. Although a chest x-ray film may show an area of infiltrate that resembles localized pulmonary edema, the heart size is within normal limits. Differentiating CHF and pulmonary edema is very difficult in cases of acute asthma associated with dyspnea and wheezing and with secondary pulmonary infection. However, acute pulmonary edema may occur with acute myocardial infarction and in patients with mitral stenosis whose heart size is often normal. Gallop rhythm may not always be audible. Acute intoxication with smoke or kerosene may be associated with diffuse pulmonary and bilateral hilar infiltration. A history of exposure to smoke or kerosene helps make the proper diagnosis.

In chronic lung diseases, dyspnea develops more gradually. Chest x-ray films show a normal heart size, absence of increased pulmonary venous markings in the upper lobes, and Kerley's B lines. Patients with cirrhosis of the liver with ascites have normal jugular venous pressures. Nephrotic syndrome and chronic venous insufficiency can be differentiated from CHF by the normal heart size, normal jugular venous pressure, and absence of an S3 gallop.

DIAGNOSIS

CHF most commonly affects renal and liver function tests and arterial blood gas studies. Proteinuria and a high specific gravity of the urine are common findings. Blood urea nitrogen and creatinine levels are often moderately elevated secondary to the reduced renal blood flow and glomerular filtration rate. Hyponatremia may result from water retention or from an excess urinary loss of sodium in response to diuretic agents. The serum potassium level is usually normal, although hypokalemia can occur either as a result of secondary aldosteronism or as a side-effect of kaliuretic diuretics. Hyperkalemia may occur in patients with severe heart failure who show a markedly reduced glomerular filtration rate and an inadequate delivery of sodium to sodium–potassium exchange sites in the distal tubules, particularly in patients receiving potassium-retaining diuretics.

Hypochloremia may also result from diuretic therapy. The results of liver function tests are often abnormal with mild-to-moderate elevations of serum bilirubin, transaminases, and alkaline phosphatase because of hepatic venous congestion. In patients with longstanding cardiac cirrhosis, albumin synthesis may be impaired with resultant hypoalbuminemia. In chronic CHF, a low arterial oxygen tension is common, and the arterial P_{CO2} is low owing to hyperventilation. The arterial pH is often alkalotic as a result of both hyperventilation and diuretic-induced metabolic alkalosis. However, in severe low cardiac output failure, the arterial pH may be acidotic because of carbon dioxide retention and anaerobic metabolism.

The electrocardiogram (ECG) may reflect the underlying pathologic cardiovascular condition or the effects of digitalis and diuretic therapy, but a completely normal ECG may occasionally be seen, making this test nonspecific to the diagnosis of CHF.

Radiography plays an important role in the diagnosis of CHF and is affected by the duration and to some degree by the severity of the heart failure. The size and shape of the cardiac silhouette provide important information concerning the underlying heart disease.

When the patient is standing and has normal pulmonary capillary and venous pressures, the lung bases are better perfused than the apices, and the vessels supplying the lower lobes are larger than those of the upper lobe. With the pressure elevated 18 to 23 mm Hg, pulmonary vascular redistribution occurs with constriction of the vessels to the lower lobes and dilation of the vessels to the upper lobes (cephalization). When the pulmonary capillary pressure increases to 20 to 25 mm Hg, interstitial pulmonary edema occurs, producing Kerley's lines and perihilar haze. When the capillary wedge pressure exceeds 25 mm Hg, alveolar edema manifests in a cloudlike appearance and concentration of fluid around the hili in a butterfly pattern. Large pleural effusions may also occur. With an elevated systemic venous pressure, the

azygos vein and superior vena cava may enlarge. Pericardial effusion as a result of CHF may also contribute to the increased heart size.

Echocardiography helps confirm the underlying pathologic cardiac condition and is useful in evaluating the dimensions of the various heart chambers, the contractility of the ventricles, and the abnormalities of localized wall motion. It may identify pericardial effusion, valve malfunction, cardiac thrombi, or tumors.

Radionuclide scanning techniques are an alternate method of evaluating ventricular function. A reasonably good determination of the ejection fraction provides an excellent index of left ventricular systolic performance.

Cardiac catheterization and ventriculography are rarely indicated to establish the diagnosis of CHF. Although not routinely necessary in managing heart failure, catheterization is at times very helpful in patients with difficult diagnostic or management problems in whom noninvasive studies provide incomplete answers. Hemodynamic findings indicating heart failure include elevated ventricular filling pressures, decreased cardiac output, decreased ejection fraction, and depressed ventricular contractility.

PRINCIPLES OF PREVENTION AND THERAPY

To treat CHF, remove the primary underlying cause and treat the precipitating factors (Table 21–5). Inotropic drug therapy is traditional to increase the contractile force of the heart, as is diuretic therapy to increase the renal excretion of salt and water. Effective inotropic therapy allows greater stroke output at any ventricular filling pressure. Diuretic agents relieve the symptoms of congestion at the expense of a fall in stroke volume. In mild CHF, digitalis and diuretic therapy are often effective in relieving symptoms.

Vasodilator therapy has emerged as an important adjunct in the management of severe heart failure. Impaired ventricular function in CHF is associated with high peripheral vascular resistance, which increases impedance to left ventricular ejection, resulting in further aggravation of ventricular dysfunction. Vasodilating agents interrupt this vicious positive feedback cycle of elevated resistance and depressed cardiac function.

TABLE 21–5.
Management of CHF

TREAT THE UNDERLYING CAUSE

Surgical Management
Acquired valvular disease
Congenital cardiac malformation
Constrictive pericarditis
Cardiac tamponade
Postmyocardial infarction complication
   Ventricular aneurysm
   Ventricular septal defect
   Mitral regurgitation
   Medical Management
Hypertension
Infective endocarditis

TREAT THE PRECIPITATING CAUSE

Noncompliance with treatment regimen
Excess of dietary sodium
Arrhythmias
Systemic infection
Pulmonary embolism
High output states (listed in Table 21–1)
Excessive intravenous fluids
Cardiac depressant or salt-retaining drugs
Increased systemic arterial hypertension

SPECIFIC TREATMENT

Reduce physical activity
Reduce sodium intake
Diuretics
Digitalis and other positive ionotropic agents
Vasodilators
   Arteriolar
   Venous
   Mixed (balanced)

Vasodilators are frequently classified according to their venous dilating (nitrates) versus arterial dilating (hydralazine) properties. Some vasodilators (prazosin and nitroprusside) have both venous and arterial effects. Venous dilators cause reduced left atrial pressure or preload, whereas arteriolar dilators augment cardiac output without substantially lowering the pulmonary capillary wedge pressure. Vasodilators have a difinite place in the therapy of New York Heart Association Class III and Class IV patients with heart failure. When conventional measures (morphine, oxygen, and diuretic agents) for treating acute pulmonary edema have failed, parenteral vasodilators frequently produce a favorable response. Recently angiotension-converting enzyme inhibitors (captopril and enalapril) have also been used successfully in resistant cases.

Preventing heart failure involves early detection and management of hypertension, coronary artery disease, and other treatable causes of heart failure.

REFERENCES

Braunwald E: Pathophysiology of heart failure. Management of heart failure, in Braunwald E (ed): *Heart Disease—A Textbook of Cardiovascular Medicine*, ed. 2. Philadelphia, WB Saunders Co, 1984, pp 447–559. *Excellent review for in-depth study.*

Firth BG: Southwestern internal medicine conference: Chronic congestive heart failure—the nature of the problem and its management in 1984. *Am J Med Science* 1984; 288(4):178–192. *Up-to-date review of the clinical approach to the management of CHF.*

Gazes RC, Assey ME: The management of congestive heart failure. *Curr Probl Cardiol* 1984; 8(11):70. *The most up-to-date and well-referenced discussion.*

Kannel WB, Savage D, Castelli WP: Cardiac failure in the Framingham study: twenty year follow-up, in Braunwald E (ed): *Congestive Heart Failure. Current Research and Clinical Applications*, New York: Grune and Stratton, 1982, pp 15–30. *Nice review of epidemiology.*

Killip T: Epidemiology of congestive heart failure. *Am J Cardiol* 1985; 56(2):2A–6A. *Good discussion of the epidemiology of CHF.*

Parmley WW: Pathophysiology of congestive heart failure. *Am J Cardiol* 1985; 56(2):7A–11A. *Well-written review of the pathophysiology of CHF.*

Schlant RC, Sonnenblick EH: Pathophysiology of heart failure; and Spann JF Jr, Hurst JW: The recognition and management of heart failure, in Hurst JW (ed): *The Heart, Arteries and Veins*, ed. 6. New York, McGraw-Hill Book Co. 1986, pp 319–369. *Reference book with nice graphs and x-ray films.*

22

CARDIOMYOPATHY

A. G. Suryaprasad, M.D.

Cardiomyopathies are diseases that primarily involve the heart muscle (myocardium) of one or both ventricles and often result in heart failure. Excluded from this definition is myocardial dysfunction due to valvular, hypertensive, congenital, pulmonary vascular, or coronary artery disease with focal myocardial involvement such as ventricular aneurysm. The World Health Organization (WHO) definition restricts cardiomyopathy to heart muscle disorders of unknown etiology, but a broader definition favoring the concept of primary myocardial disease with a pluricausal etiology is clinically more useful.

CLINICAL SIGNS AND SYMPTOMS

Three broad clinical groups can be characterized. (A summary of the important clinical features of each is presented in Table 22–1.)

1. Dilated (congestive) cardiomyopathy with predominant systolic (pump) dysfunction manifested by ventricular dilatation and congestive heart failure
2. Hypertrophic cardiomyopathy characterized by inappropriate left ventricular hypertrophy, asymmetric (disproportionate) septal hypertrophy with or without left ventricular outflow obstruction and with diminished compliance with diastolic dysfunction of the left ventricle
3. Restrictive cardiomyopathy with primary impairment of diastolic filling often due to endocardial scarring and/or infiltration of the myocardium

The symptoms of dilated cardiomyopathy are due to low cardiac output, congestive heart failure, arrhythmias, or emboli (Table 22–1).

The patient should be questioned carefully to exclude the role of toxic, metabolic, or infectious agents, such as alcohol, viral infections, psychotropic drugs such as tricyclic antidepressants, and nutritional deficiencies. Table 22–2 lists an etiologic classification.

The most common dilated cardiomyopathy in North America is due to coronary artery disease—"ischemic" cardiomyopathy. Alcoholic cardiomyopathy is the second most common dilated cardiomyopathy. Peripartum cardiomyopathy is rare and appears in the last trimester and first 3 months postpartum. It occurs frequently in black multiparous women with multiple nutritional deficiencies. In rare cases of postpartum cardiomyopathy a history of viral infection may be obtained. Hypertension is a significant risk factor associated with dilated cardiomyopathy. Diabetes mellitus may be associated with subclinical or clinically evident dilated cardiomyopathy with or without coronary artery disease. Diabetes mellitus rarely gives rise to restrictive cardiomyopathy.

The family history is important in distinguishing dilated cardiomyopathy from neuromuscular disorders including Duchenne type muscular dystrophy, myotonic dystrophy, and Friedreich's ataxia. A careful metabolic history is important in excluding thyroid dysfunction or phosphate or other electrolyte depletion. Anthracycline derivatives such as doxorubicin are well known for their dose-related myocardial toxicity and are associated with dilated cardiomyopathy.

The cardinal symptoms of hypertrophic cardiomyopathy are dyspnea (in 95% of patients), angina (in 58% to 86%), and syncope. One important subgroup of patients presents before age 30 years and has a history of sudden death in family members with or without other symp-

TABLE 22–1.
Clinical Features of Cardiomyopathies

DILATED	HYPERTROPHIC	RESTRICTIVE
SYMPTOMS		
Congestive heart failure (35%–70%)* (particularly of the left side)	Dyspnea (95%)	Dyspnea
Fatigue, weakness	Angina pectoris (58%–86%)	Fatigue
Arrhythmia (38%–55%) (palpitations, atrial fibrillation, premature ventricular contractions, atrioventricular block)	Fatigue	Congestive heart failure (predominantly of the right side)
Emboli (18%–22%) (systemic or pulmonary)	Syncope	Signs and symptoms of systemic diseases such as hemochromatosis or amyloidosis
	Palpitations (atrial fibrillation, ventricular arrhythmia)	
	Sudden death	
PHYSICAL EXAMINATION		
Low blood pressure, narrow pulse pressure	Blood pressure normal	Blood pressure normal
Mild elevation of diastolic blood pressure	Mild cardiomegaly	Postural hypotension
Moderate or severe cardiomegaly	"a" wave in jugular veins	Loud P_2 heart sound wide (right bundle branch block)
Loud P_2 heart sound, occasional paradoxical split	Brisk carotid pulse	Mild cardiomegaly
Atrial and ventricular gallop (S_3, S_4 heart sounds)	Apical systolic murmur (80% of idiopathic hypertrophic subaortic stenosis)	Pulmonary or systemic congestion
Summation gallop (25%–50%)	Thrill and heave	S_3 heart sound often on the right side
Left ventricular heave (30%–40%)	Palpable S_4 heart sound	Atrioventricular valvular regurgitation
Right ventricle (parasternal lift in 10%)	Systolic murmur at left sternal border (crescendo–decrescendo)	Inspiratory increase in jugular venous pressure (Kussmaul's sign)
Mitral regurgitation (pansystolic murmur at apex in 20%)	Increased with Valsalva, standing	Ascites
Tricuspid regurgitation (pansystolic murmur at left sternal border increases with inspiration in 5%)	Decreased with squatting	Resembles constrictive pericarditis
Jugular venous distention, pulsatile liver	Occasional S_3 heart sound (left)	
Hepatomegaly, edema (anasarca)	Paradoxical split S_2 heart sound (28%)	

* Percentage of patients with this type of cardiomyopathy with the feature.

TABLE 22–2.
Etiologic Classification of Cardiomyopathies

	Resultant Type(s) of Cardiomyopathy
IDIOPATHIC (PRIMARY) CARDIOMYOPATHIES	
Idiopathic dilated	
Hypertrophic cardiomyopathy	
Restrictive (endomyocardial fibrosis)	
SECONDARY CARDIOMYOPATHY	
Associated Factor	
Infections	Dilated
Viral, bacterial, fungal, protozoan	
Metabolic	Dilated
Toxic	Dilated
Alcohol, drugs (doxorubicin, phenothiazines), radiation, cobalt	
Infiltrative	Dilated, restrictive
Amyloidosis, sarcoidosis, hemochromatosis, neoplasm	
Connective tissue disorders	Dilated
SLE, scleroderma, polyarteritis nodosa, rheumatoid arthritis	
Neuromuscular disorders	Dilated
Muscular dystrophy, myotonic dystrophy,	
Freidreich's ataxia	Hypertrophic, dilated
Deficiencies	Dilated
Hypophosphatemia, thiamine or selenium deficiency (electrolytes and nutritional)	
Familial storage disorders	Dilated, restrictive
Glycogen storage disease, mucopolysaccharidosis	
Peripartum heart disease	Dilated
Endocardial fibroelastosis	Restrictive

toms. Autosomal dominant inheritance and HLS-linkage are genetic expressions of this disorder. Symptoms are usually secondary to diastolic dysfunction.

The symptoms of restrictive cardiomyopathy are those of predominant right heart failure, and they mimic constrictive pericarditis closely. They are also primarily due to diastolic dysfunction of the ventricles.

Physical examination of patients with dilated cardiomyopathy may show a spectrum of signs from mild cardiomegaly to severe biventricular congestive heart failure. In hypertrophic or restrictive cardiomyopathy, the predominant finding is a crescendo–decrescendo systolic murmur which intensifies with maneuvers that decrease left ventricular volume such as a Valsalva maneuver or administration of amyl nitrite and which diminishes when the patient squats. This reflects dynamic obstruction. Important associated features are left ventricular hypertrophy and diminished compliance (a loud S_4 sound). The clinical signs in restrictive cardiomyopathy closely mimic constrictive pericarditis, but no pericardial knock is present.

Studies of dilated cardiomyopathy are hard to compare because of differences in patient selection, in diagnostic criteria, and in the stage at which patients were accepted into the study. Fuster and associates (1981) followed up 104 patients for 6 to 20 years. Their findings showed that 87% had cardiomegaly and 73% had heart failure. Within the first year 30% died, and within the first 2 years 48% died. The survival of 24 living patients was comparable to that of the control group.

The average annual mortality rate in all these studies ranged from 5.7% to 9.8%. Factors contributing to poor prognosis include excessive preload or afterload (cardiac dilatation) or imparied myocardial structure or function (Table 22–3). Overall, 30% to 40% of patients die suddenly, presumably due to ventricular arrhythmias. Patients with coronary artery disease have the worst prognosis.

The clinical course of hypertrophic cardiomyopathy is highly variable. Symptomatic patients may be stable for 5 to 10 years, but the overall annual attrition may be 4%. The 7.6% rate of sudden death jumps to 22% in patients with ventricular arrhythmias. Prognosis is poor

TABLE 22–3.
Prognostic Factors in Cardiomyopathies

TYPE	FAVORABLE FACTORS	UNFAVORABLE FACTORS
Dilated cardiomyopathy	Reversible cause Alcohol abuse, hypertension, thyrotoxicosis, thiamine deficiency Transient precipitating factors amenable to treatment Infection, pregnancy, arrhythmias Early detection Minimal-to-slight structural changes in endomyocardial biopsy specimen	Significant cardiomegaly Severe pump dysfunction with frank chronic congestive heart failure Marked structural changes in cardiac biopsy specimen Coexistence of heart disease from another cause (e.g., coronary artery disease) Noncompliance Arrhythmias Complex premature ventricular contractions, ventricular tachycardia, atrial fibrillation
Hypertrophic cardiomyopathy	Late age at diagnosis Negative family history Absence of arrhythmias No history of syncope	Age under 30 years at diagnosis Family history of sudden death History of syncope, arrhythmias, ventricular and atrial fibrillation
Restrictive cardiomyopathy	Reversible or remediable cause Hypereosinophilic syndrome with eosinophilic endomyocardial fibrosis	Systemic defects not amenable to treatment (e.g., amyloidosis)

in patients younger than 30 years and in patients with a family history of sudden death and syncope. Sudden death often occurs during severe exertion, as in young athletes. Symptoms are not related to the severity of the obstruction. In rare cases, hypertrophic cardiomyopathy may progress to dilated cardiomyopathy, usually after a septal myotomy-myomectomy or a myocardial infarction.

The course and outlook in restrictive cardiomyopathy depend primarily on the underlying pathology. Prognosis is poor in specific heart disorders such as amyloidosis, but the course in nonspecific restrictive cardiomyopathy may be benign.

PATHOPHYSIOLOGY

Dilated cardiomyopathy is the end result of myocardial damage produced by a variety of toxic, metabolic, or infectious agents. Idiopathic, or primary dilated cardiomyopathy is the diagnosis when the etiology is not identified, and secondary cardiomyopathy is the diagnosis when the dilated cardiomyopathy is associated with factors such as hypertension or coronary artery disease.

Four major conditions lower the threshold for development of myocardial damage: the presence of alcohol, pregnancy, systemic hypertension, and a variety of infections. The role of viral myocarditis and the contributions of endocrine or immunologic abnormalities to idiopathic cardiomyopathy are speculative. Microvascular spasm may also contribute to the disorder. The end result is systolic pump dysfunction.

The location and degree of hypertrophy vary in hypertrophic cardiomyopathy, sometimes extending to the anterolateral wall and rarely to the right ventricle. Five major hemodynamic subsets of this condition are latent obstruction, resting obstruction, labile obstruction, midventricular obstruction, and a nonobstructive variety. Latent obstruction is associated with localized subaortic hypertrophy involving the lower third of the septum in 53% of patients. Of these patients, the hypertrophy extends to the papillary muscles in 35%, and to the whole length of the septum in 12%.

In resting obstruction and in nonobstructive hypertrophic cardiomyopathy, the entire length of the septum is involved in 72% of the patients. Anterolateral wall extension is seen in 91% of this group. In the familial varieties of both subsets, autosomal dominance or HLA-linkage is seen. The main histologic feature is a high degree of myocardial disarray with short, plump myocardial fibers in loose intercellular connective tissue. The ratio of septum to free wall is usually 1.5:1 or more. Although asymmetric septal hypertrophy is characteristic, it is not specific.

Left ventricular outflow obstruction and mitral regurgitation are best explained by systolic anterior motion of the anterior leaflet of mitral valve. Table 22–4 lists macroscopic and microscopic features of all cardiomyopathies. Possible causes of hypertrophy include abnormal sympathetic stimulation or supersensitivity to cathecholamines, abnormal intramural coronary arteries, accelerated conduction, primary collagen abnormality, and subendocardial ischemia.

Systolic function is supernormal. Most symptoms result from diastolic dysfunction. Dynamic obstruction is a cardinal feature.

In restrictive cardiomyopathy, the primary pathophysiology involves diastolic dysfunction due to decreased compliance of ventricles associated with high filling pressures, and pulmonary and systemic congestion. In some situations, the right side of the heart is more involved. The cause (Table 22–3) is often well defined, as in amyloid heart disease, hemachromatosis, neoplastic infiltration, eosinophilia, and sarcoidosis.

CLINICAL–PATHOLOGIC CORRELATIONS

Clinical-pathologic correlations (Table 22–5) may be summarized as poor systolic function in dilated cardiomyopathy, supernormal systolic function with decreased compliance in hypertrophic cardiomyopathy, and primary diastolic dysfunction with normal or slightly diminished systolic function plus cavity obliteration and scarring causing atrioventricular valve insufficiency in some cases, with or without myocardial infiltration in restrictive cardiomyopathy.

TABLE 22–4.
Macroscopic and Microscopic Features of Cardiomyopathies

TYPE	MACROSCOPIC FEATURES	MICROSCOPIC FEATURES
Idiopathic dilated cardiomyopathy	Dilated ventricular and atrial chambers Marked left ventricular hypertrophy (average weight: 600 gm) Mural thrombi (35%)* Systemic and pulmonary emboli (50%) Normal (widely patent) coronary arteries Nonspecific endocardial thickening	Extensive interstitial and perivascular fibrosis with or without calcification Necrotic area with cellular infiltrates Myocardial cell degeneration; cellular hypertrophy Abnormal mitochondria and myocytes Reduced enzyme activity (nonspecific) and elevated LDH activity
Cardiomyopathy secondary to coronary artery disease	Ventricular aneurysm Multiple infarcts Severe multivessel coronary artery disease	
Hypertrophic cardiomyopathy	Marked increase in myocardial mass Asymmetric septal hypertrophy (95%) (septum to free left ventricular wall = 1.3 to 1.5) Concentric hypertrophy Apical left ventricular hypertrophy Small left ventricular cavity (95%) Dilated atria (100%) Abnormal intramural coronary arteries (50%) Contact lesions—mural plaques in outflow tract (75%) Thickened mitral valve (75%)	Myocardial cellular disarray (95%) mainly in the septum Foci of disorganized cells MI disarray; markedly hypertrophic, abnormal-looking cells
Restrictive cardiomyopathy	External myocardial fibrosis with stiff, rubbery ventricles Relatively minor hypertrophy and dilatation Mural thrombi Small pericardial effusion Focal thickening or deposits on valves (in amyloidosis) Sarcoidosis Predominant involvement of the right side of the heart Extreme inflow tract and apical thickening and obliteration of cavity	Severe hyalinized fibrosis Amyloid deposits in myocardium, sinoatrial and atrioventricular nodes, and bundle branches Interstitial edema Calcific foci Noncaseating granulomas (in sarcoidosis) Eosinophilic infiltrates (early stages of Löffler's endocarditis) Glycogen deposits Iron deposits

* Percentage of patients with this type of cardiomyopathy with the feature.

TABLE 22–5.
Clinical–Pathologic Correlations of the Cardiomyopathies

CLINICAL FINDINGS	PATHOLOGIC FINDINGS
DILATED CARDIOMYOPATHY	
Congestive heart failure (left or biventricular)	Marked ventricular dilatation and hypertrophy (average weight: 560 gm; range: 200–850 gm)
Atrial and ventricular gallop	
Ventricular arrhythmias (syncope, sudden death)	Myocardial fibrosis (76%)*
Fatigue, dizziness	Systolic dysfunction (EF < 0.40)
Severe congestive heart failure	Low cardiac output
Systemic and pulmonary emboli (18%–22%)	Endocardial thickening
ECG: Left ventricular hypertrophy, pseudoinfarction patterns, atrial fibrillation	Mural thrombosis (35%)
Anginal chest pain	Severe left ventricular hypertrophy (average weight: 634 gm)
Mitral and tricuspid regurgitation	Atrial dilatation, fibrosis of conduction system with marked cardiomegaly
Diabetes mellitus	
Anginal pain, multiple myocardial infarctions	Multivessel coronary artery disease with cardiomyopathy
Mitral regurgitation	
HYPERTROPHIC CARDIOMYOPATHY	
Normal or supernormal systolic function (EF = 0.60 to 0.90)	Marked left ventricular hypertrophy
	Diastolic dysfunction
Dyspnea, increased filling pressures, atrial gallop, prominent "a" wave in jugular venous pressure	Asymmetric septal hypertrophy and systolic anterior motion of mitral valve
ECG: Left ventricular hypertrophy, pseudoinfarction pattern (deep Q waves in Leads II, III, aVF or V_5, V_6)	Increased left ventricular mass with imbalance of oxygen supply and demand
Dynamic subaortic gradient	Arrhythmias (ventricular or atrial fibrillation)
Mitral regurgitation	Accessory pathway
Angina pectoris	
Myocardial infarction with or without coronary artery disease	
Sudden death, syncope (7.6%–29%)	
ECG: Short P–R interval, Wolff-Parkinson-White pattern	
RESTRICTIVE CARDIOMYOPATHY	
Dyspnea	Diastolic dysfunction (with or without hypertrophy) due to:
Marked systemic venous congestion	
Hepatomegaly, ascites, edema	Myocardial fibrosis
ECG: Conduction disturbances (left or right bundle branch block, atrioventricular block)	Myocardial infiltration or deposits (e.g., amyloid, iron, glycogen)
Low voltage QRS complex	Eosinophilia with necrosis
ST–T changes, atrial fibrillation	Endomyocardial fibrosis
Atrioventricular regurgitation (mitral and tricuspid) and atrial fibrillation	Granulomas (sarcoid)
	Endocardial scarring or thickening
Restrictive physiology, early diastolic dip, square root sign	Mural thrombi
Systemic and pulmonary emboli	

* Percentage of patients with this type of cardiomyopathy with the finding.

DIFFERENTIAL DIAGNOSIS

Although the diagnosis of cardiomyopathy is one of exclusion, a positive diagnosis is possible because of sufficiently distinctive clinical and hemodynamic features.

Coronary artery disease with focal or diffuse myocardial involvement ("ischemic" cardio-myopathy) must commonly be distinguished from cardiomyopathy. Chest pain, arrhythmia, conduction disturbance, and heart failure may be seen in both idiopathic dilated cardiomyopathy and ischemic cardiomyopathy, but classic angina pectoris or evidence of an old myocardial infarct or a ventricular aneurysm favor the diagnosis of coronary artery disease.

RHEUMATIC (VALVULAR) HEART DISEASE

Dilated cardiomyopathy may mimic valvular heart disease because of functional mitral or tricuspid regurgitation. Treatment of heart failure that reduces ventricular size and increases the murmur of regurgitation (mitral) favors a diagnosis of organic mitral disease. Aortic valve stenosis with advanced heart failure may be mistaken for dilated cardiomyopathy because the murmur may be insignificant. Echocardiography and fluoroscopy are valuable in differentiating these two conditions. Hypertrophic cardiomyopathy with obstruction should be carefully differentiated from aortic stenosis. For this, echocardiography and hemodynamic studies are helpful, as are the clinical differences in the behavior of murmur when the patient squats or performs the Valsalva maneuver.

CONGENITAL HEART DISEASE

Artrial septal defect, anomalous pulmonary veins, and Ebstein's anomaly are rarely confused with cardiomyopathy. Echocardiography, cardiac catheterization, and angiography help in the final differentiation.

HYPERTENSIVE HEART DISEASE

The myocardial abnormality in hypertension does not always correlate with the degree of hypertension. End-stage hypertensive cardiovascular disease (HCVD) may closely mimic idiopathic cardiomyopathy.

CONSTRICTIVE PERICARDITIS

Constrictive pericarditis is difficult to differentiate from restrictive cardiomyopathy because both conditions result from impaired diastolic filling. Constrictive pericarditis is etiologically related to idiopathic or viral pericarditis, radiation, tuberculosis, or neoplastic disease, or may be post-traumatic disease. The differentiation is crucial from a therapeutic standpoint. In constrictive pericarditis, gastrointestinal symptoms predominate. Pericardial calcification is a useful clue, and echocardiography demonstrates a thick pericardium, systolic retraction, or a scintillating pattern in amyloidosis. Diastolic equilibration of pressure is seen in both disorders, but left ventricular end-diastolic pressure and pulmonary capillary wedge pressure usually exceed the right atrial pressure in restrictive cardiomyopathy. The pulmonary artery pressure is usually normal in constrictive pericarditis, whereas it may exceed 50 mm Hg during systole in restrictive cardiomyopathy. Endomyocardial biopsy or thoracotomy may be the only means of exact differentiation.

DIAGNOSIS

The major laboratory features for the three categories of cardiomyopathy are presented in Table 22–6.

M-mode and two-dimensional echocardiography are valuable noninvasive techniques for characterizing the ventricular chamber size, function, and location and the distribution of the hypertrophy and valve motion. An ECG might provide helpful clues. The ultimate differentiation can be precisely made by invasive hemodynamic and angiographic studies.

In dilated cardiomyopathy, filling pressures are elevated, and, in the idiopathic variety there is poor global systolic function with normal coronary arteries. In hypertrophic cardiomyopathy, small left ventricle with vigorous contraction, cavity obliteration, septal hypertrophy, systolic anterior motion, and mitral regurgitation are seen. In restrictive cardiomyopathy, the picture resembles constrictive pericarditis, but, in contrast to constrictive pericarditis, the pulmonary artery pressure is over 50 mm Hg during systole. Systolic function is relatively good; the pulmonary capillary wedge pressure is greater than the right atrial pressure; and the diastolic dip may be absent.

The ultimate diagnosis can be precisely made with invasive hemodynamic and angiographic studies. Endomyocardial biopsy is valuable and is indicated in differentiating restrictive cardiomyopathy from constrictive pericarditis, or evaluating the involvement with systemic disease, myocarditis, or toxicity due to antitumor agents such as doxorubicin.

PRINCIPLES OF PREVENTION AND THERAPY

The purpose of treating cardiomyopathy is fivefold: maximize cardiac function, reduce the workload, prevent secondary damage to the

TABLE 22–6.
Distinctive Laboratory Features of the Cardiomyopathies

LABORATORY TEST	DILATED	HYPERTROPHIC	RESTRICTIVE
Chest x-ray film	Moderate or marked cardiomegaly Predominantly left ventricular changes Pulmonary venous hypertension Pulmonary congestion Large heart, clear lung fields simulating pericardial effusion	Mild cardiomegaly Left ventricle often with prominent left atrium	Mild cardiomegaly Pulmonary venous hypertension
Electrocardiogram	Sinus tachycardia Atrial fibrillation, ventricular ectopy Intraventricular conduction defect (left-bundle branch block) ST–T changes	Left ventricular hypertrophy Abnormal Q waves (pseudoinfarction) Accelerated conduction (Wolff-Parkinson-White) Atrial and ventricular arrhythmias	Low voltage Intraventricular conduction defect (right-bundle branch block) Atrioventricular conduction defects
Echocardiogram	Left ventricular dilatation Global or regional left ventricular dysfunction (decreased ejection fraction) Abnormal diastolic mitral valve motion secondary to abnormal compliance and filling pressures Mural thrombus	Asymmetric septal hypertrophy Small hypercontractile left ventricle with decreased distance between "E" point and septal tracing Systolic anterior motion	Increased left ventricular thickness and mass Small or normal left ventricular cavity Normal systolic function Small pericardial effusion Specific patterns (scintillating pattern in amyloidosis)
Radionuclide studies	Left ventricular dilation (radionuclide ventriculogram or multiple-gated acquisition scan) Left ventricular EF ($<$ 0.40) Global or wall motion abnormalities	Vigorous hypercontractile left ventricle (radionuclide ventriculogram) Asymmetric septal hypertrophy Left ventricular ejection fraction (0.60–0.90)	Left ventricular ejection fraction (0.40–0.60) Small or normal left ventricle (radionuclide ventriculogram or multiple-gated acquisition scan)
Cardiac catheterization	Left ventricular dilatation Left ventricular dysfunction Mitral regurgitation Tricuspid regurgitation Elevated right and left filling pressures Diminished cardiac output Filling defects due to mural thrombus Widely patent coronary arteries (idiopathic) Extensive coronary artery disease (ischemic cardiomyopathy)	Diminished compliance (increased left ventricular end-diastolic pressure) Vigorous systolic function Systolic anterior motion Mitral regurgitation Dynamic left ventricular outflow gradient Spike and dome pattern in aortic and carotid pulse	Diminished left ventricular compliance Diastolic pressure = 1/3 Systolic pressure in left or right ventricle (square root sign) Increased left ventricular end-diastolic pressure, right ventricular end-diastolic pressure Pulmonary capillary wedge pressure $>$ right atrial pressure by 10 mm Hg or more Pulmonary hypertension (Systolic blood pressure $>$ 50 mm Hg)

myocardium, prevent damage to crucial organs such as the brain and kidneys, and promote healing and recovery of function. In addition to the conventional treatment of congestive heart failure with rest, diuretics, and inotropic agents (digitalis), vasodilator therapy with parenteral agents such as nitroprusside, or long-term administration of oral hydralazine, nitrates, or captopril (or enalapril) should be considered in refractory heart failure. Infusions of inotropic agents such as dobutamine for 48 to 72 hours may be lifesaving. Antiarrhythmic agents and long-term anticoagulation therapy to prevent systemic or pulmonary embolism are other important adjuncts. Cardiac transplantation is promising.

In cases with clearly reversible causes such as alcoholic cardiomyopathy, early intervention may prevent irreversible myocardial damage, and strict abstinence from alcohol may result in an 80% likelihood of living at least 42 months. In peripartum cardiomyopathy, avoiding another pregnancy and aggressive management of heart failure and hypertension may return the heart size to normal in more than half the patients. In "beer drinker's" cardiomyopathy, eliminating cobalt from beer additives has resulted in an excellent outcome. The prognosis of patients undergoing cardiac transplantation seems favorable, and 50% to 60% survive 3 years.

Beta-adrenergic blocking agents and calcium-channel blocking agents are the cornerstones of medical treatment in hypertrophic cardiomyopathy. Digitalis, inotropic agents, and nitrates should be avoided. Digitalis is used when there is atrial fibrillation. A septal myotomy-myomectomy is indicated for severely symptomatic patients refractory to medical treatment and may prolong life. Beta-adrenergic blocking agents may improve symptoms, but they do not prevent sudden death. Effective antiarrhythmic therapy such as with amiodarone seems promising, but has not been established as improving survival.

In restrictive cardiomyopathy, digitalis should be used with caution as exquisite sensitivity may be present, especially with amyloidosis. Calcium-channel blocking agents may help diastolic dysfunction. In eosinophilic myocarditis, corticosteroids may be helpful early in the course of the disease. Surgical treatment for valve regurgitation is valuable in improving and controlling severe symptoms and may result in a better prognosis. Pacemakers may be lifesaving in conduction disorders. The outlook is grim in amyloidosis and disorders for which no effective therapy is available.

Primary prevention is the most desirable goal and involves recognizing and eliminating cardiotoxins such as cobalt and drugs (doxorubicin) and immunizing against viral infections. Cardiomyopathy is a pluricausal disorder. Many risk factors can contribute to the myocardial insult, and eliminating these might mitigate the damage. Control of nutrition, systemic disease, hypertension, diabetes mellitus, anemia, and infections and avoidance of cardiotoxins such as alcohol, radiation, and cigarettes are important preventive measures.

REFERENCES

Abelmann WA: Classification and natural history of primary myocardial disease: Progress in cardiovascular disease. *Prog Cardiovasc Dis* 1984; 27(2):73–94. *Succinct, current overview of cardiomyopathies.*

Fuster V, Gersh BJ, Guiliani ER, Tajik AJ, Brandenburg RO, Frye RL: The natural history of idiopathic dilated cardiomyopathy. *Am J Cardiol* 1981; 47:525–531. *Good description of the natural history of dilated cardiomyopathy.*

Johnson RA, Palacios I: Dilated cardiomyopathies of the adult, Parts 1 and 2. *N Engl J Med* 1982; 307(18):1051–1057, 1119–1126. *Best review of current concepts and pathophysiologic aspects.*

Report of the WHO/ISFC task force on the definition and classification of cardiomyopathies. *Br Heart J* 1980; 44:672–673. *Internationally accepted classification and definition of cardiomyopathies.*

Segal JP, Stapleton JF, McClellan JR, Waller BF, Harvey WP: Idiopathic cardiomyopathy—clinical features, prognosis and therapy. *Curr Probl Cardiol* 1978; 3(6):9–48. *Best description of clinical aspects.*

Wynne J, Braunwald E: The cardiomyopathies and myocarditides, in Braunwald E (ed). *Heart Disease. A Textbook of Cardiovascular Medicine,* ed 2, vol 1. Philadelphia, WB Saunders Co, 1984, pp 1399–1456. *Exhaustive review of the topic.*

23

VENTRICULAR ARRHYTHMIAS

Joseph Askenazi, M.D.
A. K. Agarwal, M.D.

Ventricular arrhythmias are commonly seen in clinical practice and may range from an isolated premature ventricular contraction to complex ventricular arrhythmias including ventricular fibrillation, an invariably fatal event, if not immediately corrected. Ventricular arrhythmias may occur in normal persons, during acute ischemic episodes, and during the natural course of various cardiovascular disorders. They assume clinical significance depending on the underlying and precipitating factors, varying from a relatively benign prognosis to a potentially catastrophic event. Early recognition and management of the ventricular arrhythmias are important.

PREMATURE VENTRICULAR COMPLEXES

The most common ventricular arrhythmia in human hearts is premature ventricular contractions (PVC), also termed ventricular premature depolarization (Fig 23–1**A**).

A premature ventricular complex in the ECG is characterized by the premature occurrence of a QRS complex having a bizarre shape and a duration usually more prolonged than the dominant QRS complex, so that it generally exceeds 120 msec. The T-wave is commonly large and opposite in direction to the major deflection of the QRS complex. A PVC is followed by a complete compensatory pause; the R–R interval produced by two sinus-mediated QRS complexes on either side of a premature complex equals twice the normally conducted R–R interval. *Bigeminy* refers to the repeated occurrence of a sinus-mediated complex followed by a premature ventricular contraction. (Fig 23–1**B**). *Trigeminy* is the repeated occurrence of two normal beats followed by a PVC, (Fig 23–1**C**), *quadrigeminy* is three normal beats followed by a PVC, and so on. Two successive premature contractions are called a couplet, while three successive premature ventricular contractions are called ventricular tachycardia. Premature ventricular complexes with a uniform appearance and uniform coupling interval (the R–R interval between the previous sinus beat and that of the PVC) are called unifocal complexes. Those with different contours and coupling intervals are called multiform complexes (Fig 23–1**D**).

CLINICAL SIGNS AND SYMPTOMS

Premature ventricular contractions are uncommon in children, but the incidence increases with age even in the absence of demonstrable heart disease. The PVCs may be present or become worse with ingestion of coffee or tea, heavy smoking, or emotional stress. They are also seen during infection, ischemia of the myocardium, surgery, or the administration of anesthesia (Zipes, 1984). Autonomic activity has a profound effect on the heart rate, which may potentiate or suppress PVCs. Various potentially reversible factors may precipitate ventricular arrhythmias (Table 23–1). Up to 80% of patients with acute myocardial infarctions will demonstrate PVCs in the first 72 hours, but their incidence decreases later in the course of the illness. Predischarge 24 hour electrocardiographic monitoring of the ECG reveals that about 50% of patients have fewer than one PVC per hour and only 20% have more than 10 PVCs per hour. In patients with more than 10 PVCs per hour, the 1-year mortality rate is 2.5 to 4 times higher than those with no PVCs. The presence of couplets and nonsustained ventricular tachycardia also potentiates the risk.

Lown and Wolf during early phases of

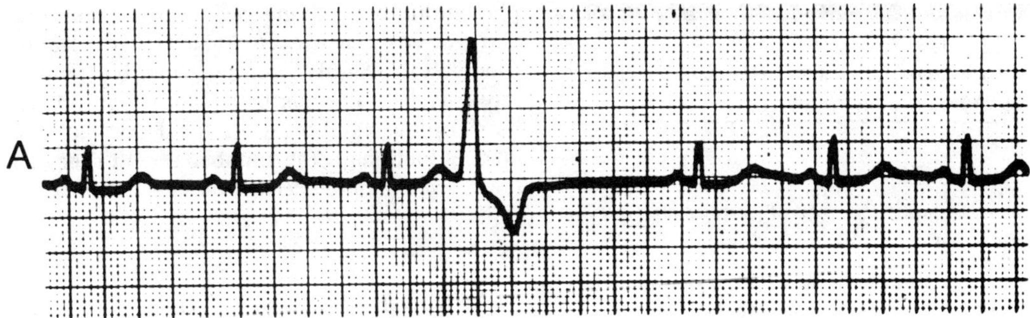

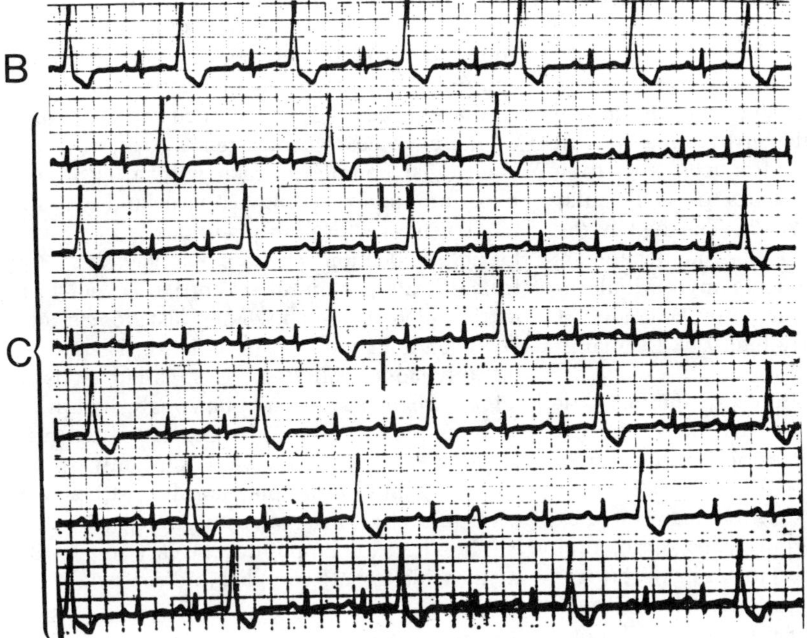

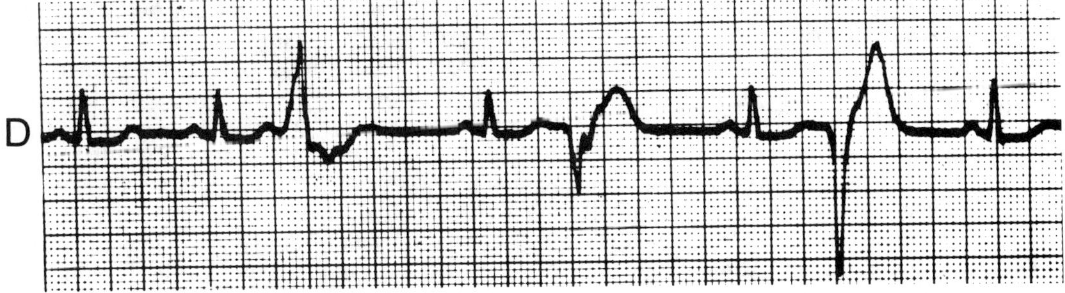

FIG 23–1.
Premature ventricular contractions: **A,** Single ventricular premature beat. The QRS shape is bizarre and the T wave is in the opposite direction to the QRS complex. The PVC is followed by a complete compensatory pause. **B,** Bigeminy. Every second ventricular response is a PVC. **C,** Trigeminy. Every third ventricular response is a PVC. **D,** Multifocal PVCs. All three PVCs have different contours, and all have different coupling intervals representing different sites of origin.

TABLE 23–1.
Potentially Reversible Factors That May Precipitate Various Ventricular Arrhythmias

Ischemia
Acidosis
Hypoxia
Hypokalemia, hypomagnesemia, hypercalcemia
Extreme bradycardia
Digitalis toxicity
Catecholamine excess (exogenous and endogenous)
Long QT interval with or without drug association
Xanthine oxidase inhibitor toxicity (aminophylline)
Hyperthyroidism
Reperfusion associated with thrombolytic therapy

coronary care unit experience observed that certain types of PVCs were precursors of malignant sustained ventricular arrhythmias (Lown and Wolf, 1971). They introduced a grading system to describe the types of ventricular premature beats (Table 23–2). The higher the grade, the higher the risk of a malignant arrhythmia. Patients with acute myocardial infarctions and ectopic beat patterns graded 4 and 5 are at a particularly high risk for malignant arrhythmias.

The PVCs may be entirely asymptomatic or may cause palpitations or discomfort in the neck or chest. Prolonged ectopic activity may precipitate angina, congestive heart failure, or hypotension in patients with impaired cardiovascular reserves. A physical examination reveals an irregular pulse, in which a premature impulse followed by a longer-than-normal pause is felt. It is often impossible to differentiate a PVC from a premature atrial contraction on clinical grounds alone. A cannon wave in a jugular vein or the presence of an abnormal V wave favors the diagnosis of PVC.

TREATMENT

If the results of a thorough history and physical examination and the necessary cardiac studies for organic heart disease show no abnormalities and the patient is relatively asymptomatic, no treatment is necessary. In patients with symptomatic ventricular ectopic activity or when associated with organic heart disease, appropriate therapy should be instituted. In hospitalized patients lidocaine still remains the initial drug of choice. Procainamide, quinidine,

phenytoin, beta-adrenergic receptor blockers, and various other newer agents can also be used (Table 23–3). Therapy should be monitored by blood levels of agents used and 24-hour Holter monitoring of the ECG. At least 80% reduction in the number of PVCs per 24 hours is considered acceptable therapeutic control.

VENTRICULAR TACHYCARDIA

Ventricular tachycardia arises in the special conduction system distal to the bifurcation of the His bundle, in ventricular muscle, or in combination of both types of tissues. Electrocardiographic diagnosis of ventricular tachycardia is suggested by the occurrence of three or more successive bizarre-shaped premature ventricular complexes each with a QRS complex duration exceeding 120 msec and with the ST–T wave vector pointing opposite to the major QRS deflection. The rate may vary from 100 to 250 beats per minute. Ventricular tachycardia is called sustained when it lasts longer than 30 seconds or requires termination because of hemodynamic collapse. It is called nonsustained when it stops spontaneously within 30 seconds. The QRS complex configurations may be identical (uniform), vary randomly (polymorphic, multiform, pleomorphic), display a cyclically changing pattern around an isoelectric line (torsade-de-pointes) or vary in polarity with each alternate complex (bidirectional).

CLINICAL SIGNS AND SYMPTOMS

The spectrum of findings in patients with ventricular tachycardia range from being entirely asymptomatic and noted only with electrophysiologic monitoring to being the primary arrhythmic event in victims of sudden death. The 24-hour Holter monitoring shortly before discharge of patients with acute myocardial infarction reveals evidence of nonsustained ventricular tachycardia in about 10% of patients. The mortality rate in this group is about three times the rate in those not exhibiting this arrhythmia during that time period. In contrast, ventricular tachycardia commonly occurs during the first 48 hours after myocardial infarction and carries no worse a prognosis than that for patients who do not have ventricular tachycardia during that time. About two-thirds of patients who have a cardiac arrest outside the hospital do not have evidence of acute myocardial infarction, and electrical events (ventricular tachycardia, ventricular fibrillation, asystole) have been demonstrated to be the most likely causes.

Zipes and co-workers (1984) have reported that in one series of 516 patients who were treated for symptomatic recurrent ventricular tachycardia, 284 had ischemic heart disease, 74 had cardiomyopathy (congestive or hypertrophic), 75 had primary electrical disease, 45 had mitral valve prolapse, 20 had valvular heart disease and 18 had miscellaneous causes. Primary electrical disease includes patients with ventricular tachycardia without any recognizable structural heart disease.

The symptoms of ventricular tachycardia depend on the rate at which the tachycardia occurs and the underlying myocardial reserve. Symptomatic patients may have a feeling of a thump, a sensation of sinking, or palpitations, or may present with evidence of cardiovascular decompensation, such as angina, congestive heart failure, or symptoms related to low cardiac output states.

PATHOPHYSIOLOGY

Ventricular tachycardia mostly affects a diseased heart, although it is known to occur in patients with no recognizable heart disease especially in younger patients. Ventricular tachycardia is most often found in patients with coronary artery disease, cardiomyopathy, and valvular heart disease, especially aortic valvular disease. Recurrent sustained ventricular tachycardia is often associated with ventricular aneurysms or broad, confluent scars from previous myocardial infarction. Up to 40% of patients after an acute myocardial infarction may exhibit episodes of nonsustained ventricular tachycardia, and most episodes occur during the first 72 hours after acute myocardial infarction. Up to 6% of patients with mitral valve prolapse may exhibit episodes of ventricular tachycardia; a worse prognosis occurs in patients with redundant mitral valve leaflet as compared with patients with a nonredundant leaflet. Ventricular tachycardia is also an important precursor of the sudden death syndrome and also a cause of significant mortality

TABLE 23–2.
Grading System of Ventricular Premature Beats (VPBs)*

GRADE	DESCRIPTION
0	No VPBs
1A	< 30 VPBs/hr and < 1/min
1B	< 30 VPBs/hr and occasionally > 1/min
2	> 30 VPBs/hr
3	Multiform VPBs
4A	Repetitive VPBs-couplets
4B	Repetitive VPBs-ventricular tachycardia (three sequential VPBs)
5	Early R-on-T VPBs

The grading system is applied to a 24-hour monitoring period and indicates the number of hours within that period during which a patient has VPBs of a particular grade, expressed as superscripts in the resulting "equation." Subscripts indicate particular aspects of the VPBs of a given grade. For example, in the equation below, the subscript for grade 2 indicates the approximate total number of grade 2 VPBs over the 24-hour period; for grade 3 it denotes the number of different forms observed in any single hour: for grade 4B the two subscripts indicate the largest number of paroxysms of tachycardia in a single hour and the maximum number of successive cycles, respectively; for grade 5 the subscript represents the largest number of early ectopic beats in any single hour. A complete translation of this particular equation is as follows:

$$0^3 \ 1A^0 \ 1B^4 \ 2^6_{760} \ 3^6_2 \ 4A^2_3 \ 4B^2_{+7} \ 5^1_3$$

0	Occurred during 3 hours
1A	No infrequent VPBs
1B	Infrequent VPBs but more than 1/min observed during 4 hours
2	Occurred during 6 hours (with a total of 760 VPBs)
3	Occurred during 6 hours; exhibited two forms
4A	Occurred during 2 hours; greatest frequency in any single hour was 3
4B	Occurred during 2 hours; there were 4 paroxysms, and the longest duration was 7 cycles
5	An early VPB observed 3 times during a single hour in the 24-hour monitoring session

* From Lown B: Cardiovascular collapse and sudden cardiac death, in Braunwald E (ed): *Heart Disease*, ed 2. Philadelphia, WB Saunders Co, 1984, pp 774–806. Used by permission.

and morbidity in hypertrophic cardiomyopathies. Ventricular tachycardia may be precipitated by any of the factors listed in Table 23–1, the correction of which may lead to the resolution of the arrhythmia.

The most important mechanisms associated

TABLE 23–3.
Vaughan-Williams Classification of Antiarrhythmic Drugs According to Electrophysiologic Effects

CLASS		SUBCLASS	EFFECT	CONVENTIONAL AGENTS
	AGENTS			
I.	Local anesthetics	A	Depresses phase 0 Slows conduction Prolongs repolarization	Quinidine Procainamide Disopyramide
		B	Depresses phase 0 in abnormal fibers Shortens repolarization	Lidocaine Mexiletene Phenytoin Tocainide
		C	Markedly depresses phase 0 Profoundly slows conduction Slight effect on repolarization	Flecainide Encainide
II.	Beta adrenergic receptor blockers		Inhibits sympathetic activity	Propranolol Timolol Acebutolol
III.	Prolonged repolarization agents		Prolongs action potential duration	Amiodarone Bretylium
IV.	Calcium-channel blockers		Blocks slow inward current	Verapamil

with ventricular tachycardia are reentry, enhanced automaticity, and triggered activity.

Reentry is the most commonly cited mechanism responsible for ventricular tachycardia. Diseased myocardial tissue juxtaposed with relatively normal tissue sets the stage for reentry. An area of focal depression of conductivity in the vicinity of an ectopic focus offers an area of localized refractoriness. The impulse traverses through normal myocardium, which is non-refractory at that point, producing a normal beat. Meanwhile the localized area of refractoriness recovers, becomes excitable again, and conducts the initial impulse retrogradely. The excitation impulse then again traverses the normal myocardium in the original normal direction. Premature depolarizations propagate slowly in abnormal regions and shorten refractoriness in normal regions, thus making reentry more likely (Fig 23–2).

Abnormal automaticity may be displayed by atrial or ventricular myocardial cells under pathologic conditions, as around an infarct. These cells take over or compete with the pacemaker function that normally results from the sinoatrial node and the atrioventricular node and results in a normal cardiac rhythm. Abnormal automaticity is probably the mechanism for accelerated idioventricular rhythm, although it probably is an uncommon mecha-

nism for recurrent sustained ventricular tachycardia.

Triggered activity is seen when a driven action potential results in a secondary after-depolarization (early or late) which reaches threshold for regenerative response (action potential) and initiates a repetitive response. Early repolarization may be seen in the presence of hypoxia, increased CO_2 concentration, or excess catecholamine in myocardial tissue. Mechanical injury or stretch as seen in congestive heart failure has also been a postulated cause. Cardiac glycoside toxicity is one of the most common recognized causes of after-depolarizaiton.

Underlying myocardial pathologic changes leads to heterogeneity of myocardial refractoriness, priming the myocardium to sustain various reenterant ventricular tachycardias. Regional wall motion abnormalities, electrolyte imbalance, and high norepinephrine levels may play a role from time to time in the genesis of ventricular tachycardia.

DIAGNOSIS

A clinical examination and an ECG will reveal evidence of this underlying cardiovascular disorder. Atrioventricular dissociation may be evident on clinical examination. It is mani-

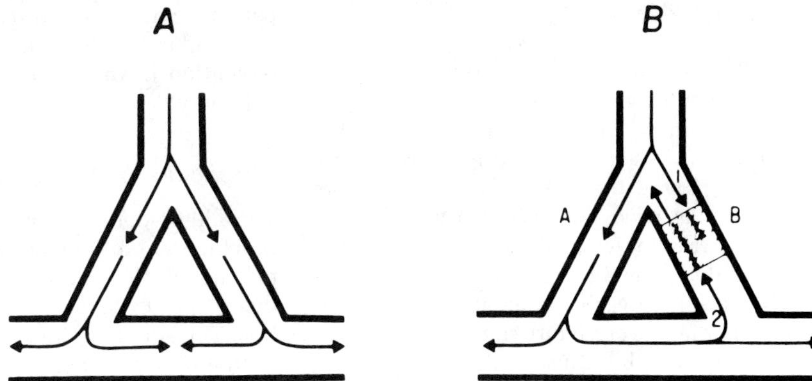

FIG 23–2.

Reentry mechanism. Pathway b has an antegrade unidirectional block and slow retrograde conduction *(shaded area)*. An activation wavefront finds pathway b refractory and activates normal myocardium (a, c). The activation impulse then activates pathway b retrogradely and after emerging activates myocardium, again producing a premature ventricular contraction. (From Rosen, MR, Danilo, Jr, P: Cellular Electrophysiologic Mechanism of Antiarrhythmic Drug Action, in Reiser, HJ, Horowitz, LN: Mechanism and Treatment of Cardiac Arrhythmias, Urban and Schwartenberg, Baltimore, 1985, p. 72.)

fested by variable intensity of the first heart sound, by an inconsistent relationship of the "a" waves in jugular venous pulse with the ventricular contractions, or by intermittent cannon waves. Paroxysmal ventricular tachycardia is often triggered by an isolated ventricular premature beat. The presence of fusion beats (simultaneous activation of the ventricle by two different foci, resulting in an intermediate fusion complex on the ECG) and capture beats (momentary activation of the ventricles by a sinus impulse during AV dissociation) is helpful in the diagnosis of ventricular tachycardia. The P waves occur independently of the QRS complex (AV dissociation), although in a small percentage of cases a retrograde P wave may be seen on the ECG (VA association). The R–R interval is usually slightly irregular. Grossly irregular cycles are very uncommon, but may be seen in torsade-de-pointes, multiform ventricular tachycardia, or in rapid atrial fibrillation conducted over an accessory pathway. Sustained ventricular tachycardia often degenerates into ventricular fibrillation.

DIFFERENTIAL DIAGNOSIS

Ventricular tachycardia may often be difficult to differentiate from supraventricular tachyarrhythmias. Supraventricular tachycardia with preexisting right- or left-bundle branch block (RBBB or LBBB), aberrant ventricular conduction, or anomalous AV conduction associated with Wolff-Parkinson-White (WPW) syndrome may mimic ventricular tachycardia. Atrial fibrillation associated with an anomalous pathway with WPW syndrome closely resembles ventricular tachycardia. The following criteria are helpful in establishing the ventricular origin of a tachycardia:

1. AV dissociation during tachycardia
2. QRS complex width greater than 0.14 seconds
3. Left axis deviation in the frontal plane
4. In patients with a RBBB pattern, a small or absent R wave in ECG lead V_6; in patients with an LBBB pattern, a QR or QS complex in lead V_6
5. QRS complexes that are all negative or all positive in all precordial leads
6. Presence of capture beats and fusion beats
7. No response to vagal stimuli

Grossly irregular R–R intervals are uncommon, which helps to differentiate ventricular tachycardia from atrial fibrillation associated with aberrant conduction. Often diagnosis may be impossible with a surface ECG, and invasive electrophysiologic studies may be necessary to differentiate the supraventricular from the ventricular tachycardia.

TREATMENT

In one study (Kennedy et al., 1985), the presence of complex ventricular ectopic activity including short, nonsustained ventricular tachycardia in the absence of organic heart disease did not increase the risk of death. Therefore such patients need not necessarily be treated with antiarrhythmic agents. Organic heart disease should be carefully excluded on the basis of clinical, noninvasive, and, if indicated, invasive studies. Every effort should be made to identify a reversible cause and, if one is present, it should be treated. The underlying cardiovascular pathologic changes should also be treated when possible. All patients with sustained ventricular tachycardia and all patients resuscitated from sudden cardiac death syndrome should receive follow-up treatment. Patients with symptomatic ventricular tachycardia, underlying coronary artery disease, or cardiomyopathy (dilated and hypertrophic) should be treated.

In patients without hemodynamic decompensation, ventricular tachycardia is usually treated with intravenous lidocaine. If a response is not obtained with maximal dosages of intravenous lidocaine, intravenous procainamide or bretylium may be attempted. Sustained ventricular tachycardia associated with hemodynamic decompensation (shock, severe congestive heart failure) or not responsive to medical treatment should be treated with synchronized DC cardioversion with a starting energy as low as 10 to 50 joules. Thump version (cardioversion from striking the sternum with the fist) is sometimes effective. Certain sustained ventricular tachycardias will respond to ventricular overdrive pacing. Paroxysmal nonsustained ventricular tachycardia can be treated with a variety of antiarrhythmic agents such as quinidine, procainamide, disopyramide tocainide, mexiletine, flecainide, amiodarone, encainide, or various investigational drugs such as propafenone, or lorcainide. Digitalis-induced ventricular tachycardia is very responsive to phenytoin. Amiodarone has been found very effective in controlling complex ventricular arrhythmias associated with New York Heart Association (NYHA) Class III and IV congestive heart failure, although its use is limited by a high incidence of pulmonary, hepatic, or dermatologic side-effects. Certain groups of patients with a life-threatening drug-resistant ventricular tachycardia will need surgical intervention in the form of an encircling ventriculotomy or an endocardial resection.

Torsade-de-Pointes

Torsade-de-pointes is a ventricular tachycardia in which a continual cyclical change in the amplitude of the tachycardia complexes makes them appear to twist around the isoelectric line. Torsade-de-pointes generally occurs in the setting of a prolonged QT interval. In contrast to other ventricular tachycardias in which an early PVC is the initiating event, in torsade-de-pointes the initiating extrasystole is usually late. The rate is usually between 200 and 250/minute, and during resolution of the episode the QRS complexes widen and become larger and the episode ends either with return to the basal rhythm, with ventricular standstill, or with a new attack of torsade-de-pointes. Precipitating factors include sinoatrial depression with bradycardia, a high degree of AV block, hypomagnesemia, hypokalemia, congenital long QT syndromes, various antiarrhythmic agents (especially type IA agents like quinidine and disopyramide), tricyclic antidepressants, and less commonly myocarditis, mitral valve prolapse, and some liquid diets.

Treatment consists of identification of the underlying cause, if possible, and withdrawal of the offending drug. Agents such as intravenous lidocaine, phenytoin, beta-adrenergic blocking agents, or bretylium are helpful in controlling this arrhythmia. Agents like isoproteronol that shorten the QT interval are more effective in control of resistant torsade-de-pointes. Rapid ventricular pacing is the treatment of choice to control the arrhythmia not responsive to pharmacologic intervention.

Ventricular flutter and fibrillation

Ventricular flutter (sine wave appearance on the ECG; large regular oscillations at the rate of 150 to 300/minute) and fibrillation (irregular undulations of various contours and amplitude on ECG; absence of distinct QRS complexes, ST segments and T waves) represent the worst arrhythmic events, which have an inevitably fatal outcome if not terminated within 3 to 5 minutes. Primary ventricular fibrillation associated with acute ischemia occurs in about 5% to 10% of patients admitted to coronary care units with acute myocardial infarction. It is also recognized as the commonest arrhythmia in patients resuscitated from an out-of-hospital cardiac arrest. Complex ventricular ectopic activity and ventricular tachycardia often precede the onset of ventricular fibrillation. Ventricular fibrillation may occur during hypoxia, ischemia, reperfusion following thrombolytic therapy, atrial fibrillation with rapid ventricular rates in patients with preexcitation syndrome and after DC countershock administered during cardioversion. The phenomenon of R on T (an early PVC falling during the vulnerable period of repolarization of the previous normally conducted beat) has been proposed as an important marker identifying the patients with acute myocardial infarction or chronic coronary artery disease who are particularly susceptible to ventricular fibrillation. Multiple asynchronous reentry phenomenon is generally considered to be the underlying mechanism.

Ventricular fibrillation is manifest by loss of consciousness, apnea, seizures, and, if uncorrected, death. All pulses are absent, and no heart sounds are audible.

Immediate defibrillation with nonsynchronized DC countershock of 100 to 400 joules is mandatory. Cardiopulmonary resuscitation should be initiated immediately if defibrillation equipment is not available. (Intravenous lidocaine, bretylium, or procainamide should be started immediately.) Efforts to prevent a recurrence should be instituted including identifying and treating the underlying condition.

REFERENCES

Bigger JT Jr: Antiarrhythmic treatment: An overview. *Am J Cardiol* 1984; 53:8B–16B. *An excellent discussion of therapeutic modalities for various cardiac arrhythmias including ventricular arrhythmias.*

German LD, Idekar RE: Ventricular tachycardia: Mechanisms, diagnosis and management. *Med Clin North Am* 1964; 68:919–928. *An overall good review article on ventricular tachycardias.*

Kennedy HL, Whitlock JA, Sprague MK, Kennedy L, Buckingham TA, Goldberg RJ: Long term follow up of asymptomatic healthy subjects with frequent and complex ventricular ectopy. *N Engl J Med* 1985; 312:193–197. *A good study of the long-term course of ventricular ectopic activity in asymptomatic healthy individuals.*

Krikler DM, Curry PVL: Torsade-de-pointes, an atypical ventricular tachycardia. *Br Heart J* 1976; 38:117–120. *A good review of the torsade-de-pointes arrhythmia.*

Lown B: Cardiovascular collapse and sudden cardiac death, in Braunwald E (ed): *Heart Disease,* ed 2. Philadelphia, WB Saunders Co, 1984, pp 774–806.

Lown B, Wolf M: Approaches to sudden death from coronary heart disease. *Circulation* 1971; 44:130–142. *A good study co-relating incidence of PVCs post MI with mortality.*

Wellens HJJ, Bar FWHM, Lie KI: Value of the electrocardiogram in the differential diagnosis of a tachycardia with a widened QRS complex. *Am J Med* 1978; 64:27–33. *An excellent article describing the electrocardiographic differentiation between supraventricular arrhythmias with wide QRS complexes and ventricular tachycardia.*

Zipes DP: Ventricular rhythm disturbances, in Braunwald E (ed): *Heart Disease,* ed 2. Philadelphia, WB Saunders Co, 1984, pp. 719–743. *An excellent overall review of the diagnostic and clinical features of various ventricular rhythm disturbances.*

Zipes DP, Heger JJ, Prystowsky EN; Treatment of patients with life threatening cardiac arrhythmias. *Ann NY Acad Sci* 1984; 427:307–318. *A good discussion of management strategies in patients with complex cardiac arrhythmias.*

Satyendra C. Gupta, M.D.

Cardiac arrhythmia refers to a disturbance of heart rhythm, rate, or conduction. Based on anatomic origin, cardiac arrhythmias are either supraventricular or ventricular. Atrial arrhythmias are a subsection of supraventricular arrhythmias. Some common atrial arrhythmias are discussed below.

MECHANISMS OF CARDIAC ARRHYTHMIAS

The common mechanisms of cardiac arrhythmias are reentry, abnormal automaticity, and triggered activity. An arrhythmia may be initiated by one mechanism and perpetuated by another. Reentry involves impulse conduction along two longitudinally dissociated pathways (Fig 24–1,A). Each pathway has different characteristics of conduction and refractoriness. For reentry to occur, these pathways join distally to form a closed loop.

The most frequent cause of paroxysmal supraventricular tachycardia is atrioventricular (AV) nodal reentry. Conduction of an atrial premature beat is blocked in the faster pathway because it has a relatively longer refractory period, but the impulse can be conducted down the slower pathway, which has a shorter refractory period. The slowness of the conduction produces enough delay to allow the faster pathway to recover and permit the impulse to

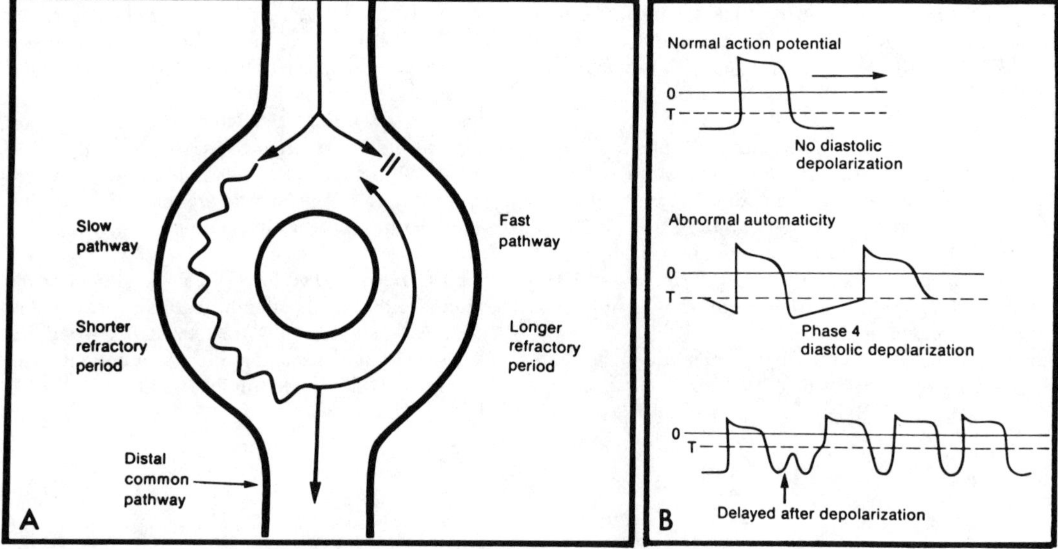

FIG 24–1.

A, Mechanisms of reentry and **B,** abnormal automaticity. See text. (Reproduced with permission from *Consultant* from page 283 of the April 1984 issue of *Consultant* in the article by Alan B. Schwartz and Melvin M. Scheinman entitled "Supraventricular Arrhythmias.")

be conducted retrograde. If conditions are just right, the circus movement will continue and tachycardia will be sustained. This explanation holds true for other supraventricular and ventricular tachyarrhythmias.

In nonpacemaker cells, such as atrial or ventricular muscle cells, the action potential does not have slow diastolic depolarization. However, in patients with ischemia, abnormal automaticity may occur when diastolic depolarization develops (Fig 24–1,**B**). When the cell voltage decays to threshold (T), another action potential is generated. When this rate of depolarization exceeds that of the sinus pacemaker, the cell may usurp the pacemaker function of the heart and determine the dominant rhythm.

Triggered automaticity depends on oscillatory potentials, which occur during diastole (Fig 24–1,**B**). Under certain circumstances, these potentials may increase in amplitude sufficiently to reach threshold voltage and trigger repetitive depolarizations. Probable electrophysiologic mechanisms responsible for atrial arrhythmias are listed in Table 24–1.

Atrial arrhythmias may originate from anywhere in the atria. They almost always are generated by active impulse formation. Common atrial arrhythmias include atrial premature contractions (APCs), atrial tachycardia, atrial flutter, and atrial fibrillation. These arrhythmias are closely interrelated in terms of mechanisms. It has been suggested that an ectopic focus in the atria that produces an isolated APC may be capable of producing atrial tachycardia, flutter, and fibrillation.

ATRIAL PREMATURE CONTRACTIONS

Atrial premature contractions originate prematurely from an ectopic focus in the atrial muscle outside the SA node. Propagation occurs through the AV junction and ventricles in a normal fashion, or aberration and block may be encountered.

DIAGNOSTIC CRITERIA

There is an early P wave which is usually more peaked than the sinus P wave, is biphasic, or is inverted. Occasionally the atrial premature contractions occur so early in the cardiac cycle

TABLE 24–1.
Probable Electrophysiology of Atrial Arrhythmias

MECHANISM	ARRHYTHMIA
Automaticity	Atrial escape beats
	Atrial tachycardia with or without block
	Multifocal atrial tachycardia
Reentry	Paroxysmal supraventricular tachycardia
	Atrial flutter
	Atrial fibrillation

that the AV conduction system has not recovered sufficiently to respond. Under these circumstances (blocked atrial premature contractions), the premature P wave is seen without the accompanying ventricular response (Fig 24–2,**A**). This is the most common cause of a pause interrupting an otherwise regular sinus rhythm. When there is an unexplained pause on the electrocardiogram (ECG), look for a hidden P wave superimposed on the T wave preceding the pause. However, for most premature P waves, the resulting QRS complex following the P wave usually has a normal contour. Atrial premature contractions may be followed by aberrant ventricular conduction (an abnormal and wide QRS complex) when the coupling interval is short and the impulse traverses the ventricle during a relative or nearly absolute refractory period of part of the intraventricular conduction system, usually the right bundle branch (Fig 24–2,**B**).

CLINICAL SIGNIFICANCE

Atrial premature contractions occur in patients with and without heart disease and may also occur following emotional excitement, excess use of tobacco, drinking large amounts of caffeinated beverages, and use of sympathomimetic drugs. Atrial premature contractions are seen in patients with cardiomyopathy, coronary artery disease, acute myocardial infarction, and chronic lung disease. When they occur repetitively in groups of two or three, they are often a precursor of atrial tachycardia, atrial flutter, or atrial fibrillation. Although atrial premature contractions may or may not affect cardiac output, their effects are less marked than those of ventricular premature beats.

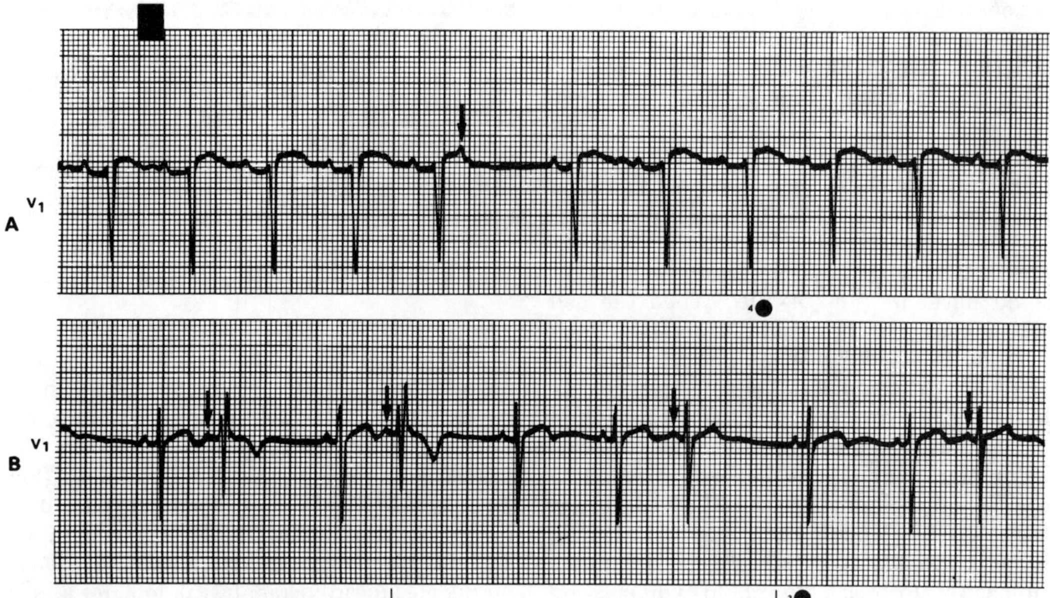

FIG 24–2.
Atrial premature complexes. **A,** Blocked atrial premature contractions *(arrow).* **B,** Atrial premature contractions with normal
ventricular conduction *(third and fourth arrows)* and aberrant ventricular conduction *(first and second arrows).*

SYMPTOMS AND SIGNS

Although premature atrial contractions usually
cause no symptoms, a patient may complain of
irregular heartbeat, skipped beat, or flip-flop.
The irregularity can be detected by feeling the
pulse, but an ECG is required to recognize
atrial premature contractions. When atrial
premature contractions occur while the patient
is standing, light-headedness or giddiness may
occasionally ensue. Brief chest pain may occur.

TREATMENT

In general, atrial premature contractions are
benign. Therapy should include reassurance
and be directed toward the underlying cause.
In the few cases in which chemotherapy is indicated, the drugs of choice for frequent or
symptomatic atrial contractions include digitalis, quinidine, procainamide, or propranolol.

PAROXYSMAL SUPRAVENTRICULAR TACHYCARDIA

Like atrial premature contractions, paroxysmal
supraventricular tachycardias (PSVTs) may originate anywhere in the atria and AV junction.

Conduction below the AV node is the same as
in normal sinus rhythm. The QRS complex in
paroxysmal supraventricular tachycardia is
usually normal, but either aberrant ventricular
conduction or preexisting bundle branch block
may widen the QRS complex. The differentiation between atrial and AV junctional tachycardia is usually not clear, hence the term
"supraventricular tachycardia" is used.

DIAGNOSTIC CRITERIA

Six or more consecutive atrial premature contractions are considered sufficient for the diagnosis of atrial tachycardia. The atrial rate is
usually 140 to 250 per minute. The P-wave
configuration, usually different from that of the
sinus P wave, is often superimposed on a portion of the ST segment, T wave, U wave, or the
QRS complex of the preceding beat, making it
difficult to recognize in an ordinary ECG (Fig
24–3,A).

CLINICAL SIGNIFICANCE

About 30% of all PSVTs may be found in apparently healthy hearts, but the paroxysm is
usually of short duration. Atrial tachycardia

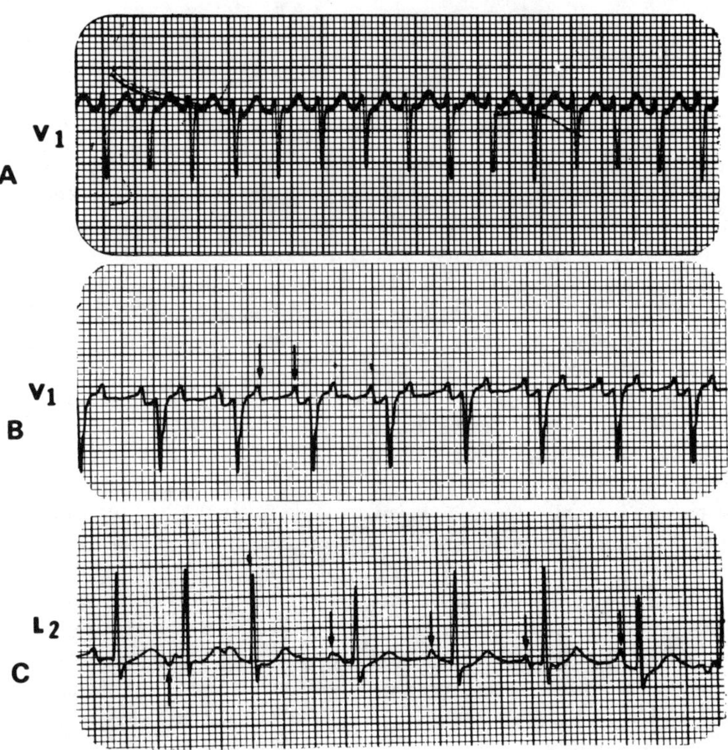

FIG 24–3.
Atrial tachycardias. **A,** Paroxysmal supraventricular tachycardia at a rate of 215/minute. The P waves are not discernable because they are most likely superimposed on the T wave or QRS complexes of the preceding beat. **B,** Paroxysmal atrial tachycardia with 2:1 AV conduction. *(Arrows point to atrial complexes.)* **C,** Multifocal atrial tachycardia. The configuration of P waves *(arrows)* varies from beat to beat with varying P–P, P–R, and R–R intervals.

may occur in digitalis intoxication and is almost always associated with AV block. Figure 24–3,**B** illustrates paroxysmal atrial tachycardia with block. This type of atrial tachycardia comprises about 10% to 15% of the total digitalis-induced cardiac arrhythmias (often in association with decreased potassium) and is frequently associated with coronary artery disease, particularly acute myocardial infarction, hypertensive heart disease, Wolff-Parkinson-White syndrome, acute or chronic cor pulmonale, acute pericarditis, thyrotoxicosis, and various congenital heart diseases including atrial septal defect and Eisenmenger's complex. States such as those induced by hyperventilating, emotional stress, exercise, or eating a heavy meal may precipitate the paroxysms in a susceptible individual.

The effect of paroxysmal supraventricular tachycardias on cardiac hemodynamics depends on the condition of the heart, the ventricular rate, and the duration of the tachycardia. PSVT at a rate of 170 to 180 beats per minute in a normal heart usually does not cause any decrease in cardiac output. At rates faster than this, cardiac output falls. In a diseased heart, this drop occurs at a heart rate of less than 170 beats per minute.

SYMPTOMS AND SIGNS

Paroxysmal supraventricular tachycardia starts and stops abruptly. Almost all patients are asymptomatic, but a few may have an occasional palpitation. In tachycardia with a rapid ventricular rate, the patient may feel giddy and become dizzy, but rarely loses consciousness. Patients with rapid rates and underlying heart disease may have either chest pain due to ischemia, or dyspnea secondary to heart failure. The pulse is rapid and weak, and heart sounds are usually identical throughout. Polyuria is typical.

TREATMENT

The decision to treat paroxysmal supraventricular tachycardia, the choice of drug, and the route of administration depend on the clinical situation. Physical maneuvers (vagal), such as Valsalva's maneuver, carotid sinus massage, attempts to retch, and extending the head backward, are often effective. The importance of carotid massage in the diagnosis and treatment of various arrhythmias is shown in Table 24–2. Digitalis, drugs that increase parasympathetic stimulation to the heart (neostigmine, edrophonium), beta-adrenergic blocking agents, and calcium-channel blocking agents (verapamil) are effective during the attacks. Some patients may respond to vagal stimulation after digitalis administration. Electrical cardioversion and override atrial pacing can be effective in terminating episodes of paroxysmal supraventricular tachycardias. Cardioversion should not be attempted in the atrial tachycardias caused by digitalis toxicity.

Digitalis is the drug of choice for preventing paroxysmal atrial tachycardias. If it is unsuccessful alone, a combination of digitalis and either quinidine, procainamide, propranolol, or a calcium antagonist such as verapamil or diltiazem may be tried.

MULTIFOCAL ATRIAL TACHYCARDIA

The mechanism of multifocal atrial tachycardia is the same as for unifocal atrial tachycardia, except that multiple atrial ectopic foci are present.

DIAGNOSTIC CRITERIA

The diagnosis of multifocal atrial tachycardia rests on an atrial rate above 100 beats per minute and three or more atrial foci with P waves of changing morphology in the same ECG lead. The baseline is isoelectric and the P–P, P–R, and R–R intervals are irregular (Fig 24–3,**C**).

CLINICAL SIGNIFICANCE

Multifocal atrial tachycardia is almost always present in seriously ill elderly patients. Chronic lung disease, especially during acute exacerbations, accounts for 60% to 85% of the cases. Excessive theophylline therapy may be a contributing factor in such patients. Other causes include coronary artery disease with severe congestive heart failure, hypoxia attributed to general anesthesia, electrolyte imbalance, pulmonary embolism, and septicemia.

TREATMENT

Because multifocal atrial tachycardia is often refractory to the usual antiarrhythmic management regimen, treating the underlying disease is more important than using antiarrhythmic agents. Bronchodilators and sympathomimetic drugs such as aminophylline and isoproterenol must be avoided. The use of digitalis in multifocal atrial tachycardia is controversial, but digitalis may be tried when a rapid rate with heart failure is present. However, especially in

---

TABLE 24–2.
Effect of Carotid Massage (Carotid Sinus Pressure) on Cardiac Arrhythmias

ARRHYTHMIA	EFFECT
Sinus tachycardia	No response or slight slowing of heart rate (a decrease of 10 to 20 beats per min)
	Return to previous rate with release of pressure
Paroxysmal supraventricular tachycardia (atrial or AV junctional)	No response or converts to normal sinus rhythm and remains at that rate on release of pressure
Atrial flutter or atrial tachycardia with block	No response or slowing of ventricular rate in mathematical order* (from 150 to 100 to 75 beats per min) due to increased AV block
	Returns to original rate on release of pressure
Ventricular tachycardia	No response

*This is the result of increasing the AV block from 2:1 to 3:1 or 4:1.

patients with acute exacerbations of their lung disease, half the usual dose should be used in most cases because such patients are unusually prone to digitalis toxicity. Verapamil also appears to be a useful drug for multifocal atrial tachycardia.

ATRIAL FLUTTER

Atrial flutter, like atrial tachycardia, may originate from anywhere in the atria outside the sinus node. Atrial flutter occurs in either chronic or paroxysmal form. Chronic atrial flutter is more common and persists for months or years.

DIAGNOSTIC CRITERIA

Atrial flutter has a rapid, absolutely regular atrial rhythm with a characteristic "sawtooth" flutter wave (Fig 24–4,**A**). The atrial rate in pure atrial flutter is 240 to 360 beats per minute (usually 300 per minute). The AV block usually is 2:1, so the ventricular rate is usually about 150 per minute. In the presence of AV node disease or after administration of drugs, especially digitalis, the degree of AV block varies. With fast ventricular rates, carotid massage is useful in establishing the diagnosis of atrial flutter. The characteristic response is an increased AV block with slowing of the ventricular rate and the appearance of characteristic flutter waves.

CLINICAL SIGNIFICANCE

Atrial flutter is almost always observed in people with diseased hearts and is commonly encountered in rheumatic (particularly mitral stenosis), coronary, and hypertensive heart disease. It has been reported to occur in 1% to 5% of patients with acute myocardial infarction and occurs less commonly with thyrotoxicosis, congenital heart disease, pericarditis, cor pulmonale, Wolff-Parkinson-White syndrome, and cardiomyopathy. Stress, infections, hypoxia, and rarely drug intoxication (with digitalis, quinidine, or epinephrine) may cause or precipitate atrial flutter in susceptible individuals.

Atrial flutter is often associated with a lowered cardiac output when the ventricular rate is rapid, but no change is noted when the ventricular rate is slow.

SYMPTOMS AND SIGNS

The symptoms and signs of atrial flutter depend on the degree of heart damage, ventricular rate, and duration of the flutter. When the ventricular rate is slow, the patient may not be aware of the flutter. When the ventricular rate is fast, palpitations are present and congestive heart failure develops, especially in elderly patients with advanced heart disease. Angina pectoris, fainting, and mental disturbances including confusion may occur.

TREATMENT

Atrial flutter is treated with certain drugs, electric countershock, and override atrial pacing. Beta-adrenergic blocking agents, calcium-channel blocking agents, (verapamil and diltiazem, but not nifedipine), and digitalis have been used to slow the ventricular rate. Digitalis increases the degree of AV block, and its administration is sometimes followed by conversion to atrial fibrillation or a sinus rhythm. Quinidine is successful two thirds of the time in converting atrial flutter to a normal sinus rhythm. The patient should be properly digitalized before administering quinidine because quinidine frequently increases the ventricular rate and may result in a 1:1 AV conduction with extremely rapid ventricular rates. Some physicians consider DC cardioversion the preferable initial treatment. Override atrial pacing can be used both in resistant cases and in cases in which electric countershock is considered dangerous, as in digitalis toxicity.

ATRIAL FIBRILLATION

Atrial fibrillation, both paroxysmal and established forms, is probably the most frequent arrhythmia associated with organic heart disease and heart failure, but it occasionally occurs when heart disease is absent.

DIAGNOSTIC CRITERIA

Atrial fibrillation may be clinically suspected in patients with an irregular cardiac rhythm. Irregular atrial oscillation waves of varying configuration and amplitude characteristically replace P waves on the ECG. The atrial rate is said to be 450 to 650 beats per minute, and the ventricular response (QRS complex) is grossly irregular because every third to sixth atrial impulse passes down the AV junction (Fig 24–4,**B**).

CLINICAL SIGNIFICANCE

Atrial fibrillation occurs most frequently in patients older than 40 years of age and is often seen in patients with heart failure. Common etiologic factors include rheumatic mitral stenosis or mitral insufficiency, coronary artery disease, hypertensive heart disease, cardiomyopathies, pericarditis, thyrotoxicosis, and respiratory decompensation. Occasionally idiopathic atrial fibrillation without evidence of underlying heart disease is seen. Hypoglycemia, emotional upset, ingestion of alcohol, and sometimes digitalis administration, electrolyte disturbance, and sympathomimetic drugs may precipitate atrial fibrillation.

The hemodynamic consequences of atrial fibrillation lead to a reduced cardiac output resulting from failure of the atria to contract with loss of that contribution to ventricular filling, an irregular ventricular rhythm, and an underlying cardiac abnormality. Chronic atrial fibrillation predisposes to pulmonary or systemic embolization.

SYMPTOMS AND SIGNS

Atrial fibrillation may occur with or without symptoms. The patient may complain of palpitation, a rapid and irregular heartbeat, dyspnea, syncope, or giddiness. Congestive heart failure may be precipitated or aggravated. Physical examination reveals an irregular rhythm with pulse deficit. The first heart sound changes in intensity on cardiac auscultation. The venous pulse has no A waves.

TREATMENT

Treating atrial fibrillation involves slowing the ventricular rate, with digitalis being the drug of choice. In patients with atrial fibrillation and Wolff-Parkinson-White syndrome, neither digitalis nor calcium antagonists should be used, because their effects on the anomalous bypass tract may lead to very rapid ventricular rates. In selected cases, treatment involves conversion to a normal sinus rhythm, which can be accomplished by either DC cardioversion or by administering quinidine. Because a sinus rhythm is difficult to maintain once established, conversion to a sinus rhythm should be considered only in selected cases, including atrial fibrillation of less than 6 months' duration with a normal or minimally enlarged heart.

The incidence of thromboembolism following conversion of atrial fibrillation to a sinus rhythm is estimated to be 1% to 3%. Thus, anticoagulation should be initiated, and elective cardioversion should be planned for about 2 weeks later. Long-term anticoagulant therapy is also recommended in selected cases of chronic atrial fibrillation when the risk of thromboemboli is especially increased, as in mitral valve disease and in congestive heart failure.

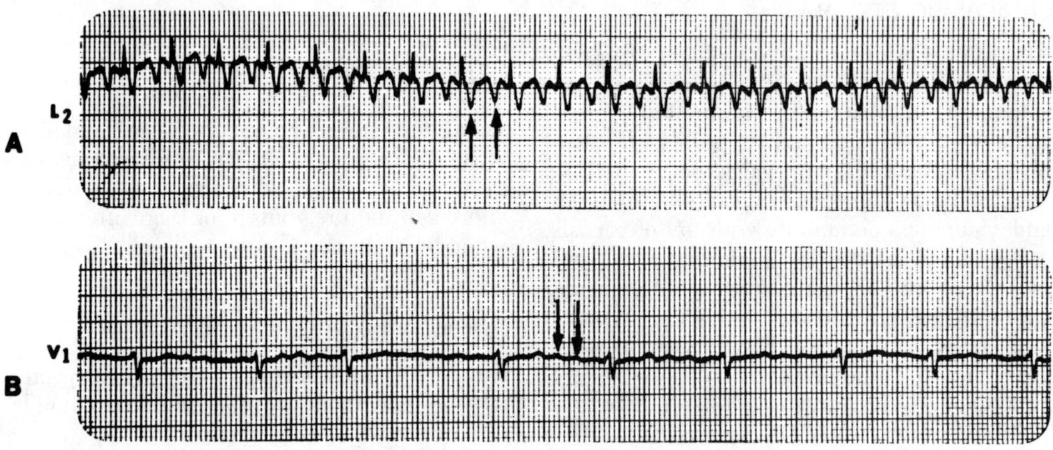

FIG 24–4.
A, Atrial flutter with 2:1 AV conduction. Atrial rate *(arrows)* is 300/minute, and ventricular rate is 150/minute. **B,** Atrial fibrillation *(arrows)* with irregular ventricular (QRS complex) response.

REFERENCES

Benditt DG, Benson DW Jr, Dunnigan A, Gornick CC, Anderson RW: Atrial flutter, atrial fibrillation, and other primary atrial tachycardias, in Zipes DP (guest ed). Symposium on cardiac arrhythmias I. *Med Clin North Am* 1984; 68(4):895–918. *Review with recent bibliography. Easy to read.*

Heger JJ: Diagnosis and management of cardiac arrhythmias. *Curr Probl Cardiol* 1985; 10(12):69. *A good, in-depth discussion of arrhythmias.*

Katz RI, Helfant RH: Paroxysmal supraventricular tachycardia, in Helfant RH (ed). *Bellet's Essentials of Cardiac Arrhythmias*, ed 2. Philadelphia, WB Saunders Co, 1980, pp 74–107. *Excellent reference book on cardiac arrhythmias.*

Lipman BS, Dunn M, Massie E: *Clinical Electrocardiography*, ed 7. Chicago, Year Book Medical Publishers, 1984, pp 376–481. *A nice book equally good for beginning and advanced electrocardiographers.*

Schwartz AB, Scheinman MM: ECG arrhythmia patterns: Part 1—Supra-ventricular arrhythmias. *Consultant* 1984; 26:275–298. *Excellent review of supraventricular arrhythmias with graphic illustrations.*

25 MITRAL VALVE DISEASE

Paul Kezdi, M.D.

Diseases of the mitral valve may lead to obstruction of blood flow from the left atrium to the left ventricle during diastole (stenosis) or to back flow from the ventricle to the atrium during systole by regurgitation (insufficiency) or to both. The cause of mitral stenosis is most frequently an acute rheumatic fever earlier in life. With acute rheumatic fever becoming much less frequent, the most common causes of chronic mitral regurgitation in the United States are now myxomatous degeneration of the valve and papillary muscle dysfunction. Acute mitral regurgitation may be the consequence of papillary muscle rupture in acute myocardial infarction, or ruptured chordae tendinea often idiopathic in origin or related to myxomatous change or due to bacterial endocarditis. Mitral stenosis in early childhood may rarely be congenital in origin.

CLINICAL SIGNS AND SYMPTOMS

Mitral stenosis is more frequently present in women (more than two thirds the cases) than men. Rheumatic fever often occurs in childhood with one or more milder relapses. Symptoms of valvular disease usually develop following a 10- to 12-year latent period after the first attack of rheumatic fever. There has been a definite decrease in the incidence of rheumatic mitral valve disease in the western hemisphere in the last 10 years subsequent to the introduction of the treatment and prevention of beta-hemolytic streptococcus infections by antibiotic agents.

The early symptom of mitral stenosis consists of mild-to-moderate dyspnea during exertion. As time passes the increasing exertional dyspnea may progress to attacks of coughing connected with shortness of breath, particularly when lying down at night (orthopnea). Rarely the first indication of severe mitral valve disease is an acute attack of pulmonary edema after severe exertional effort. However, in todays more frequent casual medical examinations, the presence of a heart murmur in children or young adults is often detected before symptoms of this magnitude become manifest. Late symptoms of mitral stenosis are usually the consequence of pulmonary hypertension and progressive right ventricular failure depending on the degree of mitral valvular orifice narrowing.

The early symptom of mitral insufficiency is predominantly exertional fatigue. As the left atrial pressure becomes elevated and the left atrial chamber distends, exertional dyspnea and later orthopnea develop. However, mitral insufficiency of mild-to-moderate degree is often well tolerated for a long period of time, even for 10 to 20 years, and with proper treatment incapacitating symptoms often can be delayed further.

Patients with mitral valve prolapse are often asymptomatic for many years. However, a high percentage of them have atypical chest pain with or without feeling of palpitations, skipping of beats, shortness of breath, and anxiety which is out of proportion to the other symptoms. The anxiety and panic syndrome is so typical that some authors tried to establish the existence of a mitral valve prolapse personality abnormality.

Occasionally, platelet microemboli can occur in mitral valve prolapse manifest in severe migrainelike headaches or transitory neurologic and pathologic syndromes such as vision disturbances, increase of arrhythmias, and mild hematuria. While there has been an association between the mitral valve prolapse and transitory ischemic attacks (TIAs) of the brain the mechanism and cause/effect relationship remain speculative.

In mitral stenosis, physical examination shows that the transverse diameter of the heart is usually not enlarged in the early stage, and the apex beat is in the normal position. When pulmonary hypertension is present, a precordial right ventricular thrust may be felt by placing the examiner's palm over the lower sternal area. Later in the disease, right ventricular enlargement and increased right ventricular thrust can be felt. On auscultation the typical diastolic rumble and a loud snapping and somewhat delayed first heart sound are present. The diastolic murmur is accentuated in presystole, both in sinus rhythm and atrial fibrillation. Following the second sound, there is a typical opening snap of the mitral valve. If some degree of mitral regurgitation is also present, a slight holosystolic murmur may be audible at the apex. Signs of pulmonary congestion with basal or generalized rales may be present on auscultation of the chest.

In mitral insufficiency, the predominant physical examination sign is the dilatation of the left ventricle with the diffusely enlarged apical pulse extending to the anterior axillary line. On auscultation the first heart sound is followed by a loud holosystolic murmur at the apex, which is transmitted toward the midaxillary line and the left side of the sternum. In sinus rhythm, a fourth heart sound may be present due to forcèful atrial contraction particularly in acute mitral regurgitation. With progressive cardiac enlargement, frequently atrial fibrillation develops with a variable ventricular rate. Right ventricular hypertrophy and increased right ventricular thrust usually appear late in the disease when secondary pulmonary hypertension increases right ventricular work. Increased right ventricular diastolic pressure and right atrial pressure may manifest themself in neck vein distension in 45-degree upright or sitting positions. When secondary tricuspid insufficiency develops due to enlargement of the tricuspid ring, a prominent systolic wave may be seen in the distended jugular vein.

In mitral valve prolapse, the specific sign is the nonejection systolic click. The nonejection systolic click may be accompanied by a brief late systolic murmur. The click is the result of a hammocking or billowing of one of the cusps, mostly of the posterior leaflet of the mitral valve.

The natural history of mitral valvular disease is at times interrupted by complications that are different for stenosis, insufficiency, and the mitral valve prolapse syndrome. The most frequent complication in mitral stenosis is systemic embolization. Left atrial thrombi, especially in the left atrial appendage, develop more frequently after the patient's cardiac rhythm has changed intermittently or permanently to atrial fibrillation. Systemic embolization can produce ischemic brain injury or kidney or other organ damage, and rarely the emboli can lodge in the coronary arteries causing myocardial ischemia and infarction. In mitral insuffiency, left atrial thrombi are infrequent and only occur in rather large atria in patients with chronic congestive heart failure and/or atrial fibrillation.

Mitral insufficiency of rheumatic fever origin is more frequent in men than women. Mitral insufficiency is now more frequently the result of other pathologic conditions such as chronic cardiomyopathy with dilatation of the mitral ring and malposition of the papillary muscles with lack of adequate closure of the valve due to separation of the opposing cusps. In mitral valve prolapse with the systolic click syndrome and late nonejection systolic murmur, the frequency of late complications is relatively low. The most frequent is the progression of the prolapse leading to increase of the regurgitation and the left atrial and ventricular enlargement. Mitral regurgitation may develop acutely as a result of a torn or ruptured chordae tendineae due to trauma to the chest or bacterial endocarditis. Bacterial endocarditis is a rare complication in mitral valve prolapse from infections with bacteremia. Sudden death from arrhythmias in mitral valve prolapse has rarely been reported. Sometimes a myocardiopathy type of cardiac enlargement with severe chronic arrhythmias develops late in the course of the disease. A more rare condition of weakness of the mitral valve may be present in Marfan's syndrome. In coronary artery disease, ischemia or infarction involving the papillary muscles can lead to chronic problems of closure of the mitral valve and, with papillary muscle rupture, to severe acute mitral regurgitation.

PATHOPHYSIOLOGY

The narrowed orifice of the mitral valve in stenosis is compensated by increased left atrial pressure to maintain the flow, resulting in a pressure gradient across the valve. The gradient is maintained by increased right ventricular work and raised pulmonary arterial pressure. The effective mitral orifice can be calculated from the pressure gradient and the flow across the valve (Gorlin formula[1]). The normal mitral orifice in diastole is 3.5 to 4.0 cm^2. In severe stenosis, this may decrease to 0.5 to 0.9 cm^2. Mitral insufficiency results in regurgitation of blood to the left atrium, which could be a significant fraction of the forward flow to the aorta. The left atrial pressure is elevated particularly in systole showing an accentuated, large V wave. Emptying of the left atrium to the left ventricle is, therefore, not hampered during the latter half of diastole. However, eventually left ventricular diastolic pressure becomes elevated as the left ventricle starts to fail.

---

[1]Valve area $= \dfrac{\text{Flow through valve}}{\text{Constant} \times \sqrt{\text{gradient}}}$.

CLINICAL–PATHOLOGIC CORRELATIONS

When valves come to pathologic examination, they are often markedly deformed, calcified, leaving only a small opening or are unable to close the orifice. Microscopically large segments are replaced by scar tissue, other areas show cellular infiltration and no resemblance to normal tissue structure.

In mitral valve prolapse, particularly the primary idiopathic variety, the primary pathologic abnormality was thought to be due to connective tissue degeneration of the leaflets and the chordae tendineae. Because this condition is often accompanied by pectus excavatum and other developmental abnormalities of the bony thorax, it has been suggested to be the result of an inherited disorder of the connective tissue. However, more recent autopsy studies indicated that a separation between the atrial-mitral valve junction (annulus fibrosus) and the left ventricular attachment may lead to hypermobility of the valve apparatus causing the prolapse of one or more of the cusps. Variations of the morphological structure of the annulus may cause the secondary disjunction and lead to the floppy valve syndrome. (See Table 25–1 for summary of clinical-pathologic correlations.)

DIFFERENTIAL DIAGNOSIS

The characteristic diastolic rumble ending in the loud first heart sound and the subsequent opening snap differentiates mitral stenosis from other defects of the mitral valve. A holosystolic murmur of mitral regurgitation on the other hand has to be differentiated from the ejection type of murmurs of the aortic and pulmonic valve or ventricular septal defect as well as from the systolic murmur of tricuspid insufficiency. The location of predominance and the characteristic of the murmur in combination with other physical findings will relatively easily separate these valve defects. Additional tests, such as chest x-ray films, and electrocardiograms and ECHO are needed to confirm the clinical impression. These provide information about predominant chamber enlargement, pulmonary vascular markings, left or right ventricular hypertrophy, and left or right atrial enlargement. Differential diagnosis

TABLE 25–1.
Clinical–Pathologic Correlations—Mitral Valve Disease: Pathophysiologic Mechanisms

ABNORMALITIES OF VALVE FUNCTION	CAUSES
Mitral stenosis	Rheumatic fever Congenital valve defect Left atrial myxoma
Mitral insufficiency	Rheumatic fever Cardiomyopathy with dilated mitral annulus Mitral valve prolapse Papillary muscle insufficiency or rupture due to coronary artery disease and trauma Rupture of chordae tendineae due to trauma or bacterial endocarditis

Mitral valve prolapse (nonejection systolic click syndrome)	Idiopathic. Separation of the annulus from left ventricular wall
	Associated with many other conditions including the following:
	    Marfan's syndrome
	    Pectus excavatum and straight back syndrome
	    Congenital heart diseases (e.g., atrial septal defect)
	    Turner's syndrome
	    Ehlers-Danlos syndrome

of complications such as pulmonary edema or atrial fibrillation in mitral stenosis, especially when occurring for the first time in a middle-aged patient, requires a careful diagnostic evaluation to determine the underlying cause.

In mitral valve prolapse, the multiple underlying conditions may have to be separated. In idiopathic mitral valve prolapse, the clinical finding of nonejection click may be present early in life accompanying the other symptoms. When the click syndrome is present in ischemic heart disease or cardiomyopathy, its secondary nature is not difficult to ascertain especially when it had not been heard earlier in life.

Mitral valve prolapse with chest pain in the presence of signs of mitral regurgitation and frequent premature ventricular contractions in a middle-aged person is often difficult to differentiate from underlying coronary artery disease. Many of these patients end up in the angiography laboratory and are found to have normal coronary arteries.

DIAGNOSIS

The key diagnostic procedures in mitral valve disease, listed in order of their usual application, include an electrocardiogram, a chest x-ray film often with barium swallow (to de-

lineate displacement of the esophagus), echocardiography, and cardiac catheterization. In pure mitral stenosis, the typical configuration of the heart is a normal transverse diameter, predominant enlargement of the left atrium, and in advanced stenosis with pulmonary hypertension prominence of the pulmonary outflow tract. There is an impression on the esophagus by the left atrium and an upward extended contact of the right ventricle with the sternum. In addition, there is increased hilar prominence (perihilar haze), Kerley's B lines and vascular redistribution markings indicating pulmonary congestion. Echocardiography (ECHO) is exceptionally useful in making the diagnosis and quantifying accurately the degree of stenosis.

In mitral insufficiency, the typical x-ray film configuration is the predominant left ventricular and left atrial enlargement. In mitral valve prolapse, the heart is normal in size and configuration, but in a certain percentage of patients there is a narrow AP diameter of the chest or even a slight pectus excavatum.

In mitral stenosis, the electrocardiogram may show signs of left atrial hypertrophy with biphasic P waves in lead V_1 and somewhat broad, tall P waves in the other leads. Different degrees of right ventricular hypertrophy may be present late in the course. In mitral insufficiency, signs of left atrial enlargement and different degrees of left ventricular hypertrophy and strain pattern are present depending on the degree of the insufficiency. Mitral valve prolapse has no typical electrocardiographic changes, though nonspecific ST&T changes are not uncommon and frequently ventricular PVCs are present (in 25%–50%).

The primary diagnostic tool in mitral valve prolapse is the M-mode and two-dimensional echocardiographic visualization of the prolapse (see Figs 25–1 and 25–2). With this technique, billowing and prolapse of the mitral valve of any degree can be seen. Sometimes there is billowing without prolapse or regurgitation, or just a prolapse with regurgitation, or both billowing and prolapse with regurgitation. Rarely, primary mitral valve prolapse is accompanied by an ostium secundum type atrial septal defect (ASD). ECHO may be useful in diagnosing ASD; it demonstrates paradoxic septal movement and small shunts may be visualized by special technique. The presence of septal defect is usually verified by cardiac catheterization.

The presence of cardiomyopathy can only be confirmed by myocardial biopsy. In recent years, myocardial biopsy has been made possible by cardiac catheterization techniques with a special catheter removing myocardial tissue from the right ventricle.

PRINCIPLES OF PREVENTION AND THERAPY

Drug treatment of mitral valve disease is restricted to treatment of the complications such as heart failure, atrial fibrillation, or other arrhythmias. Treatment of the anatomic defect requires surgical repair or replacement of the valve. In mild mitral stenosis, moderate sodium and fluid restriction and mild diuretic treatment often delay the necessity for surgical correction. Beta-blockers may be useful because they decrease rapid heart rate response with exercise, thereby prolonging diastolic filling time and thus decreasing the mitral valve gradient. However, if progressive, severe symptoms develop, the present treatment of choice is relatively early open-heart surgical correction of the valve, namely, under direct vision, separation of the fused cusps or, if the valve is markedly scarred or calcified, replacement by a valve prosthesis or heterograft porcine valve.

Atrial fibrillation early in the disease can often be converted to a sinus rhythm by digitalis treatment and maintained by additional quinidine treatment. Sinus rhythm is preferred, and, if necessary, electrical conversion is used even after valve repair or replacement. Patients with mitral stenosis usually respond well to

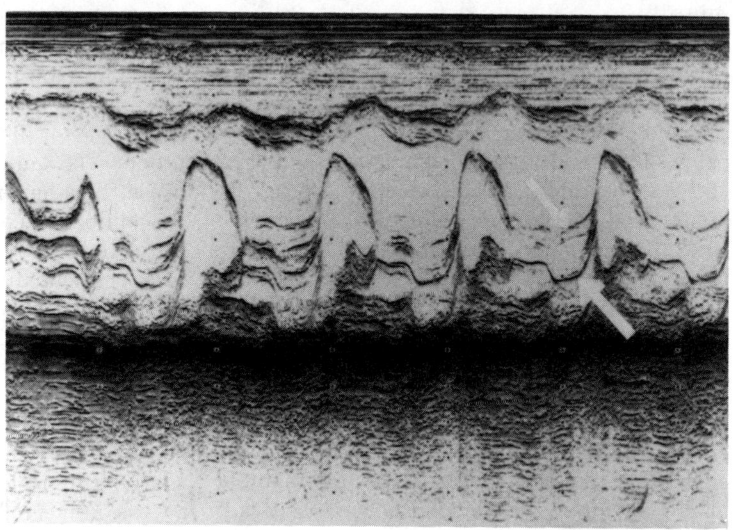

FIG 25–1.
M-mode echocardiogram of the mitral valve in mitral valve prolapse. *Upper arrow:* Anterior leaflet in normal position. *Lower arrow:* Markedly prolapsed posterior leaflet. Normally the two leaflets are close together.

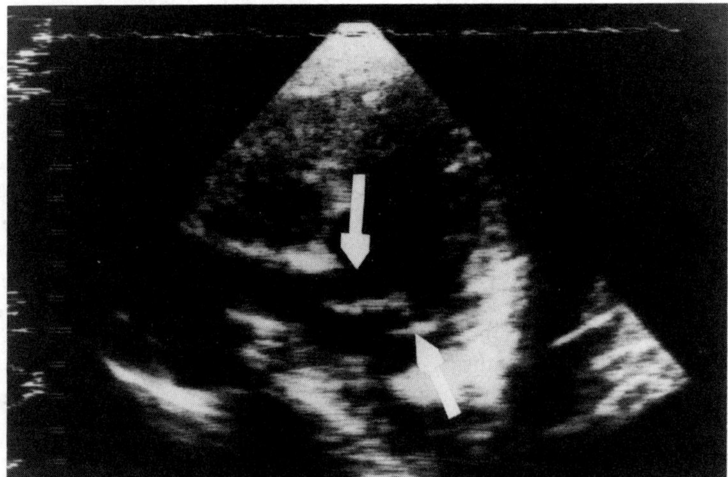

FIG 25–2.
Two-dimensional echocardiogram of the mitral valve. *Lower arrow:* Posterior leaflet prolapsed. *Upper arrow:* To the left of the arrow is the tricuspid valve; below the arrow the anterior leaflet of the mitral valve is somewhat prolapsed also. Normally the two mitral leaflets would only be somewhat below the horizontal line of the tricuspid valve.

surgical correction. Left ventricular and right ventricular function usually return close to normal unless significant secondary myocardial damage already exists.

Mitral insufficiency is usually tolerated for long periods of time, particularly with support treatment of diuretic agents and, if necessary, digitalis and antiarrhythmic drugs. Timing of the surgery for mitral regurgitation is more difficult than for stenosis. A good method to determine the optimal time for surgery is the echocardiographic evaluation of the ejection fraction and the end-diastolic and end-systolic diameters. When ejection fraction is decreased below 40%, end-diastolic diameter is 39 mm and end-systolic diameter is approaching 26 mm/m² body surface area, it seems to be advisable to recommend surgical correction of the valve defect to prevent irreversible myocardial damage. This seems to be the case, according to recent studies (Fowler & Van Der Bel-Kahn, 1979), even if symptoms are relatively few.

In mitral valve prolapse, the usual treatment is the control of the hyperadrenergic state and ectopic activity with low doses of a beta-adrenergic blocking agent such as propranolol. Often reassurance is the most effective treatment. In a small percentage of patients with primary mitral valve prolapse who have marked mitral insufficiency later in life, surgical correction of the valve or ruptured chordae tendineae may be necessary. In secondary mitral valve prolapse such as occurs in cardiomyopathy, the problem is similar to that in rheumatic mitral insufficiency, but complicated by the more advanced myocardial disease, which may preclude adequate cardiac function even when the valve is replaced.

Prevention of mitral valve disease relates to prevention of its multiple etiology. As indicated before, rheumatic fever and chronic rheumatic valve disease are decreasing due to proper recognition and treatment of their cause, beta-hemolytic streptococcus infection. Prevention of coronary artery disease by risk factor reduction will also prevent valvular defects occasionally associated with it. In mitral valve prolapse, the general consensus is that prevention of subacute bacterial endocarditis by antibiotic coverage of dental work and other potential infections will to some extent reduce the subsequent valve scarring and tendency for mitral insufficiency. Mitral valve prolapse itself as well as most forms of cardiomyopathies cannot be prevented because their cause is generally unknown.

REFERENCES

Barlow JB, Pocock WA; The mitral valve prolapse enigma—two decades later. *Mod Concepts Cardiovasc Dis* 1984; 53:13–17. *An up-to-date review.*

Bonchek LI: Current status of cardiac valve replacement: Selection of a prosthesis and indications for operation. *Am Heart J* 1981; 101:96–106. *A review of valve replacement, well referenced.*

Fowler NO, Van Der Bel-Kahn JM: Indications for surgical replacement of the mitral valve. With particular reference to common and uncommon causes of mitral regurgitation. *Am J Cardiol* 1979; 44:148–157. *A useful analysis of decision making.*

Hurst JW: *The Heart.* New York, McGraw-Hill Book Co, 1982, p 892. *In-depth discussion.*

Hutchins GM, Moore G, Skoog DK: The association of floppy mitral valve with disjunction of the mitral annulus fibrosus. *N Engl J Med* 1986; 314:535–540. *A discussion of pathology.*

Rackley CE: Valvular heart disease, in Wyngaarden JB, Smith LH, Jr (eds): *Cecil Textbook of Medicine.* Philadelphia, WB Saunders Co, 1985, pp 242–252. *Brief discussion in a standard textbook.*

Ross JO: Afterload mismatch in aortic and mitral valve disease: Implications for surgical therapy. *J Am Coll Cardiol* 1985; 5:811–826. *Correlations between pathophysiology and therapy.*

Wei JY, Fortuin NJ: Diastolic sounds and murmurs associated with mitral valve prolapse. *Circulation* 1981; 63:559–564. *A careful description of the auscultatory findings.*

26 AORTIC VALVE DISEASE

Satyendra C. Gupta, M.D.

Aortic valve disease may be subdivided into two categories: aortic stenosis and aortic regurgitation. Each will be discussed separately.

AORTIC STENOSIS

Valvular aortic stenosis may be congenital (unicuspid or bicuspid aortic valve), a residual of rheumatic inflammation, or secondary to cusp calcification of unknown cause. The most likely cause of aortic stenosis in patients younger than 30 years old is a congenitally abnormal aortic valve. Rheumatic heart disease and calcification of congenitally bicuspid aortic valves may play a role in patients from age 30 to age 70 years, and calcification of a tricuspid aortic valve is the usual cause in patients more than 70 years old. Multivalvular lesions are still considered to be rheumatic in origin. Table 26–1 lists these and rare causes of aortic stenosis.

CLINICAL SIGNS AND SYMPTOMS

A patient with aortic stenosis remains asymptomatic for a long period, during which obstruction gradually increases across the aortic valve. The classic triad of symptoms is angina, dyspnea, and syncope or dizziness. Angina occurs in two-thirds of those with critical aortic stenosis. Dyspnea on exertion is initially a diastolic dysfunction probably due to increased left ventricular end-diastolic pressure secondary to decreased compliance. Decreased compliance, in turn, is secondary to left ventricular hypertrophy. Effort syncope is another typical symptom which occurs with or immediately after physical exertion. Once these symptoms develop, the patient's condition deteriorates rapidly.

A slowly rising pulse with an anacrotic notch, delayed peak, and diminished amplitude (pulsus parvus et tardus) is characteristic of aortic stenosis. The pulse contour is altered

TABLE 26–1.
Etiology of Aortic Valvular Disease

AORTIC STENOSIS

Congenital abnormalities
Rheumatic
Degenerative (senile) calcification
Rare causes
    Hyperlipidemia
    Infective endocarditis
    Fabry's disease
    Ochronosis
    Systemic lupus erythematosis
    Rheumatoid involvement

AORTIC REGURGITATION

Chronic
Rheumatic
Congenital abnormalities (bicuspid valve)
Syphilis
Ankylosing spondylitis
Rheumatoid arthritis
Systemic lupus erythematosis
Systemic hypertension
Marfan's syndrome
Ehlers-Danlos syndrome
Osteogenesis imperfecta
Associated with ventricular septal defect
Myxoid degeneration of the aortic valve
Aneurysm of Valsalva sinus

Acute
Infective endocarditis
Dissecting aortic aneurysm*
Trauma

* Systemic hypertension, Marfan's syndrome, or idiopathic cystic medial necrosis are the usual bases of this pathologic change.

even by mild aortic regurgitation. The pulse pressure is typically narrow. The apical pulse is well localized, forcible, and sustained throughout systole. A systolic thrill is often present over the base of the heart and the second right intercostal space. The auscultatory findings include the diamond-shaped crescendo–decrescendo murmur and delayed closure of the aortic valve. This delayed closure may result in paradoxical splitting of the second heart sound. An aortic ejection click is audible in congenital aortic stenosis if the leaflets are mobile. As the aortic valve becomes fibrosed and calcified, the ejection click disappears and the intensity of the aortic component of the second sound is reduced or absent.

The murmur is usually loudest in the aortic area in the second right intercostal space and often radiates to the carotid vessels and apex of the heart. A late peaking of this diamond-shaped murmur indicates severe stenosis. An audible fourth heart sound in younger patients is also an indicator of severe aortic stenosis, with a peak systolic pressure gradient of more than 50 mm Hg across the aortic valve.

Patients with congenital aortic valve stenosis come to the attention of the physician at two different ages: (1) in childhood or early adulthood because of a murmur or symptoms, and (2) in their fifties, sixties, or seventies when the malformed valve calcifies, producing stenosis. Hemodynamically severe aortic valve disease is well tolerated for a number of years without symptoms, but once symptoms appear, the course is progressively downhill. Clinical studies have demonstrated an average life expectancy of 3 to 4 years from the onset of syncope, 2 to 3 years from the onset of angina, and 1.5 to 2 years after the onset of dyspnea and heart failure. Sudden death usually occurs in symptomatic patients and accounts for 20% of all deaths from aortic valve stenosis.

PATHOPHYSIOLOGY

Table 26–2 lists the major gross and microscopic findings of aortic stenosis. In aortic stenosis, left ventricular outflow is gradually obstructed. The heart compensates for such an increased hemodynamic burden mainly by left ventricular hypertrophy, without left ventricular dilatation, development of symptoms, or reduction in cardiac output. The elevated left ventricular end-diastolic pressure, which is characteristic of aortic stenosis, does not necessarily mean that left ventricular dilatation or failure is present, but reflects decreased compliance of the hypertrophic left ventricular wall. In aortic stenosis, atrial contraction is critical in filling the left ventricle. Loss of vigorous atrial contraction, as occurs in atrial fibrillation, may result in rapid clinical deterioration. Late in the course of the disease, as the myocardium gradually weakens, the pressure generated in the left ventricle decreases, with a reduced cardiac output and stroke volume. This also leads to a reduced pressure gradient across the aortic valve, whereas mean left atrial and pulmonary arterial pressures rise. In addition, left ventricular dilatation may produce mitral regurgitation.

TABLE 26–2.
Pathologic Features of Aortic Stenosis

	PATHOLOGIC FEATURES	
ANATOMIC STRUCTURES	MACROSCOPIC FINDINGS	MICROSCOPIC FINDINGS
Aortic valves		
Congenital	Unicuspid, bicuspid, or tricuspid	NA*
	Commissural fusion	Fibrotic changes
	Calcification	Calcification
Rheumatic	Adhesions and commissural fusion	Vascularization of cusp leaflets and valve ring (stigmata of rheumatic heart disease in other valves)
	Retraction and stiffening of free cusps	
	Calcific nodules on both free surfaces of cusps	Calcification
Degenerative (senile, calcific)	Calcium deposits along flexion lines of the cusps	Loss of myofibrils; large nuclei; large cytoplasmic areas devoid of contractile material; proliferation of fibroblasts and collagen fibers in the interstitial spaces
Myocardium	Left ventricular hypertrophy and dilatation	
	Left atrial enlargement	
Coronary arteries	Narrowing of coronary ostia	NA
	Calcium emboli	NA
Aorta	Dilatation of ascending aorta (poststenotic dilatation)	NA

* NA = Not applicable

TABLE 26–3.
Clinical–Pathologic Correlations in Aortic Stenosis

CLINICAL FINDINGS		PATHOLOGIC FINDINGS
Systolic thrill Crescendo–decrescendo ejection murmur	Severe outflow obstruction at the aortic valve	Turbulent blood flow
Paradoxic or reversed splitting of S^2 heart sound		Delayed A_2 closure
Decreased pulse pressure		Decreased systolic arterial blood pressure, and low cardiac output, peripheral vasoconstriction, and increased diastolic pressure*
Syncope and dizziness		Cardiac arrhythmias and decreased cardiac output
Ejection sound absent	Commissural fusion	Shortening of cusps
S_2 heart sound reduced or inaudible	Extensive calcification	Impaired cusp movement
Possible aortic regurgitant murmur		
A–V heart block		Aortic annulus calcification extending into membranous portion of intraventricular septum, region of His bundle, and proximal left bundle branch
Dyspnea	Left ventricular hypertrophy and dilatation	Increased left ventricular end-diastolic pressure
Paroxysmal nocturnal dyspnea		Decreased ejection fraction
Orthopnea		
Pulmonary edema		Increased end-systolic volume
		Increased left atrial pressure
Angina	Left ventricular hypertrophy	Increased myocardial oxygen demand Increased LV pressure Increased LV systolic end-diastolic tension
Angina	Narrowing of coronary ostia	Decreased blood supply; excessive compression of intramyocardial coronary vessels
	Calcium emboli enter coronary vascular bed	Increased intercapillary distance by myocardial hypertrophy
	Associated arteriosclerotic heart disease	

* Exception: Independent systemic hypertension.

CLINICAL–PATHOLOGIC CORRELATIONS

The clinical features of aortic stenosis are the result of left ventricular hypertrophy and dilatation and of severe outflow obstruction at the aortic valve. Table 26–3 summarizes the major clinical-pathologic correlations.

DIFFERENTIAL DIAGNOSIS

Aortic stenosis enters into the differential diagnosis of all patients with a systolic murmur at the base of the heart. It is important to rule out the possibility of aortic stenosis in patients with congestive heart failure or a history of syncope, dizziness, and angina. Table 26–4 lists common conditions and differentiating features.

DIAGNOSIS

Most patients with a significant hemodynamic gradient across the aortic valve have electrocardiographic evidence of left ventricular hypertrophy, which may precede the development of symptoms. Except in advanced cases, the heart is normal size on chest x-ray films. This finding is deceptive because a thick chamber wall does not give rise to significant radiographic abnormality.

Poststenotic dilatation of the ascending aorta is a common feature in aortic stenosis. Calcification of the aortic valve is found in almost all adults with hemodynamically significant aortic stenosis, but such calcification can be confirmed only by fluoroscopy of the heart. Phonocardiogram and carotid pulse tracings not only confirm the physical signs, but also provide measurements to assess ventricular function. Narrowing of the aortic valve and calcification can be readily appreciated on echocardiogram. The normal boxlike opening of the aortic cusps is replaced by heavy multilayered echoes. A bicuspid aortic valve may sometimes also be recognized in an echocardiogram by the eccentric position of the aortic cusps in diastole. Doppler echocardiography is a recent means of identifying the severity of aortic stenosis.

In preparing for surgical intervention, cardiac catheterization should be performed to (1)

TABLE 26–4.
Conditions That May Mimic Valvular Aortic Stenosis

CONDITION	DIFFERENTIATING FEATURES
Supravalvular aortic stenosis	Congenital condition
	Peculiar facies (Elfin)
	High location of murmur
	Unequal pulses and blood pressure in both arms
	Signs of stenosis coexisting in both branches of peripheral pulmonary artery
Subvalvular aortic stenosis (discrete membranous or tunnel)	Congenital condition
	Maximum intensity of murmur to the left of sternum with poor transmission to aortic area and carotid arteries
	Absence of ejection click
	Usually recognized in childhood
Hypertrophic obstructive cardiomyopathy	Characteristic brisk arterial pulse
	Murmur best heard at left lower sternal border
	Accentuation of murmur with Valsalva's maneuver
	Bifid apical impulse in systole
	Echocardiogram shows asymmetric septal hypertrophy and systolic anterior motion of mitral leaflet
Aortic atherosclerosis (aortic root murmur)	Occurs after age 65 years
	Aortic second sound normal
	Normal aortic valve echocardiogram
Mitral regurgitation	Murmur holosystolic
	Murmur best heard at apex, radiating to axilla
	Murmur decreased with amylnitrite inhalation*
Bruit arising in carotid or subclavian arteries	Bruit louder in neck or supraclavicular fossae
	Bruit decreased or inaudible by subclavian artery pressure
	Normal A_2

* Murmurs of hypertrophic obstructive cardiomyopathy and aortic stenosis increase with amylnitrite inhalation.

confirm the severity of aortic stenosis, (2) assess left ventricular function, (3) determine the presence or absence of other valve disease, and (4) ascertain the coronary artery anatomy, especially in patients over 40 years old. Figure 26–1 shows the typical simultaneous pressure changes in the left ventricle and brachial artery obtained during cardiac catheterization in a patient with aortic stenosis.

PRINCIPLES OF THERAPY

Patients with aortic stenosis should be informed of the hazards of endocarditis, and prophylactic antibiotics should be given for elective dental and surgical procedures. Patients with multivalvular involvement should receive rheumatic prophylaxis. After the onset of symptoms, patients with aortic stenosis require immediate evaluation and surgical correction, and there is little justification for medical therapy. In younger patients with mobile, noncalcified valves, commissurotomy may effectively relieve obstruction, but this is rarely possible when the valve is calcified. Calcified valves are replaced by prostheses. For patients who for a number of reasons are not suitable surgical candidates, valvuloplasty is now seen as an alternative to surgery. Bypass of signifi-

cantly obstructed coronary arteries is usually performed at the time of aortic valve replacement.

AORTIC REGURGITATION

Unlike aortic stenosis, aortic regurgitation is a disease of many causes and occurs in both acute and chronic forms. It may be caused by primary disease of either the aortic valve leaflets or the wall of the aortic root, or both. Table 26–1 lists the important etiologic factors of both acute and chronic aortic regurgitation.

CLINICAL SIGNS AND SYMPTOMS

In chronic aortic regurgitation, the patient usually remains asymptomatic for many years, during which the left ventricle gradually enlarges. The earliest symptom is often an uncomfortable awareness of the heartbeat or palpitation, particularly while lying on the left side. This is caused by the large stroke volume and rapid diastolic runoff. In the fourth or fifth decade of life, when considerable cardiomegaly has occurred, symptoms of myocardial dysfunction become apparent, and patients complain of exertional dyspnea, orthopnea, and

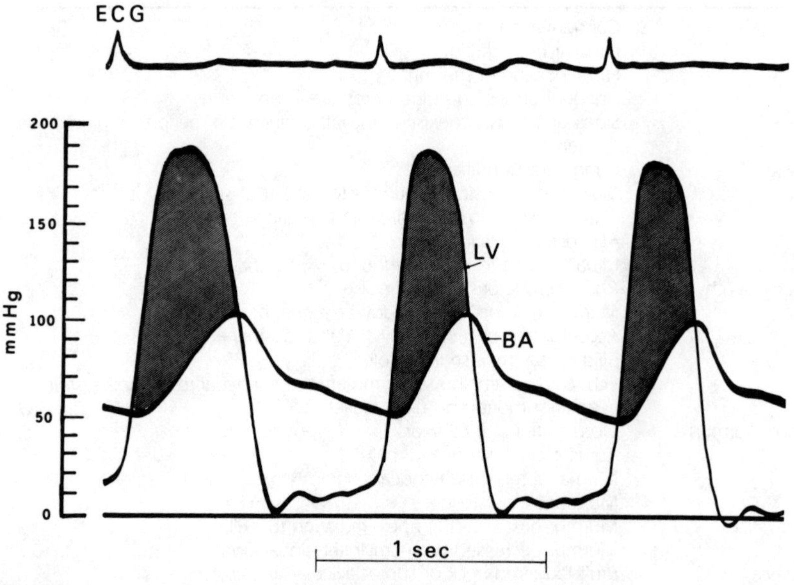

FIG 26–1.
Simultaneous left ventricular (LV) and brachial artery (BA) pressure recordings. The 75-mm Hg LV–BA pressure gradient indicates severe aortic stenosis.

paroxysmal nocturnal dyspnea. Angina pectoris is less frequent, and syncope is rare. In acute regurgitation, patients often develop symptoms of cardiovascular collapse with weakness, hypotension, and severe dyspnea.

In the early stages of aortic regurgitation, the physical findings may be normal except for the characteristic diastolic blowing murmur. The impressive peripheral vascular findings in severe aortic regurgitation include a collapsing pulse (water-hammer pulse, Corrigan's pulse), pulsating capillaries in the nailbed, and systolic head bobbing. The systolic blood pressure is elevated with an abnormally low diastolic pressure. Korotkoff sounds often persist to 0 mm Hg on the sphygmomanometer. The heart may be normal size or extremely enlarged, depending on the duration and severity of the regurgitation. The second heart sound (A_2) is variable in intensity. A systolic ejection click may be heard and is probably related to sudden distension of the aorta.

The characteristic auscultatory finding is a high-pitched diastolic blowing murmur, heard best along the left sternal border. In patients with aortic regurgitation secondary to disease of the aortic root, the murmur is often best heard to the right of the sternum. In the early stages, the murmur is best heard with the patient seated and at full expiration. In addition, a diastolic rumble (Austin Flint murmur) is heard at the apex in moderate and severe aortic regurgitation. In severe aortic regurgitation, a short midsystolic murmur may be present at the base of the heart from increased flow across the aortic valve, even though no obstruction exists.

Chronic aortic regurgitation is marked by a fairly long asymptomatic period. Once the diagnosis is made, the survival rate is about 75% for 5 years, and 50% for 10 years. Without surgical intervention, the survival of patients with aortic regurgitation and congestive heart failure is less than 2 years. Patients with angina will often die within 4 years. Without timely aortic valve replacement, mortality in acute aortic regurgitation is often extremely high.

PATHOPHYSIOLOGY

The major gross and microscopic findings of aortic regurgitation are shown in Table 26–5. Severe aortic regurgitation places a large volume load on the left ventricle, which dilates, in order both to accommodate the increased volume of blood and to increase stroke volume, which is necessary to maintain an adequate forward flow. Systolic pressure rises because of increased stroke volume. Aortic diastolic pressure falls because of backward leak, and the pulse pressure is therefore wide. Peripheral vascular resistance decreases to help forward blood flow. This, along with increased stroke volume, manifests in characteristic hyperkinetic circulatory signs.

Although left ventricular compliance increases, eventually left ventricular diastolic pressure rises and may become very high, resulting in left ventricular failure. In acute aortic regurgitation, the left ventricle is not able to increase compliance or distensibility. This results in marked elevation of filling pressure and rapid development of pulmonary vascular congestion.

CLINICAL–PATHOLOGIC CORRELATIONS

The clinical features of aortic regurgitation, shown in Table 26–6, are the result of a hypertrophic left ventricle, increased stroke volume, and increased left ventricular diastolic volume because of regurgitation.

DIFFERENTIAL DIAGNOSIS

The murmur of aortic regurgitation can easily be confused with the murmur of pulmonary regurgitation in patients with severe pulmonary hypertension. Other conditions can cause characteristic peripheral physical signs of rapid runoff because blood enters from the aorta into some low-pressure area or into other areas of circulation. These conditions include patent ductus arteriosus, aortopulmonary window, arteriovenous fistula, Paget's disease, and pregnancy.

DIAGNOSIS

Electrocardiograms of patients with significant aortic regurgitation show a pattern of left ventricular hypertrophy and diastolic volume overload. Chest x-ray films reveal cardiac enlargement with dilatation of the left ventricle. In acute aortic regurgitation, cardiac enlargement is generally absent, yet pulmonary venous congestion and pulmonary edema may be seen. The echocardiogram shows increased left

TABLE 26–5.
Pathologic Features of Aortic Regurgitation

ANATOMIC STRUCTURES	PATHOLOGIC FEATURES	
	MACROSCOPIC FINDINGS	MICROSCOPIC FINDINGS
Aortic Valves		
Congenital	Bicuspid (one cusp may be redundant and prolapsed)	Myxomatous changes may be present
Rheumatic	Contractures, retraction, and malalignment of cusps	Vascularization and fibrosis of cusps Rheumatic stigmata
Endocarditis	Vegetations Cusp destruction with perforation and detachment	Bacterial inflammatory changes
Aorta		
Syphilis	Dilatation Aneurysm	Thickened adventitia Degeneration of media Intimal proliferation Abnormal vasa vasorum
Trauma	Laceration of ascending aorta	May be associated with cystic medial necrosis

TABLE 26–6.
Clinical–Pathologic Correlations in Aortic Regurgitation

CLINICAL FINDINGS		PATHOLOGIC FINDINGS
Decrescendo diastolic blowing murmur	Rapid runoff with backflow from aorta to left ventricle	Decreased diastolic pressure
Midsystolic ejection murmur		Increased stroke volume
Ejection click		Increased systolic pressure
Bounding pulse and other peripheral signs		Increased pulse pressure
Angina	Left ventricle hypertrophy and dilatation	Increased myocardial oxygen demands
		Increased pressure-volume overload of left ventricle
	Low aortic diastolic and left ventricle filling pressures	Decreased coronary blood supply
		Decreased pressure gradient between aortic root and intramyocardial and subendocardial coronary vessels
		Calcification or obstruction of coronary ostia (syphilitic aortitis)
Congestive heart failure	Dilatation of left ventricle	Decreased stroke volume
		Decreased ejection fraction
		Increased left ventricular filling pressure
		Increased left atrial pressure
Mitral regurgitation	Marked left ventricular dilatation	Enlargement of mitral annulus
		Displaced or overly long papillary muscles

ventricular systolic and diastolic dimensions and diastolic fluttering of the anterior mitral leaflet. In hemodynamically significant acute aortic regurgitation, premature closure of the mitral valve before the onset of the QRS complex may be seen. Echocardiograms can be helpful in identifying the cause of aortic regurgitation (e.g., vegetations of infective endocarditis). A Doppler ultrasound study can also identify aortic regurgitation by recording the jet with reversed velocity in the left ventricular outflow tract in diastole.

In severe, chronic aortic regurgitation, left ventricular size and performance should be assessed at intervals using noninvasive methods such as echocardiography or radionuclide angiography or both. Cardiac catheterization assesses the severity of aortic regurgitation (with injection of contrast material at the aortic root), evaluates left ventricular function, and identifies additional cardiac abnormalities including coronary artery anatomy.

PRINCIPLES OF THERAPY

Prophylaxis against bacterial endocarditis is important in all cases of aortic regurgitation. Patients with aortic regurgitation secondary to syphilitic aortitis should receive a full course of penicillin therapy. Although medical treatment including salt restriction, digitalis, diuretics, and vasodilators may be useful temporarily in controlling congestive heart failure, the primary form of treatment is valve replacement, particularly for patients who are symptomatic.

COMBINED AORTIC STENOSIS AND AORTIC REGURGITATION

The combination of aortic stenosis and aortic regurgitation results from thickened, deformed valve leaflets that cannot open or close properly. The disease is most often due to rheumatic endocarditis, but also frequently results from a congenitally malformed valve. The clinical and hemodynamic picture depends on whether stenosis or regurgitation is the predominant lesion. Surgical treatment is indicated when the patient is disabled by symptoms. Valve replacement is almost always required.

REFERENCES

Braunwald E: Valvular heart disease, in Braunwald E (ed): *Heart Disease—A Textbook of Cardiovascular Medicine*, ed 2, vol 2. Philadelphia, WB Saunders Co, 1984, pp 1063–1135. *Good review with recent bibliography.*

Frank S, Johnson A, Ross J Jr: Natural history of valvular aortic stenosis. *Br Heart J* 1973; 35:41–46. *Good source for review of the natural history of aortic stenosis.*

Goldschlager N, Pfeifer J, Cohn K, Popper R, Selzer A: The natural history of aortic regurgitation. A clinical and hemodynamic study. *Am J Med* 1973; 54:577–588. *A nice review on the natural history of aortic regurgitation.*

Harries AD, Griffiths BE: Assessment of chronic aortic valve disease in adults. *Postgrad Med J* 1982; 58:1–5. *Easy-to-read article on chronic aortic valve disease.*

Perloff JK: Acute severe aortic regurgitation: Recognition and management. *J Cardiovasc Med* 1983; 8:209–218. *A good article to read for understanding acute regurgitation.*

Rackley CE, Edwards JE, Wallace RB, Katz NM: Aortic valve disease, in Hurst JW (ed): *The Heart—Arteries and Veins*, ed 6. New York, McGraw-Hill Book Co, 1986, pp 729–754. *Excellent reference book on valvular diseases.*

Waller BF: Morphologic aspects of valvular heart disease: Part 1. *Curr Problems Cardiol* 1984; 9(7):1–66. *A good in-depth discussion.*

Moshen Sakhaii, M.D.
Sylvan L. Weinberg, M.D.

27 TRAUMATIC HEART DISEASE

Throughout the centuries and until relatively recently penetrating cardiac trauma has been equated with death. In 1709 Boerhaave stated "all wounds to the heart were mortal." In 1896 Paget was convinced "surgery of the heart has probably reached the limits set by nature of all surgery; no new method, and no new discovery can overcome the natural difficulties that attend a wound to the heart" (Symbas, 1982). Only one year later in 1897, Rehn performed the first successful cardiorrhaphy in a human. Since that time there have been great discoveries and refinements of surgical technique, anesthesiology, intensive care units, diagnosis, and extracorporeal perfusion. In spite of all these, the mortality still remains high.

Cardiac trauma has classically been divided into contusion due to blunt injury and penetrating wounds of the heart. In the era of invasive cardiology, probably a third category should be added, injuries occurring in the catheterization laboratory as the result of cardiac catheterization, both diagnostic and therapeutic. Although these procedural injuries are increasing in frequency, they are considered outside the scope of this discussion.

Traumatic disorders of the heart and the great vessels are becoming increasingly important. For example, over 5 million cases of bodily injury of moderate severity and 56,000 deaths resulted from 25 million automobile accidents in 1973. An estimated 900,000 cases of cardiac trauma were among these injuries. Among trauma victims in 1982, 41% died of head injury, 23% of chest injury, and 15% of thoracoabdominal injury. Unfortunately, there is no evidence that the frequency of these injuries is declining or even reaching a plateau. According to another statistic, violent injuries account for most deaths of persons under 40 years of age, and among these victims cardiac trauma is one of the leading causes of death.

CLINICAL SIGNS AND SYMPTOMS

A patient with traumatic heart disease usually has a history of a violent accident. The signs and symptoms may be delayed and not present when the patient is first seen, especially in the case of nonpenetrating cardiac injury. The absence of overt cardiac injury following a major trauma does not necessarily exclude the possibility of such an event. Historically, the most common cause of blunt trauma to the heart is vehicular accidents, usually resulting in "steering wheel syndrome." A blow to the chest by a clenched fist or different types of sporting equipment, as well as kicks of animals, falls, fracture of the bony structure of the anterior chest, and, ironically, cardiopulmonary resuscitation may lead to significant cardiac trauma.

Penetrating injuries are usually diagnosed more easily. An exception is the apparently innocuous penetrating blow to the chest, neck, or abdomen resulting in an obscure cardiac injury without significant initial manifestations.

MYOCARDIAL CONTUSION

Symptoms and signs of myocardial contusion usually depend on the extent of injury. Often there is no initial cardiac symptom. Anginal pain, early signs of congestive failure, arrhythmias, and heart block may be the prevailing manifestations. Rarely, murmurs and a gallop sound will be heard. Pericarditis and at times postpericarditis syndrome may become a problem. The most common cause of death in this group of patients is cardiac arrhythmias.

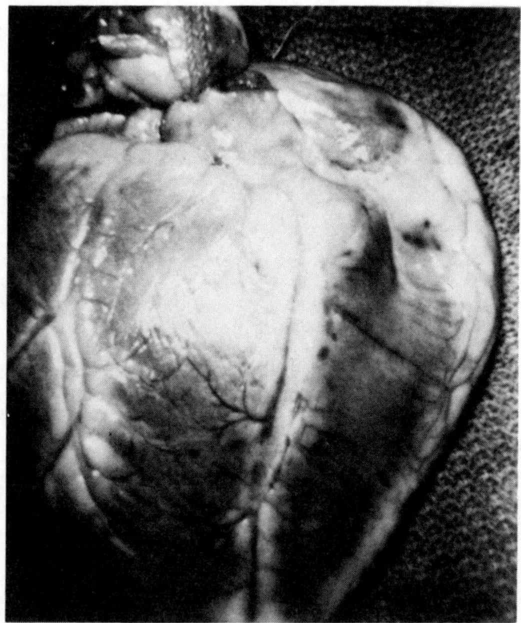

FIG 27–1.
Cardiac contusion of the posterior wall injury due to blunt trauma (From Symbas PN: *Traumatic Injuries of the Heart and Great Vessels.* Springfield, Ill; Charles C Thomas, Publisher, 1972; p 41. Reproduced by permission.)

PENETRATING INJURIES

Penetrating cardiac trauma in civilian life is usually caused by bullets, pellets, knives, fractured ribs or sternum, and rarely ice picks and other projectiles. Penetrating cardiac injury in military life is almost always the result of high-speed projectiles.

The pathophysiology of penetrating cardiac injury is relative to the size, site, and mode of penetration. From a practical point of view, one should determine whether an open pericardial wound is producing signs of hemorrhage and shock or of an obliterated pericardium with intrapericardial bleeding, which may rapidly lead to fatal cardiac tamponade. Primary penetrating wounds may occur in the chest, neck, or upper abdomen. The mortality rate from penetrating cardiac trauma remains between 60% and 80%.

PATHOPHYSIOLOGY

The pathophysiology of traumatic heart disease is complex because cardiac structures are numerous and varied.

MYOCARDIAL CONTUSION

Myocardial contusion usually occurs from either sudden acceleration or deceleration of the heart, causing the cardiac structure to be thrust against the sternum, ribs, or vertebrae. The force may be applied directly against the chest or may be bidirectional against the thorax. Increased intravascular pressure, decelerative, blast, concussive forces, or a combination of any or all of these factors may be responsible for the cardiac injury. The most common specific cause is the chest hitting the steering wheel, which results in the "steering wheel syndrome."

Pathologic study may reveal subendocardial or subepicardial hemorrhage (Fig 27–1). Not infrequently intramural bleeding results in myocardial dysfunction and, rarely, congestive failure. Myocardial rupture may occur after cardiac contusion as a consequence of the rapid increase in thoracic or intra-abdominal pressure. Subepicardial hemorrhage usually occurs near the large coronary arteries. The myocardium or pericardium may be lacerated; the conduction system may be damaged; the normal cardiac rhythm may be disrupted; and the valvular structures may be injured.

CLINICAL–PATHOLOGIC CORRELATIONS

MYOCARDIAL CONTUSION

Nonpenetrating injuries may result in myocardial laceration, intramural hemorrhage, and, less frequently, damage to epicardial coronary arteries. Any of these lesions may produce angina. There may be chest pain due to pericardial irritation (Table 27–1).

Rupture of the heart in nonpenetrating injury is possible, but rare. The signs and symptoms of rupture of the heart are catastrophic, with manifestations of refractory shock and at times electromechanical dissociation.

Nonpenetrating injuries may produce symptoms of myocardial infarction, but a typical electrocardiographic evolution of infarction is rare. Other electrocardiographic changes are usually limited to repolarization abnormalities. Serial electrocardiograms are essential; the initial electrocardiograms may be negative. Conduction abnormalities and arrhythmias are not uncommon. Symptoms typical of pericarditis may result from pericardial irritation. Symptoms associated with the so-called Dressler's syndrome occur rarely. A variety of cardiac murmurs may result from valvular injury.

PENETRATING INJURIES

In patients with penetrating cardiac trauma the clinical picture is usually impressive. A variety of lesions result from stab or bullet wounds. The structures most damaged, in order of frequency, are the right ventricle, left ventricle, right atrium, left atrium, and the coronary arteries. Bullet wounds most commonly cause disruption of the left ventricle, right ventricle, right atrium and left atrium, and coronary arteries (Table 27–2). Symptomatically, there may be an insidious initial presentation. If the patient survives the injury itself, complications such as permanent disorders of the cardiac conduction system, arrhythmias, endocarditis, and pericarditis may occur (Fig 27–2).

Soft heart sounds (at times absent cardiac sounds) may be the initial manifestation. Paradoxic pulse may be difficult to determine because of the combination of hypovolemia and tamponade. Central venous pressure is important but may be difficult to measure.

Delayed sequelae of traumatic heart disease are related to the segment of the heart that is damaged. Aortocardiac, aortopulmonary, coronary AV, and coronary–cardiac chamber fistulas may occur. A ventricular aneurysm (true or false) may develop. A ventricular septal defect, valvular defects, relapsing pericarditis, and neurotic manifestations are considered late sequelae.

DIFFERENTIAL DIAGNOSIS

The differential diagnosis includes any catastrophic trauma. It is imperative to identify traumatic heart damage because it drastically affects the course of early treatment. The most important study to differentiate penetrating cardiac trauma from other causes of shock is a meticulous search for cardiac tamponade. Preexisting cardiovascular disorders may pose problems in accurate evaluation. An important differentiating point is the presence of tamponade.

TABLE 27–1.
Pathologic Findings in Cardiac Trauma

Myocardial injury
  Contusion (most common)
  Rupture
  Laceration
  Infarction or aneurysm
Conduction system disorder
Pericardial injury
  Rupture
  Laceration
  Pericarditis
  Hemopericardium
Coronary artery injury
Valvular damage
Great-vessel injury
  Rupture
  Aneurysm or fistula
  Thrombosis

TABLE 27–2.
Penetrating Cardiac Trauma

Myocardial injury
  Myocardial damage and infarction
  Myocardial rupture and tamponade
  Aneurysmal formation
  Ventricular septal defect
  Fistula
  Rupture of papillary muscle or chordae tendineae
  Valvular cusp injury
Pericardial injury
  Laceration
  Perforation
  Hemopericardium or pneumopericardium
  Pericarditis
  Constrictive pericarditis
Coronary artery injury
  Rupture or laceration (could cause acute myocardial infarction)
  Thrombosis (could cause acute myocardial infarction)
  Fistula or aneurysm
Retained foreign object (missile in the heart)
  Endocarditis
  Thromboembolism
Disturbances of the conduction system (temporary or permanent)

DIAGNOSIS

When clinical events suggest possible cardiac contusion, serial electrocardiograms are the key diagnostic studies. A typical elevation of serum creatinine kinase–myocardial band (CK–MB) followed by a rapid decline, if present, is a helpful finding, especially if the rise is followed by a subsequent rise in levels of SGOT and hydroxybutyric dehydrogenase (HBD). An echocardiogram, especially a two-dimensional echocardiogram, could be beneficial. At times, cardiac angiography and radionuclide studies are required for a more objective diagnosis.

PENETRATING INJURIES

Small wounds, particularly stab wounds, may cause slow bleeding leading to defibrination of the blood with no clot formation. Larger wounds cause the clotting of blood within the pericardial sac, hence pericardiocentesis has limited benefit. If the rate of accumulation is very rapid, volumes of as little as 60 ml to 100 ml of blood within the pericardial sac could cause tamponade. This is especially likely if there is a preexisting low-output state, severe left- and right-ventricular disease, dehydration, or anemia. On the other hand, the development of cardiac tamponade could be delayed if the accumulation is gradual (over days or weeks); in this circumstance, several liters of fluid and blood may accumulate in the pericardium.

The clinical manifestation of tamponade includes a state of shock plus specific features of tamponade: agitation, confusion, air hunger, cold and clammy skin, distention of the jugular veins (Kussmaul's sign), paradoxical pulse, and soft heart sounds. Kussmaul's sign, distention of the neck veins during inspiration, is a result of compression of the right side of the heart during inspiration from the excessive rise in intra-pericardial pressure. Normally, the negative intrathoracic pressure generated during inspiration causes collapse of the cervical veins. With tamponade, accelerated flow to the heart during inspiration is not well tolerated because of constriction of the right side of the heart secondary to increased intrapericardial pressure. This increases jugular venous pressure during inspiration, in essence a paradoxical phenomenon, and thereby distends the neck veins.

Paradoxical pulse, on the other hand, is not a truly paradoxical phenomenon because normally there may be a 5- to 10-mm Hg drop in arterial blood pressure during inspiration. By definition, paradoxical pulse is present when arterial pressure decreases more than 10 mm Hg during inspiration. The best way to measure paradoxical pulse is to let the patient breathe normally while inflating the blood pressure cuff until the Korotkoff sounds and the arterial pulse completely disappear. The cuff is then very slowly deflated. The first few Korotkoff sounds that are heard will be intermittent because there is a significant drop in blood pressure during inspiration. This number is registered and deflation of the cuff continued gently until there is one-to-one transmission of the arterial pulse and regular Korotkoff sounds. The difference between these two readings is defined as the measure of paradoxical pulse.

A paradoxical pulse of 30 mm Hg or more (normal <10) when there is tamponade is not

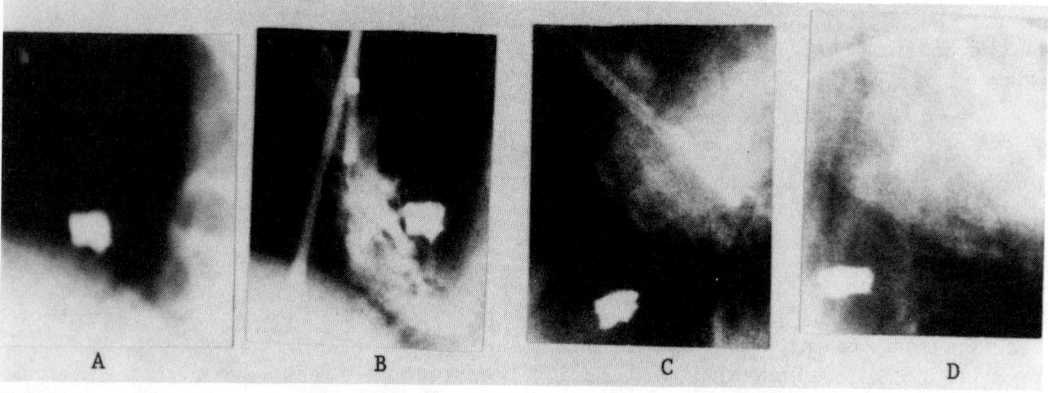

FIG 27–2.
Angiogram made in 1985 showing shrapnel fragment embedded in the inferior myocardium during World War II. Forty years later the patient needed cardiac catheterization because of unstable angina and was found to have severe multivessel coronary artery disease. He underwent coronary artery bypass surgery and did well. The shrapnel fragment was left in place (personal collection).

unusual. Chronic obstructive pulmonary disease, constrictive pericarditis, and cardiomyopathy may cause confusion because they can lead to a significant degree of paradoxical pulse.

It is imperative for both diagnosis and treatment to establish an intravenous line to measure central venous pressure, usually a subclavian or internal jugular line (Table 27–3). The pressure line should be adjusted to read 0 cm of H_2O with the transducer in midaxillary line at the fourth intercostal space. The saline solution should fluctuate freely with respiration. The measurement should be done when the patient is quiet. If the central venous pressure in a hypotensive patient is about 12 cm H_2O and rapidly rises with IV infusion of crystalloids, there is cardiac tamponade (Table 27–4). If the central venous pressure does not increase with a significant fluid challenge, the patient is hypovolemic, which commonly reflects significant hemorrhage into the pleural space, abdomen, or other compartments.

The intravenous line for measuring the central venous pressure may also be used for the rapid administration of fluids, blood, and pharmacologic agents.

PRINCIPLES OF PREVENTION AND THERAPY

While prevention of cardiac trauma is very difficult if not impossible, control of drunk driving, mandatory use of seat belts, and installation of air bags may reduce the incidence and extent of cardiac trauma caused by vehicular accidents. Prevention or reduction of cardiac damage inflicted by sharp objects, bullets, and projectiles is difficult if not impossible. In

TABLE 27–3.
Treatment of Traumatic Heart Disease

1. Establish a central intravenous line.
   a. Measure CVP.
   b. Administer fluids and blood.
2. Pericardiocentesis if patient in tamponade (while preparing operating room)
3. Thoracotomy under general (or no) anesthesia to establish acceptable vital signs and vital function
4. Repair intracardiac defect during emergency operation only if patient would not survive without it.

TABLE 27–4.
Hemodynamic Alterations in Tamponade

CVP

1. Zero level in midaxillary line, 4th intercostal space.
2. Saline solution column should fluctuate freely with respiration.
3. Measure when the patient is quiet.

If the CVP in a hypotensive patient is about 12 cm water and rapidly rises with IV infusion of crystalloids, tamponade is most likely.

peacetime, some feel gun control would be a positive step.

Hypovolemia not associated with tamponade is treated with rapid administration of crystalloids, colloids, and blood. Prompt treatment of tamponade with pericardiocentesis may provide the necessary time for emergency surgical intervention.

The goal of an acute thoracotomy is to establish acceptable vital signs and vital function. The repair of complex intracardiac defects during the acute phase is not usually well tolerated. These defects are best repaired electively after the patient recovers and appropriate angiographic studies have been made.

REFERENCES

Bland EF, Beebe GW: Missiles in the heart: A 20 year follow-up report of World War II cases. *N Engl J Med* 1966; 274:1039–1047. *Reports EKG findings and discusses selected cases.*

Braunwald E (ed): *Heart Disease.* Philadelphia, WB Saunders Co, 1984. *In-depth well-referenced discussion.*

Breaux EP, Dupont JB, Albert HM, et al.: Cardiac tamponade following penetrating mediastinal injuries: Improved survival with early pericardiocentesis. *J Trauma* 1979, 19:461–466. *A high index of suspicion is required.*

Hurst W (ed): *The Heart.* New York, McGraw-Hill Book Co, 1986. *A comprehensive discussion.*

Jones JW, Hewitt RL, Drapanas T: Cardiac contusion: A capricious syndrome. *Ann Surg* 1975; 181:567–574.

Moncure AC, McEnany MT: Cardiovascular emergencies, in Wilkins EW (ed): *MGH Testbook of Emergency Medicine*. Baltimore, Williams & Wilkins Co, 1983. *Diagnosis and treatment in the emergency room.*

Sugg WL, Rea WJ, Ecker RR, et al.: Penetrating wounds of the heart: An analysis of 459 cases. *J Thorac Cardiovasc Surg* 1968; 56:531–545. *A detailed clinical analysis.*

Symbas PN: Traumatic heart disease. *Curr Probl Cardiol* 1982; 1:7–35. *A discussion of the major presentations and diagnosis.*

Symbas PN, Harlaftis N, Waldo WJ: Penetrating cardiac wounds: A comparison of different therapeutic methods. *Ann Surg* 1976; 183:377–381. *A comprehensive discussion of therapy.*

Weinberg SL, Schoenwetter A: Auricular flutter and indirect cardiac trauma. *Arch Intern Med* 1951; 83:252–257. *A complication of indirect cardiac trauma.*

28   PERIPHERAL ARTERY DISEASE

Margaret M. Dunn, M.D.

Peripheral arterial disease most commonly affects the lower extremities and most often is arteriosclerotic in origin. The usual patterns of arteriosclerotic lesions, the greater circulatory demand of the lower extremities, and relative abundance of arterial supply to the upper extremities all contribute to the usual presentation of arterial insufficiency in the legs. In obstructive arterial disease the clinical picture will depend on the duration and distribution of lesions. The development of collateral arterial pathways as a result of chronic insufficiency as well as the exercise limitations imposed by concomitant cardiopulmonary disease may allow extensive obstructive arterial disease to be clinically asymptomatic. Therapy is not indicated in cases without significant flow reduction and symptomatic tissue ischemia, despite multiple anatomic lesions. Atherosclerosis and diabetes mellitus will underlie the vast majority of arterial insufficiency. The following discussion will focus on lesions of the major peripheral arteries. Vasospasm and endarteritis, both often associated with collagen vascular diseases, may also produce peripheral arterial insufficiency, particularly in the hand. Aneurysms, the second most common problem of the aorta and its branches, are often asymptomatic, but when discovered deserve treatment before the development of catastrophic complications such as rupture and thrombosis.

CLINICAL SIGNS AND SYMPTOMS

In chronic occlusive disease, claudication, from the Latin *claudicare* "to limp," will be an early symptom. Claudication is defined as the onset of crampy discomfort in the calf, thigh, or buttock muscles which is relieved by rest. The onset of claudication with a set distance walked and its relief with a discrete period of rest is predictable. "Rest pain," a burning sensation of the toes or forefoot often requiring narcotics for relief, is a sign of arterial inflow insufficient for basal perfusion demands. The onset of rest pain may be induced by assumption of the supine position. Dependency, which produces a normally insignificant augmentation in blood flow from gravity, often brings relief. Impotence together with thigh and buttock claudication constitute Leriche's syndrome of aortoiliac insufficiency.

On physical examination, there may be no signs of arterial insufficiency in the claudicating extremity at rest. Distal pulses may even be present, though immediately after exercise they will be diminished. Atrophic hairless skin below midcalf, dependent rubor, pallor on elevation, and cool skin are associated with more advanced ischemia. In aortoiliac occlusive disease the femoral pulses will be diminished, absent, or have a thrill or bruit. Absence of the popliteal pulse indicates occlusion of the superficial femoral artery in the absence of aortoiliac disease. Absence of the distal pulses alone is a pattern seen in the diabetic patient in whom severe disease may start just below the trifurcation of the popliteal artery with preservation of the arterial tree above. Skin ulceration of arterial origin will be deep, with irregular edges and poor granulation tissue. Gangrene obviously represents end-stage ischemia. Scattered, discrete petechial lesions suggest an embolic origin. Necrosis may be limited to part or all of a digit or extend further. In "wet" gangrene, cellulitis is present in adjacent viable tissue.

In acute occlusion the patient will present a cool, pale, painful extremity. After a few hours, parethesias will progress to analgesia and paralysis, and the limb may become mottled. The signs and symptoms of pain, pallor, pulselessness, paresis, paralysis, and poikilothermy or coolness constitute the classic "Ps" of acute arterial ischemia. The level of changes will be far distal to the level of arterial obstruction. Femoral artery occlusion will produce findings to the midthigh level, whereas popliteal occlusion will demarcate in midcalf. The development of paralysis and tense, tender swelling of involved muscle indicate the onset of irreversible ischemia.

Abdominal aortic aneurysms may be asymptomatic or may be initially detected by leak or rupture. Abdominal and back pain together with hypotension and pulsatile abdominal mass represent a ruptured abdominal aortic aneurysm until proven otherwise. Aortic aneurysm may also appear with distal embolization, rarely with fistulization into the inferior vena cava and congestive failure, or ureteral obstruction. The most common site of peripheral arterial aneurysm is the popliteal artery. About half of these patients will be asymptomatic. Symptoms may result from acute thrombosis, embolization, and venous or nerve compression. The majority of popliteal aneurysms will be bilateral as well as associated with other aneurysms, usually aortic. A popliteal pulse that is easily felt should raise the suspicion of a popliteal aneurysm. When a popliteal aneurysm presents with thrombosis, no mass may be felt, and the clinical picture is simply that of acute ischemia.

Mild-to-moderate claudication is associated with little increased risk of limb loss. Typically two-thirds of these patients will remain stable or improve, and only 5% will ultimately require amputation. In diabetic patients who continue to smoke, the ultimate risk of amputation is higher. In the face of rest pain or tissue necrosis the immediate risk of amputation is approximately 20%. Because of the systemic nature of the atherosclerotic process, the overall survival rate for patients with intermittent claudication is only 72% at 5 years and 50% at 10 years in contrast to 90% at 5 years for age-matched control subjects with no peripheral arterial disease.

Acute arterial ischemia will begin to produce irreversible nerve and muscle damage after 6 to 8 hours. Occasionally spontaneous improvement may be seen in the patient who sustains an acute thrombosis in the face of chronic ischemia and has previously developed collaterals. However, progressive untreated tissue necrosis will result in limb loss. Renal failure secondary to myoglobinuria and cardiac dysrhythmias from hyperkalemia are possible complications of late untreated acute necrosis.

The natural history of abdominal aortic aneurysms was studied prior to the advent of aortic surgery. The 5-year survival of patients presenting with nonleaking abdominal aortic aneurysms is about 30%, with 40% dying of other largely arteriosclerotic problems and 40% from rupture of their aneurysms. The survival rate after surgical correction of a leaking or ruptured aneurysm is less than 50%. The risk of rupture in abdominal aortic aneurysm is less than 15% for a 4-cm aneurysm and greater than 75% for an 8-cm aneurysm. The major catastrophic complication of popliteal aneurysms is thrombosis with resultant limb loss rather than rupture. In a study that followed 100 cases of popliteal aneurysms, only about 20% were asymptomatic over 5 years. The risk of limb loss, however, is far greater after acute thrombosis. The incidence of acute thrombosis is not affected by aneurysm size and is not necessarily preceded by any chronic symptoms.

PATHOPHYSIOLOGY

Atherosclerosis is the leading cause of occlusive and aneurysmal. vascular disease. The three major risk factors contributing to atherosclerosis are hypertension, hypercholesterolemia, and smoking. Diabetes mellitus is a minor risk factor for atherosclerosis. However, the increased risk of infection in diabetes together with peripheral neuropathy and any major arterial obstruction produces the difficult clinical problem of the diabetic foot.

Atheromas are characterized by intimal smooth muscle proliferation and lipid infiltration. An atherosclerotic plaque can ulcerate and embolize platelet debris or atheromatous material as well as produce stenosis. Complete occlusion will generally result from superimposed thrombosis or hemorrhage into the plaque. Atheromas most often occur at arterial bifucations, at the sites of major arterial branches, or at points such as the adductor canal where an artery passes through a muscle sling. The flow alteration induced by all these situations produces turbulence and some intimal damage, predisposing to plaque formation. The most common sites of occlusive disease are the superficial femoral artery and the aortic bifurcation.

Atherosclerotic lesions producing sufficient stenosis to reduce flow can produce chronic arterial insufficiency. Flow within an artery (Q) will be directly proportional to arterial pressure (D) and inversely proportional to peripheral resistance (R) or

$$Q = P/R$$

The Poiseuille equation expresses the pressure–flow relationship within a length of a rigid cylindrical tube.

$$Q = (P_1 - P_2) \cdot \pi r^4/8L\eta$$

where $P_1 = P_2$ is the pressure differential, r is the radius, L is the length, and η is the viscosity. Pulsatile in vivo arterial flow is only roughly described by this equation, but obviously the radius of a stenotic segment is the major factor limiting flow. The relationship between the radius of a stenotic segment and the flow is exponential. A "critical stenosis" or one that significantly affects hemodynamics must reduce the cross-sectional area by at least 75%.

In the face of chronic stenosis, collateral vessels will develop. The pressure differential created by a significant arterial occlusion contributes to reversal of the flow direction in minor arterial branches that arise distal but course proximally. The development of a collateral bed will decrease total peripheral resistance and will tend to mitigate the effects of arterial occlusive disease.

Acute occlusion results from thrombosis or embolism. Emboli most commonly arise from the heart. Emboli from arteriosclerotic ulcerations or of aneurysm content will be small enough to progress distally in the absence of obstruction and produce punctate distal necrosis. Larger emboli will often lodge at bifurcations or branches where the arterial lumen is abruptly reduced. If acute occlusion occurs in presence of chronic disease, the developed collateral circulation may often compensate.

The distal abdominal aorta is the most common site of aneurysm formation, and more than 90% of these aneurysms will be atherosclerotic in origin. The arteriosclerotic process extends into the media with disruption of collagen and elastin. There is some evidence to suggest an inherited collagen defect in some patients with arteriosclerotic aneurysms. Other causes include mechanical factors as in poststenotic aneurysms as well as infection, congenital diseases such as Marfan's syndrome, and conditions producing mural degeneration such as pregnancy. The tension of the aneurysm wall (T) will be directly proportional to the pressure (P) and radius (r) as in Laplaces' law.

$$T = Pr$$

in accordance with the observation that larger aneurysms have a greater risk of rupture.

CLINICAL–PATHOLOGIC CORRELATIONS

The major signs and symptoms of insufficiency with the corresponding noninvasive pressure data are reviewed in Table 28–1.

DIFFERENTIAL DIAGNOSIS

In occlusive arterial disease, diagnosis can almost always be made on the basis of the patient's history and physical examination. The differential diagnoses of extremity pain and ulceration are reviewed in Tables 28–2 and 28–3. In a few patients with claudication, no signs of arterial insufficiency may be found on routine examination, and evaluation during and after exercise may be required. In contrast, evidence of arterial insufficiency on examination may be seen in patients with extremity pain from other causes such as diabetic neuropathy or causalgia. The presence of sensory neu-

rologic changes as well as the lack of arterial occlusive disease severe enough to produce rest pain would suggest that symptoms might not be ischemic in origin, despite some arterial compromise.

In the abdomen, an ectatic aorta as well as an abdominal mass overlying the aorta and transmitting its impulse such as a pancreatic malignancy can be confused with an aneurysm. In the popliteal fossa a Baker's cyst must be excluded. In both cases, ultrasonography or computed tomography (CT scanning) should be helpful in establishing a diagnosis.

DIAGNOSIS

The Doppler stethoscope can be used to detect flow in vessels without palpable pulses. Audibly pulsatile and nonpulsatile arterial flow, as well as venous flow, can be differentiated from each other. Systolic pressure measurements can be obtained using a proximal cuff. Distal lower extremity pressures are often expressed as a ratio or index between the pressure measured at the brachial level and pressures at the popliteal, posterior tibial, or dorsalis pedis levels. When the ankle pressures are used, this is referred to as the ankle-systolic index or ASI. The normal index is 1.10. Rest pain or tissue necrosis will usually be associated with an index of less than 0.3 and an absolute pressure of less than 50 mm Hg (Table 28–1).

In some diabetic patients, calcification of the media will falsely elevate these pressures to give indices of greater than 1.0 in the face of advanced ischemia. More sophisticated devices available can determine the direction of flow

TABLE 28–1.
Clinical–Pathologic Correlations for Peripheral Arterial Disease*

	PATHOLOGIC FINDINGS	
CLINICAL FINDINGS	FLOW CHARACTERISTICS	ANKLE SYSTOLIC INDEX MEAN ± SEM
Claudication	Normal resting flow diminished; increased with exercise	0.59 ± 0.15
Rest pain	Diminished resting flow	0.26 ± 0.13
Impending gangrene	Insufficient nutrient flow	0.05 ± 0.08

* Adapted from Yao ST: Hemodynamic studies in peripheral arterial disease. *Br J Surg* 1970; 57:761. By permission of the publishers, Butterworth & Co.

TABLE 28–2.
Differential Diagnosis of Painful Extremity

	CHARACTERISTICS OF PAIN FROM VARIOUS SITES				
CONDITION	ARTERY	VEIN	MUSCLE	JOINT	NERVE
Dependency	Decrease	Increase	No change	No change	No change
Onset with exercise	Yes	No	Yes	Yes	No
Relief with exercise	Yes	No	Yes or no	Yes or no	No
Noctural	Yes	No	No	No	Yes
Reproducibility	Yes	No	No	No	Yes

and can produce wave-form tracings for analysis. The pulse–volume recorder, which measures changes in the volume of the extremity with flow, can also be used for noninvasive assessment of the arterial and venous circulation. All these techniques can be used for quantitation of baseline status and for follow-up and postoperative assessment. Wave-form and pressure analysis can help determine additional distal levels of obstruction when distal pulses are absent from a proximal lesion (e.g., the additional presence of femoral popliteal disease when all pulses are absent from aortoiliac occlusion).

ULTRASONOGRAPHY

Because aneurysms typically have a normal-sized lumen through an organized clot that fills the aneurysm sac, ultrasonography (or CT scanning) rather than angiography is the procedure used for establishing the presence of an aneurysm and quantitating its dimensions. Because angiography only defines intraluminal anatomy rather than the external arterial wall, aneurysms can be completely missed on angiography. Ultrasonography or CT scanning can also demonstrate an acute leak into the aneurysm wall or the retroperitoneum.

ANGIOGRAPHY

Angiography by the transfemoral or translumbar route will document the basic vascular anatomy and the levels of obstruction and will define vessels reconstituted by collateral flow distal to occlusive lesions. Without biplanar views, assessment of the iliac and profunda femoris arteries is limited because the often-posterior plaques in these vessels may simply attentuate rather than narrow the contrast

column. Noninvasive testing rather than angiography is far more useful in determining the actual changes in flow produced by occlusive arterial disease. Angiography in general should be reserved for the patient with indications for vascular reconstruction who is a surgical candidate.

PRINCIPLES OF TREATMENT

The management of chronic arterial ischemia depends on the degree of functional compromise. Mild to moderate claudication will initially be treated by a program of exercise to tolerance and cessation of smoking. Exercise therapy can provide relief by encouraging collateral dilation. Trental, a xanthine derivative, has recently been introduced as a rheostatic agent, but has had only limited clinical use in the United States. The available oral vasodilators have little to no effect on either plaque or collateral vessels and so are ineffective.

Surgery may be considered for patients with claudication limiting their ability to work or unacceptably altering their life-style. Patients with rest pain or tissue necrosis should be evaluated for limb-salvage reconstruction. Inability to ambulate for other reasons (e.g., hemiplegia following a stroke) constitutes a relative contraindication to aggressive vascular reconstruction. Improvement in perioperative management and the development of lower-risk extra anatomical procedures have lowered the operative mortality of reconstruction, so it is often lower than the operative mortality of major amputation. Angiography is reserved for candidates for reconstruction and is performed in a well-hydrated patient to prevent renal injury. Balloon angioplasty by a percutaneous route can be useful on selected lesions, particu-

TABLE 28–3.
Differential Diagnosis of Common Leg Ulcers*

FEATURE	CHARACTERISTICS OF ULCERS FROM VARIOUS CAUSES		
	ARTERIAL	VENOUS	DIABETIC
Location	Distal dorsal foot or toes	Lower third of leg (gaiter area)	Under calluses or pressure points (plantar aspect of 1st or 5th metatarsal-phalangeal joint)
Pain	Severe, particularly at night, relieved by dependency	Mild, relieved by elevation	None
Bleeding with manipulation	Little or none	Venous ooze	Brisk
Wound characteristics	Irregular edge, poor granulation tissue	Shallow, irregular shape, granulating base, rounded edges	Punched out deep sinus
Associated	Trophic changes of chronic ischemia	Stasis dermatitis	Neuropathy

* Adapted from Rutherford RB: *The Vascular Consultation in Vascular Surgery,* ed 2. Philadelphia, WB Saunders Co, 1984, p 10.

larly in the iliac arteries. Bypass of obstructing arterial lesions can be accomplished with saphenous or cephalic vein grafts as well as a variety of synthetic conduits. Long-term patency of distal below-knee bypass grafts is significantly higher with an autogenous vein graft.

Amputation is performed for control of infection, necrosis, or pain. It should be performed at a level where there is sufficient blood supply to allow healing of the amputation site itself. Local amputation, limited to the foot, should be performed only when the presence of distal pulses or when favorable noninvasive test results suggest a possibility of healing, or when it is combined with reconstruction. Similarly, the decision to perform below- or above-knee amputation should be based on the presence of pulses or on noninvasive pressure measurements supporting the expectation of healing. Compared with above-knee amputations, below-knee amputations allow better mobility with a prosthesis and ambulation.

In acute ischemia, treatment will depend on whether the limb is threatened and whether it is still viable. Usually angiography will be necessary to determine whether the cause is an embolus or a thrombus superimposed on chronic disease. Heparin is administered intravenously to halt further proximal propagation of thrombosis. Surgical correction will not be indicated if the limb improves sufficiently with heparin to not be in danger of immediate loss or if the limb is no longer viable. Results of revascularization done after 6 to 8 hours of ischemia will be poor, and the return of the venous blood with the ischemic limb can cause severe cardiac arrhythmias and arrest. Embolectomy can be performed with a balloon catheter often under local anesthesia. Thrombosis of previously diseased vessels will require correction or bypass of the underlying obstruction as well as thrombectomy.

Abdominal aortic aneurysms of 5-cm diameter or more should be treated surgically because at this size the risk of rupture and death is greater than the operative mortality. Symptoms of any sort or rapid growth are also indications. Popliteal or peripheral aneurysms of any size should be repaired. For both aortic and popliteal aneurysms, the current treatment consists of bypass of the aneurysm with ligation proximally and distally and placement of the graft within the opened aneurysmal artery.

REFERENCES

Barnes RW: Hemodynamics for the vascular surgeon. *Arch Surg* 1980; 115:216–223. *A good summary of this area.*

Blaisdell FW, Steele M, Allen RE: Management of acute lower extremity arterial ischemia due to embolism and thrombosis. *Surgery* 1978; 84:822–834. *A now-classic paper on this subject.*

Imparato A: Intermittent claudication: Its natural course. *Surgery* 1975; 78:795–799. *A review of the natural history with angiographically defined lesions.*

Kempczinski RF, Bernhard VM: The management of chronic ischemia of the lower extremities, in Rutherford RB (ed): *Vascular Surgery*, ed 2. Philadelphia, WB Saunders Co, 1984, pp 547–557. *Excellent introduction to a complex topic.*

Rutherford RB: The vascular consultation, in Rutherford RB (ed): *Vascular Surgery*, ed 2. Philadelphia, WB Saunders Co, 1984, pp 1–10. *Good overview of the initial clinical evaluation in vascular disease.*

Walker WF: *Color Atlas of Peripheral Vascular Diseases.* Chicago, Year Book Medical Publishers, 1980. *A thorough review of physical and angiographic findings in vascular disease.*

29 VENOUS INSUFFICIENCY

James B. Peoples, M.D.

Venous insufficiency is the condition arising when venous blood flow from an organ or body part is less than arterial blood flow to the organ or part. Although the condition can occur both systemically and locally secondary to another disease, such as with congestive heart failure or cirrhosis of the liver, its occurrence as a primary disease is restricted nearly always to the lower extremities.

CLINICAL SIGNS AND SYMPTOMS

Venous insufficiency of the lower extremities is a disease with a spectrum ranging from simple varicose veins to tissue necrosis. The initial signs and symptoms depend both on the stage of the disease at the time the patient seeks medical attention and also on whether the superficial, the deep, or both venous systems of the legs are involved.

Simple varicose veins are the most common and least serious form of this disease. Patients may complain only of unattractive bulges on their legs, or they may be affected with calf pain, ankle swelling, or both. The pain and swelling are characterized as worsening with prolonged standing or sitting and improving with elevation of the legs or lying down. The pain is described as aching. Frequently, a family history of similar problems is obtained.

Physical examination may disclose only dilated, tortuous subcutaneous veins. These will empty with leg elevation and fill with leg dependency. A tourniquet placed on the thigh while the leg is elevated will prevent filling of the veins when the patient stands (Trendelenburg's test). There is no tenderness of either the skin, muscles, or veins themselves. A pitting edema of the postmalleolar area may be demonstrated. Rarely, such varicosities may be ignored by the patient until rupture with hemorrhage or overlying skin necrosis with ulceration occurs. The natural history of varicosities is variable. In men, they seem to slowly progress in size and symptomatology with age. In women, they more frequently fluctuate in severity with the menstrual cycle and quite often regress following menopause.

Varicose veins/venous insufficiency of the deep venous system, usually because of chronic obstruction, leads to a more serious situation. People so afflicted present early with moderate-to-severe aching pain, marked swelling, and, frequently, early skin changes. Although the pain is identical to that due to only superficial disease, the severity is more marked. It occurs earlier on after standing and takes longer to abate when the legs are elevated. Edema behaves similarly. Unlike with superficial disease, the varicose veins are generally not visible. Skin changes due to pigmentation from the iron in trapped red cells leads to the typical appearance of venous stasis dermatitis. The skin also becomes thickened and coarse. As the disease progresses, multiple confluent ulcerations occur with repeated episodes of supervening cellulitis. Prolonged leg elevation lasting several days may be required to reduce the swelling. Eventually, untreated limbs will succumb to either a life-threatening invasive infection or blood flow reduction to the point that limb death results. In either case, amputation is generally required.

PATHOPHYSIOLOGY

In most cases, superficial venous disease is due to venous valve incompetency, whereas deep venous disease is due to venous obstruction. Valvular incompetency is due in some cases to congential absence of a specific valve or valves and in other cases to destruction of the valve leaf by phlebitis or to dilatation of the valve annulus due to obesity or pregnancy. Venous obstruction is nearly always due to recurrent episodes of thrombophlebitis, but occasionally is clearly related to a long-bone fracture or other similar injury. In either case, the resulting inflammatory reaction leads to progressive thrombosis and fibrosis of the vein. In rare cases, obstruction may be caused by extrinsic vein compression by either a neoplasm or inflammatory reaction. Macroscopically, varicose veins are characterized as elongated in their longitudinal axis with lumen dilatation. Occluded veins have no lumen and appear shrunken and fibrosed. Microscopically, varicosities display thickening of the media, whereas the normal tissue walls of occluded veins are nearly completely replaced by fibrotic tissue.

More important is the pathophysiology. Increases in the resting pressure of either the superficial or deep venous systems result in dilatation of the veins, and edema is produced according to Starling's equation. Increases in either the venous pressure or the resistance tend to decrease capillary blood flow proximally. This leads to blood stagnation and reduction in oxygen delivery by the arterioles. It also results in thrombosis of capillary beds and venules with a further increase in resistance and further decrease in oxygen delivery. Ultimately, reduced oxygenation will lead to cell death, skin necrosis, ulceration, and gangrene. The problem is compounded when secondary infection occurs by the inability of leukocytes to reach the site through the arterioles.

CLINICAL–PATHOLOGIC CORRELATIONS

The clinical features of venous insufficiency are the results of (1) venous obstruction or valvular imcompetency leading to (2) increased venous pressure or resistance or both causing (3) decreased venous blood flow and inadequate tissue oxygenation. A summary of the clinical–pathologic correlations are shown in Table 29–1.

DIFFERENTIAL DIAGNOSIS

Differential diagnosis of superficial venous disease is relatively simple. The major pitfall is to ascribe erroneously the symptoms of pain or swelling to visible, obvious varicosities. Diseases such as lumbar disc herniation, arthritis, spinal stenosis, muscular spasms, sprains, strains, and contusions may all have pain similar to that in a patient with varicose veins. Spinal disease generally produces pain that is aggravated by sitting and relieved by standing, whereas venous insufficiency pain is always made worse by standing. The various traumatic conditions of the musculoskeletal system produce pain that is reproduced by passive motion or palpation of the extremity. Venous insufficiency pain is not reproducible. Arterial insufficiency pain may also be confused with venous insufficiency pain, but is usually made worse with walking and leg elevation and is relieved by simple standing or leg dangling, which is exactly the reverse of venous insufficiency pain. Edema also must not be assumed to be due to varicose veins. Other causes, such

TABLE 29–1.
Clinical–Pathologic Correlations for Venous Insufficiency

CLINICAL FINDINGS	PATHOLOGIC FINDINGS
Dilated, tortuous superficial veins	Increased superficial venous pressure
Edema	Increased deep venous pressure
Pain	
Stasis dermatitis	Decreased venous blood flow
Thrombosis, micro	
Skin ulceration	Reduced oxygen extraction
Cellulitis	
Necrosis	

as congestive heart failure, myxedema, and hypoproteinemia must be excluded.

Deep venous insufficiency may also be quite obvious, but frequently is quite difficult to differentiate. The major diseases with which it is confused are primary cellulitis of the leg and acute deep venous thrombophlebitis. Because chronic deep venous insufficiency is often complicated by supervening infection, it is sometimes literally impossible to ascertain whether cellulitis alone is present or whether both conditions are present until the infection has been adequately treated. In either case, cellulitis itself is characterized by the signs and symptoms of systemic infection such as fever and chills, a hot, tender leg, and leukocytosis. Likewise, acute deep venous thrombophlebitis and chronic deep venous insufficiency are inexorably intertwined. Many investigators believe that acute, recurrent deep venous thrombophlebitis causes chronic deep venous insufficiency. As with cellulitis, the correct diagnosis may not be possible with the initial examination, but may require treatment for suspected thrombophlebitis on an empirical basis.

DIAGNOSIS

Laboratory testing may be useful for excluding other diseases, but is not useful for proving venous insufficiency. The only definitive test for conclusively demonstrating venous insufficiency is direct ambulatory venous pressure measurement of the affected limb. Normally, in the absence of insufficiency, the pressure will be low at rest and will further decrease with exercise. Patients with obstruction will have at rest a high pressure, which will rise with exercise. Those with incompetent valves will have at rest a high pressure, which will decrease with exercise, but not to normal. Venography, either with radiocontrast material or with radioactive imaging techniques, is useful to determine obstruction, but does not assess either pressure or flow characteristics. Noninvasive techniques of venous assessment such as Doppler examination and plethysmography should be considered.

PRINCIPLES OF THERAPY

The primary goal of therapy is to improve blood flow and reduce stagnation. Superficial vein stripping will completely resolve problems related to this system alone. Rarely, it is possible to surgically bypass segmental deep venous occlusions. For the occasional patient suffering from valvular incompetency of the deep system, it is possible to transplant a functional valve from an arm vein. Most patients with deep venous occlusion are, however, best treated with graded, measured external pressure stockings, which act to increase deep system flow by occlusion of the superficial collaterals. Stockings also reduce edema and prevent superficial blood stagnation. Good patient compliance with support hose and good personal hygiene coupled with early medical therapy for cellulitis and ulceration will generally arrest the disease progression. Reduction in aggravating factors such as obesity, prolonged sitting, or standing are also helpful.

REFERENCES

Cranley JJ: Vascular surgery, in Cranley JJ (ed): *Peripheral Venous Disease*. Philadelphia, JB Lippincott Co, 1975, vol 2, pp 1–350. *Excellent review article.*

DeCamp PT, Schramel RJ, Ray CJ, Feibleman ND, Ward JA, Ochsner A: Ambulatory venous pressure determinations in postphlebitic and related syndromes. *Surgery* 1951; 29:44–70. *Historical interest.*

Hoare MC, Nicolaides AN, Miles CR, Shull K, Jury RP, Needham T, Dudley HAF: The role of primary varicose veins in venous ulceration. *Surgery* 1982; 92:450–453. *Excellent review of recent treatment of venous ulcer pathophysiology.*

Linton RR: The post-thrombotic ulceration of the lower extremity: Its etiology and surgical treatment. *Ann Surg* 1953; 138:415–432. *Historical interest.*

McLachlin AD: Venous disease of the lower extremity. *Curr Prob Surg* Jan 1967; 3–44. *Comprehensive overview.*

Warren R, Thayer TR: Transplantation of the saphenous vein for post-phlebitic stasis. *Surgery* 1954; 35:867–876.

30 DEEP VEIN THROMBOSIS

Steven M. Cohen, M.D.

Deep vein thrombosis (DVT) refers to partial or complete occlusion of one or more deep veins by a thrombus and is usually accompanied by inflammation of the vein and surrounding tissue. In this chapter, discussion is limited to thrombosis of the thigh and leg, which accounts for 95% of all cases of venous thrombosis.

Pulmonary embolism, the major complication of DVT, is one of the leading causes of morbidity and mortality in hospitals and accounts for about 50,000 deaths annually in the United States. About 500,000 nonfatal but clinically significant pulmonary emboli from DVT are estimated to occur yearly in the United States. Clearly the prevention, early diagnosis, and prompt treatment of DVT carries important health and financial implications.

CLINICAL SIGNS AND SYMPTOMS

Basing the diagnosis of DVT on clinical grounds only is extremely unreliable. Objective testing indicates no thrombosis in half the patients thought to have DVT by clinical impression, and there may be few or no symptoms or signs in almost half the documented cases of DVT.

The three most frequent clues to thrombosis are lower extremity pain, tenderness, and unilateral swelling. The pain is typically a dull, heavy ache, often evoked only after exertion. The pain may be located over the site of the thrombus, distal, or even proximal to it. Pain in the gastrocnemius region on dorsiflexion of the foot (Homans' sign) may be a useful clue, but can also be present in a variety of other conditions, particularly muscle strain or hematoma, and may be absent in a large proportion of DVTs.

Pitting edema secondary to venous congestion may be fairly localized to the distal part of the leg or may involve the entire limb in massive ileofemoral thrombosis. A palpable thrombus or cord in a superficial vein with localized erythema, swelling, and tenderness is pathognomonic of superficial phlebitis, but diagnosing an extension of the condition to the deep venous circulation usually requires objective testing. Deep vein cords are only occasionally palpable.

Skin changes frequently accompany DVT. Erythema of all or part of the leg indicates soft tissue inflammation. In severe cases, profound venous congestion with tissue anoxia causes the skin to become cyanotic. If arterial spasm is present, the limb will be cool, pale, and pulseless.

Extensive, potentially fatal DVT can be present with few or no physical signs or symptoms. A high index of suspicion is paramount in all cases of thigh or leg pain, swelling, or erythema.

Left untreated, 20% to 30% of large proximal (above the knee) thrombi may give off emboli that go to the lungs. Between 10% and 30% of calf vein thrombi may propagate above the knee. Thrombi limited to the calf veins rarely embolize or lead to significant postthrombotic sequelae.

The postphlebitic syndrome is a complication in which one or more episodes of DVT destroys the valves of the veins and causes venous congestion. The loss of normal circulation causes chronic swelling, pain, and occasionally ulceration of the skin.

PATHOPHYSIOLOGY

The superficial venous collecting system in the leg drains into the deep system by way of communicating veins. Blood flow is maintained by precapillary arteriolar contraction, the bellows action of the thorax, and right ventricular contraction. Contraction and relaxation of the calf muscles help propel the blood. Unidirectional blood flow is maintained by a series of one-way semilunar valves. Alterations of any of these mechanisms predisposes to the formation of venous thrombi. The clinical conditions that may lead to DVT are listed in Table 30–1.

Venous stasis, hypercoagulability, and injury to the venous endothelium constitute Virchow's triad and are the pathogenic basis of DVT. Table 30–2 lists the clinical risk factors associated with the triad. The risk factors for venous stasis common to DVT and Virchow's triad are immobilization, outflow obstruction secondary to trauma, extrinsic venous compression, previous DVT, congestive heart failure, obesity, and pregnancy.

Hypercoagulability is now recognized as a major factor in the genesis of DVT. Inadequate circulation during venous stasis leads to the retention of activated serum coagulation factors and provides the substrate for thrombus formation. Hypercoagulability is difficult to test objectively, except in the rare cases of a deficiency of protein C, protein S, and antithrombin III. Clinical conditions associated with hypercoagulability and DVT include malignancy, intake of estrogen compounds, surgery, previous DVT, and pregnancy.

When associated with venous stasis or hypercoagulability, injury to the venous endothelial lining may provide a nidus for thrombus formation. Surgery, trauma, fracture, and scarring from previous DVT are all associated with thrombogenesis. After orthopedic procedures of the hip and knee, the lower extremity becomes especially prone to thrombus formation.

Whatever the precipitating event or predisposing factor, the process of thrombus formation is essentially the same. The clotting cascade is activated at a site of vessel injury or venous pooling. Exposure of the endothelial lining stimulates platelet adherence and fibrin deposition, which attracts more platelets. A loose fibrin–platelet mass develops and ensnares leukocytes and erythrocytes. Propagation is rapid and may occur in minutes. Embolization is most likely to occur during the first 3 days of thrombosis because of the weak proximal attachment of the enlarging clot. Organization and recanalization are then established, and the clot becomes more firmly attached. The course of DVT is a balance between factors that promote propagation of the thrombus and those that lead to its removal. Extensive vessel damage or persistent venous congestion leads to further thrombus formation.

Once active thrombosis ceases, fibrinolysis and further organization with recanalization occur, usually within 7 to 10 days. Although partial recanalization after the clot becomes organized results in return of some blood flow through the area, this process commonly involves scarring of the vein and loss of competent semilunar valves. If a large segment of the venous system is involved, blood flow becomes bidirectional and gravity emerges as the

TABLE 30–1.
Clinical Risk Factors for Deep Vein Thrombosis

COMMON	UNCOMMON
Surgery	Deficiencies of
Trauma	Antithrombin III
Immobilization	Protein C
Previous DVT	Protein S
Acute myocardial infarction	Homocystinuria
Paralysis	Systemic lupus erythematosus
Obesity	Polycythemia
Estrogen compounds	
Pregnancy	
Malignancy	
Varicose veins	
Congestive heart failure	
Volume depletion	

TABLE 30–2.
Correlation of Clinical Risk Factors to Virchow's Triad

STASIS

Immobilization due to
  Surgery
  Trauma/fracture
  Prolonged bedrest
  Prolonged sitting
  Paralysis
Congestive heart failure
Acute myocardial infarction
Volume depletion
Obesity
Varicose veins
Extrinsic venous pressure
Previous DVT
Pregnancy

INJURY TO VESSEL WALL

Trauma
Surgery
Previous DVT
Infection/inflammation

HYPERCOAGULABILITY

Estrogen compound intake
Pregnancy
Surgery
Malignancy
Hemolytic anemia
Polycythemia vera
Systemic lupus erythematosus
Previous DVT

primary force directing circulation. This results in chronic swelling and pain in the leg, and occasionally the postphlebitic syndrome.

CLINICAL–PATHOLOGIC CORRELATIONS

Correlations of the clinical signs and symptoms with the underlying pathologic processes are presented in Table 30–3.

DIFFERENTIAL DIAGNOSIS

The differential diagnosis of the acutely painful and swollen thigh or leg encompasses a wide variety of conditions both common and rare. The most common illnesses confused with DVT are orthopedic problems, which account for about 40% of all cases. Strained or torn muscles or tendons may be difficult to differentiate from DVT because pain after exertion, lo-

calized tenderness, and erythema are common to both conditions. A palpable gap produced by a muscle tear may be a useful differentiating point, but further objective testing is usually required.

A ruptured popliteal cyst (Baker's cyst) often mimics venous thrombosis of the calf and not uncommonly coexists with it. Because arthritis or trauma to the knee commonly precedes rupture of a popliteal cyst, a good history may help in making the diagnosis. A muscle hematoma can be hard to diagnose, particularly if the patient is on warfarin for previous DVT.

Cellulitis is associated with erythema and swelling, but fever and an obvious source of infection, such as an abscess, insect bite, or trauma, help distinguish this from DVT. Lymphangitis, myositis, and vasculitis are more problematic to diagnose.

DIAGNOSIS

In all suspected cases, DVT should be confirmed or ruled out by objective testing. Contrast venography is generally accepted as the standard of diagnosis against which all other tests are compared. In most institutions in which noninvasive studies are unavailable, contrast venography is and should be the test of choice. Radiopaque dye is injected into a vein of the dorsal part of the foot. The test result is positive when a constant intraluminal defect is found on two or more projections. A true negative result requires adequate visualization of the common iliac vessels, which may be difficult. Other drawbacks to the procedure include discomfort and induction of phlebitis in 1% to 3% of the patients. In addition, it does not differentiate old from new thromboses in most cases, making the diagnosis of acute, recurrent DVT difficult.

Impedance plethysmography (IPG) has rapidly gained favor as the noninvasive test most commonly used and studied. When a pneumatic cuff on the thigh is inflated and deflated, the blood volume in the leg changes, altering impedance or electrical resistance as measured by skin electrodes. IPG is specific and sensitive, both around 95%, for popliteal, ileal, and femoral thromboses and is as diagnostically informative as contrast venography for these vessels. However, its relative insensitivity to calf vein thrombosis limits its usefulness.

TABLE 30–3.
Clinical–Pathologic Correlations of Deep Vein Thrombosis

CLINICAL FINDINGS	PATHOLOGIC FINDINGS
Palpable cord	Thrombus in superficial or deep vein
Swelling	Obstruction to venous outflow
	Increased venous pressure
	Inflammation of soft tissue
Pain/tenderness/erythema	Vascular and perivascular inflammation
	Distension of veins secondary to obstruction
Pallor/cool skin	Arterial spasm (usually temporary)
Cyanosis	Tissue anoxia secondary to venous stasis

Nevertheless, when IPG is combined with ^{125}I-labeled fibrinogen scanning, the accuracy equals that of ascending venography. IPG does not differentiate among the causes of venous outflow obstruction, such as extrinsic mass compression, congestive heart failure, and an inadequate position of the patient.

Another noninvasive technique, Doppler ultrasonography, measures changes in the velocity of blood flow induced by normal respiration. Ultrasound microphones are used to monitor the changes in circulation during vein compression. This technique is very sensitive to proximal thrombosis, and, in skilled hands, is as accurate as IPG. It is, however, fairly insensitive to calf thrombosis.

The accuracy of ^{125}I-labeled fibrinogen scanning depends on active clot formation. Intravenous radioisotope-labeled fibrinogen is incorporated into an actively accreting thrombus, and the radioactivity is measured by an isotope counter placed over the leg. Scanning is used to diagnose active thrombosis in calf veins and to screen high-risk surgical patients. Its sensitivity in calf vein thrombosis approaches 95%, but definitive diagnosis is often delayed 48 to 72 hours to allow sufficient labeled fibrinogen to accumulate. Proximal vein clots may go undetected, and hematomas and cellulitis cause false-positive results. Scanning must be used in conjunction with a test more sensitive to proximal thrombosis, such as IPG or Doppler ultrasonography.

Phleborrheography has been advocated as a useful, noninvasive test for proximal vein thrombosis and may approach IPG in accuracy. Radionuclide scanning has yet to be fully evaluated in large, controlled studies. Its major usefulness appears to be in its ability to visualize the pelvic veins well.

In summary, the diagnostic approach in a case of suspected DVT is determined by which tests are available and the reliability of their interpretation. IPG or Doppler ultrasonography combined with ^{125}I-labeled fibrinogen scanning appears to be a safe and reasonable alternative to contrast venography. Phleborrheography might also be substituted for IPG or Doppler ultrasonography, but it is not yet widely used. In most small, community hospitals where adequate noninvasive tests are not available, contrast venography is the test of choice.

PRINCIPLES OF PREVENTION AND THERAPY

The goal of prophylaxis is to modify Virchow's triad by a variety of mechanical and pharmacologic methods. Studies using ^{125}I-labeled fibrinogen scanning and IPG in longitudinal tracking of high-risk medical and surgical patients have shown a reduced incidence of DVT (if not pulmonary embolism) in certain subgroups using low-dose or mini-dose heparin given subcutaneously every 8 to 12 hours. It carries minimal risk of hemorrhage. This regimen has been proposed in the following high-risk situations:

1. Patients over the age of 40 years undergoing major abdominal, thoracic, or gynecologic surgery and continuing until they are ambulatory.
2. Patients with acute myocardial infarction, particularly if the condition is complicated by CHF, obesity, venous insufficiency, or previous DVT.

Low-dose heparin has not been shown to be effective in preventing DVT in patients who have hip fractures or who have had hip or knee surgery, or urologic procedures. Dextran infusion or warfarin has been advocated for these high-risk patients. Aspirin has not been shown to be consistently useful in preventing DVT.

Mechanical maneuvers to reduce venous stasis include early ambulation, leg elevation, pneumatic compression, and compression stockings. Correction of underlying hypovolemia, shock, and anemia is also mandatory for reducing the risk.

Anticoagulation with full doses of heparin is the mainstay in treating cases of DVT with or without pulmonary embolism. Heparin inhibits active clot formation by binding and activating antithrombin III. It does not directly lyse thrombi but allows the fibrinolytic arm of the coagulation system to act unimpeded. Most clinicians prefer continuous intravenous infusion of heparin, but intermittent bolus injection is also acceptable.

The goal of therapy is to maintain the partial thromboplastin time at one-and-one-half to two times the control value. Full anticoagulation treatment should be maintained for 7 to 10 days, at which time the clot will have become organized and more firmly adherent to the vessel wall. Bedrest and leg elevation are recommended until pain and tenderness resolve, usually during the first week. Elastic support hose are recommended after the acute symptoms subside.

If warfarin is used, administration of it may be started after the first 2 or 3 days. Warfarin decreases the levels of factors II, VII, IX, and X. The prothrombin time, used to monitor therapy, should be kept between 1.2 and 1.5 times control. No exact guidelines are available regarding the length of chronic anticoagulation therapy. If DVT is secondary to an acute insult such as surgery, anticoagulation therapy should be continued until the patient is ambulatory and the acute condition resolves. If a pulmonary embolism is present, anticoagulation therapy for 6 months or longer is recommended. In patients with thrombotic tendencies and a chronic predisposing medical condition, the risk of repeated DVT and possible pulmonary embolism should be weighed against the risk of possible hemorrhagic complications caused by warfarin.

Fibrinolytic therapy with streptokinase or urokinase enhances the resolution of DVT and pulmonary embolism, but neither short- nor long-term improvement in morbidity or mortality has been satisfactorily documented. These agents work by activating plasmin, which is the body's natural fibrinolytic agent. Thrombolytic therapy is acceptable treatment for massive ileofemoral DVT or for DVT complicated by pulmonary embolism, particularly in cases where a high risk of a second pulmonary embolism would be catastrophic.

Thrombectomy or venacaval ligation or plication and transvenous insertion of vena cava filters are uncommon because of disappointing outcomes. These procedures are reserved for patients with documented recurrent, serious pulmonary embolism while taking full-dose heparin or patients in whom anticoagulation is absolutely contraindicated.

REFERENCES

Bernstein E (ed): *Noninvasive Diagnostic Techniques in Vascular Disease*, ed 2. St Louis, CV Mosby Co, 1982. *A comprehensive evaluation of the various techniques for diagnosing DVT.*

Classen J, Richardson JB, Koontz C: A three-year experience with phleborrheography. *Ann Surg* 1982; 195(6):800–803. *A good discussion advocating phleborrheography.*

Hirsh J, Genten E, Hull R: *Venous Thromboembolism.* New York, Grune & Stratton, 1981. *A concise, in-depth, definitive approach to all aspects of DVT.*

Hull R, Hirsh J, Carter CJ, et al: Diagnostic efficacy of impedance phlethysmography for clinically suspected deep-vein thrombosis. *Ann Intern Med* 1985; 102:21–28. *The latest large-scale study by Hull and Hirsh advocating the efficacy and safety of the noninvasive approach to DVT.*

Hull R, Raskob GE, LeClerc JR, Jay RM, Hirsh J: The diagnosis of clinically suspected venous thrombosis. *Clin Chest Med* 1984; 5(3):439–455. *A good review of the techniques for diagnosing DVT.*

Moser K: Pulmonary thromboembolism, in Petersdorf R, Adams R, Braunwald E, Isselbacher K, Martin J, Wilson J (eds): *Harrison's Principles of Internal Medicine*, ed 10. Minneapolis, McGraw-Hill, 1983, pp 1561–1567. *Currently ac-*

cepted approach to diagnosis and treatment of DVT.

Moser KM, LeMoine JR: Is embolic risk conditioned by location of deep venous thrombosis? *Ann Intern Med* 1981; 94(Part 1): 439–444. *An often-cited article raising the question of the need for anticoagulation treatment of calf-vein thrombosis*

and advocating the noninvasive diagnosis of deep vein thrombosis.

Thomas D: Venous thrombogenesis. *Annu Rev Med* 1985; 36:39–50. *An excellent review of recent advances in elucidating the pathogenesis of venous thrombosis.*

part III

Respiratory Disorders

CHRONIC AIRFLOW OBSTRUCTION

Charles B. Payne, Jr., M.D.

The most common cause of chronic airflow obstruction is cigarette smoking. The older term chronic obstructive pulmonary disease (COPD) was defined to include three entities: emphysema, chronic bronchitis, and asthma. Chronic bronchitis is clinically defined as the presence of a chronic productive cough on most days for 3 consecutive months for not less than 2 years in the absence of other causes of coughing. Emphysema is a disease of the lung parenchyma characterized by destruction of alveolar walls, blood vessels, and interstitium. Asthma is a distinctive disease entity which has airflow obstruction and occurs over a long period of time but is usually reversible and results from such distinctive pathogenetic mechanisms that it is discussed separately. Patients with hyperreactive airways and asthma, however, have been shown to be at particularly high risk for developing pulmonary morphologic changes from cigarette smoking. They may, therefore, develop emphysema, chronic bronchitis, and abnormal structure of the airways leading to mixtures of diseases characterized by airflow obstruction. These mixtures may cause great confusion to both the patient and physician.

Chronic bronchitis and emphysema usually occur together, but a number of studies now show that airway irritation, marked by cough and sputum production, may occur as an occupational response to a myriad of inhaled irritants, as well as cigarette smoke. Moreover, the peak incidence of chronic bronchitis occurs well before the peak incidence of severe emphysema. Morphologic and physiologic information also indicates that the clinical entity of chronic bronchitis is not responsible *per se* for airflow obstruction. Chronic airflow obstruction is now felt to be a result of the changes in the smaller airways resulting from the development of emphysema in susceptible individuals who smoke.

CLINICAL SIGNS AND SYMPTOMS

Most patients are asymptomatic in the early states of chronic airway obstruction. Because this disorder is strongly associated with tobacco smoking, screening programs involving pulmonary function testing of smokers frequently detect abnormal airflow before patients notice any problem beyond "smoker's cough" and sputum production, which they often ignore or consider to be normal.

Late in the disease the major presenting symptom is dyspnea on unusual exertion. Lingering or unusually frequent respiratory infections also prompt the patient to seek medical attention. Patients with cough and sputum production have been shown to have a higher than normal incidence of respiratory infections. Continued smoking produces worsening exertional dyspnea with an inexorable reduction in exercise tolerance and eventual exhaustion from performing activities of daily living.

Eventually the patient notices wheezing and prolonged expiration. Sleep disturbances are common. Although the appetite may be normal, patients find it difficult to eat normal meals because of breathlessness. Muscle mass is lost, but, in some, weight loss may be masked by edema. Somatic concern, hypochondria, anxiety, and depression are frequently detected.

Early in the disease there are no specific physical signs for chronic airway obstruction. Early skin wrinkling, tar staining of the fingers, staining of the teeth, and dental problems such as periodontitis mark the chronic smoker.

Late in the disease the patient speaks in phrases. Exhalation is prolonged and interrupted by paroxysms of cough. Tachypnea is apparent, and breathing may be through pursed lips. Wheezing and central cyanosis may be present. Scleral hyperemia may be present with facial puffiness if hypercarbia is present. The anteroposterior diameter of the thorax is increased, and breathing is more comfortable while sitting up or leaning forward with the arms extended and fixed. The suprasternal and supraclavicular fossae sink on inspiration, and jugular venous filling and distention are visible during expiration. The lower rib cage margin moves inward throughout inspiration (Hoover's sign), and the normal upward and outward rib motion on inspiration is lost. The intercostal muscles retract on inspiration.

Palpation in the posterior cervical triangle elicits hardening and contraction of the scalene muscles, and the sternomastoid muscles are also used in inspiration. With the tip of the index finger on the thyroid cartilage, the trachea can be felt to descend on inspiration. The thorax is generally hyperresonant to percussion, and diaphragmatic excursion during inspiration decreases to one interspace or less. The normal width of hepatic dullness is decreased. The liver edge may be palpated below the costal margin and may be tender with right heart failure, which also produces dependent edema.

Auscultation over the trachea in forced expiration indicates prolongation of exhalation beyond the normal 1:3 inspiration/expiration (I/E) ratio, and exhalation may exceed 3 seconds. Breath sounds are diminished bilaterally. Crackles are most frequently heard late in inspiration in various locations, usually at the lung bases. Wheezes and ronchi are frequently heard. The decreased heart sounds are best heard over the xiphoid process.

Disease manifestations range from severe hypoxemia and cyanosis, pulmonary hypertension, carbon dioxide retention, secondary polycythemia, and cor pulmonale in the so-called blue bloaters to less hypoxemic, late carbon dioxide retention, and fewer symptoms at rest in the so-called pink puffers, who are more dyspneic, slender, and barrel-chested.

With continued smoking, viral or bacterial infections, use of respiratory depressant drugs, heart failure, or pulmonary emboli frequently produce steplike decrements of functions, leading to respiratory failure. One out of two patients with hypercapnea and severe disease dies within 5 years. The prognosis may be predicted from the forced expiratory flow over the middle half of the spirogram (FEF_{25-75}). In 91 patients, the average annual rate of decline

in the FEF_{25-75} was 11.4%. The FEF_{25-75} halved every 7.1 years.

Respiratory failure is defined as a $PaCO_2$ more than or equal to 50 torr and a PaO_2 less than or equal to 50 torr, with respiratory acidosis present. Failure leads to progressive somnolence, confusion, personality changes, headaches, cardiac arrhythmias, seizures, asterixis, stupor, and death.

PATHOPHYSIOLOGY (Table 31–1)

Smoke inhalation initiates an inflammatory reaction in the airways and lung parenchyma, with earliest lesions probably being respiratory bronchiolitis with clusters of pigmented alveolar macrophages. A small but significant increase in denuded epithelium and inflammatory cells (polymorphonuclear leukocytes) is present in the membranous bronchioles of young smokers as opposed to nonsmoking control subjects. These inflammatory cells produce qualitatively and quantitatively different patterns of elastase-type proteolytic enzymes in the lungs of smokers as opposed to nonsmokers and mediate greater lymphocyte responsiveness to soluble antigens than autologous, nonpulmonary macrophages. Smoke also paralyzes the cilia of the airway mucosa and damages the protective mucociliary transport mechanism.

The process of inflammation and the destruction by enzymes are opposed by the antielastase and antiproteinase properties of the lungs. Individuals who are homozygous for alpha$_1$-antitrypsin deficiency are particularly prone to develop an accelerated form of panlobular emphysema. The genetic system of alpha$_1$-antitrypsin is described by the "Pi system" (protease inhibitor) of alleles at the Pi gene locus. There are approximately 30 alleles of which PiM is the most common. In the proposed model of multiple codominant alleles at one locus, Pi- variants with either low or chemically abnormal levels of alpha$_1$-antitrypsin include PiZ, Pi (with a silent allele and no gene product), PiS, PiI, and others. There are conflicting data as to whether or not the development of emphysema is accelerated in heterozygotes, but in homozygotes the evidence is clear that smoking is associated with rapidly progressive, panlobular emphysema. Smoking may also partially inactivate alpha$_1$-antitrypsin

TABLE 31–1.
Pathophysiologic Correlations in Chronic Airflow Obstruction

MAJOR SMOKING-RELATED DERANGEMENTS	CLINICAL AND LABORATORY ABNORMALITIES
Destruction of parenchymal lung tissue (emphysema)	Loss of elastic recoil (increased lung compliance). Hyperinflation. Increased chest and lung volume results in mechanical disadvantage for thoracic muscles. Enlarged CO_2 reservoir. Loss of respiratory surface area with few vascular markings on chest x-ray film. Loss of radial support for airways. Increased work and oxygen cost of breathing. Heterogeneity of lung unit time constants.
Inflammation and distortion of bronchioles leading to altered airflow (bronchitis)	Increased resistance to airflow with air trapping. Decreased FEV_1, $FEV_1/FVC\%$, and airflow measurements. Wheezing and ronchi. Increased closing volume and capacity. Abnormal distribution of ventilation with heterogenous emptying of lung units. Increased work and oxygen cost of breathing.
Damage to lung defense mechanisms	Hypertrophy of bronchial mucous glands with cough and sputum production. Impaired muco-ciliary clearance and macrophage function with increased susceptibility to infections. Increased levels of superoxide dismutase and other enzymes.
Disturbances in gas exchange	Alteration in both high and low ventilation and perfusion ratios leads to hypoxemia not corrected by hyperventilation. CO_2 retention produces acidosis. PaO_2 falls and $D(A-a)O_2$ increases. Loss of alveolar capillary units in emphysema is reflected by decreased D_LCO. Preserved vasculature with decreased ventilation leads to physiologic shunting, worse in chronic bronchitis. Destruction of vasculature and reactive, hypoxemic vasoconstriction increase pulmonary vascular resistance, causing pulmonary hypertension, cor pulmonale, and right heart failure.

through oxidation. Although it is not yet clear that the emphysema is directly caused by the lack of inhibition or destruction of elastases produced by inflammatory cells in the lungs of smokers, the protective nature of alpha$_1$-antitrypsin is unquestioned. The cellular defense mechanisms of the lung produce the increased quantity of mucus and mucosal hypertrophy measurable in chronic bronchitis. Denudation of irritant receptors may encourage bronchospasm and wheezing. Epidemiologic studies strongly suggest that asthmatic patients whose airways are sensitive to histamine and methacholine are more susceptible to the damaging effects of smoking.

Two physical factors, elastic recoil of the lung, measured by static lung compliance ($\Delta V/\Delta P$), and resistance to airflow (R), determine the ease with which gas is expelled from the lungs. Remember that exhalation is normally passive, while inflating the lungs requires muscular force. Smoking alters both compliance and airway resistance. Elastic recoil is decreased by the digestion and destruction of alveolar walls, elastic fibers, and parenchyma which enlarges the terminal air-

spaces. This both reduces the tractive forces that keep the airways open and also increases lung compliance. Increased secretions, tortuosity, and narrowing of the bronchioles increases the resistance to airflow in the small airways. Changes in recoil and in resistance usually proceed simultaneously. The predominance of one over the other is responsible for the variable clinical features seen initially.

The chest enlarges because the natural tendency for the chest wall to expand (thoracic compliance) is progressively less opposed by the compliance of the lungs. Enlargement increases the mechanical disadvantage of the respiratory muscles. Loss of radial tethering of the airways allows them to collapse during the expiratory increase in transpulmonary pressure, producing obstruction with both increased work and oxygen cost of breathing. Where parenchymal destruction predominates, proportional loss of alveolar spaces and pulmonary capillaries occurs. Ratios of alveolar ventilation ($\dot{V}_A$) to pulmonary capillary perfusion ($\dot{Q}_c$) are disturbed across a spectrum. The spectrum ranges from relatively little mismatching when alveoli and capillaries are detroyed approximately equally, to marked mismatching when impaired ventilation to areas of the lung which remain well perfused occurs. Preservation of ventilation to poorly perfused alveoli also disturbs $\dot{V}_A/\dot{Q}_C$ ratios. The first case produces the so-called pink puffer for whom exertion is required to unmask the mechanical muscular disadvantage and the loss of gas-exchange surface area usually resulting in dyspnea.

Increases in resistance characterize the *chronic bronchitic* patient. High airflow resistance increases muscular work and oxygen cost of breathing and obstructs ventilation. Because more highly obstructed alveoli empty at slower rates, heterogenous ventilation results, although blood flow remains relatively undisturbed, leading to a greater disturbance of $\dot{V}_A/\dot{Q}_c$ ratios than in *pure emphysema.* The poorly ventilated areas produce "physiologic shunting," which lowers the PO_2 in the systemic circulation. This PO_2 reduction cannot be compensated by the areas of high $\dot{V}_A/\dot{Q}_c$ ratios. Hypoxemia produces pulmonary hypertension, leading to cor pulmonale, which is more common in the edematous, oxyhemoglobin-desaturated "blue bloater."

When progressive mechanical disadvantage, hypoxemia, hypercapnea, and increased work and oxygen cost of breathing exceed the capacity of the diaphragm and other respiratory muscles, respiratory muscle failure occurs, resulting in further increases in $PaCO_2$ and hypoxemia even though the central respiratory drive is actually high.

DIFFERENTIAL DIAGNOSIS

Entities that mimic or may coexist with chronic airway obstruction are listed in Table 31–2. Thorough historic, laboratory, and radiologic investigations are often required for precise diagnosis of the existence or proportional contribution of these conditions to the overall clinical picture.

DIAGNOSIS

Except for secondary polycythemia or an elevated serum bicarbonate level in patients with chronic respiratory acidosis, routine laboratory studies are not useful. Determining the phenotype of patients suspected to be deficient in alpha$_1$-antitrypsin (by antigen–antibody crossed immunoelectrophoresis or polyacrylamide gel isoelectric focusing techniques) is di-

---

TABLE 31–2.
Differential Diagnosis of Chronic Airflow Obstruction

DISEASE	DIFFERENTIAL DIAGNOSTIC POINTS
Bronchial asthma	History of childhood/adolescent attacks, bronchitis, or intractable cough. Relief by bronchodilator medications. Family history of atopy. May coexist with chronic airway obstruction if subject smokes. Large reversible bronchospastic component on lung function testing. Eosinophilia in nasal secretions.
Congestive heart failure	History of hypertension, coronary artery disease, cardiomyopathy, or myocardial infarction. Cardiomegaly on chest x-ray film. Obstruction without significant hyperinflation on lung function testing. Clinical response to treatment for heart failure.
Bronchiectasis	History appropriate to various causes of bronchiectasis. Changes in chest x-ray films or bronchograms demonstrating bronchiectasis, Kartagener's syndrome, Swyer-James-Macleod's syndrome, or allergic bronchopulmonary aspergillosis. Classical layering of sputum. Localized wheezing.
Chronic granulomatous diseases	Tuberculosis, histoplasmosis, and sarcoidosis produce parenchymal fibrosis, bullae, and airways scarring. Bronchiectasis produces cough, sputum, and chronic airway obstruction.
Tumors of lungs and upper airways	Early benign and malignant tumors in the trachea and airways may be invisible in chest x-ray films, but depending on the site of the tumor, may produce wheezing, dyspnea, and cough, as well as airflow obstruction on lung function tests.

agnostic of the homozygous genetic deficiency. The family history and the youth of the patient suggest these tests.

Spirometry shows a reduced forced expiratory volume (FEV_1) and an FEV_1/FVC ratio of less than 70%, with reduced airflow measurements such as the FEF_{25-75} and FEF_{50}. Lung volume measurements show a hyperinflated residual volume and functional residual capacity. The alveolar-arterial oxygen pressure gradient or $P(A–a)O_2$ is abnormally wide. In advanced cases, respiratory acidosis with carbon dioxide retention is present.

Increases of 15% or more in FEV_1 with corresponding increases in airflow rates after administering a bronchodilator aerosol are commonly accepted as indicating asthma or an asthmatic bronchospastic component of chronic airway obstruction.

The diffusing capacity for carbon monoxide (D_LCO) is usually normal or nearly so in asthma and chronic bronchitis. The reduction in D_LCO has been shown to correlate well with the amount of emphysema quantitated at autopsy.

The chest x-ray film may be normal. There are associated, but not pathognomonic, changes in the film showing hyperaerated (dark) lung fields, enlarged hilar vessels, a vertical heart, and a flattened diaphragm with an increased retrosternal airspace in the lateral chest x-ray.

The electrocardiogram may be normal or show signs of right ventricular loading, such as P pulmonale, right axis deviation, incomplete right bundle branch block, right ventricular hypertrophy, and right ventricular strain.

PRINCIPLES OF PREVENTION AND THERAPY

Both prevention and therapy are based on NO SMOKING! Studies of the effects of all therapies show no slowing of progressive functional decline as long as smoking continues. Palliative treatment includes the use of theophylline, beta-adrenergic bronchodilator medications both orally and by aerosol, along with antibiotics as indicated for infections. Influenza vaccine and amantadine are useful to prevent and ameliorate influenza, and pneumococcal pneumonia vaccine should be given. Steroid therapy is usually of little benefit, but a brief trial may reveal an occasional patient with a reversible bronchospastic component.

Home oxygen therapy, when significant hypoxemia is present as indicated by a PaO_2 less than 55 to 60 mm Hg, and when given for at least 14 to 18 hours daily, will retard pulmonary hypertension and cor pulmonale, and will also reduce the frequency of hospitalization and prolong life.

REFERENCES

Campbell EJM: Physical signs of diffuse airways obstruction and lung distension. *Thorax* 1969; 24:1–3. *An old but fundamental discussion of the generation of physical signs and their relationship to disordered lung mechanics.*

Fletcher C, Peto R: The natural history of chronic airflow obstruction. *Br Med J* 1977; 1:1645–1648. *The summation of many years of work with data indicating that smoking cessation retards the decline of lung function in chronic airway obstruction.*

Idell S, Cohen AB: Alpha-1-antitrypsin deficiency. *Clin Chest Med* 1983; 4(3):359–375. *This is an excellent review and summary of a very complex literature that provides both historic background on the pulmonary and hepatic abnormalities of this genetic disorder and discusses plans for replacement therapy.*

Niewoehner DE: Clinical aspects of chronic airflow obstruction, in Baum GL, Wolinsky E (eds): *Textbook of Pulmonary Diseases*, ed 3. Boston, Little, Brown & Co, 1983, pp 915–948. *A well-referenced, detailed, and readable account that fleshes out the bare bones of this introductory text.*

Sharp JT: The respiratory muscles in emphysema. *Clin Chest Med* 1983; 4(3):421–432. *A review article that supplies the vocabulary and concepts in the study of why respiration fails and efforts to train and improve muscle function.*

Stone PJ: The elastase-antielastase hypothesis of the pathogenesis of emphysema. *Clin Chest Med* 1983; 4(3):405–412. *A brief, readable exposition of the evidence for and direction of research in the enzymatic production of emphysema up to 1983.*

32 LUNG CANCER

Charles B. Payne, Jr., M.D.

Lung cancers are malignant growths arising from the cellular structures of the lung. These growths have the capacity to spread either by direct invasion or by vascular or lymphatic dissemination to other organ systems. Cancers arising from the epithelial or glandular cells of the bronchi are called bronchogenic carcinoma. These bronchogenic neoplasms, squamous cell (epidermoid) carcinomas, adenocarcinomas, small cell anaplastic carcinomas (including "oat cell" carcinoma), and large cell carcinomas, compose the great bulk of lung cancers.

Other cell types in the lung parenchyma, such as the alveolar lining cells and bronchial cartilage, may undergo malignant change and produce cancers such as alveolar cell carcinoma and chondromas. These less frequent neoplasms may be of various degrees of malignancy and may be benign. Unfortunately even benign enlarging new growths within the thorax may create mischief by compression or obstruction of essential structures. For this and other reasons involving diagnostic techniques, we will discuss all of these lesions under the heading lung cancer.

CLINICAL SIGNS AND SYMPTOMS

The patient is usually a middle-aged man or woman who began smoking in adolescence. Frequently there is a change in the usual cough associated with smoking, expectoration of sputum mixed with flecks, streaks, or clots of blood. There may be unexplained weight loss. There is often chest pain of a dull, poorly localized but unremitting nature. Poorly resolving respiratory infections and pneumonias often lead to a diagnosis of lung cancer after investigation. Less frequently, clubbing of the fingers and toes is detected by an associate of the patient. A lump or nodule may be felt in the neck,

supraclavicular fossae, axillae, or elsewhere. A variety of symptoms such as headaches, bone pain, hoarseness, or seizures may occur in association with metastases.

A number of lung cancers produce paraneoplastic syndromes, which are usually associated with specific cancer cell types. The syndromes, cell types, and some information about the relative frequencies of occurrence are listed in Table 32–1.

Physical examination may be totally unrewarding. The findings of recent weight loss, clubbing of the digits, and palpable lymph nodes or masses are nonspecific. On auscultation of the chest, a localized expiratory wheeze occasionally gives away the location of a neoplasm that partially obstructs a bronchus. On occasion, light percussion over a painful rib or other bone will produce painful evidence of metastatic involvement. Hoarseness should lead to laryngoscopic examination of the vocal cords. Paralysis of the left vocal cord is an accepted sign of inoperability if associated with lung cancer. Patients with tumors of the superior sulcus of the lung (Pancoast's tumors) usually have a long history of arm and shoulder pain that has been unsuccessfully treated as cervical arthritis or other degenerative condition. When the syndrome is complete, these patients have neurologic signs of thoracic nerve root irritation and Horner's syndrome and may have unilateral clubbing of the fingers on the affected side. In any patient with suspected lung cancer, a thorough neurologic examination and careful palpation of the abdominal viscera for metastases are indicated.

The standard chest x-ray, contrary to commonly held opinion, does not detect lung cancer during its early stages of development. Calculations of the signal-to-noise ratio of x-ray films show that lung lesions less than 1.0 cm in

TABLE 32–1.
Paraneoplastic Syndromes of Lung Cancer

SYNDROME	CAUSE
Cushing's syndrome	Small cell cancer (rarely anaplastic carcinoma); ACTH-like substance not, or only partially, suppressible by dexamethasone
Hyperpigmentation	Small cell cancer (rarely adenocarcinoma); a subset of Cushing's syndrome; increased levels of 17-ketosteroids, ketogenic steroids, and hydroxycorticoids
Syndrome of inappropriate production of antidiuretic hormone (SIADH)	Small cell cancer; tumor secretes ADH or ADH-like substance.
Gynecomastia	Anaplastic or poorly differentiated cancers; tumor produces LH and FSH.
Hypercalcemia (May occur in epidermoid tumors other than in the lung)	Squamous cell cancer (rarely adeno-large cell anaplastic cancers); most common paraneoplastic syndrome; usually associated with bone metastases; when not, may be caused by parathormone-like substance.
Hypoglycemia	Fibrosarcomas of thorax, retroperitoneum; very rarely from the lung; insulin or insulin-like secretion from tumor
Miscellaneous	Oat cell, anaplastic tumors frequently secrete calcitonin. Tumors secreting alkaline phosphotase, amylase, and epinephrine have been reported.
Carcinoid syndrome	Adenomas of bronchus, occasionally in oat cell carcinoma; may also occur from intestinal carcinoid tumors with hepatic metastases; tumor produces 5-hydrosytryptamine, rarely 5-hydroxytryptophan, and serotonin.
Nonmetastatic neuromyopathic carcinomatous manifestations Encephalopathy Myelopathy Neuropathy Myopathy	One of these abnormalities occurs in 40% of all bronchogenic carcinomas; the myopathies include myasthenia gravis, Eaton-Lambert syndrome, dermatomyositis, and carcinomatous neuromyopathy.
Clubbing of fingers and toes	Of unknown etiology; clubbing is quite common.
Hypertrophic pulmonary osteo-arthropathy (HPO)	HPO is more unusual but not rare.

diameter are seldom detectable against the "noise" of other information on the x-ray film. In order to reach a diameter of 1 cm a single malignant cell has to have doubled approximately 30 times. Because growth in mass is a cubic exponential function, after 40 doublings there will be a 10-cm, 1-kg tumor and death. It is apparent therefore that the chest x-ray film detects late disease. In addition, a tumor growing within an airway may produce no visible changes until it has obstructed a bronchus producing distal atelectasis or infection. The Philadelphia Pulmonary Neoplasm Research Project (Weiss et al., 1982) demonstrated that x-ray screening of high-risk populations for the early detection of lung cancers was neither clinically nor economically effective in reducing the morbidity and mortality of lung cancer.

The usual diagnostic studies such as chest x-ray films and computerized tomography (CT scans) only identify the presence and location of lesions, not their nature, unless serial studies are available. Whenever possible, previous studies must be sought for comparison. In general, a period of 2 or 3 years without change in size of a lesion strongly suggests that it is benign. A detailed description of the radiologic changes of the various malignancies is beyond the scope of this text. Figure 32–1 provides general information about x-ray manifestations of various tumors. There are many exceptions to these rules. A cytologic or tissue diagnosis cannot be made from the x-ray film or CT scan.

The natural history of these diseases is one of a preclinical phase during which the neoplasm grows unnoticed. Studies indicate that the biologic behavior of the tumor establishes the prognosis. Simply stated, if you have a rapidly growing bronchogenic carcinoma, it will kill you rapidly. If it is slow growing, chances for a 5-year survival are between 5% and 8%. Considerably longer survival figures are occasionally reported when a slowly growing neoplasm is detected when it is small. The dating of these

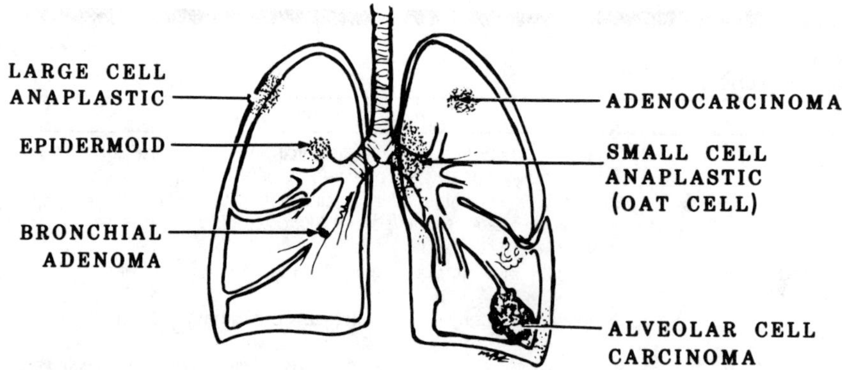

FIG 32–1.

Common radiographic features of various lung cancer types.

Epidermoid (squamous cell) cancers appear as lesions causing bronchial obstructions, though much of the tumor is parenchymal and outside the bronchus. They occur almost entirely in smokers. About 10% may have central cavitation.

Adenocarcinomas compose 1/5 of all tumors, but the incidence is increasing. They are the most common type of "scar" cancers and tend to metastasize early.

Small cell anaplastic (oat cell) cancers are approximately one-third of all primary tumors. About 20% may arise in the lung periphery, but most are central in origin. They are derived from Kulchitsky-type APUD cells.

Bronchial adenomas may be benign or of low-grade malignancy and are locally obstructing, bleed easily, and are destructive of lung tissue.

Large cell anaplastic carcinomas are of variable incidence depending on the pathologic criteria. They behave like oat cell carcinomas in terms of metastases and growth, but are not of unique cellular origin.

Alveolar cell carcinoma accounts for up to 8% of all tumors. They appear as a solitary nodule, as multiple nodules, or as diffuse pneumonic infiltrate. They arise from alveolar Type II lining cells. The classic description of production of copious, watery sputum occurs in 10% to 20% of cases. Fewer than 50% of patients produce any sputum at all in early stages of the cancer.

lung cancers of long duration is often made during a retrospective review of chest x-rays. The steps involved in the medical diagnostic and staging processes tend to select those patients with slow growing tumors so that it is very difficult to show that surgical excision of the neoplasms actually extends life over the normal 5% to 8% survival percentage. Nonetheless, complete removal of the tumor offers the best theoretical basis for cure and should be the goal of treatment whenever possible.

PATHOPHYSIOLOGY

Exclusive of paraneoplastic syndromes, lung cancer produces effects by the presence of a mass that may invade, press upon local tissue, or create vascular anastomoses such as from bronchial arteries. In addition, metastases may spread to adjacent structures primarily by way of lymphatic vessels to nodes. The variety of abnormalities caused by distant, blood-borne metastases defies categorization. Anemia, bone pain, pathologic fractures, seizures, and jaundice, are only a few of these effects. Local abnormalities and those caused by regional lymphatic spread are shown in Table 32–2.

CLINICAL–PATHOLOGIC CORRELATIONS

Major clinical findings which arise from the growth, spread, and anatomical location of lung cancers are summarized in Table 32–2.

DIFFERENTIAL DIAGNOSIS

The special case of the solitary pulmonary nodule (frequently incorrectly called the "coin lesion") requires attention. This is a nodular density on x-ray film that is less than 3 cm in diameter and that is not contiguous with other thoracic structures. It is important to attempt to differentiate benign from malignant nodules to avoid unnecessary thoracotomy. The most important diagnostic step, after a careful history

TABLE 32–2.
Clinical–Pathologic Correlations for Lung Cancer*

PATHOLOGIC FINDINGS	CLINICAL FINDINGS
Partial bronchial obstruction	Cough, hemoptysis, dyspnea, and ventilation/perfusion mismatch; poorly resolving infections
Complete bronchial obstruction	Distal atelectasis, infection; pleural effusion from infection or atelectasis; asphyxia if lesion at the carina
Pleural and chest wall invasion	Sanguineous pleural effusion with positive findings from biopsy and cytologic studies; compression of lung with dyspnea; rib pain, fractures, and bone destruction
Pulmonary vasculature invasion	Hemoptysis; bleeding from the tumor, pulmonary vessels, or bronchial artery anastomoses with systemic blood vessels
Spread to lymphatics	Pleural effusion from lymphatic obstruction; may be chylous or pseudochylous
Mediastinal involvement	Obstruction of superior vena cava; pericardial involvement with tamponade

* Effects of lung cancer exclusive of those associated with paraneoplastic syndromes and distant metastases.

and physical examination, is to find old x-ray films to establish whether or not the lesion has been present or has changed over a 2- or 3-year period. Special x-ray views such as tomography (laminography) or CT scans are useful to determine whether or not the lesion is truly solitary and whether or not it has a central calcified core. Tumors that appear as densities with concentric, calcified cores are benign. Age and smoking history assist in estimating the patient's risk. A solitary nodule in a nonsmoking patient younger than age 35 years has a small risk of being malignant. The risk increases with age and smoking. If the lesion is new or has increased in size, if there is adequate lung function and no demonstrable calcification and the lesion is truly solitary, then surgical excision is indicated. Here, too, radionuclide scans are of little diagnostic value and are not cost-effective. The role of CT scans and nuclear magnetic resonance examinations in both assessing the solitary pulmonary nodule and staging of tumors in general is not yet clear.

Lesions that may appear as solitary nodules include tuberculomas, histoplasmomas or other mycetomas, small inflammatory lesions, benign tumors such as hamartomas, and congenital vascular anomalies.

DIAGNOSIS

Diagnostic studies produce two kinds of information. The first kind establishes the nature of the lesion and may or may not provide the second kind of information. The second kind of diagnostic information is the staging of the degree of tumor involvement. With few exceptions, treatment requires histologic diagnosis of malignancy. Commonly used biopsy procedures include examination of the sputum for malignant cells, fiberoptic or rigid bronchoscopy with brushing, washing, and forceps or needle biopsies, percutaneous needle aspirations, or surgical excision of lung or other tissue such as lymph nodes likely to harbor tumor cells.

Knowledge of the cell type assists in the selection of chemotherapeutic agents and radiation therapy portals and doses and, in the case of oat cell carcinomas, excludes surgical attempts at cure. There are, however, terminally ill patients for whom, because of the added morbidity and discomfort, diagnostic procedures are not indicated. Unless treatment will be altered by the diagnostic procedure, it is not indicated. Consultation from specialists in pulmonary medicine, thoracic surgery, radiology, and oncology is usually required to select and perform appropriate diagnostic procedures and to plan therapy.

Staging of the disease involves determining whether or not the tumor has spread beyond the confines of the thorax or has other indices of inoperability. The schema for staging is briefly outlined in Table 32–3. In addition to anatomic and cellular definition of the neoplasm, nutritional and immunologic assessments of the patient are useful to assist in estimating his or her response to therapy and to gain some information about the likely prog-

TABLE 32–3.
TNM Staging System for Lung Cancer*

T (primary tumor)
  T_0: No evidence of primary tumor
  T_X: Malignant cells in secretions, but no x-ray or bronchoscopic evidence of tumor
  T_1: Tumor less than 3.0 cm in greatest diameter, located distal to a lobar bronchus
  T_2: Tumor larger than 3.0 cm in greatest diameter, or any tumor extending to hilum; at bronchoscopy
    the tumor is at least 2 cm from the carina; no pleural effusion; atelectasis or obstructive pneumonia,
    if present, involves less than an entire lung
  T_3: Tumor of any size extending to chest wall, diaphragm, or mediastinum; within less than 2 cm of
    carina at (bronchoscopy) or with effusion or atelectasis of entire lung
N (regional lymph nodes)
  N_0: None involved
  N_1: Metastases to ipsilateral hilar region
  N_2: Mediastinal nodes involved
M (distant metastases)
  M_0: None
  M_1: Any metastases to distant sites

* From Mountain CF, Carr DT, Anderson WAD: A system for the clinical staging of lung cancer. *Am J Roentgenol Radium Ther Nucl Med* 1974; 120:132. Used by permission of authors and the American Roentgen Ray Society.

nosis. Clinical studies should include measuring the hemoglobin and hematocrit values and a urinalysis. Additional studies should include measurement of the levels of serum calcium, phosphorus, alkaline phosphatase, serum aspartate aminotransferase (AST, SGOT), alanine aminotransferase (ALT, SGPT), urea nitrogen, creatinine, and electrolytes and serum protein determinations to detect gross protein deficiency as well as paraneoplastic disturbances of the electrolytes. The ideal body weight should be determined. Nutritional and immunologic competences in the response to various injected antigens have been shown to be positively correlated with survival and positive responses to various therapies.

Hypercalcemia is frequently seen in sqamous cell neoplasms and is one of the paraneoplastic syndromes when not due to bone metastases (Table 32–1). Elevation of the alkaline phosphatase by more than 150 IU/L approaches 100% in its sensitivity as a detector of hepatic metastases but has an 85% false-positive rate when compared to liver biopsy. Studies of hepatic enzymes are very important because radionuclide scans of the liver, spleen, bone, and brain have been shown to be of little diagnostic value and not cost-effective in staging the disease in patients who have no abnormal findings in a review of systems or a physical examination and have normal results in laboratory studies.

PRINCIPLES OF PREVENTION AND THERAPY

The United States Surgeon General has set a goal of a "smoke-free society by the year 2000" to reduce the epidemic of approximately 140,000 annual deaths from lung cancer. If national smoking cessation was immediate, 7 to 15 years would pass before an appreciable decline would be recorded in the number of cases of lung cancer. After a smoker quits, approximately 7 years are required for his risk of developing lung cancer to decline to that of a nonsmoker of the same age. Certain occupations, such as uranium mining, asbestos work, and certain kinds of welding, multiply the risk for developing lung cancer in smokers. Malignant mesothelioma is directly related to asbestos exposure. The risk of developing neoplasms of the upper respiratory tract, esophagus, and upper gastrointestinal tract is multiplied three- to fourfold by smoking alone and even more by the combination of asbestos exposure and smoking.

Surgical excision of the neoplasm offers the best theoretical opportunity for complete cure of lung cancer except for small cell (oat cell) cancers of the lung. Oat cell tumors are presumed to have metastasized at the time of diagnosis and are currently best treated by some combination of chemotherapy and radiation. Almost all reported surgical series have a selection bias because of the possibility of cure. Nevertheless, when staging criteria are applied

TABLE 32–4.
Results of Surgical Therapy of Lung Cancer at Various Stages

STAGE OF DISEASE AT THE TIME OF SURGICAL THERAPY	FIVE-YEAR SURVIVAL RATE* (% OF CASES)
Stage I (except $T_1N_1M_0$)	70–80
Modified Stage II	50
Visceral pleura involved	32
Stage III	
T_3N_0 (chest wall)	54
T_3N_0 (other)	40
Squamous cell cancer with node involvement observed at surgery	36
All other N_2	20
Pneumonectomy for adenocarcinoma	5

* Data courtesy of Dr. Howard Liss.

to surgical patients, 5-year survival data (Table 32–4) indicates the value of staging. Accurate and intelligent staging is the foundation for the development of all management strategies for lung cancer.

In light of the good prognosis for slow-growing neoplasms, it is not surprising that radiation therapy alone has resulted in some 5-year survivals without either surgery or chemotherapy. Chemotherapy has been most beneficial in improving both the quality of life and the average survival from small cell (oat cell) carcinoma of the lung. Chemotherapy is minimally useful against epidermoid tumors or adenocarcinomas.

Treatment is primarily directed toward palliation in the 75% of patients who are incurable at the time of diagnosis. Relief of pain and dyspnea and preservation of a tolerable quality of life with avoidance of ill-advised or fraudulent therapies form the cornerstone of successful palliation.

REFERENCES

Cohen MH: Natural history of lung cancer. *Clin Chest Med* 1982; 3:229–241. *From the beginning, as a preclinical tissue abnormality, to autopsy correlations and prognostic factors, this brief paper and the bibliography thoroughly describe the natural history of lung cancer.*

Hooper RG, Beechler CR, Johnson MC: Radioisotope scanning in the initial staging of bronchogenic carcinoma. *Am Rev Respir Dis* 1978; 118:279–286. *This report presents good prospective and retrospective data about the cost and clinical efficacy of the large battery of expensive and time-consuming tests that are available.*

Margolis R, Hansen HH, Muggia FM, Kanhouwa S: Diagnosis of liver metastases in bronchogenic carcinoma. *Cancer* 1974; 34:1825–1829. *This article presents a detailed comparison of biopsy-proven liver metastases in 111 patients to the results of liver function tests, liver scans, and peritoneoscopy.*

McKenna RJ, Haynie TP, Libshitz HI, et al: Critical evaluation of the gallium-67 scan for surgical patients with lung cancer. *Chest* 1985; 87:428–431. *This good, prospective study shows the specificity, accuracy, predictive value, and worthlessness of the gallium scan in staging.*

Morgan WKC, Andrews CE: Extrapulmonary syndromes associated with tumors of the lung, in Baum G, Wolinsky E (eds): *Textbooks of Pulmonary Diseases*, ed 3. Boston, Little, Brown, & Co, 1983, pp 1125–1143. *This is a recent, scholarly review of what is known and unknown about the potential ability of lung cancer cells to alter body function through endocrine and as yet unknown mechanisms.*

Morgan WKC, Hales MR: Bronchogenic carcinoma, in Baum G, Wolinsky E (eds). *Textbook of Pulmonary Diseases*, ed 3. Boston, Little, Brown & Co, 1983, pp 1045–1086. *This and the subsequent chapter on tumors other than bronchogenic carcinoma cover the epidemiology and the evidence for smoking as the major cause. There is also an excellent discussion of staging.*

Mountain CF, Carr DT, Anderson WAD: A system for the clinical staging of lung cancer. *Am J Roentgenol Radium Ther Nucl Med* 1974; 120:130–138. *This paper explains the detailed application of the TNM staging system to lung cancer.*

Weiss W, Boucot KR, Seideman H: The Philadelphia Pulmonary Neoplasm Research Project. *Clin Chest Med* 1982; 3:243–256. *This report represents the distillation of 30 years of clinical and radiographic evaluation of lung neoplasms in a well-defined, carefully studied population.*

ACUTE BACTERIAL PNEUMONIA

Jorge Crespo, M.D.

Pneumonia is a broad term used to describe microbial-induced inflammatory changes occurring in the terminal airways and alveolar spaces. While *pneumonia* denotes a relatively well-demarcated area of parenchymal involvement, *bronchopneumonia* usually implies a patchy distribution; qualitatively, the inflammatory process is indistinguishable.

CLINICAL SIGNS AND SYMPTOMS

Collection of historical data must be oriented to define the epidemiologic and clinical setting as well as the predisposing factors and lung-defense mechanisms involved (Table 33–1). The history may also unmask other clinical entities that mimic pneumonia such as tumors, atelectasis, and pulmonary infarction (Table 33–2).

Abruptly or towards the end of an upper respiratory infection, the patient has a single or multiple rigors that may last up to 30 minutes. A severe chest pain, worsened by deep inspiration and coughing, appears and may radiate to the shoulder or the upper abdomen or may be more prominent on the affected side. Cough, initially dry but soon productive of usually purulent sputum, appears next, and both the temperature and the pulse rate raise rapidly. Fever greater than 38.5°C is present in over 75% of patients, and tachypnea of 30 to 40 respirations per minute is also common; relative bradycardia (an increase of less than 10 beats/min for every degree Celsius) is found in viral and other atypical pneumonias and in *Legionella* pneumonia.

The patient looks anxious, the eyes are bright, and the skin, while flushed over the face, may show acral cyanosis; a fine perspiration is the rule. In patients with pneumococcal pneumonia, jaundice may be present. The patient is observed to prefer shallow breathing, splinting the affected side while resting on it; early on the pulse is full and bounding and later may appear feeble. Frequently, herpes labialis is present.

Examination of the lungs reveals a consolidation syndrome (dullness, increased vocal fremitus, bronchial breathing, e to a changes, decreased breath sounds), but it may be masked, totally or partially, by a pleural effusion. In severely ill patients, the alae nasi dilate with inspiration, marked cyanosis is present, and sternal retraction is seen. Postural changes in pulse rate and blood pressure should be sought. On occasion, a paralytic ileus and upper abdominal tenderness are found.

As the process evolves, the cough becomes frankly productive, with a rusty or bloody character, or it may appear purulent; signs of dehydration become apparent, and the temperature remains elevated. The initial disorientation and confusion of the patient may give way to overt psychotic behavior, particularly in alcoholic patients. Depending on the microorganism involved, the clinical course may follow a progressive, slow resolution as it does in most patients (pneumococcal pneumonia), or it may evolve rapidly into a septic picture with shock, disseminated intravascular coagulation, respiratory insufficiency, and death (gram-negative bacillary pneumonias).

Metastatic infections (meningitis, arthritis, endocarditis) are rare in the antibiotic era. More commonly, empyema, particularly with anaerobic microorganisms and *Staphylococcus aureus*, still poses a problem. Hyponatremia due to inappropriate secretion of antidiuretic hormone is relatively common.

TABLE 33–1.
Pathophysiologic and Etiologic Relationships in Acute Bacterial Pneumonias

PREDISPOSING FACTORS*	DEFENSE MECHANISM AFFECTED	AGENTS, COMMUNITY-ACQUIRED*	AGENTS, HOSPITAL-ACQUIRED
Alcohol, anesthesia, unconsciousness, CNS depression, esophageal disorder, periodontal infection	Defective or overwhelmed epiglottal and/or cough reflexes	Pneumococci; *Klebsiella pneumoniae;* mixed, predominantly anaerobic oral flora	GNEB,† *Staphylococcus aureus,* pneumococci, oral anaerobes
URI, alcohol, tracheal intubation, chronic bronchitis, immotile cilia	Impaired mucociliary system	Pneumococci, *Hemophilus influenzae, K. pneumoniae*	GNEB, pneumococci
URI, anesthesia, bronchiectasis, toxic inhalants	Increased airway secretions	Pneumococci, oral flora	Pneumococci, GNEB
Mucous plugging, after surgery, intraluminal tumor or foreign body	Stasis of airway secretions	Pneumococci, oral flora	Pneumococci, oral flora, GNEB
CHF, liver cirrhosis, aspiration trauma	Accumulation of alveolar fluid	Pneumococci	Pneumococci, GNEB
Neutropenia, sickle-cell disease, asplenia	Defective phagocytosis	Pneumococci, *H. influenzae, K. pneumoniae*	Pneumococci, GNEB
Hypogammaglobulinemia (congenital, multiple myeloma, CLL, malnutrition)	Defective opsonization	Pneumococci, *H. influenzae*	Pneumococci, *H. influenzae*

* In approximate order of frequency.
† GNEB: gram-negative enteric bacilli.

TABLE 33–2.

Clinical, Laboratory and Radiologic Differentiation of Causes of Pulmonary Infiltrates and Fever

DIFFERENTIATING FACTOR	BACTERIAL PNEUMONIA	PULMONARY INFARCTION	TUMOR	ATELECTASIS	"COLLAGEN" DISORDERS
Predisposing factor(s)	URI, alcoholism, critical illness, immunosuppression	Surgery, immobility, trauma, CHF	Smoking	Thoracic or abdominal surgery	Unknown
Fever, sweating	Yes, usually >39.5°C	Yes, usually <39.5°C	Yes, variable	Yes, usually <39.5°C	Yes, usually <39.5°C
Cough, sputum	Yes, purulent, bloody	Yes, bloody	Yes, bloody	No	Rare
Hemoptysis	Yes, rusty sputum	Yes, fresh blood	Yes, blood streaks	No	No
Pleuritic pain	Yes	Yes	Variable	No	Variable
Pleural effusion	Yes, clear to purulent	Yes, bloody	Yes, bloody	No	Yes, usually clear
Dyspnea, cyanosis	Common	Common	Frequent	Common	Rare
Leukocytosis	Yes	Yes	No	No	No
Bilirubin level	May be elevated	May be elevated	Normal	Normal	Normal
PaO_2	Decreased	Decreased	Normal	Decreased	Usually normal
Gram's stain of sputum	Neutrophils predominate	Normal flora, RBCs, few leukocytes	Normal flora	Normal flora, no leukocytes	Normal flora, no leukocytes
Chest x-ray films	Variable infiltrate, commonly lobar or segmental or patchy	Pleural-based, wedge-shaped, segmental infiltrate	Variable	Volume loss, plate-like lines	Nodular or diffuse infiltrates
Radionuclide scans	Matched V̇/Q defects	Matched V̇/Q defects	Unmatched V̇/Q defects	Unmatched V̇/Q defects	Unmatched V̇/Q defects
Pulmonary angiogram	Normal	Intraluminal filling defect	Variable	Normal	Normal

PATHOPHYSIOLOGY

Microorganisms may reach the lung parenchyma by inhalation, microaspiration, gross aspiration, hematogenous spread, or direct implantation (e.g., penetrating chest injuries or surgery). A host of defensive mechanisms is operative: air-suspended organisms can be inhaled into alveolar spaces only if they are present in particles between 0.5 and 3 microns in diameter; larger particles adhere to mucus lining the respiratory epithelium and are removed by ciliary clearance. When nonparticulate material reaches the airways, the cough reflex effectively removes the bulk of it, the remaining being cleared by the mucociliary apparatus. Should this barrier prove inadequate, invading microorganisms will find in the alveoli surfactant, immunoglobulins, and complement components which, jointly or independently, will opsonize them and enhance resident alveolar macrophage or polymorphonuclear phagocytosis.

Microbes that are inhaled and have appropriate pathogenic characteristics will produce disease in exposed susceptible individuals. Microorganisms present in the oropharynx (e.g., pneumococci in normal hosts, gram-negative bacili in hospitalized or immunocompromised patients) are carried into the alveoli by microaspirates (common even in normal individuals) during periods of mucociliary apparatus dysfunction such as viral upper respiratory infections, smoke inhalations, and so forth. When the cough mechanism is defective or simply insufficient to deal with the volume of aspirated material (as occurs with a decreased epiglottal reflex), the microorganisms locate in the most dependent portion of the airway, with frank predominance of anaerobic oral flora. Historical data, can, therefore, be extremely helpful in pointing out likely candidate organisms. Similarly, mechanical problems of the airway, such as increased secretions, atelectasis, alveolar fluid collection, and endobronchial masses, are also factors favoring microbial stasis and multiplication. Finally, inadequate phagocytosis (such as in neutropenia and asplenia) or defective opsonization (such as in hypogammaglobulinemia and sickle-cell disease) also represent a higher infection risk.

The presence of microorganisms in the alveoli triggers a predictable sequence of events: an outpouring of fluid into the alveoli, as leukocytic enzymes increase capillary permeability, brings to the site serum factors such as complement, which is activated directly by microbial polysaccharide capsular material or endotoxin, or with the assistance of specific antibodies; chemotactic factors generated in this process attract polymorphonuclear leukocytes, which together with red blood cells leaking from damaged capillaries produce an almost solid area of consolidation, facilitating phagocytosis of the microbes, which is limited only by anatomical barriers like the pleura. Inflammation of the visceral pleura produces loss of its normal smoothness, and, with respiratory movements, contact with the parietal pleura produces pleuritic pain and an audible rub; a protein-rich fluid commonly accumulates in the pleural space. As polymorphonuclear phagocytosis becomes more efficient, aided by a more solid environment and increasing levels of opsonizing antibodies, the inflammatory process recedes and macrophages make their appearance to "clean up" the battlefield.

When pneumococci are the causative bacteria, alveolar architecture is preserved as a rule, and there is complete healing; however, particularly with anaerobic and gram-negative enterobacteria, variable degrees of permanent parenchymal damage will occur. On occasion, the inflammatory process is not clearly circumscribed, and multiple, smaller areas are involved usually following a bronchial distribution, therefore, the designation *bronchopneumonia*. Also, invasion of the bloodstream and metastatic infections occur with variable frequency depending on the characteristics of the microbe and of the host.

CLINICAL–PATHOLOGIC CORRELATIONS

The clinical manifestations of bacterial pneumonias represent the expression of an acute, extensive inflammatory process; host factors such as underlying disease(s) and the ability to mount an appropriate response interplay with microbial characteristics, like intrinsic resistance to phagocytosis, production of histotoxic substances, and antibiotic susceptibility. Table 33–3 summarizes some of the salient relationships between the causative agent and the clinical syndrome.

TABLE 33–3.
Etiologic and Clinical–Pathologic Correlations for Acute Bacterial Pneumonia

AGENT	SETTING	CLINICAL FEATURES	X-RAY FILM APPEARANCE	SPUTUM FINDINGS
Streptococcus pneumoniae	Any person after URI; alcoholism; sickle-cell disease; asplenia	Acute onset, single shaking chill, pleuritic pain	Homogeneous lobar or segmental consolidation, pleural effusion	Rusty, abundant neutrophils, predominantly lancet-shaped, gram-positive diplococci
Mixed anaerobic bacteria	Episodes of unconsciousness; after anesthesia; esophageal disorders	Insidious onset, night sweat, weight loss, slow progression	Abscess in dependent lung segment, empyema in 30% of cases	Foul-smelling, copious on awakening, abundant neutrophils, mixed gram-positive and gram-negative cocci and rods, cultures, show "normal flora"
Gram-negative enteric bacilli	Immunosuppression tracheal intubation, alcoholism	Acute severe illness, pleuritic pain, multiple rigors, septic shock	Lobar or segmental consolidation, pleural effusion, necrosis, and cavitation	"Currant jelly" (*Klebsiella pneumoniae*), predominant bacterium or mixed with normal flora in Gram's stain
Legionella group	Middle age to elderly, endemic or in outbreaks	Prodromal period, multiple rigors, diarrhea, pulse–temperature dissociation	Nodular or interstitial pattern, progress to multisegmental or multilobar, pleural effusion	Mucoid or blood-tinged, few neutrophils, normal flora in Gram's stain and cultures
Staphylococcus aureus	Post-influenza, intravenous drug abuse	Acute severe illness, multiple rigors, metastatic infections	Nodular bronchopneumonias, pneumatoceles, empyema, pyopneumothorax	Abundant, numerous neutrophils; predominant gram-positive cocci in clusters
Hemophilus influenzae	Elderly patients, chronic obstructive lung disease, alcoholism, hypogammaglobulinemia	Acute onset, pleuritic pain	Bronchopneumonic or lobar consolidation, pleural effusion	Numerous neutrophils, gram-negative coccobacilli or normal flora

DIFFERENTIAL DIAGNOSIS

Bacterial pneumonia is initially seen as a febrile illness with variable degrees of respiratory distress, productive cough, and radiologic evidence of pulmonary infiltrates and, frequently, pleural effusion. Table 33–2 depicts distinguishing features that are helpful in separating several clinical conditions with these findings. Distinguishing among these conditions is, however, complicated by the dynamic interaction of different factors, such as tumors predisposing to pneumonia by obstructing the bronchial tree, bedrest in patients with pneumonia predisposing to pulmonary embolism and infarction, or thick purulent sputum producing atelectasis. Continuous and painstaking observation is necessary throughout the disease course in a patient with pneumonia, and ancillary diagnostic methods must be undertaken only when it is predicted that the information gained will significantly alter the therapeutic program or the anticipated course of the disease.

DIAGNOSIS

The clinical and radiologic diagnosis of pneumonia is usually not difficult. However, the most relevant aspect in the diagnostic approach to pneumonia is to elucidate the cause because critical decisions regarding therapy, prognosis, and isolation measures are dictated by this information. The physician must also decide the degree of diagnostic invasiveness appropriate for each individual situation. Important diagnostic testing includes a combination of information derived from the following test categories: blood, radiologic evaluation, evaluation of respiratory secretion, and evaluation of pleural fluid.

BLOOD

The WBC count is commonly elevated, between 15,000–35,000/mL, with a shift toward immature forms; when present, leukopenia indicates a poor prognosis. The hematocrit and RBC indices are usually normal. At least three blood cultures should be collected prior to antibiotic therapy; these will be positive in about 25% of cases of pneumococcal pneumonia,

10% of *Staphylococcus aureus* pneumonia, and about 8% of enteric gram-negative pneumonias. Positive results are incontrovertible evidence of the cause of the pneumonic process. In cases where the clinical suspicion centers on atypical pneumonias or *Legionella* infections, an acute serum[1] specimen should be obtained for serologic studies. Various techniques for bacterial antigen detection (in sputum, blood, urine) are available, but their role in diagnosis is not clearly defined.

RADIOLOGIC EVALUATION

X-ray films of the chest, ideally posteroanterior and lateral views, are extremely helpful in defining the presence of infiltrates and their characteristics and distribution and the presence of pleural effusion. Determination of the cause cannot, however, be made on the basis of radiologic examinations, although some clues, together with other clinical and diagnostic findings, may suggest a certain cause. Homogeneous lobar consolidation is common in pneumococcal pneumonia, but also occurs in *Hemophilus influenzae* infection. Consolidation of a lower lobe, cavitation, and large pleural effusions are frequently seen in gram-negative bacillary pneumonia. A patchy interstitial or nodular infiltrate that rapidly progresses to involve two or more lobes is found in *Legionella* infections. Upper lobe consolidation with bulging fissure lines and central necrosis points to a *Klebsiella pneumoniae* infection. Necrotizing features, cavitation, and empyema, all in dependent areas of the lung, raise the suspicion of an anaerobic infection. Finally, thin-walled cavities (pneumatoceles) and multiple nodular infiltrates are present in cases of *Staphylococcus aureus* hematogenous infection.

EVALUATION OF RESPIRATORY SECRETIONS

The oropharynx is the source of the infecting agent in most cases of bacterial pneumonia and harbors multiple potential agents. When failure of the mucociliary system (microaspiration) or of the epiglottal and cough reflexes (gross as-

---

[1]Serum sample for determination of specific antibodies; this will be compared with a "convalescent" serum sample obtained 2 to 4 weeks later.

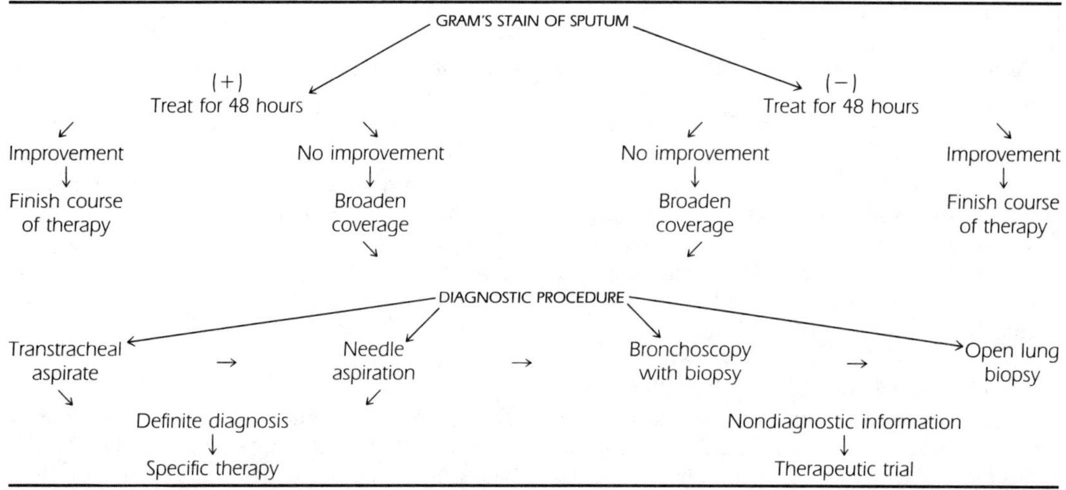

(+): Predominant organism present.
(−): No predominant organism present.
(a): Patient receiving antibiotics for other indication; immunocompromised host.

FIG 33–1.
Algorithm for the Diagnosis and Management of Acute Pneumonia.

piration) allows these microorganisms to reach the alveoli, an active infection may ensue depending on the balance between inoculum size, bacterial pathogenicity, and host factors. As a result of the inflammatory process that follows, exudates containing the offending microorganism are expectorated in the form of sputum. Unfortunately, this material must pass through the oropharynx, which results in contamination by the resident flora. Although it is possible to identify the responsible agent from this exudate, it also contains numerous other likely candidates. Few issues in diagnostic testing have generated as much controversy as the usefulness, or the lack of it, of evaluating expectorated sputum, but because the sample is easily obtained, this evaluation continues to play an important role in the initial evaluation of a patient with pneumonia. Certainly once antibiotic therapy has been initiated, interpretation of sputum tests is unreliable.

For an adequate evaluation, careful attention to procedure is paramount. The patient should be instructed to rinse the oral cavity and then cough deeply, bringing up sputum from the airway and not the mouth. Prompt transport to the microbiology laboratory is critical. If the patient is unable to produce sputum, cough induction with ultrasonic nebulization of hypertonic saline may help. The sputum is usually mucopurulent in cases of bacterial pneumonia, but is also purulent in up to half of patients with mycoplasmal or adenoviral infections. Rusty sputum is common in pneumococcal pneumonia, whereas dark-red, mucoid (current jelly), tenacious sputum occurs in *Klebsiella pneumoniae* infections. Anaerobic infections produce foul-smelling sputa.

The most obviously purulent portions of the specimen are selected for Gram's staining, ignoring organisms adherent to flat, large epithelial cells and establishing the presence or absence of a clearly predominant type of bacterium. With this information, the algorithm in Figure 33–1 can be used. Sputum cultures can offer valuable information when specimens are processed rapidly following preselection by strict criteria, such as fewer than 10 epithelial cells and more than 25 neutrophils per high-power field.

Alternative methods that bypass the oropharynx (transtracheal aspiration, bronchoscopic brushings with or without transbronchial biopsy, percutaneous lung aspiration, open lung biopsy) represent variable levels of invasiveness. Their use depends on consideration such as indications, availability, local expertise, cost, and patient risk.

EVALUATION OF PLEURAL FLUID

Accumulation of exudates (in which the ratio of lactic dehydrogenase (LDH) concentration in the pleural fluid to that in the serum is greater than 0.6; and the protein concentration ratio is greater than 0.5) is a common complication of enteric gram-negative pneumonias (50%–70%), pneumococcal pneumonia (10%–20%), *Legionella* pneumonia (25%–30%), and is almost the rule in group A streptococcal pneumonia (more than 95%). While most effusions resolve with appropriate therapy of the infectious process, a small number (less than 5%) progresses to empyemas (frankly purulent or culture-positive effusions). An exception is anaerobic lung infections in which empyemas may develop in up to one-third of cases. In early states, empyemas can be drained with a tube thoracostomy, whereas organized, loculated empyemas may require partial rib resection for drainage. All large effusions and those in patients with a poor clinical response to therapy should be studied further. In addition to protein and LDH determinations and aerobic and anaerobic cultures, the pH (using the same technique employed for blood gas analysis) should be measured. Effusions with a pH lower than 7.0 need to be treated by tube thoracostomy because they almost invariably evolve into empyemas.

PRINCIPLES OF PREVENTION AND THERAPY

Community-acquired pneumonias commonly follow upper respiratory infections, and the excess mortality[2] rates following influenza outbreaks have been attributed to pneumonia-related deaths. Pneumococcal polysaccharide vaccines (e.g., Pneumovax 23) contain antigens from the most common pneumococcal serotypes (those responsible for up to 90% of infec-

------

[2]Death rate above the expected normalized rate for a given time period.

tions) and produce adequate protection in about 80% of recipients. High-risk patients such as asplenic or sickle-cell disease patients as well as those with chronic cardiac and respiratory disorders should be vaccinated. Revaccination no more frequently than every 5 years is recommended.

Aspiration pneumonias can be prevented by adequate control of convulsive or other disorders compromising consciousness, avoidance of alcohol intoxication, and diligent postanesthetic care. In the care of the immunoincompetent and the critically ill patient, careful handwashing and appropriate cleaning of respiratory equipment is essential.

The initial selection of antibiotic therapy is empiric; it is based on the clinical interpretation of historic, epidemiologic, and radiologic data together with information derived from a Gram's stain of sputum. By necessity, the antibiotic therapy must include adequate coverage for the worst possible situation likely in each individual case. The clinical response or the microbiologic data may prompt modification of the antibiotic program. Causes other than a failure to respond to antibiotics produce fever, such as atelectasis due to mucous plugs, development of empyema, and drug fever. Physical chest therapy, including postural drainage, is an important adjunct. Supportive therapy directed to ensure proper oxygenation, adequate nutrition, and maintenance of a balanced fluid status is important.

Bacterial pneumonias continue to carry a grave prognosis. The overall mortality rate for pneumococcal pneumonia treated with penicillin is around 5%, but bacteremic cases have a mortality rate of 20%. In gram-negative bacillary pneumonias the mortality rate averages 50%, whereas in appropriately treated *Legionella* infections, it is about 5%.

Pneumococcal pneumonia patients have a rapid defervescence with return to normal temperatures within the first 48 hours after penicillin. A feeling of well-being usually appears before the normal temperature returns. Recurrence of fever should initiate the search for a complication. On the other hand, gram-negative pneumonias have a much slower clinical recovery and may take 7 to 10 days before significant clinical improvement can be observed. Anaerobic lung infections also resolve slowly.

REFERENCES

Davidson M, Tempest B, Palmer DL: Bacteriologic diagnosis of acute pneumonia. Comparison of sputum, transtracheal aspirates, and lung aspirates. *JAMA* 1976; 235:158–163. *Exposes the limitations of sputum cultures as a diagnostic tool. An eye-opener.*

Donowitz GR, Mandell GL: Acute pneumonia, in Mandell GL, Douglas RG, Bennett JE (eds). *Principles and Practice of Infectious Diseases,* ed 2. New York, Wiley Medical Publication, 1985, pp 394–404. *An up-to-date exhaustive review with 152 references.*

Lerner AM, Jankauskas K: The classic bacterial pneumonias. *DM,* February 1975, pp 1–46. *Comprehensive discussion of the clinical course, diagnosis, therapy, and complications of pneumococcal* pneumonia as well as of other common bacterial pneumonias.

Light RN, Girard WM, Jenkinson, SJ, et al: Parapneumonic effusions. *AM J Med* 1980; 69:507–512. *Reviews experience with relationship between pleural fluid parameters and the natural course of parapneumonic effusions.*

Reynolds HY: Lung host defenses—status report. *Chest* 1979; 75 (suppl):239–242. *A thorough review of the mechanisms of lung defense.*

Stulbarg MS: Problems in diagnosing pneumonia. (Medical Staff Conference) *West J Med* 1984; 140:594–601. *Discusses the practical clinical application of diagnostic techniques with emphasis on the microbiologic evaluation of lower respiratory secretions.*

34   ATYPICAL PNEUMONIA

Charles B. Payne, Jr., M.D.

The term *atypical pneumonias* originated to describe pulmonary infections with a bronchopneumonic infiltrate seen in chest x-ray films and from which no specific or predominant organism could be identified with gram-negative staining or bacteriologic culture of the sputum. Today, the viral pneumonias are excluded from this group. We will discuss psittacosis (once known as "parrot fever") caused by *Chlamydia psittaci,* primary atypical pneumonia caused by *Mycoplasma pneumoniae,* and pneumonia caused by *Legionella* species. These nonviral organisms are poorly detected or not detected by Gram's stain. Their identification is important because they respond to antibiotic treatment. Another member of this group, Q fever, will not be discussed because of its infrequent occurrence in the United States, the only recent cases being in laboratory workers exposed to sheep. *Psittacosis* is used as a term because of the desire to restrict the term *ornithosis* to mean the disease as it occurs in birds.

CLINICAL SIGNS AND SYMPTOMS

PSITTACOSIS

The usual incubation period for psittacosis is 7 to 15 days, although periods up to 2 months have been reported. About 75% of the patients report contact with a bird. The bird may or may not be sick and may or may not be a member of the psittacine birds, such as parakeets and parrots, as cases have been reported after contact with chickens, turkeys, pigeons, and ducks. Human-to-human infection also occurs. About 25% of cases have no known source.

The onset is severe with fever, myalgia, and a

mild-to-moderate cough. Shaking chills may occur in one-third of patients. As a rule, not much sputum is produced, but it may be either blood-tinged or frankly bloody. Pleurisy may occur.

Physical examination of the chest may reveal patchy crackles or areas of consolidation in several lobes of the lung. On occasion, the chest physical examination may be normal. Pleural effusion may occur. The general examination may show severe lymphadenopathy, jaundice, or bradycardia disproportionate to the height of the fever. Splenomegaly is found in 10% to 30% of patients. Pleuropericardial friction rubs and pharyngitis are found occasionally and meningoencephalitis is reported.

Psittacosis has a protracted course in both the flulike form in which respiratory symptoms predominate and the "typhoidal" form in which systemic fever, myalgia, and headache predominate. Before effective therapy was available, the mortality rate was as high as 30% to 40% in reported epidemics. Listed complications include thyroiditis, myocarditis, pericarditis with rubs, acquired valvular heart disease, endocarditis, encephalitis with seizures, anemia, usually hemolysis with a negative cold-agglutinin test but occasionally with a positive Coombs' test, disseminated intravascular coagulation, hepatitis, pancreatitis, oliguria, and proteinuria. With treatment, the reported mortality rate is between 1% and 4%. The disease is unusual before adolescence.

MYCOPLASMA (PRIMARY ATYPICAL) PNEUMONIA

Mycoplasma pneumonia may be sporadic or epidemic. It has been reported to cause 20% of all adult pneumonias and more than 50% of pneumonias in college students and military recruits. Only 3% to 10% of persons infected with *M. pneumoniae* will develop pneumonic symptoms with pharyngitis and tracheobronchitis being the predominant complaint in other symptomatic patients. The incubation period is 7 to 21 days. The onset of illness may be acute or insidious with an unremitting hacking cough, the hallmark of the disease. The cough is usually nonproductive. More than 50% of symptomatic patients have severe headache and 80% have a temperature over 38.4°C. Influenza-like symptoms of myalgia and

nasal congestion are common. Pleurisy is said to occur in fewer than 5% of patients, with pneumonia and shaking chills in 25%.

Mycoplasma pneumonia is usually self-limited with fatal cases being rare. In 10% of pneumonic patients with fever, headache, and malaise, the generalized symptoms resolve within 3 to 10 days. The cough and crackles resolve in an average of 4 to 6 weeks, paralleling the improvement in the chest x-ray films. Musculoskeletal and gastrointestinal complaints are common. In pneumonic cases, earache, sore throat, and rhinorrhea may occur in half the patients. Bullous and hemorrhagic myringitis occur infrequently. Complications may be severe in patients who have sickle cell disease. The adult respiratory distress syndrome has been reported as a complication of *M. pneumoniae* infections. Treatment with antibiotics is known to alleviate the symptoms and hasten radiographic resolution of pneumonic infiltrates, but does not eradicate the organism from the sputum. Relapses within 7 to 10 days after the completion of treatment are not uncommon.

LEGIONELLA PNEUMONIA

In 1977, legionnaire's disease, a severe, epidemic multisystem disease involving the lungs (pneumonia), the central nervous system, and the gastrointestinal tract led to the identification of the organism *Legionella pneumophila*. The number of species in the genus and the clinical picture of disease produced by these organisms continue to expand. *L. pneumophila* is also implicated as a cause of Pontiac fever, a flulike illness characterized by fever, myalgia, and chest pain. Its incubation period is between 5 and 66 hours, versus 2 to 10 days for legionnaires' disease. *L. pneumophila* has been implicated in pneumonia epidemics dating back to 1947. Both sporadic and epidemic cases of hospital-acquired pneumonia caused by various species of *Legionella* have been reported. Pericarditis without pneumonia, infections in immunosuppressed patients, and cutaneous abscesses have been described, and the species *L. micdadei*, *L. bozemanii*, *L. dumoffi*, and *L. wadsworthii* have been shown to cause disease in humans.

The organisms live in water. Epidemics from contaminated water-cooling towers and shower heads have been reported, and transmission by potable water has been documented. Because of the great variation in and incomplete description of the clinical picture, high awareness is necessary to initiate the appropriate diagnostic studies for determining whether or not *Legionella* plays a role in the pathogenesis of an atypical pneumonic infection.

The course of *Legionnella* pneumonia (legionellosis) may be extraordinarily variable. One variant, Pontiac fever, is an acute, self-limited gastrointestinal illness which may last up to 3 days. Individuals may develop serum antibodies to the organism without symptoms. In contrast, during the explosive outbreak of legionnaires' disease in Philadelphia in July 1976, 29 of 182 reported cases were fatal. All of these patients had acute chills, fever up to 39°C, and x-ray evidence of pneumonia. Approximately 50% of patients have central nervous system involvement. Abdominal pain, tenderness, nausea, and vomiting occur in about 15% of patients.

In nosocomial outbreaks, the disease has been more common in male smokers and in those with alcoholism, immunosuppression, and underlying disease such as renal insufficiency or cancer. Because of the marked variability of clinical findings and the existence of seropositive patients without disease, the effects of treatment are difficult to assess. Antibiotic therapy does shorten the course of disease and results in earlier defervescence and clearing of infiltrates shown on x-ray films. Relapses are reported.

CLINICAL–PATHOLOGIC CORRELATIONS

The clinical–pathologic correlations for the atypical pneumonias are listed in Table 34–1.

TABLE 34–1.
Clinical–Pathologic Correlations for the Atypical Pneumonias

CLINICAL FINDINGS	PATHOLOGIC FINDINGS
PSITTACOSIS	
Pneumonia	Disease begins in the hilum; capillary leak leads to fluid-filled interstitial spaces and alveoli; polymorphonuclear leukocytes respond to early inflammation; mononuclear leukocytes rapidly follow; patchy consolidation and minor hemorrhage may occur.
Hepatosplenomegaly	Nonspecific splenic inflammation and reactive hepatitis; focal hepatic necrosis in fatal cases
Bradycardia Myocarditis Valvular heart disease	Fatty degeneration and lymphocytic infiltration of the myocardium; subendocardial hemorrhage, especially near the mitral and aortic valves; intracytoplasmic myocardial inclusion bodies
Headache Confusion	Fibrinous or gelatinous arachnoiditis around the sylvian fissures; meningeal and cerebral congestion; perivascular hemorrhages in brain and cord; lymphocytic infiltrates
Oliguria Proteinuria	Glomerular capillary hyaline occlusions; acute tubular necrosis occurs rarely.
MYCOPLASMA PNEUMONIA	
Pneumonia	Lungs show interstitial inflammatory reaction, predominantly lymphocytic with plasma cells; alveolar lining cells may become cuboidal and desquamate.
Pleural fluid	Exudative; serous or serosanguinous; normal glucose level; cells are mixed polys and lymphs up to 10,000/ml.
Tracheitis Tracheobronchitis	Polymorphonuclear leukocytes in the tracheal and bronchial lumen, with an interstitial mononuclear infiltrate
Carditis	Myocardium and pericardium involved; tissue information scarce
LEGIONNAIRES' DISEASE	
Pneumonia	Neutrophils combine with macrophages and fibrin to form dense, nonspecific, fibrinopurulent, intralveolar infiltrates; inflammatory cell lysis is common; fibrinous pleuritis is also common.

DIFFERENTIAL DIAGNOSIS

Diseases that produce fever of unknown origin, bronchopneumonia, or influenza-like symptoms are included in the differential diagnosis of atypical pneumonias. Patients with either a *M. pneumoniae* infection or the Pontiac-fever type of *Legionella* infection are asymptomatic or only mildly symptomatic. *C. psittaci* infections may cause systemic signs, and symptoms predominate. A great many diseases could be included in the differential diagnosis of *C. psittaci* infection; the most common ones include lung cancer, lymphangitic cancer spread in the lungs, lymphomas, cystic fibrosis, and tuberculosis.

A diagnosis depends on a high index of suspicion, epidemiologic evidence of the disease in the community, and a thorough history that should include queries about exposure to birds. The diagnosis is often made retrospectively after laboratory testing.

The radiographic features of each disease are described in the section on diagnosis. Because the pulmonary infiltrates are bronchopneumonic, it is not possible to make the specific or differential diagnosis of any of the atypical pneumonias by x-ray evidence alone.

DIAGNOSIS

PSITTACOSIS

A chest x-ray film shows extremely variable bronchopneumonic infiltrates, predominantly involving the lung bases and frequently radiating from the hilum. Focal areas of consolidation occur in 10% to 20% of cases. X-ray findings may be more extensive than is suggested by physical examination.

The leukocyte count is usually normal. Gram's stain of the sputum usually shows few polymorphonuclear leukocytes and no predominant organism. The sputum is rarely purulent. *Chlamydia* is readily isolated from sputum, lung, or other tissue, but because this procedure is hazardous for laboratory technicians, it is seldom done.

Cold-agglutinin titers occasionally rise in psittacosis. Complement-fixing antibodies appear in the serum 2 to 4 weeks after infection, although antibiotic therapy may cause a 2-week delay. The antibody level usually occurs at about 21 days. A fourfold rise in the antibody titer is diagnostic. Serum samples taken during the acute and convalescent phases are normally required.

MYCOPLASMA PNEUMONIA

In the chest x-ray film, the infiltrates may be nodular, patchy, or perihilar. Most cases are unilateral, involving one or two lobes, but are bilateral in 10% to 40% of cases. Lung abscesses are rare. The incidence of pleural effusions is controversial. Large effusions are reported. Resolution of infiltrates usually occurs in 10 to 21 days, but may take as long as 6 weeks.

The leukocyte count may be elevated in one-fourth of cases, with counts as high as 25,000/mL reported in severe cases (Yow, Brennan, Preston, and Levy, 1959). The ESR is elevated. Occasionally elevations of the transaminase level, biologic false-positive VDRL tests, and tuberculin anergy have been reported. Hemolytic anemia with positive Coombs' tests and reticulocytosis is common. A severe, cold-agglutinin autoimmune hemolytic anemia occurs rarely. The ECG may show changes of the myocarditis.

Cold agglutinins occur in 70% to 85% of patients with pneumonia between 1 and 4 weeks after infection. The agglutinins are nonspecific and may not accompany the development of specific antibodies against *M. pneumoniae;* hence measuring cold agglutinins is not recommend as a specific diagnostic test. Syringes warmed to 37°C and special handling are required for complete detection of cold agglutinins. Cold agglutinins are a useful screening test but should be supported by specific antibody studies for precise diagnosis.

The first of two preferred diagnostic methods for isolating *M. pneumoniae* from sputum, throat washings or swabs, requires 7 to 10 days. If available, body fluids, such as pleural fluid, skin and middle ear vesicle fluid, should also be sent to the laboratory for attempted isolation of the organism. The second method is the detection of complement-fixing antibodies in the serum. A fourfold increase in titer in the sera collected during the acute and convalescent phases is diagnostic. A titer of 1:64 or greater in serum collected during the convalescent phase is highly suggestive of *M. pneumoniae* infection. The responsible antibody appears 7 to 9 days after infection, reaches peak levels at 4 to 6 weeks, and begins to decline 4 to 6 months later, falling to levels of 1:16 in 2 to 3 years.

LEGIONELLA PNEUMONIA

The bronchopneumonic x-ray picture is not characteristic. Small, unilateral pleural effusions may appear 6% to 59% of the time, depending on the series reported and how carefully the effusion was sought. A number of cases may not have abnormal findings in the x-ray films. Occasional lung abscesses have been reported.

The leukocyte count may be normal or elevated. The ESR is often markedly elevated. Serum abnormalities including azotemia, elevated transaminase levels, hyponatremia, high levels of antidiuretic hormone from inappropriate secretion, and hypophosphatemia have been reported. Although proteinuria is frequent, microscopic hematuria is rare. A Gram's stain of sputum rarely shows bacteria identifiable as *Legionella* species, although gram staining of lung tissue from biopsy specimens may be useful. The modified Dieterle staining of lung tissue is preferred.

Current diagnostic tests on sputum include direct fluorescent antibody (DFA) staining and serologic testing. Culture of the sputum using improved methods is reported to be positive earlier in the course of the disease than are DFA techniques, but each laboratory generally has a preferred method. When available, pleural fluid should be sent for examination by either or both techniques. Specimens may be secured by transtracheal aspiration and sleeved bronchial brushes during fiberoptic bronchoscopy.

Serologic testing requires sera from both the acute and convalescent phases. Seroconversion begins as early as 1 week after the onset of pneumonia. Because existing methods produce both false-negative and false-positive results, improved diagnostic techniques are under development.

PRINCIPLES OF PREVENTION AND THERAPY

Public health measures directed toward examination, quarantine, and elimination of infected birds are the most effective preventative for *C. psittaci* infections. There is currently no effective prevention for *M. pneumoniae* infections and no known preventive strategy for sporadic cases of Legionellosis. Epidemics of Legionellosis traceable to potable water sources have been controlled either by superheating or hyperchlorinating the water. Because *Legionella* infections are spread by aerosolized infectious droplets, the preventing of exposure of people at risk, such as immunocompromised patients or hotel dwellers, requires careful engineering design. Existing as well as proposed public places must be constructed with prevention of *Legionella* species outbreaks in mind.

C. psittaci infections respond to tetracyclines, which should be given in doses of 1 gm to 2 gm per day for 10 to 14 days after defervescence. Relapse may occur. Chloramphenicol is also an effective drug, and although penicillin in large doses may be beneficial, its efficacy has not yet been well established.

M. pneumoniae responds to either erythromycin or tetracycline in doses of 2 gm per day for 10 to 14 days. Resistance to oxytetracycline has been reported. Up to half the patients may remain culture-positive for 6 to 13 weeks after treatment. The efficacy of retreatment is controversial.

L. pneumophila and other species are best treated with intravenous erythromycin, 2 gm to 4 gm per day. Oral erythromycin therapy in doses of 500 mg to 1 gm at 6-hour intervals may be used in those less seriously ill. Recommended durations of therapy vary from 14 to 21 days. Optimal doses and duration are as yet unknown.

REFERENCES

Fraser DW, Tsai RT, Orenstein W, et al: Legionnaires' disease. *N Engl J Med* 1977; 297:1189–1197. *This is the earliest detailed description of the epidemic which brought this disease to everyone's attention.*

Louria DB: Pneumonia due to viruses, *Chlamydiaceae*, and mycoplasmas, in Baum GL, Wolinsky E (eds): *Textbook of Pulmonary Diseases.* Boston, Little, Brown & Co, 1983, pp 431–443.

Mangione EJ, Remis RS, Tait KA, et al: An outbreak of Pontiac fever related to whirlpool use, Michigan 1982. *JAMA 1985; 253(4):535–539. This is an excellent description of the milder, epidemic form of infection with epidemiologic studies implicating a whirlpool bath used by a church group.*

Murray HW, Tuazon C: Atypical pneumonias. *Med Clin North Am 1980; 64:507–527. This is a detailed and extremely well-referenced survey of the atypical pneumonias by a recognized authority on M. pneumoniae.*

Shands KN, Ho JL, Meyer RD, et al: Potable water as a source of legionnaires' disease. *JAMA 1985; 253:1412–1416. This report of a 3-year epidemic in a hospital illustrates the epidemiologic and engineering work required to control this nosocomial infection.*

Yow EM, Brennan CJ, Preston J, Levy S: The pathology of psittacosis. *Am J Med 1959; 27(5):739–749. This older but detailed and pertinent reference work describes the pathologic changes in Chlamydia psittaci infections very well. Contains useful clinical information.*

Zuravleff JJ, Yu VL, Shonnard JW, Davis BK, Rihs JD: Diagnosis of legionnaires' disease. *JAMA 1983; 250:1981–1985. This is a 1983 update on the various laboratory methods for isolation and clinical diagnostic studies for legionnaires' disease.*

35 LUNG ABSCESS

Timothy B. Sorg, M.D.

Lung abscess is a suppurative pulmonary infection that destroys lung parenchyma. The most common cause is aspiration of anaerobic bacteria that normally colonize the upper respiratory tract, but a number of other pathogenic bacteria can cause lung abscess. The lesion consists of an area of central necrosis surrounded by inflamed tissue and fibrosis. The necrotic process eventually causes communication with a bronchus and partial drainage of liquefied material by way of the tracheobronchial tree. Air enters the abscess cavity and forms the characteristic air–fluid level.

CLINICAL SIGNS AND SYMPTOMS

Lung abscess occurs most frequently in patients whose risk of aspiration is increased by altered consciousness, as in alcoholic stupor, cerebral vascular accident, drug overdose, general anesthesia, or seizure disorder. Esophageal obstruction and neuromuscular disease may also lead to aspiration. Factors other than aspiration, such as bacteremia, bronchiectasis, septic emboli, and gingivitis also predispose to development of lung abscess.

The illness commonly begins as a subacute

aspiration pneumonia. Patients usually have symptoms for 2 to 4 weeks prior to presentation. The most frequent complaints are low-grade fever, malaise, weight loss, and cough. The cough is often productive of copious amounts of sputum. About half of the patients with anaerobic lung abscess report foul-smelling sputum.

Lung abscess may sometimes be associated with a more fulminant infection called anaerobic necrotizing pneumonitis, which begins with an acute onset of chills, fever, cough, hemoptysis, shortness of breath, and pleuritic chest pain. This infection is more severe and destructive than classic lung abscess and is sometimes referred to as pulmonary gangrene. Abscess formation that complicates pneumococcal, staphylococcal, and gram-negative bacterial pneumonias also has an acute onset.

Patients often appear chronically ill on initial presentation. Weight loss, low-grade fever, and periodontitis are common findings. Initially, the findings on examination of the chest are consistent with pneumonia and include rales, egophony, and dullness to percussion. After cavitation, there may be amphoric or cavernous breath sounds. Decreased breath sounds and splinting of the chest usually indicate an empyema as a complication. Occasionally cyanosis or clubbing of the fingers is noted. When lung abscess is secondary to hematogenous spread from endocarditis, pelvic thrombophlebitis, or central venous catheters, the patient may also have signs and symptoms related to the primary infection.

The earliest manifestation of this disease is pneumonia. Without therapy, or with inadequate therapy, the infection may progress to lung abscess or necrotizing pneumonia. The average time required for a cavity to appear on chest x-ray film is 12 days, but may be seen as early as the seventh day. The abscess may drain into the pleural space and produce an empyema. Brain abscess and bronchopleural fistula may also occur as late complications. If untreated, the patient gradually deteriorates, and death ensues within weeks or months. Occasionally, death is sudden due to asphyxiation from rupture of a large abscess and discharge of pus into the airway. Mortality rates prior to the development of surgical drainage procedures and antibiotics exceeded 90%. The mortality rate with therapy is 10% to 20%. Prognosis is worst in patients with cancer or necrotizing pneumonia.

PATHOPHYSIOLOGY

The main routes by which pyogenic bacteria gain access to the lung are aspiration, hematogenous seeding, and direct extension from contiguous structures such as a ruptured esophagus or intra-abdominal infection. Aspiration is the most common. Healthy people aspirate small quantities of respiratory secretions during sleep, but large amounts of secretions are prevented from reaching the lung by the cough and gag reflexes and by mucociliary transport in the trachea. Alveolar macrophages are able to remove the low numbers of bacteria that penetrate beyond the cilia. In patients with neuromuscular disease, viral illness, chronic obstructive disease, or altered level of consciousness, these defense mechanisms are compromised. Normal mouth flora can be carried to the alveoli with the aspirated materials in sufficient numbers to overwhelm the macrophages. Some pathogens possess a capsular polysaccharide or cell-wall protein that enables the organism to avoid phagocytosis by the macrophages.

Abscess formation is the result of the host response to invasion of the lung by pyogenic bacteria. Neutrophils infiltrate the area and release proteolytic enzymes and other toxic substances that produce tissue necrosis. In lung abscess, granulation tissue surrounds the necrotic center and limits the infection to one or two large cavities. In necrotizing pneumonia, these barriers are absent or ineffective, and multiple small cavities form within an expanding infiltrate.

Anaerobic bacteria, either alone or mixed with aerobes, can be isolated from up to 90% of community-acquired lung abscesses. There are usually multiple isolates from the same abscess, with an average of three. The most common anaerobes are *Bacteroides melaninogenicus, B. fragilis, Fusobacterium necrophorum,* and anaerobic and microaerophilic streptococci. Some anaerobes produce butyric acid, methane, and other putrid by-products that cause the foul smell often noted. In lung abscess caused by hospital-acquired aspiration, nosocomial pathogens such as *Klebsiella, Pseudomonas, Escherichia coli,* and *Staphylo-*

coccus are found more frequently, although anaerobes still predominate.

Lung abscesses caused by hematogenous seeding are usually multiple small lesions distributed through different lobes of the lung. Right-sided endocarditis, intravenous (IV) drug abuse, pelvic thrombophlebitis, and nosocomial bacteremia are potential sources. *Staphylococcus aureus* is the most common cause, especially in children and IV drug abusers. Abscesses secondary to contiguous spread from the esophagus or abdomen contain bowel flora and are usually solitary lesions.

CLINICAL–PATHOLOGIC CORRELATIONS

Many of the clinical and pathologic features of lung abscess are common to deep-seated abscesses in other organs. A summary of the major clinical–pathologic correlations are listed in Table 35–1.

DIFFERENTIAL DIAGNOSIS

The most important diseases to distinguish from bacterial lung abscess are pulmonary neoplasm, tuberculosis, and cavitary fungal infection. Lung carcinoma can develop a necrotic center that cavitates and looks like an abscess on chest x-ray films. Bacterial abscess can also develop within or behind a lung tumor. Sputum cytologic studies should be done for all patients with an undiagnosed lung cavity. The level of suspicion for carcinoma should increase when the cavity wall is thick and irregular, the lesion is located in a nondependent lung segment, and when the patient is edentulous. Tuberculosis can generally be distinguished from lung abscess on the basis of history of contact, location of the cavity, purified protein derivative (PPD) reaction, and sputum AFB smear. Cavitary histoplasmosis and coccidioidomycosis should be considered in endemic areas, but often can be excluded on the basis of history and x-ray film findings.

DIAGNOSIS

The diagnosis should be suspected on the basis of history and physical findings and confirmed by chest x-ray film. Pneumonia is the initial feature of lung abscess to appear in the x-ray film, followed by cavitation and formation of an air–fluid level. Aspiration lung abscess occurs more frequently in the right lung than the left, and in the most dependent segment of the lung. The apical segment of the lower lobe is the most frequent location of lung abscess when the patient aspirates in the supine position, and the posterior segment of the upper

---

TABLE 35–1.
Clinical–Pathologic Correlations for Lung Abscess

CLINICAL FINDINGS	PATHOLOGIC FINDINGS
Fever and signs of chronic inflammation such as weight loss, anemia, and elevated erythrocyte sedimentation rate (ESR)	Release of interleukin I (endogenous pyrogen) from activated macrophages
Cough, signs of consolidation, dullness to percussion, egophony, increased transmission of breath sounds	Edema and infiltration of fibrin and neutrophils at the site of infection; alveoli filled with exudate
Cavity with air–fluid level, cough producing copious sputum	Release of proteases from neutrophils results in central liquefaction necrosis and drainage of pus into tracheobronchial tree
Fetid sputum	Production of butyric acid, H_2S, methane, and other by-products of some anaerobes
Pleuritic chest pain, pleural rub	Inflammation of pleura adjacent to the infiltration
Pleuritic chest pain, decreased breath sounds on auscultation, dullness to percussion, pleural fluid on chest x-ray film	Drainage of abscess contents into pleural space; empyema
Pneumothorax and empyema, air–fluid level in pleural cavity	Communication of the abscess cavity with both the pleural space and a bronchus; bronchopleural fistula

lobe when the patient aspirates while lying on his or her side. Aspiration abscess usually causes one or two large cavities. Necrotizing pneumonitis produces consolidation and multiple small cavities in a single lobe, which may spread to a contiguous lobe. Abscesses produced by hematogenous spread often appear as multiple small cavities in diffuse areas of lung. Laboratory values in patients with lung abscess are nonspecific; the WBC count is mildly elevated, the erythrocyte sedimentation rate is elevated, and the patient may be anemic.

Identification of anaerobes in a lung abscess requires an invasive procedure because coughed-up sputum specimens are contaminated by normal oral flora as they pass through the mouth. Transtracheal aspiration, percutaneous aspiration of the cavity, or bronchoscopy is necessary to isolate the anaerobic pathogens. Fortunately empiric therapy for the anaerobes is generally effective, and these invasive procedures are unnecessary in most cases. Routine sputum cultures should be obtained to detect the presence of *Staphylococcus*, pneumococcus, and gram-negative organisms.

PRINCIPLES OF PREVENTION AND TREATMENT

Prevention of lung abscess depends on good supportive care for those at high risk for aspiration, prevention and care of periodontal disease, and early treatment for aspiration pneumonia.

The incidence of lung abscess has decreased over the last five decades due in part to the use of antibiotics, advances in anesthesiology, better care of unconscious patients, and improved feeding techniques for the chronically ill.

Penicillin has long been the drug of choice for community-acquired aspiration lung abscess. Increasing penicillin resistance has been noted among *Bacteroides* species, especially *B. melaninogenicus*. A recent study reported that the cure rate for penicillin has decreased to 60%, and the efficacy of clindamycin was superior to penicillin. The cure rate for penicillin in this study was considerably lower than that experienced by many clinicians, and some continue to use penicillin initially and switch to clindamycin if the patient does not respond. In hospital-acquired lung abscess, an aminoglycoside should be added to penicillin, or an extended-spectrum cephalosporin can be used. When staphylococcal infection is suspected, a penicillinase-resistant penicillin should be used.

Most patients can be cured with medical management alone, but 10% to 20% require surgical drainage. The procedures employed include closed drainage via bronchoscopy, open drainage, or lobectomy. The indications for surgery are delayed closure of the abscess, disease that progresses despite adequate therapy, and massive hemoptysis. Chest tube placement is required for treatment of empyema. Bronchoscopy should be performed on patients suspected of having a lung cancer as a predisposing cause of the abscess.

REFERENCES

Alexander JC, Wolfe WG: Lung abscess and empyema of the thorax. *Surg Clin North Am* 1980; 60(4):835–849. *A review of lung abscess including the surgical approaches to the disease.*

Brooks SJD, Braude AI: Bacterial lung abscess, nocardial lung abscess and aspiration pneumonia, in Braude AI, David CE, Fierer J (eds): *Infectious Diseases and Medical Microbiology*, ed 2. Philadelphia, WB Saunders Co, 1986, pp 823–831. *Good description of the pathophysiology.*

Estrara AS, Platt MR, Mills LJ, Shaw RR: Primary lung abscess. *J Thorac Cardiovasc Surg* 1980; 79:275–282. *A review of the authors' experiences with lung abscess not involving carcinoma.*

Finegold SM: Lung abscess, in Mandell GL, Douglas RG, Bennett JE (eds): *Principles and Practice of Infectious Diseases*, ed 2. New York, John Wiley & Sons, 1985, pp 407–411. *A well-referenced and complete review of lung abscess.*

Finegold SM: *Anaerobic Bacteria in Human Disease.* New York, Academic Press, 1977, pp 223–256. *A discussion of the microbiology.*

Levison ME, Mangura CT, Lorber B, et al: Clindamycin compared with penicillin for treatment of anaerobic lung abscess. *Ann Intern Med* 1983; 98:466–471. *The most recent study comparing clindamycin with penicillin.*

Osler W: *The Principles and Practice of Medicine.* New York, D Appleton and Co, 1892, pp 550–553. *An early description of lung abscess in the pre-antibiotic era by the best-known clinician of his day.*

36 ASTHMA

Glenn C. Hamilton, M.D.

Asthma is characterized by an increased responsiveness of the airways to various stimuli manifested by diffuse narrowing of the bronchi. This narrowing may change spontaneously or as a result of therapy. Asthma is common, appearing in 2.5% of the population. Asthma causes about 5,000 deaths in the United States annually, but most of these could be prevented.

CLINICAL SIGNS AND SYMPTOMS

Asthma may occur at any age. Management is usually more difficult than diagnosis. The history includes episodic cough, dyspnea, and wheezing. Cough may be an early complaint or the only symptom. The symptoms may occur spontaneously or be triggered by cold, exercise, or inhaled irritants. Wheezing is the most common finding in asthma, but in severe attacks, airflow may be so reduced that the wheezing disappears. Therefore, the disappearance of wheezing may be a good or an ominous sign. Late in an attack, severe dyspnea and "air hunger" are the main symptoms. The initial interrogation may be limited by patient anxiety and breathlessness so a thorough history may need to be done later. The information necessary for evaluating and treating the asthmatic patient is listed in Table 36–1.

The physical examination has proved to be a useful predictor of the clinical outcome in acute asthma. Table 36–2 groups physical examination findings according to a suggested severity scale. The wide range of patient presentation and tolerance, as well as the rapidity of change in asthma, makes overcommitment to this scale hazardous. The initial appearance of the patient correlates with the airflow as measured in clinical studies. Nondiaphoretic recumbent patients, sitting patients, and diaphoretic sitting patients were found to have peak expiratory flow rates (PEFR) of 225 ($\pm$ 7.5), 134 ($\pm$ 21), and 73 ($\pm$5) L/min, respectively.

The vital signs information in asthma is not consistently helpful. The respiratory rate varies with patient fatigue. The pulse rates have a wide range, though initial rates greater than 130/min that persist despite therapy are associated with severe asthma. Blood pressure measurements are unreliable in assessing severity, though some studies relate a pulsus paradoxus of greater than 15 mm Hg to a 1-second forced expiratory volume (FEV_1) of less than 1.0 L.

TABLE 36–1.

Historical Information to Obtain from the Patient with Acute Asthma

1. The length of the present episode
2. The patient's pattern of response to therapy, identifying effective therapies
3. The severity of this attack in context of the asthma pattern
4. The medications being taken for asthma before this attack. Changes, if any, in the amount or frequency of dose in response to this episode. Time of the most recent dose
5. Any different features of this attack. Symptoms other than cough, dyspnea, or wheezing
6. The potential precipitating factors (e.g., allergies, respiratory infection, exercise, cold, emotions, medications)
7. The medical history including the present episode, smoking history, and cardiac history
8. Before discharge, determine the patient's compliance, knowledge of medications, environment, and follow-up arrangements

TABLE 36–2.
Methods of Assessing the Severity of Asthma

DEGREE OF SEVERITY	PHYSICAL FINDINGS	PULMONARY FUNCTION TESTS	ARTERIAL BLOOD GAS LEVELS (BREATHING ROOM AIR)		
			PaO_2	Pa_{CO_2}	pH
Mild	Tachypnea <30/min define, > 1.5 L Patient tolerance good when recumbent Accessory musculature not used Pulsus paradoxus not present Wheezing audible	FEV_1* not precisely defined PEFR* >100 L/min	Normal	Slight decrease	Slight increase
Moderate	Tachypnea 20–40/min Patient tolerance fair with sitting Accessory musculature not used Pulsus paradoxus not present Wheezing diffuse, E>I, may be higher pitched	$FEV_1$1–1.5 L PEFR 80–100 L/min	Slight or moderate decrease	Slight or moderate decrease	Slight or moderate increase or normal
Severe	Tachypnea greater than 40/min Patient tolerance poor with sitting, diaphoresis Accessory muscles active Pulsus paradoxus present, > 15 mm Hg Wheezing may be high pitched, low intensity, or absent ("silent chest")	FEV_1 <1 L PEFR <80 L/min	Moderate to severe decrease	Normal or increased	Normal or slight decrease or increase

	PHYSICAL FINDINGS	PULMONARY FUNCTION TESTS	ARTERIAL BLOOD GAS LEVELS (BREATHING ROOM AIR)
Drawbacks of Assessment Method	Assessment varies with examiner and patient	Not immediately available	Do not relate well to pulmonary function test values. PO_2 may paradoxically drop with improvement
	Provides only late signs	Flow rates are effort-dependent	Painful
	Accessory musculature and pulsus paradoxus related to FEV_1 <1 L not always present	Values altered by changes in lung volume	Expensive if serial studies done

* FEV_1 = 1-second forced expiratory volume; PEFR = peak expiratory flow rate.

This finding is effort-dependent and not a key determinant of severity or predictor of outcome.

Sternocleidomastoid muscle use has a good correlation with an FEV_1 of less than 1.0 L. Breath sounds on auscultation have a fair correlation with severity but are not predictive because of rapid changes. The percentage of wheezing during the cycle, inspiratory/expiratory ratios, and the pitch of the wheeze have a variable examiner-influenced correlation with spirometric severity indexes. In severe airway obstruction, an urgent finding is the "silent chest," indicating flow rates too low to generate breath sounds.

Altered mental status of the patient is the hallmark of inadequate oxygenation and ventilation. It is a late finding and should be anticipated by other physical and laboratory findings. Cyanosis, an unreliable and late finding in hypoxemia, is influenced by the patient's race and hemoglobin level.

The severity of asthma symptoms correlate well with the patient's age at onset and the persistence of the disease. Asthma newly diagnosed or persistent in adulthood has a greater chance of being recurrent and severe.

Three types of asthma predominate. Chronic persistent asthma requires constant therapy to maintain airflow. Patients with this type may require corticosteroids, have a high sensitivity to aeroallergens/irritants, and have an increased incidence of progressive respiratory failure. Patients with acute intermittent asthma have symptom-free periods without respiratory infection and are managed without corticosteroids. Undiagnosed asthma may be first seen with cough or "shortness of breath" precipitated by exercise or occupational exposure. It may also be caused by nocturnal gastroesophageal reflux and aspiration.

Untreated asthma is unpredictable. It can spontaneously resolve, but more often is persistent with exacerbations and can rapidly progress to respiratory failure and death. Associated complications include atelectasis, pneumonia, pneumothorax, pneumomediastinum, and mucous plugging.

PATHOPHYSIOLOGY

Asthma is a disease of the pulmonary airways, involving the bronchial smooth muscle, mucosa, and mucous glands. This change in airway resistance leads to reduced airflow rates, air trapping, a ventilation–perfusion mismatch, changes in intrathoracic pressure, increased pulmonary vascular resistance, and right ventricular systolic overload. The concept of extrinsic and intrinsic asthma is useful in discussing the pathophysiology despite the complex overlap between the two conditions.

Extrinic asthma is reversible bronchospasm due to allergens. One underlying mechanism is the involvement of the antibody IgE in an immediate hypersensitivity response. The IgE reacts with an antigen and begins a cascade that forms a precursor of the leukotrienes. A combination of leukotrienes is thought to form the "slow reactive substance of asthma." Mast cells are also stimulated and release multiple preformed and secondary mediators. The mast cell may have a central role in allergic asthma because the mediators influence bronchoconstriction, mucus production, leukocyte chemoattraction, and cholinergic reactivity. The result is bronchospasm, bronchial edema, production of viscid mucus, and mucous plugging.

Intrinsic asthma may involve similar pathways but with a nonallergenic origin. It is associated with infection, ingestion of aspirin and other cyclooxygenase inhibitors, exercise, emotional stress, air pollution, and respiratory infection. Underlying both extrinsic and intrinsic asthma is an imbalance between the adrenergic and the cholinergic systems, and the influence of these systems on bronchial muscle tone and mucous secretion. The precise pathophysiology of asthma is unclear because the influences of immunologic, emotional, physical, hormonal, and infectious stimuli continue to complicate a "unified theory" for asthma.

Macroscopically, bronchial smooth muscle spasm is the major determinant of the reversible airway obstruction. Microscopically, this bronchoconstriction is complicated by mucosal edema from increased capillary permeability. In patients who have died to status asthmaticus, cellular infiltrates of neutrophils, eosinophils, and desquamated epithelial cells are mixed with abundant secretions. Mucous plugging, that is, complete or partial obstruction of the airway with plugs of mucus, is a significant component of the airway obstruction in these patients. The mucous component of these secretions comes from hypertrophied goblet cells and parasympathetic-innervated submucous glands.

TABLE 36–3.
Clinical–Pathologic Correlations for Asthma

CLINICAL FINDINGS	PATHOLOGIC FINDINGS
Cough	Increased mucus production, bronchial irritant cough receptor stimulation, and/or mucosal edema
Wheeze	Turbulent airflow through narrowed airways
Dyspnea	Increased work of breathing
Retractions/accessory muscle use	Increased negative intrapleural pressure from recruitment of mechanism to maintain inspiratory force in setting of hyperinflated lungs
Pulsus paradoxus	Accentuation of normal respiratory variation in blood pressure, caused by lung hyperinflation and wide variations in intrapulmonary pressure
Anxiety	Air hunger, increased work of breathing, adrenergic substance release, hypoxemia, and drug administration
Cardiac arrhythmia	Hypoxemia, adrenergic autonomic system stimulation and drug administration, acid–base disturbance (usually CO_2 retention and lactic acidemia)
Cyanosis	Late finding, 5.0 gm of reduced hemoglobin necessary. Hypoxemia from ventilation/perfusion mismatch, possible hypoventilation
Positive skin test	Patient has mast cell and basophil IgE specific for the antigen being tested

CLINICAL–PATHOLOGIC CORRELATIONS

The pathologic bases for the clinical manifestations of asthma are airway obstruction and the compensatory mechanisms recruited to maintain adequate airflow and exchange. A list of symptoms and signs with their pathophysiologic correlates is given in Table 36–3.

DIFFERENTIAL DIAGNOSIS

Asthma, though common, has a large number of imitators. The adage "all that wheezes isn't asthma" continues to hold true. Table 36–4 lists a differential diagnosis of asthma, in order of catastrophic potential. Those diagnoses listed as potentially catastrophic conditions should be considered early in the evaluation because missing the diagnosis could be life-threatening for the patient. An important corollary is "asthma doesn't always wheeze." Asthma must be included in the differential diagnosis of episodic or persistent cough, cold- or exercise-induced dyspnea, or episodic "shortness of breath" of unknown cause.

Bronchospasm is a common response of the lung to many stimuli, and an "asthmatic component" may be part of a number of lung diseases, particularly infection, bronchitis, and emphysema. The diagnosis of "asthma" should

be given only after a thorough examination and a clinical pattern of reversible airway disease has been established

DIAGNOSIS

The diagnosis is asthma involves evaluation during two stages of the disease: the documentation of hyperreactivity, reversible airway obstruction, or both when the disease is relatively stable; and assessing the severity of the process during an acute attack.

Clinical laboratory evaluation has a limited usefulness in diagnostic assessment of asthma. Table 36–5 lists a number of laboratory tests considered useful in stable or acute asthma and comments on their present role. Arterial blood gas levels in acute asthma deserve special comment because they have long been viewed as an accurate discriminator of asthma severity using the standards listed in Table 36–2. Several studies done in emergency departments indicate that arterial blood gases are not the accurate standard they were once considered to be. The following guidelines are recommended for performing arterial blood gas determinations in acute asthma:

1. Usually unnecessary if patient is awake, alert, recumbent, and nondiaphoretic, or if the PEFR is greater than 130 L/min
2. Necessary in patients appearing to have

severe asthma on physical examination or from spirometric studies

3. Necessary in all patients with a history of a recurrent complicated clinical course
4. Necessary in corticosteroid-dependent asthmatic patients
5. Necessary in patients not responding or worsening, despite maximum therapeutic measures given for more than 30 to 60 minutes.

A number of diagnostic procedures may be performed in the stable and the acute stages (Table 36–6). Spirometric studies in the acute stage deserve more attention than they have received because they help distinguish between mild, moderate, and severe asthma at different times during therapy (Table 36–2). Spirometry is painless, can be used repetitively, can be cost-efficient, and with appropriate training of both patient and physician can give reproducible results.

PRINCIPLES OF PREVENTION AND THERAPY

The management of the asthmatic patient is a complex task which requires a combination of preventive measures, emotional support, and medication. Education of the patient about all three is necessarily a continuing process.

Once asthma is diagnosed, information gained from the history, physical examination, and laboratory and procedural testing is directed toward the prevention of an exacerbation. Sensitivity to aspirin, foods, and aeroallergens is explored, and behavioral patterns are modified to increase avoidance of known precipitants. Emotional support has proved to be an important aspect of the prevention of asthmatic attacks. Stress-management techniques, physical conditioning, and detailed education all improve the patient's sense of well-being, reduce the frequency of attacks, and increase tolerance of acute bronchospastic episodes. The diurnal cycle of asthma and the propensity toward complications in the early morning should be discussed with the patient and anticipated with appropriately timed medication. With the side range of medication available for treatment of bronchospasm, it is essential that the preventive and emotional aspects of caring for the asthmatic patient not be neglected.

Medication use varies depending on whether

TABLE 36–4.
Differential Diagnosis of Asthma

POTENTIALLY CATASTROPHIC CONDITIONS
Anaphylaxis
Aspiration
Chemical or smoke inhalation (sulfur dioxide)
Chronic obstructive pulmonary disease with asthmatic component
Congestive heart failure
Epiglottitis
Foreign body obstructing airway
Infections (bronchitis, pneumonia)
Noncardiogenic pulmonary edema
Pneumothorax
Pulmonary embolism

USUALLY LESS URGENT CONDITIONS
Airborne irritants (cotton, detergents)
Allergic response to infection (aspergillosis) or infestation (Ascaris)
Allergic vasculitis
Beta-adrenergic blocker effect
Carcinoid syndrome
Endobronchial tumor
Hyperventilation
Löffler's syndrome
Psychogenic

stable asthma or an acute attack is being treated. Table 36–7 gives the underlying principles and basic medication regimens for each condition.

Ten to fifteen percent of asthmatics will require hospital admission. The criteria for admission include respiratory failure, failure to respond to optimum therapy, pneumonia, pneumothorax, cardiac toxicity (tachyarrhythmias, frequent ventricular ectopic beats, angina), frequent visits to the emergency department, and spirometric criteria for admission.

The expanded use of spirometry has provided the basis for admission on spirometric criteria. Testing 20 to 30 minutes after initiating therapy has been found to be particularly useful. Selected spirometric criteria for admission are listed in Table 36–8.

Eighty-five to ninety percent of asthmatic patients presenting to the hospital emergency department or outpatient clinic will be discharged. Their recovery is usually discernible during 4 to 6 hours of observation and follows a pattern of lessened air hunger, decreased chest wall retractions, subjective disappearance of wheezing symptoms, and objective confirmation of being "wheeze-free." After acute intervention and improvement a "wheeze-free"

TABLE 36–5.

Use of Laboratory Tests in Stable and Acute Asthma

TEST	FINDINGS	
	STABLE (DIAGNOSTIC)	ACUTE (ASSESSING SEVERITY)
Complete blood count	Gross assessment of degree of infection and/or inflammation	Helps assess degree of infection and/or inflammation. May be influenced by epinephrine-induced demargination
Total eosinophilic count (blood)	Useful in identifying allergic component; normally less than 85 cells/mm	Helps identify allergic component. More than 400 cells/mm. May predict responsiveness to corticosteroids. Count should go to zero with effective treatment.
Eosinophilia (nasal and sputum samples)	Useful in identifying allergic component	30% to 40% eosinophils or smear may predict responsiveness to corticosteroids.
Arterial blood gas levels	Not routine, unless COPD complicates condition	Selected use (Table 36–7). Poor to fair differentiation of severity (Table 36–2).
IgE level or radioallergosorbent (RAST)	Helpful in identifying the allergic asthmatic patient	Not useful
Cold agglutinins	Not useful	Selected use for diagnosis of *Mycoplasma pneumoniae;* wide differential is positive
Aminophylline level	Important to maximize therapy, assess compliance, prevent complications of overdose	Use to diagnose *M. pneumoniae;* wide differential is positive
Erythrocyte sedimentation rate	Not useful	Not useful
Sputum cultures	Not useful	Only 10% of cases associated with respiratory infection; less than 50% of these are bacterial

TABLE 36–6.

Procedures for Assessment in Stable and Acute Asthma

PROCEDURE	FINDINGS	
	STABLE (DIAGNOSTIC)	ACUTE (ASSESSING SEVERITY)
Spirometry (pulmonary function testing)	Full testing; decreased flow rates, decreased maximum voluntary ventilation, increased tidal volume, increased residual volume; may improve with bronchodilator therapy	PEFRs are standard; fair-to-good delineation of severity; serial studies better than single
Chest x-ray film	Limited usefulness for finding complications of asthma: hyperinflation, atelectasis, pneumonia, air in chest cavity	Limited use in finding complications. Findings change therapy in less than 10% of adult patients; order if symptoms warrant.
Electrocardiogram	Limited usefulness for finding complications of asthma	May have reversible changes of right ventricular strain in 30%–40%; continuous cardiac monitoring for arrhythmia is more useful
Skin testing for allergic reactions	Use to determine the IgE allergens the patient reacts to	Not useful
Metacholine- or histamine-inhalation challenge test	Used if baseline spirometric values are normal; graded inhalations used to measure degree of bronchospasm; reversal with bronchodilation documents variability	Not useful

TABLE 36–7.
Medical Management of Stable and Acute Asthma

	STABLE	ACUTE
PRINCIPLES	Prevention of acute attacks	Oxygenation (essential, monitor with arterial blood gas levels)
	Normalization of activities	Hydration (if complicated asthma, 1.5 L over 6–8 hr)
		Reversal of bronchospasm
		Prevention of cardiopulmonary arrest
MEDICATIONS	Theophylline or methylxanthines	Beta-adrenergic agents, aerosol or parenteral (Patients with acute asthma may have adverse response.)
	Beta-adrenergic agents	Theophylline, oral and inhaler
	Prevention therapy with chromolyn sodium	Corticosteroids (Give early in acute asthma that does not respond to bronchodilators.)
	Corticosteroids, particularly in chromolyn or inhaler form	Avoid chromolyn or inhaled corticosteroids
	Calcium antagonists in selected cases	Anticholinergic agents (may be combined with beta-adrenergic aerosols)
		Avoid sedation
ADJUNCT PROCEDURES	Desensitize patients with allergic asthma	Oxygen
		Cardiac monitor
		Hydration
		In severe cases, stabilize acid–base; intubate and begin mechanical ventilation; do bronchial lavage; bronchoscopy

TABLE 36–8.
Spirometric Criteria for Hospital Admission (If any indication is present, consider patient admission.)

TIMING OF ASSESSMENT	INDICATION FOR ADMISSION
Initial presentation	Fischl index ≥ 4*
	Inability to perform spirometry FEV_1 <0.6 l
Response to first treatment	Unresponsive to epinephrine and PEFR <60 L/min
	Unresponsive to bronchodilators and <16% change in PEFR plus <0.15-L increase in FEV_1 after subcutaneous administration of broncodilator
	PEFR >100 L/min initially and >160 L/min after 0.25 mg terbutaline
	FEV_1 >30% of predicted value; not improving to >40% of predicted value; < 4 hours therapy needed
Response to full treatment	PEFR <100 L/min initially and <300 L/min after full treatment
	FEV_1 <0.6 L initially and <1.6 L after full treatment plus FEV_1 increased by 4 L after bronchodilator administration
Other	Deterioration of PEFR by 15% after initial good response to bronchodilator therapy

* See Table 36–9.

asthmatic has an FEV_1 that is 65% of that predicted and may take 1 week of therapy before reaching the best spirometric baseline values obtainable.

Though there are no specific proven criteria for discharge, the best therapy minimizes the risk of an out-of-hospital relapse. Spirometric values greater than 60% of those predicted, a PEFR greater than 300 L/min or FEV_1 greater than 1.6 L are reasonable criteria for discharge. Appearing to be asymptomatic does not always correlate well with outcome; up to 25% of such patients return with a relapse within 10 days of treatment.

The Fischl index, if supported by the clinical evaluation, was designed to predict the potential for relapse and readmission after discharge (Table 36–9). The index was developed for a

TABLE 36–9.
Criteria (Fischl Index) for Predicting Relapse*

Pulse ≥ 120 beats/minute
Respiratory rate ≥ 30/minute
Pulsus paradoxus ≥ 18 mm Hg
PEFR ≤ 120 L/min
Moderate or severe dyspnea
Moderate or severe use of accessory muscles
Moderate or severe wheezing

* Patients with scores greater than or equal to 4 (one point for each criterion the patient meets) are high risk for relapse.

patient given 8 to 12 hours of aminophylline intravenous infusion, inhaled and parenterally administered beta-adrenergic agonists, and no glucocorticoids. Although the usefulness of the index has been questioned by later work, patients with a score greater than or equal to 4 should be considered at high risk for relapse on discharge.

Finally, the following points must be considered at the time of discharge:

1. Is the patient returning to an environment that may precipitate bronchospasm?
2. Does the patient understand the appropriate dose, use, and administration technique of the prescribed medication?
3. Have the following pharmacologic issues been considered? With the use of glucocorticoids, the rate of relapse and occurrence of respiratory symptoms can be decreased by a glucocorticoid bolus followed by ever-decreasing doses over the next 7 to 10 days. This regimen should be considered for asthmatic patients with complex disease patterns or whose reversal of bronchospasm has taken a long time. If an inhaler is prescribed, does the patient know how to use it? Has the effect of analgesics, particularly aspirin, on the course of the asthma been discussed? Has the timing of the next dose of methylxanthines (e.g., aminophylline) been decided? A slow-release form is optimally given at the time of discontinuing the intravenous administration.
4. Have follow-up arrangements been made for the patient to contact the physician within 24 to 48 hours after discharge? Telephone contact may help lessen the two common causes of relapse, patient noncompliance with medication instructions and not filling prescriptions.

REFERENCES

Benatar SR: Fatal asthma. *N Engl J Med* 1986; 314(7): 423–429. *Up-to-date review of a small subset of the asthmatic population which needs to be better understood.*

Brenner BE: Bronchial asthma in adults: Presentation to the emergency department. *Am J. Emerg Med* 1983; 1(1):50–70 and 1(3):306–333. *This two-part article is a complete recent review of acute asthma from the perspective of emergency medicine. It somewhat discourages the use of epinephrine. Over 700 references.*

Fischl MA, Pitchenik A, Gardner LB: An index predicting relapse and need for hospitalization in patients with acute bronchial asthma. *N Engl J Med* 1981; 305(14):783–789. *A well-done study with continued viability. Read and compare with later work critical of its findings.*

Goldstein RA: Advances in the diagnosis and treatment of asthma. *Chest* 1985; 87(1 Supp):1–135. *An excellent series of short monographs discussing basic mechanisms, clinical evaluation, treatment, and self-management programs.*

McFadden ER, Kiser R, DeGroot WJ: Acute bronchial asthma. *N Engl J Med* 1973; 288(5):221–225. *One of the best papers to correlate physical findings and airflow status.*

McFadden ER, Lyons HA: Arterial blood gas tension in asthma. *N Engl J Med* 1968; 278(19):1027–1032. *An early paper providing the basis for blood gas use in assessing severity. Read with the Nowak paper (cited below).*

Nowak RM, Tomlanovich MC, Sarkar DD, Kvale PA, Anderson JA: Arterial blood gases and pulmonary function testing in acute bronchial asthma: Predicting patient outcomes. *JAMA* 1983; 249(15):2043–2046. *A paper supporting the selective use of ABGs in acute asthma.*

Turner ES, Greenberger PA, Patterson R: Management of the pregnant asthmatic patient. *Ann Intern Med* 1980: 93(6)905–908. *An excellent authoritative review of a topic not covered in the preceding discussion.*

37 ADULT RESPIRATORY DISTRESS SYNDROME

Jorge Crespo, M.D.

The adult respiratory distress syndrome is the clinical expression of a pathophysiologic process that occurs in subjects with previously healthy lungs with no left ventricular failure and that is characterized by a rapid onset, progressive dyspnea and hypoxemia, increased lung stiffness, and diffuse bilateral pulmonary infiltrates which result in life-threatening respiratory failure. Although it is associated with a wide range of unrelated clinical entities, the pathophysiologic, radiologic, and clinical features are remarkably constant regardless of the initiating process (Table 37–1).

CLINICAL SIGNS AND SYMPTOMS

Clinically, adult respiratory distress syndrome evolves with some variation in time and intensity depending on the nature of the triggering mechanism. However, four sequential phases are observed.

Phase I is the period immediately following the initiating event. Unless direct pulmonary damage is present, the lungs are normal at examination and chest x-ray films are normal. The most significant features, and the ones that direct attention to the respiratory system, are persistent hyperventilation, tachypnea, and dyspnea. The resulting respiratory alkalosis is frequently aggravated by a metabolic component such as that resulting from oxidation of citrate in transfused blood, excessive amounts of sodium bicarbonate, or loss of chloride through gastric suction. Although hyperventilation in response to pain may add to the respiratory alkalosis, some patients develop a coexisting mild lactic acidemia.

Phase II is a deceptive period of 24 to 72 hours in which the patient is hemodynamically stable and has an adequate urinary output, proper mobilization of resuscitation fluids, and clearing of lactic acidemia. Physical examination reveals only mild tachypnea. However, an increased alveolar-arterial oxygen tension difference, D $(A–a)O_2$, a moderately reduced arterial oxygen tension (PaO_2), and an increased intrapulmonary arteriovenous shunt are present. Radiologic examination of the lungs is unrewarding.

Phase III is heralded by progressive severe respiratory insufficiency with a shunt fraction in excess of 0.20 and the need for high concentrations of inspired oxygen, both of which culminate in the need to provide the patient with mechanical ventilatory support (Table 37–2). Arterial carbon dioxide tension (Pa_{CO_2}) remains low and, once again, lactic acid concentration rises. The patient is cyanotic and dyspneic; diffuse rales and ronchi are present; the heart sounds remain normal. Lung compliance rapidly decreases, and x-ray films of the chest reveal the classic picture of widespread bilateral interstitial and intra-alveolar infiltrates, which are centrally confluent and spare the apices and costophrenic angles. With increasing hypoxemia, cerebral dysfunction may become apparent.

Phase IV is characterized by the onset of marked respiratory acidosis, which appears toward the end of phase III with an increase in physiologic dead space and respiratory muscle fatigue. This acidosis, combined with the worsening arterial hypoxemia and intrapulmonary shunt (greater than 30%), establishes an irreversible state of myocardial dysfunction which in turn produces inadequate cerebral and renal perfusion. Death is usually the result of the ventricular dysrhythmias that trigger cardiopulmonary arrest.

TABLE 37–1.
Disorders Associated with Adult Respiratory Distress Syndrome

CARDIOCIRCULATORY	
Shock	Septic
	Anaphylactic
	Hemorrhagic
	Hypovolemic
Embolism	Fat
	Fibrin clots
	Amniotic fluid
	Cellular aggregates
INFECTION	
Pulmonary	Bacterial (staphylococcal, streptococcal, legionellosis)
	Fungal
	Pneumocystis carinii
	Miliary tuberculosis
Extrapulmonary	Septicemia
TRAUMA	
Thoracic	
Extra-thoracic	
INHALATION	
Gases	Irritant (nitric oxide, smoke, phosgene)
	Nonirritant (oxygen)
	Liquids (gastric juice, salt and fresh water)
HEMATOLOGIC	
Disseminated intravascular coagulation	
Massive blood transfusion	
METABOLIC	
Diabetic ketoacidosis	
Uremia	
DRUGS	
Heroin	
Methadone	
Aspirin	
Propoxyphene	
Ethchlorvynol	
NEUROGENIC	
Cerebral edema	
Intracranial hemorrhage	
OTHER	
Pancreatitis	
High altitude	
Radiation pneumonitis	

PATHOPHYSIOLOGY

Almost surprisingly, the morbid anatomical changes in adult respiratory distress syndrome show homogeneity despite the heterogeneity of initiating conditions. Depending on the duration of illness, the lungs may appear heavy and beefy or liver-like or light, gray, and fibrotic. Similarly, two microscopic phases have been recognized. The acute exudative phase has interstitial edema, widespread capillary en- dothelial damage, and necrosis of type I alveolar epithelial cells. Thrombi made up of platelets and fibrin are found in the capillaries. In more severely affected areas, the edema is predominantly perivascular, peribronchiolar, and intra-alveolar, and alveolar hemorrhage may also be present. Fibrin, other plasma proteins, and necrotic type I alveolar cells are matted together and form the typical hyaline membranes that extend from the alveoli to alveolar ducts and respiratory bronchioles. The chronic

TABLE 37–2.
Mechanical Ventilation in Adult Respiratory
Distress Syndrome: Indications and Management

INDICATIONS

Alveolar–arterial oxygen tension difference > 300 m Hg
(FIO_2 = 1.0)
Venoarterial shunt fraction ($\dot{Q}_s/\dot{Q}_T$) > 15% of cardiac
  output
Dead space fraction ($V_D.V_T$) > 0.6
Respiratory acidosis with pH < 7.35
Respiratory rate > 35/minute
Static compliance < 30 ml/cm H_2O

MANAGEMENT

Volume cycled ventilator
Maintain/keep FIO_2 < 0.5
Maintain tidal volume between 10 and 15 ml/kg
Maintain PEEP between 10 and 15 cm H_2O or as guided
  by best lung compliance/mixed venous O_2
  saturation/cardiac output

proliferative phase shows regeneration of the capillary endothelium and alveolar epithelium, with lymphocytes, fibroblasts, and collagen fibers present in the interstitium. Fibrosis may also be present. The alveoli are lined by cuboidal type II alveolar cells, and surfactant produced by type I cells is not found.

The balance of transmembrane fluid flux, which determines the production of interstitial and alveolar edema, results from the interplay between hydrostatic pressures in the capillaries and interstitium, the oncotic pressures of plasma and interstitium, and the filtration or membrane permeability coefficient of the pulmonary capillaries. Of these potential pathogenetic variables, there is ample evidence supporting a central role for an increase in capillary permeability ("leaky capillaries") as the major cause of adult respiratory distress syndrome. Pathogenesis of this phenomenon is complex and probably involves multiple mechanisms, the initial event appearing to be an inappropriate activation of the alternative pathway of the complement cascade, which induces formation of leukocytic aggregates, which embolize the pulmonary capillary bed. Increased capillary permeability results from the additive effects of lysosomal enzymes and toxic oxygen radicals released by polymorphonuclear leukocytes, of arachidonic acid derivatives (leukotrienes, prostaglandins, thromboxanes) activated by platelets, mast cells, and leukocytes recruited by the activation of the complement system (particularly C_{5a}, a potent chemotactic product), and of histamine and serotonin, released from microaggregates of platelets, erythrocytes, and fibrin. All these elements combine to mediate further capillary injury which results in intravascular fluid leakage into the interstitium and alveolar spaces. (See Fig 37–1.)

CLINICAL–PATHOLOGIC CORRELATIONS

Two problems are operative in adult respiratory distress syndrome. Both correlate with the described pathologic features.

1. *Changes in lung mechanics:* Lung compliance depends on tissue elasticity and alveolar surface tension directly and on lung volume indirectly. Inadequate surfactant activity produces extensive microatelectasis, which decreases elasticity and reduces all lung volumes. As volumes decrease, the functional residual capacity (FRC) reaches a critical value beyond which the small airways close and further atelectasis impairs gas exchange. In addition, an increase in the dead space/tidal volume ratio together with decreased lung compliance will significantly increase the work of breathing.

2. *Alterations in gas exchange:* Three mechanisms coincide to produce hypoxemia: (a) a ventilation-perfusion mismatch resulting from perfusion of poorly ventilated alveoli, particularly at the bases where peribronchial edema interferes with effective ventilation, (b) perfusion of nonventilated alveoli (a true shunt), which may account for up to 70% of the cardiac output and is due to diffuse atelectasis, (c) impaired diffusion, resulting from an increased thickness of alveolar septa and a decreased vascular volume, which produces a fast transit time of blood through the pulmonary capillary bed.

DIAGNOSIS AND DIFFERENTIAL DIAGNOSIS

The onset of the adult respiratory distress syndrome is dramatic and reasonably easy to recognize. Because of the severity and catastrophic nature of the syndrome, the attention of the physician is often directed entirely to-

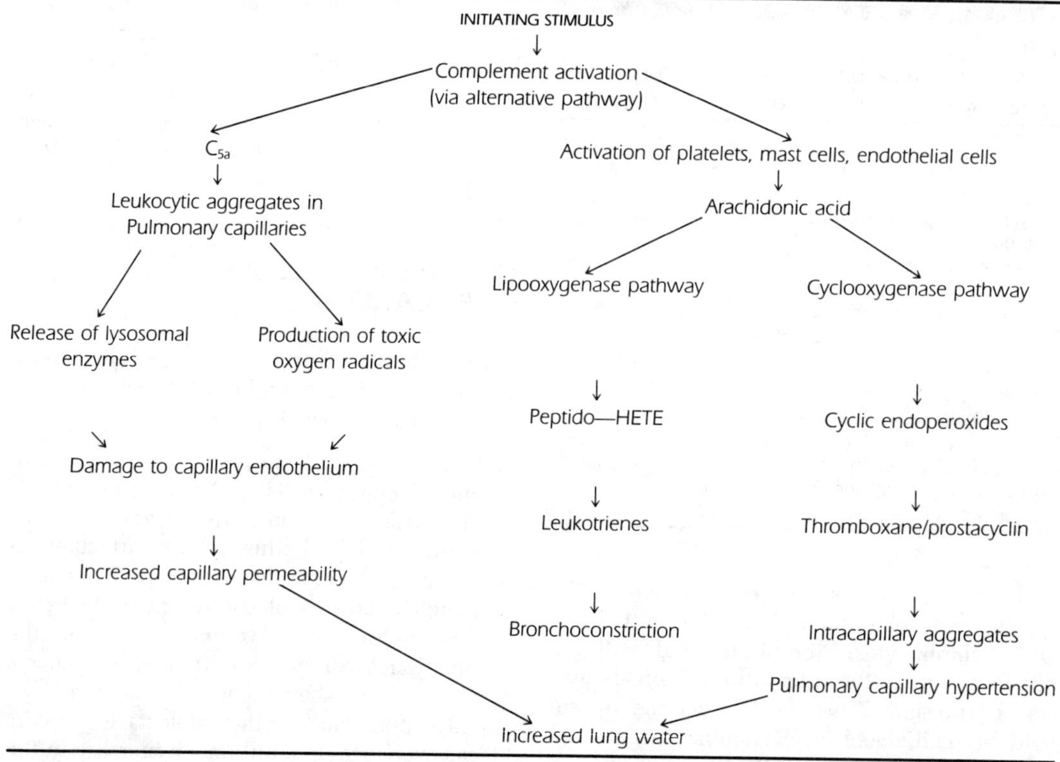

FIG 37–1.
Pathophysiological interactions in adult respiratory distress syndrome.

ward treating the severe and acute respiratory failure. There is a substantial risk that the underlying cause may go undiagnosed and untreated.

Although increased pulmonary capillary permeability, and therefore increased lung water content is pivotal in the pathogenesis of the adult respiratory distress syndrome, direct measure of lung water is not available clinically and research methods have proven cumbersome. Recent studies that compare dye and radioactive isotope dilution with other methods show that knowledgeable interpretation of the chest x-ray is the simplest and most clinically reliable method for determining pulmonary water at this time.

Because of the absence of a reliable predictive test for the onset of pulmonary edema in patients at risk to develop the syndrome, minor alterations in clinical signs such as tachypnea, dyspnea, and cough are very important in providing early recognition of the onset of adult respiratory distress. Early recognition and therapy may lead to a better prognosis.

In practice, measurement of the pulmonary capillary wedge pressure (PCWP) using a pulmonary artery balloon flotation catheter will help elucidate the cause of the pulmonary edema, and the adult respiratory distress syndrome is diagnosed by exclusion if the PCWP is too low (less than 18 mm Hg) to serve as evidence for left ventricular failure. Of course, on some occasions the adult respiratory distress syndrome may occur simultaneously with left ventricular dysfunction.

Radiologically, the findings in adult respiratory distress syndrome are nonspecific, and the patterns reflect the timing of the examination. Acute pulmonary edema is seen early, as occurs with cardiogenic pulmonary edema, but without cardiomegaly, pleural effusion, or vascular changes. With time, patchy, ill-defined nodular, or miliary densities replace the pulmonary edema, and progression into a more confluent, advancing interstitial pattern follows. As the clinical process evolves, chest x-ray films may reflect the presence of infection (pneumonic consolidation, not infrequently with evidence of parenchymal necrosis) and barotrauma (pneumothorax, pneumomediastinum, soft-tissue emphysema, pneumoperitoneum). Similarly, the use of positive end-expiratory pressure (PEEP) may produce radiographic changes such as vesicular rarefactions, lucent lines streaking toward the hila, lucent halos around vessels or bronchi, pneumatoceles, and subpleural emphysema manifested by blebs or lucent lines.

PRINCIPLES OF PREVENTION AND THERAPY

The correction of the physiologic abnormalities in the period following the initiating insult is theoretically important, but appropriate studies have not firmly demonstrated an improved outcome. Corticosteroids and prophylactic PEEP (5–8 cm H_2O) have also not been conclusively shown to be beneficial.

Correction of tissue hypoxia is the ultimate goal of therapy in adult respiratory distress syndrome because it seems that at this time we cannot reverse the pathophysiologic changes already present. A host of other supportive measures is also necessary.

1. *Maintenance of oxygenation:* As lung mechanics and gas exchange worsen, mechanical ventilation is necessary for most patients. The criteria for ventilatory support are listed in Table 37–2. There is evidence suggesting a better prognosis with early ventilatory assistance. Volume-cycled ventilation is most commonly used, with tidal volumes around 12 to 15 ml/kg and fraction of inspired oxygen (FIO_2) adequate to maintain the PaO_2 above 60 mm Hg (90% hemoglobin saturation); the Pa_{CO_2} should be kept below 50 mm Hg and the pII between 7.35 and 7.45. All this requires close monitoring; for monitoring of cardiac output and PCWP, a pulmonary artery catheter is necessary especially if an FIO_2 greater than 0.5 is needed to maintain the PaO_2 above 60 mm Hg because PEEP will be needed to improve lung mechanics. The use of PEEP increases the FRC by preventing end-expiratory alveolar collapse and by recruiting hypoventilated alveoli. However, PEEP reduces cardiac output by interfering with venous return, and the circulating

blood volume must be optimized, and the amount of PEEP adjusted to the value resulting in an adequate mixed venous PO_2, cardiac output, and unchanged or increased lung compliance.

Alternative approaches to oxygenation such as high-frequency positive-pressure ventilation and extracorporeal membrane oxygenation have not gained wide use.

2. *Adequate delivery of oxygen to the tissues:* The amount of oxygen delivered to tissues depends on the cardiac output, the oxygen-carrying capacity of the blood, and the ability to unload oxygen from hemoglobin. In addition to changes in FIO_2 and PEEP to achieve a PaO_2 greater than 60 mm Hg, adequate filling of the vascular compartment, judicious use of inotropic drugs and vasoactive drugs, correction of anemia, and avoidance of alkalosis are paramount in the management of adult respiratory distress syndrome.

3. *Avoidance of oxygen toxicity:* Histologic and functional changes similar to those in other causes of adult respiratory distress syndrome are produced by oxygen when, in practical terms, an FIO_2 above 0.8 is administered for more than a few hours. The goal of PEEP therapy and other maneuvers is to reduce the FIO_2 below 0.6.

4. *Fluid management:* Close monitoring of the fluid status is important because the adverse effects of a decreased effective circulating volume in the systemic and pulmonary beds and those of fluid overload are separated by a fine line. Measurements of the PCWP serve as a useful guideline for fluid replacement. The type of fluid replaced is yet another consideration. While crystalloids are generally used, fresh red blood cells are required to maintain a hemoglobin level above 10.0 gm/dl and, if a documented reduction in oncotic pressure (absolute reduction in plasma proteins or hemodilution) is present, solutions of purified protein fractions or albumin (25% solution) can be used.

5. *Suppression of putative mediating mechanisms:* Increased surfactant production, stabilization of lysosomal membranes, and improved tissue perfusion are allegedly possible modes of action for high doses (30 mg/kg) of methylprednisolone. However, clear-cut evidence for increased survival

with corticosteroid use is still absent. Cyclooxygenase blockers are being studied in animal models, but until evidence of their efficacy is produced, they are not indicated in the therapy of adult respiratory distress syndrome.

6. *Nutritional support:* A significant nutritional depletion occurs in most, if not all, patients with adult respiratory distress syndrome. Immediate effects such as muscle weakness (particularly respiratory muscles) and impaired immunity make adequate nutritional support mandatory.

7. *Control of infection:* Colonization of the nasopharynx by enteric gram-negative organisms is an almost constant feature in adult respiratory distress syndrome patients. Their upper airway defense mechanisms are impaired by endotracheal or tracheostomy tubes; monitoring and intravascular access lines may be easily infected; and immunologic compromise is a common feature. Established infections significantly decrease survival in adult respiratory distress syndrome, and prompt, effective antibiotic therapy guided by appropriate studies is important. Determination of the etiologic diagnosis of respiratory infections is a major challenge. Prophylactic antibiotics are not recommended.

Despite constant improvements in therapeutics and improved means of supportive approaches, about 50% of patients with adult respiratory distress syndrome die. The development of hypercapnia signals severe pulmonary damage. Lactate accumulation leading to metabolic acidosis heralds a steady downhill course. Infection usually complicates adult respiratory distress syndrome in its late stages. Surprisingly, survivors show little clinical evidence of late sequelae and most can be expected to be free of significant pulmonary problems.

REFERENCES

Bernard GR, Brigham KL: The adult respiratory distress syndrome. *Annu Rev Med* 1985; 36:195–205. *A concise review presented in a very clear format.*

Brigham KL: Mechanisms of lung injury. *Clin Chest Med* 1982; 3:9–24.

Hudson LD: Causes of the adult respiratory distress syndrome: Clinical recognition. *Clin Chest Med* 1982; 3:195–212. *Comprehensive reviews, part of a whole volume devoted to adult respiratory distress syndrome.*

Shoemaker WC, Appel PL: Pathophysiology of adult respiratory distress syndrome after sepsis and surgical operations. *Crit Care Med* 1985; 13:166–172. *Close hemodynamic and respiratory monitoring of postsurgical and septic patients helps delineate the natural history of adult respiratory distress syndrome. Identifies changes that antecede adult respiratory distress syndrome and discusses perspectives for early recognition and intervention.*

38 INTERSTITIAL LUNG DISEASE

Charles B. Payne, Jr., M.D.

Interstitial lung diseases have a variable mixture of alveolitis, vasculitis, and disordering of lung collagen as common features. Although there are many and diverse causes, the majority of which are unknown, the diseases are classified together because of great similarities in clinical, radiologic, pathophysiologic, and pathologic features. The heterogenous causes invoke pathologic responses in the lung leading to fibrosis and consequent distortion of lung architecture. Sarcoidosis is commonly classified as an interstitial pulmonary disease, but is discussed in Chapter 39.

CLINICAL SIGNS AND SYMPTOMS

Most patients first complain of exertional dyspnea; nonproductive cough is the second most common complaint. Tachypnea is present. Occasionally, when the pulmonary involvement is secondary to a systemic illness, the symptoms of the primary disease predominate. Hemoptysis is not common, but may occur in certain types of interstitial disease such as Goodpasture's syndrome. Physical examination shows clubbing of the fingers in 60% or more of most reported series. Auscultation of the lungs characteristically shows end-inspiratory fine crackles which have been called "Velcro" or "cellophane" crackles. Examination of the heart may show an accentuated second heart sound at the pulmonic area and a right ventricular heave indicative of cor pulmonale. With progression of disease, tachypnea increases, and dyspnea, central cyanosis, dependent edema, hepatomegaly, and other signs of right ventricular failure may occur.

Approximately one-third of the cases of interstitial lung diseases may be traced to specific causes (Table 38–1). The prognosis and natural history of these known diseases are extremely variable. Nonsmoking patients with pneumoconioses such as simple silicosis or stannosis (tin-dust inhalation) may have normal life spans. Prompt diagnosis and treatment of infections such as tuberculosis may reduce morbidity and mortality to a minimum. On the other hand, despite successful diagnosis of hypersensitivity pneumonitis secondary to exposure to a specific pathogen, the inflammatory process in the lung may continue even without further exposure to the inciting agent.

The prognoses of the interstitial lung diseases of unknown causes are also extremely variable (Table 38–2). When first described by Hamman and Rich in 1944, idiopathic pulmonary fibrosis ("usual" interstitial pneumonitis, cryptogenic fibrosing alveolitis) was considered to be a rapidly progressive, uniformly fatal disease with a life expectancy of less than a year. Although the overall prognosis is still poor, the course is now known to vary from an

TABLE 38–1.
Known Causes of Interstitial Lung Disease

Environmental and occupational inhalation diseases
    Inorganic dust inhalation
        Pneumoconioses (e.g., silicosis, anthracosis, stannosis)
        Organic dust inhalation
        Hypersensitivity pneumonitis (Farmer's lung, air-conditioner's lung)
    Aerosol, vapor, or fume inhalation
Infectious diseases
Drug-induced diseases
Radiation-induced diseases
Poisons
Cardiac disease associated with chronic pulmonary edema
Chronic renal failure

TABLE 38–2.
Some Interstitial Lung Diseases with Unknown Causes

Idiopathic pulmonary fibrosis ("usual" interstitial pneumonitis, fibrosing alveolitis)
Sarcoidosis
Diseases associated with collagen-vascular disorders
Inherited disorders
Eosinophilic granuloma (histiocytosis X)
Ankylosing spondylitis
Chronic eosinophilic pneumonia
Lymphocytic infiltrative disorders
Pulmonary veno-occlusive disease
Goodpasture's syndrome, idiopathic hemosiderosis, and other hemorrhagic disorders
Lymphangioleiomyomatosis
Hypersensitivity angiitis, overlap vasculitides, Churg-Strauss syndrome
Diffuse pulmonary amyloidosis

acute, fulminating process to a gradual deterioration or to healing. The average life expectancy is about 5 years, but 15-year survival is recorded. In sarcoidosis, the disease may improve spontaneously or as a result of treatment.

PATHOPHYSIOLOGY

The initial insult to the lung produces an alveolitis, which frequently is shown by an inflammatory exudate in the alveolar spaces, a loss or dedifferentiation of the alveolar type I lining cells, and an inflammatory infiltrate that involves the endothelium of the vessels, the alveolar spaces, and the interstitium. Mediators of inflammation such as factors that inhibit macrophage migration, lymphokines, and similar substances then stimulate the production of abnormal amounts and types of collagen and connective tissue, leading to fibrosis.

The composite picture of the interstitial diseases is that of a restrictive ventilatory disorder with derangement of gas exchange. The total lung capacity is normal or reduced, and the vital capacity is usually the most seriously reduced volume. Lung elastic recoil is increased (decreased compliance) so that the static deflation compliance curve is shifted to the right and down. This increased lung stiffness reduces the lung volumes, in contrast to obstructive disease in which the lungs are hyperinflated. Although rarely performed clinically, the frequency-dependent dynamic lung

compliance is also abnormal, suggesting involvement of the smaller airways in the inflammatory process. Airflow is not usually obstructed, but in diseases such as sarcoidosis, which may have granulomatous endobronchitis, or in advanced histiocytosis X and inhalation diseases associated with bronchiolitis, airflow obstruction and air-trapping in cystic lesions may occur. Bronchodilator aerosols usually produce little response. Except for the Churg-Strauss syndrome of allergic granulomatosis and angiitis, which only occurs in atopic individuals, asthma and marked bronchodilator responsiveness are not features of these diseases.

Both the reduction in lung volume and the decrease in compliance are caused by the alterations in lung architecture and the increase in fibrous tissue stemming from the inflammatory response of the lung to injury. This alteration in length–tension relationships of the lung parenchyma is involved in the production of stimuli to the mechanoreceptors of the lung and vessels leading to the production of exertional dyspnea (see Chapter 9, Dyspnea), which is a cardinal symptom in interstitial lung diseases.

The inflammatory processes and repair leading to fibrosis occur in patchy but widespread distribution throughout the lungs. As a result, because of varying pressure–volume (compliance) relationships which allow variable airway closure and vascular remodeling in the fibrotic parenchyma, the lung no longer behaves in homogenous fashion. Surface area available for gas transport from the alveolae to the pulmonary capillary blood is diminished. This loss of surface area is measurable, in part, by the diffusing capacity ($D_L CO$). The heterogenous distribution of lesions produces lung units with poor alveolar ventilation ($\dot{V}_A$) but good perfusion ($\dot{Q}_c$), and units with excellent ventilation and poor perfusion. In other words, areas of high and low $\dot{V}_A/\dot{Q}_c$ ratios occur. As fibrosis worsens, significant amounts of shunted flow through the lung may also occur. The net result is a widened alveolar–arterial oxygen difference ($D[A–a]O_2$). The response of the cardiac output and redistribution of ventilation and blood flow during exercise is unpredictable, but the older concept of an alveolar-capillary block caused by a thickened alveolar-capillary membrane is no longer felt to be tenable. Diffusion impairments cannot be excluded, but current evidence suggests that impaired diffusion plays at most a minor role in the production of hypoxemia. As interstitial disease progresses, hypoxemia worsens and pulmonary hypertension of the reflex vasoconstrictive type and also secondary to the vascular remodeling recently reported by Reid and associates (Jones et al, 1985), probably occurs. Cor pulmonale with right ventricular failure and secondary polycythemia are frequent causes of death.

DIAGNOSIS

A detailed history is the single most useful noninvasive tool in making a diagnosis. Careful interrogation should include a detailed occupational history, inquiry as to possible environmental exposures, a thorough history of medication ingestion or radiation therapy for illnesses, and a history of a connective tissue disorder diagnosis or any family history of interstitial lung disease. In the hypersensitivity lung diseases and in those caused by drugs, obtaining the history may prevent repeated exposures to the offending agent. This may prevent further loss of lung function and is necessary in making determinations of compensation and disability.

Chest x-ray films may be entirely normal or show a variety of interstitial patterns varying from a ground-glass homogenous haze over the lungs through nodular, reticular, and reticulonodular patterns to full-blown "honeycombing."

When the clinical history and radiologic findings strongly suggest that the differential diagnosis includes miliary tuberculosis or disseminated fungal or protozoal diseases, sarcoidosis, eosinophilic pneumonia, and histiocytosis X, transbronchial lung biopsy using the fiberoptic bronchoscope has an 80% to 90% success rate.

When the diagnosis is not evident from the history and when granulomatous or infectious lung disease is excluded, most cases of interstitial lung disease require an open lung biopsy. The usual biopsy of the lingula, done because of surgical convenience and ease, is not recommended because the tissue from the subpleural area may not be representative of the lung as a whole. It is recommended that biopsies from areas only moderately involved be taken rather than from the most obvious areas of disease indicated by the chest x-ray film. Biopsies from less fibrotic areas are more suitable both for making an accurate diagnosis and for establishing the cellularity, intensity, and type of inflammatory infiltrates.

DIFFERENTIAL DIAGNOSIS

The differential diagnosis of interstitial pulmonary infiltrates is extensive. An accurate and detailed history, including an occupational history, will detect a substantial number of the diseases of known etiology. When the interstitial infiltrate is associated with a disease such as one of the collagen-vascular diseases in which interstitial lung involvement is common, the diagnosis may be reasonably presumed without biopsy confirmation. Miliary infections, such as tuberculosis, aspergillus, and *Pneumocystis carinii*, may present as interstitial infiltrates on the chest x-ray. Because these diseases are treatable and life-threatening, prompt diagnostic efforts which may include lung lavage, bronchial brushing, and open or transbronchial lung biopsy are required. The selection of diagnostic techniques should include the principle of preserving as much functioning lung tissue as possible while still making an accurate diagnosis.

Differential diagnosis is complicated by the fact that patients may present with symptoms before there are recognizable radiologic changes. It is also not uncommon for patients with established diseases, such as rheumatoid arthritis, to develop pulmonary infiltrates during the course of their illness raising the specter of infection. Although an experienced pulmonologist or radiologist may be able to detect characteristic findings in specific patients, lung biopsy is the tool most certain to establish the diagnosis, prognosis, and treatment possibilities.

CLINICAL–PATHOLOGIC CORRELATIONS

A theoretical model for the production of interstitial lung diseases is shown in Figure 38–1. The nature of the inciting insult is variable, but all causes lead to damage of the alveolae, capillaries, or interstitium. This damage triggers

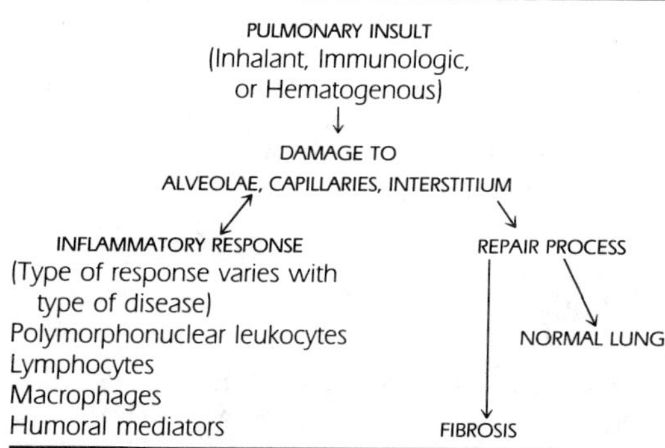

FIG 38–1.
Model of the pathogenesis of interstitial lung disease

repair processes that restore the normal lung or leave areas of fibrosis and triggers an inflammatory response, which can itself cause further damage.

The development of silicosis exemplifies the process initiated by inhaled particles. Inorganic particles of respirable size such as silica dust reach the alveolar space where they are engulfed by pulmonary macrophages. The duration and intensity of exposure, the type of silica (quartz, cristobalite, and so forth), particle size, genetic background of the patient, and the presence or absence of associated infection such as tuberculosis, all interact to produce various manifestations of the disease silicosis. Current evidence suggests that silica-bearing macrophages produce mediators or cytokines responsible for altering the behavior of adjacent cells.

As lymphocytes and macrophages accumulate at developing silicotic nodules, the helper-T cell becomes involved in the inflammatory response. Neutrophils are attracted and together with activated macrophages may be intimately involved in the perpetuation of tissue injury and fibroblastic proliferation.

In nonparticulate injury, damage to capillary endothelium and alveolar type I lining cells initiates the inflammatory response. Depending on the nature of the injury, an alveolitis results with variable involvement of the vascular, cellular, and connective tissue structures. Alveolar type I lining cells are replaced by hyperplastic type II cells during attempts at repair. An inflammatory response with increased numbers of neutrophils, histiocytes, and lymphocytes occurs, and, if the inflam-

matory process becomes chronic, abnormal fibrosis ensues. The details of various models of injury are beyond the scope of this chapter but are well detailed in the references. Using the fiberoptic bronchoscope for bronchoalveolar lavage enables the clinician and investigator to sample the cell populations in the alveolar spaces. Idiopathic interstitial fibrosis yields predominantly polymorphonuclear leukocytes, while sarcoidosis yields mononuclear cells in the lavage fluid. Studies have shown that there is a large population of sequestered inflammatory cells circulating in the lung that may not be reflected in the peripheral blood count. Patients with sarcoidosis, for example, are usually lymphopenic, but have a rich population of lymphocytes in the material recovered by lavage. Bronchoalveolar lavage is still an investigative tool at this time. Work is going forward on recovery of the cytokines and the elucidation of the inflammatory process. Lavage is not generally recommended as a clinically useful procedure. The general clinical–pathologic correlations for interstitial fibrosis are shown in Table 38–3.

PRINCIPLES OF PREVENTION AND THERAPY

There is a growing list of substances known to cause lung injury. New, complex inhalants are by-products of the rapid growth of technology. In addition, the lag time between exposure to a substance such as asbestos fibers and the development of clinical illness hinders efforts at prevention. This same lag time may exist for other substances that are not yet known to be capable of producing disease. Where possible, avoidance, protective equipment, and other environmental controls are essential to the prevention of interstitial lung diseases. Publicized exposures to chlorine gas show that injury may occur in the home and community as well as in the workplace. Public education and adequate training of public safety forces are essential to limit potentially disastrous exposures to toxic substances that may produce lung injury.

Treatment of the interstitial diseases usually involves the use of adrenocorticosteroids, commonly prednisone, in doses of sufficient size and duration to suppress the inflammatory

TABLE 38–3.
Clinical–Pathologic Correlations for Interstitial Lung Disease

CLINICAL FINDINGS	PATHOLOGIC FINDINGS
Dyspnea and tachypnea at rest or with exertion; nonproductive cough	Deranged interstitial collagen (fibrosis); chronic or subacute inflammatory reaction involving alveoli, interstitium, and vessels leads to decreased lung compliance and to stimulation of length–tension reflex receptors in the lung.
Cyanosis; pulmonary hypertension; reduced Pa_{CO_2} and PaO_2; increased work and oxygen cost of breathing	Inflammatory disease of small airways in many conditions; disordered alveolar-capillary relations because of fibrosis; vasculitis in some conditions. All lead to abnormal gas transport.
End-inspiratory fine crackles	Small lung volume with fibrotic small airways; increased transpulmonary pressure causes small airways to open and produce the "crackle" sound.
Clubbing of the fingers	Mechanism unknown

reaction and consequent fibrosis. Other immunosuppressives such as azothioprine, chlorambucil, methotrexate, cyclophosphamide, vincristine, vinblastine, and antimalarials are either under study or have been reported to be of value. Most reports involving these agents suffer from either being anecdotal or involving small numbers of patients without adequate controls.

The success or failure of suppressive therapy may be judged by a variety of means. Among these are serial gallium lung scans and bronchoalveolar lavage to assess the activity of the alveolitis; serial measurements of lung function, including the diffusing capacity; serial determinations of blood-gas transport such as measurements of the $D(A–a)O_2$; and in unusual situations serial biopsies. In most situations, serial chest x-ray films are not sufficiently sensitive to be useful. Sufficient time has not passed and well-controlled studies have not yet been performed to assess the correlation of these studies with outcome. Because most of the drugs used and the follow-up procedures listed are associated with significant risk and morbidity, judicious, individualized therapy and follow-up are required.

Much can be done to improve both the life-style and survival of patients with interstitial disease by providing oxygen and treatment of infections. In addition, pneumococcal and influenza vaccines are recommended, as is the prophylactic use of isoniazid where tuberculosis is a consideration, such as in silicosis.

REFERENCES

Davis GS: The pathogenesis of silicosis: State of the art. *Chest* 1986; 89:166–169S. *Although silicosis is an old disease, much is currently being learned about the nature of the effects of silica in the lung.*

Fraser RG: The radiology of interstitial lung disease. *Clin Chest Med* 1982; 3:475–484. *This succinct description by an experienced radiologist of the various x-ray film appearances is based on sound anatomical and pathophysiologic information.*

Fulmer JD: An introduction to the interstitial lung diseases. *Clin Chest Med* 1982; 3:457–473. *This overview and its accompanying bibliography will quickly bring the reader up to speed.*

Fulmer JD, Crystal RG: Interstitial lung disease, in Simmons DH (ed): *Current Pulmonology.* Boston, Houghton Mifflin, 1979, vol 1, pp 1–65. *This chapter contains a particularly good discussion of therapy.*

Hamman L, Rich AR: Acute diffuse interstitial fibrosis of the lungs. *Bull Johns Hopkins Hosp* 1944; 74:177–212. *Although the first case was reported in 1935 by these authors, it is commonly accepted that this report directed attention to idiopathic pulmonary fibrosis.*

Jones R, Langleben D, Reid LM: Patterns of remodeling of the pulmonary circulation in acute and subacute lung injury, in Said SI (ed): *The Pulmonary Circulation and Acute Lung Injury.*

Mount Kisco, Futura Publishing Co, 1985, pp 137–188. *The response of pulmonary vascular beds to various clinical and laboratory models of lung injury is described to illustrate potential mechanisms in the development of pulmonary hypertension.*

Snider GL: Interstitial pulmonary fibrosis. *Chest* 1986; 89:115–121S. *This superb review describes the findings from animal models of lung injuries other than particulate inhalation that produce fibrosis.*

39 SARCOIDOSIS

Alvin L. Stein, M.D.

Sarcoidosis is a multisystem, granulomatous disorder of unknown etiology, most commonly affecting young adults and presenting most frequently with bilateral hilar adenopathy, pulmonary infiltration, skin or eye lesions. Diagnosis is established most securely when clinical and radiographic findings are substantiated by histologic evidence of widespread noncaseating epitheloid cell granulomas in more than one organ.

Signs and symptoms of sarcoidosis vary widely. In 12% to 34% of the patients, asymptomatic pulmonary disease is detected through a routine chest x-ray film. Common initial symptoms of sarcoidosis are constitutional symptoms such as weight loss, fever, fatigue, malaise, and night sweats.

Respiratory symptoms are probably the most common with 90% to 100% of the patients with sarcoidosis having pulmonary involvement. The initial symptoms may include shortness of breath, dyspnea on exertion, cough, and chest pain. The stages of sarcoidosis are mainly for radiologic classification. Stage 1 disease is defined as the presence of bilateral hilar adenopathy with no involvement of any lung parenchyma. Stage 2 is characterized by bilateral hilar adenopathy and pulmonary infiltrates. Stage 3 is characterized by extensive interstitial infiltrates without hilar changes.

Because sarcoidosis is a multisystem disease (Table 39–1), the patients may present with ocular findings of uveitis, chorioretinitis, and retinal perivasculitis. Neurologic disease usu-

TABLE 39–1.
Frequency of Organ System Involvement in Sarcoidosis*

ORGAN SYSTEM	FREQUENCY OF INVOLVEMENT (% OF CASES)
Lungs	94
Upper airways	11
Lymph nodes	73
Skin	32
Erythema nodosum	8
Eyes	21
Liver	21
Spleen	18
Bones	14
Salivary glands	6
Heart	5
Nervous system	5
Joints	5
Endocrine	5
Kidneys	4
Lacrimal glands	3
Breast	1
Uterus	< 1
Stomach and intestines	< 1

* From Thrasher DR, Briggs DD: Pulmonary sarcoidosis. *Clin Chest Med* 1982; 3:546.

ally occurs after the involvement of other systems, but may occasionally cause the initial symptom. Erythema nodosum is a common skin finding in sarcoidosis. Cardiac involvement may be first seen as congestive heart failure symptoms or arrhythmias. In endocrine involvement the patient may have symptoms of diabetes insipidus, impotence, amenorrhea, or visual field defects. Table 39–2 lists the manifestations of sarcoidosis that involve a single organ system.

Physical findings vary depending on the organ system involved. Patients with pulmonary involvement may have no physical findings, but may present with tachypnea, rales, wheezes or signs of respiratory failure, pulmonary hypertension, or cor pulmonale. Clinically significant pleural effusions are rare. Skin involvement may be heralded by a wide variety of papules, rashes, and other lesions. Visual complaints are common when the eye is involved. Myalgias may suggest musculoskeletal involvement. Parotid enlargement and dry mouth may suggest Sjögren's syndrome. In Heerfordt's disease (uveoparotid fever), facial paralysis occurs with bilateral parotid swelling and uveitis. Manifestations of cardiac involvement may include palpitations or clinical findings suggestive of congestive heart failure. Peripheral lymphadenopathy occurs in 75% of the patients with acute or chronic disease. Splenomegaly occurs in 10% to 25% of the patients. The natural history of the disease varies widely.

TABLE 39–2.
Sarcoidosis with Initial Dominant Symptoms or Signs in a Single Organ System

SYSTEM	MANIFESTATIONS
Pulmonary	Shortness of breath
	Dyspnea on exertion
	Hemoptysis
	Cough
	Chest pain
	Hilar adenopathy, bilateral
	Pulmonary fibrosis
Cardiac	Sudden death
	Arrhythmias (ventricular tachycardia, heart block, conduction system, premature ventricular contractions)
	Congestive heart failure
	Pericardial effusion
	Papillary muscle dysfunction
Neurologic	Peripheral neuropathies
	Leptomeningitis
	Olfactory dysfunction
	Facial palsy
	Seizures
Dermal	Erythema nodosum
	Maculopapular rashes
	Keloids
	Plaques
Renal	Nephritis
	Hypercalcemic nephropathy
Ocular	Uveitis
	Chorioretinitis
	Conjunctival granulomas
	Sjögren's syndrome
Endocrine	Diabetes insipidus
	Amenorrhea
	Visual disturbances
Hepatic	Elevated values for liver function tests
	Hepatic granulomas
Musculoskeletal	Myositis
	Bone cysts (hands and feet)

PATHOPHYSIOLOGY

Histopathologic correlations are noted in Table 39–3. The hallmark of sarcoidosis is a noncaseating granuloma found in the affected organs. The granulomas usually have multiple epithelial cells and Langerhans' giant cells surrounded by lymphocytes and other mononuclear cells. Within the giant cells, inclusion bodies such as Schaumann's bodies consisting of calcium carbonate, phosphate, and iron are found, as are asteroid bodies containing lipoprotein. Residual bodies represent lipomucoprotein, the end product of activated liposomes.

The cause of sarcoidosis remains unknown. A variety of antigenic insults are felt to initiate the cellular response to injury in sarcoidosis. Anergy to delayed hypersensitivity skin tests such as the tuberculin test (or PPD) is evident from the depressed cellular immunity of peripheral tissues and blood. Stimulated B-cell activity as evidenced by spontaneous secretion of immunoglobulins is also noted.

Bronchoalveolar lavage has led to a major breakthrough in the understanding of the immunopathogenesis of sarcoidosis. Focal areas of accumulated inflammatory cells and immunoeffector cells appear within the interstitium and alveoli. Bronchoalveolar lavage studies have demonstrated increased numbers of mononuclear cells in active pulmonary sarcoidosis. There appears to be a reduction in circulating blood lymphocytes with an increase in lung T-lymphocytes. An abnormal proliferative response to mitogens and antigens is noted. Abnormal lymphokine production along with hyperactivity of the humoral immune system occurs. Granulomas in sarcoidosis have a high "turnover" and require supplementation of the effector cells such as macrophages and monocytes. These effector cells are derived predominantly from the accumulating pool of monocytes in the blood.

The differential diagnosis of sarcoidosis includes diseases in which noncaseating granulomas may be found (Table 39–4).

Laboratory findings in sarcoidosis include hypercalcemia and hypercalciuria and, in the active stages of the disease, an elevated erythrocyte sedimentation rate. Hypergammaglobulinemia is seen in 20% to 25% of the patients, and approximately 10% will have elevated values for liver function tests. The ECG findings include bundle branch block, arrhythmias, PVCs, and nonspecific ST–T segment changes. The angiotensin-converting enzyme level may be elevated in a significant number of patients with active disease. This test is not as specific and sensitive as it once was thought to be in the diagnosis of sarcoidosis. The level may be elevated in a wide variety of conditions. A Kveim test entails an intradermal injection of sarcoid tissue gen-

TABLE 39–3.
Histopathologic Correlations

ORGAN SYSTEM	PATHOLOGIC FEATURES
Pulmonary	Alveolitis—inflammatory immunoeffector cells, noncaseating granuloma primarily perivascular and in interstitium
	Fibrosis—border of granuloma, interstitial with honeycomb lung at end stage
Cardiac	Noncaseating granulomas in left ventricular free wall, pericardium, endocardium, and conduction system
Musculoskeletal	Noncaseating granuloma
	Granulomatous synovitis
	Bone cysts
Renal	Granulomatous nephritis
	Nephrocalcinosis
Vascular	Perivasculitis
Hepatic	Granulomas
	Chronic intrahepatic cholestasis of sarcoidosis
Dermal	Septal panniculitis (erythema nodosum)
	Granulomas, nodular lesions

erally obtained from spleens. Three to six weeks later the presence of typical sarcoid granulomas in a skin biopsy at the site of injection is interpreted as a positive result. However, because of the lack of validated material and the questionable sensitivity and specificity of the test, the Kveim test is not widely used.

A patient suspected of having sarcoidosis should have a complete physical examination, chest x-ray film, eye examination including slit lamp testing, an ECG, measurement of the angiotensin-converting enzyme level, electrophoresis of plasma proteins, and skin tests for anergy evaluation. At times, pulmonary function tests may be indicated including measurement of the diffusing capacity and a gallium scan, although the latter is highly sensitive and is not specific for inflammation caused solely by sarcoidosis. Histologic confirmation is required, and the biopsy site needs to be carefully selected. Biopsy sites may include lung, conjunctivae, peripheral lymph nodes, minor salivary glands, and peripheral muscle.

Invasive procedures include bronchoscopy, mediastinoscopy, and thoracotomy. Bronchoscopy and transbronchial biopsy reveal disease in 60% to 80% of the cases. Biopsy of the mediastinal nodes, when successful, has led to a diagnosis of sarcoidosis in 98% to 100% of the cases. Thoracotomy may rarely be indicated. Liver biopsy may be also considered if other sites fail to confirm the diagnosis. Bronchoalveolar lavage with evaluation of the immunoeffector cells should be regarded as a research tool at this time and has been used by some to follow the response to treatment.

The basic treatment for progressive or life-threatening sarcoidosis has been corticosteroids. Corticosteroids are thought to be efficacious in treating the active alveolitis seen in sarcoidosis. Pharmacologic management of sarcoidosis with corticosteroids is still somewhat controversial, because data from many studies fail to substantiate a long-term efficacy of corticosteroid therapy. Similarly the value of corticosteroids in preventing the development of pulmonary fibrosis has not been shown. Corticosteroids are usually given in high (suppressive) doses for 6 to 8 weeks, then, after reevaluation of clinical response using a gallium-scan and angiotensin-converting enzyme level determination, they are tapered to maintenance doses for 6 months to 1 year.

TABLE 39–4.
Diseases with Noncaseating Granulomas*

Sarcoidosis
Tuberculosis
Atypical tuberculosis
Fungal infections
Leprosy
Syphilis
Cat-scratch disease
Berylliosis
Hypersensitivity pneumonitis
Foreign-body reactions
Lymphoma
Carcinoma
Biliary cirrhosis
Regional enteritis
Hypogammaglobulinemia
Granulomatous arteritides

* From Thrasher DR, Briggs DD: Pulmonary sarcoidosis. *Clin Chest Med* 1982; 3:538.

MANAGEMENT

Serum angiotensin-converting enzyme levels have been used by some to assess the progression of the disease and the response to therapy. If gallium scanning is combined with bronchoalveolar lavage or measurement of serum angiotensin-converting enzyme levels, valuable information may be provided about the degree of inflammation of the parenchyma.

PROGNOSIS

Many patients with sarcoidosis do well, most likely in stage 1 disease, without therapy. Clearing of the disease may occur in 1 to 2 years without any residual functional defects. Some patients, however, develop progressive lung disease leading to pulmonary fibrosis and eventually death. Between 90% and 100% of sarcoid patients will have parenchymal lung involvement, 25% will have permanent functional loss, and 10% will die from the unrelentingly progressive disease. An overwhelmingly large percentage of the deaths due to sarcoidosis are caused by pulmonary involvement leading to respiratory failure. Cardiac involvement may produce sudden death from heart block, an arrhythmia, an aneurysm, and heart failure. Blindness may result from ocular involvement. The prognosis in each individual case of sarcoidosis is difficult to predict at this time.

REFERENCES

James DG: Sarcoidosis, in Wyngaarden JB, Smith LH Jr (eds): *Cecil Textbook of Medicine.* Philadelphia, WB Saunders Co, 1985, pp 432–439. *Concise textbook discussion.*

Kerdel FA, Moschella SL: Sarcoidosis. *J Am Acad Dermatol* 1984; 11:1–19. *Updated review of sarcoidosis.*

Lazarus AA: Sarcoidosis. *Otolaryngol Clin North Am* 1982; 15(3):621–633. *Well-referenced discussion.*

McCarty DJ: *Arthritis.* Philadelphia, Lea & Febiger, 1979, p 920. *Good discussion of sarcoid arthropathy.*

Rohatgi PK, Goldstein RA: Immunopathogenesis, immunology and assessment of activity of sarcoidosis. *Ann Allergy* 1984; 52:316–323. *Excellent detailed discussion of immunopathogenesis.*

Thrasher DR, Briggs DD Jr: Pulmonary sarcoidosis. *Clin Chest Med* 1982; 3(3): 537–563. *Concise review of the subject.*

40 CYSTIC FIBROSIS

Howard P. Liss, M.D.

Cystic fibrosis is a lethal, genetic disorder of infants, children, adolescents, and young adults, and is characterized mainly by chronic pulmonary disease, pancreatic enzyme deficiency, and elevated levels of electrolytes in sweat. It is believed to be an autosomal recessive trait that occurs in one of 2,000 live white births and in one of 17,000 live black births. It is the most common cause of chronic airflow obstruction and pancreatic insufficiency up to age 30 years.

CLINICAL SIGNS AND SYMPTOMS

Over 60% of patients with cystic fibrosis are diagnosed before age 1 year. Meconium ileus, failure to thrive, and rectal prolapse are often the initial features. Twenty percent of patients with cystic fibrosis are now diagnosed after age 15 years. The clinical signs and symptoms are not as severe in these patients. Chronic airflow obstruction usually dominates the clinical picture. A dry, chronic cough develops into chronic bronchitis and bronchiectasis after repeated pulmonary infections. Eventually cough, sputum production, dyspnea, and limitation of exercise develop.

Symptoms of pancreatic and gastrointestinal disease include bulky stools, steatorrhea, diarrhea, flatus, and abdominal pain. Patients without major pulmonary or gastrointestinal symptoms may present with sinusitis, heat stroke, infertility (in men and women), or nasal obstruction from polyps.

The general appearance of a cystic fibrosis patient depends on the severity of the disease. Although only 7% of patients are below the third percentile for height and weight, many appear chronically undernourished. Others are indistinguishable from normal subjects and may even be obese.

Hyperinflation and airflow obstruction are present in severe pulmonary involvement from cystic fibrosis. Intercostal retractions, accessory muscle use, cyanosis, and clubbing are seen. Auscultation of the lungs reveals diminished breath sounds and rales. Late in the course, signs of cor pulmonale such as sternal heave, a loud P_2 heart sound, jugular venous distention, and edema of the lower extremities are present. Sinusitis, chronic otitis media, and nasal polyps are seen with upper airway involvement.

Abdominal examination may reveal a palpable mass of bowel contents. Rectal prolapse is common in infants, but rare after age 15 years. A firm nodular liver may be palpable, and the spleen may be palpable if portal hypertension exists. The incidence of inguinal hernia is increased, and an absent vas deferens noted during hernia repair is pathognomonic for cystic fibrosis. Women may have cervical polyps and abnormal cervical mucus.

In the 1950s, most patients with cystic fibrosis died by age 5 years. Today, the median age of death is 15 to 20 years. Beyond the neonatal period, the progression of the lung disease determines survival. Recurrent bacterial and viral infections lead to bronchiectasis and colonization of the airways by *Staphylococcus aureus* and mucoid strains of *Pseudomonas aeruginosa*. Other gram-negative rods encountered less frequently include *Hemophilus influenza*, *Escherichia coli*, *Klebsiella pneumonia*, *Proteus* and *Enterobacter* species. Some fungi, notably *Aspergillus fumigatus*, may be seen.

Complications of the pulmonary disease include hemoptysis (which is common but rarely life-threatening), lobar atelectasis, pneumothorax, lung abscess, and cor pulmonale. Almost all patients with heart failure die within 2 to 3 years.

Gastrointestinal complications include the adult equivalent of meconium ileus, which appears as a small-bowel obstruction from inspissated bowel contents and may be mistaken for an abdominal mass. Intussusception and gallstones occur more often than in the general population. Multilobular cirrhosis is uncommon in cystic fibrosis, but accounts for most nonrespiratory deaths in adults because of hypersplenism and bleeding esophageal varices.

As the pancreatic disease progresses, abnormal results of glucose tolerance tests, hyperglycemia, and insulin-dependent diabetes mellitus appear. Diabetic ketoacidosis is not seen. The clinical signs and complications and their incidence are listed in Table 40–1.

PATHOPHYSIOLOGY

The basic genetic defect in cystic fibrosis is unknown. Five percent of the white population are asymptomatic heterozygous carriers and are detected only when their offspring are noted to have cystic fibrosis.

Elevated levels of sweat electrolytes are the major diagnostic finding in cystic fibrosis. Normally sodium is pumped out of the sweat duct

TABLE 40–1.
Signs and Symptoms of Cystic Fibrosis

PROBLEM OR ORGAN	ABNORMALITY	INCIDENCE (%) OF PATIENTS
Lungs	Chronic obstructive pulmonary disease	97
	Hemoptysis	67
	Minor (60)	
	Major (7)	
	Pneumothorax*	16
	Atelectasis	4
Upper airway	Sinusitis (by x-ray)	100
	Nasal polyps	
	Adults	48
	Children	10–15
Pancreatic insufficiency	Total achylia	85–90
	Abnormal glucose tolerance test	20–30
	Diabetes mellitus	2–8
Intestinal disorders	Meconium ileus equivalent*	24
	Meconium ileus	10–15
	Rectal prolapse	20
	Intussusception	1–5
Liver	Biliary cirrhosis	2–5
	Cholelithiasis	4–12
Miscellaneous	Heat prostration	5
	Male infertility	95–98
	Female infertility	Unknown

* Uncommon in patients younger than 10 years old.

producing hypotonic sweat. In cystic fibrosis, the duct is impermeable to chloride, and both the sodium and chloride concentrations of sweat become elevated. This is usually not a problem unless large quantities of salt are lost from fever or other causes of excess sweating. Heat prostration and vascular collapse may occur. Chloride permeability also appears to be impaired in the respiratory epithelium, although the significance of this is not clear.

At birth, the lungs appear normal, but abnormal mucus and mucociliary clearance lead to repeated pulmonary infections, colonization with various bacteria, and progressive lung destruction. As bronchitis and bronchiectasis develop, ventilation-perfusion mismatch worsens and chronic hypoxemia develops, leading to pulmonary hypertension, cor pulmonale, and death. In cystic fibrosis, the overall immune system is intact but the lungs are susceptible to recurrent bacterial and viral infections because the defenses which normally clear pathogens from the lung are defective.

Inspissation of pancreatic secretions in the pancreatic ducts leads to autolytic destruction of the pancreas and malabsorption. As damage to the pancreas progresses, its endocrine function is affected. Abnormal results to glucose tolerance tests and hyperglycemia are seen, and insulin may be required.

CLINICAL–PATHOLOGIC CORRELATIONS

Although the basic genetic defect of cystic fibrosis is unknown, the pathogenesis and pathologic changes of many of the clinical findings have been described (Table 40–2).

DIFFERENTIAL DIAGNOSIS

Cystic fibrosis is responsible for most of the chronic airway obstruction and pancreatic insufficiency in patients up to age 30 years, most of the intestinal malabsorption in children, and all of the pancreatic insufficiency and meconium ileus in the newborn. As patients are diagnosed at older ages, the differential diagnosis expands.

Bronchiectasis may be due to Young's syndrome (obstructive azoospermia and pulmonary disease), immotile cilia syndrome, or Kartagener's syndrome. An occasional patient who is thought to have obstructive lung disease related to cigarette smoking is discovered by aware practitioners to have cystic fibrosis because of reduced fertility. Sweat electrolytes are elevated only in cystic fibrosis.

Diseases of malabsorption may be confused with cystic fibrosis. Celiac disease, disaccharidase deficiency, lymphangectasia, and abetalipoproteinemia can be differentiated by normal levels of sweat electrolytes and by response to dietary manipulation. In other illnesses, the level of sweat sodium may be elevated. Adrenal insufficiency, ectodermal dysplasia, malnutrition, hereditary nephrogenic diabetes insipidus, fucodosis, hypothyroidism, mucopolysaccharidosis, and glucose-6-phosphatase deficiency are easily distinguished from cystic fibrosis on clinical grounds.

DIAGNOSIS

The diagnosis of cystic fibrosis is based on elevated levels of sodium and chloride in the sweat and either (1) typical pancreatic involvement, (2) typical pulmonary involvement, or (3) a family history of cystic fibrosis.

Meconium ileus of the newborn, mucoid *P. aeruginosa* in the sputum, or a sibling with cystic fibrosis are absolute indications for a sweat test. Other conditions often due to cystic fibrosis include recurrent bronchiolitis or pneumonia prior to age 1 year, rectal prolapse, clubbing or nasal polyps in a child, radiographic evidence of pansinusitis, a young adult with bronchiectasis, or colonization of the respiratory tract with *Pseudomonas cepacia*, *S. aureus*, or *A. fumigatus*.

The sweat test is done by pilocarpine iontophoresis. The sweat is either absorbed onto a previously weighed filter paper or gauze or collected in a disposable coiled capillary tube. At least 100 mg of sweat must be collected for accurate analysis. The test is technically difficult and should be performed by experienced personnel. In order to ensure accurate results, both the sodium and chloride concentrations of the sweat should be within 20 mEq/L of each other. A duplicate test should be done to confirm a positive or negative result. Ninety-nine percent of patients with cystic fibrosis have a chloride

TABLE 40–2.
Clinical–Pathologic Correlations for Cystic Fibrosis

CLINICAL FEATURES	PATHOLOGIC FEATURES
Chronic obstructive pulmonary disease, bronchiectasis	Hyperplasia of mucous glands; increased number of goblet cells; inspissated secretions; recurrent pulmonary infections
Pneumothorax	Multiple subpleural blebs in areas of (1) bronchiectasis, (2) emphysematous alveoli, or (3) isolated interstitial cysts unrelated to alveoli or bronchi
Discolored teeth	Tetracycline therapy in childhood
Male sterility	Anatomical absence of vas deferens, epididymis, seminal vesicles; ejaculate has decreased volume and fructose concentration and increased acidity
Female sterility	Menstrual abnormalities of chronic disease; cervical polyps; abnormal cervical mucus acts as barrier to sperm
Cholelithiasis	Loss of bile acids from malabsorption leads to lithogenic bile
Heat prostration	Excess salt loss through sweat from extreme heat or fever
Meconium ileus equivalent	Inspissated bowel contents in ileocecal region
Firm nodular liver	Fatty liver due to malnutrition, which is reversible with treatment; obstruction of bile ducts leads to focal biliary fibrosis and multinodular cirrhosis

concentration greater than 60 mEq/L. While sweat electrolyte concentration does increase with age, the sweat of adults rarely exceeds this level and the test has excellent positive and negative predictive value.

Other tests of pancreatic insufficiency have been used to diagnose cystic fibrosis, but none is as specific as the sweat test. If cystic fibrosis is suspected, a sweat test should be done.

PRINCIPLES OF PREVENTION AND TREATMENT

Cystic fibrosis cannot be prevented or cured. Treatment is directed at minimizing the malabsorption from pancreatic disease and at aggressive treatment of pulmonary infections.

Nutritional support consists of adequate caloric intake, vitamin supplementation, and pancreatic enzyme replacement. The number of capsules of enzymes used is that which controls symptoms and is not based on metabolic studies. Cimetidine may be useful to decrease stomach and duodenal acidity, thereby increasing the bioavailability of exogenous enzymes. Supplemental salt should be given during times of excess sweating, such as exercise, fever, or hot weather.

Because pulmonary disease accounts for most of the morbidity and mortality in cystic fibrosis, aggressive treatment of pulmonary infections is indicated. Antibiotics are given orally or intravenously for 2 to 4 weeks and should be directed against *Pseudomonas aeruginosa* and other pathogens present in the sputum. Eradication of the pathogens is desirable but often not possible, and patients remain colonized with virulent organisms. As the pulmonary disease progresses, oral antibiotics may be needed continuously. Aerosolized antibiotics may be beneficial.

Removal of pulmonary secretions is also important in patients with cystic fibrosis. This is accomplished with percussion, postural drainage, or directed coughing along with oral, intravenous, or aerosolized bronchodilators.

Yearly influenza vaccine is recommended because of the increased risk to develop complications from influenza.

Many affected women are infertile, but pregnancy can occur and has a deleterious effect on maternal health. Some form of contraception should be used by all female cystic fibrosis patients. Birth control pills appear to be safe in women with cystic fibrosis.

Cystic fibrosis is a chronic, lifelong disease that causes psychosocial stress, and counseling should be available to patients and their families. Cystic fibrosis patients are now finishing college, entering the work force, marrying, and raising families. Their psychosocial needs should not be ignored while their varied medical problems are being treated.

REFERENCES

Davis PB (ed): Cystic fibrosis. *Semin Respir Med* 1985; 6:243–333. *Collection of 10 articles on genetics, diagnosis, pathophysiology, complications, and treatment of cystic fibrosis.*

Davis PB, Del Rio S, Muntz JA, Dieckman L: Sweat chloride concentrations in adults with pulmonary disease. *Am Rev Respir Dis* 1983; 128:34–37. *Reports that 96% of an adult population with lung disease (not including cystic fibrosis) had sweat chlorides less than 60 mEq/L.*

Davis PB, di Sant'Agnese PA: Diagnosis and treatment of cystic fibrosis: An update. *Chest* 1984; 85:802–809. *Reviews diagnosis, complications, and treatment of cystic fibrosis.*

Matthews LW, Dearborn DG, Tucker AS: Cystic fibrosis, in Fishman AP (ed): *Pulmonary Diseases and Disorders.* New York, McGraw-Hill Book Co, 1980, pp 600–613. *Reviews all aspects of cystic fibrosis in the adult patient.*

Matthews LW, Drotar D: Cystic fibrosis—A challenging long-term chronic disease. *Pediatr Clin North Am* 1984; 31:133–152. *Reviews all aspects of cystic fibrosis.*

Palmer J, Dillon-Baker C, Tecklin JS, et al: Pregnancy in patients with cystic fibrosis. *Ann Intern Med* 1983; 99:596–600. *Reviews 11 pregnancies in eight patients with cystic fibrosis and discusses the clinical course of their cystic fibrosis as a result of the pregnancies.*

Park RW, Grand RJ: Gastrointestinal manifestations of cystic fibrosis: A review. Gastroenterology 1981; 81:1143–1161. *Reviews the gastrointestinal, pancreatic, and liver complications of cystic fibrosis.*

Tomashefski JF, Bruce M, Stern RC, Dearborn DG, Dahms B: Pulmonary air cysts in cystic fibrosis. *Hum Pathol* 1985; 16:253–261. *Demonstrates pathologic changes with the various types of subpleural blebs seen in cystic fibrosis patients.*

41   PNEUMOTHORAX

Howard P. Liss, M.D.

Pneumothorax, or air in the pleural cavity, may be spontaneous (primary or secondary), traumatic, or iatrogenic.

CLINICAL SIGNS AND SYMPTOMS

A sharp, pleuritic pain on the affected side occurs in 90% of patients with spontaneous pneumothorax, even if the pneumothorax is small. Over several hours, the pain becomes dull and aching, but is severe in only 20% to 30% of patients. Dyspnea is the second, major complaint in spontaneous pneumothorax. The patient feels unable to inspire fully, and this may be associated with an inspiratory, nonproductive cough.

Secondary spontaneous pneumothorax occurs in patients with underlying lung diseases, such as bullous emphysema, congenital cysts, alph1-antitrypsin deficiency, cystic fibrosis, eosinophilic granuloma, or *Staphylococcus aureus* pneumonia with pneumatocele formation. Symptoms of the underlying disease predominate, and the spontaneous pneumothorax may be relatively asymptomatic. With severe lung disease, a small pneumothorax may precipitate respiratory decompensation.

Iatrogenic pneumothorax is often asymptomatic and detected in a chest x-ray film made after an invasive procedure.

Eighty to ninety percent of patients with primary spontaneous pneumothorax are tall, thin, healthy men, 20 to 40 years old. Diminished breath sounds, diminished vocal and tactile fremitus, and increased resonance to percussion are present on the affected side. With a left pneumothorax, a pericardial knock or clicking sound may be heard best over the lower retrosternal area with the patient in the left lateral decubitis position. The respiratory rate is increased. In severe cases, cyanosis and accessory muscle use are evident, and the trachea is shifted away from the affected side.

In about 2% to 3% of patients, air continues to leak into the pleural space and tension pneumothorax develops. During expiration, pleural pressures exceed atmospheric pressure. Respiration appears labored and rapid, and the patient looks exhausted and diaphoretic. The affected hemithorax appears larger than the unaffected side, and hypotension may be present.

Primary spontaneous pneumothorax is a benign disease. Symptoms resolve in a few days, although complete resolution of the pneumothorax may take several weeks. Pneumothorax recurs on the ipsilateral side in 20% to 30% of patients and occurs on the contralateral side in another 10%. Less than 5% of patients have simultaneous bilateral pneumothorax. Aggressive treatment of iatrogenic and traumatic pneumothorax is necessary to prevent respiratory decompensation or tension pneumothorax.

PATHOPHYSIOLOGY

Air leaks out of the lung spontaneously when the pressure gradient between the air-filled alveolus and the surrounding interstitial tissue causes alveolar rupture. Pneumomediastinum and occasionally, subcutaneous emphysema are present, if the air dissects into the mediastinum. The air can also dissect into the subpleural space and form blebs, which may eventually rupture into the pleural cavity causing pneumothorax.

CLINICAL–PATHOLOGIC CORRELATION

Air may be introduced into the pleural space from alveolar spaces spontaneously, by trauma, or by procedures violating the chest wall and parietal pleura. Table 41–1 lists the pathologic findings in various, clinical situations associated with pneumothorax.

DIFFERENTIAL DIAGNOSIS

Patients presenting with dyspnea and chest pain may have spontaneous pneumothorax, acute myocardial infarction, dissecting aortic

TABLE 41–1.
Clinical–Pathologic Correlations of Pneumothorax

CLINICAL FINDINGS	PATHOLOGIC FINDINGS
Spontaneous pneumothorax without underlying lung disease in young adults	Apical fibrosis surrounded by one or more subpleural cysts (1 to 2 cm in diameter)
Spontaneous pneumothorax with concomitant conditions (rare)	
Marfan's syndrome	Abnormal connective tissue in interstitium and subpleural space
Ehlers-Danlos syndrome	Abnormal connective tissue in interstitium and subpleural space
Boerhaave's syndrome	Esophageal rupture into thorax
Catamenial pneumothorax (in women only)	Endometrial implants on pleura or diaphragm (in 25% of patients)
	Fenestrations (1–5 mm in diameter) in diaphragm (in 19% of patients)
	Concurrent with menses
Underlying lung disease	Subpleural blebs or other cysts rupture into pleural space
Traumatic pneumothorax	Tear in pleura and lung from rib or foreign body
Penetrating trauma	Tear in pleura and lung from shear forces at a point of adhesion of parietal pleura
Nonpenetrating trauma	
Iatrogenic pneumothorax	Puncture of lung (thoracentesis, CVP line placement)
	Air enters pleural cavity during an invasive procedure (needle biopsy of pleura)
Mechanical ventilator use	Blebs or alveoli overdistended by high pressure in airway

aneurysm, or pulmonary embolus. A chest x-ray film and a physical examination should easily distinguish pneumothorax from these more serious illnesses.

Pneumothorax may be mistaken for a large bulla or cyst, for which chest-tube drainage is inappropriate. Thoracentesis must be done if a large pleural effusion is present with spontaneous pneumothorax. Hemothorax, esophageal rupture, and empyema with bronchopleural fistula must be ruled out. When a small, traumatic pneumothorax is associated with a large amount of pneumomediastinum or subcutaneous emphysema, a ruptured main-stem bronchus must be considered while seeking the cause of the pneumothorax (e.g., fractured ribs).

DIAGNOSIS

The diagnosis of pneumothorax rests on the chest radiograph. The visceral pleura of the collapsed lung is visible and separated from the chest wall by a hyperlucent area without lung markings. Fat lines, skin folds, and even long hair can mimic the visceral pleural line, but these other lines often extend beyond the thoracic cage. Because even a very small pneumothorax takes up a larger percentage of the thoracic cage in expiration, it may be visible only on an expiratory film when the normal lung appears more dense.

PRINCIPLES OF THERAPY

The pressure in the pleural space is about 5 cm H_2O below atmospheric pressure, while gases in venous blood have partial pressures totaling 73 cm H_2O below atmospheric pressure. Because a large pressure gradient favors absorption of gas from the pleural space, a small pneumothorax that does not continue to leak air into the pleural space may be allowed to resolve spontaneously over a few weeks. This is the recommended treatment of primary spontaneous pneumothorax in young adults. Symptoms may be relieved by simply aspirating the air. A large or unresolving spontaneous pneumothorax requires drainage with a chest tube. Reexpansion pulmonary edema of unknown

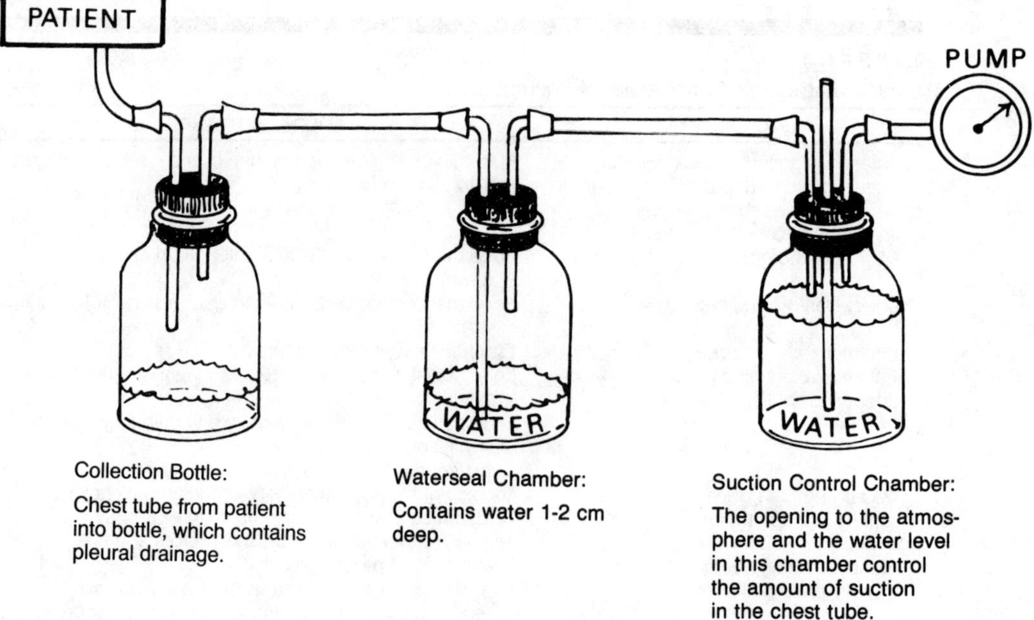

Collection Bottle:
Chest tube from patient into bottle, which contains pleural drainage.

Waterseal Chamber:
Contains water 1-2 cm deep.

Suction Control Chamber:
The opening to the atmosphere and the water level in this chamber control the amount of suction in the chest tube.

FIG 41–1.
Three-bottle system for evacuation of pneumothorax and pleural effusions.

etiology is a rare complication of this therapy, which is more likely if the pneumothorax has been untreated for more than a few days.

Tube drainage is required in many iatrogenic pneumothoraces, because the lung puncture may take several days to close and air accumulates faster than it can be absorbed throughout the pleura. Tension pneumothorax requires immediate chest tube placement. The standard, three-bottle chest tube drainage system is shown in Figure 41–1.

Barotrauma from a mechanical ventilator needs aggressive treatment. Any sudden drop in blood pressure, unexplained worsening of blood values, decrease in compliance (i.e., increase in peak airway pressure), or development of subcutaneous emphysema should prompt an immediate search for pneumothorax. Airway pressures must be brought down by decreasing the tidal volume, reducing PEEP, or sedating the patient. For recurrent spontaneous pneumothorax, pleurodesis or surgical removal of blebs can be considered.

REFERENCES

Boisset GF: Subpleural emphysema complicating staphylococcal and other pneumonias. *J Pediatr* 1972; 81:259–266. *Describes pneumatoceles that pathologically are subpleural blebs formed as air escapes from the alveoli into interstitial interlobular tissue.*

Johnston RF, Green RA: Pneumothorax, in Baum GL, Wolinsky E (eds): *Textbook of Pulmonary Diseases*, ed 3. Boston, Little, Brown & Co, 1983, pp 1327–1341. Thorough review of pathophysiology, clinical course, differential diagnosis, complications, and treatment of pneumothorax.

Kernodle DS, DiRaimondo CR, Fulkerson WJ: Re-expansion pulmonary edema after pneumothorax. *South Med J* 1984; 77:318–322. *Two case reports and discussion of the pathophysiology of this complication of pneumothorax.*

Lichter I, Gwynne JF: Spontaneous pneumothorax in young subjects. *Thorax* 1971; 26:409–417. *Describes young adults with spontaneous pneumothorax who have apical lung cysts.*

Macklin MT, Macklin CC: Malignant interstitial emphysema of the lungs and mediastinum as an important occult complication in many respiratory diseases and other conditions: An interpretation of the clinical literature in the light of laboratory experiment. *Medicine (Baltimore)* 1944; 23:281–358. *Interesting historical review of pneumothorax and pneumomediastinum.*

Shearin RPN, Hepper NGG, Payne WS: Recurrent spontaneous pneumothorax concurrent with menses. *Mayo Clin Proc* 1974; 49:98–101. *Discusses the unusual entity of pneumothorax associated with the menstrual cycle. Endometrial implants and diaphragmatic defects have been demonstrated in some patients, but the syndrome is idiopathic in most.*

Stradling P, Poole G: Conservative management of spontaneous pneumothorax. *Thorax* 1966; 21:145–149. *Discusses spontaneous pneumothorax which in most cases resolve in a few weeks and can be treated conservatively.*

42 PLEURAL EFFUSION

Howard P. Liss, M.D.

A pleural effusion is the accumulation of any fluid (blood, serum, pus, lipid, intravenous fluids, urine) in the pleural space. The fluid may be free-flowing or loculated and may have an associated pneumothorax.

CLINICAL SIGNS AND SYMPTOMS

Patients with small pleural effusions are often asymptomatic. As the effusion increases in size, symptoms appear and worsen. Dyspnea, the most common symptom, can be quite severe with a massive effusion. Pleuritic chest pain may be present and contributes to dyspnea when it limits inspiration. The symptoms of the underlying disease predominate in many illnesses.

Pleural effusion decreases the transmission of lung sounds through the fluid, resulting in dullness to percussion, decreased breath sounds, and decreased tactile and vocal fremitus. Egophony and bronchial breath sounds may be heard if the effusion causes atelectasis of the underlying lung. If the pleural surfaces rub together during the ventilatory cycle, a pleural friction rub may be heard or palpated.

The natural history of untreated pleural effusion depends on the underlying disease. Tuberculous effusions often resolve spontaneously. Effusions associated with rheumatoid arthritis are often small and stable, and require no treatment. Effusions caused by congestive heart failure continue to increase if the congestive heart failure is not treated.

PATHOPHYSIOLOGY AND CLINICAL–PATHOLOGIC CORRELATIONS

Although 5 to 10 liters of fluid enter and exit the pleural space daily, less than 10 ml are present at any time in normal circumstances (Fig 42–1). Protein-free fluid leaks into the pleural space from the parietal pleural capillaries and is almost completely absorbed by the visceral pleural capillaries because of their lower hydrostatic pressure. The small amount of protein in the pleural space is cleared by the lymphatic system.

Changes in the pleural capillary hydrostatic, colloid oncotic, or intrapleural pressures can lead to the formation of pleural fluid. Such ef-

	PARIETAL PLEURAL CAPILLARIES	PLEURAL SPACE	VISCERAL PLEURAL CAPILLARIES
PLASMA PRESSURES			
Colloid oncotic pressure	← 34		34 →
Capillary hydrostatic pressure	30 →		← 11
PLEURAL SPACE PRESSURES			
Intrapleural pressure		→ 5 ←	
Colloid osmotic pressure		→ 8 ←	
	9 →		10 →

* All pressures expressed in centimeters of water.

FIG 42–1.
Pressures involved in fluid shifts across the pleural space.*

fusions are called *transudates*. The underlying pleura is normal; the pressures affecting fluid flow are not.

Systemic illnesses that cause changes in the pleural surfaces can cause effusions in spite of normal hydrostatic, oncotic, and intrapleural pressures. These are called *exudates*.

DIFFERENTIAL DIAGNOSIS

When the clinical picture or a known underlying disease suggests the cause of a pleural effusion, the underlying disease can be treated and the effusion followed clinically. In all other cases, a diagnostic thoracentesis is advised.

Differentiating transudates from exudates requires measurement of the total protein and lactic dehydrogenase levels of the fluid and serum (Table 42–1). Transudates fulfill all three of the criteria listed in Table 42–1. Transudates accumulate because of changes in the hydrostatic, oncotic, or extrapleural pressures. Table 42–2 lists diseases having transudates and the mechanism by which the transudate forms. Congestive heart failure is the most common cause of transudative effusions.

If any one of the three criteria for transudates in Table 42–1 is not met, the fluid is an exudate. The two most common causes of exudates are neoplasms and infections, but many illnesses are associated with exudative effusions (Table 42–3). The work-up in each of

these conditions depends on the differential diagnosis.

If tuberculosis is suspected, a closed pleural biopsy is indicated in addition to a culture of the pleural fluid. The diagnostic yield of mycobacterial stains and culture together with histologic study of pleural biopsy specimens is 80%, while pleural fluid cultures are often negative.

If malignancy is suspected and the results of the initial thoracentesis are not diagnostic, a closed pleural biopsy or a second thoracentesis should be done. The first thoracentesis yields a diagnosis of malignancy in 60% of malignant effusions. This percentage increases to 90% if three separate thoracenteses are done.

Cytologic studies and culture of the pleural fluid are the only specific tests available for pleural fluid. All other tests merely suggest

TABLE 42–1.
The Three Criteria for Diagnosis of a Transudate*

$$\frac{\text{Pleural Fluid LDH Level}}{\text{Concomitant Serum LDH Level}} < 0.6$$

$$\frac{\text{Pleural Fluid Total Protein Level}}{\text{Concomitant Serum Total Protein Level}} < 0.5$$

Pleural Fluid LDH Level <200IU/ml†

* From Light RW, MacGregor MI, Luchsinger PC, Ball WC Jr: Pleural effusions: The diagnostic separation of transudates and exudates. *Ann Intern Med* 1972; 77:507–513.
† In this study, the upper normal limit of LDH level was 300 IU.

TABLE 42–2.
Clinical–Pathologic Correlations of Transudates

DISEASE	MECHANISM
Congestive heart failure	Increased hydrostatic pressure in the pulmonary capillary vasculature from increased left ventricular pressure
Nephrotic syndrome	Decreased oncotic pressure from albuminuria
Superior vena cava obstruction	Increased hydrostatic pressure in parietal pleural capillaries
Ascites 　Cirrhosis 　Peritoneal dialysis 　Meigs' syndrome	Fluid passes from abdomen into pleural space through defects in the diaphragm or through the diaphragmatic lymphatics
Ex vacuo effusions 　Acute atelectasis 　Pneumothorax	Decreased intrapleural pressure eliminates pressure gradient that removes fluid by way of visceral pleura
Urinothorax	Associated with obstructive uropathy. Retroperitoneal urine leaks into pleural space similar to ascites
Misplaced subclavian catheter	Intravenous fluids accumulate in pleural space
Myxedema	Unknown. Exudative effusions also occur

TABLE 42–3.
Differential Diagnosis of Exudates

INFECTION

Tuberculosis
Parapneumonic effusions
Viral pneumonia
Fungal pneumonia
Mycoplasma pneumoniae
Empyema
Paragonimiasis
Hydatid cyst
Amoeba

NEOPLASM

Carcinoma
Multiple myeloma
Lymphoma
Leukemia
Sarcoma
Mesothelioma
Hypernephroma

PULMONARY EMBOLUS/INFARCTION
IMMUNOLOGIC-MEDIATED DISEASES

Systemic lupus erythematosus
Rheumatoid arthritis
Wegener's granulomatosis
Dressler's syndrome
Familial paroxysmal polyserositis

CHYLOTHORAX

Tumor invading thoracic duct
Trauma
Iatrogenic rupture
  Surgical
  Intravenous pacemaker placement

HEMOTHORAX

Traumatic
Iatrogenic intercostal artery laceration
Bleeding diathesis

GASTROINTESTINAL DISEASE

Pancreatitis
Peritonitis
Esophageal rupture
Subdiaphragmatic abscess

MISCELLANEOUS

Asbestosis
Postirradiation
Yellow nail syndrome
Milroy's disease
Uremia

possible diagnoses. The more common tests and their significance are listed in Table 42–4.

Bilateral effusions are usually transudates or caused by immune-related diseases. These effusions are often not the same size, so care must be taken not to miss a small effusion on one side.

If the initial work-up is not diagnostic and tuberculosis is suspected, antituberculous chemotherapy may be given. Computed tomography (CT scan) of the chest might reveal mediastinal lymphadenopathy; other organs, such as a palpable lymph node, may be investigated. Invasive procedures such as pleuroscopic examination or thoracotomy with open biopsy should be reserved for patients in whom malignancy or tuberculosis is strongly suspected because the results of these procedures are otherwise not diagnostic. If the clinical picture is nonspecific, observation and close follow-up are recommended.

DIAGNOSIS

The physical signs of dullness to percussion and decreased or absent breath sounds are found in most, if not all, clinically significant effusions. The radiographic diagnosis of pleural effusion relies on the silhouette sign. A very small pleural effusion may obliterate the posterior diaphragmatic surface and be visible only on lateral chest x-ray films. On an upright PA film, costophrenic angle blunting occurs when 300 ml of fluid has accumulated. By the time symptoms appear, the effusion has obliterated the entire diaphragmatic border, tracing an upward-curving meniscus on the lateral chest wall. Cardiac and other mediastinal borders are eventually obliterated as the effusion fills the hemithorax.

Effusions may have an atypical appearance. Fluid may accumulate in the subpulmonic, paramediastinal, and apical areas, especially if prior pleural adhesions cause the fluid to become loculated. Fluid may also accumulate in the major and minor fissures, causing pseudotumors of the lung.

Once effusion is suspected, right and left lateral decubitus x-ray films are usually taken to demonstrate the fluid moving within the thoracic cage, but any two views in different positions can be used. When enough fluid has accumulated to cause blunting of the lateral costophrenic angle on an upright PA film, a supine film will show evidence of fluid movement also. Findings on a supine film include increased homogeneous density superimposed over the lung fields, obliteration of the dia-

TABLE 42–4.
Diagnostic Tests of Pleural Fluid

TEST	FINDING	POSSIBLE CAUSES
Levels of LDH and of total protein	(See Table 42–1.)	(See Table 42–2.)
Appearance	Grossly bloody* (> 100,000 RBC/μl)	Trauma, pulmonary embolus, malignancy
	Purulent	Empyema
	Milky	Empyema, chylothorax
WBC differential count	> 50% lymphocytes	Tuberculosis, malignancy
	> 50% polys	Early tuberculosis, any inflammatory illness
	> 10% eosinophils	Viral pleuritis, trauma
pH	< 7.20	Potentially infected effusion associated with pneumonia (parapneumonic effusion), empyema, rheumatoid arthritis, malignancy
Glucose	< 60 mg/dL	Same as for pH. In rheumatoid effusion, glucose is often less than 30 mg/dL.
Amylase	Elevated (Normal not established)	Pancreatitis, esophageal rupture, malignancy
Culture	Positive	Bacterial, tuberculous, or fungal infection
Cytologic studies	Positive	Malignant mesothelioma, other tumors metastatic to pleura (lung, breast, kidney)

* Traumatic taps may be blood-tinged. Even 1 ml of blood in 500 ml of pleural fluid will give the effusion fluid a serosanguinous appearance.

phragm silhouette, apical capping, and accentuation of the right minor fissure. If free fluid is still suspected but is not seen, an ultrasound of the chest will localize the fluid and direct the thoracentesis.

The radiographic pictures of parenchymal atelectasis, parenchymal consolidation, pleural thickening, or elevated hemidiaphragm must be distinguished from effusion. Segmental and lobar atelectasis have distinctive x-ray patterns easily distinguished from pleural effusion. In massive effusion the mediastinum is shifted *away* from the affected side, while massive atelectasis of an entire lung causes volume loss and shifting *toward* the affected side.

Air bronchograms are the hallmark of consolidation. This and bronchial breath sounds rather than diminished breath sounds separate consolidation from pleural effusions. Pleural effusion can be differentiated from pleural thickening only by demonstrating fluid in the thorax. Pleural plaques are thin, calcified, needle-like dense areas in the x-ray films of the diaphragm and chest wall. These areas are characteristic of both asbestosis and old hemothorax and indicate pleural thickening.

An elevated hemidiaphragm can be distinguished from a subpulmonic effusion by the absence of free-flowing fluid.

PRINCIPLES OF THERAPY

Exceptions to treating a pleural effusion by treating the underlying disease include recurrent malignant pleural effusion and empyema. If a recurrent malignant effusion cannot be controlled with repeated thoracentesis, pleurodesis should be considered. Pleurodesis consists of complete chest tube drainage, followed by the instillation of an irritating agent such as tetracycline into the pleural space. Pleural inflammation results in adhesions, obliterating the space and preventing a recurrence of the pleural effusion.

Drainage is indicated for empyema. The infection in the pleural space will not resolve with antibiotics alone. Depending on the extent of the infection, tube thoracostomy, minithoracotomy with rib resection, or Eloesser flap may be done. Complicated parapneumonic effusions should also be drained. Their pH is often less than 7.20, but a decision to drain should not be based on the pH value alone. Other factors to consider include the purulence and viscosity of the fluid, the results of a Gram's stain and culture of the fluid, and whether the fluid is flowing freely or is loculated. Drainage can be accomplished by tube thoracostomy or repeated thoracentesis.

REFERENCES

Gunnels JJ: Perplexing pleural effusion. *Chest* 1978; 74:390–393. *Reports that invasive diagnostic procedures are indicated if neoplasm or granulomatous diseases are strongly suspected; otherwise observation is appropriate.*

Hills BA: The pleural interface. *Thorax* 1985; 40:1–8. *Reviews the physiology of the pleura and how it functions to allow ventilation.*

Johnston RF, Green RA: Pleural inflammation and pleural effusion, in Baum GL, Wolinsky E (eds). *Textbook of Pulmonary Diseases*, ed 3. Boston, Little, Brown & Co, 1983, pp 1299–1325. *A thorough review of all physiologic and clinical aspects of pleural effusions.*

Light RW, MacGregor MI, Luchsinger PC, Ball WC Jr: Pleural effusions: The diagnostic separation of transudates and exudates. *Ann Intern Med* 1972; 77:507–513. *Defines the accepted criteria for transudates and exudates.*

Potts DE, Levin DC, Sahn SA: Pleural fluid pH in parapneumonic effusions. *Chest* 1976; 70:328–331. *Prospective study demonstrating that pleural fluid pH can separate complicated from uncomplicated parapneumonic effusions.*

Sahn SA: The differential diagnosis of pleural effusions. *West J Med* 1982; 137:99–108. *Reviews physiology, differential diagnosis, and work-up of pleural effusions.*

Sahn SA: Pleural effusion in lung cancer. *Clin Chest Med* 1982; 3:443–452. *Discusses clinical features, pathogenesis, and management of pleural effusions in patients with bronchogenic carcinoma.*

Woodring JH: Recognition of pleural effusion on supine radiographs: How much fluid is required? *AJR* 1984; 142:59–64. *Reports that when 175 to 525 ml of pleural fluid accumulates and causes blunting of the lateral costophrenic angle on an upright PA film, increased density of the lower lung zone is noticeable on a supine film.*

part IV

Infectious Diseases

UPPER RESPIRATORY INFECTION: STREPTOCOCCAL PHARYNGITIS AND THE COMMON COLD

Toni I. Evans, M.D.
Kim Goldenberg, M.D.

STREPTOCOCCAL PHARYNGITIS

Streptococcal pharyngitis is an acute bacterial inflammation of the pharynx and tonsils caused by group A beta-hemolytic streptococci (*Streptococcus pyogenes*).

CLINICAL SIGNS AND SYMPTOMS

The symptoms of streptococcal pharyngitis include sore throat, malaise, fever, and headache, all of abrupt onset. Nausea, vomiting, and abdominal pain are common in children.

Upon physical examination, the posterior pharynx is red and edematous and usually has enlarged tonsils. About 50% of the time, a grayish-white exudate is also present. Enlarged, tender anterior cervical lymph nodes are also common. A low-grade fever may be present. Palatal petechiae or a diffuse red macular rash (as associated with scarlet fever) with the above findings is suggestive of streptococcal pharyngitis, but this combination is not often present.

Untreated steptococcal pharyngitis may be self-limited, but the incidence of suppurative and nonsuppurative complications is increased, so treatment is necessary. In addition, some studies have shown shortening of the symptomatic period with antibiotic treatment, especially if instituted early.

Suppurative complications include entities such as peritonsillar or retropharyngeal abscess, acute sinusitis, otitis media, and suppurative cervical lymphadenitis. Other, less common complications include meningitis, brain abscess, and thrombosis of the intracranial venous sinuses. If bacteremia develops, other complications including endocarditis, arthritis, osteomyelitis, or liver abscess can occur. These complications are very unusual now that antibiotics are routinely used. Nonsuppurative complications include acute rheumatic fever and acute glomerulonephritis. The risk of development of rheumatic fever from untreated streptococcal pharyngitis varies from 0.6% to 2.9% depending on the population studied. In the United States the risk is less than 1%.

PATHOPHYSIOLOGY

Streptococcal pharyngitis is spread by close person-to-person contact by way of saliva or nasal secretions. Initially, the group A *Streptococcus* must attach to mucosa cells before either colonization or infection can occur. Mucosal penetration is probably accomplished by the action of the many cellular and extracellular products of S. pyogenes.

From studies of the inoculation of S. pyogenes on the mucosa of volunteers, there appears to be a latent period of 36 to 72 hours before infection occurs. Sore throat with its accompanying inflammation of the pharynx and tonsils then appears. The severity of disease varies widely for unclear reasons. Probably host factors play a role.

During the period of acute infection, large numbers of M-typable group A streptococci can be found in the nose and throat. The M protein appears to be the major virulence antigen of the group A *Streptococcus*. The M protein contributes to the resistance to phagocytosis by polymorphonuclear cells (PMNs), enables the *Streptococcus* to multiply rapidly in blood, and appears capable of initiating disease.

There are many extracellular products of group A streptococci that also contribute to its virulence. Streptolysins O and S are capable of damaging the membranes of PMNs. DNAases A, B, C, and D degrade DNA, thus facilitating the spread of streptococci through tissue planes. Hyaluronidase degrades hyaluronic acid, which is part of the ground substance of connective tissue.

CLINICAL–PATHOLOGIC CORRELATIONS

The clinical manifestations are the result of the inflammatory reaction that occurs after the streptococci penetrate the mucosa. Table 43–1 presents the clinical–pathologic correlations for streptococcal pharyngitis.

DIFFERENTIAL DIAGNOSIS

The differential diagnosis includes tonsillopharyngitis caused by other bacteria or viruses. Diphtheria, caused by *Corynebacterium diptheriae*, is an uncommon disease today because of immunizations, and can be differentiated clinically by the formation of a whitish pharyngeal membrane, as well as by cardiac and neurologic involvement. Vincent's angina, which is pharyngitis caused by oral anaerobes, is accompanied by oral ulcers and fetid breath as well as a membranous exudate. *Neisseria gonorrhea* may also cause an exudative pharyngitis, but the patient will have a history of oral sex. *Mycoplasma pneumoniae* is another bacterial cause of pharyngitis, usually accompanied by pneumonia. Viral causes include adenovirus, herpes simplex virus, Coxsackievirus, and Epstein-Barr virus. Herpes virus infection is usually accompanied by vesicular or ulcerated lesions, and Epstein-Barr pharyngitis is accompanied by other signs and symptoms of infectious mononucleosis. Table 43–2 presents methods of diagnosis of some of the organisms mentioned.

DIAGNOSIS

A positive throat culture for group A beta-hemolytic *Streptococcus* remains the standard for diagnosis. However, 5% to 20% of healthy people can carry group A *Streptococcus* in their pharynx without infection (false-positives). In addition, a single culture may miss 7% to 10% of streptococcal pharyngitis infections (false-negatives).

A fourfold increase in antistreptolysin O titer in the convalescent stage compared with that in the acute stage also indicates recent streptococcal infection, but is not clinically useful because of the delay in obtaining convalescent titers.

Several clinicians have used clinical criteria to attempt to diagnosis streptococcal pharyngitis and therefore obviate the need to wait for culture results. Fever, pharyngeal exudate, tender anterior cervical lymphadenopathy, and lack of cough are common accompaniments of streptococcal pharyngitis but are not diagnostic. As previously mentioned, palatal petechiae or a diffuse, red macular rash are helpful but are not very common.

Commercial tests for rapid diagnosis of streptococcal pharyngitis by detecting group A streptococcal antigen directly from a throat swab have recently become available. Sensitivity varies from 77% to 95%, and specificity from 86% to 100%. These tests make cultures unnecessary, can be as accurate as cultures, and enable immediate treatment if positive, but they require a lot of staff time if run individually.

PRINCIPLES OF TREATMENT

Penicillin orally or intramuscularly is the treatment of choice. Erythromycin may be used in patients allergic to penicillin.

COMMON COLD

The common cold is a viral infection of the upper respiratory tract that is mild and self-limited. Table 43–3 lists the viruses that can cause colds.

CLINICAL SIGNS AND SYMPTOMS

The patient's symptoms may include nasal discharge, sneezing, cough, sore throat, low-grade fever, and nasal "stuffiness." In addition, decreased ability to smell and taste, burning eyes, and a feeling of pressure in the ears or sinuses may be present.

The typical patient has a mildly inflamed nasal and erythematous mucosa with a clear-to yellowish nasal discharge.

TABLE 43–1.
Clinical–Pathologic Correlations for Streptococcal Pharyngitis

| | PATHOLOGIC FEATURES | |
CLINICAL FEATURES	MICROSCOPIC	MACROSCOPIC
Sore throat	Polymorphonuclear cells, congested microvasculature, increased vascular permeability to group A streptococci	Inflammation of pharynx and tonsils with erythema, edema, and exudate
Enlarged lymph nodes and tonsils	Possibly reactive reticuloendothelial tissue in the lymphoid germial centers	Lymphoid hyperplasia
Rash with scarlet fever	Erythrogenic toxin	Hyperemia

TABLE 43–2.
Methods of Identifying Organisms That Cause Pharyngitis

ORGANISM	IDENTIFICATION METHODS
BACTERIA	
Corynebacterium diptheriae	Throat culture (Löffler's medium)
Neisseria gonorrhea	Throat culture (Thayer-Martin medium or Transgrow)
Oral anaerobes (Vincent's angina)	Gram-stained smear (crystal violet) of the exudate to demonstrate fusobacteria and spirochetes
Mycoplasma pneumoniae	Serologic tests (during acute and convalescent stages)
VIRUSES	
Epstein-Barr	Complete blood count (lymphocytosis with atypical lymphocytes) Monospot test (hetrophile antibodies) 95% sensitive Epstein-Barr antibody titers
Other viruses (herpes simplex virus, adenovirus, Coxsackievirus, rhinovirus, coronavirus, influenza)	Throat cultures and serologic tests, available in some laboratories

After 1 to 2 weeks, the symptoms resolve, but complications such as otitis media and bacterial sinusitis can occur in a small percentage of cases.

PATHOPHYSIOLOGY

Colds are transmitted by suspension of viral particles in droplets that are passed during coughing or sneezing as well as by close hand contact (or fomites) with autoinoculation. The mechanism that predominates probably varies with the virus. After an incubation period of several days, the epithelium of the nasal passages become infected. The virus is spread contiguously, resulting in inflammation and edema of the submucosa. The virus presence stimulates the release of serum proteins into the nasal secretions and attracts polymorphonuclear cells and sloughed epithelium cells, causing the nasal discharge to become purulent. The peak of viral shedding occurs during the time of clinical symptoms.

TABLE 43–3.
Causes and Occurences of Common Cold

VIRUS	TIME OF YEAR
Rhinoviruses	Fall, spring
Influenza	Winter (in epidemics)
Parainfluenza	Fall, spring
Respiratory syncytial virus	Winter, early spring
Adenovirus	Year-round
Coronavirus	Winter
Enterovirus	Summer, fall
Other	Unknown

TABLE 43–4.
Clinical–Pathologic Correlations for Common Cold

CLINICAL FINDINGS	PATHOLOGIC FINDINGS
Rhinorrhea	Irritation of the mucosa with increased mucus production
Cough	Hyperirritable airways
Edema, erythema with nasal stuffiness and congestion	Increased vascular permeability, congested microvasculature cholinergic stimulation

CLINICAL–PATHOLOGIC CORRELATIONS

The pathologic changes during a cold occur during the time of viral and epithelial cell shedding. Table 43–4 presents the clinical-pathologic correlations.

DIFFERENTIAL DIAGNOSIS

Allergic and vasomotor rhinitis can have the same nasal symptoms as colds, but they tend to be chronic conditions. Allergic rhinitis can often be linked to environmental exposures. Sore or scratchy throat is another symptom of colds, so pharyngitis (both viral and bacterial) should also be considered in the differential diagnosis. Otitis media and bacterial sinusitis can occur (in 2% and 0.5% of cases, respectively) as complications of colds. Examinations of the tympanic membranes of the ears should show if otitis media is present. The diagnosis of sinusitis is suggested by headache and tenderness over the involved sinus accompanied by a yellowish nasal discharge and a fever. Transillumination of the sinuses is helpful, looking for opacification of the involved sinus. X-ray films of the sinuses will usually make the diagnosis but are not cost-effective in the initial evaluation of uncomplicated cases.

DIAGNOSIS

The signs and symptoms of colds are so common that most patients diagnose themselves. Many viruses can be isolated by cell cultures, but cell cultures are expensive and not widely available at this time. In addition, a fourfold increase in the titers of some viruses from the acute to the convalescent stage (3 weeks later) can be done and may be diagnostic but are not clinically useful because of the time lag.

PRINCIPLES OF TREATMENT

Because there is no definitive treatment for most viruses, symptomatic measures are the mainstay of therapy. Local decongestants can be used to relieve nasal "stuffiness" but may cause rebound congestion if used for more than 3 to 4 days. Saline nose drops can be used to clear nasal passages in children. Warm saline gargles can be used for sore throat, and cough suppressants can be used if a dry cough is present. Bedrest, acetaminophen, and aspirin can be used for constitutional symptoms.

Infections by two viruses, influenza and respiratory syncytial virus (RSV), are exceptions because treatment is currently available for them. Influenza can be prevented with vaccine and prevented as well as treated with amantadine. For severe RSV infections, ribavirin is available.

REFERENCES

Abramowicz M (ed): Rapid office diagnostic tests for streptoccocal pharyngitis. *The Medical Letter* 1985; 27(689):49–51. *A concise discussion of rapid diagnostic tests for streptococcal pharyngitis.*

Dillion HC Jr, Votsi KL: Streptococcal diseases, in Hoeprick PD (ed): *Infectious Disease.* Philadelphia, Harper & Row, 1983, pp 288–289. *Good discussion of the pathogenesis of streptococcal pharyngitis.*

Fulginiti VA: Still more on streptococcal pharyngitis: An important disease with yet unresolved clinical issues. *JAMA* 1985; 253(9):1302. *A good editorial on the current controversies in the diagnosis and management of streptococcal pharyngitis.*

Gwalty JM Jr: The common cold; Douglas RG, Betts RF: Influenza virus; Hall CB: Respiratory syncytial virus; Bisno AL: Streptococcal pyogenes, in Mandell GL et al (eds): *Principles and Practice of In-*

fectious Diseases. New York, John Wiley & Sons, 1985, pp 351–359, 860–861; 885; 1124–1129. *Excellent reference for both the common cold and streptococcal pharyngitis.*

Hall CV, McBride JT: Upper respiratory tract infections, in Pennington JE (ed). *Respiratory Infections: Diagnosis and Management.* New York, Raven Press, 1983, pp 79–84. *A good, brief summary about the common colds and pharyngitis.*

Hendley JO: Rhinovirus colds: Immunology and pathogensis. *Eur J Respir Dis* 1983; 64(suppl 128):340–343. *A good discussion of the pathogenesis of colds.*

Levy ML, Ericson CD, Pickering LK: Infections of the upper respiratory tract. *Med Clin North Am* 1983; 67(1):153–158. *A good discussion of pharyngitis.*

Lowe R, Hedges J: Early treatment of streptococcal pharyngitis. *Ann Emerg Med* 1984; 12(6):440–448. *A good discussion of the diagnosis and early treatment of streptococcal pharyngitis.*

44 INFECTIOUS MONONUCLEOSIS

Jack M. Bernstein, M.D.

Infectious mononucleosis is an infectious disease characterized by fatigue, fever, pharyngitis, lymphadenopathy,and splenomegaly. The proliferation of atypical lymphocytes in the peripheral blood is responsible for the syndrome's name. The etiologic agent responsible for the syndrome is Epstein-Barr virus (EBV). Cytomegalovirus (CMV), and *Toxoplasma gondii* can produce similar syndromes.

CLINICAL SIGNS AND SYMPTOMS

Infectious mononucleosis has an insidious onset over 1 to 2 weeks, during which time the patient experiences fatigue, malaise, and anorexia. Pharyngitis, fever, and lymphadenopathy follow soon after. In an occasional case, the onset of disease is heralded by a sudden fever. The incidences of common symptoms of infectious mononucleosis are listed in Table 44–1.

By the time the patient has reached healthcare personnel, the disease is near its peak. There is usually diffuse lymphadenopathy involving the cervical, axillary, and inguinal nodes. Other lymph node regions are less commonly involved. Exudative pharyngitis and tonsillar enlargement are almost always appreciated. The pharyngitis seen bears a striking resemblance to that found in "strep throat" and, as such, the two syndromes are frequently confused. Moreover, persons with mononucleosis often have concomitant "strep throat."

TABLE 44–1.
Signs and Symptoms of Infectious Mononucleosis*

SYMPTOM OR SIGN	OCCURRENCE (% OF PATIENTS)
Malaise	100
Fever	98
Sore throat	76
Lymphadenopathy	100
Fever	98
Pharyngitis	85
Splenomegaly	75
Jaundice	10

* Adapted from Fleisher GR: Epstein-Barr virus, in Belshe RB (ed): *International Textbook of Human Virology.* Littleton, Mass, PSG Publishing Co, 1984, pp. 853–886 and Sugden B: Epstein-Barr virus: A human pathogen inducing lymphoproliferation in vivo and in vitro. *Rev Infect Dis* 1982; 4:1048–1061.

A differentiating feature is the characteristic maculopapular rash which develops in response to ampicillin in patients with infectious mononucleosis. Splenomegaly can be found in 40% to 75% of patients with infectious mononucleosis; in some cases, the spleen is massively enlarged. Jaundice is frequently seen, although significant hepatomegaly is unusual. However, even in the absence of jaundice, the liver function studies are still abnormal. Because splenomegaly is unusual in hepatitis A or B infections, the combination of splenomegaly, jaundice, pharyngitis, and lymphadenopathy points strongly to infectious mononucleosis.

The acute phase of the illness usually lasts for several weeks to a month or two. Older persons are more severely ill than younger and may be ill for longer periods of time. Patients are usually extremely fatigued and may have to remain in bed. Splenomegaly can become so massive that splenic rupture may occur with minimal provocation. Other complications seen during the course of the disease are listed in Table 44–2. Recently, it has been shown that EBV-induced infectious mononucleosis may not be self-limiting. In these studies, some patients with persistent illnesses consistent with infectious mononucleosis had evidence of continuing active EBV infection.

PATHOPHYSIOLOGY

Infection with EBV is initiated in the oropharynx. The early stage(s) of infection are unclear, however, infection of B-lymphocytes probably takes place at this site. In response to the foreign viral antigens expressed on the B-cell's surface, T cells become stimulated and divide. These activated "killer" T cells are the atypical lymphocytes seen in the peripheral blood smear. Infected B cells may infiltrate any organ. Cytotoxic T cells, in an effort to control the infection, destroy infected B cells; injury to uninvolved tissue may occur as a sequelae.

In unusual cases, such as the X-linked lymphoproliferative syndrome, the body is unable to mount an effective cell-mediated immune response against the virally infected cells. These persons either die of overwhelming infectious mononucleosis or aplastic anemia, or hemolytic anemia or hematologic malignancies develop.

Both nasopharyngeal carcinoma and Burkitt's lymphoma have been linked with EBV infection. In these cases, the virus becomes latent within the cell and eventually causes or poten-

TABLE 44–2.
Complications of Infectious Mononucleosis

ORGAN OR SYSTEM	COMPLICATION
Spleen	Tenderness
	Rupture
Hematologic	Aplastic anemia
	Hemolytic anemia
	Thrombocytopenia
Neurologic	Encephalitis
	Neuropathy
Cardiac	Abnormal conduction
Dermatologic	Maculopapular exanthems
	Jaundice
	Petechiae

TABLE 44–3.
Clinical–Pathologic Correlations in Infectious Mononucleosis

CLINICAL FINDINGS	PATHOLOGIC FINDINGS
Painful splenomegaly; hepatomegaly; lymphadenopathy	Infection of B cells; invasion of organs with organomegaly and lymphadenopathy
Pain in all organs in which there is lymphocytic infiltration	Atypical lymphocytes (transformed T cells) proliferate
Seizures	Immunologic injury secondary to host response (neuropathy, carditis, orchitis)
Peripheral neuropathy	
Tachycardia	
Orchitis	
Cancer-like syndrome with eventual death	Uncontrolled lymphoproliferation (seen only in X-linked lymphoproliferative syndrome and in patients with abnormal cell-mediated immune responses)

TABLE 44–4.
Differential Diagnosis of Infectious Mononucleosis

SYMPTOM, SIGN OR LABORATORY FINDING	EBV INFECTION	CMV INFECTION	T. GONDII INFECTION	STREPTOCOCCAL PHARYNGITIS	LEUKEMIA (ALL)	HEPATITIS
Age (years)	8–18	20–30	All ages	All ages	<15	All ages
Fever	+*	+	+	+	+/−	+
Pharyngitis (exudative)	+	−	−	+	−	−
Lymphadenopathy	+ Generalized	+ Generalized	+ Generalized	+ Cervical	+/− Generalized if present	−
Splenomegaly	+	+/−	+/−	−	+/−	−
Atypical lymphocytosis (present/% of WBCs)	+(>30)	+(10–20)	+(10–20)	−	+(blast cells)	−
Elevated values for liver function tests	+	+	−/+	−	−/+	++
Heterophile tests	+	−	−	−	−	−

* + = present; − = absent; +/− = + may or may not be present.

tiates transformation of the cell to a malignant state.

CLINICAL–PATHOLOGIC CORRELATIONS

The clinical features of infectious mononucleosis are due to EBV infection of the B cell and the body's cell-mediated immune response to control the infection. A summary of these correlations is shown in Table 44–3.

DIFFERENTIAL DIAGNOSIS

Infectious mononucleosis the disease must be distinguished from infectious mononucleosis the syndrome, which is caused by other agents, such as CMV and *Toxoplasma gondii*. Similarly, drugs such as phenytoin are responsible for hypersensitivity-induced infectious mononucleosis. Diseases confused with infectious mononucleosis and differentiating points are listed in Table 44–4.

DIAGNOSIS

The classic test for infectious mononucleosis was the Paul-Bunnell heterophile agglutination test. This test relied on the agglutination of sheep red cells by the sera of persons suffering from infectious mononucleosis. Of the heterophile tests, this test is the least sensitive and must be "absorbed" with guinea pig kidney or beef red blood cells in order to ensure specificity. Horse red blood cells are more sensitive

than sheep cells (90% vs 50% in 6- to 10-year-old children) and have replaced them in some assays. These red cell agglutination assays are the basis for the frequently used "mono spot" test.

Serologic tests directed against EBV viral antigens are more sensitive and specific than the mono spot tests. The presence of IgM-antibody directed against the viral capsid antigen (VCA) confirms an acute infection. Later in the course of the illness, antibodies directed against early antigen and Epstein-Barr nuclear antigen appear.

PRINCIPLES OF PREVENTION AND THERAPY

There are no vaccines presently available for preventing EBV infectious mononucleosis. In general, persons with infectious mononucleosis should rest as much as possible. Antipyretics may afford some relief from fever and malaise. Contact sports are prohibited for at least 6 weeks after onset to lessen the chance of rupturing the spleen.

Corticosteroids have been advocated for the symptomatic treatment of infectious mononucleosis. Studies have shown some benefit from their use in severely ill patients (e.g., those with impending airway obstruction, hemolytic anemia, prolonged significant symptoms); however, complications such as peritonsillar abscesses and diabetes mellitus have been observed during or following treatment. We would recommend the use of steroids in only those who have severe symptoms or have serious complications.

REFERENCES

Fleisher GR: Epstein-Barr virus, in Belshe RB (ed): *International Textbook of Human Virology.* Littleton, Mass, PSG Publishing Co, 1984, pp 853–886. *Well-written textbook chapter with much clinical information.*

Hoagland RJ: The clinical manifestations of infectious mononucleosis: Report of two hundred cases. *Am J Med* 1960; 240:21. *A clinical synopsis of symptoms and disease manifestations in infectious mononucleosis.*

Horwitz CA, Henle W, Henle G et al: Clinical and laboratory evaluation of elderly patients with heterophil-antibody postive infectious mononucleosis. *Am J Med* 1976; 61:333–339. *Description of infectious mononucleosis in the "elderly"; an atypical population.*

Jones JF, Ray CG, Minnich LL et al: Evidence for active Epstein-Barr virus infection in patents with persistent, unexplained illnesses: Elevated anti-early antigen antibodies. *Ann Intern Med* 1985; 102:1–7. *This important article answers a question that had plagued clinicians for years.*

Purtillo DT, Yang JPS, Allegra S et al: Hematopathology and pathogenesis of the X-linked recessive lymphoproliferative syndrome. *Am J Med* 1977; 62:225–234. *Discussion of the "fatal form" of infectious mononucleosis and what happens when EBV-induced B-cell proliferation remains unchecked.*

Sugden B: Epstein-Barr virus: A human pathogen inducing lymphoproliferation in vivo and in vitro. *Rev Infect Dis* 1982; 4:1048–1061. *Good overview of EBV-induced diseases from infectious mononucleosis to Burkitt's lymphoma.*

45 INFLUENZA

Jack M. Bernstein, M.D.

Flu is a term used to describe an illness ascribed to infection by viruses that cause systemic disease characterized by respiratory complaints. The term *flu* has also been attached to any viral illness, thus the commonly used phrase *stomach flu.* In spite of these misrepresentations, influenza is a specific disease caused by a member of the influenza virus family (single-stranded, segmented RNA viruses). Manifestations of this disease are predominantly attributable to respiratory tract involvement, but systemic complaints such as malaise and fever may be equally troublesome. Influenza is amenable to both prophylaxis (e.g., vaccine) and chemotherapy (e.g., amantadine).

CLINICAL SIGNS AND SYMPTOMS

Influenza is seen in both localized epidemics and in pandemics that may involve the entire world. Thus, one usually entertains the diagnosis of influenza in the milieu of an ongoing outbreak. Influenza may be caused by either influenza A virus, influenza B virus, or influenza C virus. While there may be some subtle differences in the clinical manifestations of illnesses due to each of these viruses, they shall be considered together in this discussion.

The onset of influenzal illness is usually abrupt. Chills, headache, and myalgias are seen in most patients, followed by cough and sore throat. Rhinorrhea is seen is a smaller number of patients, as are gastrointestinal complaints (Table 45–1).

The duration of influenza illness is usually from 5 to 7 days. In spite of an absence of complaints, alterations in small-airway function and bronchial reactivity may be detected for as long as 4 to 6 weeks following illness. In addition, debilitated patients with preexisting chronic respiratory disease may develop superinfecting bacterial pneumonias, which are frequently fatal.

Patients are usually febrile, with temperatures reaching as high as 41°C. Lymphadenopathy is unusual. The pulmonary signs include rhonchi and rales; occasionally, these signs may be almost entirely absent. Conjunctival suffusion, nasal discharge, and hyperemia of the mucous membranes may be seen occasionally. In spite of the presence of headache and myalgias, neurologic signs are absent in uncomplicated influenza.

In uncomplicated influenza, the clinical disease abates after a period of 4 to 10 days. Asymptomatic illness is the exception. Several complications of influenza have been noted. Primary influenzal pneumonia has been observed and was seen extensively during the pandemic of 1918–1919. Since then, pneumonic influenza has been limited to patients with underlying cardiopulmonary disease and the elderly. Myositis and myoglobinuria, with

TABLE 45–1.

Comparison of Symptoms in Uncomplicaated Infections by Influenze A, B, and C Viruses*

SYMPTOM	INCIDENCE (%) OF CASES		
	TYPE A	TYPE B	TYPE C
Myalgia-arthralgia	60–80	60–80	50
Headache	90	75	80–100
Chills	70–90	55–80	
Rhinorrhea	25	80	90
Cough	75	80	50
Sore throat	44	40–70	60–100
Gastrointestinal	10–25	10–45†	0

* Adapted from Van Voris LP, Young JF, Bernstein JM et al: Influenza virus, in Belshe RB: *Textbook of Human Virology*. Littleton, Mass, PSG Publishing, 1984, p 276.

TABLE 45–2.

Clinical–Pathologic Correlations for Influenza

CLINICAL FINDINGS	PATHOLOGIC FINDINGS
Cough	Destruction of columnar epithelial cells
Sore throat	
Pulmonary function abnormalities	
Fever	Activation of cytotoxic T cells. Production of interleukins and interferon.
Malaise	
Myalgias	
Headache	

elevated creatinine phosphokinase levels, are rarely seen, but may be associated with renal failure. Guillain-Barré syndrome has been associated with influenza and, especially, with vaccination with the inactivated influenza vaccine directed against "swine flu." No other inactivated influenza vaccines have been associated with Guillain-Barré since the ill-fated campaign to immunize against swine flu.

Influenza B and, less frequently, influenza A infections have been associated with occurrences of Reye's syndrome. The Centers for Disease Control's (Atlanta, Georgia) criteria for the diagnosis of Reye's syndrome is the occurrence of a noninflammatory encephalopathy in association with (1) fatty metamorphosis of the liver, (2) an SGOT level three times greater than normal with a blood ammonia level 1.5 times greater than normal, and (3) no other explanations for the neurologic or hepatic abnormalities.

PATHOPHYSIOLOGY

The influenza viruses have a tropism for the ciliated epithelial cells lining the trachea, bronchi, and bronchioles. In severe cases, the virus may also be found in the parenchyma of the lung.

Bronchoscopy of persons with influenza reveals diffuse inflammation of the larynx, trachea, and bronchi. In severe cases, a hemorrhagic pneumonia with hyaline membranes involving the terminal bronchioles and alveoli is seen.

Within 24 hours after the onset of infection, respiratory columnar epithelial cells become vacuolated and edematous, and they lose their cilia. As infected cells die, they desquamate into the bronchiolar lumen. Under the light microscope, areas in which the basal cell layer is only one cell thick can be seen to be interspersed with areas of naked basement membrane. Submucosal edema is present in association with an infiltration of neutrophilic and mononuclear cells.

CLINICAL–PATHOLOGIC CORRELATIONS

The clinical features of influenza are the result of the destruction of respiratory epithelial cells by the virus (Table 45–2). Further damage may

TABLE 45–3.
Relative Importance of Viruses Associated With Respiratory Syndromes in Adults*

VIRUS	COMMON COLD	PHARYNGITIS		TRACHEOBRONCHITIS	PNEUMONIA	
		CIVILIAN	MILITARY		CIVILIAN	MILITARY
Rhinovirus (>100 types)	+ + + +†	+ +	+	+	+	+
Influenza virus type A	+	+ +	+	+ + +	+ +	+ +
Influenza virus type B	+	+ +	+	+ +	+	+
Coronavirus	+	+	+	+	+	+
Adenovirus types 4 and 7	+	+	+ + + +	+	+	+ + + +
Adenovirus types 1, 2, 3, and 5	+	+	+	+	+	+
Herpes simplex virus	−	+ +	+	−	−	−
Respiratory syncytial virus	+	+	+	+	−	−
Parainfluenza virus types 1, 2, and 3	+	+ +	+	+	−	−

* Adapted from Douglas RG: Respiratory disease, in Galasso CJ, Merigan TC, Buchanan RA (eds): *Antiviral Agents and Viral Diseases of Man.* New York, Raven Press, 1984, p. 315.

† Relative frequency: + = occasional case; + + = small proportion of cases; + + + = substantial proportion of cases; + + + + = majority of cases; − = not involved.

result from cell-mediated immunity (e.g., cytotoxic T cells) directed against infected cells. It is unclear why influenza causes a myriad of systemic manifestations. Similarly, the exact correlation between influenza B virus infection and Reye's syndrome is unknown.

DIFFERENTIAL DIAGNOSIS

Influenza may be confused with many other respiratory viral infections, both in symptoms and in the spectrum of diseases they cause. Table 45–3 differentiates influenza from other respiratory viral syndromes.

DIAGNOSIS

Influenza may be suspected on epidemiologic grounds, given the occurrence of classic symptoms during an ongoing epidemic. Immunofluorescent (IF) techniques will detect infected epithelial cells within several hours of obtaining a specimen. Similarly, ELISA (enzyme-linked immunosorbent assays) may detect the presence of influenza antigen within clinical specimens, although this test has not proven as sensitive as IF tests. Tissue culture remains the "gold standard" for the diagnosis of influenza infections. Alternately, the virus may be isolated by injecting the specimen into 7- to 8-day-old embryonated eggs. In tissue culture, viral growth is detected by the hemadsorption assay using guinea pig or chick red blood cells. Serologic techniques require considerably longer periods

of time to confirm infection and should be used solely for epidemiologic studies.

PRINCIPLES OF PREVENTION AND THERAPY

Influenza vaccines have been available for more than two decades. Vaccines are classified as either "whole virus" or "split" (subunit) vaccines. Vaccines are reformulated on a yearly basis according to recommendations from the Centers for Disease Control regarding likely epidemic strains. Recently the vaccine has been composed of equal proportions of influenza A (H1N1), influenza A (H3N2), and influenza B. These vaccines are approximately 60% to 80% effective in preventing disease. As previously noted, no significant vaccine side-effects have been noted since the end of the swine flu program.

Amantadine is an effective drug for both the chemoprophylaxis and chemotherapy of influenza virus A infection. When taken prophylactically, amantadine is 28% to 100% (mean approximately 70%) effective in preventing influenza virus A infection. Therapeutically, amantadine has been shown to decrease the number of febrile days, allow earlier return to work or school, and ameliorate influenza-related pulmonary function abnormalities. Side-effects such as nervousness, nightmares, and insomnia have been reported and are related to amantadine's actions on the central nervous system. Amantadine is ineffective against influenza virus B infections.

REFERENCES

Corey L, Rubin RJ, Hattwick MAW et al: A nationwide outbreak of Reye's syndrome: Its epidemiologic relationship to influenza B. *Am J Med* 1976; 61:615–625. *Analysis of the correlation of Reye's syndrome with influenza B virus infection.*

Douglas RG: Respiratory disease, in Galasso CJ, Merigan TC, Buchanan RA (eds): *Antiviral Agents and Viral Diseases of Man.* New York, Raven Press, 1984. *Excellent discussion of viral respiratory disease.*

Meiklejohn G, Eickhoff TC, Allan ID et al: Antigenic

drift and efficacy of influenza virus vaccines: 1976–77. *J Infect Dis* 1978; 138:618–624. *Discussion of the relationship between antigenic drift and the efficacy of influenza vaccines.*

Murphy B, Webster RG: Influenza virus, in Fields B (ed): *Textbook of Virology.* New York, Raven Press, 1985. *Excellent discussion, especially about molecular biology, genetics, and vaccines.*

Van Voris LP, Young JF, Bernstein JM et al: Influenza virus, in Belshe RB: *Textbook of Human Virology.* Littleton, Mass, PSG Publishing, 1984, pp

267–297. *Good overview of the influenza viruses, especially with respect to diagnosis and clinical findings.*

Younkin SW, Betts RF, Roth FK et al: Reduction in fever and symptoms in young adults with influenza A/Brazil/78 H1N1 infection after treatment with aspirin or amantadine. *Antimicrob Agents Chemother* 1983; 23:577–582. *One of the first papers to show effectiveness of amantadine in naturally occurring influenza.*

46 ACUTE SINUSITIS

Steven M. Cohen, M.D.

Sinusitis is an inflammation of the mucosal lining of the paranasal sinuses. Acute suppurative sinusitis results from microbial invasion of the mucosa of the sinus environment. Chronic sinusitis is a persistent obstruction or infection or both due to irreversible alteration of the normal mucosal lining.

CLINICAL SIGNS AND SYMPTOMS

Acute suppurative sinusitis is usually preceded by a viral upper respiratory infection. The symptoms of each are similar. The brisk, clear rhinorrhea of the common cold changes to a mucopurulent discharge if secondary bacterial invasion occurs. Early in the illness (1 or 2 days), one experiences nasal congestion and discharge with mild malaise, headache, and low grade fever <37.8°C. There may be a slight pressure sensation over the affected sinus, which often becomes severe in 2 to 4 days.

Sinus pain is usually exacerbated by bending forward. The location of the pain is often a clue to which sinus is involved. Frontal sinusitis causes forehead pain, and maxillary sinusitis causes cheek and upper molar pain. Ethmoiditis is associated with pain of the bridge of the nose, and sphenoid sinusitis may cause pain deep behind the eyes radiating to the vertex of the skull.

The fever, if present, is usually mild, 37.8°C occasionally up to 38.9°C but rarely higher. Nasal obstruction with mucopurulent discharge and systemic symptoms are almost invariably present. Cough and sore throat due to purulent postnasal drainage are frequently present.

In most cases, tapping or pressing over the frontal or maxillary sinus that is acutely infected will elicit pain. Tapping the upper molars will often produce pain under the offending maxillary sinus. Transillumination may be helpful because a nonvisualized maxillary or frontal sinus usually indicates a problem; however, this examination is not sensitive enough to be reliable by itself.

There may be ecchymosis and swelling of the skin over the affected sinus.

Examination of the nose often reveals hyperemic and edematous nasal mucosa and turbinates. A mucopurulent discharge is usually found in the middle or superior meatus once the swollen turbinates are shrunken using topical vasoconstriction. A posterior pharyngeal or lateral wall exudate is often seen in the oropharynx.

Untreated, the majority of acute sinus infections will last 4 to 5 days followed by mild symptoms for up to 14 days. With antibiotics, complications of acute suppurative sinusitis are rare, but are potentially dangerous.

Chronic sinusitis results from an inadequately treated or persistent infection that may irreversibly alter the normal epithelium resulting in chronic obstruction and anaerobic bacterial overgrowth. Patients suffering from chronic sinusitis occasionally complain of constant dull headaches and intermittent purulent nasal discharge. This condition is difficult to treat medically and may require surgical drainage. Acute suppurative sinusitis may complicate chronic sinusitis. Other complications are less common but more dangerous. Cellulitis or orbital abscesses may occur as a result of extension of the infection through the bone or by way of the venous circulation. Osteomyelitis is a rare but serious complication. Infection of the frontal bone causes tenderness and doughy edema over the sinus, the so-called Pott's puffy tumor.

Extension of the acute infection by the phlebitic diploic veins to the meninges may result in cavernous sinus thrombus, or meningitis, as well as subdural, epidural, or brain abscess.

The correlation of signs and symptoms with underlying pathophysiologic changes is listed in Table 46–1.

PATHOPHYSIOLOGY

The paranasal sinuses are four pairs of air-filled cavities within the skull. The maxillary sinuses are located in the cheeks, below each orbit. In the frontal bone, the frontal sinuses form the medial portion of the orbit. The ethmoid sinuses are located slightly deeper in the skull and compose the medial wall of the orbits. The sphenoid sinus is bordered laterally by the cavernous sinus and lies below the pituitary gland.

At birth, only the maxillary and ethmoid sinuses are present. The frontal sinuses develop during the first and second year of life whereas the sphenoid sinus appears in the third year.

The exact purpose and function of the sinuses are not known. Each sinus is lined with pseudostratified, ciliated columnar epithelium with goblet cells. This mucosal lining is continuous with the nasal epithelia. Mucus is constantly being secreted, blanketing the sinus walls. Cilia divert the mucus toward the opening of each sinus and into the nose by way of the middle and superior meatuses. By this means, the sinuses are constantly being "cleansed."

Viral infection of the upper respiratory tract causes cilial dysfunction, increased secretion, and swollen nasal turbinates, all of which impede the drainage of the sinuses. This altered defense mechanism allows secondary bacterial invasion. Many other factors may contribute or predispose to impaired sinus drainage including foreign bodies, overuse of topical decongestants, a deviated nasal septum, a hypertrophied adenoid, polyps, and allergic rhinitis. Another cause of acute sinusitis is forced injection of water during diving or swimming.

Streptococcus pneumonia or *Hemophilus influenzae* account for 60% to 80% of acute sinus infections. *Streptococcus pyogenes*, *Staphylococcus aureus*, anaerobic bacterial organisms, and various gram-negative organisms account for the remainder.

Chronic sinusitis with persistent mucous accumulation and obstructed drainage results in local tissue anoxia, a decreased pH, and an in-

TABLE 46–1.
Clinical–Pathologic Correlations of Acute Sinusitis

CLINICAL FINDINGS	PATHOLOGIC FINDINGS
Nasal congestion	Edema and inflammation of turbinates and nasal mucous membranes
Mucopurulent discharges	Inflammation of the mucosa causes increased serum secretion mixed with epithelial debris, bacteria, and mucus. Coagulation of the serum fibrin changes the initially watery discharge to a thick and tenacious one.
Headache	Edema and congestion of the sinus ostia
Erythema	Periostitis and soft-tissue inflammation

creased temperature allowing for anaerobic overgrowth, particularly *Bacteriodes*, *Peptostreptococcus*, and *Fusobacterium* organisms.

In the immunocompromised host, fungal infections of the sinuses may be rapidly fatal. *Aspergillus* is the usual organism seen but *Actinomycetes*, *Nocardia*, and *Candida* may be found. Mucormycosis is a rare fungal necrotizing infection seen in diabetic patients. This infection is aggressive and if untreated is uniformly fatal. Timely biopsy for examination and culture is necessary.

DIFFERENTIAL DIAGNOSIS

The symptoms of nasal congestion and discharge are very common and are usually due to noninfectious causes. Acute suppurative sinusitis is probably overdiagnosed. Most causes of sinus symptoms are due to allergic or vasomotor rhinitis.

Allergic or seasonal rhinitis can usually be differentiated from acute suppurative sinusitis by obtaining a history of recurrent bouts of sneezing, nasal congestion, and clear rhinorrhea. Microscopic examination of the discharge will often reveal eosinophils. Facial tenderness will usually be absent.

Vasomotor rhinitis is a common cause of chronic recurring nasal congestion and discharge and may be confused with chronic sinusitis. A variety of common medical conditions can be associated with vasomotor rhinitis including anxiety, pregnancy, and hypothyroidism.

Neoplasms of the paranasal sinus present initially as progressive nasal obstruction and drainage. Because the symptoms may mimic acute sinusitis, an infection that fails to respond to appropriate therapy should raise the possibility of an underlying neoplasm. Other conditions in the differential diagnosis include polyps, cysts, foreign bodies, and vasculitis (Wegener's). Appropriate ear, nose, and throat evaluation and sinus x-ray or computerized tomography may be necessary for proper diagnosis.

One entity that should not be overlooked is a dental abscess or root canal disease as a cause of maxillary sinus symptoms. Sinus symptoms following a dental procedure should alert one to the possibility of rupture or erosion into the floor of the maxillary sinus.

DIAGNOSIS

The diagnosis of acute suppurative sinusitis can usually be made on clinical grounds. In particularly severe cases or when the diagnosis is in doubt, sinus x-ray films should be obtained. The acutely infected sinus may show an air–fluid level or may be completely opaque. Significant mucosal thickening is common to both acute and chronic sinusitis. A CT scan and an ultrasound study may be of benefit, but their use should be restricted to unusual cases.

Gram's stain and culture of the nasal discharge are not routinely helpful. If the exact etiologic agent must be known, as in the immunocompromised host, then direct aspiration of the sinus is of greatest value. If fungal invasion is suspected, the culture needs to be done as rapidly as possible.

The leukocyte count in most cases of acute suppurative sinusitis is normal or even slightly decreased. A high leukocyte count with a high fever (>38.9°C) should alert the physician to a diagnosis other than uncomplicated acute suppurative sinusitis.

PRINCIPLES OF THERAPY

Most cases of acute sinusitis will resolve spontaneously. When severe pain and tenderness are present, antibiotics are indicated. Because most infections are due to *S. pneumonia* or *Hemophilus influenzae*, empiric therapy with ampicillin is appropriate. Trimethoprim-sulfamethoxazole or cefaclor are adequate alternatives. A response is usually seen within 48 hours, but treatment should be continued for 7 to 14 days. Topical or oral decongestants are advocated to aid in reducing the drainage and obstruction, but patients should be cautioned to avoid chronic use of topical decongestants, which may cause rebound mucosal edema (rhinitis medicamentosa).

Antihistamines are contraindicated because of their drying effect, which often causes secretions to thicken. Locally applied moist heat and analgesics are employed for symptomatic relief, and cool mists may help loosen tenacious mucus.

If, after adequate antibiotic therapy, the patient does not respond, direct aspiration for a definitive diagnosis is recommended. Failure to respond to medical treatment usually requires surgical drainage of the sinus.

Chronic sinusitis is much more difficult to treat. Bacterial colonization tends to become resistant to antibiotic therapy, and decongestants are only minimally effective. In severe cases, surgical drainage is necessary.

REFERENCES

Ballenger JJ (ed): *Diseases of the Nose, Throat, Ear, Head, and Neck*, ed. 13. Philadelphia, Lea & Febiger, 1985, pp 205–248. *A very in-depth, comprehensive review of sinus diseases.*

Deweese DD, Saunders WH: *Textbook of otolaryngology*, ed 6. St Louis, CV Mosby Co, 1982, pp 177–188, 223–252. *A popular text with an excellent review of acute sinusitis.*

Evans FO Jr, Sydnor B, Moore WEC et al: Sinusitis of the maxillary antrum. *N Engl J Med* 1975; 293(15):735–739. *A study confirming the etiologic agents responsible for acute sinusitis.*

Friedman WH, Salvin RG: Diagnosis and medical and surgical treatment of sinusitis in adults. *Clin Rev Allergy* 1984; 2:409–428. *A recent, comprehensive review with emphasis on surgical treatment.*

Hamory BH, Sande MA, Sydnor A Jr, Seale DL, Gwaltney JM Jr: Etiology and antimicrobial therapy of acute maxillary sinusitis. *J Infect Dis* 1979; 139(2):197–202. *A large-scale study using direct needle aspiration to determine the cause of the sinusitis and the response to treatment.*

Kern EB: Sinusitis. *J Allergy Clin Immunol* 1984; 73 (1, Part 1):25–31. *A recent overview of the current concepts regarding etiology, diagnosis, and treatment of sinusitis.*

Quick CA, Payne E: Complicated acute sinusitis. *Laryngoscope* 1972; 82:1248–1263. *An excellent review of the complications with treatments and outcomes of acute sinusitis.*

47   URINARY TRACT INFECTION

Adel N. Shenouda, M.D.

Urinary tract infection is one of the most common infections. Upper urinary tract infection can be acute or chronic. Lower urinary tract infection can involve the bladder (cystitis), urethra (urethritis), or both. A majority of females who live to age 70 years will have one or more urinary tract infections. The role of the physician for these patients is to examine and culture the urine, treat accordingly with an appropriate antibiotic, and attempt to determine the predisposing factor(s) for the infection.

Urinary tract infection is more common in females at all ages after infancy (Table 47–1). This higher incidence is, in major part, due to the shorter female urethra. In infancy the incidence is higher in males because of congenital abnormalities of the lower urinary tract (e.g., urethral stricture). The incidence in men increases after age 65 years due to varying degrees of prostate enlargement and urethral obstruction. Other factors that appear to be related to urinary tract infection are: (1) in preschool children vesicoureteral reflux, (2) in teenagers the initiation or an increase in sexual activity, (3) in women of childbearing age, pregnancy, (4) in menopausal women a decrease in the vaginal acidity and increased bacterial colonization of the vaginal introitus, and

TABLE 47–1.
Incidences of Bacteriuria and Pyelonephritis in Male and Female Patients in the United States*

	PERCENT INCIDENCE	
	MALE	FEMALE
Preschool children	0.03	1.2
School children	0.03	5.0
Adults		
Middle-aged	0.5	4.4
Elderly	7.0	30.0
Pregnant women		
With bacteriuria		7.0
Without bacteriuria		93.0
Hospital patients		
(age > 60 years)	12–14	16.35

* Data from Brenner and Rector, 1986.

TABLE 47–2.
Clinical–Pathologic Correlations of Urinary Tract Infection

CLINICAL FINDINGS	SIGNS AND SYMPTOMS	PATHOLOGIC FINDINGS
Acute pyelonephritis	CVA tenderness, abdominal pain, fever and chills	Edema and congestion of the renal parenchyma
	Nocturia and suprapubic pain may be present.	Stretching of the capsule
	Renal function may be impaired.	
Simple cystitis	Nocturia and suprapubic pain	Edema and congestion of the bladder
	Burning sensation on micturition	
Chronic pyelonephritis	Nonspecific symptoms, including cystitis symptoms, low-grade fever, occasional backache	Small, scarred kidneys with ectasia of the caliceal system without obstruction
	Hypertension and chronic renal failure may be associated.	

(5) in hospitalized patients catheterization especially in the elderly.

CLINICAL SIGNS AND SYMPTOMS

The clinical picture depends on the location of the infection (Table 47–2). Patients with an upper urinary tract infection usually present with costovertebral angle pain and tenderness associated with fever and chills. Those with lower urinary tract infection typically have a burning sensation on urination and micturition frequency as well as suprapubic pain. These symptoms may be self-limited (2–3 days). However, these clinical manifestations do not always differentiate between an upper and lower tract or combination infection.

The urinalysis typically reveals bacteriuria and pyuria often with white blood cell casts.

Urine culture and sensitivity will usually identify the responsible organism and direct therapy. Blood cultures should be drawn if an upper urinary tract infection is suspected, especially for elderly patients.

After antibiotic treatment is started additional tests may be useful in determining further management. Renal function can be evaluated by measuring the amount of protein in the urine (24 hour) and the creatinine clearance. Hypertension is found in 22% to 70% of patients with chronic pyelonephritis with the highest incidence in those patients with advanced renal failure. Progressive renal failure and end-stage renal disease with uremia may result from chronic pyelonephritis, but this issue continues to be debated. An intravenous pyelogram or renal scan may be useful in identifying predisposing anatomic factors. A renal biopsy is rarely indicated.

PATHOPHYSIOLOGY

A number of host factors appear to predispose to urinary tract infection such as poor blood circulation, congenital anomalies, hypertonicity, and a high ammonia concentration in the renal medulla which impedes complement activity against bacterial growth.

Normally the ureter enters the bladder wall at an oblique angle and functions like a sphincter. A defect in this sphincter-like function can cause vesicoureteral reflux and increase the risk of repeated urinary tract infection and occasionally lead to chronic pyelonephritis.

The hypertonicity and acidity of the urine suppresses bacterial growth. Adequate hydration and high volume urine flow with frequent micturition will also decrease the rate of bacterial growth in the bladder. The bladder wall itself may also have a bacteriostatic effect.

The short female urethra appears to be the major factor that increases the incidence of urinary tract infection in women. The rate of bacterial colonization around the vaginal introitus is normally inhibited by the acidity of the vaginal secretions and other factors (e.g., hygienic habits). In men, prostatic fluid secretion (spermine) is bactericidal thus helping to prevent bacteria from ascending up the urethra to the bladder.

Obstruction that impedes urine flow, leaving a greater residual urine volume in the bladder, fosters bacterial growth. This process reduces the bladder wall/urine volume ratio which appears to decrease the bladder wall's bacteriostatic effect. Hematogenously routed acute pyelonephritis is also more common in patients with an obstructive uropathy than those without an obstruction. *Calculi* may produce varying degrees of obstruction as well as serve as a locus for bacterial trapping and growth.

Beginning in childhood, *vesicoureteral reflux* tends to predispose to recurrent urinary tract infection and may result in chronic pyelonephritis. Bladder and ureteral anatomic or neurologic abnormalities (e.g., bladder neck obstruction, neurogenic bladder, congenital ureteral stricture, and bladder diverticulae) also appear to predispose to urinary tract infection. Instrumentation of the genitourinary tract, such as cytoscopy, catheterization, and retrograde pyelography, also increases the risk of ascending urinary tract infection. *Pregnancy* tends to produce a partial obstruction and atony of the ureters due to the effect of high levels of progesterone and the mechanical pressure of the uterus. It has also been suggested that vesicoureteral reflux may occur during pregnancy.

Noninfectious renal injury, such as acute tubular necrosis, glomerulonephritis, collagen vascular disease, atherosclerosis, analgesic abuse, sickle cell disease, sickle cell trait, and hypokalemic nephropathy, appears to predispose patients to urinary tract infection. Whether diabetes mellitus predisposes to urinary tract infection is controversial. An association between hypertension and chronic pyelonephritis has been documented. Hypertension may be secondary to chronic pyelonephritis, or urinary tract infection may be due to the hypertension because hypertensive patients with renal involvement appear to have a higher incidence of urinary tract infection. Diarrhea and constipation may also be predisposing factors for urinary tract infection. Upper respiratory tract infection, especially when caused by a virus may increase the susceptibility to bacterial urinary tract infection.

The routes of infection are (1) ascending, with the infection moving up the tract from the urethra, (2) hematogenous, starting as acute pyelonephritis and spreading down the urinary tract, and (3) lymphatic, with bacteria moving from the bowel to the urinary tract. Most patients with hematogenous infection have a septic focus such as an abscess or infective endocarditis. The most common organism in these settings is *Staphylococcus aureus*. Renal tuberculosis is a result of hematogenous spread.

In chronic pyelonephritis, the kidneys are usually small, contracted, and scarred. Fibrosis produces nonobstructive localized dilations of the caliceal system. Histologic examination typically reveals interstitial fibrosis with an infiltration of chronic inflammatory cells (e.g., lymphocytes and plasma cells). The tubules are scarce and dilated. Scarring can be explained by the following mechanisms: (1) the healing process following acute inflammation, (2) renal parenchymal damage resulting from an autoimmune response to the high antibody concentration against a bacterial endotoxin(s), and (3) vascular ischemia, which produces ischemic renal tissue necrosis.

BACTERIOLOGY

The organisms that infect the urinary tract are many (Table 47–3). The most common organisms producing an ascending infection are *E. Coli*, *Proteus* species, and *Klebsiella* species. Other organisms include enterococci, *Pseudomonas*, and *Serratia*. *Stapholococcus aureus* is the most common organism in hematogenous spread followed by tuberculosis. Some organisms cause a nonspecific urethritis (e.g., *Mycoplasma*, *Chlamydia*, adenovirus, or anaerobic bacteria.

DIAGNOSIS

The clinical picture may help localize the infection. An analysis of urine collected at three different times during a voiding may also provide a clue as to whether the infection involves the upper or lower urinary tract. If the first 2.5 ml of urine voided is the only sample showing pyuria, this suggests urethritis. If the urine collected during midpoint voiding is predominantly affected, this suggests cystitis. If all three aliquots of urine are affected, this suggests acute pyelonephritis.

A test in which fluorescent antibodies coat the bacteria suggests an upper urinary tract infection; however, false-positive results may occur as in prostatitis. A high erythrocyte sedimentation rate with positive C-reactive protein also suggest upper urinary tract infection.

PRINCIPLES OF PREVENTION AND THERAPY

In preparing a treatment plan for the patient with a urinary tract infection, the following questions should be answered: (1) Where is the site of infection? (2) Is the patient septic? and (3) Are there predisposing factors for a urinary tract infection?

Patients with a lower urinary tract infection can be treated with an appropriate oral penicillin, cephalosporin, or sulfa preparation. Other

TABLE 47–3.
Microorganisms Associated with Urinary Tract Infection in Humans

COMMON
Escherichia coli
Proteus spp.
Klebsiella spp.
Enterobacter spp.
Pseudomonas spp.
Serratia spp.
Staphylococcus saprophiticus
Enterococcus *(Streptococcus faecalis)*
Candida spp.
UNUSUAL
Staphylococcus aureus
Coagulase-negative staphylococci
Mycobacterium tuberculosis
RARE
Actinomyces spp.
Fungi (non-candida)
Brucella spp.
Anaerobic bacteria
Adenovirus
Mycoplasma
Chlamydia

agents such as nitrofurantoin and methenamine mandelate may also be used, but are not first-line choices.

The patient with an upper urinary tract infection (i.e., acute pyelonephritis) may be treated with an appropriate parenteral penicillin, cephalosporin, and/or aminoglycoside for 7 to 14 days. Some infections, especially enterococcal, cannot be eradicated with this approach, and longer periods of treatment with combinations of the above antibiotics may be required. If the patient is septic, intravenous antibiotics are recommended for the full course or until the patient is afebrile and asymptomatic.

Prophylactic measures may need to be taken in certain high-risk patients. Women should be instructed to void after sexual intercourse and for selected patients one tablet of a sulfa preparation may also be prescribed. At-risk patients scheduled for genitourinary instrumentation should have a short course of antibiotics (i.e., 12 hours before and 3 days after the procedure) to decrease the potential of an induced urinary tract infection.

REFERENCES

Montgomerie JZ: *Renal infections*, in Massry S, Glassock R (eds): *Textbook of Nephrology*. Baltimore, Williams and Wilkins, 1983, pp. 668–678. *Pathogenesis of UTI.*

Ronald AR, Harding GKM: Urinary infection prophylaxis in women. *Ann Intern Med* 1981; 9:268. *Prophylaxis of UTI in women.*

Rubin RH: Infection of the urinary tract, in Rubenstein E, Federman DD (eds): *Scientific American Textbook of Medicine*, section 7. New York, Scientific American 1983, pp. 1–10. *Clinical–pathologic correlations of UTI.*

Rubin RH: Urinary tract infection, in Brenner B, Rector F (eds): *The Kidney*. Philadelphia, WB Saunders Co, 1986, p. 1085. *General review of UTI.*

Stamey TA: Urinary tract infections in the female: A perspective, in Remington JS, Swartz MN (eds): *Current Clinical Topics in Infectious Disease*. New York, McGraw-Hill Book Co, 1981, vol 2, p. 31. *Management of UTI.*

48   BACTEREMIA AND SEPTIC SHOCK

Jorge Crespo, M.D.

Bacteremia is self-defined. Sepsis is a term employed to describe a state of "toxicity" resulting from bacterial products and/or from the host's response to infection. Although septic shock, sometimes referred to as endotoxic shock, more commonly complicates gram-negative bacillary infections, it also occurs in gram-positive and fungal infections.

CLINICAL SIGNS AND SYMPTOMS

There is ample variation in the clinical manifestations of bacteremia, from the totally asymptomatic (e.g., bacteremias following dental procedures) to the rapidly progressive and catastrophic. The determinants of this variability are, for the most part, not well-established. The best studied of the bacteremic pictures is that caused by gram-negative bacteria.

Following the manipulation of infected tissues, such as debridement of infected wounds or drainage of abscesses; following the introduction of instruments into an organ system that harbors an abundant normal resident flora or infection, particularly the gastrointestinal and genitourinary tracts; during the course of an established localized infection (meningitis, pneumonia, peritonitis); or for no apparent reason, a patient experiences a sudden onset of multiple severe chills and rigors, with a rapid elevation of the temperature. Obvious hyperpnea, mental confusion in either a delirious or lethargic patient, warm, dry skin, a fast but full pulse, and a state of general prostration all point toward the presence of a severe systemic physiologic derangement. Conversely, otherwise unexplained arterial hypotension, oliguria or anuria, or evidence of bleeding, in patients that remain afebrile, particularly in the elderly and the debilitated, are frequently intitial signs of bacteremia and sepsis.

Cutaneous manifestations of septicemia are variable, ranging from the acute, rapidly progressive petechial and ecchymotic lesions seen in acute meningococcemia and in disseminated intravascular coagulation to well-circumscribed necrotic and ulcerated patches (ecthyma gangrenosum) observed in *Pseudomonas aeruginosa* infections. Occasionally, cellulitis (red-bluish facial cellulitis in children caused by *Hemophilus influenzae*), diffuse erythema, showers of petechial lesions (bacterial endocarditis, typhoid fever), and vesicular or bullous lesions may also be found.

Because for the most part bacteremia is intermittent, the phenomena secondary to it such as fever, chills, and rigors also show periodicity. The fever may be as high as 41.6°C and may follow varied patterns, usually fluctuating widely. The patient may remain normotensive, but the systemic pressures may drop significantly early in the clinical course even with evidence of a hyperdynamic cardiovascular state. The changes in urinary output parallel the changes in blood pressure.

Although the clinical course is affected and may initially be overshadowed by the underlying infection at the source of the bacteremia, the patient with established septicemia continues to deteriorate. Metabolic acidosis, which is secondary to lactic acid overproduction resulting from tissue hypoxia and a shift to anaerobic metabolism, supervenes. The hypotensive state gives way to a frank state of shock, and cerebral hypoperfusion gives rise to further changes in mentation. The skin becomes cold and clammy with acral cyanosis. Frank bleeding from mucosal surfaces or intravascular access sites may be apparent. If the patient does not succumb at this stage, progressive pulmonary insufficiency follows, resulting in yet deeper tissue hypoxia, worsening of the acidosis, and eventually cardiorespiratory standstill, usually secondary to a cardiac dysrhythmia.

PATHOPHYSIOLOGY

The mechanism(s) responsible for the clinical manifestations of bacteremia and septic shock is still not completely defined. In gram-negative sepsis, endotoxin has been the central focus of attention, and although the syndrome of septic shock can be duplicated by endotoxin administration in animal models, microorganisms devoid of endotoxin also are capable of inducing septic shock in the clinical setting. Other factors and initiating mechanisms remain areas of active research.

Pathophysiologic changes induced by the presence of circulating bacteria, and particularly of endotoxin include fever, shock, and disseminated intravascular coagulation.

In the pathophysiology of fever, phagocytosis of circulating particulate matter by a variety of cells (polymorphonuclear leukocytes, eosinophils, monocytes, tissue macrophages) results in release of a factor called endogenous pyrogen. Endotoxin is an even more potent promoter of endogenous pyrogen production and release. Endogenous pyrogen, now characterized as interleukin-1, acts on the hypothalamus to reset the thermostat to a higher point; heat-producing muscular activity in the form of shivering and heat-conserving peripheral vasoconstriction follows. Clinically, the onset of fever and chills occurs 60 to 90 minutes after the bacteremic episode.

Severe infections with any bacterial species may be complicated by shock. Distinguishing the mechanisms responsible for cardiovascular dysfunction is difficult because changes associated with the primary infectious process and bacteremia-induced changes may not be easily separated. Shock is not a common feature in gram-positive bacteremias (occurring in 10% of pneumococcal bacteremias, in 5% of *Staphylococcus aureus* bacteremias). On the other hand, shock is present in about 35% to 45% of gram-negative bacteremias and appears between 4 and 10 hours after the bacteremic episode.

The earliest demonstrable change during prospective monitoring of patients with sepsis is a fall in peripheral vascular resistance, which is compensated by an increase in cardiac output with essentially no change in mean arterial pressure. The capillary beds may be uncontrollably dilated, in effect bypassing blood flow through peripheral tissues. Despite the high cardiac output, tissue oxygen extraction is decreased, as evidenced by an elevated hemoglobin saturation in mixed venous blood. These findings indicate that a metabolic insult is occurring at the cellular level such that even a hyperdynamic circulatory state (the "warm stage" of septic shock) is not sufficient to supersede the maldistribution of blood flow nor the attendant inadequate oxygen extraction by the tissues. Eventually, systemic resistance decreases further and is not matched by a compensatory increase in cardiac output, resulting in a drop in arterial pressure. All indices of myocardial performance demonstrate a progressive impairment, and, if therapeutic interventions are not taken, the falling cardiac output is inadequate to maintain appropriate levels of tissue perfusion despite late elevation of the sytemic resistance in an attempt to sustain the arterial pressure. This results in worsened tissue perfusion, the "cold stage" of septic shock.

In the pathophysiology of disseminated intravascular coagulation, endotoxin can activate Hageman factor, which in turn can trigger the intrinsic pathway of the coagulation system. As intravascular fibrin clotting occurs, the fibrinolytic system may also be activated, again by the effect of Hageman factor which activates plasminogen. The resulting degradation of fibrin produces fibrin-split products which exert anticoagulant activity, helping sustain the bleeding tendency initiated by the consumption of coagulation factors (II, V, VIII) resulting from the activation of the coagulation cascade. Frequently these changes are mild, and though there is evidence of thrombocytopenia and prolonged prothrombin time and partial thromboplastin time, progression to frank bleeding is not a constant feature. Gram-positive bacteria as well as viral and fungal organisms can also induce disseminated intravascular coagulation.

The interaction of these multiple pathophysiologic changes is depicted in Figure 48–1. Alternative initiating factors are being sought because it is becoming evident that endotoxin-related effects do not explain all the derangements observed in septic shock.

CLINICAL–PATHOLOGIC CORRELATIONS

The hallmark of septic shock is a complex multifaceted physiologic derangement involving a variety of vasoactive substances, the coagulation and complement systems, the kinin cascade, as well as some as yet elusive myocardial depressant factor(s). The possibly important role of the products of arachidonic acid metabolism (such as prostaglandins and thromboxanes) is currently being investigated.

Because physiologic changes are most prominent, there is a relative paucity of pathologic changes. In patients dying from septic shock, the most significant findings are in the lungs, which show the characteristic features of adult respiratory distress syndrome; in the kidneys, which may evidence changes secondary to acute tubular necrosis and, rarely, cortical necrosis; and in the microvasculature, particularly in the venous side, which frequently shows microthrombi. Hemorrhagic changes accompanied by necrosis can also be found in various organs; the lung and then the intestine and the liver are most commonly affected. A particularly catastrophic form of hemorrhage and necrosis occurs in the adrenal cortices, most commonly with acute meningococcemia. Metastatic infections are rare in gram-negative bacteremia, but men-

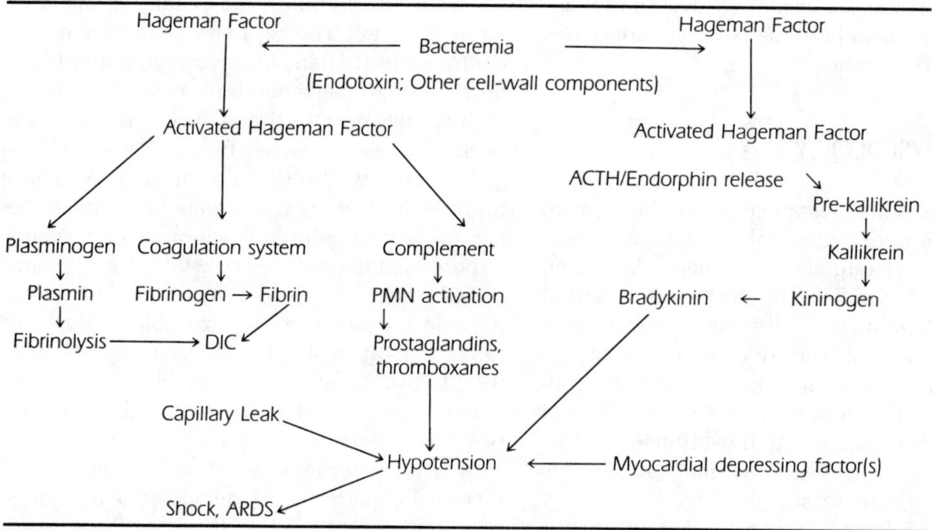

FIG 48–1.
Pathophysiologic events in septic shock

TABLE 48–1.
Initial Clinical Features of Gram-Negative Bacteremia*

Hypotension following chills and fever
Fever in immunosuppressed patients (particularly in acute leukemia,
    after chemotherapy, in hematologic malignancies)
Fever in patients with intravascular lines and/or mechanical ventilation
Fever following insertion or removal of urinary catheters
Fever following urogenital instrumentation
Hyperpnea, respiratory alkalosis
Oliguria or anuria
Thrombocytopenia, prolonged PT/PTT
Hypotension without recognized cause
Agitation, confusion, stupor
Metabolic acidosis
Hypothermia
Ecthyma gangrenosum
Fall in systemic vascular resistance ⎤
Increase in mixed venous blood   ⎬ In patients with pulmonary artery catheter in place
Hemoglobin saturation   ⎦

* Adapted from McCabe WR: Gram-negative bacteremia. *DM* 1983; Dec:1–38.

ingitis, osteomyelitis, pneumonia, and splenic, renal, and hepatic abscesses occur frequently in gram-positive bacteremias.

DIFFERENTIAL DIAGNOSIS

Septic shock is a diagnosis made on clinical grounds after the exclusion of cardiogenic, hypovolemic, and neurogenic causes. Although the clinical setting (such as with the introduction of instruments into the urinary tract) many times suggests septic shock, only careful hemodynamic monitoring can provide data that allow the recognition of the characteristic features of septic shock (see Pathophysiology). Table 48–1 lists the clinical features that may appear as the initial manifestations of sepsis. Physicians caring for immunosuppressed patients, for patients in intensive care units, and for burned patients keep the possibility of sepsis high in their list of possible diagnoses when facing patients presenting with otherwise unexplained changes such as those in Table 48–1. This high index of suspicion is important for initiating diagnostic and therapeutic measures that may have an impact on mortality.

Gram-positive and gram-negative septic shock have somewhat different hemodynamic profiles, but these features are not helpful in the management of the individual case.

DIAGNOSIS

The clinical features of bacteremia and sepsis are not specific, and the frequent coexistence of active infections in organs that may produce changes similar to those triggered by bacteremia makes the diagnosis more elusive. Gram-negative bacteremia may be suggested by the presence of a constellation of historic data including immunosuppression, instrumentation, multiple invasive organ-support systems (e.g., mechanical ventilation), and of clinical findings such as unexplained hyperventilation or hypotension, oliguria, metabolic acidosis, or evidence of coagulopathy.

Although monitoring of hemodynamic performance provides information that is many times almost pathognomonic of septicemia, the definitive diagnosis of bacteremia still rests on the demonstration of bacteria in the blood. Efforts to detect bacterial "markers" such as endotoxin are fraught with technical difficulties. The yield of blood cultures is variable depending on the timing and number of cultures obtained, the growth requirements of bacteria, and the presence in serum of inhibiting factors such as antibiotics. Of course, the clinician suspecting a bacteremic episode should also obtain appropriate cultures from other potential sites of infection. When skin lesions are present, cultures and staining with Gram's stain of aspirated material may prove helpful on occasion. When no obvious source of infection is apparent, bacteremia and septic shock represent a challenging entity which tests the clinician's skills and diagnostic acumen.

PRINCIPLES OF PREVENTION AND THERAPY

It seems reasonable that the simplest measure to decrease the occurrence of bacteremia and septic shock is to minimize the number of events that are clearly associated with this problem. The lessons learned from adequate decontamination of respiratory therapy equipment point to the importance of this approach.

In the hospital setting, the hazards of Foley catheterization and prolonged intravascular catheterization cannot be overemphasized. Although most infections in immunosuppressed patients are caused by bacteria harbored in the patient's gastrointestinal tract, handwashing by medical and paramedical personnel continues to be an effective means of reducing spread of nosocomial organisms. Prompt and technically careful drainage of abscesses and handling of infected tissues are also important.

The value of antimicrobial prophylaxis is still controversial, but data are starting to emerge pointing to significant reduction in the number of infections in critically ill patients receiving antibiotics directed to reduce the population of enteric gram-negative aerobic flora without affecting the ecology of anaerobic organisms. Research regarding the factors that promote colonization of the oropharynx by gram-negative bacilli, the role of immunization against bacterial products, and means for earlier recognition of septic shock is badly needed.

Early clinical suspicion, prompt physiologic assessment, effective antimicrobial therapy, control of sources of infection, and comprehensive supportive care are the fundaments of therapy in bacteremia and septic shock. In general, intravascular lines and recently implanted prosthetic devices in place during an episode of bacteremia need to be removed. Antibiotic selection should be guided by appropriate knowledge of the patient's underlying disorder(s) or predisposing factors, and the antici-

pated antibiotic susceptibility of bacteria (which varies considerably with geographic locale). Bactericidal compounds are usually employed, and advantage is taken of potential synergistic effects; most antibiotic regimens include a cephalosporin and an aminoglycoside. Individualization of antibiotic selection is necessary when variables such as drug allergy, the presence of renal failure, bleeding tendencies, or other factors intervene.

Patients with a suspected diagnosis of septic shock should be cared for in an intensive care unit, with adequate facilities to provide appropriate and continuous physiologic assessment and prompt nursing care. The use of high doses of corticosteroids has been disputed for a long time. The cornerstone of management of the hemodynamic alterations is the administration of fluids with the goal of maximizing cardiac function by optimizing the filling pressure (preload) of the left ventricle. This is best accomplished by the use of a pulmonary artery catheter, which will also provide very useful information about cardiac performance and the status of the peripheral vasculature, and which allows monitoring of tissue oxygen utilization. The judicious use of vasoactive drugs to modify the role of the peripheral circulation may also play an important role.

The management of disseminated intravascular coagulation has proven difficult; adequate control of bacteremia is probably the best way to correct the coagulopathy. Naloxone, an opiate and beta-endorphine antagonist, has been reported to reverse arterial hypotension; the effect seems transient and its role is not as yet defined. Passive immunization with antisera directed against common determinants present in the core portion of the cell wall of gram-negative enteric bacteria has been found to increase survival among patients in septic shock, particularly those in more advanced stages; more experience is needed with this approach. In spite of continued improvements in antibiotic therapy, direct assessment of hemodynamic function, and in supportive care, septic shock continues to carry a high mortality rate. Although the major determinant of mortality seems to be the nature of the underlying process, an overall mortality rate for established septic shock between 30% and 40% attests to the severity of this process.

REFERENCES

Abraham E, Shoemaker WC, Blaud RD, Cobo JC: Sequential cardiorespiratory patterns in septic shock. *Crit Care Med* 1983; 11:799–803. *Study of early and sequential hemodynamic events occurring in septic shock.*

Hess ML, Hastillo A, Greenfield LJ: Spectrum of cardiovascular function during gram-negative sepsis. *Prog Cardiovasc Dis* 1981; 23:279–298. *Summary of the extent of our present understanding of the physiologic changes operative in septic shock.*

McCabe WR, Treadwell TL, DeMaria A: Pathophysiology of bacteremia. *Am J Med* 1983; 75(1B): 7–18. *Summary of all aspects related to bacteremia.*

Sprung CL, Caralis PV, Marcial EH et al: The effects of high-dose corticosteroids in patients with septic shock: A prospective, controlled study. *N Engl J Med* 1984; 311:1137–1143. *High-dose methylprednisolone or dexamethasone were prospectively and randomly compared to a control group in patients with established septic shock. Steroid-treated patients had shock reversed more promptly and frequently, and early mortality was* also decreased in this group. *Late mortality was nevertheless comparable in both groups.*

Young LS: Gram-negative sepsis, in Mandell GL, Douglas RG, Bennett JE (eds): *Principles and Practice of Infectious Diseases*, ed 2. New York, Wiley Medical Publications, 1985, pp 453–475. *An encyclopedic review by one of the most authoritative experts on the subject. Includes 260 references.*

Young LS, Martin WJ, Meyer RD et al: Gram-negative rod bacteremia: Microbiologic, immunologic and therapeutic considerations. *Ann Intern Med* 1977; 86:456–471. *Reviews blood culture results, bacterial-host relationship, and delineates principles of antibiotic therapy.*

Ziegler EJ, McCutchan JA, Fierer J et al: Treatment of gram-negative bacteremia and shock with human antiserum to a mutant *Escherichia coli. N Engl J. Med* 1982; 307:1225–1230. *Describes a mortality rate in untreated patients of 39%, and in immunized patients of 22% (p = 0.011). For patients with "profound shock" the mortality rates were 77% in the control group and 44% in the immunized group (p = 0.003).*

49 INFECTIVE ENDOCARDITIS

H. Bradford Hawley, M.D.

Infective endocarditis is defined as infection of the endocardial surface of the heart. A heart valve is most frequently involved, but a septal defect or the mural endocardium may be the site of infection. Infection of vascular shunts, such as patent ductus arteriosus, and aortic coarctations are more properly termed endarteritis, but may be considered under endocarditis because the clinical manifestations are often identical and the pathogenesis and treatment are similar. Infective endocarditis is preferable to the term *bacterial endocarditis* because it includes other organisms, especially fungi, which are now recognized as etiologic agents in this disorder.

Infective endocarditis accounts for approximately one case in every 1000 hospital admissions in the United States. The incidence has remained fairly constant over the last 30 years, but the type of patient has changed. Heroin addicts, the elderly, and patients with prosthetic intravascular devices compose an increasing percentage of endocarditis cases.

CLINICAL SIGNS AND SYMPTOMS

The clinical manifestations of endocarditis are varied and often nonspecific. Early on, the symptoms are similar to those encountered in most infections: fever, malaise, and fatigue. As the disease progresses, more cardiovascular and renal-related symptoms may appear: dyspnea, chest pain, and stroke. Fever and heart murmurs are found in most patients. Splenomegaly, skin lesions, and evidence of emboli are commonly present. The small, painful, modular skin lesions usually found on the pads of the fingers or toes (Osler's nodes) are not pathognomonic of endocarditis and are seen in a maximum of 10% to 25% of patients with endocarditis. Splinter hemorrhages are also nonspecific and are frequently found in the elderly patient or the patient with nail-bed trauma often related to occupation. The hemorrhagic, painless macules found on the palms or soles (Janeway lesions) are found more commonly when endocarditis is caused by staphylococci. Roth's spots, pale retinal lesions surrounded by hemorrhage, are now uncommon and are most frequently seen in fungal endocarditis. A summary of some of the signs and symptoms is in Table 49–1.

Endocarditis is one of the few infections that is nearly always fatal if untreated. In the preantibiotic era the usual progression to death of the untreated disease was used to classify bacterial endocarditis as acute (death in less than 6 weeks), subacute (death in 6 weeks to 3 months), or chronic (death in more than 3 months). Advances in clinical microbiologic isolation and identification procedures, antimicrobial agents, and cardiovascular surgery make it more useful to classify cases by the causative organisms rather than the clinical course. These classification schemes are not mutually exclusive, however, because the most virulent organisms, such as *Staphylococcus aureus*, typically produce the acute form of the disease.

PATHOPHYSIOLOGY

Much of our current knowledge concerning the pathogenesis of infective endocarditis is derived from an experimental model in rabbits produced by introducing an intravenous polyethylene catheter into the right heart followed by inoculation of microorganisms. Microscopic examination of the lesions of the rabbit endocardium show the microorganisms adhering to underlying fibrin-platelet thrombi deposited on the damaged endocardial surface. Bacteria have been shown to vary in their ability to adhere to endocardial thrombi. In the case of oral streptococci the dextran elaborated appears to be an important virulence factor in endocarditis by allowing thrombotic adherence much as it does in dental caries by allowing adherence to dental enamel. Transient bacteremia with virulent bacteria, especially oral/dental bacteria, may result in the colonization (infection) of valvular thrombi, which produces clinical disease in about 2 weeks.

The vegetative lesions of endocarditis are found juxtaposed to areas of turbulence. The decrease in pressure laterally downstream from the flow is associated with turbulence and with the lowered intimal perfusion that creates conditions for platelet-fibrin deposition and colonization. When preexisting valvular disease has resulted in regurgitant flow, the term downstream usually refers to the regurgitant direction. Thus, in the case of the aortic insufficient valve, the vegetation is located on the ventricular side of the valve.

Prosthetic valve endocarditis may be divided into early (within 2 months) and late (more than 2 months) endocarditis relative to surgical placement of the valve because pathogenesis,

TABLE 49–1.
Incidence of Selected Symptoms and Signs of Infective Endocarditis*

SYMPTOM	PERCENTAGE OF CASES
Fever	80
Sweats	25
Chills	40
Weakness	40
Dyspnea	40
Malaise	25
Weight loss	25
Chest pain	15
Stroke	20
Hemoptysis	10
Abdominal pain	10
Back pain	10

SIGN	PERCENTAGE OF CASES
Fever	90
Heart murmur	85
Splenomegaly	40
Cutaneous signs	40
Embolic phenomena	40
Retinal lesions	5
Edema	15

* Modified from Scheld and Sande, 1985.

TABLE 49–2.
Microbial Etiology of Endocarditis

| CAUSATIVE ORGANISM | PERCENTAGE OF CASES | | | |
| | WITH NATIVE VALVES | | WITH PROSTHETIC VALVES | |
	NONADDICTS	ADDICTS	EARLY INFECTION	LATE INFECTION
Streptococci				
viridans	35	5	5	30
group D	20	5	< 5	5
Staphylococci				
S. epidermidis	< 5	< 5	30	25
S. aureus	20	55	20	10
Diphtheroids	< 5	< 5	10	5
Gram-negative bacilli	5	15	15	10
Candida	5	10	10	5

etiologic agents, and prognosis are different. Cases of early endocarditis are thought to be a result of intraoperative contamination, particularly with skin bacteria such as *Staphylococcus epidermidis* and diphtheroids. Later cases appear to develop as a result of transient bacteremia in the same manner as native valve endocarditis. The infection of prosthetic valves involves the securing sutures and the sewing ring. In cases of porcine or bovine heterografts the infection spills out from the ring onto the leaflets rather than beginning at the leaflet margin as in native valve cases. The result is often the same, destruction of the leaflet and valvular insufficiency. Myocardial abscesses are unusual in native valve endocarditis (20% of cases) and are found primarily in cases of *S. aureus* infection, but abscesses associated with the ring sutures and extending into the myocardium occur in over half the prosthetic valve infections, particularly infections of mechanical valves.

Intravenous drug addiction traumatizes the endocardium with chemical and particulate matter resulting in endocardial damage allowing deposition of platelets and fibrin. This process occurs primarily on the right side of the heart, which is unprotected by the pulmonary circulation resulting in the predominance of tricuspid valve disease. Infection of the valve is a result of bacteremia associated with cellulitis, phlebitis, or direct intravenous injection of contaminated material.

Gram-positive cocci remain the most common cause of endocarditis, although different species predominate in the various conditions/situations: viridans streptococci in native

TABLE 49–3.
Frequency of Site of Valvular Infection

| VALVE | PERCENTAGE OF CASES | |
	NONADDICTS	ADDICTS
Tricuspid	< 5	55
Pulmonic	< 5	< 5
Mitral	50	30
Aortic	40	35
Multiple valves	20	25

valves, *S. aureus* in drug abusers, and *S. epidermidis* in prosthetic valves (Table 49–2). Gram-negative bacilli and *Candida* are seen more commonly in association with prosthetic valves and intravenous drug addiction.

In the drug addict the tricuspid valve is most commonly involved (Table 49–3). The nonaddict with native valve endocarditis nearly always has involvement of the valves on the left side of the heart. Multiple valvular infection is not rare.

CLINICAL–PATHOLOGIC CORRELATIONS

The clinical features of endocarditis result from the valvular infection and accompanying bacteremia, emboli to various organ systems, and immune complex deposition. Some of the manifestations are not entirely understood and may be a result of a combination of these processes; for example, Osler's nodes probably are a result of minute septic emboli combined with immune-complex vasculitis. A summary of these correlations can be found in Table 49–4.

TABLE 49–4.
Clinical–Pathologic Correlations for Infective Endocarditis

CLINICAL FINDINGS	PATHOLOGIC FINDINGS
	Endocardial infection
Heart murmur	Valvular incompetence/obstruction
Dyspnea	
Dysrhythmias	Abscesses
Fever, chills	Bacteremia
Splenomegaly	
	Emboli
Abdominal pain	Spleen
Back pain	Kidney
Hematuria	
Chest pain	Lung
Dyspnea	
Hemoptysis	
Petechiae	Skin
Osler's nodes	
Janeway lesions	Nails
Splinter hemorrhage	
Blindness	Eye
Stroke	Brain
Osler's nodes	Immune complexes
Edema	

TABLE 49–5.
Conditions Mimicking Infective Endocarditis

IMMUNOLOGIC
Acute rheumatic fever
Systemic lupus erythematosus
Drug reactions
Postcardiotomy syndrome

NEOPLASTIC
Leukemia
Lymphoma
Atrial myxoma

INFECTIONS
Meningococcemia
Miliary or disseminated tuberculosis
Brain abscess
Herpes encephalitis

VASCULAR
Pulmonary thromboembolism
Myocardial infarction
Cerebral thrombosis
Sickle-cell disease

DIFFERENTIAL DIAGNOSIS

Table 49–5 lists some of the disorders that may be confused with infective endocarditis. Perhaps more important, however, is to emphasize the necessity of suspecting endocarditis in any patient with positive blood cultures, particu-

larly if they are multiple and contain organisms commonly known to cause valvular infection. Daily examination of the patient for petechiae, heart murmur, splenomegaly, and retinal lesions is beneficial in establishing the diagnosis.

DIAGNOSIS

The key to the diagnosis of infective endocarditis is to suspect the illness and obtain blood cultures. Febrile patients who have a heart murmur, cardiac failure, a prosthetic heart valve or other intravascular device, a history of intravenous drug abuse, preexisting valvular disease (including mitral valve prolapse), stroke (especially in young adults), multiple pulmonary emboli, sudden arterial occlusion, unexplained prolonged fever, or lastly, multiple positive blood cultures are likely to have endocarditis. The hallmark of infective endocarditis is continuous bacteremia; thus, nearly all blood cultures will be positive. The so-called culture-negative endocarditis has been nearly eliminated by modern culture techniques and the avoidance of masking by prior antibiotic therapy. Three pairs (for aerobic and anaerobic culture) of blood cultures should be obtained at the same time during the first 24 hours. If the patient has received prior antibiotic therapy, there may be a slightly increased yield if the cultures are obtained using the Antimicrobial Removal Device (Marion Scientific, Kansas City). The Castaneda principle (bottle with broth and agar) may help in isolating fungi from the blood.

A variety of other nonspecific laboratory tests helpful in establishing a diagnosis of endocarditis are listed in Table 49–6. Other more specific serologic tests such as introduced acid antibodies (S. aureus), Q fever antibodies, and mannan antigenemia (Candida) are somtimes helpful.

Electrocardiography may show arrhythmias or conduction defects suggesting surrounding inflammation and edema or abscess formation. Echocardiography can visualize vegetations in 50% to 90% of patients, but is not sensitive enough to exclude the diagnosis if negative.

PRINCIPLES OF PREVENTION AND THERAPY

Endocarditis has never been shown to be preventable by administration of antibiotics because of the inherent difficulties in performing such a study; however, prophylactic antibiotics are routinely employed. Patients with known valvular disease (including mitral valve prolapse) or with prosthetic valves should be given antimicrobial agents immediately prior to any procedure (such as dental extraction) known to be associated with bacteremia. Studies using the previously mentioned rabbit model of endocarditis show maximum efficacy with antibiotics given intravenously. Guidelines have been established and are periodically updated by the American Heart Association.

Because nearly all patients will have organisms isolated from the blood, antimicrobial therapy should be targeted to the specific microorganism using susceptibility tests to aid in selection of the agents. In order to ensure proper selection, tube-dilution susceptibility testing must be performed on the causative microorganism establishing a minimum inhibitory concentration (MIC) and minimum bactericidal concentration (MBC) for all of the possibly useful antibiotics. In endocarditis, bactericidal, not just inhibitory, concentrations of antibiotics are needed to produce a bacteriologic cure. During therapy the bactericidal activity of the serum can be monitored. A recent study has shown that a peak serum bactericidal titer of 1:64 or greater or a trough serum bactericidal titer of 1:32 or greater predicted bacteriologic cure in all patients. The duration of therapy is from 2 to 6 weeks (usually 4) depending on the causative agents and the antibiotics used.

In some cases it may be necessary to start antibiotic therapy prior to the availability of

---

TABLE 49–6.
Laboratory Findings in Infective Endocarditis*

LABORATORY FINDING	PERCENT OF PATIENTS
HEMATOLOGIC	
Anemia	70–90
Peripheral intragranulocytic bacteria	50
Leukocytosis	20–30
Ear lobe histiocytes	20–30
Thrombocytopenia	5–15
URINARY	
Proteinuria	50–65
Microscopic hematuria	30–50
Red cell casts	10–15
CHEMISTRIES	
Elevated erythrocyte sedimentation rate	90–100
Positive rheumatoid factor	40–50
Hypergammaglobulinemia	20–30
Increased serum creatinine	10–20
Hypocomplementemia	5–15

* Modified from Mandell in Kaye, 1976.

results from cultures and sensitivity tests. In the acutely ill patient without a prosthetic valve, including drug abusers, therapy may be initiated with nafcillin and gentamicin. If the patient is allergic to penicillin, vancomycin can be used in place of nafcillin. For prosthetic valve endocarditis, therapy can be initiated with vancomycin and gentamicin. Culture-negative endocarditis should be treated with high doses of penicillin or ampicillin along with streptomycin or gentamicin, assuring adequate therapy for the hard-to-culture enterococcus. It should be emphasized that in all cases three sets of blood cultures should be obtained prior to commencing antibiotic treatment.

Surgical intervention with replacement of the involved valve may be necessary if there is moderate-to-severe heart failure or if antibiotic treatment proves unsuccessful. Laboratory indicators of failing medical therapy are "breakthrough" bacteremia (positive blood cultures while receiving therapy) and poor bactericidal serum titers.

The availability of antimicrobial agents and cardiac surgery has resulted in a cure for the majority of patients. Old age, heart failure, left-sided heart disease (especially acquired aortic valve disease), poor general condition, and long duration of infection before treatment are all adverse prognostic factors.

REFERENCES

Bisno AL (ed): *Treatment of Infective Endocarditis.* New York, Grune & Stratton, 1981. *Best current reference for therapy.*

Freedman LR, Valone J Jr: Experimental infective endocarditis. *Prog Cardiovasc Dis* 1979; 22:169–180. *Description of the rabbit model of infective endocarditis by the original investigator.*

Gould K, Ramirez-Ronda CH, Holmes RK et al: Adherence of bacteria to heart valves in vitro. *J Clin Invest* 1975; 56:1364–1370. *In vitro studies correlating the ability of bacteria to adhere to heart valves with their incidence as causative agents of endocarditis.*

Kaye D: Prophylaxis for infective endocarditis: An update. *Ann Intern Med* 1986; 104:419–423. *Most recent guidelines for antibiotic prophylaxis to prevent endocarditis.*

Kaye D (ed): *Infective Endocarditis.* Baltimore, University Park Press, 1976. *Easy-to-read general reference.*

Kerr A Jr: *Subacute Bacterial Endocarditis.* Springfield, Ill, Charles C Thomas, 1955. *Classic clinical descriptions and natural history.*

Scheld WM, Sande MA: Endocarditis and intravascular infections, in Mandell GL, Douglas RG Jr; Bennett JE (eds): *Principles and Practice of Infectious Diseases,* ed. 2. New York; John Wiley & Sons, 1985, pp. 504–530. *Well-written chapter in current standard reference textbook of infectious diseases.*

Scheld WM, Valone JA, Sande MA: Bacterial adherence in the pathogenesis of endocarditis. *J Clin Invest* 1978: 61:1394–1404. *More in vitro studies showing the importance of dextran elaboration by streptococci in adherence.*

Weinstein MP, Stratton CW, Ackley A et al: Multicenter collaborative evaluation of a standarized serum bactericidal test as a prognostic indicator in infective endocarditis. *Am J Med* 1985; 78:262–269. *A multicenter study of 129 endocarditis patients that shows the ability of a serum bactericidal test to predict bacteriologic cure.*

50 CLOSTRIDIAL INFECTIONS

Michael J. Markus, M.D.
H. Bradford Hawley, M.D.

TETANUS

Tetanus is an acute, frequently fatal disease caused by *Clostridium tetani* and preventable by immunization. The word is derived from the Greek verb *teino* which means "to stretch." The disease is most commonly seen in underdeveloped nations, especially tropical; in the United States it is most common in the rural South. Narcotic addicts are also common victims in the United States.

CLINICAL SIGNS AND SYMPTOMS

There are three basic forms of clinical manifestation: (1) generalized (most common, approximately 80% of patients), (2) localized, and (3) cephalic.

Generalized tetanus characteristically appears initially with trismus (tonic contraction of the muscles of mastication, "lockjaw") 1 to 2 weeks after injury. Later manifestations include spasm of the voluntary musculature, first of the face and then the trunk. This gives rise to a stiff neck, dysphagia, and rigidity of the abdominal wall. In severe forms, persistent trismus progresses to risus sardonicus, and the severe back muscle spasm called *opisthotonos*. The appearance of seizures indicates a poor prognosis. Autonomic manifestations (seen more often in elderly patients and narcotic addicts) include episodic tachycardia, labile hypertension, hypotension, arrhythmias, and other symptoms such as cardiovascular instability and sympathetic overactivity. Complications may include sepsis, coma, or fracture of the spine or long bones secondary to powerful and prolonged muscle spasm. Prolonged illness may give rise to pulmonary embolism, pneumonia, flexion contractions, or decubitus ulcers secondary to prolonged bedrest.

Neonatal tetanus is a type of generalized tetanus seen almost exclusively in primitive countries. The disease usually strikes the infant during the first week of life and the first symptom is inability to suck. Facial twitching progresses rapidly to muscular rigidity, convulsions, and respiratory embarrassment.

Cephalic tetanus is an unusual disease which may sometimes be seen with chronic otitis media or after a head injury. It may remain local or may progress. Isolated or multiple cranial nerve dysfunction may be seen, cranial nerve VII being the most frequently affected.

The overall mortality rate of tetanus is approximately 40%, but may be as high as 60% in neonates and the elderly. The mortality is lower in children and young adults, ranging from 15% to 30%. A poorer prognosis is seen if symptoms ensue less than 1 week after the inciting injury.

PATHOPHYSIOLOGY

C. tetani is a gram-positive, motile, spore-forming, anaerobic rod-shaped bacterium. It is found in the feces of human and domestic animals. The spores are widespread in soil and are more numerous when the earth is manured and cultivated. Disease is caused by the elaboration (by the vegetative form only under proper conditions) of a potent neurotoxin, tetanospasmin. Tetanospasmin acts in the nervous system to (1) interfere with neuromuscular transmission by inhibiting acetylcholine release from nerve endings in muscle and (2)

TABLE 50–1.
Clinical–Pathologic Correlations for Clostridial Infections

DISEASE	ORGANISM	PATHOLOGIC CHANGES	CLINICAL FINDINGS
Tetanus	C.tetani	Elaboration of neurotoxin with interruption of neuromuscular transmission and of inhibitory (primarily) spinal reflexes (cholinergic)	Severe voluntary muscle spasm; sympathetic dysinhibition; respiratory failure; seizures
Botulism	C. botulinum	Ingestion of, or intoxication with, neurotoxins, interrupting acetylcholine-mediated neuromuscular transmission; some parasympatholytic effects	Descending paralysis; cranial nerve deficits; fixed, dilated pupils; ileus; dry mouth; respiratory failure; floppy baby syndrome. Possible cause of sudden infant death syndrome.
Gas gangrene	C. perfringens C. novyi C. septicum C. bifermentans	Myonecrosis with gas formation and systemic toxicity; due to wound infection of hypoxic tissue by clostridial species capable of elaborating histotoxic lecithinases and collagenases, primarily	Myonecrosis; wound crepitance; fever; fluid shifts and loss with resultant hypovolemic shock, hemolysis, renal failure, and massive tissue necrosis
Pseudomembranous colitis	C. difficile	Cytotoxins produced by C. difficile overgrowth in colon; likely caused by antibiotic-induced alterations in normal bowel flora	Acute febrile colitis; fluid and electrolyte depletion; hypoalbuminemia; pseudomembrane formation in colon

296

interfere with synaptic reflexes in the spinal cord, especially inhibitory spinal interneurons at the presynaptic terminals. Consequently, muscle spasm and tetany result, as well as loss of sympathetic inhibition. Seizures are likely, secondary to attachment of the toxin to cerebral gangliosides. Antitoxin can only neutralize toxin before it combines with receptor nerve fibers. The toxin cannot normally cross the blood–brain barrier.

Disease is caused when spores are introduced into the body by way of puncture wounds ("skin popping" in narcotic addicts), burns, or cuts. In the presence of necrotic tissue and other organisms, the lowered redox potential locally enhances reversion of the spores to the vegetative form, which are capable of toxin production. The incubation period ranges from several days to 3 weeks, longer periods corresponding to inoculation sites more distal to the central nervous system.

CLINICAL–PATHOLOGIC CORRELATIONS

The clinical–pathologic correlations for tetanus are presented in Table 50–1.

DIFFERENTIAL DIAGNOSIS

The differential diagnoses may include meningitis, phenothiazine reaction, hypocalcemic tetany, epilepsy, drug withdrawal, retroperiotoneal hemorrhage, and decerebrate posturing. Trismus may be seen in patients with dental abscesses, a fractured mandible, temporomandibular joint degeneration, mumps, diphtheria, retropharyngeal abscesses, and other infections. Opisthotonos may also be seen in patients with rabies, strychnine poisoning, a perforated peptic ulcer, and septicemic spondylitis.

DIAGNOSIS

The diagnosis of tetanus usually is made on the basis of the clinical manifestations combined with a history of recent injury or other important epidemiologic factors. Occasionally the diagnosis may be confirmed by microscopic or cultural evidence of *C. tetani* in material obtained from the wound. Frequently, such efforts at bacteriologic confirmation are unrewarding.

PRINCIPLES OF PREVENTION AND THERAPY

Treatment revolves around supportive measures and attempts to prevent further production or absorption of toxin. Antitoxin is indicated, as well as high doses of penicillin. Wound debridement and foreign body removal are recommended. Mild spasm may be controlled with barbiturates or diazepam; seizures or severe spasm may need curare-like drugs. Mechanical ventilatory support may be necessary secondary to seizures or severe spasm, or for paralysis of the respiratory musculature caused by drugs used in treatment. A tracheostomy early in the disease course is recommended; visual and auditory stimuli should be minimized. Morphine and labetalol are reported to be useful in controlling sympathetic effects. Prevention is the "gold standard" in treatment and is possible with proper immunization.

Current recommendations for tetanus immunization include tetanus toxoid boosters every 10 years for minor uncontaminated wounds once primary immunization is completed. Combined diphtheria-tetanus toxoids (Td) are preferred to tetanus toxoid alone in persons over 7 years of age. Passive immunity with tetanus immune globulin (TIG) is the recommended treatment for severe wounds in persons with uncertain or one or no prior immunizations.

There are generally no permanent sequelae to tetanus. Microscopically, the local injury site shows only nonspecific inflammatory changes. In the nervous system, changes are likewise nonspecific, with some nuclear swelling and chromatolysis in the motor ganglion cells of the spinal cord and medulla.

BOTULISM

Botulism is a life-threatening illness caused by the potent neurotoxins produced by *Clostridium botulinum*. The mortality ranges from 17% to 40% depending on the toxin type, the amount of toxin, and the time appropriate therapy is begun. There are three major types of clinical disease: (1) food-borne botulism, (2) wound botulism, and (3) infant botulism.

CLINICAL SIGNS AND SYMPTOMS

Food-borne botulism occurs 12 to 36 hours after the ingestion of preformed toxin in contaminated foodstuffs. The toxin is absorbed mainly in the stomach and small bowel and is not destroyed by digestive enzymes. Ingestion of raw or home-canned foods can often be implicated as the cause.

Wound botulism (the rarest form) presents the same clinical syndrome as the food-borne disease. The toxin is made by organisms in an infected wound. Young men are most often affected.

Infant botulism is the most commonly encountered form in the United States and is also known as the *floppy baby syndrome*. It has been postulated as one of several causes of sudden infant death syndrome (SIDS). Affected infants are usually the product of a normal gestation and delivery and range from 3 to 20 weeks old.

Early symptoms include weakness, lassitude, and dizziness. A dry mouth and a sore throat, both unrelieved by drinking water, may be seen as secondary to decreased saliva production. Ileus, urinary retention, and constipation can also occur due to interrupted parasympathetic transmission. Focal neurologic signs may appear at the onset or up to 3 days later. The cranial nerves are usually affected first. Blurred vision, diplopia, and photophobia are frequent. Bulbar effects include dysphonia, dysarthria, and dysphagia. A symmetrical, usually descending weakness of the extremities, accompanied by weakness of the respiratory musculature, occurs with variable speed. Nausea and vomiting are common with type E toxin, but only in approximately one-third of the patients with disease due to types A and B.

On physical examination, the patient is afebrile, alert, and oriented. Mandell cites a constellation of signs suggesting botulism: (1) unexplained postural hypotension, (2) dilated, unreactive pupils, (3) dry mucous membranes, (4) descending paralysis with progressive respiratory weakness, and (5) absence of fever. The results of the sensory examination are normal, and there is absence of pathologic reflexes. In wound botulism, fever may be present due to the usual polymicrobial nature of the infection.

The first symptom of infant botulism is generally mild constipation, followed by a weak cry and depressed gag reflex. The disease may progress to include cranial nerve defects, general muscle weakness, hypotonia, and areflexia. Respiratory arrest may occur in up to one-half of the affected infants. Affected infants are afebrile with normal CSF laboratory studies. The electromyogram may be useful in diagnosis, revealing abnormalities in post-tetanic facilitation (prolonged), muscle fibrillation, and small amplitude polyphasic motor unit potentials.

PATHOPHYSIOLOGY

C. *botulinum* is a gram-positive, anaerobic, spore-forming organism, ubiquitous in soil and marine sediments. The neurotoxin is produced in the vegetative state and released on autolysis. There are eight types of neurotoxin known, only three of which (Types A, B, and E) produce illness in humans. The toxins are heat labile, and thorough heating of food can prevent illness. The neurotoxin binds to the synaptic vesicles of cholinergic nerve fibers at the myoneural junction, of the synaptic ganglia, and of the parasympathetic motor endplates peripherally located in the autonomic nervous system. The toxin interrupts neurotransmission by blocking the calcium-mediated acetylcholine release. In infant botulism, the GI tract is apparently colonized from environmental sources (contaminated honey has been implicated as a possible source) with toxin production in vivo. Organisms and toxins have been recovered for up to 8 weeks, despite antibiotic therapy. Recovery can occur in the face of continued colonization, though this phenomenon is not well-understood.

CLINICAL–PATHOLOGIC CORRELATIONS

The clinical–pathologic correlations for botulism are presented in Table 50–1.

DIFFERENTIAL DIAGNOSIS

The differential diagnosis varies with the stage of illness. Early pharyngitis may be confused with a streptococcal infection. Ileus may mimic intestinal obstruction. Atropine, belladonna, or jimson weed poisoning cause fixed, dilated pupils and dry mucous membranes, but are accompanied by CNS excitation and hallucinations. Guillain-Barré syndrome appears with weakness and respiratory embarrassment, but an ascending paralysis with muscle cramps and paresthesias. Guillian-Barré syndrome also has classic late CSF findings. Myasthenia gravis responds well to edrophonium, whereas only a slight response is noted in botulism. Tick paralysis appears with an ascending neuropathy, perioral paresthesias, and an entry wound. Polio is a febrile disease with asymmetric, neurologic findings and CSF abnormalities.

DIAGNOSIS

A diagnosis of botulism may be confirmed by identifying the toxin in the blood or by identifying the toxin or organism in the stool, gastric contents, or food. Pathologic findings on a cellular level are minimal. Both *C. botulinum* organisms and the toxin can be recovered from the stool of affected infants.

PRINCIPLES OF PREVENTION AND THERAPY

Treatment centers on intensive, supportive care. Mechanical ventilation may be necessary. Administration of trivalent antitoxin is recommended (available through the U.S. Centers for Disease Control). Aminoglycosides may potentiate the neuromuscular paralysis and are, therefore, contraindicated. Prevention of illness involves avoidance of contaminated foodstuffs and care to avoid injury in potentially contaminated environments.

GAS GANGRENE

Clostridial myonecrosis (gas gangrene) is a rapidly progressive disease caused primarily by *Clostridium perfringens* with resultant muscle destruction, crepitance, and signs of systemic toxicity. The untreated disease is usually fatal, and the mortality rates vary from 15% to 60%, depending on the site of the infection.

CLINICAL SIGNS AND SYMPTOMS

Gas gangrene typically follows a traumatic injury that has significant tissue devitalization, but may follow inadequate wound debridement or biliary and colorectal surgery. The incubation period averages 4 days and ranges from 8 hours to 20 days. The first sign of illness is the sudden onset of excruciating pain in the wound. The overlying skin becomes tense and edematous and may take on a magenta discoloration. Large surrounding hemorrhagic bullae may be seen. Then there is a serous discharge with a foul/sweet odor. An initial tachycardia that is out of proportion to the fever or circulatory changes may be seen. Shock, intravascular hemolysis, and renal failure may ensue. The fever may be quite high, up to 41°C. The surviving patients generally require amputation and extensive debridement.

PATHOPHYSIOLOGY

The disease is caused by the "histotoxic" clostridia (including *C. perfringens, C. novyi, C. septicum,* and *C. bifermentans*), with 90% of the cases due to infection with *C. perfringens.* The organisms must be introduced into tissue where they can germinate and elaborate toxin. Tissue anoxia, due to trauma or vascular disease, and a low redox potential are necessary for toxin production. In the United States, approximately 60% of cases are related to trauma and 40% to surgery, usually abdominal. Patients with diabetes mellitus, malignancies, or vascular disease may develop gas gangrene spontaneously, that is, without a traumatic wound.

C. perfringens is an anaerobic, gram-positive, spore-forming, rod-shaped bacterium found in soil, human feces, and on clothing. Once introduced into a wound with a sufficiently low redox potential, it elaborates a variety of toxins. The alpha toxin, a lecithinase, is the principal agent of destruction in gas gangrene. It disrupts cell membranes and probably mitochondria, resulting in tissue destruction and hemolysis. Other lethal toxins include a collagenase, necrotizing toxins, hemolytic cardiotoxin, and proteolytic toxin.

CLINICAL–PATHOLOGIC CORRELATIONS

The clinical–pathologic correlations for gas gangrene are presented in Table 50–1.

DIFFERENTIAL DIAGNOSIS

Gas gangrene is differentiated from other necrotizing and subcutaneous skin infections by its characteristic destruction of muscle tissue and severe systemic toxicity. Nonclostridial anaerobic cellulitis and simple clostridial cellulitis are further set apart by the absence of severe pain or skin discoloration in these conditions.

DIAGNOSIS

Cultures are of limited diagnostic value in gas gangrene due to its rapid course and the usual polymicrobial nature of the infection. The affected muscle must be viewed surgically to diagnose clostridial myonecrosis. Initially, the muscle appears pale and edematous, later becoming beefy red and noncontractile. Frankly gangrenous muscle tissue shows histologic evidence of liquefactive necrosis and is black and friable. At this stage the patient is near death. Gas bubbles and necrosis, dissecting along tissue planes, are noted with thrombosis of local vessels. Gram's stain of wound exudate reveals numerous gram-positive bacilli and few WBCs. Blood cultures will be positive in approximately 15% of patients. Classically, gas may be seen dissecting deeply along muscle fiber bundles on x-ray film.

PRINCIPLES OF PREVENTION AND THERAPY

Treatment must include rapid and thorough surgical wound debridement, high doses of penicillin given intravenously, and, in the case of extreme toxemia, antitoxin therapy. Hyperbaric oxygen therapy is indicated and may reduce mortality and the need for amputation. Careful attention should be paid to fluid balance, and the underlying causes of poor tissue oxygenation should be addressed.

PSEUDOMEMBRANOUS COLITIS

Clostridium difficile is recognized as the most frequent cause of antibiotic-associated colitis. The disease can occur in all age groups, but is uncommon in infants. Increased incidence is found in elderly patients, debilitated patients with malignancies, women, and in intensive care unit patients. Although the original reports focused on the disease's occurrence after clindamycin, it can follow even a short course of nearly all commonly used antibiotics given by any route. Exact figures are lacking, but the mortality rate is low. Recurrence of the disease occurs in 10% to 20% of treated patients.

CLINICAL SIGNS AND SYMPTOMS

The illness is an acute colitis. The affected patient typically experiences watery or mucoid, green, foul-smelling diarrhea (10 to 20 stools per day), with cramping abdominal pain 4 to 9 days after antibiotic therapy is initiated. Up to one-third of patients are affected days to weeks after therapy is discontinued. A high fever (39.4°C–40.5°C), peripheral leukocytosis (up to 35,000 WBCs/mm^3), a tender abdomen, and hypoalbuminemia are commonly seen. The WBCs are present in the stools of about 50% of patients. Less often, the disease involves little diarrhea and appears with symptoms of an acute abdomen, peritonitis, a toxic megacolon, or a perforated colon.

PATHOPHYSIOLOGY

C. difficile is a anaerobic, gram-positive, sporeforming bacillus. It normally inhabits soil, water, intestinal tracts of animals, and colonizes a low percentage of human adults. Greater colonization rates may be found in asymptomatic, hospitalized patients.

Antibiotic-associated colitis caused by *C. difficile* has as its hallmark the formation of a pseudomembrane formed of fibrin, mucus, necrotic epithelial and inflammatory cells and found only in the colon. Pseudomembranes may be extensive or absent, but are diagnostic when found. The disease and lesion are caused by two major toxins elaborated in the intestinal lumen, both of which are cytotoxic, attacking cell membranes and microfilaments. There is subsequent necrosis, inflammation, and increased fluid and electrolyte loss to the lumen. There is also an associated increase in peristalsis and myoelectric responses. Microscopically, there is necrosis of colonic epithelial cells superficially, with mixed, inflammatory infiltration of the lamina propria and pseudomembranes overlying the epithelial cells.

Thrombosis of superficial venules is characteristic.

CLINICAL–PATHOLOGIC CORRELATIONS

The clinical–pathologic correlations for pseudomembranous colitis are presented in Table 50–1.

DIFFERENTIAL DIAGNOSIS

The differential diagnosis must include other infections that produce diarrhea, (*Shigella* infections especially produce membranous lesions), inflammatory bowel disease, and ischemic colitis. Patients with inflammatory bowel disease have higher rates of *C. difficile* colonizations (up to 20%), and this may further confuse the diagnosis. Toxin assay may be particularly useful in these patients.

DIAGNOSIS

Diagnosis is made by direct endoscopic visualization of colonic lesions and recovery of *C. difficile* or toxin from stools. Late abnormalities may be noted on barium enema, which carries the risk of several complications, including toxic megacolon and perforation.

Treatment is directed at eradication of *C. difficile* and supportive measures. Oral vancomycin is currently the drug of choice. Metronidazole is an alternative therapy. Opiates and other antiperistaltic agents should not be used. Mild cases may respond to discontinuing the inducing antibiotic, and to replacing fluid and electrolytes. Severe cases may be complicated by toxic megacolon and bacteremia necessitating specific antibiotic therapy for the bacteremia in addition to the antibiotic therapy for *C. difficile*.

REFERENCES

Allen SD: Clostridium, in Lennette EH, Balows A, Hausler WJ Jr, Shadomy HJ (eds): *Manual of Clinical Microbiology*, ed 4. Washington, DC, American Society for Microbiology, 1985, pp. 434–444. *An up-to-date reference with a clinical laboratory emphasis.*

LeFrock JG, Molavi A: Necrotizing skin and subcutaneous infections. *J Antimicrob Chemother* 1982; 9(suppl. A):183–192. *A review giving the differential diagnosis of necrotizing infections of skin and subcutaneous tissues.*

Mandell GL, Douglas RG Jr, Bennett JE (eds): *Principles and Practice of Infectious Diseases*, ed 2. New York, John Wiley & Sons, 1985. *The definitive reference work on infectious diseases.*

MMWR 1978; 27:17–23. *A follow-up on infant botulism in the United States. A summary of reported cases up to 1978.*

Niinikoski J, Aho AJ: Combination of hyperbaric oxygen, surgery, and antibiotics in the treatment of clostridial gas gangrene. *Infections in Surgery*, 1983; 2:23–37. *A good review on clostridial myonecrosis and treatment.*

Silva J, Fekety R: Clostridia and antimicrobial enterocolitis. *Annu Rev Med* 1981; 32:327–333. *A good review article by the discoverers of the disease.*

Swartz MN: Anaerobic spore-forming bacilli: The clostridia, in Davis BD, Dulbecco R, Eisen HN, Ginsberg HS, (eds): *Microbiology*, ed 3. Hagerstown MD, Harper & Row, 1980, pp 704–722. *An excellent textbook on microbiology with clinical correlations.*

51

INFECTION IN THE IMMUNOCOMPROMISED HOST

Howard F. Wunderlich, M.D.

Fever in an immunosuppressed host often signals infection. The causes of immunosuppression are variable and include the underlying disease's effect on the immune system or the iatrogenic results of chemotherapy or radiation treatments. Advances in the treatment of cancer have added productive years to the lives of patients with a once rapidly fatal disease, but therapy has a double-edged effect. It creates febrile illnesses and opportunistic infections in patients with little ability to fight back. Additionally, these often-neutropenic patients lack the customary signs of inflammation making diagnosis and localization of infection difficult.

CLINICAL SIGNS AND SYMPTOMS

Often the postchemotherapy course of cancer patients who seem to be doing well is suddenly punctuated by fever or chills. Little else may indicate an infection or untoward problem. In other instances, patients may present with fever and a wasting syndrome as an initial manifestation of their underlying immunosuppressive illness. This may be accompanied by symptoms related to the site of infection or by complications from pancytopenia, obstruction, or mucosal damage secondary to a malignancy.

One of the important principles to remember is that these patients will not always manifest any of the classic symptoms of disease. The pain may not be as severe. A cough may not be productive. Discharges may be serous or serosanguinous instead of purulent. Of special interest are symptoms evolving from sites along the upper respiratory system and alimentary canal. Epistaxis, or nasal discharge, along with painful gingiva, buccal mucosa, or teeth may focus attention to a nasopharyngeal or oral cavity source. Dysphagia or odynophagia may be associated with esophagitis. Pain on defecation, an anal discharge, or swollen hemorrhoids may lead to the diagnosis of proctitis or a perirectal abscess.

A conscientious physical examination is perhaps more critical in finding a focus of fever in the immunocompromised patient than in seeking the cause of a fever of undertermined origin in a patient who is not immunosuppressed. Inspection of the integument should include the axillae and inguinal areas for lesions or evidence of a rash. Ecthyma gangrenosum (Fig 51–1), a cutaneous *Pseudomonas* endarteritis, and other necrotic lesions or nodules may be found. A good funduscopic evaluation is important. Finding *Candida* endophthalmitis (Fig 51–2) or choroid tubercles associated with miliary tuberculosis would require antibiotic therapy with drugs not used in the usual clinical setting.

A good oral evaluation is always in order. Evidence of thrush, gingivitis, or ulcers may be a clue to the source or cause of fever. Pulmonary signs of consolidation are often negligi-

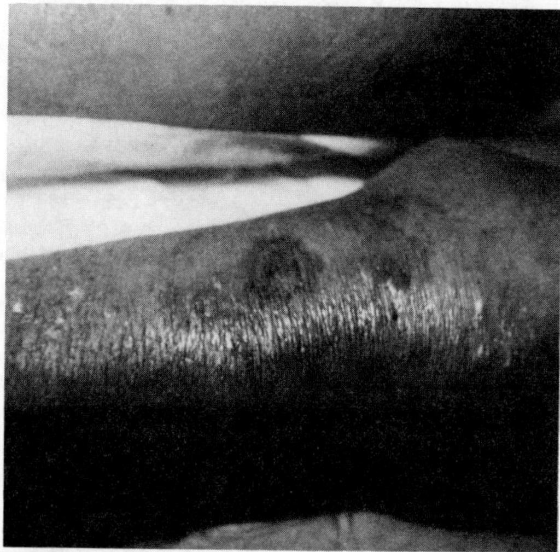

FIG 51–1.
Ecthyma gangrenosum.

ble, and a few crackles may be all that are heard. Palpation of the abdomen may reveal tenderness or enlargement of the liver or spleen, but this is less likely than in the normal host to yield much help in the diagnosis of fever. Examination of the anus, rectum, and genitalia may be very rewarding because rectal induration, tenderness, or discharge may be noted though a frank, fluctuant abscess is usually lacking in a neutropenic patient. Lastly, inspection for previous or current catheter sites may yield a source of infection and culture. These sites may not issue the usual signs of inflammation but may be tender, indurated, or slightly erythematous.

PATHOPHYSIOLOGY

Although fever in the immunosuppressed host may be due to one of many factors, infection is the most common and most likely cause of mortality. The common denominator in all cases is a lesion in the immune system predisposing to a microbial foothold and often to a soft-tissue, pulmonary, or septicemic infection. Selected immunologic impairment will influence the type of microbial opportunist that gains a foothold.

Joschi and Schimpff (1985) list seven defects of the immune system that may lead to infection. Table 51–1 lists the immune defects, associated immunocompromised states or neoplastic diseases, and associated microorganisms.

The most common defect is a quantitative decrement in phagocytic ability caused by granulocytopenia or neutropenia. Between 50% and 60% of septicemias in immunocompromised patients are caused by gram-negative bacteria, especially the Enterobacteriaceae and *Pseudomonas* species (Schimpff, Young, Greene, Vermuelen, Moody, and Wiernik, 1972). Infections from *Staphylococcus*, *Candida*, *Aspergillus*, and occasionally *Pneumocystis* organisms also occur. The J.K. bacillus of the *Corynebacterium* genus has been found to be associated with cellulitis, pneumonia, and sepsis and is most susceptible to vancomycin treatment. The more days the patient's granulocyte count is less than 500 cells per microliter the more days spent with infection; and if the count is less than 100 cells per microliter, the more serious the infection. Many of these infections are caused by endogenous flora and are

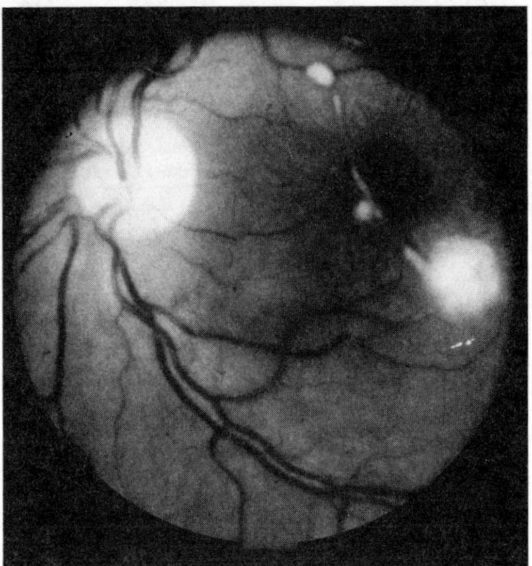

FIG 51–2.
Candida endophthalmitis.

preceded by colonization of the gastrointestinal tract.

Dysfunction in cellular immunity also predisposes to infection. This may be a quantitative decrease in lymphocytes such as that found in the acquired immunodeficiency syndrome (AIDS) or a qualitative difference in functional capacity due to leukemia or the use of immunosuppressive drugs and glucocorticoids. These drugs are often used in the chemotherapy of cancer or in the suppression of transplant rejection. This defect usually predisposes to intracellular opportunists. Infections of this type may produce disseminated disease in the reticuloendothelial system, pneumonias, or central nervous system infections.

A defect in the humoral immune system may predispose to infection by disallowing opsonization of encapsulated bacteria. The humoral antibodies aid in the phagocytosis of *Hemophilus influenzae* and *Streptococcus pneumoniae*. Diseases such as chronic lymphocytic leukemia, multiple myeloma, and acquired or congenital hypogammaglobulinemia are examples. Asplenic individuals are also predisposed to these types of infections.

Two other defects create susceptibility to infection secondarily either by obstruction or by impaired neurologic function. In the former instance, an obstructing neoplasm may lead to infection by the stasis of secretions. Broncho-

TABLE 51–1.
Immunologic Defects Predisposing to Infection in Various Immunocompromised and Disease States

IMMUNE DEFECT	ASSOCIATED IMMUNOCOMPROMISED OR NEOPLASTIC DISEASE	COMMON INFECTING ORGANISM
Decreased phagocytosis		
Granulocytopenia	Bone marrow aplasia	Gram-negative bacilli
Qualitative neutrophilic	Chemotherapy	*Staphylococcus aureus*
defect	Acute leukemia	Yeasts
		Aspergillus
Decreased cellular immunity		
Reduction in helper	AIDS	*Pneumocystis carinii*
lymphocytes	Corticosteroid therapy	*Toxoplasma*
Decreased macrophages	Lymphomas	*Cryptococcus*
		Deep mycoses
		Mycobacterium
		Listeria
		Salmonella
		Nocardia
		Strongyloides
		Herpes simplex virus
		Varicella-zoster virus
		Cytomegalovirus
Decreased humoral immunity		
Opsonization of bacteria	Malnutrition	*Streptococcus pneumoniae*
Neutralization of virus	Splenectomy	*Hemophilus influenzae*
	Chronic lymphocytic leukemia (CLL)	Gram-negative bacilli
	Multiple myeloma	
	Chemotherapy	
Anatomic-barrier damage		
Mucosal ulceration	Chemotherapy	*Staphylococcus aureus*
Integumentary bypass or	Tumor invasion	Gram-negative bacilli
damage	Decubitus ulcers	Anaerobes
Obstruction		
Stasis	Bronchogenic carcinoma	Pneumonia
	Ovarian carcinoma	Urinary tract infection (UTI)
	Common bile duct blockage	Cholangitis
CNS lesion		
Depressed gag reflex	CNS or brainstem tumor or	Aspiration pneumonia
Neurogenic bladder	hemorrhage	Urinary tract infection (UTI)
	Spinal cord tumor	
Iatrogenic		
Indwelling catheter	Foley catheter	Gram-negative bacilli
Intravenous needle		
Parenteral	Broviak, Hickman catheter	*Staphylococcus epidermidis*
hyperalimentation	Broad-spectrum antibiotic	*Candida*
Antibiosis	Chemotherapy	*Corynebacterium*
Chemotherapy	Irradiation·	
Radiation therapy		

genic carcinoma, prostatic cancer, and intrinsic or extrinsic biliary stasis by a tumor may lead to pneumonia, a urinary tract infection, or cholangitis, respectively. In the latter instance, a lesion in the nervous system can increase the propensity toward infection by decreasing the gag reflex or by bladder retention. Aspiration or a urinary tract infection may then result.

The final defect predisposing to infection is iatrogenic, which often involves the bypass of defense barriers to allow organisms an easy portal of entry. The integumentary and mucous membrane barriers require intact surfaces. These may be violated with catheters, surgical wounds, tubes into orifices, and wires used in the advanced care of the oncology patient. Chemotherapy drugs and radiation therapy may cause ulceration and denudation of mucous membrane surfaces in the oral cavity and along the alimentary canal, leading to invasion and septicemia with endogenous flora (i.e., bacteria and fungi). Lastly, the very antibiotics that are used to treat many of these infections can result in the selection of more resistant organisms which colonize and superinfect a host.

DIFFERENTIAL DIAGNOSIS

Fever in the immunosuppressed patient should always signify the probability of infection. Empirical therapy with broad-spectrum antibiotics may often be necessary. Because patients may present with little or no localizing signs, a special emphasis on gram-negative bacilli has been the standard of care. The underlying disease, the neutrophil count, the type of indwelling catheter, and the clinical presentation are factors that aid in determining the differential diagnosis.

Several scenarios will be presented for illustration. In a patient who has been on chemotherapy for a solid tumor, a fever develops 10 days after receiving antineoplastic drugs; a neutrophil count of 200 cells per microliter is found; the patient complains of pain on defacation. Examination reveals a tender old intravenous site that has a serous discharge. There is perirectal induration and tenderness. This patient has a high likelihood of bacterial infection and potential bacteremia from either the old intravenous site or a perirectal abscess. Both gram-negative aerobes and anaerobes as well as staphylococci would be potential pathogens. If the patient were receiving parenteral hyperalimentation therapy or had a permanent indwelling catheter (e.g., a Broviak or Hickman catheter), then septicemia with *Candida* species or bacteremia with *Staphylococcus epidermidis* would also be possible.

In a neutropenic patient with acute leukemia and receiving aggressive chemotherapy, the development of cough, dyspnea, fever, and bilateral pulmonary infiltrates with significant hypoxia indicates a gram-negative pneumonia until proven otherwise. Schimpff and co-workers found in a 1972 series of leukemic patients that *Pseudomonas aeruginosa* was the most frequent cause of bacteremia (Schimpff et al., 1972). Even though other gram-negative bacilli or fungi may colonize the individual, it is colonization with *Pseudomonas aeruginosa* that most often leads to bacteremic consequences in the lung, anorectal area, skin, pharynx, or urinary tract. There is a good correlation between colonization with *P. aeruginosa* in the stool, nares, throat, or skin and the degree of neutropenia in leukemic patients who develop bacteremia with this organism.

An individual with impaired cell-mediated immunity as seen in patients with Hodgkin's disease may have a different set of opportunistic pathogens, depending to some degree on whether splenectomy has been performed. Notter and co-workers found *Streptococcus pneumoniae* to be the most frequent cause of serious infection in 21% of these patients (Notter, Grossman, Rosenberg, and Remington, 1980). *Escherichia coli, Hemophilus influenzae,* and *Staphylococcus aureus* were also found. Surprisingly, there were few cases of *Pneumocystis carinii,* invasive pulmonary aspergillosis, disseminated candidiasis, or herpes simplex infection. Tuberculosis, nocardiosis, and toxoplasmosis were also infrequent. The rate of infection rose immediately after a laparotomy and if relapse of the Hodgkin's disease occurred. The extent of the Hodgkin's disease and the concomitant use of chemotherapy and radiation therapy also increased the risk of serious infection unless the patient remained in an initial remission.

The last scenario involves the transplant patient. In this situation the incidence of infection is directly related to the net immunosuppressive effect achieved and to the duration of time over which therapy is administered (Rubin, Wolfson, Cosimi, and Tolkoff-Rubin, 1981). Transplant rejection versus infection is often present when fever develops, and cytomegalovirus is often a cause of both.

A renal transplant patient has been receiving azathioprine (150mg/day) and prednisone (40 mg/day) for 3 months when fever, headache, and confusion develop over a 2-day period leading to an obtunded state with nuchal rigidity. The patient has evidence of meningitis on examination of the cerebrospinal fluid. In this situation an acute meningitis has developed in the early post-transplant period. The most likely cause of fever is *Listeria monocytogenes.* Other causes of central nervous system (CNS) infection are *Cryptococcus neoformans,* but this occurs in the late post-transplant period (after 4 months), and CNS toxoplasmosis or *No-*

cardia or *Aspergillus* infection if evidence of disease with focal neurologic signs occurs in the early period (1–4 months).

Pulmonary infiltrates in the transplant patient may be differentiated by the chest x-ray pattern and the duration of symptoms (Rubin, 1980). If the chest x-ray pattern is focal or multinodular and develops within 1 day, then a bacterial infection can be suspected. If the infiltrate is subacute or chronic, then a fungal, mycobacterial, or nocardial process may be occurring. A diffuse x-ray pattern developing over days to weeks may be caused by a fungus, virus, or *Pneumocystis carinii*. A subacute nodular pattern indicates a fungal or nocardial process. Acute lobar consolidation portends bacterial infection while over a more extended period could point toward fungal or nocardial disease.

Finally, not all patients with fever have an infection. The underlying neoplasm may be a source of fever, and the use of naproxen could aid in differentiating neoplastic fever from a fever from another cause. Chang and Gross (1984) reported that the fever in 14 out of 15 patients with neoplastic fever was relieved with naproxen. Pulmonary infiltrates and fever may be caused by drugs, such as bleomycin, or by leukocyte transfusions. Blood or platelet transfusions may also produce febrile episodes during or shortly after the transfusion. Pulmonary emboli and pulmonary hemorrhage have been associated with pulmonary infiltrates and fever. Radiation therapy may also cause fever related to radiation-induced colitis, proctitis, or pneumonitis.

DIAGNOSIS

Cultures of blood, urine, sputum, skin lesions, and if appropriate spinal fluid should be performed prior to instituting therapy. Bacteremias occur in 30% to 45% of immunocompromised patients (Schimpff et al., 1972). A chest x-ray film should always be made and repeated in the dehydrated or neutropenic patient. Serologic tests for cytomegalovirus, toxoplasmosis, and deep mycoses (e.g., histoplasmosis or coccidioidomycosis) may be helpful, but only if the baseline status is known. A serum and cerebrospinal fluid latex agglutination test for cryptococcal antigen may be valuable, as are bacterial agglutination or counter-

immunoelectrophoresis methods for detecting the bacterial antigens of the pneumococcus, *Hemophilus influenzae*, or *Pseudomonas aeruginosa*.

The most informative procedure in the diagnosis of fever in immunosuppressed patients is the appropriate culture of biopsied tissue or fluid. There should be no hesistancy to perform an invasive procedure in order to collect tissue or a specimen for culture in a critical situation. Hypoxia and coagulation deficiencies are the major hindrance, but can be circumvented with supportive measures.

In patients with pulmonary infiltrates, bronchoscopy with or without transbronchial biopsy is the procedure of choice if coagulation is sufficient (Williams, Krick, and Remington, 1976). Transtracheal aspiration has been disappointing. An aspirate taken with a sheathed bronchoscope may avoid mouth flora contamination, and bronchial lavage without biopsy also gives a good diagnostic yield especially in cases of diffuse infiltrates associated with *Pneumocystis carinii* or cytomegalovirus. A closed needle biopsy runs a high risk of complication (30% of cases). An open biopsy of the lung is useful in patients with coagulation problems or in those already on a ventilator who have a high risk of barotrauma. There is a high yield (80%) especially for fungal disease. Stains and cultures for *Legionella* as well as cultures for bacteria, fungi, acid-fast organisms, and viruses should be done. A methenamine silver stain for *Pneumocystis* should be performed along with routine histologic studies and special stains for fungal and acid-fast organisms. A cytology stain may identify neoplastic cells or viral inclusions.

Other occasionally useful procedures include computerized tomography of the head for focal cerebral processes and gallium-labeled leukocyte scans to identify sites of infection or tumor. A bone scan may be helpful in locating osteomyelitis or a metastatic tumor that is available for biopsy.

PRINCIPLES OF PREVENTION AND THERAPY

The prevention of infectious complications is most important in the immunosuppressed host because this is a common problem and is the most frequent cause of mortality in these patients. Reducing the risk of infection can take one of several approaches. Avoiding damage to body barriers such as the skin and mucous membranes with venipunctures and decubitus ulcers is important. Intravenous catheters should be rotated frequently and metal "butterfly" needles used where possible. Attention should also be directed to good urinary catheter care and avoidance of the use of urinary catheters.

Reducing the acquisition of new potential pathogens by the use of protective environments and of oral gastrointestinal decontamination regimens is controversial at best (Pizzo, 1985). Reverse isolation offers no advantage over careful handwashing. Positive-pressure rooms with laminar air flow do not reduce the risk of bacterial colonization sufficiently. A totally protected, or "life island," enviroment with sterile food and laminar, filtered air flow removing particles greater than 0.3 μm and the use of oral nonabsorbable antibiotics, skin disinfectants, and aerosols can reduce the risk of infection in neutropenic patients. It is costly, cumbersome, and not without its failures, however. The use of oral nonabsorbable antibiotics has largely been ineffective and may cause emergence of resistant bacteria.

The suppression of colonizing organisms with selective decontamination is another route to reduce the risk of infection. The principle of colonization resistance is used to produce bacterial interference in the gastrointestinal tract with anaerobic flora. One can selectively suppress aerobic gram-negative growth with trimethoprim sulfamethoxazole (TS), nalidixic acid, or polymyxin B. Nystatin is used to inhibit yeast growth, while anaerobic bacteria are allowed to flourish. This may decrease the incidence of opportunistic pathogens such as *Pseudomonas aeruginosa* in gaining a foothold.

The use of TS has gained popularity both as an agent for selective decontamination and monoprophylaxis in neutropenic hosts. There has been evidence to support its efficacy in patients with acute nonlymphocytic leukemia at high risk for infection, but overall the success has been marginal and may cause emergence of TS-resistant organisms.

The last method of attempting to prevent infection in the immunosuppressed host involves the augmentation of host defenses. In some instances this involves granulocyte transfusions

in the very neutropenic patient with proven bacterial or fungal infection. This approach has had variable success, and the success may be temporary. The risks include graft-versus-host disease, the transmission of cytomegalovirus, and the development of the adult respiratory distress syndrome especially when amphotericin B is given concurrently. Further efforts at bolstering host defenses include active immunization with pneumococcal vaccine or an experimental *Pseudomonas* vaccine or specific passive immunization with zoster immune globulin for those exposed to the varicella-zoster virus. A gram-negative immune globulin for *Pseudomonas*, which is made from antisera to nonvirulent *E. coli* mutants in human volunteers, is also being developed.

The management of immunosuppressed patients with actual or presumptive infection often takes the empirical route. Prior to receiving culture reports and knowing the frequency of gram-negative bacillary infections, therapy should initially be broad and aimed at *Pseudomonas aeruginosa*. Most regimens include both an antipseudomonal penicillin or cephalosporin and an aminoglycoside. This kind of therapy is intended to be both bactericidal and, if possible, synergistic against the putative gram-negative bacillus. Although many combinations are employed, they are all similar in efficacy as long as the aminoglycoside dose maintains peak levels of that drug in a high therapeutic range (6 to 8 μg/mL). Therapy for *Pneumocystis carinii* infections may be initiated if diffuse pulmonary infiltrates are evident on chest x-ray film, and treatment for legionnaires' disease should be used if acute, diffuse, and progressive infiltrates are developing. If the individual has not responded within 48 to 72 hours after beginning empirical treatment, antifungal therapy may be instituted. If a pulmonary infiltrate is present or worsening, a bronchoscopic specimen should be obtained. Antifungal therapy with amphotericin B can be used when systemic candidiasis, aspergillosis, or mucomycosis is suspected. Esophagitis, *Candida* endophthalmitis, and mucositis are such instances. Finding pulmonary infiltrates and multiple cultures of *Candida* growing in specimens from the oral cavity, sputum, urine, stool, or other sites is another clue supporting the use of systemic amphotericin B.

The duration of therapy depends on the length of the neutropenia, and whether the cause has been determined. Febrile neutropenia of less than 1-week duration can be treated with specific therapy aimed at the isolated pathogen. If the neutropenia has lasted more than 1 week, broad-spectrum antibiotic therapy should be continued until the neutropenia improves. If fever persists, therapy can be discontinued before resolution of the neutropenia only with close monitoring. Prompt initiation of empiric antibiotic therapy with early antifungal modification using amphotericin B may be life-saving in the neutropenic or immunosuppressed host with fever.

REFERENCES

Chang JC, Gross HM: Utility of naproxen in the differential diagnosis of fever of undetermined origin in patients with cancer. *Am J Med* 1984; 76:597–603. *The use of naproxen (250 mg bid) is associated with relief of the fever in 14 of 15 cancer patients and 0 of 5 patients ultimately shown to have an infectious cause of fever.*

Joshi JH, Schimpff SC: Infections in the compromised host, in Mandel GL, Douglas RG Jr, Bennett JE (ed): *Principles and Practice of Infectious Diseases*, ed 2. New York, John Wiley & Sons, 1985, pp 1644–1649. *An overview from a major textbook chapter on the factors predisposing to infection in the compromised host as well as the pathophysiology and etiology of infection.*

Notter DT, Grossman PL, Rosenberg SA, Remington JS: Infections in patients with Hodgkin's disease. A clinical study of 300 consecutive patients. *Rev Infect Dis* 1980; 2:761–800. *An elegant study delineating the types of infections, etiologic agents, and predisposing factors of infection in the patient with Hodgkin's disease.*

Pizzo P: Empiric therapy and prevention of infection in the immunocompromised host, in Mandel GL, Douglas RG Jr, Bennett JE (ed): *Principles and Practice of Infectious Diseases*, ed 2. New York, John Wiley & Sons, 1985, pp 1680–1688. *This text details the pros and cons in the prevention of infection in the immunosuppressed host and provides guidelines of therapy.*

Rubin RH: Infection in the immunosuppressed host. *Sci Am* 1980; 1–27. *A well-written general review of the pathophysiology of immunosuppression and its relationship to the etiology of infection; also included is a discussion of pneumonitis and x-ray patterns.*

Rubin RH, Wolfson JS, Cosimi AB, Tolkoff-Rubin NE: Infection in the renal transplant recipient. *Am J Med* 1981, 70:405–411. *A classic review of the causes of infection in the renal transplant patient with attention to the chronologic sequence related to the operation date and type of infection.*

Schimpff SC, Young VM, Greene WH, Vermuelen GD, Moody MR, Wiernik PH: Origin of infection in acute nonlymphocytic leukemia. *Ann Intern Med* 1972; 77:707–714. *A landmark study correlating the endogenous colonization of gram-negative bacilli in hospitalized leukemic patients with microbiologically documented infection.*

Williams DM, Krick JA, Remington JS: Pulmonary infection in the compromised host. *Am Rev Respir Dis* 1976; 114:359–394. *This first of a two-part review on respiratory infections in the compromised host discusses the relative merits of invasive pulmonary procedures and the specific causes of pulmonary infiltrates.*

52

SEXUALLY TRANSMITTED DISEASES

Dennis D. Barber, M.D.

Sexually transmitted diseases are infections that are acquired through sexual contact with an infected partner. Although we commonly think of sexually transmitted disease as the traditional syphilis and gonorrhea, they have been joined by many new entities which have been appearing in increasing numbers in the offices of primary care practitioners and in ambulatory care centers. These include infection with *Trichomonas*, or herpes and condyloma acuminatum, just to name a few. Patients with one sexually transmitted disease may have simultaneous infections with others. Rein (1981) found gonorrhea in 23% of women with *Trichomonas* infection, but in only 13% of women without it. Also, Judson (1979) found *Chlamydia trachomatis* in 27% to 63% of women with acute gonorrhea infection. Of patients with veneral warts, 13% will have gonorrhea.

VAGINITIS

Although discharges are a common symptom bringing a woman into the doctor's office, not all discharges are from infections, and not all of the infections are caused by the same organism (Table 52–1). One of the more common complaints that brings the patient to a physician is a vaginal discharge that may or may not be associated with a corresponding vulvar irritation (Table 52–2). Whether the latter is primary or secondary needs to be determined by a careful history. While a vaginal discharge may be the reason for seeking medical attention, the underlying concerns about the discharge may be related to something entirely different. Such unspoken concerns may be: Is it cancer? Is it a veneral disease? Is it normal? Total care should address these unspoken fears by a thorough explanation of the physiology of normal discharge as well as an explanation of the diagnosis in terms the patient can understand.

Not all discharges necessarily imply infection. It is not uncommon to have a change in the normal vaginal secretions just before or after menses as well as at midcycle, all reflecting the changing hormonal milieu within the patient. The physiologic response to psychosexual stress, anxiety, or sexual arousal may manifest itself by an increasing amount of transudate from the vaginal walls secondary to

TABLE 52–1.
Clinical–Pathologic Correlations in Sexually Transmitted Disease

PATHOLOGIC FINDINGS	CAUSATIVE ORGANISM	CLINICAL FINDINGS
Vaginal discharge	*Gardnerella vaginalis*	Odorous, white to gray discharge
Vaginal discharge	*Trichomonas*	Odorous, gray to green discharge with or without vulvar irritation
Vaginal discharge	*Candida*	White, thick discharge with or without vulvar irritation
Vaginal discharge	Gonococcus	Creamy white to yellow discharge
Vaginal discharge	*Chlamydia*	Yellow, puslike discharge from the cervix
Ulcerated lesion	Herpes simplex II	Painful ulcer of the vulva, vagina, or cervix
Ulcerated lesion	*Treponema pallidum*	Painless ulcer with hard raised border

TABLE 52–2.
Clinical and Laboratory Features of Vaginal Discharge

CONDITION ASSOCIATED WITH DISCHARGE	SYMPTOMS	pH	COLOR	CONTENTS
Physiologic	None	3.8–4.2	Pasty white	*Lactobacillus* squamous debris
Gardnerella Vaginalis infection	Watery discharge, musty odor	5.0–5.5	Gray to slate	Squamous epithelial cells stippled with gram − bacteria (clue cell)
Trichomonas infection	Profuse discharge, odor, vulvar irritation	5.5–5.8	Gray or green	Motile flagellated parasite, many WBCs
Candida infection	Vulvar irritation, discharge	4.2–5.0	White, thick	Branching pseudo-hyphae
Atrophic vaginitis	Slight irritation, discharge	6.0–7.0	Serous or mucopurulent	Mixed bacteria, WBC

the increased vascular engorgement resulting in "vaginal sweat." Hormonal medications such as estrogen stimulate cervical glands resulting in a clear watery discharge. One must thus approach each complaint as though it were a primary event rather than assume it is "the same old past infection."

CLINICAL–PATHOLOGIC CORRELATIONS

The organisms found in approximately 90% of vaginitis cases are *Candida* species, *Trichomonas*, and *Gardnerella vaginalis*. The most common organism found is *Candida albicans*, although other species of this group have also been reported. Candidiasis is not considered a veneral disease in the usual sense, although it can be sexually transmitted by contact with infected persons. *C. albicans* is a transmigrant from the gut and can commonly be present asymptomatically in the vaginal tract. It is not uncommonly found during pregnancy or after antibiotic administration. It is usually associated with a pruritic vulva and a thick white "cheesy" discharge. The vulva may be inflamed and edematous. The discharge is usually not malodorous. The pH of the vagina is 4.2 to 5.0, and budding hyphae are observed in a saline wet-mount or 10% KOH wet-mount slide preparation.

Patients with *Trichomonas* often have a profuse gray or greenish discharge with a burning sensation in the vagina or have vulvar irritation or both. The vagina may demonstrate submucosal hemorrhage, the so-called strawberry spots. The discharge is malodorous and may have a frothy appearance. The pH of the vagina is usually 5.5 to 5.8, and motile parasites the size of a WBC are found in a saline wet-mount slide preparation.

Patients with *G. vaginalis* may be relatively asymptomatic with a profuse watery gray-to-white discharge with an unpleasant "fishy" odor. In a saline wet-mount slide preparation, the epithelial cells are stippled with gram-negative bacteria, the "clue cell."

PRINCIPLES OF THERAPY

Whether the complaint is new or recurrent, a review of normal vaginal physiology and hygiene is helpful in patient education, particularly for those individuals in whom no patho-

gens are found. In many cases the reassurance may be all the patient requires. *Trichomonas* responds very well to metronidazole (500 mg bid) in most cases. In those rare cases that do not respond, doubling the dose of metronidazole (1.0 gm bid) has usually been successful. A regimen of 2 gm in a single daily dose is effective, but the associated nausea is occasionally disconcerting. The treatment of *Candida* infection has been aided immensely by the development of miconazole nitrate and clortrimazole in cream or suppository form. Intravaginal candicides in 3- or 7-day courses are usually successful, however, the persistent or chronic-recurrent cases may require additional measures such as longer treatment periods of up to 4 to 6 weeks and premenstrual use as well as treatment through the menstrual period. Improvement of diabetic control in diabetic patients with vaginitis will be followed by a marked improvement in the recurrence pattern of the vaginitis. A 1% aqueous solution of gentian violet applied to the infected tissues may be very efficacious. However, occasionally contact allergy reactions may impair its effectiveness. In some patients with chronic recurrence an oral course of nystatin may be helpful in reducing an intestinal reinfecting source. The therapy for *G. vaginalis* with topically applied vaginal agents has largely been abandoned. Pfiefer and co-workers found metronidazole (500 mg bid for 7 days) to be very effective in eradicating symptoms (Pfeifer et al., 1978). Fleury (1981) found metronidazole (250 mg tid) to be successful in over 90% of cases.

HERPES

Many viruses can be transmitted to the genital tract and can produce symptoms and lesions. Herpes simplex belongs to a group of DNA viruses that can be transmitted by contact, produce intranuclear inclusions in infected cells, and produce symptoms at various intervals throughout the life of the infected host. Although there are two antigenic types, HSV-2 usually causes genital infections. After a 3- to 5-day incubation period, the characteristic herpes lesion is a vesicle surrounded by erythema. It is usually very painful. Several lesions may form and be associated with a secondary bacterial infection. The ulcer may be painful enough to require hospitalization. This ulcer is unlike the syphilitic ulcer, which is usually hard, raised, and painless. The primary attack of herpes may produce systemic symptoms including chills, fever, malaise, myalgia, adenopathy, and headache. Recurrent attacks will usually occur at the same site. The rate of recurrent attacks is extremely variable; the attacks can be triggered by such things as stress and menses.

DIAGNOSIS

Most cases can be diagnosed by the characteristic appearance of the herpetic ulcer. The most reliable laboratory procedure is a viral culture. The greatest number of isolates will be obtained from a lesion in the vesicular stage. Seriologic studies on sera from patients in an acute and a convalescent stage are useful, but many laboratories do not distinguish between type I and type II antibody.

PRINCIPLES OF THERAPY

Because herpes infections may coexist with other sexually transmitted diseases, they must be sought and concurrently treated. With the primary attack of herpes, supportive measures such as pain relief, combating secondary infection, bladder drainage, and occasionally hospitalization may be needed. Acyclovir both topically as well as systemically has been extremely helpful in aborting attacks and providing relief. Pregnant patients should have weekly virus cultures from 36 weeks until delivery. The presence of a positive culture within 1 week of delivery or active lesions at the time of labor may necessitate a cesarean section delivery for the safety of the infant. Because of the lifelong implications of herpes infection, patient education and support should be given. Because there is the implication of an association between HSV and genital cancer, annual Pap smears are strongly recommended.

GONORRHEA

In the United States in 1980 over 1 million cases of gonorrhea were reported, and it is estimated that another 1 to 1.5 million cases were not reported. It is found in association with *Chlamydia* in 15% to 25% of heterosexual men and in 30% to 40% of women infected with gonorrhea. In women the highest attack rate is in the 20- to 24-year age group with the second highest attack group in the 15- to 19-year age group.

The causative organism is the gram-negative, nonmotile diplococcus, *Neisseria gonorrhoeae*. The organism is aerobic, relatively fragile, and requires a pH of 7.2 to 7.6.

CLINICAL–PATHOLOGIC CORRELATIONS

After initial inoculation from an infected partner, the gonococci appear to attach to columnar epithelial cells by pili. They are engulfed by endocytosis and come to lie within the cell in membrane-enclosed vacuoles from which they are eventually expelled. This engulfment is less complete in the cervix than in the tubal epithelium. After movement toward the mucosal epithelium, damage to the tubal epithelium becomes evident with eventual formation of submucosal abscess and eventual transportation of the organism by blood or lymphatic systems. The average incubation period is 3 to 5 days. The presentation of symptomatic individuals depends on the organ involved and the degree of involvement. Over 60% of the infected women are asymptomatic. Symptoms in the lower genital tract may include dysuria and frequency as well as a creamy occasionally odorous mucopurulent cervicovaginal discharge. After 3 to 5 days, upper tract disease may become evident with lower abdominal pain, fever, adenexal tenderness, and an elevated WBC count. If untreated, the infection may progress to extensive tubal damage, pyosalpinx, pelvic abscess, and widespread involvement of the abdominal cavity including the upper abdomen and liver. Symptoms of gonorrhea infection may be difficult to differentiate from such entities as appendicitis, ovarian torsion, genitourinary infection, endometriosis, and dysmenorrhea. Long-term sequelae may include increased incidence of ectopic pregnancy, infertility, and chronic pelvic pain.

PRINCIPLES OF THERAPY

Many antibiotic regimens have been used in the treatment of uncomplicated gonococcus infection (Table 52–3). However, the common association of gonococcus infection with

TABLE 52–3.
Treatment Schedule for Syphilis and Gonorrhea

STAGE	TREATMENT ALTERNATIVES
SYPHILIS	
Primary, secondary, or latent, < 1 year	Benzathine penicillin G 2.4 million units, IM once or Aqueous procaine penicillin G 600,000 units, IM qid for 8 days or Tetracycline 500 mg PO for 15 days or Erythromycin 500 mg qid PO for 15 days
Latent, > 1 year, with cardiovascular effects	Benzathine penicillin G 2.4 million units, IM weekly for 3 weeks or Aqueous procaine penicillin G 600,000 units, IM OD for 15 days or Tetracycline 500 mg PO qid for 30 days or Erythromycin 500 mg PO qid for 30 days
Neurosyphilis	Crystalline penicillin G 12 million units per day for 10 days
Pregnancy	Same as in nonpregnant persons. Alternative is erythromycin stearate in schedule for nonpregnant persons
GONORRHEA	
Urethral/cervical	Aqueous procaine penicillin G 4.8 million units, IM plus probenecid 1 gm PO or Tetracycline 500 mg PO qid for 5 days
Penicillinase-producing *N. gonorrhoeae*	Spectinomycin 2 gm IM STAT

Chlamydia infection, as well as the emergence of penicillin-resistant strains, has led to the development of treatment strategies that have proved to be more successful. In culture-proven cases, aqueous procaine penicillin G (4.8 mU IM) with probenecid (1 gm orally 1 hour prior to penicillin therapy) has been effective in most cases. In those found to have a resistant penicillinase-producing strain, spectinomycin (2gm IM) is recommended. Because of the high association of *N. gonorrhoeae* and *Chlamydia*, many authorities recommend the addition of 7 days of tetracycline or doxycycline to the regimen. Follow-up cultures should be taken 4 to 5 days after the last dose of tetracycline or doxycycline. Rectal cultures should be taken from women following therapy because 30% of treatment failures are detected only by rectal culture regardless of whether anorectal infection was detected prior to therapy.

SYPHILIS

CLINICAL–PATHOLOGIC CORRELATIONS

Syphilis is the classic example of a sexually transmitted disease. Caused by *Treponema pallidum*, the infection occurs by inoculation from sexual contact with an infected person, entering through an abrasion in the skin or a moist mucous membrane. The earliest lesion is a chancre, which develops after an incubation period of 10 to 90 days with a mean of 21 days. It usually first appears as an indurated painless ulcer with associated regional lymphadenopathy. The chancre is usually single but may be multiple in atypical cases. The ulcer usually heals within 2 to 6 weeks if it is untreated.

If untreated, syphilis can progress to other stages. Secondary syphilis appears in several different forms within a few weeks to months. Variable systemic symptoms may appear including malaise, low-grade fewer, sore throat, headache, and adenopathy. The most striking manifestation is a generalized maculopapular rash with lesions that are circumscribed and sharply defined with a hyperpigmented or erythematous border. The rash may involve the palms and soles of the feet. Mucoid lesions are common. These secondary lesions reveal the treponema on dark-field microscopy examination and are infectious. Other manifestations include nephrotic syndrome, mild hepatitis, exudative tonsillitis, chorioretinitis, and diffuse lymphadenopathy. Patchy alopecia may appear, and raised, flat-topped lesions called condyloma lata may appear on the perineum. Although not seen very much in the antibiotic era, latent syphilis evidenced by serologic studies but having none of the traditional clinical manifestations may appear in various ways years later. Cardiac lesions of the aorta and heart may occur 10 to 30 years later with neurologic manifestations present in 1% to 2% up to 30 years later.

DIAGNOSIS

The differential diagnoses of ulcerated lesions include furuncles, staphylococcal pyodermas, abrasions, chancroid, herpes infection, granuloma inguinale, lymphogranuloma venereum, drug reaction, and cancer. The diagnosis of syphilis is made most accurately by examination of the exudate utilizing dark-field microscopy. Serologic studies are not much help in early stages of the infection. If the initial test for nonspecific VDRL is negative, it should be repeated at 1 week, 1 month, and 3 months. If it remains negative, syphilis can be exluded from the diagnosis. If the nonspecific venereal disease research laboratory (VDRL) test is positive, the more specific fluorescent treponemal antibody absorption (FTA-ABS) test is indicated to distinguish syphilis from other false-positive reactions caused by such conditions as lupus erythematosus. Patients with typical lesions and a VDRL either greater than or equal to 1:16 are considered to have secondary syphilis.

PRINCIPLES OF THERAPY

The main antibiotic in the treatment of syphilis continues to be penicillin (Table 52–2). In those allergic to penicillin, tetracycline or erythromycin may be used. The standard treatment for primary syphilis is benzathine penicillin G (2.4 million units, IM) at one time. For pregnant patients with penicillin allergy, erythromycin stearate should be used. The infants born of those mothers treated with erythromycin during pregnancy should be treated with penicillin after delivery.

CHLAMYDIA INFECTION

Although human diseases caused by *Chlamydia trachomatis* have been known since antiquity, only recently has the development of successful culture techniques allowed large-scale screening studies to be done. Because the *Chlamydia* organism is an obligatory intracellular parasite, it requires a replicative cycle that kills the host cells. Thus these organisms are considered pathogens and not part of the natural flora of either the male or female reproductive tracts. They do not, however, always produce clinically apparent infections.

CLINICAL–PATHOLOGIC CORRELATIONS

Chlamydia trachomatis has been found in less than 2% of asyptomatic men, but it has been found to be the causative organism in one-third to one-half of men with symptomatic nongonococcal urethritis. Other infections caused by this organism in men include epididymitis, prostatitis, proctitis, and Reiter's syndrome. *Chlamydia trachomatis* has been found in the cervical secretions of 60% to 70% of female partners of men with chlamydial nongonococcal urethritis, and therefore treatment of it should be included in treatment strategies. Infants who pass through an infected birth canal may develop conjunctivitis or pneumonia. Sexually active teenagers may have the highest rate of infection of any age group. An estimated 3 to 4 million Americans develop chlamydial infections each year.

In women, infected sites may include the urethra, cervix, and rectum. The organism appears to attack only squamocolumnar cells. Clinically the infection appears as a yellow mucopurulent discharge that may or may not be symptomatic. Examination of a vaginal smear of infected patients does not present a distinctive picture except for the abundance of WBCs. *Chlamydia trachomatis* is increasingly identified in pelvic inflammatory disease. The clinical symptoms often overlap with those of this gonococcus infection. There seems to be a species difference between the organisms that cause pelvic inflammatory disease (PID) and those that cause lymphogranuloma venereum.

DIAGNOSIS

The development of culture techniques has allowed the accurate identification of *Chlamydia* infections. However, they are expensive and time-consuming. An important item often overlooked is the use of calcium alginate swabs in the collection of specimens which improves accuracy of organism pick-up and transfer to culture plates. Cellular change in the Pap smear has been used as a diagnostic clue, but its accuracy is too low to be used for definitive diagnosis. The development of fluorescein monoclonal antibody testing of cervical secretions has proved to be an exciting advance with a specificity of 96% to 98% and a sensitivity of 93%. The rapid return of laboratory results makes the antibody testing a valuable tool for screening clinic patients.

PRINCIPLES OF THERAPY

Clinical trials have demonstrated the superior effectiveness of tetracycline hydrochloride, doxycycline, minocycline, erythromycin, and trimethoprim-sulfamethoxazole in achieving a cure rate of 85% to 95% in relieving symptoms. A treatment of at least 1 week is usually sufficient. Tetracycline (500 mg qid for 7 days), doxycycline (200 mg qid for 24 hours then 100 mg bid for 6 days), or erythromycin (500 mg every 12 hours for 14 days) seem to be very effective in eliminating cervicitis caused by *Chlamydia trachomatis*.

TOXIC SHOCK SYNDROME

The toxic shock syndrome was introduced to the public in the spring and summer of 1980 when the term was used to describe a syndrome that seemed to preferentially affect young menstruating women using tampons. Although thought to be related to a single brand of tampon, subsequent events have shown it to be related to other brands as well. In addition 16% of cases have been reported to have occurred in children, men, and women not menstruating. As of June 1983, 2204 cases had been reported with 92% associated with menstruation and 98% with tampon use. Among cases in nonmenstruating persons, skin lesions, surgical wound infection, and postpartum infections have been found.

DIAGNOSIS

The criteria for the diagnosis of a "definite case" of toxic shock included fever, rash, hypotension, and involvement of at least three organ systems with desquamation of skin 1 to 2 weeks after the illness (Table 52–4). A "probable" case lacked one of the above criteria. The cultures of blood, throat, and cerebrospinal fluid were negative. Strains of *Staphylococcus aureus* found in patients with this syndrome are generally of bacteriophage type 1 and are resistant to penicillin, cadmium, and arsenate. Two toxins found in over 90% of strains associated with toxic shock syndrome are pyrogenic exotoxin C and staphylococcal enterotoxin F.

CLINICAL–PATHOLOGIC CORRELATIONS

The typical clinical picture begins with an abrupt onset of fever often above 39°C accom-

---

TABLE 52–4.
Case Definition of Toxic Shock Syndrome

Fever: Temperature ≥ 38.9°C
Rash: Diffuse macular erythroderma
Hypotension: Systolic BP ≤ 90 mm Hg or orthostatic drop in diastolic BP ≥ 15 mm Hg from lying to
    sitting position, or orthostatic syncope
Multisystem involvement—three or more of the following:
    Gastrointestinal: Vomiting or diarrhea at the onset of illness
    Muscular: Severe myalgia or creatine phosphokinase level at least twice the upper limit of normal
    Mucous membrane: Vaginal, oropharyngeal, or conjunctival hyperemia
    Renal: Values for BUN or creatine at least twice the upper limit of normal or urinary sediment with
        pyuria (5 WBC/HPF) in the absence of urinary tract infection
    Hepatic: Total bilirubin, AST,* or ALT† values at least twice the upper limit of normal
    Hematologic: Platelet count ≤ 100,000/ml
    Central nervous system: Disorientation or alterations in consciousness without focal neurologic signs
        when fever and hypotension are absent
Negative† results of the following tests: Blood, throat, or cerebrospinal fluid cultures; rise in titer to Rocky
    Mountain spotted fever, leptospirosis, or rubeola

---

* AST = aspartate aminotransferase; ALT = alanine aminotransferase.
† Except for *Staphlococcus aureus.*

panied by vomiting or watery diarrhea. Complaints of headache, myalgia, sore throat, and abdominal pain are common. Severe illness is manifest by a rapid drop of blood pressure with the appearance of a diffuse sunburn-like rash. Peeling of the skin, most prominent on the palms and soles of the feet begins 5 to 14 days after the onset of the illness. The WBC count is usually elevated with a left shift, toxic granulation, and Döhle's inclusion bodies. There is a urinary pyuria and proteinuria, but urine cultures are generally sterile. Cervical secretions contain WBC with sparse gram-positive cocci. The liver function test values (BUN, creatine, and creatine phosphokinase) are elevated. Disseminated intravascular coagulation may occur as well as adult respiratory distress syndrome and cardiac dysfunction.

PRINCIPLES OF THERAPY

Treatment should consist of a search for focal staphylococcal infections. In women the vagina should be examined carefully looking for lesions and ulcers as well as removing any tampons and flushing out the vagina with saline or povidone-iodine to reduce the amount of organisms or toxins present. Aggressive therapy with colloidal fluids and electrolytes and other vigorous supportive therapy should be undertaken. Penicillinase-resistant semisynthetic penicillins such as nafcillin, methicillin, or oxacillin are of value in reducing local and systemic infection. Dopamine hydrochloride may be needed to maintain a low or normal blood pressure. Other supportive measures may include ventilatory support, hemodialysis, and digoxin.

REFERENCES

Cunningham F, Hauth J, Gilstrap L et al: The bacterial pathogenesis of acute pelvic inflammatory disease. *Obstet Gynecol* 1978; 52:161–164. *Good review of bacteriology of pelvic inflammatory disease.*

Davis JP, Chesney PJ, Wand PJ et al: Toxic-shock syndrome: Epidemiologic features, recurrence, risk factors and prevention. *N Engl J Med* 1980; 303:1429–1435. *Good discussion of toxic shock syndrome.*

Fleury FJ: Adult vaginitis. *Clin Obstet Gynecol* 1981; 24:407. *Treatment of gardnerella vaginitis with metronidazole.*

Gardner HL: Infectious vulvovaginitis, in Monif, G (ed): *Infectious Diseases in Obstetrics and Gynecology*, Hagerstown: Harper & Row, 1982, pp 515–541. *Excellent coverage of vulvovaginitis.*

Judson FN: The importance of coexisting syphilitic, chlamydial, mycoplasmal and trichamonal infections in the treatment of gonorrhea. *Sex Transm Dis* 1979; 6:112. *Points out the associations of these infections in sexually transmitted diseases.*

Knox JM, Rudolph AH: Acquired infectious syphilis, in Holmes KK, Mardh PA, Sparling PF, Wiesner PJ (eds): *Sexually Transmitted Diseases.* New York, McGraw-Hill Book Co, 1982, pp 305–313. *Excellent review of infectious syphilis.*

Lee R: Sexually transmitted infections, in Burrows G, Ferris T (eds): *Medical Complications During Pregnancy.* Philadelphia, WB Saunders Co, 1975. *Excellent overview of sexually transmitted diseases.*

Oriel JD: Genital warts. *Sex Transm Dis* 1977; 4:153–159. *Review article on genital warts.*

Pfeifer TA, Forsyth PS, Durfee MA et al: Nonspecific vaginitis. *N Engl J Med* 1978; 298:1429–1434. *Treatment of nonspecific vaginitis with metronidazole.*

Rein MF: Therapeutic decisions in the treatment of sexually transmitted diseases: An overview. *Sex Transm Dis* (suppl) 1981; 8:93–99. *Discusses treatment considerations in sexually transmitted diseases.*

Westrom L: Incidence, prevalence and trends of acute pelvic inflammatory disease and its consequences in industrialized countries. *Am J Obstet Gynecol* 1980; 138:880–892. *Reports from an international symposium on pelvic inflammatory disease.*

53 ACQUIRED IMMUNODEFICIENCY SYNDROME (AIDS)

Timothy B. Sorg, M.D.

The acquired immunodeficiency syndrome (AIDS), first reported in the United States in 1981, is caused by a retrovirus infection which damages the host's immune system. The degree of immunologic damage varies from no detectable change to almost total ablation of cellular immune function. Patients whose immune systems are severely impaired develop the opportunistic infections and malignancies, which define the clinical diagnosis of AIDS. The criteria for the diagnosis are listed in Table 53–1. AIDS is the most severe and possibly the least common clinical manifestation of this retroviral infection.

ETIOLOGY

The virus that causes AIDS was first isolated in 1983. French researchers at the Pasteur Institute named it lymphadenopathy-associated virus (LAV), while researchers in the United States at the National Institutes of Health called it human T-cell leukemia virus-III (HTLV-III). A subcommittee of the International Committee on the Taxonomy of Viruses recently recommended the name human immunodeficiency virus (HIV). Although the taxonomy and nomenclature of HIV are controversial, there is little doubt about its etiologic role in AIDS. Some investigators have suggested that cofactors such as drugs, cytomegalovirus, Epstein-Barr virus, and antigen overload are also involved, but it is clear that these factors are not necessary for the induction of AIDS. At most, these factors may increase the risk of an HIV infection developing into AIDS.

Human immunodeficiency virus has both a tropism for T_4- lymphocytes and a cytopathic effect (lysis) on these cells. It can also infect B-lymphocytes, macrophages, and brain tissue, and these cells may act as a reservoir for the virus in some patients. Like other retroviruses, HIV carries an enzyme called reverse transcriptase in its core along with the viral RNA. After the virus penetrates the host cell, the reverse transcriptase uses the viral RNA as a template to synthesize double-stranded DNA. This proviral DNA is then integrated into the host cell nuclear DNA. Expression of the viral DNA impairs the function of the cell by mechanisms that are under investigation. Unintegrated proviral DNA is also found in the cytoplasm of some lymphocytes and has been associated with the cytopathic effect. Therefore HIV infection can produce impaired T_4-lymphocyte function or lysis of the cell or an asymptomatic proviral state.

EPIDEMIOLOGY

The incidence of AIDS has continued to rise since the disease was first described, and its spread to the United States, Canada, Western Europe, central Africa, the Carribean, South America, and Australia has produced a pandemic. Lack of reporting from many Eastern European and African countries has made tracking difficult in those parts of the world.

The demographic characteristics of the epidemic vary in different areas of the world. Most of the cases in the United States and other Western countries have occurred in homosexual or bisexual males, intravenous (IV) drug abusers, and hemophiliacs who receive factor VIII concentrates. These high-risk groups were identified very early. Additional cases have occurred in patients who received blood transfusions from donors in the high-risk groups, and in children born to infected mothers. Heterosexual transmission has recently been reported in the United States, and the number of cases associated with heterosexual transmission is slowly increasing.

TABLE 53–1.
Definition of AIDS

1. The presence of a reliably diagnosed disease at least moderately predictive of cellular immunodeficiency

CANCERS

Kaposi's sarcoma
Primary lymphoma of brain
Non-Hodgkin's lymphoma of high-grade pathologic type and of B cell or unknown immunologic phenotype

PROTOZOAL AND HELMINTHIC INFECTIONS

Cryptosporidiosis, intestinal: Causing diarrhea for over 1 month
Isosporiasis: Causing diarrhea for over 1 month
Pneumocystis pneumonia
Strongyloidosis: Pneumonia, CNS infection, or disseminated infection*
Toxoplasmosis: Pneumonia or CNS infection

FUNGAL INFECTIONS

Aspergillosis: CNS or disseminated infection
Candidiasis: Esophagitis, bronchitis, or pneumonia
Cryptococcosis: CNS or disseminated infection
Histoplasmosis: Disseminated

BACTERIAL INFECTION

"Atypical" mycobacteriosis (species other than *Mycobacterium tuberculosis* or *M. leprae*): disseminated infection

VIRAL INFECTION

Cytomegalovirus: Pulmonary, gastrointestinal tract, or CNS infection
Herpes simplex virus: Chronic mucocutaneous ulcers persisting more than 1 month, or pulmonary, gastrointestinal tract, or disseminated infection

PROGRESSIVE MULTIFOCAL LEUKOENCEPHALOPATHY (PRESUMED PAPOVAVIRUS)

2. The absence of an underlying cause for immunodeficiency or of any defined cause for reduced resistance to the disease

3. Exposure to HIV, as evidenced by history or a positive serum-antibody test. In the absence of positive antibody test results, patients who satisfy all other criteria in the definition will continue to be diagnosed as AIDS.

*"Disseminated infection" is infection of lungs and multiple lymph node regions or other internal organs.

In contrast, less than 20% of the patients in central Africa and Haiti are in the high-risk groups identified in the West. Heterosexual contact is believed to be the primary mode of transmission in central Africa and the Carribean, where the disease is largely confined to the young, sexually promiscuous urban population and their children. Cases are almost equally divided between men and women, and infection is particularly prevalent among female prostitutes. Medical practices that involve re-use of unsterilized needles have also been implicated as a possible mode of transmission in these developing countries.

The epidemiologic data indicate that transmission is by exchange of blood or infected body secretions through intimate contact or intravenous infusion as follows: (1) homosexual and heterosexual intercourse, (2) the use of contaminated intravenous needles, (3) transfusion of contaminated blood or clotting factor concentrates, and (4) vertical transmission in utero or at birth. There is also one report of vertical transmission through maternal milk. The route of transmission of HIV is similar to that of hepatitis B, and control measures to prevent its spread are identical.

CLINICAL SIGNS AND SYMPTOMS

Human immunodeficiency virus infection produces a broad spectrum of clinical disease. Most persons infected with the virus are asymptomatic. Others develop a chronic, progressively debilitating disease. In others, the course is rapidly fatal after a prolonged incubation period. From ongoing serologic studies and clinical observations, four distinct clinical entities have been proposed: (1) acute viral syndrome, (2) asymptomatic infection, (3) AIDS-related complex (ARC), and (4) AIDS.

ACUTE VIRAL SYNDROME

Several investigators have described an acute illness resembling mononucleosis that is associated with HIV antibody seroconversion. Although only 14 cases of this syndrome have been reported, many others may have been missed or attributed to other viruses. Based on cases in which a probable inoculation date was identified, the incubation period appears to be 1 or 2 weeks.

Patients present with acute onset of fever, sweats, sore throat, myalgias, anorexia, headache, photophobia, and general malaise. The most common physical findings are generalized lymphadenopathy, splenomegaly, pharyngeal erythema, and a macular erythematous rash on the trunk. The acute illness lasts from 3 to 14 days and is followed by seroconversion in 2 to 8 weeks. Most patients recover completely, but their long-term prognosis remains uncertain.

ASYMPTOMATIC INFECTION

Serologic studies have identified a large population of patients in high-risk groups who are antibody-positive but who have no clinical evidence of disease. These patients often have mildly abnormal immunologic laboratory features such as low numbers of T_4-lymphocytes, but they lack the constitutional symptoms, weight loss, malignancies, and opportunistic infections, which characterize AIDS-related conditions.

Antibody seroconversion does not correlate with clearance of the virus. Several studies have shown that up to 80% of seropositive patients have had at least one blood culture positive for HIV. The 20% of seropositive patients who have negative cultures may have levels of viremia below the limits of detection, latent infection without viremia, or aborted infection and subsequent immunity. Because the retrovirus integrates its genetic code into the genome of the host cell and because brain cells are infected in addition to circulating blood cells, it is likely that many seropositive, culture-negative patients harbor the virus. The rate of virus recovery is higher among asymptomatic patients than among those with AIDS, probably because infected T_4 cells are more abundant in asymptomatic patients. Asymptomatic seropositive patients should be considered carriers and represent an important reservoir of the virus in the community. Unaware of their infection, they may continue their usual sexual activity.

AIDS-RELATED COMPLEX (ARC)

In the years before antibody testing was available, a narrow definition of AIDS was needed to exclude other causes of immunodeficiency from the epidemiologic data. It soon became evident that people infected with the virus present with syndromes that do not fit the current definition of AIDS. These patients present with lymphadenopathy and the chronic constitutional symptoms seen in AIDS, but they lack the malignancies and opportunistic infections necessary for a diagnosis of AIDS. The definition of AIDS may eventually be broadened to include these patients, but at present the term ARC is used to describe their condition.

The most common clinical manifestations of ARC are listed in Table 53–2. The clinical spectrum of ARC ranges from lymphadenopathy

TABLE 53–2.
Common Manifestations of AIDS-Related Complex (ARC)

CLINICAL FEATURES
Generalized lymphadenopathy
Fever > 38°C
Diarrhea (intermittent or constant)
Weight loss (>10% of normal body weight)
Night sweats
Oral candidiasis (recurrent or persistent)
LABORATORY FEATURES
Serum antibodies to HIV
Decreased numbers of T_4 cells
Decreased T_4/T_8 cell ratio
Lymphopenia, anemia, or thrombocytopenia
Elevated serum immunoglobulin levels
Skin-test anergy
Decreased lymphocyte proliferation response to lectins

alone to lymphadenopathy plus fever, refractory diarrhea, extreme fatigue, and progressive weight loss. ARC patients may be more susceptible to a broad range of infections that are not specific enough for cellular immunodeficiency to be included in the case definition of AIDS. These infections include reactivated or disseminated tuberculosis, shingles, oral candidiasis, amoebiasis, giardiasis, and persistent enteritis due to *Salmonella* or *Shigella*.

ACQUIRED IMMUNODEFICIENCY SYNDROME (AIDS)

AIDS is the end-stage result of profound damage to the immune system caused by HIV infection. The diagnosis of AIDS is a clinical one based on the presence of one of the diseases listed in Table 53–1 in a patient with no other cause for cellular immunodeficiency. The laboratory features of AIDS are given in Table 53–3.

AIDS was first recognized due to an outbreak of two rare diseases, pneumocystis pneumonia and Kaposi's sarcoma, in previously healthy homosexual males. These two diseases remain the most common initial presentations in AIDS patients, with pneumocystis pneumonia occurring in about 60% and Kaposi's sarcoma, either alone or with an opportunistic infection, in about 30% of AIDS patients. Kaposi's sarcoma is seen more frequently in homosexuals, whereas pneumocystis pneumonia is more prevalent among IV drug users and other high-risk groups. Patients who present with Kaposi's sarcoma alone seem to have higher T_4 cell counts and longer survival than those who present with opportunistic infections.

The clinical manifestations of AIDS in its more advanced stages are protean and reflect the many microbes against which these patients are defenseless. Many of these infections, especially *Pneumocystis carinii, Mycobacterium avium-intracellulare,* and *Cryptosporidium,* occur much more frequently in AIDS than in other types of cellular immunodeficiency. Some additional diseases that commonly occur in AIDS patients but are not part of the definition are listed in Table 53–4. Many diseases in AIDS patients, such as tuberculosis, cytomegalovirus infection, and toxoplasmosis result from reactivation of latent infection.

Knowledge of the natural history of AIDS is incomplete due to the relatively recent recognition of the syndrome and the long incubation period. The present information suggests that in most patients, seroconversion occurs 4 to 10 weeks after infection and may be associated with an acute viral syndrome. A small percentage of patients may be seronegative, healthy carriers for prolonged periods before seroconversion. Seroconversion is followed by an asymptomatic, seropositive carrier state. Preliminary studies of stored serum specimens from cohorts of seropositive patients have shown that 60% have remained asymptomatic for 4 to 6 years. Of the remaining patients, 20% to 25% have developed ARC, and 10% to 20% have developed AIDS. The average latency period between infection and the onset of AIDS is about 2 years, but the upper limit is unknown. Among the patients who do not develop clinical immunodeficiency, there may be long-term CNS effects of HIV infection that are not yet apparent.

At first ARC was considered to be a prodromal state of AIDS and was called "pre-AIDS." Many AIDS patients give a history of ARC symptoms for several months before the

TABLE 53–3.
Immunologic and Laboratory Abnormalities in AIDS

Serum antibody to HIV
Markedly decreased numbers of T_4 cells and T_4/T_8 cell ratio
Absolute lymphopenia
Elevated serum immunoglobulin levels with an inability to mount a serologic response to new infection
Skin-test anergy
Anemia
Thrombocytopenia
Circulating immune complexes
Antilymphocyte antibodies

TABLE 53–4.
Clinical–Pathologic Correlations for the Presumed Findings Primary Manifestations of HIV Infection

CLINICAL FINDINGS	PATHOLOGIC FINDINGS
Susceptibility to opportunistic pathogens	Depletion and dysfunction of T_4-lymphocytes resulting in decreased lymphokine production; macrophages have diminished ability to kill parasites, and B-lymphocytes are unable to mount a serologic response to new infection
Susceptibility to unusual tumors	Decreased cytotoxic lymphocyte and natural killer-cell function
Fever	Spontaneous secretion of interleukin-1 by macrophages
Lymphadenopathy	*Early:* Follicular hyperplasia with plasmacytosis *Late:* Lymphoid depletion
Diarrhea: Weight loss	Malabsorption with jejunal villous atrophy, crypt hyperplasia, and increased intraepithelial lymphocytes
Anemia	Findings consistent with anemia of chronic disease
Nephrotic syndrome	Focal and segmental glomerular sclerosis
Dementia	Cortical atrophy; perivascular and parenchymal inflammatory cell infiltration

first opportunistic infection is recognized. Other patients have had ARC as a stable condition for years, and there have been anecdotal reports of improvement. Patients occasionally succumb to the debilitating effects of ARC, even though malignancy or opportunistic infection are not found on autopsy.

There have been no reports of recovery from AIDS. Given effective therapy, most patients have a good prognosis for recovery from the initial infection, but progressive deterioration and death due to malnutrition and multiple infections usually follow within 2 years. Patients who present with Kaposi's sarcoma alone may survive up to 5 years.

PATHOPHYSIOLOGY

T-lymphocytes play a central role in regulating the immune system. Most mature T cells can be divided into subsets based on antigens expressed on the cell surface. These antigens are identified by monoclonal antibodies directed against them. Two of these antigens are mutually exclusive; the OKT_4 antigen is expressed on cells with helper/inducer function (T_4 cells), and the OKT_8 antigen is expressed on cells with suppressor/cytotoxic function (T_8 cells). Although the correlation between surface antigens and cell function is not absolute, in general T_4 cells function by recognizing specific antigens and stimulating the effector cells (B cells, cytotoxic T cells, macrophages, and natural killer cells) of the immune system.

AIDS patients suffer from a number of immunologic abnormalities including a decreased lymphocyte proliferative response to a specific antigen, decreased lymphokine production by T cells, decreased cytoxic lymphocyte function, decreased natural killer-cell function, decreased serologic response to new infection, and decreased killing by macrophages. All of these abnormalities may be explained by selective HIV infection of the essential regulatory cell, the T_4 lymphocyte. On the other hand, the defects in B cell and macrophage function may be the direct result of HIV infection of these effector cells. These hypothetical mechanisms are the subject of intense investigation.

CLINICAL–PATHOLOGIC CORRELATIONS

The pathologic features and clinical manifestations of AIDS are the result of both the direct effects of HIV infection and the effects of multiple opportunistic infections and unusual malignancies. Tables 53–4 and 53–5 represent an attempt to make the difficult distinction between the primary and secondary effects. Only the more common clinical findings and pathogens are listed.

TABLE 53–5.
Clinical–Pathologic Correlations for the Manifestations Presumed to be Secondary to Immunodeficiency

CLINICAL FINDINGS	PATHOLOGIC FINDINGS
Diffuse pulmonary infiltrates	*Pneumocystis carinii, Mycobacterium avium-intracellulare, Mycobacterium tuberculosis, Cryptococcus,* Kaposi's sarcoma, *Legionella,* cytomegalovirus (CMV)
Skin lesions	
Purple macules	Kaposi's sarcoma
Vesicles	Herpes zoster
Mucocutaneous ulcers	Herpes simplex
Fever	Multiple infections
Lymphadenopathy	Kaposi's sarcoma, lymphoma, disseminated *Mycobacterium avium-intracellulare, Cryptococcus,* CMV
Esophagitis	*Candida,* herpes simplex, CMV
Diarrhea: Enteritis	*Cryptosporidium, Entamoeba histolytica, Giardia, Shigella, Salmonella, Campylobacter, Isospora belli,* Kaposi's sarcoma, *Mycobacterium avium-intracellulare*
Meningitis, encephalitis, dementia	*Cryptococcus, Toxoplasma gondii,* papovavirus (progressive multifocal leukoencephalopathy), CMV, primary large-cell lymphoma, Kaposi's sarcoma, aspergillosis, *Strongyloides*
Decreased visual acuity, retinal exudates	CMV, *Toxoplasma gondii, Cryptococcus*

DIFFERENTIAL DIAGNOSIS

Other causes of immunodeficiency that lead to similar opportunistic diseases and preclude the diagnosis of AIDS include corticosteroid therapy, malnutrition, immunosuppressive or cytotoxic chemotherapy, organ transplantation, lymphoma, and leukemia. The congenital immunodeficiencies that most closely resemble AIDS in pediatric patients are adenosine deaminase and purine nucleoside phosphorylase deficiency. In infants, congenital infections with *Toxoplasma gondii,* herpes simplex virus, and cytomegalovirus must be excluded to diagnose AIDS.

DIAGNOSIS

The diagnosis of any clinical syndrome associated with HIV infection is aided by a history of sexual contact with an AIDS patient or high-risk individual, IV drug use, blood transfusion from an infected donor, or the use of factor VIII concentrates. Several commercial ELISA (enzyme-linked immune sorbent assay) tests for antibody to HTLV-III (HIV) are now available to help confirm contact with the virus. Culture of the virus is not routinely available, and there are no tests for viral antigen in the blood. The currently licensed ELISA tests for antibody are estimated to be 95% sensitive and 99% specific for HIV infection. When false-positive results are suspected, the more specific Western blot assay may be done for confirmation. It must be stressed that a positive ELISA or Western blot test does not diagnose ARC or AIDS.

ARC remains a clinical diagnosis based on the presence of two or more of the signs and symptoms listed in Table 53–2 in the context of exposure to HIV. The symptoms should be present for 3 months or more without another identified cause. The laboratory tests in Table 53–2 are characteristic, but, other than the serum antibody test, are nonspecific. The clinical diagnosis of AIDS is also based on the presence of any disease listed in Table 53–1, the absence of another cause for immunodeficiency, and exposure to HIV. The laboratory tests in Table 53–3 are helpful in the diagnosis, but are not yet part of the definition of AIDS.

PRINCIPLES OF PREVENTION AND THERAPY

Present therapy for AIDS consists of supportive care and treatment for the secondary infections and tumors. There is no effective treatment for

HIV infection or the immune deficiency, but research is being done to find inhibitors of viral replication, immune modulators, and a vaccine. Preliminary clinical trials with azidothymidine, an inhibitor of reverse transcriptase, have produced encouraging results, but bone marrow toxicity is a common side-effect of the drug. Regular injections of gamma globulins appear to prolong life in pediatric AIDS patients.

At this point, prevention rests on educating the public on modes of transmission of the virus.

REFERENCES

Cooper DA, Gold J, Maclean P et al: Acute AIDS retrovirus infection: Definition of a clinical illness associated with seroconversion. *Lancet* 1985; 1:537–540. *The most complete description of the acute viral syndrome.*

DeVita VT Jr, Hellman S, Rosenberg SA (ed): *AIDS; Etiology, Diagnosis, Treatment and Prevention.* Philadelphia, JB Lippincott Co, 1985. *The most recent and complete textbook on the subject.*

Gallin GI, Fauci AS (eds): *Advances in Host Defense Mechanisms: Acquired Immunodeficiency Syndrome.* New York, Raven Press, 1985. *A recent textbook with good chapters on the epidemiology and the immunology of AIDS and the opportunistic infections and Kaposi's sarcoma in AIDS.*

International Conference on Acquired Immunodeficiency Syndrome. April 14–17, 1985, Atlanta, Georgia. *Ann Intern Med* 1985; 103(5):653–773. *The most recent comprehensive review of AIDS with particularly interesting articles on virology, natural history, immunology, and antibody tests.*

Kotler DP, Gaetz HP, Lange M et al: Enteropathy associated with the acquired immunodeficiency syndrome. *Ann Intern Med* 1984; 101(4):421–428. *A description of the enteropathy thought to be a primary manifestation of infection with the AIDS virus.*

Krensky AM, Lanier LL, Engleman EG: Lymphocyte subsets and surface molecules in man. *Clin Immunol Rev* 1985; 4(1):95–138. *An overview of lymphocyte surface antigens and their functional correlations.*

Norman C: AIDS therapy: New push for clinical trials. *Science* 1985; 230:1355–1358. *The sixth in a series of articles on AIDS research in Science, this article reviews current strategies for developing treatment and a vaccine.*

Pardo V, Aldana M, Colton RM et al: Glomerular lesions in the acquired immunodeficiency syndrome. *Ann Intern Med* 1984; 101(4):429–434. *A description of the renal lesions seen in AIDS.*

Seligmann M, Chessl, Fahey JL et al: AIDS—an immunologic reevaluation. *N Engl J Med* 1985; 311(20):1286–1292. *A review of the immunologic abnormalities in AIDS.*

Welch K, Finkbeiner W, Alpers CE et al: Autopsy findings in acquired immune deficiency syndrome. *JAMA* 1984; 252(9):1152–1159. *The most complete review of autopsy and histologic findings.*

54

PARASITIC DISEASES

Barrett H. Bolton, M.D.

Parasitic diseases are widespread and are caused by a wide variety of micro- and macroorganisms that live off their hosts, damaging them in the process. The damage is done in three major ways: first, by competing with the host for nutrients or by consuming host tissues; second, by damaging host tissues in the process of penetration, migration, or taking up residence; and third, by inducing immunologic reactions which result in consequent tissue damage.

The ability of parasites to damage the host, and the specific nature of that damage, depends on their number, size, life cycle, migratory habits, persistence, and capacity to reproduce and multiply in the host, on the host's response to their presence, and on their ability to resist the host's attempt to destroy or get rid of them.

The host's age and general nutritional status, as well as repeated exposure, influence the pathogenicity of many parasites. Although few parasitic diseases are common in most of the United States, they are almost universal in most of the less affluent areas of the world. Table 54–1 lists the estimated prevalence of some common parasitic diseases and infections.

CLINICAL SIGNS AND SYMPTOMS

The patient's history varies with the nature of the invading parasite. Infestations may be found incidentally as a result of routine screening examinations of blood or feces. Initial complaints by the patient such as of diarrhea, abdominal cramps or pain, nausea, vomiting,

TABLE 54–1.
Prevalence and Common Drug Treatments of Some Common Parasitic Diseases

PARASITIC DISEASE	CASES WORLDWIDE (MILLIONS)	DRUG TREATMENT
Ascariasis	650–1,000	Mebendazole or pyrantel pamoate
Hookworm infection	450–750	Mebendazole or pyrantel pamoate
Enterobiasis	450	Mebendazole or pyrantel pamoate
Trichuriasis	350–600	Mebendazole
Amebiasis	300	Iodoquinole with or without metronidazole
Filariasis	250–500	Diethylcarbamazine
Schistosomiasis	200	Praziquantel
Malaria	177	Chloroquine or quinine, primaquine, or pyrimethamine
Cestodiasis	65	Niclosamide
Dracunculosis	50	Niridazole or metronidazole
Strongyloidiasis	35	Thiabendazole
Opisthorchosis	19	Praziquantel
American trypanosomiasis	10	Nifurtimox
Fasciolopsiasis	10	Praziquantel, bithionol, or tetrachloroethylene
Trichostrongyliasis	5.5	Thiabendazole or pyrantel pamoate
Paragonimiasis	3.2	Praziquantel or bithionol

anorexia, weight loss, fever, cough, hemoptysis, various rashes, headache, seizures, somnolence, edema, and dyspnea can be attributed to many common illnesses, as well as to parasitic infestation. The geographic location, living situation, and dietary habits of the patient are the factors most likely to lead the physician to suspect a parasite as a cause of a patient's symptoms.

Most parasitic exposure is endemic. In areas of endemic malaria, this disease may be the most likely cause of fever. Chagas' disease (South American trypanosomiasis) may be the cause of acute heart failure, dyspnea, acute pulmonary edema, peripheral edema, and 30% of acute deaths in young patients in areas where this disease is endemic. Worldwide, the most common cause of iron-deficiency anemia with its attendant signs and symptoms is hookworm infestation.

Pruritis ani in children is likely caused by enterobiasis. Infestation with *Giardia, Isospora, Strongyloides, Schistosoma, Fasciolopsis* (intestinal flukes), or tapeworms may cause diarrhea that persists past the few days more commonly found with toxins or gastrointestinal viral illness. Paragonimiasis is a leading cause of hemoptysis in endemic areas.

Physical signs of infestation include periorbital edema (from trichinosis or other immunologically stimulating infestation), unilateral edema of the eyelid (Romaña's sign) in Chagas' disease, chorioretinitis from toxoplasmosis, and conjunctivitis from onchocerciasis. Subcutaneous swellings occur with *Loa loa* infestation (Calabar swellings) and with *Echinococcus* infestation. Lymphatic swelling in the posterior cervical nodes (Winterbottom's sign) is seen in African trypanosomiasis.

Onchocerciasis may lead to hyperpigmentation of the face and ears, whereas kala-azar (visceral leishmaniasis) is characterized by hyperpigmentation over the cheeks, mouth, and temples. Dermatitis is characteristic of schistosomal infestations immediately after the cercariae penetrate the skin; *Ancyclostoma, Strongyloides, Dracunculus,* and *L. loa* infestations may cause local skin reactions early or late in the course of the disease.

Splenomegaly is often seen in malaria, the trypanosomiases, filariasis, and leishmaniasis, and occasionally in a great many other parasitic diseases.

TABLE 54–2.
Some Potentially Lethal Parasitic Diseases

OFTEN FATAL
Malaria
Trypanosomiasis
American
African
Amebiasis
Leishmaniasis
Mucocutaneous
Visceral
Schistosomiasis
Philippine capillariasis
OCCASIONALLY FATAL
Ascariasis
Trichinosis
Liver flukes
Tapeworms
Echinococcosis
Angiostrongyliasis
SOMETIMES FATAL IN IMMUNOCOMPROMISED HOSTS
Pneumocystis carinii infection
Toxoplasmosis
Strongyloidiasis

The natural history of parasitic diseases varies from death at one extreme to spontaneous disappearance of the disease as reinfection ceases or as the patient's defenses control the disease and the patient leaves the endemic area. Table 54–2 lists potentially lethal parasitic infections.

PATHOPHYSIOLOGY

All organ systems can be infected by one or another parasite. Particular organs are affected by the penetration of the host (skin, gastrointestinal (GI) tract), by the migration of the parasite within the host (GI tract, lung), by the final residence (all organs), and by the body's reaction to the parasite (skin, reticuloendothelial system, lymphatics). Table 54–3 lists the organs affected and the parasites commonly involved with each system. Because all organs may occasionally be affected by many different parasites in individual patients, this table cannot be a comprehensive treatment.

The clinical–pathologic correlations are described in Table 54–3, the manifestation of each disease depending on the organ involved.

TABLE 54–3.
Clinical–Pathologic Correlations for Parasitic Diseases

CLINICAL FINDINGS	PATHOLOGIC FINDINGS	
	PARASITES	PATHOGENESIS
GENERAL		
Fever	*Plasmodium* (malaria), leishmaniasis (kala-azar), amebiasis, fascioliasis, trypanosomiasis (Chagas' disease), filiariasis	Hemolysis, tissue invasion and necrosis, migration of parasites, secondary bacterial infection, lymphangitis, destruction of parasites, rarely hypothalamic damage
Weight loss	Most parasites at some stages	Consumption of nutrients in the GI tract, hypermetabolic state with fever, anorexia with less food intake
Anorexia	Most parasites	Elaboration of toxic breakdown—metabolites from parasite or tissue destruction, swelling of liver or edema of GI tract
EYE		
Blindness	*Onchocerca, Ascaris, Toxocara, Cysticercus*	Ocular tissue invaded; opacification of humors; choroid and retinal infestation with inflammatory reactions such as iritis and keratitis
Pain	*Loa loa* and parasites that cause blindness	Migrates across conjunctiva
Conjunctivitis	*Onchocerca;* fly maggots (myiasis)	Microfilariae invade conjunctivae; deposition of larvae
Periorbital swelling	*Trypanosoma cruzi*	Chagas' disease produces unilateral lid swelling or Romaña's sign.
	Trichinella	Bilateral periorbital edema may be due to vasculitis.
Chorioretinitis	*Toxoplasma, Entamoeba histolytica*	Choroid and retina infected and heal with scarring and atrophy
EAR, NOSE, THROAT		
Sinusitis	*Naegleria*	Protozoan penetrates paranasal sinuses of swimmers and divers; may penetrate brain.
CARDIOVASCULAR		
Myocarditis	*Trypanosoma cruzi* (Chagas' disease)	American trypanosomes invade myocardium producing inflammation and heart failure.
Tachycardia	African and American *Trypanosoma,* malaria, most parasites causing fever or anemia	Direct myocardial invasion, especially involving cardiac conduction; producing fever or anemia
PULMONARY		
Asthma	*Ascaris,* visceral larva migrans, *Strongyloides*	Migration through lungs; hypersensitivity to parasite
Hemoptysis	*Paragonimus westermani*	Infiltration and cyst formation in lungs with erosion of blood vessels
Cough	*Schistosoma* (all three types), *Echinococcus, Strongyloides*	Irritate bronchial mucosa
Pneumonia	*Ascaris, Pneumocystis carinii*	Migration or interstitial invasion in immunocompromised host
GASTROINTESTINAL		
Diarrhea	*Amoeba, Balantidium coli, Giardia*	Invasion and ulceration of intestinal mucosa
	Leishmania donovani	In kala-azar, invades submucously
	Taenia solium and *Taenia saginata* (tapeworm)	Invade villi and irritate mucosa

TABLE 54–3.
Clinical–Pathologic Correlations for Parasitic Diseases *(continued)*

CLINICAL FINDINGS	PATHOLOGIC FINDINGS	
	PARASITES	PATHOGENESIS
GASTROINTESTINAL		
	Necator americanus (hookworm), *Trichurus trichiura* (whipworm)	Mechanical irritation from mucosal invasion
	Strongyloides	Local irritation of bowel
	Trichinella	Invade submucosa and intestinal wall
	Schistosoma mansoni, Schistosoma japonicum	Migrate to intestinal mucosal and submucosal tissues; egg deposition especially irritating
	Fasciolopsis buski	Attach and grow on mucosa producing local mechanical and toxic irritation
Melena	*Strongyloides*	Duodenal and jejunal irritation with heavy infestation, rarely causes upper GI bleeding to the point of melanotic stools
Pruritis ani	*Enterobius vermicularis* (pinworms)	Nocturnal perianal migration of worms leads to itching, scratching, and reinfection
Jaundice	*Plasmodium* (malaria)	Hemolytic jaundice
	Schistosoma, Fasciola hepatica	Blockage of biliary passages by heavy infestation with liver flukes or schistosomes may lead to obstructive jaundice
Intestinal obstruction	*Ascaris*	Heavy infestation may lead to intestinal blockage from a bolus of worms, local irritation, and intestinal edema; occasional peritonitis from perforation
Hepatitis	*Entamoeba histolytica*	Infiltrates liver, retrograde from duodenum; rarely produces hepatitis from local reactive inflammation
Hepatomegaly	*Plasmodium* (malaria), *Leishmania donovani, Echinococcus, Schistosoma, Fasciola*, any parasite that invades the liver	Diffuse biliary invasion by *Schistosoma* and *Fasciola*; parenchymal invasion by *L. donovani, Toxoplasma*, and malaria; cyst formation by hydatid disease *(Echinococcus)*
Nausea and vomiting	Most parasites	Toxicity from tissue destruction or death of parasites systemically or in GI tract
Abdominal pain	Any intestinal parasite	Systemic toxic reactions and tissue invasion
Ascites	*Schistosoma mansoni, Schistosoma japonicum*	Liver invasion leads to fibrosis and portal hypertension.
	Leishmania donovani	Kala-azar leads to hepatomegaly and fibrosis or nutritional cirrhosis.
Steatorrhea	*Giardia*	Upper intestinal inflammatory reactions lead to fat malabsorption.
GENITOURINARY		
Hemoglobinuria	*Plasmodium* (malaria)	Severe hemolysis in blackwater fever
Hematuria	*Schistosoma haematobium*	Bladder invasion
Chyluria	*Filaria*	Disruption of obstructed lymphatic varices with lymph spillage into urine
Proteinuria	*Plasmodium* (malaria)	May occur in blackwater fever or in nephrotic syndrome; rarely associated with malaria
Orchitis, funiculitis, epididymitis	*Filaria*	Invasion of lymphatics with consequent lymphangitis
Urethritis, vaginitis	*Trichomonas vaginalis*	Heavy infestation of vagina (or urethra in men) causes local inflammatory reaction

TABLE 54–3.
Clinical–Pathologic Correlations for Parasitic Diseases *(continued)*

CLINICAL FINDINGS	PATHOLOGIC FINDINGS	
	PARASITES	PATHOGENESIS
DERMATOLOGIC		
Ulcers	*Leishmania*	Several species of *Leishmania* produce ulcers; *Leishmania tropica* causes "Oriental sore."
	African *Trypanosoma*	Ulcers may appear at sites of inoculation
Nodules	*Dermatobia hominis* (botflies)	Burrowing into skin produces myiasis.
	Taenia solium, Echinococcus	Subcutaneous cysts in some patients
	Trypanosoma	Winterbottom's sign with lymphadonitis in posterior neck
Dermatitis	*Sarcoptes scabiei, Pediculus, Schistosoma, Loa loa, Ascaris, Leishmania, Dracunculus*	Mechanical irritation, hypersensitivity to parasite; penetration of skin or residence in skin and subcutaneous tissues leads to local inflammatory reaction.
Urticaria	*Schistosoma, Strongyloides,* most parasites causing eosinophilia	Hypersensitivity reaction
LYMPHATIC		
Edema	*Trichinella spiralis, Filaria, Trypanosoma, Necator* (hookworm), *Fasciolopsis, Taenia* (tapeworm)	Orbital edema due to hypersensitivity (Chagas' disease, trichinosis); leg, scrotal, and vulvar edema by *Filaria* late in disease course; many parasitic infections that interfere with ingestion or absorption of nutrients result in edema of legs and body because of hypoproteinemia and malnutrition.
Lymphadenopathy	*Filaria*	Invade lympathics and migrate centripetally
Lymphangitis	*Trypanosoma*	May lead to generalized lymphadenopathy
HEMATOLOGIC		
Anemia	*Necator, Ancylostoma* (hookworm)	Most common cause of iron-deficiency anemia worldwide; worms ingest blood from intestinal wall
	Plasmodium (malaria)	Hemolysis
	Taenia (tapeworm), *Fasciola, Schistosoma*	Cause anemia by interfering with nutrition
Leukopenia	*Leishmania*	Kala-azar involves the reticuloendothelial system and often causes leukopenia.
	Plasmodium (malaria)	During afebrile periods, associated with some leukopenia; hypersplenism may contribute.
Splenomegaly	*Plasmodium* (malaria)	Related to hemolysis and stimulation of reticuloendothelial system, phagocytosis of abnormal RBCs and fragments
	Leishmania, Trypanosoma	Generalized lymphatic hypertrophy includes the spleen.
	Schistosoma	Leads to portal hypertension and consequent splenomegaly
Eosinophilia	Helminths [*Strongyloides, Trichinella,* visceral larva migrans, *Necator, Ancylostoma* (hookworm), *Filaria, Schistosoma, Fasciolopsis, Toxocara, Trichurus, Ascaris, Taenia* (tapeworm)]	Eosinophilia is to some degree immunologically induced; tissue-dwelling worms stimulate greater degree of esophilia than gut-dwelling parasites.

TABLE 54–3.
Clinical–Pathologic Correlations for Parasitic Diseases *(continued)*

| CLINICAL FINDINGS | PATHOLOGIC FINDINGS | |
	PARASITES	PATHOGENESIS
NEUROLOGIC		
Coma	*Plasmodium* (malaria), *Trypanosoma, Amoeba naegleria,* cysticercosis, *angiostrongylus*	Parasites that invade the CNS may produce cerebral edema from cerebritis or meningoencephalitis, leading to coma
Convulsions	Organisms that cause coma; *Schistosoma, Ascaris, Trichinella, Echinococcus, Coenurus*	Parasites whose eggs embolize to the CNS may form cysts in the CNS, which may cause seizures; seizures may accompany coma.
Headaches	Organisms that cause coma or convulsions	Parasites that cause fever, systemic toxicity, or hypersensitivity reactions may cause headache as a nonspecific response to illness.

DIFFERENTIAL DIAGNOSIS

The differential diagnosis of parasitic disease includes virtually all medical diseases because parasitic infestation may be confused with, and coexist with, other infections and with neoplastic, toxic, or degenerative diseases.

DIAGNOSIS

The diagnosis of parasitic diseases is based on identification of the parasite or of its serologic or other effects. Stool examinations for intestinal protozoa and helmithic worms, larvae, or eggs may be by flotation or sedimentation concentrations, or stained specimens on microscopic slides. In general, stool examinations need to be carried out by experienced technologists. Stool specimens obtained after purging may be more likely to provide diagnosis.

Blood films stained with Wright's or Giemsa stains are used to identify malaria parasites, trypanosomes, and microfilariae.

Biopsy specimens of spleen, liver, or bone marrow are often used to establish a diagnosis for leishmaniasis, of rectal mucosa for schistosomiasis, of lung for *Pneumocytis carinii,* of nodules for trypanosomiasis, and of muscle for *Trichinella spiralis.*

Aspirations of the duodenal contents may be needed to establish a diagnosis of giardiasis or *Strongyloides* or *Ancylostoma* infestation.

Cellophane tape is used to collect eggs from the perianal area for recognition of *Enterobius* and *Taenia* infestation.

Vaginal or urethral smears may be diagnostic for *Trichomonas vaginalis.*

Intradermal skin tests have been developed for filarial leishmaniasis and trichinosis as well as for echinococcosis (Casoni's intradermal test). Only the *Trichinella* skin test is available commercially; the others, prepared by individual laboratories in endemic areas, have variable reliability.

The immunologic reactions of the host to the invading parasite are not only part of the problem of infestation causing immunologic symptoms such as urticaria, glomerulonephritis, fever, hypotension, and other systemic toxicity, but have been exploited in the development of diagnostic tests measuring nonspecific and specific changes in serum. The nonspecific tests include quantitating the level of euglobulins which are increased in kala-azar, malaria, trypanosomiasis, schistosomiasis, and mycobacterial infections. The more specific tests include complement fixation tests used in the diagnosis of toxoplamosis, Chagas' disease (Machado test), schistosomiasis, trichinosis, leishmaniasis, and paragonimiasis and hemagglutination tests which are of value in amebiasis, malaria, echinococcosis, hydatid disease cysticercosis, fascioliasis, filariosis, and strongyloidiasis.

Indirect immunofluorescence may be used to diagnose African trypanosomiasis, leishmaniasis, malaria, pneumocytis, schistosomiasis, and toxoplasmosis. Enzyme-linked immune sorbent assay (ELISA) tests are used for diagnosing ascariasis, and toxocariasis. Bentonite flocculation, cholesterol-lecithin flocculation, immunodiffusion, and counter-current electrophoresis are also serologic techniques available for the investigation of some parasitic as well as some bacterial diseases. Availability of these tests depends on the endemicity of the parasitic disease and the sophistication of the local laboratory. In the United States, the Centers for Disease Control in Atlanta, Georgia, and some state public health laboratories have the widest number of tests available with evaluations of their specificities and sensitivities.

PRINCIPLES OF PREVENTION AND TREATMENT

Some drug treatments of the more common parasitic infections are outlined in Table 54–1. Many patients will have more than one parasite, and some of the drugs will effectively treat several infestations. Some parasites have to be removed surgically, such as *Anisakis* and the filariae, *L. loa*, and *Onchocerca*, or by filtration of portal blood, such as schistosomes. Encysted parasites may require surgical excision when located in critical areas such as cysticercosis of the central nervous system. Surgery

may be used to relieve edema in elephantiasis from filarial infections.

Prophylactic treatment is conventional and valuable in preventing malaria, but the cost and risk–benefit considerations of prophylactic treatment are disputed or uncertain in other diseases. Because of the nature of parasitic diseases, small populations such as families or large populations such as countries or regions have been considered suitable for mass, universal treatment without establishing a diagnosis in each person. These decisions to treat large groups of patients have been very complex, and the knowledge necessary to implement them with confidence is often unavailable and practically unobtainable. The prevalence of infection, risk, and effectiveness of treatment, consequences of failed treatment, cost, and compliance of populations all influence treatment decisions.

For personal prevention, the time-honored principles of caution include adequate cooking of meats, avoidance of both raw fruits that cannot be peeled and leafy vegetables, avoidance of biting insects such as mosquitoes, fleas, sandflies, and lice, and avoidance of swimming or wading in fresh waters that harbor cercariae of *Schistosoma*. These measures and others are included in advice to travelers, are different for each area of travel or residence, and may change as old diseases decrease in prevalence and new infestations are introduced or spread.

REFERENCES

Beck JW, Davies JE: *Medical Parasitology*, ed 3. St Louis, CV Mosby Co, 1981. *Another well-illustrated and brief textbook with tables; chapters on specimen preparation.*

Benenson AS (ed): *Control of Communicable Diseases in Man*, ed 14. Washington, D.C., The American Public Health Association, 1985. *The classic handbook outlining identification, transmission, occurrence, incubation periods, and methods of control of all communicable diseases.*

Drugs for parasitic infections. *The Medical Letter on Drugs and Therapeutics*, Jan 31, 1986; 28(Issue 706):9–16. *An authoritative, periodically updated source of currently recommended drugs that are treatments for parasitic diseases.*

Markell EK, Voge M: *Medical Parasitology*, ed 5. Philadelphia, WB Saunders Co, 1981. *An excellent brief text describing clinically important parasitic diseases with memorable illustrations.*

Strickland GT (ed): *Hunter's Tropical Medicine*, ed 6. Philadelphia, WB Saunders Co, 1984, part VI, Protozoa infections; part VII, Helmenthic infections. *A major text with discussions of each parasitic infection: life cycle, pathologic changes, and treatment.*

Warren KS, Mahmoud AAF (eds): *Tropical and Geographical Medicine*. New York, McGraw-Hill Book Co, 1984. *A recent excellent text with clinical, pathophysiologic, and therapeutic treatment of the parasitic diseases.*

55

TUBERCULOSIS

Howard P. Liss, M.D.

Tuberculosis is a systemic infection that primarily affects the lungs and is caused by the bacterium *Mycobacterium tuberculosis*. Although any organ system can be infected, the most common extrapulmonary sites are the lymph nodes, pleura, genitourinary tract, and bone. About 15% of tuberculosis cases have only extrapulmonary infections.

The distinction between tuberculous infection and disease rests in the presence or absence of clinical disease. In a tuberculous infection, there is no clinical evidence of disease and no positive culture after exposure to *M. tuberculosis*, but delayed hypersensitivity to a protein component develops and is indicated by an induration of at least 10 mm in response to an intermediate purified protein derivative (PPD) skin test. Tuberculosis, the disease, exists when there is clinical evidence of disease involving one or more organ systems, with or without symptoms.

CLINICAL SIGNS AND SYMPTOMS

Most patients with tuberculosis are symptomatic, although the symptoms are not necessarily bothersome. The onset of the illness is usually insidious with cough and sputum production. Eventually fever, night sweats, weight loss, and malaise develop and may last weeks to months. Patients who develop hemoptysis usually seek medical attention.

The medical history may reveal illnesses that increase the risk of tuberculosis, such as uncontrolled diabetes mellitus, alcoholism, malnutrition, or silicosis. The latter may result from occupational exposure to silica as in such jobs as sandblasting, coal mining, and rubber and insulation manufacturing.

Examination of the chest may reveal rales or bronchovesicular or bronchial breath sounds. Even with far advanced disease, the physical findings of a lung examination may be minimal or absent. Fever, malnutrition, weakness, or a toxic appearance may be present. If pleuritic chest pain, decreased breath sounds, and dullness to percussion are present, pleural tuberculosis should be suspected.

Signs and symptoms of extrapulmonary tuberculosis usually reflect the organ system involved. In addition, fever and weight loss may be present. The sites involved in extrapulmonary tuberculosis and their frequency are listed in Table 55–1.

Tuberculosis develops in only 5% to 15% of those infected with *M. tuberculosis*. Reactivation of an old tuberculous infection accounts for 85% to 90% of cases. The remaining patients have a progressive primary infection. Clues that an active case is a primary infection include (1) a known, new, significant (> 10-mm induration) response to PPD tuberculin

TABLE 55–1.
Sites of Extrapulmonary Tuberculosis*

SITE	EXTRAPULMONARY CASES (%)
Lymph nodes	20
Miliary	20
Genitourinary tract	18
Bones and joints	15
Meninges	9
Gastrointestinal tract and peritoneum	8
Adrenal gland	3
Pericardium	3
Miscellaneous	4
(Larynx, skin, otitis media, female genitalia, male genitalia)	

* Based on Alvarez S, McCabe WR: Extrapulmonary tuberculosis revisited: A review of experience at Boston City and other hospitals, *Medicine* 1984; 63:25–55.

skin test within the last 2 years, (2) pleural effusion, (3) hilar adenopathy, (4) isolated lower-lobe disease, and (5) a history of recent contact with someone known to have pulmonary tuberculosis.

M. tuberculosis may reactivate in infected patients at any time. The risk of reactivation varies with the extent of the primary infection, the adequacy of treatment, how recently the person was infected, and other underlying illnesses (Table 55–2).

PATHOPHYSIOLOGY

Virtually all infections occur by inhaling droplet nuclei that contain three or fewer bacteria, which are produced when a patient with active tuberculosis coughs, sneezes, sings, or talks. The airborne droplet nuclei are less than 10 μ in diameter and settle in a respiratory bronchiole or alveolus. Alveolar macrophages phagocytize the inhaled bacilli but may not be able to kill them. The organisms then remain viable and multiply within the macrophages. Four to six weeks after the initial infection, caseous necrosis occurs, leaving a focus composed of lipids and proteins from dead macrophages and bacilli. *M. tuberculosis* cannot grow well within the caseous focus but continues to grow intracellularly in the macrophages surrounding the necrotic area. During this early stage, a small number of bacilli disseminate throughout the body via the lymphatics and bloodstream. Usually at this stage, immunity develops, resulting in a decreased number of organisms and eventual scarring of the granuloma. Because the organisms may not be completely eradicated, pulmonary and extrapulmonary sites of infection may remain inactive for years.

Delayed hypersensitivity develops simultaneously with caseation and is responsible for the induration resulting from intracutaneous injection of PPD tuberculin. This is the earliest evidence of a tuberculous infection. Because the initial infection is usually asymptomatic, it is only discovered if the patient has periodic skin tests.

Tuberculosis develops when a primary focus of infection is not contained or a dormant focus reactivates and begins to grow. When either progression or reactivation occurs, the caseous focus liquefies with intense multiplication of

---

TABLE 55–2.
Risk for Reactivation and Indications for Preventive Therapy of Tuberculosis

CATEGORY	REACTIVATION PER YEAR (%)	PREVENTIVE THERAPY
Significant skin test (induration of ≥ 10-mm diameter) and chest x-ray films compatible with active tuberculosis (includes those with past history of tuberculosis who received inadequate chemotherapy)	0.5–5.0	Yes
New Infection a. Skin test conversion from non-significant to significant within 2 years b. Induration of 5–10-mm diameter in a person in close contact with someone with a recently diagnosed case of active tuberculosis	2.0–4.0*	Yes
Significant skin test of unknown duration and normal chest x-ray films	0.07	Only if younger than 35 years
Significant skin test plus a clinical situation with increased risk of tuberculosis (silicosis, diabetes mellitus, malnutrition or rapid weight loss, immunosuppressive drugs such as corticosteroids, immunosuppressive disease such as lymphoma, chronic hemodialysis, acquired immunodeficiency syndrome (AIDS), AIDS-related complex, or presence of antibody to human T-lymphocyte virus type III)	Unknown	Yes

* Highest risk present 1 to 2 years after infection.

M. tuberculosis. At this point, spread of the infection can take place in several ways. Contiguous spread within an organ occurs primarily in the lung. The softened material is coughed into a bronchus and spread to other airways, leaving a residual cavity with a tremendous number of viable, extracellular, rapidly growing bacilli. The disease can also spread from one organ to another, such as from the lungs to the pleura or to a paravertebral abscess, from the cerebral cortex to the meninges, or from the mediastinal lymph nodes to the pericardium. Epithelial spread may take place as *M. tuberculosis* is shed from a site of active infection and seeds other epithelial surfaces, for example, spread to the larynx and pharynx via infected sputum. Dissemination can also occur through the lymphatics to hilar, mediastinal, or cervical nodes. Finally, a caseous focus can erode into a blood vessel, resulting in miliary tuberculosis.

TABLE 55–3.
Clinical–Pathologic Correlates of Common Sites of Tuberculosis

SITE	CLINICAL FINDINGS	PATHOLOGIC FINDINGS
Lymph nodes	Localized or generalized adenopathy (especially cervical and supraclavicular), draining sinuses, asymptomatic neck mass	Most common sites are cervical and supraclavicular nodes. Liquifecation in nodes causes fluctuance and "cold" abscess which may drain into neck or throat producing chronic draining sinus tracts.
Miliary	Fever, weakness, malaise, coma, abdominal pain (variable presentation)	Hematogenous spread of organisms throughout body, lodging in alveolar septae. Seen on chest x-ray as 2-mm discrete nodules by 6 weeks. Bacterial emboli occur in many tissues and organs.
Genitourinary tract	Hematuria, pyuria, flank pain, costovertebral angle tenderness, frequency, urgency	Infection begins in renal cortex. Foci of organisms spread to tubules, renal papilla, ureter, and bladder. Cortical abscess, papillary necrosis, ureteral scarring, hydronephrosis, and ulceration of trigone area.
Bones and joints	Leg weakness, paraplegia, back pain, gibbous deformity of thoracic spine	In the spine, fusing of vertebral bodies and loss of joint space are seen. Collapse of vertebral bodies leads to spinal deformities. Granulomatous inflammation of bones (marrow, cortex, periosteum, and epiphyseal plate) and joints (synovium).
Central nervous system, meninges	Seizures, bizarre behavior, stiff neck, lethargy, ataxia, confusion	Cerebral cortex, cerebellum, or spinal cord involved. Any lesion undergoing liquefaction necrosis can slough into an adjacent ventricle or subarachnoid space, leading to meningitis. Lesions often seen at base of brain, circle of Willis, optic chiasm, and sylvian fissures.
Gastrointestinal tract	Nausea, vomiting, and abdominal distention, small bowel obstruction, diarrhea, ascites, anal fistula	Granulomatous inflammation may cause either ulcerative disease in the lower ileum or thickened wall and narrowed lumen in the cecum.
Pleura	Shortness of breath, pleuritic chest pain, pleural friction rub	Exudative, high protein, lymphocytic pleural effusion. Rarely empyema. Pleural fluid often sterile. Granulomatous inflammation seen on pleural biopsy.
Lung	Fever, cough, sputum, hemoptysis	Ghon complex—Healed primary infection along with calcified hilar or paratracheal lymph node Cavity—Area of liquefaction necrosis. Material is expectorated.

CLINICAL–PATHOLOGIC CORRELATIONS

The characteristic finding in tuberculosis is the caseating granuloma. This is an area of necrosis surrounded by epithelioid histiocytes, Langerhans' giant cells, and an outer ring of lymphocytes. Special stains may show acid-fast bacilli. Tuberculous granuloma of the liver are noncaseating and do not have a central area of necrosis. This pattern may occasionally be seen in other tissues. Table 55–3 lists the clinical signs and pathologic findings of the common sites of extrapulmonary tuberculosis.

DIFFERENTIAL DIAGNOSIS

The incidence of tuberculosis is declining. In addition, its clinical presentation may mimic many other illnesses. Because turberculosis has a vast differential diagnosis, its diagnosis is often missed or delayed.

Cavitary bacterial pneumonias and septic pulmonary emboli are usually seen as acute illnesses. Tuberculosis, especially when it presents in the lower lobe, is more readily confused with anaerobic lung abscess. A negative reaction of sputum to stains for acid-fast bacilli and a response to penicillin indicate a nontuberculous infection. Tuberculosis may also be confused with fungal pneumonias, especially those caused by *Histoplasma capsulatum*, *Blastomyces dermatitidis*, and *Cryptococcus neoformans*. Fungal cultures, serologic studies, and stains of bronchoscopy specimens may be necessary to confirm the diagnosis. Differentiation from *Mycobacterium kansasii* and *M. avium intracellular*, the common atypical mycobacteria causing lung disease, rests on studies of the cultured sputum or bronchoscopy specimens. Tuberculosis can also mimic many noninfectious pulmonary diseases. Necrotizing bronchogenic carcinoma, pulmonary metastases from extrapulmonary sites, Wegener's granulomatosis and other systemic vasculidites, eosinophilic pneumonia, and sarcoidosis are diagnosed by examination of sputum cytology or lung biopsy.

Chest x-ray findings of a pleural effusion, miliary pattern, hilar or mediastinal lymphadenopathy, pericardial effusion, kyphoscoliosis, and upper-lobe fibrosis can all be seen with thoracic tuberculosis, but each pattern suggests other diseases as well. An upper lobe infiltrate, with or without cavitation, is seen in only two-thirds of patients.

Catastrophic results may occur if miliary tuberculosis is not recognized. Patients are often quite ill, and the results of the skin tests and sputum examination may not be diagnostic. Treatment should be started immediately if the

TABLE 55–4.
Fluid Smear and Culture in Tuberculosis

SOURCE OF FLUID	POSITIVE AFB SMEAR (% OF CASES)	POSITIVE AFB CULTURE (% OF CASES)	CHARACTERISTICS
Peritoneal cavity	0–2	63–69*	Protein > 3.0 gm/dL Lymphocytes > 50% of cells WBC > 100 cells/mm³
Urine	Not done†	76–90	Pyuria and/or hematuria
CSF	20–37	40–69	Protein > 60 mg/dL Glucose < 40 mg/dL WBC > 40 cells/mm³ Lymphocytes > 50% of cells
Pleural cavity	7–20	24–36*	Protein > 3.0 gm/dL LDH > 200 IU Glucose > 50 mg/dL Lymphocytes > 50% of cells

* At least 500 to 1000 ml of fluid should be concentrated for culture.
† Urine AFB smears are not recommended because saprophytes in the urine yield false-positive findings.

diagnosis is suspected. With severe spinal involvement, immediate neurosurgical intervention is indicated because of the risk of cord compression and severe neurologic sequelae.

DIAGNOSIS

The definitive diagnosis of tuberculosis rests on the culture of *M. tuberculosis* from a body fluid or tissue. The usefulness of sputum smear and culture depends on the severity of the lung involvement. In mild cases, multiple samples of sputum may be negative, whereas in severe, cavitary disease, negative samples of sputum eliminate tuberculosis from consideration.

A presumptive diagnosis of extrapulmonary tuberculosis can be made if caseating or noncaseating granuloma are seen on tissue biopsy in the appropriate clinical setting. Caseating granuloma or acid-fast organisms in tissue or fluid are stronger evidence of tuberculosis. Noncaseating granulomas are less specific and can be seen in sarcoidosis, syphilis, berylliosis, histoplasmosis and other fungal illnesses, and brucellosis. If acid-fast bacilli are seen in fluid or tissue, tuberculosis can also be strongly suspected. Cultures of fluid and tissue are important to differentiate tuberculosis from infections with atypical mycobacteria. Tables 55–4 and 55–5 list commonly biopsied tissues and fluids and their usefulness in diagnosing extrapulmonary tuberculosis.

Skin testing identifies more than 90% of those infected with *M. tuberculosis*. A significant reaction is defined as an induration of at least 10 mm diameter at 48 to 72 hours after intracutaneous injection of 0.1 ml (5 units) of PPD tuberculin. Induration less than 10 mm may be caused by delayed hypersensitivity to the atypical mycobacteria that cross-react with PPD. Induration of 5 to 10 mm diameter is significant in known contacts of a patient with active tuberculosis.

However, a significant response to a skin test implies infection with *M. tuberculosis*, not active disease. Between 5% and 25% of patients with active tuberculosis have nonsignificant skin tests, and up to 5% have selective anergy to PPD. Other factors that cause anergy include immunosuppression by drugs or steroids, malnutrition, malignancy such as lymphoma, and overwhelming infection. Thus a nonsignificant skin test, with or without positive controls (*Candida*, mumps) does not rule out active tuberculosis, and a significant response to a skin test does not mean active disease. The response to intermediate-strength PPD (5 units) must always be interpreted in light of the clinical situation. Table 55–6 lists the clinical–immunologic correlations of different reactions to PPD.

Standard posterior-anterior and lateral chest x-ray films indicate the location, extent, and activity of disease. In two-thirds of the cases of advanced disease, upper-lobe cavitary lesions are present with marked parenchymal destruction. The patterns in the films of the remaining

TABLE 55–5.
Tissue Culture and Histopathology in Tuberculosis

SITE OF EXTRAPULMONARY DISEASE	GRANULOMA AND/OR AFB IN BIOPSY SPECIMEN (% OF CASES)	POSITIVE AFB CULTURE (% OF CASES)
Pleura	56–64	55–88
Peritoneal cavity	64–100*	67
Liver†‡ (miliary)	76–100	0–8
Bone marrow† (miliary)	15–40	40–50

* The yield of positive results with peritoneal biopsies is lowest with Cope biopsies and reaches 100% if done with peritoneoscopy or laparotomy.
† Liver and bone marrow biopsies should be considered if miliary tuberculosis is suspected.
‡ Caseation necrosis is more specific for disseminated tuberculosis. Noncaseating granulomas are formed in a variety of nontuberculous diseases such as sarcoidosis, syphilis, berylliosis, histoplasmosis, or brucellosis. In addition, noncaseating granulomas of the liver are present in 25% of patients with isolated pulmonary tuberculosis.

TABLE 55–6.
Clinical–Immunologic Correlations of PPD Tuberculin Skin Tests in Tuberculosis and Tuberculosis Infections

CLINICAL FINDINGS	IMMUNOLOGIC FINDING
Significant skin test (> 10 mm induration)	Delayed hypersensitivity to a protein component of the tubercle bacillus Microscopic capillary dilatation, fluid exudation, perivascular infiltrate of lymphocytes and macrophages
Doubtfully significant skin test (induration of 5–9-mm diameter)	Delayed hypersensitivity to a protein component of an atypical mycobacterium with cross-reaction to PPD
Nonsignificant skin test reaction: Specific anergy to PPD	Inhibited response of sensitized T-lymphocyte due to circulating adherent suppressor mononuclear cells in active disease
Other causes of negative reaction	No infection Poor antigen, administration, or reading of skin test
Generalized anergy to PPD and other skin tests	Overwhelming infection (miliary tuberculosis) Malnutrition Waning hypersensitivity of old age Immunosuppression by drugs (corticosteroids) Immunosuppression by disease (lymphoma, viral infection, lymphoma)
Booster effect (nonsignificant skin test becomes significant with repeated testing 1 week later)	Waning delayed hypersensitivity of old age First test may stimulate an immune response and increase the reaction of the repeat test. This does *not* indicate a new infection.

cases show pleural effusion, lower- or middle-lobe disease, solitary or multiple tuberculoma, hilar or mediastinal lymphadenopathy, or a miliary pattern.

Between 10% and 40% of patients with extrapulmonary tuberculosis have concomitant pulmonary tuberculosis. The incidence is lowest in osseous and genitourinary tuberculosis and highest in pleural and peritoneal disease. Another 30% to 50% of patients have chest x-ray film evidence of a previous tuberculosis infection.

PRINCIPLES OF PREVENTION AND THERAPY

Patients with suspected pulmonary tuberculosis, especially if cavitary, should be isolated until the diagnosis is confirmed and treatment is started. Isolation consists of a private room and the use of face masks by the patient and personnel entering the room. Ultraviolet light in the patient's room will diminish the aerosolized bacillary load.

Infectivity diminishes rapidly once therapy is started, and patients need not be hospitalized until smears and cultures are negative. The usual length of stay is 2 weeks, although patients who are well and excreting small numbers of bacilli in their sputum need to be hospitalized for a short time, if at all. Patients who are quite ill may require 1 to 2 months of hospitalization. Patients with extrapulmonary tuberculosis may require hospitalization but do not need isolation unless concomitant pulmonary tuberculosis exists.

The goal of treatment in cases of tuberculous infection or tuberculosis is eradication of the organism with antituberculosis chemotherapy. Two factors play a role in therapy. First, the mutation rate to drug-resistant forms of *M. tuberculosis* is 10^{-5} to 10^{-7} per drug. In active cavitary disease, at least 10^8 bacilli are present, so therapy must include at least two drugs to prevent an overgrowth of resistant organisms. Second, *M. tuberculosis* grows slowly and can remain dormant but viable within the macrophages. To ensure killing all the pathogens, standard therapy with two bactericidal drugs (isoniazid, 300 mg qd, and rifampin, 600 mg qd) must be given for 9 months. With this regimen, the sputum smears and cultures of 95% of patients should convert to negative by 4 months, and the relapse rate should be 0% to 2%.

Certain patients with a tuberculous infection who have an increased risk of developing tuberculosis are candidates for preventive therapy with isoniazid, 300 mg qd for a year. Because fewer bacilli are involved in infection than in active disease, one-drug therapy does not lead to drug-resistant organisms. Table 55–2 lists candidates for preventive therapy. The benefits of administering isoniazid is counterbalanced by the risk of isoniazid hepatitis, which ranges from 0.3% in adults up to age 35 years, to 2.3% in adults older than 50 years. Patients with a significant skin test of unknown duration and a normal chest x-ray are not given preventive therapy. An exception is made if the patient is age 35 years or younger. This group has minimal risk for isoniazid hepatitis, while their risk of developing tuberculosis, although small, is lifelong. They should receive preventive therapy.

REFERENCES

Alvarez S, McCabe WR: Extrapulmonary tuberculosis revisited: A review of experience at Boston City and other hospitals. *Medicine* 1984; 63:25–55. *An excellent clinical review of extrapulmonary tuberculosis.*

American Thoracic Society: Treatment of tuberculosis and other mycobacterial diseases. *Am Rev Respir Dis* 1983; 127:790–796. *Guidelines for treatment of active tuberculosis and preventive therapy.*

Khan MA, Kornat DM, Bachus B, Whitcomb ME, Brody JS, Snider GL: Clinical and roentgenographic spectrum of pulmonary tuberculosis in the adult. *Am J Med* 1977; 62:31–38. *Reviews the variety of x-ray film presentations of tuberculosis in the chest.*

Reichman LB: Tuberculin skin testing. *Chest* 1979; 76:7645–7705. *Explains how to do, read, and interpret tuberculin skin tests.*

Sahn SA, Neft TA: Miliary tuberculosis. *Am J Med* 1974; 56:495–505. *Review of clinical features, pathogenesis, diagnosis, and therapy of miliary tuberculosis.*

Stead WW: Pathogenesis of the sporadic case of tuberculosis. *N Engl J Med* 1967; 22:1008–1012. *Discusses the concept that sporadic cases of tuberculosis are due to reactivation of an endogenous focus, not reinfection.*

Stead WW, Dutt AL (eds): Tuberculosis. *Clin Chest Med* 1980; 1:167–284. *A series of articles on all aspects of tuberculosis, including epidemiology, pathogenesis, treatment, immunology, and extrapulmonary tuberculosis.*

Wolinsky E: Tuberculosis, in Baum GL, Wolinsky E (eds): *Textbook of Pulmonary Diseases,* ed 3. Boston, Little, Brown & Co, 1983, pp 507–572. *A thorough review of all aspects of tuberculosis.*

56

HISTOPLASMOSIS

H. Bradford Hawley, M.D.

Histoplasmosis is an illness caused by infection with the dimorphic fungus *Histoplasma capsulatum*. The organism was first recognized as a cause of disease in humans by a U.S. Army pathologist, Samuel Taylor Darling, in 1905 while performing an autopsy on a Panama canal worker thought to have died from miliary tuberculosis. Darling observed small, round or oval bodies, mostly intracellular, in tissue smears from lungs, spleen, and bone marrow. He believed the organism was a protozoan. A few years later Henrique de Rocha-Lima noted that the microorganism was more similar to a yeast than to *Leishmania donovani*. *Histoplasma capsulatum* was first isolated from a soil sample obtained at the entrance to a rat hole next to a chicken house in West Virginia by C. W. Emmons in 1948. Subsequent studies confirmed the association between bird droppings and also bat droppings and positive soil cultures. Several large epidemics have been described; a recent epidemic in Indianapolis associated with the construction of a major sports complex is estimated to have involved as many as 100,000 people.

Primary infection occurs in the lung following the inhalation of spores from the soil. By correlating radiographic pulmonary calcification and skin tests, Amos Christie, a Vanderbilt University pediatrician, concluded that the vast majority of infected patients have a benign pulmonary illness which heals without treatment. In some patients, however, the infection can become disseminated and progressive in multiple organ systems.

CLINICAL SIGNS AND SYMPTOMS

Light exposure usually results in a totally asymptomatic illness. Inhalation of greater numbers of spores may result in a respiratory illness with fever, myalgias, headache, and nonproductive cough commencing about 2 weeks after infection. Exposure to construction sites, chicken houses, bird roosts, and bat-infected caves or attics may have occurred 10 to 23 days prior to the onset of symptoms. If the acute form assumes a more severe course with dissemination, the patient may complain of high fever, chills, abdominal distention, diarrhea, and dyspnea.

Chronic disease may develop. Cavitary pulmonary disease and mediastinal fibrosis can result in complaints of chronic cough, dyspnea, chest pain, weight loss, and the superior vena cava obstruction syndrome. Ocular involvement can lead to decreased vision.

A reactivation type of disseminated disease can occur in the immunocompromised patient. The symptoms are similar to those previously described as associated with the more severe, acute histoplasmosis.

In acute pulmonary histoplasmosis, the results of the chest examination are usually normal. Basilar rales are occasionally present, and dullness to percussion may be noted if a small pleural effusion occurs as a result of pulmonary infection or as a complication of pericarditis. In more severe, acute cases, hepatosplenomegaly will often occur. Gastrointestinal involvement may be heralded by abdominal distention, hyperactive bowel sounds, and positive stool guaiac tests. Erythema nodosum or erythema multiforme occasionally occur and are more often observed in young women.

The results of the physical examination in chronic cases depend on the organs involved, with weight loss or oropharyngeal ulcers being particularly common findings. Hepatosplenomegaly is unusual, and fever is either nonexistent or intermittent.

Over 90% of *Histoplasma* infections are asymptomatic. Symptomatic primary infection is occasionally recognized in young children and only rarely in adults. These individuals usually recover in a few days to 3 weeks without significant clinical sequelae. Radiographic signs in the form of small calcifications may be observed later particularly in the lung fields, mediastinal lymph nodes, and spleen. Although rare, primary infection may progress, particularly if the exposure is heavy, the patient is immunocompromised, or chronic pulmonary disease is present. Disseminated disease is usually fatal in the immunocompromised patient and is occasionally fatal in normal hosts if no treatment is given. The chronic pulmonary disease appears to progress more in association with the underlying pulmonary disease than with the *Histoplasma* infection.

Amphotericin B and ketoconazole are curative for severe or disseminated disease in most instances. Chronic cavitary pulmonary disease may benefit from chemotherapy with these agents or from surgical resection.

Mediastinal fibrosis occurs rarely following infection with *Histoplasma* and can obstruct bronchi, the superior vena cava, pulmonary veins, pulmonary arteries, or esophagus in decreasing order of frequency. The complications can be serious, particularly bilateral pulmonary venous obstruction. Surgical relief of the symptomatic obstruction can sometimes be helpful.

A form of chorioretinitis has been attributed to the immunologic response occurring as a result of earlier *Histoplasma* ocular infection. The cause of this illness remains controversial. The course of retinal involvement is quite variable; progressive disease can be treated using laser techniques.

DIAGNOSIS

Histoplasmosis can be easily overlooked if a history of exposure is not elicited and the possibility is not considered in the febrile patient. In the United States the illness is endemic to the Central states following the Ohio and Mississippi Rivers, and the possibility of infection should be considered more strongly in natives or travelers in these states. A febrile illness in an immunocompromised patient should also arouse suspicion.

The histoplasmin skin test is a useful epidemiologic indicator, but it is not helpful in disease diagnosis. Furthermore, it may falsely elevate the serologic antibody titers for several weeks making the interpretation of these important tests impossible.

Chest x-ray films in cases of acute disease may reveal scattered pulmonary infiltrates, hilar adenopathy, and, rarely, pleural effusion. Hepatosplenomegaly may be evident with scanning procedures.

Direct observation of the yeast-phase in silver methenamine-stained tissue smears can provide immediately useful diagnostic information. Mediastinal lymph nodes and liver are most useful for such histopathologic studies. The yeast can occasionally be seen in Giemsa or Wright's stains of peripheral blood from patients with disseminated infection. Culture for fungus of biopsy specimens of any organs and the bone marrow provides the specific diagnosis in up to 70% of the patients with disseminated histoplasmosis. It is rare for the organism to be isolated from blood, but newer lysis-centrifugation culture methods are increasing the detection rate and decreasing the recovery time. Cerebrospinal fluid, preferably 8 ml or more, should be cultured if meningitis is suspected. Cultured material is usually placed on Sabouraud agar or other enriched media and takes 10 to 14 days to grow.

Infection can usually be documented by serologic evidence. Fungal immunodiffusion tests are positive in 88% of patients, and complement-fixing antibodies are found in 94% of patients. The immunodiffusion tests detect precipitating antibodies against the H and M protein antigens of histoplasmin. H bands are associated with acute infection, and M bands are associated with both acute and chronic infection. The complement-fixation tests detect titratable antibodies directed against both yeast and mycelial forms. Antibodies develop in 4 weeks. Titers of 1:8 or greater against either phase are considered presumptive evidence of histoplasmosis. Titers above 1:32 or those showing a fourfold or greater rise are considered strongly presumptive. As previously stated, skin tests can produce falsely elevated antibody titers as detected by either immunodiffusion or complement fixation.

DIFFERENTIAL DIAGNOSIS

As was the case with Darling's original patient, histoplasmosis is often confused with tuberculosis and other mycobacterial diseases. Neoplasms, particularly lymphomas, can result in febrile illnesses with lymphadenopathy, pulmonary infiltrates, and organomegaly, which can be difficult to distinguish from the findings in histoplasmosis on the basis of clinical and radiographic information. Immunologic pulmonary illnesses, especially sarcoidosis, mimic histoplasmosis. Acquired immune deficiency syndrome and its associated neoplasms and infections can be confused with or complicated by histoplasmosis. Lastly, histoplasmosis must be considered in the differential diagnosis in any immunocompromised patient with a fever or in any patient with a fever of unknown origin particularly if there is a history of recent exposure, residence, or travel in an endemic area.

PATHOPHYSIOLOGY

Spores from fungus growing in the soil or in droppings are inhaled and deposited in human alveoli and bronchioles. In a few days the spores germinate into yeasts, which are ingested by macrophages. In the nonimmune host the yeast proliferate within the macrophages. Spreading then occurs via the lymphatic channels, bloodstream, bronchi, and direct extension to adjacent tissue.

Cellular immunity develops in about 2 weeks, and healing begins. A granulomatous hypersensitivity develops similar to that seen in tuberculosis. There are all gradations of severity in both the infection and the immunologic response. Inhalation of relatively few spores and a normal immune response results in asymptomatic illness without residual disease. Heavy exposure or poor immune responsiveness can allow for progression and dissemination of the infection. An overly zealous immune system may produce mediastinal fibrosis.

Reinfection or reactivation of infection occasionally occurs. Reactivation of infection in a patient who is immunosuppressed as a consequence of illness or therapy can occur resulting in a febrile, multisystem illness.

TABLE 56–1.
Clinical–Pathologic Correlations for Histoplasmosis

CLINICAL FINDINGS	PATHOLOGIC FINDINGS
Fever	Endogenous pyrogens from macrophages stimulate hypothalmic thermoceptors
Cough	*Acute:* Infection results in alveolar exudate stimulating cough reflex
	Chronic: Cavity infection with exudate fibrosis with obstruction
Malaise and weakness	Altered metabolic state with infection rarely
	Addison's disease if adrenal severely involved (decreased cortisol secretion)
Abdominal distention	Hepatosplenomegaly with disseminated infection
	Intestinal ulceration from spread of infection by macrophages
	Occasionally, peritonitis secondary to bowel perforation from ulceration
	Rarely, obstructive at terminal ileum
Diarrhea (stool often positive for occult blood)	Intestinal ulceration
Disorientation	Central nervous system infection (meningitis)
Dyspnea	Pulmonary parenchymal infection with exudate
	Pulmonary fibrosis
	Obstruction of bronchi by enlarged mediastinal lymph nodes or fibrosis
	Hepatosplenomegaly with decreased diaphragmatic excursion
	Pleural effusion (rarely significant)

CLINICAL–PATHOLOGIC CORRELATIONS

The clinical signs and symptoms result both from infection with *Histoplasma* and the immunologic response to the infection (see Table 56–1).

PRINCIPLES OF THERAPY

The usual asymptomatic or mild primary infection requires no specific therapy. Progressive or disseminated histoplasmosis is treated with amphotericin B or ketoconazole. Obstructive complications may occasionally benefit from surgical treatment.

REFERENCES

Bonner JR, Alexander WJ, Dismukes WE, et al: Disseminated histoplasmosis in patients with the acquired immune deficiency syndrome. *Arch Intern Med* 1984; 144:2178–2181. *A descriptive review of an opportunistic infection in AIDS patients.*

Goodwin RA, Jr, Des Prez RM: Histoplasmosis. *Am Rev Respir Dis* 1978; 117:929–956. *Excellent general discussion.*

Goodwin RA, Loyd JE, Des Prez RM: Histoplasmosis in normal hosts. *Medicine* 1981; 60:231–266. *An extensive review including the pathogenesis, with 290 references.*

Goodwin RA, Nickell JA, Des Prez RM: Mediastinal fibrosis complicating healed primary histoplasmosis and tuberculosis. *Medicine* 1972; 51: 227–246. *A retrospective study of 38 cases.*

Goodwin RA, Jr, Owens FT, Snell JD, et al: Chronic pulmonary histoplasmosis. *Medicine* 1976; 55: 413–452. *A summary of a 20-year prospective study.*

Goodwin RA, Jr, Shapiro JL, Thurman GH, et al: Disseminated histoplasmosis: Clinical and pathologic correlations. *Medicine* 1980; 59:1–33. *The most complete review of disseminated disease.*

Lennett EH, Balows A, Hausler WJ, Jr, Shadomy HJ (eds): *Manual of Clinical Microbiology*, ed 4. Washington, DC, American Society of Microbiology, 1985. *Excellent reference for microbiology and serology.*

National Institute of Allergy and Infectious Diseases Mycoses Study Group: Treatment of blastomycosis and histoplasmosis with ketoconazole: Results of a prospective randomized clinical trial. *Ann Intern Med* 1985; 103(6 Pt 1):861–872. *The most recent summary of ketoconazole therapy.*

Sarosi GA, Davies SF: Histoplasmosis, in Braude AI, Davis CE, Fierer J (eds) : *Infectious Diseases and Medical Microbiology*, ed 2. Philadelphia, WB Saunders Co, 1986, pp 863–867. *A succinct review in a standard text.*

Swantz J: *Histoplasmosis.* New York, Praeger, 1981. *A complete textbook covering all aspects of histoplasmosis.*

Wheat LJ, Slama TG, Eitzen HE, et al: A large urban outbreak of histoplasmosis: Clinical features. *Ann Intern Med* 1981; 94:331–337. *A description of an epidemic involving 100,000 people.*

part V

Gastrointestinal Disorders

57

ESOPHAGEAL REFLUX

Christopher J. Barde, M.D.

Gastroesophageal reflux occurs when liquid from the stomach enters the esophagus. It is associated with a spectrum of clinical manifestations. Heartburn is due to irritative material in the esophagus, often producing a hot or burning sensation. Esophagitis is inflammation of the esophagus with defined histologic changes.

CLINICAL SIGNS AND SYMPTOMS

The patient history is valuable in cases of symptomatic reflux. A normal person will have reflux 1% of the time in the supine position and 2% in the upright position. The vast majority of these normal people are asymptomatic. Of those with symptomatic gastroesophageal reflux, heartburn is the initial complaint for 85% of patients, gastroesophageal dysphagia for 8%, and cricopharyngeal dysphagia for 5%. Bleeding and aspiration are infrequent complaints. Over 95% of patients with symptomatic gastroesophageal reflux have heartburn. Reflux up to the mouth occurs in 70%, and symptoms of night aspiration may be present in 25%. Intermittent dysphagia is a frequent complaint (78%), most likely secondary to a motility disorder (e.g., diffuse spasm) because of the waxing and waning nature. Almost everyone identifies a type or amount of food that precipitates gastroesophageal reflux. Over 70% will note a relationship to posture, such as lying supine or bending over, and occasionally exercise (15%) or hunger (17%). Most patients have tried antacids for relief. Certain medications and medical conditions are associated with reflux esophagitis (chronic obstructive pulmonary disease, scleroderma, peptic ulcer, and pregnancy). Weight loss may be secondary to odynophagia, dysphagia, or malignancy.

The physical examination is not very revealing in gastroesophageal reflux. Examination of the pharynx may demonstrate herpetic or monilial lesions that can be confused with peptic esophagitis. There may be nonspecific epigastric pain or rarely a succession splash as with delayed gastric emptying. Examination of the lungs may reveal wheezing or findings suggestive of an aspiration pneumonia. The fingers may show sclerodactyly, and the face may show a tightening of the mouth, both signs of scleroderma.

Our knowledge of the natural history of gastroesophageal reflux is limited by the lack of longitudinal studies. The symptoms and findings of gastroesophageal reflux may resolve in some patients without treatment. How the disease course relates to the frequency and duration of reflux is not known. The development of esophageal ulcers is predominantly seen in patients with swallowing disorders and delayed gastric emptying, though the explanation for this is unknown. The patients are usually over the age of 30 years. Stricture formation is most common between the ages of 50 and 70 years and may be seen in 10% to 15% of patients. Reduction of inflammatory swelling causes slight improvement, but dilation is usually required.

Bleeding occurs in 3% of patients and usually requires surgery. While bleeding is usually slow and chronic, some patients with esophageal ulcers will have massive amounts. Over 50% of patients having antireflux surgery had pulmonary complaints before the operation. Most of these patients smoked, and in only 8% of cases was the reflux thought to be a cause of the symptoms. These patients present with morning hoarseness, aspiration pneumonia, fibrosis, and asthma. The development of Barrett's esophagus is now felt to be secondary to chronic gastroesophageal reflux, though the frequency of this development is not known. Barrett's esophagus is defined as the extension

TABLE 57–1.
Agents Altering The Lower Esophageal Sphincter Pressure (LESP)

AGENT	INCREASES LESP	DECREASES LESP
Hormone	Gastrin	Secretin
	Prostaglandin F_{2a}	Progesterone
		Estrogen
		Glucagon
		Prostaglandin E_2
Drug	Urecholine	Epinephrine
	Edrophonium	Isoproterenol
	Metoclopramide	Nitroglycerin
		Theophylline
		Calcium-channel
		blocking agents
		Nicotine
		Alcohol
Food		Fats
		Chocolate
		Carminatives

of columnar mucosa above the lower esophageal sphincter. It may be associated with ulcerations (68%), strictures (50%), and an increased risk of adenocarcinoma (30- to 40-fold increase over normal).

PATHOPHYSIOLOGY

The role of the lower esophageal sphincter pressure (LESP) is crucial in gastroesophageal reflux. The LESP is an ill-defined family of pressures preventing gastric contents from reaching the stomach. The pressure fluctuates over time, and episodes of spontaneous relaxation can be seen. Hormones, drugs, and certain foods may alter this pressure (Table 57–1).

A hiatal hernia, in which the proximal portion of the stomach is in the thorax, is associated with a decreased LESP. Inflammation of the distal esophagus by itself may decrease the LESP. The measurement of the LESP has shown that a low LESP does not always produce gastroesophageal reflux or esophagitis and that other factors may play a role.

The material refluxed may be acid, pepsin, or alkaline bile. They all decrease the mucosal resistance by acting on the cell membrane. If reflux occurs and the material is not rapidly cleared from the esophagus, irritation and inflammation of the mucosa then occur. At night, gastrointestinal clearance is decreased in patients with a hiatal hernia or with a motility

disorder like scleroderma. Delayed gastric emptying of solid food is also present in 41% to 57% of patients with gastroesophageal reflux and esophagitis. Most of these patients have histologic gastritis, and the inflammation may cause the delayed gastric emptying.

Endoscopy has led to a standarized grading of esophagitis by the microscopic appearance of the esophagus: grade 0 (normal-appearing mucosa), grade 1 (hyperemia), grade 2 (granularity), grade 3 (erosions), and grade 4 (ulcerations and strictures). Barrett's esophagus appears similar in color to gastric mucosa and may be associated with strictures, ulcerations, or tumor. This columnar epithelium may resemble intestinal metaplasia, the gastric cardia, or the gastric fundus. Biopsy of normal-appearing mucosa will often show histologic evidence of esophagitis in symptomatic patients. Microscopically, the key points in esophagitis are (1) basal-layer thickening composing more than 15% of the epithelium and (2) the lamina propria (rete pegs) extending over 50% of the epithelial thickness. In addition, 20% of patients with reflux may have polymorphonuclear leukocytes in the lamina propria. Superficial erosions may be seen, and some ulcers will extend into the muscular layers.

CLINICAL–PATHOLOGIC CORRELATIONS

The clinical symptoms are related to mucosal inflammation, motility disorders secondary to the irritation, stricture formation, or reflux severe enough to cause aspiration. The pathologic changes correlate well with the clinical findings (Table 57–2).

DIFFERENTIAL DIAGNOSIS

The symptoms of heartburn must be differentiated from angina. The latter is uncommon in younger patients and is usually associated with activity. An abnormal ECG or stress test suggests angina. Atypical chest pain (that differing from classic angina) can be esophageal in origin or related to other adjacent structures in the chest. Provocative esophageal manometric testing in addition to evaluation for other diseases may help in defining the cause of pain. Gas-

TABLE 57–2.
Clinical–Pathologic Correlations For Esophageal Reflux

| | PATHOLOGIC FINDINGS | |
CLINICAL FINDINGS	MECHANISM	PATHOLOGIC FEATURES
Heartburn	Acid reflux	Esophagitis +/−
	Hyperosmolar substance	Abnormal potential difference
	Esophageal spasm	
Pain	Unknown	Ulcerations with penetration to muscular layers
Dysphagia	Motor disorder	Esophagitis, ulcer
	Stricture	Fibrosis
Bleeding	Acid or bile reflux	Esophagitis, ulcer
Cough	Reflux at night	Pulmonary fibrosis or pneumonia
Weight loss	Diet limited to liquids	Stricture
	Learned response to dysphagia	Motility disorder or stricture

TABLE 57–3.
Tests For Gastroesophageal Reflux and Its Complications*

TEST	REFLUX	ESOPHAGITIS	ULCER	BARRETT'S ESOPHAGUS	ALTERED MOTILITY
24 hour pH	+ + + +				
Barium swallow	+	+	+ +		+
GE scintigraphy	+ +				+
Endoscopy with biopsy		+ + +	+ + + +	+ + + +	
Manometry					+ + + +
Bernstein	+ †				

* Accuracy of tests, + (poor) to + + + + (excellent).
† Based on the reproduction of symptoms but low sensitivity and specificity.

troesophageal reflux is not the only cause of esophagitis. Ingestion of caustic agents or certain medications, radiation therapy, and infection with herpes virus or *Candida* may produce esophagitis detected endoscopically. This can be differentiated from peptic esophagitis by history, culture, or cytology. An esophageal stricture from chronic gastroesophageal reflux must be distinguished from cancer. Radiographically the peptic stricture is smooth, but an endoscopic biopsy is usually needed to rule out either gastric cancer from the cardia or esophageal cancer.

detecting the complications of inflammation, stricture, and Barrett's formation, but cannot detect actual acid reflux or its pattern. Even tests with low sensitivities have a role in diagnosing gastroesophageal reflux. Nuclear scintigraphy may demonstrate gastroesophageal reflux or delayed gastric emptying, and esophageal manometry can evaluate the lower esophageal sphincter pressure and motility of the esophagus. Table 57–3 summarizes the value of various tests. Patients who do not respond to conservative treatment or have dysphagia, bleeding, or aspiration should undergo testing.

DIAGNOSIS

There is no one perfect test to evaluate gastroesophageal reflux. While the 24-hour monitoring of esophageal pH in an ambulatory patient is specific and sensitive for gastroesophageal reflux, it is unable to detect possible complications. Endoscopy is excellent for

PRINCIPLES OF THERAPY

A conservative approach to uncomplicated gastroesophageal reflux should be tried first. This includes elevation of the head of the bed on (6-in) blocks or wedge pillows, weight reduction in the obese patient, cessation of smoking, and dietary manipulation (remain upright for 1 hour after meals and avoid caffeine, chocolate, mints, and fats). Medicines that lower the LESP should be discontinued if they are no longer needed or if substitutes can be found. Antacids may be used after meals and at bedtime. Only 20% of patients with moderate to severe esophagitis will respond to this conservative approach.

Medical therapy is the next step for patients who are still symptomatic or have esophagitis. Reduction of gastric acid output by histamine H_2-receptor antagonists has had varied success in both symptomatic and histologic improvement. Metoclopramide enhances lower esophageal sphincter pressure, and gastric emptying has led to symptomatic, but not to histologic, improvement. Similar results have also been found for antacids, alginic acid, and sucralfate. Combination therapy with an H_2-receptor antagonist and metoclopramide has shown greater symptomatic and histologic improvement than with either agent alone.

The complication of stricture can be managed with bougienage. Bleeding is usually self-limited and may respond to intensive medical therapy. Pulmonary aspiration is a serious complication but may be managed with metoclopramide. Surgical treatment is reserved for these complications when they cannot be managed medically. In the repair of a hiatal hernia, the esophagus is pulled into the abdominal cavity and usually anchored with a fundoplication. The success rate is about 80% for those having this surgery.

REFERENCES

Jenkins AF, Cowan RJ, Richter JE: Gastroesophageal scintigraphy: Is it a sensitive screening test for gastroesophageal reflux disease? *J Clin Gastroenterol* 1985; 7:127–131. *A critical look at the limitations of nuclear medicine for detecting gastroesophageal reflux.*

Johnson LF: New concepts and methods in the study and treatment of gastroesophageal reflux disease. *Med Clin North Am* 1981; 65:1195–1222. *An in-depth look at 24-hour pH monitoring.*

Knuff TE, Benjamin SB, Worsham GF, et al: Histologic evaluation of chronic gastroesophageal reflux. *Dig Dis Sci* 1984; 29:194–201. *Shows limitation of endoscopy in detecting histologic esophagitis.*

McCallum RW, Berkowitz DM, Lerner E: Gastric emptying in patients with gastroesophageal reflux. *Gastroenterology* 1981; 80:285–291. *Discusses role of delayed gastric emptying in gastroesophageal reflux.*

Pope CE: Gastroesophageal reflux disease (reflux esophagitis), in Sleisenger M, Fordtran JS (eds): *Gastrointestinal Disease.* Philadelphia, WB Saunders Co, 1983, pp 449–476. *A in-depth review of gastroesophageal reflux.*

Richter JE, Castell DO: Drugs, foods and other substances in the cause and treatment of reflux esophagitis. *Med Clin North Am* 1981; 65:1223–1234. *A well-referenced review of the general approach to treating gastroesophageal reflux.*

Spechler SJ, Goyal RK: Barrett's esophagus. *N Engl J Med* 1986; 315:362–371. *Excellent review of the pathogenesis, complications, and treatment of Barrett's esophagus.*

58

PEPTIC ULCER DISEASE

N. Gopalswamy, M.D.

Benign ulcers occurring in the distal non-acid-secreting area of the stomach and in the duodenal bulb are referred to as peptic ulcers. They can also occur less frequently in the proximal portions of the stomach, distal esophagus, distal duodenum, jejunum, and Meckel's diverticulum. Peptic ulcers are believed to result from the imbalance of acid, pepsin, and mucosal resistance.

Duodenal ulcers are three to four times more common than gastric ulcers and on the average occur a decade earlier and more often in men than in women. About 10% of the population of the United States will have the disease in their lifetime. The incidence and prevalence of peptic ulcer vary markedly with geographic location and season. The incidence of peptic ulcer in the United States is about 18 per 10,000 population. The rates of hospitalization and mortality are diminishing in the United States.

CLINICAL SIGNS AND SYMPTOMS

The clinical features of peptic ulcer and its complications are summarized in Table 58–1. Epigastric pain or burning or upper abdominal

TABLE 58–1.
Clinical Features of Peptic Ulcer

CLINICAL DIAGNOSIS	SIGNS AND SYMPTOMS	CONFIRMATORY TESTS
Uncomplicated duodenal or gastric ulcer	Intermittent epigastric pain lasting 3 to 4 weeks with asymptomatic intervals of variable length. Pain relieved by food or antacids.	Barium study or endoscopy
Complications:		
Mild bleeding	Melena, stool positive for occult blood without significant drop in hemoglobin	Upper GI series
Moderate to severe bleeding ulcer	Moderate to severe GI bleeding with postural hypotension, tachycardia, etc., and no stigmata of chronic liver disease	Endoscopy
Perforation	Acute onset of severe abdominal pain in a patient with known ulcer disease and obliteration of preexisting liver and splenic dullness	Plain x-ray films of the abdomen Laparotomy
Peritonitis due to perforation	Fever, sepsis, diffuse abdominal pain, guarding, rigid abdomen with absent bowel sounds in a patient with known ulcer disease	Laparotomy
Penetration	Atypical ulcer pain with incomplete or no relief by antacids; radiation of pain to the back	Elevated serum amylase and lipase levels Laparotomy
Acute obstruction	Nausea, vomiting, atypical abdominal pain in a patient with known ulcer disease	Endoscopy revealing an active ulcer with narrow lumen Pylorus
Chronic obstruction	Vomiting, weight loss, abdominal pain	Upper GI series or endoscopy confirming pyloric stenosis

discomfort occurring 1 to 3 hours after eating, often occurring during the night, and relieved by ingestion of food, antacids, or milk is the most common initial manifestation of both duodenal and gastric ulcer. Gastrointestinal (GI) bleeding occurs in 15% to 20% of the cases. Blood loss may be mild, as in minor bouts of melena, and may be detectable only by stool examination for occult blood. Slight bleeding may go on over a long period without giving rise to the symptoms of anemia until a late stage. If the blood loss is acute, dizziness and shortness of breath can occur.

The pattern of pain may change in 5% to 10% of the cases to last longer than usual, with incomplete relief, no relief, or even exacerbation after antacids or food. The pain may radiate to the back, as in the case of a penetrating duodenal ulcer or a combination of gastric and duodenal ulcers. Acute, severe pain suggests a perforating ulcer. Atypical pain, vomiting, and weight loss suggest gastric outlet obstruction.

The physical findings are usually normal in uncomplicated cases, except for slight tenderness elicited in the epigastric area. Slight amounts of GI bleeding or chronic GI bleeding resulting in significantly low hemoglobin values could be asymptomatic until the late stages. Rapid, acute blood loss results in significant postural hypotension, tachycardia, and black or maroon stools on rectal examination. These findings signify an intravascular volume loss of 20% or more.

Patients may occasionally present with obvious shock. Severe, diffuse abdominal tenderness, tympanitic note on percussion, and obliteration of the previously existing hepatic or splenic dullness on percussion indicate a perforated peptic ulcer. If left untreated, this condition progresses to boardlike rigidity of the abdomen, fever, and sepsis. Significant blood volume loss (as shown by postural hypotension) without anemia and with a history of vomiting suggests gastric outlet obstruction either due to an acute ulcer or to chronic pyloric stenosis. Peristaltic waves can sometimes be seen on abdominal inspection, and a succession splash elicited in a patient who is fasting (has not eaten or drunk anything for 4 hours or more) is indicative of gastric outlet obstruction; occasionally peristaltic waves in the left upper abdomen seen on close inspection also signify gastric outlet obstruction.

Information obtained from the few longitudinal studies of patients with benign peptic ulcers and from many of the double-blind placebo-controlled studies in the last 20 years have shown that untreated benign ulcers have mortality rates of less than 1% in patients under age 60 years and less than 5% in patients over age 60. The higher mortality in elderly patients is related to coexistent diseases such as coronary artery disease, chronic obstructive pulmonary disease, and complications of peptic ulcer. Both gastric and duodenal ulcers recur often (greater than 50%) with variable symptom-free intervals.

In general, about 75% of the ulcers have a benign course, with the remainder complicated by GI bleeding, gastric outlet obstruction, perforation, penetration, or occasional fistula. In a small percentage of cases, the ulcer may be asymptomatic. The initial manifestation may be one of the complications of ulcers.

PATHOPHYSIOLOGY

In the absence of gastric acidity, ulcers are almost nonexistent. Gastric ulcer has been reported with achlorhydria, but if this occurs gastric carcinoma should be suspected. Most patients with duodenal ulcer secrete at least 12 mEq of hydrochloric acid per hour after stimulation with either pentagastrin or histamine. An increased parietal cell population, increased sensitivity of the parietal cells to stimuli such as food and gastrin, increased pepsinogen secretion, diminished bicarbonate secretion, rapid gastric emptying of liquids, an impaired feedback mechanism to shut off gastrin and acid production, and diminished mucosal resistance have all been implicated as causes of duodenal ulcers. In an individual case, one or more of these factors act to cause duodenal ulcer.

A number of factors have been cited as causes of gastric ulcer. These include pyloric dysfunction giving rise to a reflux of bile and pancreatic secretions from the duodenum into the stomach, back diffusion of acid, injury to the mucosa by barrier-breaking agents such as alcohol, aspirin, nonsteroidal anti-inflammatory drugs, and associated gastritis.

TABLE 58–2.
Clinical–Pathologic Correlations in Peptic Ulcer

CLINICAL FINDINGS	PATHOLOGIC FINDINGS	
	MACROSCOPIC	MICROSCOPIC
Epigastric pain and tenderness	Round or punched-out oval	Break in epithelium
	Denuded epithelium with yellowish exudate or necrotic base	Lesion extending beyond the muscularis mucosa with fibrinous exudate and fragmented leukocytes
		Chronic inflammatory cells and granulation tissue in later stages
Hematemesis and melena with hemodynamic changes	Blood clot or visible vessel in the base of the ulcer	Ulcer with hemorrhagic base
		Occasional bare arteriole
Persistent atypical pain	Ulcer burrowing into adjacent organs	Ulcer bed formed by inflamed adjacent organ
Atypical pain Vomiting	Active ulcer with spasm and edematous mucosal folds obliterating the GI lumen	Edema and congestion with active ulceration
Atypical pain Weight loss Vomiting	Narrow lumen of stomach or duodenum that cannot be made to open with insufflation by air or use of antispasmodics	Dense fibrosis No active ulceration
	No active ulcer seen	

CLINICAL–PATHOLOGIC CORRELATIONS

The clinical–pathologic correlations of peptic ulcer are summarized in Table 58–2. Exactly how pain is caused by ulcers is not clear. Popular explanation is irritation of the nerve endings by acid and pepsin in the area of the ulcer. Pain relieved by placebos in one-third to one-half of the patients with ulcers is difficult to explain on these grounds. Pain produced by penetrating or perforated ulcer is better understood because the pain-sensitive parietal peritoneum is involved.

Clinical signs and symptoms correlate well with the degree of GI bleeding, as well as with the acute or chronic nature of the bleeding. Acute rapid loss of blood from peptic ulcer is more symptomatic than is chronic slow bleeding. Symptoms and signs of anemia and postural hypotension indicate significant bleeding. In the case of upper GI bleeding, hematemesis or maroon-colored stools indicate moderate to severe bleeding from the ulcer. Severe blood loss is defined as 1 ml/min or three or more units of blood in 24 hours.

In a patient with a known ulcer, an acute onset of severe abdominal pain followed by signs of peritonitis correlates well with perforation. Atypical pain or a changing pattern of pain could be due to (1) penetrating ulcer resulting in mild pancreatitis, (2) multiple ulcers, (3) combined duodenal and gastric ulcers, or (4) ulcer with obstruction. Vomiting food eaten 24 hours earlier correlates well with gastric outlet obstruction, which may be either due to acute ulcer with edema and spasm or to chronic fibrotic process; weight loss with vomiting points to the latter. Recent endoscopic studies show that pain may persist despite complete healing of the ulcer and that, in contrast, some ulcers may remain unhealed but without symptoms even after full treatment.

DIFFERENTIAL DIAGNOSIS

Table 58–3 summarizes the differential diagnoses of peptic ulcer. Though gastric and duodenal ulcers have different pathogeneses, they have similar biologic behaviors. On the basis of clinical features alone, it is very hard to differentiate duodenal from gastric ulcer, duodenitis from duodenal ulcer, and gastritis from gas-

TABLE 58–3.
Differential Diagnosis of Peptic Ulcer

Duodenal ulcer
Gastric ulcer
Duodenitis
Gastritis
Esophagitis
Pancreatitis
Irritable bowel syndrome
Gastrinoma (Z-E syndrome)
Gastric cancer
Inferior wall myocardial infarction or ischemia
Anastomotic ulcer

tric ulcer. A single-contrast barium study helps to diagnose ulcer, and double-contrast barium study or an endoscopy establishes an exact diagnosis, though these procedures are often not absolutely needed.

A diagnosis of esophagitis is suggested by retrosternal heartburn that worsens in the supine position accompanied with regurgitation or dysphagia.

A diagnosis of pancreatitis is established by radiation of pain to the back, elevated serum amylase or lipase levels, and diffuse pancreatic involvement shown by an ultrasound examination of the abdomen.

Irritable bowel syndrome should be diagnosed by exclusion. Patients with either alternating constipation and diarrhea, or anxiety, or both can have upper abdominal pain without ulcers.

Symptoms and signs of perforation are nonspecific in that perforation of any organ, the intestine, colon, uterus, or gallbladder, can give rise to similar findings. A history of peptic ulcer allows a tentative diagnosis of perforated ulcer.

Zollinger-Ellison (Z-E) syndrome or gastrinoma is suggested by strong family history of ulcer disease or the presence of a duodenal ulcer with unexplained diarrhea, or features of malabsorption or association with hypercalcemia. High serum gastrin levels and the paradoxical rise of gastrin levels after intravenous secretin would clinch the diagnosis.

Dyspepsia occurring for the first time in an elderly person suggests cancer. Upper GI series would show pictures characteristic of either a benign or a malignant ulcer, and endoscopy would confirm or refute the diagnosis of cancer.

A burning pain in the epigastrium could be of cardiovascular origin. Pain brought on by exertion or emotional disturbance in an elderly patient with risk factors for coronary artery disease may not be from peptic ulcer. Definitive electrocardiographic abnormalities and elevated CPK and SGOT levels should establish the diagnosis of a cardiovascular problem.

An anastomotic ulcer is suggested by a history of previous gastric surgery for ulcer disease followed by a recurrence of symptoms. An endoscopy should be done to confirm the diagnosis.

DIAGNOSIS

A single-contrast barium study is of diagnostic help in about 70% of the cases of uncomplicated duodenal ulcer. In chronic duodenal ulcer disease, the duodenal bulb is deformed, so repeated barium studies are not helpful; in many cases, an acute ulcer in a deformed bulb will not be revealed by barium studies. It is not necessary to perform an endoscopy each time symptoms recur in patients with known duodenal ulcer disease. Thus, the clinical diagnosis alone is enough to treat recurrence, unless complicating features of the ulcer necessitate endoscopy.

Barium studies can confirm the diagnosis of benign gastric ulcer. It is customary, however, to perform an endoscopy in all such cases and to take biopsy specimens of the ulcer, because gastric cancer is not diagnosed in 1% to 5% of the cases in which the diagnosis of benign gastric ulcer is based on radiologic data alone.

In cases complicated by bleeding, barium studies can reveal ulcer; they cannot determine the source of the bleeding. When bleeding necessitates a blood transfusion, endoscopy must be done to find the source of bleeding. If the source is not found, angiographic studies or radionuclide studies with tagged red cells may be helpful.

An x-ray film of the abdomen or chest showing free air under the diaphragm suggests a perforated viscus. A laparotomy is needed to make the final diagnosis.

In many cases of anastomotic ulcer, barium studies are singularly unhelpful, and endoscopy is needed to establish the diagnosis.

The advantages and disadvantages of barium studies and endoscopy in diagnosing peptic

TABLE 58–4.
Diagnostic Tests in Peptic Ulcer

| | DIAGNOSTIC TEST | | |
| | SINGLE-CONTRAST | DOUBLE-CONTRAST | |
FEATURE	BARIUM STUDY	BARIUM STUDY	ENDOSCOPY
Availability	Universal	Low	High
Accuracy*	60%–70%	80%–85%	90%–95%
Morbidity	< 1%	< 1%	1–2%
Mortality	0	0	Rare
Cost	Low	Variable	High

* Accuracy is the percentage of correctly diagnosed cases in the total number of cases.

TABLE 58–5.
Medical Treatment for Peptic Ulcer

| | TREATMENT | |
EFFECT	ANTACIDS	H_2-RECEPTOR BLOCKERS
Healing efficacy	60%–70%	80%–85%
Side-effects	Well known	Known for 20 years
	Safe	Long-term safety undocumented
Compliance	Poor	Very good
	a. Multiple doses	a. Limited doses
	b. Hard to carry liquids	b. Tablet form
Cost (4-plus scale)	+ +	+ + +
Prevent recurrence	No	Yes

ulcer are shown in Table 58–4. Though endoscopy helps establish an accurate diagnosis, it is not needed in uncomplicated cases of benign duodenal ulcer or ulcer with mild bleeding. Endoscopy is indicated in cases of ulcers with obstructive features or significant bleeding and in cases with unsatisfactory response to treatment or in which ulcer symptoms and normal results of the barium studies occur.

PRINCIPLES OF TREATMENT

The aims of treatment are (1) to relieve symptoms, (2) to heal ulcers, (3) to prevent complications, and (4) to prevent recurrence. The average duration of treatment for duodenal ulcer is 4 to 6 weeks and for gastric ulcer, 6 to 8 weeks or longer if the ulcer is large.

Bringing the gastric pH to 3.5, where 80% of the pepsin is inactivated, is the goal of medical treatment. In the 1980s, the mainstays of medical treatment of peptic ulcer are antacids and H_2-blockers. In addition, recent studies have shown sucralfate, a sulfated disaccharide that coats the ulcer, to be as effective as H_2-receptor blockers in healing both gastric and duodenal ulcers. Promising drugs on the horizon are analogues of prostaglandin E_2 and a proton pump inhibitor called omeprazole. Anticholinergic agents by themselves are not very effective primary therapy.

Compared to placebo, antacids and H_2-receptor blockers are very effective during the first 2 weeks of treatment. In the later stages, the differences between the two groups fall to a minimum. In general, 85% of the benign ulcers heal with H_2-receptor blocker therapy, and 60% to 70% of such ulcers heal with antacid treatment (Table 58–5). The unhealed ulcers from the antacid of H_2-receptor blocker treated group can be treated effectively with either omeprazole or colloidal bismuth compound.

A single daily nocturnal dose of H_2-receptor blocker effectively prevents recurrences of duodenal ulcer. A few studies also show blockers effective in preventing recurrent gastric ulcers.

There is no place for a Sippy or bland diet. Patients may be instructed to eat a regular diet and avoid foods that produce abdominal pain. Though no convincing data exist showing that either caffeine or alcohol interferes with healing, in common practice patients are instructed to restrict consumption of these products.

Though it has been known for many years that stopping smoking helps heal gastric ulcers, its role in treating duodenal ulcers was controversial until recent studies showed that smoking delays healing of duodenal ulcers, too. Patients should be instructed to stop smoking or to cut down to fewer than 10 cigarettes per day.

Surgical treatment is definitely indicated for a perforated ulcer, a penetrating ulcer, ulcers with significant recurrent bleeding (especially in elderly patients), gastric outlet obstruction caused by chronic peptic ulceration, and ulcers refractory to medical management.

REFERENCES

Berk JE (ed): *Bockus Gastroenterology*, vol. 2, ed 4. Philadelphia, WB Saunders Co, 1985, pp 1013–1254. *Exhaustive coverage of all aspects of peptic ulcer. Good reference volume.*

Elashoff J, Van Deventer G, Reedy TJ et al: Long-term follow-up of duodenal ulcer patients. *J Clin Gastroenterol* 1983; 5:509–515. *Recent article describing a good 4- to 6-year follow-up of 245 patients with duodenal ulcers.*

Fry J: Peptic ulcer: A profile. *Br Med J* 1964; 2:809. *Overview of natural history and complications.*

Gibinsky K: Step by step towards the natural history of peptic ulcer disease. *J Clin Gastroenterol* 1983; 5(4):299–302. *A good editorial covering seasonal variation in ulcer disease.*

Grossman MI (ed): *Peptic Ulcer—A Guide for the Practicing Physician.* Chicago, Year Book Medical Publishers, 1981. *An excellent short monograph covering all aspects of peptic ulcer, written in simple and elegant style.*

Isenberg JI, Johansson C (eds): Peptic ulcer disease. *Clin Gastroenterol* 1984; 13(2):287–654. *In-depth discussions about the epidemiology, pathophysiology, and management of peptic ulcers.*

Myren J: The natural history of peptic ulcer—Views in the 1980s. *Scand J Gastroenterol* 1983; 18(8):993–997. *Many of the facts in this article are also applicable to the US population.*

Richardson CT: Peptic ulcer disease, in Stein JH (ed): *Textbook of Internal Medicine.* Boston, Little, Brown & Co, 1983, pp 93–104. *Succinct, up-to-date information about peptic ulcer. Easy to read.*

59 GASTRIC CARCINOMA

N. Gopalswamy, M.D.
Christopher J. Bard, M.D.

Carcinoma of the stomach is the most common malignant tumor of the stomach (Table 59–1). It is the third most common malignancy of the gastrointestinal tract and the sixth most common cause of deaths from cancer in the United States. It occurs more commonly in men, blacks, persons above 50 years of age, and immigrants from Japan, Russia, and Northern Europe. Persons with the following conditions fall into the increased-risk group for developing stomach cancer: (1) atrophic gastritis, (2) pernicious anemia, (3) blood group A, (4) gastric polyps, and (5) patients who had gastric surgery for benign ulcers 15 to 20 years earlier.

The incidence of carcinoma of the stomach in the United States has decreased in the last 50 years.

CLINICAL SIGNS AND SYMPTOMS

About 70% to 80% of patients with both early and advanced cancer of the stomach have weight loss and a history of abdominal pain that mimics a peptic ulcer and responds variably to antacids. Chronic gastrointestinal bleeding, vomiting, dysphagia, jaundice, and ascites occur in the late stages but can also be the initial symptoms.

The results of a physical examination are usually normal in the early stages. Weight loss, signs of anemia, abdominal mass, hepatomegaly, ascites, a palpable, hard lymph node in the left supraclavicular area, acanthosis nigricans, and a palpable mass in the rectum may be found in the later stages.

The prognosis for cancer confined to the mucosa or submucosa of the stomach, that is, early gastric cancer or superficial spreading cancer, is excellent, with a 5-year survival rate of 25% to 50%. Unfortunately, fewer than 10% of the tumors are diagnosed in the early stages in the United States, whereas 25% to 30% of the tumors are diagnosed early in Japan. Carcinomas that occur on the lesser curvature of the stomach have a relatively better prognosis than those that occur in the cardia or on the greater curvature.

Fewer than 50% of the Stage 2 and 3 gastric carcinomas are resectable, and the 5-year survival rate with curative resection is 10% to 15%. Patients who have palliative resections survive up to 10 months after surgery.

Complications of gastric cancer include malnutrition, perforation, and massive gastrointestinal bleeding.

PATHOPHYSIOLOGY

The exact cause of carcinoma of the stomach is not known. Interesting epidemiologic studies show that the cancer rate for the first American-born generation of immigrants from Japan is higher than the average for other Americans, but less than that for the Japanese. The incidence of stomach cancer in subsequent generations decreases markedly, pointing to the change in environment and dietary habits as relevant factors. A high-starch or high-salt diet, the use of substances such as talc to preserve the flavor of rice in Japan, nitrosamines formed in the stomach, and low intake of fresh vegetables with a high vitamin C content have been cited as possible etiologic agents.

On gross appearance, gastric carcinomas can be polypoid, fungating, ulcerative, infiltrative, or of the superficial spreading type. The staging of stomach carcinomas is based on the spread of the tumor from the mucosa to serosa or adjacent organs, involvement of regional lymph nodes, and distant metastatic lesions. Stage 0 is in situ carcinoma, and Stage 4 is cancer with distant metastases (Table 59–2).

TABLE 59–1.
Frequency Distribution of Primary Tumors of the Stomach

TYPE OF TUMOR	PERCENTAGE OF CASES
BENIGN	
Hyperplastic polyps	40
Adenomatous polyps	10
Leiomyoma	25
Other	25
MALIGNANT	
Carcinoma	90
Lymphoma	5
Sarcoma	2
Other	3

TABLE 59–2.
Staging of Carcinoma of the Stomach

Stage 0	Carcinoma in situ (Superficial tumor in the mucosa with intact muscularis mucosa)
Stage 1	Tumor confined to the mucosa or submucosa. No spread to lymph nodes. No metastases.
Stage 2	Tumor spread to the serosa. No spread to lymph nodes. No metastases.
Stage 3	Tumor inside the stomach or spread to contiguous organs such as omentum, duodenum, and transverse colon. Lymph nodes within 3 cm of the stomach lesion are involved. No metastases.
Stage 4	Involvement of intra-abdominal lymph nodes more than 3 cm from the gastric lesion. Distant metastases.

CLINICAL–PATHOLOGIC CORRELATIONS

The clinical–pathologic correlations for carcinoma of the stomach are given in Table 59–3. Blood loss from the tumor and insufficient iron intake result in iron-deficiency anemia. Early satiety or anorexia give rise to malnutrition and weight loss. Dysphagia results from tumors in the cardia obstructing the lumen near the esophagogastric junction. Tumors in the antrum involving the whole circumference obstruct the pylorus and cause vomiting and weight loss. Metastases to the liver or peritoneum may lead to jaundice, ascites, or in the terminal stages, hepatic failure.

DIFFERENTIAL DIAGNOSIS

The differential diagnosis for carcinoma of the stomach includes benign gastric ulcer, gastric polyps, leiomyoma, and lymphoma. Clinical symptomatology lasting over a period of years favors the diagnosis of benign gastric ulcer. Barium studies are 70% accurate, with both false-positive and false-negative findings. The error rate increases if the ulcer cannot be classified either as benign or malignant on the basis of radiologic criteria. Hence, it is customary to endoscope all patients with benign gastric ulcer and perform multiple biopsies to make sure malignancy is not missed.

Gastric polyps are less frequent, and 70% to 80% of them are hyperplastic, measure less than 1 cm in length, and are not precancerous. About 15% to 20% of the polyps are adenomas, and 1% to 5% of these may become malignant. In 25% to 30% of patients with gastric polyps, carcinoma of the stomach coexists; hence, polyps should alert the endoscopist to look for coexistent cancer in the rest of the stomach. Polyps more than two cm in size should be removed endoscopically.

Leiomyoma, a benign tumor of the stomach, is often well defined with smooth mucosa over it and can be detected by radiologic techniques or by endoscopy. Mucosal biopsies are unhelpful. Only complete excision of the tumor is helpful in establishing a diagnosis.

Lymphoma is either primary in the stomach or secondary to a generalized process. The presence of lymphadenopathy, hepatosplenomegaly, and anemia indicates a generalized process, and a gastric lesion could be secondary to this process. Primary lymphoma of the stomach constitutes 2% of the tumors of the stomach and can be diagnosed by endoscopy and biopsy.

TABLE 59–3.
Clinical–Pathologic Correlations For Carcinoma of the Stomach

| CLINICAL FINDINGS | PATHOLOGIC FINDINGS | |
	MACROSCOPIC	MICROSCOPIC: ADENOCARCINOMA
Dysphagia, weight loss	Infiltrating or polypoid tumor of the cardia of the stomach	Mucus-producing
Vomiting, weight loss, visible peristalsis, succussion splash	Tumor extensively involving the stomach antrum or polypoid tumor of the antrum	Mucus-producing Well or poorly differentiated
Anorexia, weight loss	Leather-bottle stomach with thick, rigid stomach walls and narrow lumen (linitis plastica)	Undifferentiated with desmoplastic reaction
Bleeding, weight loss	Polypoid or fungating tumor	Necrotic
Bleeding	Ulcer with raised margin and irregular base; nodular, friable mucosa	Ulcerative
Hard; nodular, enlarged liver; jaundice; ascites	Foci of metastatic lesions of liver, variable in size and number	Islands of adenocarcinoma amidst normal liver tissue

DIAGNOSIS

Laboratory studies are nonspecific but may reveal anemia due to iron deficiency, abnormal liver function tests due to liver metastases, and achlorhydria even after pentagastrin stimulation. Single-contrast barium studies of the stomach can detect mass lesions, irregularities of the mucosal pattern, linitis plastica, and ulcerative cancers with an accuracy of 70%, with a false-positive rate of 5% to 10%. Double-contrast barium studies of the stomach are more sensitive than single-contrast studies and can detect cancer in the earlier stages. In experienced hands, gastroscopy with biopsy can establish the diagnosis with an accuracy of 90% to 95%. Where endoscopic findings are equivocal and there is a high index of suspicion of cancer, gastric cytologic studies can be done. The likelihood of a firm diagnosis is high when an experienced pathologist or cytologist reads the sample. Computed tomography (CT scan) of the abdomen is helpful to exclude metastatic lesions outside the stomach.

PRINCIPLES OF THERAPY

Every effort should be made to detect the lesions early. Unfortunately, periodic endoscopic surveillance in subjects who are at high risk for developing carcinoma is not cost-effective. This nonetheless seems to be the only effective way of detecting early cancers. Cancers that have not spread to the serosa may be treated by curative resections. Palliative resections can be done even for advanced cancer of the stomach to prevent or treat significant gastrointestinal bleeding or obstructive symptoms.

Combination chemotherapy with 5-fluorouracil (5-Fu) plus doxorubicin and mitomycin C is marginally more effective than chemotherapy with 5-Fu alone. Supportive care is the mainstay of treatment both perioperatively and for patients who cannot have surgery. It consists of correcting malnutrition with enteral or parenteral alimentation, correcting fluid and electrolyte imbalance, and treating symptoms.

REFERENCES

Bedikian AY, Chen TT, Khankhanian N et al: The natural history of gastric cancer and prognostic factors influencing survival. *J Clin Oncology* 1984; 2(4):305–310. *Data on 783 patients with gastric cancer from the M.D. Anderson Cancer Institution.*

Carter KJ, Schaffer HG, Ritchie WP Jr: Early gastric cancer. *Ann Surg* 1984; 199(5):604–609. *Retrospective review of the curative surgical resection of carcinoma of the stomach, comparing the survival rates of early gastric cancer in the United States and Japan.*

Kurtz RC, Sherlock R: Carcinoma of the stomach, in Berk JE (ed):*Bockus Gastroenterology*, vol 2, ed 4. Philadelphia, WB Saunders Co, 1985, pp 1278–1304. *Up-to-date, comprehensive review.*

Schein PS, Sherlock P: Gastric cancer. *Semin Oncol* 1985; 12(1):1–53. *Good discussion about epidemiology, staging, and management.*

60 GALLBLADDER DISEASE

James B. Peoples, M.D.

Gallbladder disease is any condition that prevents the gallbladder from performing its normal function. The normal function of the gallbladder is to collect, store, and concentrate hepatic bile and to expel it into the duodenum on demand. Conditions that affect this function are broadly subdivided into obstructive and inflammatory.

CLINICAL SIGNS AND SYMPTOMS

Clinically, signs and symptoms of gallbladder disease do not appear until the process has progressed to the point where either emptying is impeded or acute infection occurs. With obstructive disease, patients first present with abdominal pain, which characteristically occurs shortly after eating a fatty meal. The pain is localized to the area overlying the gallbladder but may radiate subcostally to the right or superiorly to the xiphoid. It is described as aching or squeezing and varies from moderate to severe. It is self-limited, lasting from a few minutes to several hours and then gradually or suddenly ceasing. It is recurrent. It may be associated with nausea and vomiting. The physical examination may demonstrate mild tachycardia, acute distress, and perhaps mild direct-palpation tenderness, but is frequently normal. Unattended, such episodes will progress in both frequency and severity as obstruction becomes more complete.

Acute infection may occur without prior symptoms, or it may develop in a person with prior obstructive complaints. The primary complaint with infection is also pain localized over the gallbladder. The onset does not necessarily correlate with eating or other activity. The pain is aching in quality and moderate to severe in quantity. Systemic signs and symptoms of infection such as fever and chills may be present. Nausea, vomiting, and anorexia are common.

The physical examination will generally elicit evidence of fever, tachycardia, moderate to marked tenderness to direct palpation over the gallbladder, and frequently also direct rebound tenderness. With more advanced infection, referred tenderness and rebound tenderness may be elicited. Gentle palpation may reveal an inflammatory mass around the gallbladder. The bowel sounds may be diminished to absent. Untreated, acute infection will progress to necrosis, perforation, localized abscess formation, generalized peritonitis, bacteremia, septic shock, and death.

DIFFERENTIAL DIAGNOSIS

Biliary colic, the label applied to pain secondary to gallbladder outlet obstruction, is easily confused with several other conditions involving the upper abdomen and lower chest. Acute peptic ulcer disease, other than with perforation, and acute gastroduodenitis, whether bacterial, viral, or chemical, all have similar symptoms and histories. The physical findings are generally unremarkable. Careful history taking is essential to determine if the pain occurs only after eating fatty food or if it occurs with any food. Inflammation of the gastroduodenal mucosa also produces more severe nausea, vomiting, and anorexia. Frequently the diagnosis of peptic ulcer disease will only be confirmed for certain by laboratory and radiologic testing. Coronary insufficiency, especially involving the diaphragmatic surface of the heart, also produces pain similar to biliary colic and may be precipitated by eating. The history and physical findings may not differentiate, and consequently an exact diagnosis usually rests on ancillary testing. Esophageal spasm, secondary to reflux esophagitis, initially appears with pain similar to that of gallbladder disease but is generally precipitated by large chunks of meat or bread or by hot or cold liquids rather than by fat. It is briefer in duration and is unassociated with nausea or vomiting but may involve regurgitation.

Acute cholecystitis, infection of the gallbladder, is often confused with a perforated peptic ulcer, acute pancreatitis, or acute appendicitis. A perforated peptic ulcer generally results immediately in diffuse peritonitis with marked generalized involuntary guarding, so-called boardlike rigidity. Although the pain may be localized, the tenderness is not. Nausea and vomiting are not prominent features, but anorexia is marked. The bowel sounds are totally absent early in the course. Acute pancreatitis, especially if localized to the head of the pancreas, results in localized evidence of peritonitis identical to that of cholecystitis. Because pancreatitis, like perforated ulcer, is not caused by bacteria, at least early in its course, it will not produce systemic signs or symptoms of infection. Fever is never more than mildly elevated. The differential diagnosis rests on laboratory determinations.

DIAGNOSIS

The definitive diagnosis of biliary colic is based on the demonstration of obstructed gallbladder emptying coupled with the exclusion of other causes for the patient's pain. Because the vast majority of cases of biliary colic are caused by impaction of gallstones in the cystic duct, diagnosis has come to equal demonstration of stones in the gallbladder. In recent years, ultrasonography for this purpose has progressed to the point where it is now 95% accurate, with a sensitivity of 98% and a specificity of 92%. Due to its costs, rapidity, and absent morbidity, it is currently the first, and frequently the only, test obtained to assess gallstone presence. Rarely, specific functional tests of actual emptying are required. Timed oral cholecystography, with cholecystokinin stimulation, is 95% specific, but only about 50% sensitive. Assay of duodenal bile for gallbladder "B" bile after cholecystokinin stimulation is accurate to a similar degree. When coupled, they raise the accuracy to 85% to 90% with a specificity of 99%, but a sensitivity of only about 75%.

The diagnosis of acute cholecystitis is similarly strengthened by the demonstration of gallstones by ultrasonography. In about 50% of cases, the sonogram will also show a thickened gallbladder wall consistent with acute inflammation. Currently, nuclear biliary imaging techniques, such as the P.I.P.I.D.A (Technetium-99m para-isopropyl-imino-diacetic-acid) scan, are the most accurate techniques for diagnosing acute cholecystitis. Absence of gallbladder imaging in the presence of adequate common duct imaging is highly accurate for making a diagnosis of acute cholecystitis. Unfortunately, the time required to obtain the study frequently precludes its use. Consequently, in practice, demonstration of gallstones coupled with leukocytosis in a patient with appropriate historic and physical evidence of acute cholecystitis is considered adequate for a diagnosis provided other causes for the symptoms have been excluded.

PATHOPHYSIOLOGY

The primary pathologic event in most cases of both obstruction and infection is the formation of gallstones. Although lithogenic bile produced by the liver is a necessary prerequisite, concentration in the gallbladder is required for precipitation to occur. Once formed, the stones may directly obstruct the cystic duct or may produce a chronic inflammatory reaction of the foreign-body type in the wall of the gallbladder. The latter sequence results in fibrosis of the musculature with poor contraction, stasis, and further stone formation with bacterial overgrowth. It also produces partial venous obstruction with decreased blood flow to the organ. When bacterial inoculum exceeds normal resistance mechanisms, acute invasive infection occurs. Initially, only the gallbladder wall is involved, but with progression it may extend to the liver or result in perforation with spillage of highly infective bile into the local area, into the peritoneal cavity, or both. Rarely, in the body's attempt to isolate such a gallbladder, a segment of intestinal tract will adhere to the organ such that perforation leads to formation of a fistulous tract between the gallbladder and the intestine.

Macroscopically, gallbladder disease ranges from a normal organ containing stones, through a fibrosed, contracted organ typical of chronic cholecystitis, to the acutely inflamed, suppurative organ, to the black, gangrenous, necrotic

TABLE 60–1.
Clinical–Pathologic Correlations for Gallbladder Disease

CLINICAL FINDINGS	PATHOLOGIC FINDINGS
None	Gallstones
Pain with contraction of the gallbladder	Cystic duct obstruction
Local pain, fever, local tenderness, leukocytosis	Bile, stasis, bacterial proliferation, invasive infection
Generalized pain and tenderness	Perforation
Shock, acidosis, mental confusion, death	Bacteremia

organ of the late infection. Microscopically, the organ may be normal; it may have mild cholesterol deposition; it may have the characteristic of chronic inflammation and fibrosis; or it may have features consistent with an acute leukocytic inflammatory reaction with patchy or diffuse necrosis.

CLINICAL–PATHOLOGIC CORRELATIONS

Biliary colic is directly related to gallbladder contraction in the face of obstruction. The factors that produce contraction correlate with production of the symptom. Because the strongest stimulus to contraction is cholecystokinin, food that stimulates cholecystokinin release also produces biliary colic. Interestingly, the severity and duration of pain parallels the expected cholecystokinin response almost exactly. A small meal with minimal fat content results in mild pain of short duration. A large meal containing large quantities of fat produces severe pain lasting several hours.

The clinical findings in acute cholecystitis also parallel the pathologic course of the infection. Early, patients have mild fever and leukocytosis with moderate, localized tenderness. At the peak of the infection, they have a high fever, marked leukocytosis, marked localized tenderness, rebound tenderness, and referred tenderness. Following perforation, hypother-

mia may supervene with leukopenia, shock, and generalized signs of peritonitis.

A summary of these correlations is presented in Table 60–1.

PRINCIPLES OF THERAPY

The treatment of gallbladder obstruction is founded on removal of the obstructing element. In the case of gallstones, removal of the stones with retention of the gallbladder results in rapid reformation of stones. This is presumably due to the damage that has already occurred to the gallbladder because of the stones. Attempts to dissolve stones chemically has had a similar outcome, although patients willing to ingest bile salts daily for life can dissolve existing stones if small and can also prevent reformation to a great degree. In most cases, however, removal of the entire gallbladder together with the stones results not only in relief of the entire process, but completely prevents further stone formation. Gallbladder absence is tolerated with no noticeable sequelae with the exception of mild, temporary diarrhea in some patients.

Acute cholecystitis may be treated successfully with appropriate antibiotics, but recurs in virtually every patient, frequently with a more fulminant course than with the first episode. Cholecystectomy is curative and prevents further possible complications of the disease.

REFERENCES

Gill PT, Dillon E, Leahy AL, Reeder A, Peel ALG: Ultrasonography, H.I.D.A. scintigraphy or both in the diagnosis of acute cholecystitis? *Br J Surg* 1985; 72:267–268. *Diagnosis using sonography and scintigraphy.*

McSherry CK, Ferstenberg H, Calhoun WF, Lahman E, Virshup M: The natural history of diagnosed gallstone disease in symptomatic and asymptomatic patients. *Ann Surg* 1985; 202:59–64. *A comprehensive review.*

Silen W: *Cope's Early Diagnosis of the Acute Abdomen*, ed 16. New York, Oxford University Press, 1983. *A classic in diagnosis.*

Spiro HM: *Clinical Gastroenterology*, ed 3. New York, Macmillan Publishing Co, 1983. *An in-depth text, well-referenced.*

Suarez CA, Block F, Bernstein D, Serafini A, Rodman G, Zeppa R: The role of H.I.D.A./P.I.P.I.D.A. scanning in diagnosing cystic duct obstruction. *Ann Surg* 1980; 191:391–396. *Diagnosing cystic duct diseases.*

Thal ER, Weigelt J, Landay M, Conrad M: Evaluation of ultrasound in the diagnosis of acute and chronic biliary tract disease. *Arch Surg* 1978; 113:500–503. *A useful, concise summary.*

61 VIRAL HEPATITIS

Dietmar V. Trulzsch, M.D.

Viral hepatitis, particularly hepatitis B, affects over 1 million individuals in the United States. Hundreds of millions are afflicted worldwide. Acute hepatitis can be caused by type A, type B with or without delta co-infection, and by non-A, non-B (NANB) infection. The same viruses, except A, may also cause chronic hepatitis or a carrier state.

CLINICAL SIGNS AND SYMPTOMS

The incubation period for hepatitis A ("short incubation hepatitis") is between 2 and 6 weeks (average 25 days); for hepatitis B ("long incubation hepatitis"), 6 weeks to 6 months (average 75 days); and for NANB, 30 to 180 days (average 50 days). It is not possible to discriminate among the various forms of hepatitis on clinical grounds.

The symptoms in the prodromal phase of hepatitis are flulike with mild fever, malaise, nausea, vomiting, joint pain, and general prostration (Fig 61–1). Macular rashes appear rarely. These symptoms, which resemble serum sickness, are thought to be caused by immune complexes. The patient is frequently unaware of hepatitis until entering the icteric phase. At this point, the symptoms usually improve despite increasing jaundice. The jaun-

diced patient has tender hepatomegaly; some patients also have a palpable spleen. In the occasional patient whose nausea and vomiting

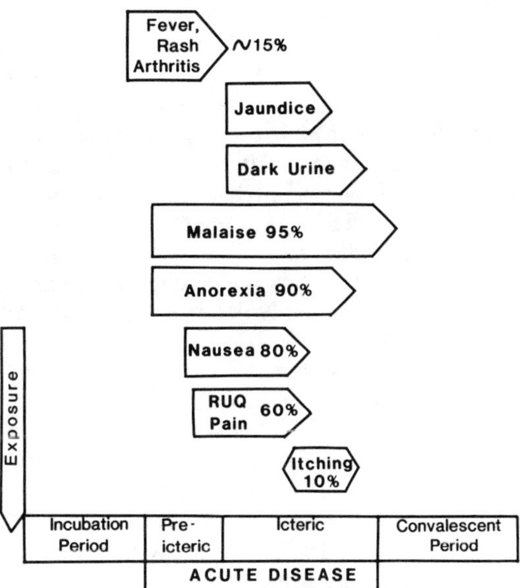

Fig 61–1.
The course of symptoms in typical acute viral hepatitis. The timing and incidence of the major symptoms during the four clinical periods of this disease are shown. [Reproduced with the permission of Abbott Laboratories, Diagnostics Division, North Chicago, Ill.]

continue at the height of the icteric phase, hospital admission and intravenous fluid replacement are needed to prevent additional liver injury from hypotension. In the overwhelming majority of cases, the jaundice subsides within 6 weeks, and the patient enters the convalescent phase with gradual normalization of serum transaminase values. In the usual benign course of hepatitis B, serum bilirubin and transaminase levels return to normal and HBsAg is cleared from the serum within 3 months (Fig 61–2, A).

The spectrum of disease includes asymptomatic infection to fulminant hepatitis, to which about 1% of icteric cases progress. An ominous sign is a liver suddenly decreasing in size, followed by hepatic coma. About 10% of the patients with hepatitis B, and probably a higher fraction with NANB, fail to recover completely within 6 months. The condition is then arbitrarily diagnosed as chronic hepatitis. HBsAg persists, and liver function tests are abnormal. Such a patient with chronic hepatitis B may have an acute exacerbation caused by the delta agent.

PATHOPHYSIOLOGY

The type A virus is a 27-nm, single-stranded RNA virus classified as picornavirus. The viral capsid is made of 32 capsomers in icosahedral order. It is similar to polio or coxsackievirus in that it can be grown in tissue culture and is noncytopathic. The IgM antibody, which develops early in the course of hepatitis A infection, can be used to establish the diagnosis. Later the presence of IgG antibody documents permanent immunity (Fig 61–3).

In contrast, the hepatitis B virus contains DNA and is therefore classified as a hepadna virus. The 45-nm Dane particles seen on electronmicroscopy represent the intact virus. The core of the particle is made of partially double-stranded DNA in circular arrangement. The gap in the incomplete DNA strand may be responsible for the virus' propensity to integrate into host DNA. The other, complete DNA strand is nicked and contains the entire message, which can be transcribed with the help of a unique DNA-dependent DNA polymerase.

Up to ten viral genomes of hepatitis B virus

may be present per nucleus. Spheres and tubules can be identified electron-microscopically in serum. Immunologic techniques have shown that these surface proteins correspond to hepatitis B surface antigen (HBsAg), which is found in serum in levels up to 50 mg/dL, unique for viral protein concentration. Another protein marker found in serum is e-antigen (HBeAg), also originating in the core (HBcAg) of the virus. Its presence is associated with infectivity.

The immune response to HBsAg (seroconversion to anti-HBs) confers permanent immunity to hepatitis B. In contrast, anti-HBc, which appears in the serum before anti-HBs, does not render protective immunity and represents a marker for ongoing infection if present without simultaneous anti-HBs (Fig 61–2). The presence of IgM–anti-HBc signals acute B hepatitis. Anti-HBe is a useful marker in chronic hepatitis and correlates with low infectivity. Its presence likewise does not equate with immunity (Fig 61–2, B).

Delta virus is a defective 36-nm RNA satellite virus that needs the hepatitis B virus to replicate. Similar viruses are found only in plants. A delta infection occurs as either a co-infection with acute hepatitis B or as a superinfection in carriers. Delta virus replaces the core antigen in the liver. Both the delta antigen and subsequently its antibody may be detected in the serum. Again IgM appears early and is used to document an acute hepatitis involving the delta virus. The subsequent IgG anti-DAg disappears within a few years of the infection.

The agent(s) of non-A, non-B (NANB) hepatitis have been very elusive and are not characterized. Because no immunologic tests are available, NANB is diagnosed by exclusion of other viruses and drugs. Epidemiologic case analysis is compatible with at least three forms of NANBV. The first causes 95% of hepatitis associated with blood transfusions and occurs most frequently between 30 and 180 days after transfusion, with the average incubation time being 50 days. The second variant has been observed 10 to 20 days after the injection of clotting factors. The third form simulates hepatitis A clinically and occurs in epidemics in the Orient. Hepatitis A, or infectious hepatitis, is spread by the fecal–oral route and consequently occurs in outbreaks related to poor hy-

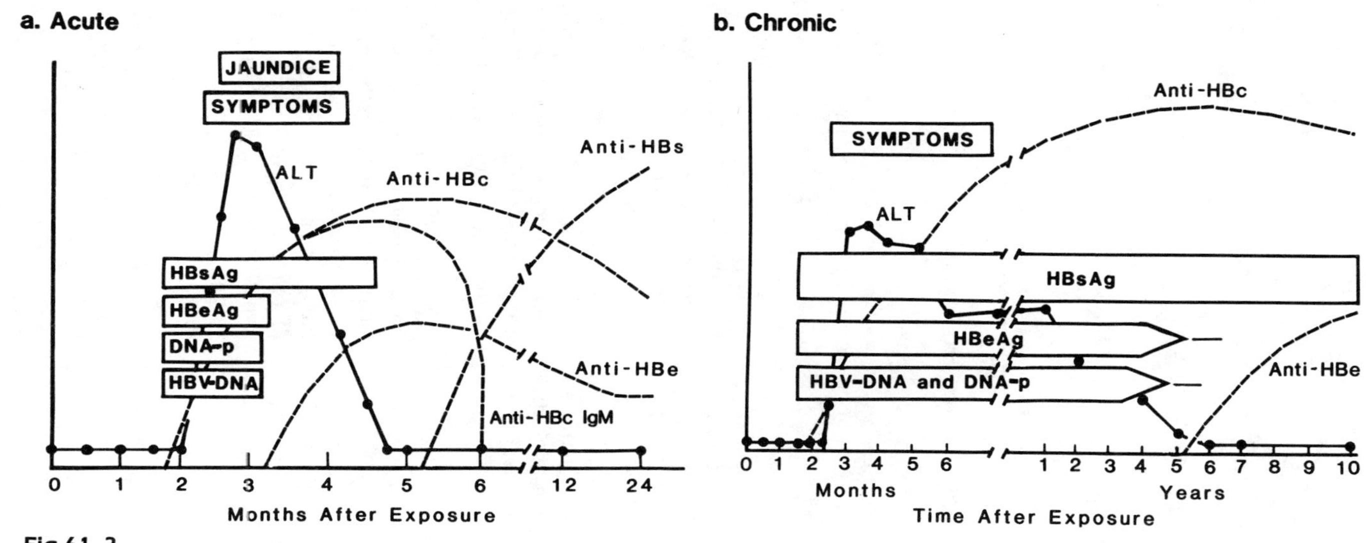

Fig 61–2.

The clinical, serologic, and biochemical course of typical type B hepatitis—*A*, acute; *B*, chronic. (ALT = alanine aminotransferase; HBsAg = hepatitis B surface antigen; HBeAg = hepatitis B e antigen; DNA-p = serum hepatitis B virus DNA polymerase activity; HBV-DNA = serum hepatitis B virus DNA; Anti-HBc = antibody to hepatitis B core antigen; Anti-HBs = antibody to HBsAg; Anti-HBe = antibody to HBeAg). [Reproduced in part with the permission of Abbott Laboratories, Diagnostics Division, North Chicago, Ill.]

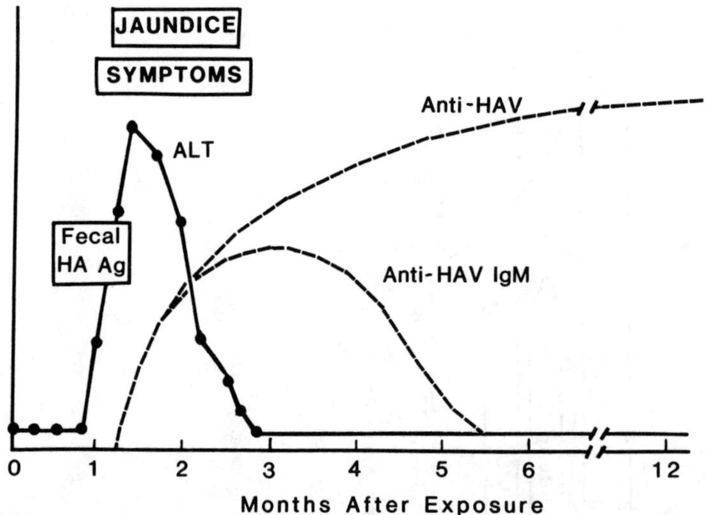

Fig 61–3.

The clinical, serologic, and biochemical course of typical type A hepatitis. (HA Ag = hepatitis A antigen; ALT = alanine aminotransferase; anti-HAV = antibody to hepatitis A virus). [Reproduced with the permission of Abbott Laboratories, Diagnostics Division, North Chicago, Ill.]

giene in day-care centers, military camps, or mental institutions. It can also be spread by close contact and through contaminated food.

Because both hepatitis B and NANB have a carrier state, parenteral infection plays a major role. The main transmission modes of "serum hepatitis" are blood transfusion or injection of blood products other than gamma globulin, contaminated hypodermic needles as occurs with drug addicts, and sexual contact.

CLINICAL–PATHOLOGIC CORRELATIONS

The clinical–pathologic correlations for various kinds of viral hepatitis are shown in Table 61–1. Biopsy specimens from patients with symptomatic or asymptomatic acute viral hepatitis show lymphocytic or histiocytic portal inflammation with periportal necrosis and lobular disarray. There is single-cell fallout with an infiltrate composed mostly of round cells with eosinophilic and neutrophilic leukocytes spread evenly throughout the lobule. The dead liver cells are transformed into acidophilic bodies (Councilman-like bodies) and are removed by Kupffer's cells, which then in-

crease in size and number. In fulminant hepatitis, the necrosis becomes confluent, resulting in massive hepatic necrosis.

Ongoing hepatitis beyond 6 months may cause the histologic picture of chronic persistent hepatitis, a mild round-cell portal infiltrate only. Because hardly any liver cell necrosis occurs, the serum transaminase levels are only mildly elevated. Symptoms, if any, include fatigue and mild jaundice. The prognosis is good.

In chronic active hepatitis, additional periportal piecemeal necrosis and erosion of the limiting plate are present. Bridges of fibrous tissue between portal tracts and central veins signal the transformation into cirrhosis. This form of chronic hepatitis occurs with B or NANB hepatitis or as an idiopathic "lupoid" form in young women that is associated with amenorrhea, acne, arthralgias, rash, fever, sicca syndrome, and other autoimmune features.

If HBsAg persists in asymptomatic subjects who have normal laboratory tests and normal liver histologic studies, a carrier state is diagnosed. Carriers may have the highest levels of circulating HBsAg. The cytoplasm of hepatocytes may be loaded with the antigen, giving a ground-glass appearance. The integration of

TABLE 61–1.
Clinical–Pathologic Correlations for Viral Hepatitis

CLINICAL FINDINGS	PATHOLOGIC FINDINGS	
	MECHANISM	PATHOLOGIC CHANGES
ACUTE VIRAL HEPATITIS (A, B, NANB)		
Heptomegaly, mild splenomegaly	Venous congestion	Lobular disarray with lobular and portal mononuclear infiltrate
Jaundice, dark urine	Transaminases markedly elevated, excretion of bilirubin decreased in bile, increased in urine	Dropout of liver cells, acidophilic bodies, apoptotic bodies
Serum sickness-like syndrome, rash, polyarteritis, glomerulonephritis	Immune complexes	Immune response to HBV*
Bleeding, petechiae	Decreased levels of coagulation factors result in increased PT	Acute viral hepatitis with confluent necrosis. Bridging hepatic necrosis (central-portal, portal-portal, central-central) with collapse; extensive dropout of liver cells
Edema, ascites	Decreased albumin levels	Acute viral hepatitis with confluent necrosis. Bridging hepatic necrosis (central-portal, portal-portal, central-central) with collapse; extensive dropout of liver cells
CHRONIC HEPATITIS		
Chronic Persistent Hepatitis (B, NANB)		
Mild hepatomegaly, fatigue	Transaminases mildly elevated	Mild portal infiltrate
Chronic Active Hepatitis (B, NANB)		
Jaundice, bleeding, edema	Excretory defect, decreased levels of coagulation factors and of albumin	Piecemeal necrosis; bridging necrosis; multilobular necrosis; portal inflammation
Portal hypertension, ascites	Fibrotic encroachment of portal blood vessels	Active cirrhosis
Chronic Active Hepatitis (autoimmune form)		
Young women with amenorrhea, acne, arthritis, arthralgias, rashes, pleurisy, fever	"Lupoid" changes: Serum gamma globulin level markedly elevated; LE preparation positive; ANA-positive; smooth muscle antibodies	Piecemeal necrosis; bridging necrosis; multilobular necrosis; portal inflammation; active cirrhosis; lymphocyte and plasma cell infiltrates in portal zones and between liver cells
Hirsutism, thyroid abnormalities, striae, sicca syndrome	Autoaggression	Nonspecific tissue antibodies
CHRONIC CARRIERS OF HBV		
Asymptomatic	High concentration of HBsAg	Ground-glass hepatocytes; no or minimal changes of architecture
	Normal Liver function tests	

* HBV = hepatitis B virus.

viral DNA into the liver nuclei creates a pre-cancerous condition, which explains the high frequency of hepatomas in carriers (perhaps aflatoxins act as co-carcinogens).

Superinfection of carriers with delta virus results in severe, frequently fulminant disease particularly in the HBeAg-negative, anti-HBe-positive individual. Portal lymphocytic infiltration with cytotoxic lesions and eosinophilic granulation of the cytoplasm is typical. Even in children, the South American variant of the disease, Labrea fever, is often fatal. The pathologic features include microsteatosis and eosinophilic necrosis.

NANB infection also shows fatty infiltration of the liver, either microvesicular or in large droplets. There are sinusoidal infiltrates and numerous acidophilic bodies. Sometimes bile duct lesions are present.

DIFFERENTIAL DIAGNOSIS

A number of viral infections may simulate acute viral hepatitis. The most frequent is infectious mononucleosis, accompanied by mild jaundice, fever, pharyngitis, lymphadenopathy, and lymphocytosis. Heterophile agglutinins (Paul-Bunnell test) are specific for infectious mononucleosis. Yellow fever and occasionally cytomegalovirus or herpes virus infections may be icteric.

Among the bacterial infections, leptospirosis deserves consideration if high fever and headaches are prominent. Drug-induced (acetaminophen, isoniazid, halothane, methyldopa, phenytoin) liver disease must be ruled out. In alcoholic hepatitis, serum transaminase levels are only moderately elevated, and cholestasis and leukocytosis are present.

Chronic active hepatitis must be differentiated from Wilson's disease in patients under age 35 years. The combination of Kayser-Fleischer corneal rings and a low serum ceruloplasmin level is diagnostic. Because Wilson's disease can be treated with penicillamine, early diagnosis may be life-saving. On rare occasions, drugs (methyldopa, INH) may be the culprit. Coexistence of emphysema with the clinical features of hepatitis in a young patient may indicate alpha$_1$-antitrypsin deficiency.

DIAGNOSIS

Liver function tests are very sensitive tools in establishing the diagnosis of acute viral hepatitis. In the typical setting, transaminase levels in the thousands, with only mildly elevated alkaline phosphatase and variable bilirubin levels, are diagnostic. The presence of antibody against hepatitis A virus (anti-HAV) IgM indicates hepatitis A, whereas the presence of HBsAg and IgM anti-HBc indicates hepatitis B. The absence of any of these markers is compatible with NANB hepatitis.

In chronic hepatitis, the transaminase levels are usually within the range of ten times normal. In B hepatitis, the e-serology is useful in assessing infectivity and prognosis. The presence of HBeAg is associated with high infectivity; anti-HBe signals low infectivity and carries a good prognosis. In young girls with "lupoid" hepatitis, a positive LE factor, antinuclear and anti-smooth muscle antibodies are common. A polyclonal hypergammaglobulinemia causes an albumin-to-globulin ratio of less than one.

A liver biopsy is usually not needed to diagnose acute hepatitis. In contrast, for the corticosteroid treatment of B-negative chronic hepatitis, a liver histologic study is a most useful guide. When marked cholestasis and high alkaline phosphatase levels are present, an ultrasound examination helps to rule out biliary duct obstruction.

PRINCIPLES OF PREVENTION AND THERAPY

When given to persons in close personal contact with infected patients, immune serum globulin protects up to 3 months against hepatitis A. To protect against hepatitis B, immune globulin pooled from donors with high anti-HBs titers must be used and should be given within hours of infection. Active immunization with hepatitis B vaccine should follow. Because the vast number of hepatitis B carriers are infected perinatally by their mothers, the newborns of HBsAg-positive mothers should be vaccinated shortly after birth using the combination of active and passive immunization. Prophylactic active immunization is recommended for health-care workers, hemodialysis patients, the sexually promiscuous, and household members in contact with carriers.

There is no rational treatment for acute or chronic viral hepatitis. "Lupoid" chronic active hepatitis in young girls responds favorably to corticosteroids. Patients with severe hepa- titis who vomit may need hospitalization for fluid and electrolyte replacement. In fulminant hepatitis, glucose infusions are given to prevent hypoglycemia. Fresh frozen plasma helps the patient overcome the severe coagulopathy. Lactulose or neomycin is useful to reverse encephalopathy.

REFERENCES

Blumberg BS: Australia antigen. The prevention of posttransfusion hepatitis. *Vox Sang* 1985; 48: 55–59. *Lucid treatise on the problem of posttransfusion hepatitis.*

Gerber MA, Thung SN: Viral hepatitis: Pathology, in Berk JE (ed): *Bockus Gastroenterology*, ed 4. vol 5, Philadelphia, WB Saunders Co, 1985, pp 2825–2855. *Comprehensive article on hepatitis from the viewpoint of a pathologist.*

Hoofnagle JH, Polesky HF, Gitnick G, Krugman S: Symposium: Hepatitis update. *Lab Med* 1983; 14(11):705–732. *Excellent survey of all relevant aspects of viral hepatitis, available through Abbott Diagnostics Division, North Chicago, Ill.*

Recommendations for protection against viral hepatitis. *MMWR* 1985; 34(22):313–335. (See also *MMWR* 1985; 34(8):105–113.) *This weekly publication of the Centers for Disease Control always contains the current recommendations for immunizations.*

Rizzetto M, Verme G, Recchia S et al: Chronic hepatitis in carriers of hepatitis B surface antigen, with intrahepatic expression of the delta antigen. An active and progressive disease unresponsive to immunosuppressive treatment. *Ann Intern Med* 1983; 98(4):437–441. *An update on delta infection from the group that discovered the agent.*

Shafritz DA, Lieberman HM: The molecular biology of hepatitis B virus. *Annu Rev Med* 1984; 35: 219–232. *An in-depth analysis of the unique features of HBV and its interaction with the liver cell.*

62 ALCOHOLIC CIRRHOSIS

Christopher J. Barde, M.D.

Alcoholic cirrhosis requires a clinical and a pathologic diagnosis. A liver biopsy is the only way to diagnose cirrhosis, but because there are several conditions that may also produce the classic findings of micronodular cirrhosis, there must be a supporting history of alcohol intake.

CLINICAL SIGNS AND SYMPTOMS

The history must concentrate on the diagnosis and the complications of alcoholic cirrhosis. It is important to obtain a history of alcohol use over a period of time. The amount of alcohol used is important in epidemiologic studies but is not easily obtained from the individual patient. Even alcohol screening questionnaires may miss 10% of patients with alcohol abuse. A strong history of alcoholism increases the likelihood of alcoholic liver disease but is not by itself diagnostic. For these reasons a search should be made for other causes of liver disease. The historian should ask about prior episodes of hepatitis, jaundice, blood transfusions, tattoos, travel, toxin exposure, and a possible family history of liver disease.

The complications frequently found with alcoholic cirrhosis are bleeding, ascites, renal involvement, and encephalopathy. The bleeding may be massive or occult and is frequently intermittent. The ascites may be associated with peripheral edema, and special attention should be paid to the presence of shortness of breath, peritonitis, or large abdominal-wall hernias. Encephalopathy may be difficult to establish but may be associated with nightmares, slower thinking, hallucinations, mood changes, and obtundation. General malnutrition may be missed if only the patient's weight is noted. Often the weight stays the same or increases secondary to ascites despite poor nutrition and muscle wasting. Unfortunately many of the patients with alcoholic cirrhosis also are active alcoholics. It is important to ask all patients or patients who are known alcoholics about their social situation and prior episodes of alcohol detoxifications, withdrawal problems, and seizure activity.

No single finding on the physical examination allows the diagnosis of alcoholic cirrhosis to be made. The physical findings are those of liver disease or its complications. The vital signs may reflect hemodynamic instability with hypotension, orthostasis, and tachycardia, all suggesting hypovolemia (secondary to bleeding or overdiuresis) or sepsis. Fever is frequently seen in association with alcoholic hepatitis or infections, though infections can occur without any elevation of temperature. The skin may show jaundice, excoriations, or vascular lesions (spider angiomas, telangiectasias, palmar erythema, ecchymosis). The head may show scleral icterus or parotid swelling. Pleural effusions are often associated with ascites. Gynecomastia and signs of feminization along with testicular atrophy may be present in male patients. The abdomen may show large abdominal collateral veins representing portal hypertension. Large amounts of ascites will grossly distend the abdomen, often causing ventral or umbilical herniation. Moderate amounts may be detected by the presence of a fluid wave or shifting dullness. The liver may be variable in size and consistency. The presence of hepar tenderness suggests alcoholic hepatitis. A bruit over the liver may also be heard on occasion (though vascular lesions may also cause bruits). The presence of splenomegaly suggests portal hypertension. A rectal examination may show hemorrhoids, which may be a manifestation of portal hypertension, although this cause is rare. Stools will frequently test positive for occult blood.

A neurologic examination may show evidence of a peripheral neuropathy or portal-systemic encephalopathy (PSE). The latter is often suspected when lethargy and asterixis are present. Early neurologic signs may include changes in personality (euphoria, depression, irritability), muscular incoordination, and an impairment of mental function. Serial hand-writing samples or the Number Connection Test are excellent methods of detecting early PSE.

A summary of the signs and symptoms of cirrhosis appears in Table 62–1. These do not vary significantly with the cause of the disease.

Cirrhosis is the fifth leading cause of death in adults. Its development revolves around the amount and duration of alcohol intake. Studies have shown that a group of patients who drank more than 160 gm of alcohol per day (the equivalent of 1 pint of whiskey) had a 9% incidence of severe liver disease after 5 years and 75% after 15 years. The patients who drank less than 160 gm per day had only a 17% incidence of severe disease after 15 years. Women develop severe liver disease with less exposure and may have a greater individual variation in their response. The role of genetic factors is to date unclear.

Alcoholic cirrhosis appears to be an end-stage of liver injury. In the majority of people with a high alcohol intake, fatty liver disease develops but does not progress to cirrhosis. Alcoholic hepatitis develops in 20% to 25% of patients, and cirrhosis develops in half of these patients.

Most patients with alcoholic cirrhosis are seen and treated either because of hepatic dysfunction or because of complications (ascites, variceal bleeding, or encephalopathy). Twenty percent of patients with cirrhosis, though, are asymptomatic and are often identified only in the course of a routine examination. A smaller number remain undetected until their death and an autopsy is performed. The percentage of unrecognized liver disease increases with age and may reach 90% in the aged. But these patients make up a minority of those with cirrhosis, and, with the onset of ascites, jaundice, or variceal hemorrhage, the 5-year survival rate is only 5% to 8%.

The prognosis for patients with alcoholic liver disease and predictions of treatment response have traditionally been based on assigning a patient to a group reflecting the severity

TABLE 62–1.
Signs and Symptoms in Cirrhosis

CLINICAL FINDINGS	FREQUENCY (% OF PATIENTS)
Hepatomegaly	67
Ascites	58
Jaundice	49
Varices	48
Weakness	43
Splenomegaly	40
Spider nevi	38
Anorexia	37
Encephalopathy	36
Abdominal pain	34
Nausea and vomiting	32
Hematemesis	28

of the liver disease. The most frequently used method is the Child-Turcotte classification (Table 62–2). Of the five factors, only the measurement of the bilirubin and albumin levels are reliable. The others are often subjective or poorly controlled. In addition the factors often overlap categories. A patient may be jaundiced with hypoalbuminemia but no ascites, thus making it difficult to place him or her in a category. These difficulties must be taken into account when reviewing studies on survival to see if the placement of patients in categories was comparable among different studies.

PATHOPHYSIOLOGY

Alcohol and its metabolite acetaldehyde are direct toxins of the liver. Together they cause a decrease in nicotinamide-adenine dinucleotide (NAD) levels, a decrease in mitochondrial function, and an alteration in the microtubules that integrate cell organelle function. These result in hypertrophy of the smooth endoplasmic reticulum and impairment of protein and lipid transport and release. The precursor of alcoholic cirrhosis is alcoholic hepatitis with hepatocyte swelling, balloon degeneration, and necrosis with polymorphonuclear cell infiltration. In cirrhosis, an increase of collagen deposition begins in the space of Disse and around the central vein. The collagen may be synthesized in fibroblasts, Ito cells, hepatocytes, circulating lymphocytes, and other cells. In addition, regeneration following cell necrosis is disordered. This and the increase in collagen

TABLE 62–2.
Child-Turcotte Classification

FACTOR	A	B	C
Serum bilirubin mg/dl	Below 2.0	2.0–3.0	Over 3.0
Serum albumin gm/dl	Over 3.5	3.0–3.5	Under 3.0
Ascites	None	Easily controlled	Poorly controlled
Neurologic disorder	None	Minimal	Advanced "coma"
Nutrition	Excellent	Good	Poor

may lead to venous obstruction and portal hypertension or ascites. Disruption of the microcirculatory unit with arteriovenous anastomosis in addition to decreased hepatocyte function leads to a decreased clearance of nitrogenous substances and to hepatic encephalopathy. The decrease in hepatic function may also lead to jaundice, coagulopathy defects, feminization, and hypoalbuminemia. The liver grossly may look yellow from fat deposition, red from congestion, or green from jaundice. The surface may resemble a pigskin, with micronodules 3 mm in diameter, or may have the larger nodules of macronodular cirrhosis that are seen in end-stage alcoholic cirrhosis.

CLINICAL–PATHOLOGIC CORRELATIONS

The correlation between clinical findings and the pathologic mechanisms behind them are listed in Table 62–3. The methods by which these features may be identified are also listed.

DIFFERENTIAL DIAGNOSIS

Twenty percent of patients with suspected alcoholic cirrhosis will have, upon liver biopsy, another disorder, despite a negative hepatitis B profile and an SGOT-to-SGPT ratio greater than 2:1. These disorders include acute or chronic hepatitis, periocholangitis, congestive failure, granulomatous infiltration, and tumors. Other patients may have alcoholic liver disease and one of the above problems concomitantly. Micronodular cirrhosis is a hallmark of alcoholic cirrhosis, but there are also other diseases with the same pathologic findings (biliary obstruction, hemachromatosis, and small-bowel bypass surgery). End-stage alcoholic liver disease

may also show a macronodular cirrhosis where the differential would have to include hepatitis.

DIAGNOSIS

The diagnosis of alcoholic cirrhosis is made by liver biopsy with a supporting history of alcohol intake. Rankin and co-workers have shown how unreliable the clinical and laboratory findings are in differentiating the types of alcoholic liver disease (Rankin et al., 1978). Alcoholic cirrhosis was found in 37% of patients with suspected fatty liver disease and 45% with presumed alcoholic hepatitis. While the diagnostic reliability of a liver biopsy is 98% in alcoholic cirrhosis, it cannot be performed on all patients. Those with ascites or coagulation disorders may have complications from a liver biopsy, and for this reason the biopsy is often deferred. In this case it is important to rule out other causes of liver disease with a hepatitis B virus profile and measurement of serum ferritin, ceruloplasmin, and alpha$_1$-antitrypsin levels. In cases with jaundice and an elevated alkaline phosphatase level, biliary obstruction should be ruled out with an ultrasound study or an endoscopic retrograde cholangiogram (ERCP)

Laboratory tests by themselves cannot make the diagnosis of alcoholic cirrhosis, but certain tests may indicate alcoholic liver disease. Whereas elevated levels of serum transaminases reflect inflammation or damage to the hepatocyte, an SGOT-to-SGPT ratio greater than 2:1 with an SGOT level of less than 500 IU/ml suggests alcoholic liver disease. The mean cell volume (MCV) and the gamma-glutamyl transferase (GGT) and alkaline phosphatase levels are often good indicators of the degree of alcohol consumption.

TABLE 62–3.
Clinical–Pathologic Correlations for Alcoholic Cirrhosis

CLINICAL FINDINGS	PATHOLOGIC FINDINGS	
	PATHOLOGIC MECHANISM	IDENTIFICATION
Ascites	Portal hypertension because lymphatic drainage unable to remove all fluid	Shifting dullness; shown on ultrasound scans and flat x-ray plate of abdomen
Hemorrhage	Portal hypertension	Varices on endoscopy, UGI, angiography
Encephalopathy	Elevated blood NH_3 False neurotransmitters	Asterixis, abnormal EEG, abnormal results of mental tests
Jaundice	Hepatic function with inability to conjugate or excrete bilirubin	Elevated bilirubin level
Coagulopathy	Decreased synthesis of vitamin K-dependent clotting factors	Prolonged prothrombin time
	Thrombocytopenia	Decreased platelet count
	Increased fibrinolysis	Prolonged PT, PTT; normal level of factor VIII; thrombocytopenia
Hepatomegaly	Fatty infiltration Cirrhosis	Physical examination or liver scan
Pain in the right upper quadrant	Hepatitis Hepatoma	Pain on physical examination
Hyponatremia	Dilution Depletion secondary to diuretics Inappropriate production of antidiuretic hormone	Serum Na^+ below 135 mEq/L
Hypokalemia	Diuretics Secondary hyperaldosteronism	Serum K^+ below 3.5 mEq/L
Hypoxemia	Arteriovenous shunting; Decreased tidal volume due to ascites	Arterial blood gas
Feminization and Hypogonadism	Hyperestrogenism	Gynecomastia Female escutcheon Testicular atrophy

Laboratory tests are useful for ruling out other causes of liver disease and for making a prognosis and monitoring the alcoholic liver disease. The prothrombin time is a good measurement of hepatic reserve because it reflects the liver's ability to synthesize factors involved in coagulation. The albumin level also reflects hepatic synthesis but may be affected by low protein intake, other chronic diseases, and loss into ascitic fluid.

PRINCIPLES OF TREATMENT

There is no specific therapy for alcoholic cirrhosis. The fibrous scars appear to be permanent. Abstinence may decrease the amount of fat in the hepatocyte. In alcoholic hepatitis, the inflammatory reaction has been initiated, and cirrhosis becomes a possibility despite further abstinence. Powell and Klatskin reported that survival improved in patients who stopped drinking, though others have failed to confirm this.

The treatment of cirrhosis is often the management of its complications. Bleeding esophageal varices carry a high mortality rate (up to 85%). Acute management is begun with blood transfusions, intravenous administration of vasopressin, or balloon tamponade. Endoscopic sclerosis of the varices and portocaval shunt surgery are effective in preventing rebleeding. Whether these procedures alter the mortality rate is questionable.

Ascites only requires treatment if it interferes with respiration or significantly limits a patient's activity. Sodium restriction is the first step in therapy followed by the use of diuretics in those who don't respond. While peritoneovenous shunts are a popular treatment, controlled studies have shown them to be no more beneficial than medical management. Encephalopathy requires a search for and removal of the possible initiating factors (infections, bleeding, high-protein diet, sedatives, metabolic abnormalities). Lactulose and neomycin inhibit the amount of ammonia absorbed from the bowel, though by different mechanisms, and are effective in the treatment of hepatic encephalopathy.

The hepatorenal syndrome has a mortality rate of over 90%. Blood flow is redistributed in an otherwise healthy kidney with a resultant decrease in urine output. Volume depletion has to be ruled out as a possible cause of the problem. Peritoneovenous shunting has occasionally been a successful treatment.

Liver transplantation is the only way to restore the terminally injured liver. Because of the expense and limited personnel, selection of patients often requires age limitations and proven abstinence from alcohol. At this point transplantation cannot be considered a possibility for the thousands of patients with alcoholic cirrhosis.

REFERENCES

Conn Ho: A peek at the Child-Turcotte classification. *Hepatology* 1981; 1:673–676. *Editorial on the development and limitations of the Child-Turcotte classification.*

Galambos JT: Alcoholic liver disease: Fatty liver, hepatitis, and cirrhosis, in Berk JE (ed): *Bockus Gastroenterology*, ed 4. Philadelphia, WB Saunders Co, 1985, pp 2985–3048. *Extensive review of the epidemiology, pathogenesis, and diagnosis of alcoholic liver disease, with supporting chapters on the complications of cirrhosis.*

Galambos JT: Portal hypertension. *Semin Liver Dis* 1985; 5:277–290. *Excellent references for aspects of medical and surgical treatment of portal hypertension.*

Geokas MC, Lieber CS, French S et al: Ethanol, the liver, and the gastrointestinal tract. *Ann Intern Med* 1981; 95:198–211. *A review of the metabolism of alcohol and its effects on several organ systems. 148 references.*

Levin DM, Baker AL, Riddell RH et al: Nonalcoholic liver disease: Overlooked causes of liver injury in patients with heavy alcohol consumption. *Am J Med* 1979; 66:429–434. *Describes the significant number of patients with suspected alcoholic liver disease that is not caused by alcohol.*

Powell WJ and Klatskin G: Duration of survival in patients with Laennec's cirrhosis. *Am J Med* 1968; 44:406–420. *Influence of alcohol withdrawal on the course of cirrhosis.*

Rankin JG, Orrego-Matte H, Deschênes J et al: Alcoholic liver disease: The problem of diagnosis. *Alcoholism* 1978; 2:327—338. *Excellent study pointing out the limitations of the physical examination in defining the type of alcoholic liver disease present.*

Stassen WN, McCullough AJ: Management of ascites. *Semin Liver Dis* 1985; 5:291–305. *A well-referenced review of the pathophysiology and treatment of ascites.*

63 HEPATOCELLULAR CARCINOMA

Larry W. Weprin, M.D.

Malignant tumors of the liver may be primary or metastatic. Primary malignant tumors may arise from hepatic parenchymal cells (hepatocellular carcinoma), bile duct epithelium (cholangiocarcinoma), mesenchymal tissue, or from a combination of the above. Of all primary malignant liver tumors, 90% are from hepatic parenchymal cells, and 10% are from bile duct epithelium and other supporting structures. *Hepatoma* is a term used interchangeably with the more recommended *hepatocellular carcinoma* (HCC).

Malignant liver tumors encountered in children are generally hepatocellular in origin rather than metastatic. In industrialized Western society, metastatic liver disease (from the breast and colon) is more prevalent than hepatocellular carcinoma. Worldwide, hepatocellular carcinoma is the most common liver tumor and is one of the most malignant of internal organ cancers in terms of prognosis.

The types and patterns of the hepatic tumors encountered depend in large part on the geographic location and age of the patient. Because of the geographic distribution and the occurrence in migrant populations, multiple etiologic agents have been suggested as possible causes (Table 63–1). Worldwide epidemiologic studies of cancer show that specific parts of Africa and Asia are the areas of highest incidence of hepatocellular carcinoma and that hepatocellular carcinoma can account for up to 70% of all malignancies in men and 20% of all malignancies in women. There are approximately 250,000 new cases worldwide per year. In California the frequency has tripled in the past 20 years. Currently the United States has a rate of 2.7 cases per 100,000 men per year.

CLINICAL SIGNS AND SYMPTOMS

Hepatocellular carcinoma has an insidious onset and runs a silent course until the end stage of the disease. Approximately one-third of the patients present with signs and symptoms of carcinoma, approximately another third present with unexplained deterioration of a patient with known cirrhosis and approximately one-third present with an abdominal catastrophe, fever of unknown origin, gallbladder disease, or some of the systemic manifestations of the tumor. Lastly, about 10% of the cases are found at the time of autopsy.

The first complaint of those presenting with symptoms of carcinoma is usually abdominal discomfort and pain. The abdominal pain is usually a dull ache and usually occurs in the right upper quadrant and may be made worse by movement.

Table 63–2 lists the common signs seen in hepatocellular carcinoma. Ascites is present in 20% to 50% of cases at the time of diagnosis and becomes more prominent as the disease progresses. Jaundice and splenomegaly also occur in approximately 50% of the cases.

Other signs and symptoms of hepatocellular carcinoma occur because of metastatic disease and paraneoplastic manifestations. The lung is the most common site of metastases. Other sites include the lymph nodes, the adrenal glands, and bone.

Ectopic hormone production can result in clinical paraneoplastic syndromes which occasionally may be the predominant symptoms and may dominate the clinical picture. The mechanisms underlying the paraneoplastic syndrome are multifactorial and include pro-

TABLE 63–1.
Possible Causes of Hepatocellular Carcinoma

Chronic infection with Hepatitis B virus (HBV)
Hemochromatosis
Alpha$_1$-antitrypsin deficiency
Exposure to chemicals: Nitrosamines, mycotoxins, vinyl
  chloride
Alcohol ingestion
Cirrhosis

TABLE 63–2.
Clinical Signs in Hepatocellular Carcinoma

SIGN	OCCURRENCE (% OF CASES)
Hepatomegaly	90
Ascites	35–60
Hepatic bruit	6–25
Jaundice	10–40
Splenomegaly	10–40
Tender liver	15–60
Fever	10–50
Edema	10–30

duction of hormone-like substances and of hormones that alter metabolism, and increasing utilization of normal serum constituents. Table 63–3 lists the paraneoplastic manifestations.

Erythrocytosis is the most common paraneoplastic manifestation. An erythropoietic factor secreted by the tumor or an inability to metabolize normal erythropoietin are two proposed mechanisms for the erythrocytosis. Hypoglycemia is thought to be secondary to overutilization of glucose by the tumor or possibly from production of an insulin-like substance by the tumor. Hypercalcemia is postulated to develop from a parathyroid hormone-like substance produced from the tumor. Other tumor-associated findings include hyperlipidemia, porphyria cutanea tarda, hypercholesterolemia, hyperglycemia, and disseminated intravascular hemolysis.

The natural history of hepatocellular carcinoma is one of rapid, progressive deterioration in the end stages. The average survival after diagnosis is about 6 months. The patient may become increasingly weak with increasing abdominal pain, anorexia, cachexia, tense ascites, and massive hepatomegaly. The most common cause of death is cachexia and weight loss. Gastrointestinal bleeding and hepatic failure are also common causes for death. Occasionally a dramatic terminal event with a hemoperitoneum can be seen secondary to rupture of the tumor into the abdomen.

Table 63–4 lists some of the common clinical manifestations and the apparent pathophysiologic mechanisms.

PATHOPHYSIOLOGY

The wide variations in the incidence of hepatocellular carcinoma in different parts of the world have been thought to be related to exposure to multiple environmental carcinogens. Table 63–1 lists some of the etiologic factors in hepatocellular carcinoma.

The high incidence of carriers of hepatitis B virus surface antigen (HBsAg) in patients with hepatocellular carcinoma has led this to be considered an etiologic association. Eighty to ninety percent of cases of hepatocellular carcinoma worldwide occur in patients who are hepatitis B virus (HBV) carriers. The antibody to HBV is rarely found in patients with hepatocellular carcinoma. Places that have high carrier rates for HBV have a high incidence of hepatocellular carcinoma, and locations that have low carrier rates have a low incidence of hepatocellular carcinoma. There are an estimated 120 million carriers of HBV in the world, with 200,000 in the United States. In areas where hepatocellular carcinoma is common, the HBV carrier state is usually seen in infants and children. The HBV is usually transmitted vertically from mother to child in these areas.

In sub-Saharan Africa the mycotoxin aflatoxin is thought to act as a co-carcinogen with HBV. The aflatoxin possibly supresses cellular immunity and allows an HBsAg carrier state.

TABLE 63–3.
Paraneoplastic Manifestations of Hepatocellular Carcinoma

	OCCURRENCE (% OF CASES)
Erythrocytosis	2–10
Hypercalcemia	7
Hypoglycemia	5–27
Hyperlipidemia	Rare
Porphyria cutanea tarda	Rare
Hypercholesterolemia	30
Disseminated intravascular hemolysis	Rare

DIAGNOSIS

The diagnosis is usually made late in the disease because of the slow and insidious onset. It can be suspected by biochemical tests as

TABLE 63–4.
Clinical–Pathologic Correlations for Hepatocellular Carcinoma

CLINICAL FINDINGS	PATHOLOGIC FINDINGS
Erythrocytosis	Erythropoietin-stimulating hormone, or the inability to metabolize erythropoietin
Hypoglycemia	Over-utilization of glucose by the tumor, or production of an insulin-type hormone
Hepatic bruit	Secondary to the vascular nature of this tumor
Hemoperitoneum	Rupture of the vascular tumor into the peritoneum
Dyspnea	Secondary to pulmonary metastases or to tumor compression of the diaphragm
Ascites	Portal vein thrombosis from blockage of the portal vein by the tumor, or portal hypertension
Pruritis	Bile stasis and deposition in the skin
Abdominal pain	Perihepatitis

well as by x-ray investigation. The differentiation of primary disease from metastatic disease to the liver can be difficult. Hepatocellular carcinoma should be considered in the differential diagnosis when there is deterioration in a person known to have cirrhosis.

Alpha-fetoprotein, an alpha$_1$ globulin normally present in the developing fetus, is present in minute amounts in adults. A high serum value of the alpha-fetroprotein in an adult usually indicates hepatocellular carcinoma. There is no obvious correlation between the elevation of the alpha-fetoprotein and the clinical or biochemical features of the disease, the size and stage of the tumor, or the survival time after diagnosis. Also, the degree of elevation of alpha-fetoprotein does not correlate with the extent of differentiation of the tumor itself. The level of alpha-fetoprotein has been used postoperatively to detect recrudescence of the disease. Alpha-fetoprotein levels are usually normal in metastatic liver disease, helping to differentiate between this and hepatocellular carcinoma. Other biochemical changes such as liver function tests are of no specific value in diagnosing hepatocellular carcinoma or for distinguishing primary from secondary liver disease.

Other diagnostic modalities include multiple radiologic investigations. Hepatic arteriography has been extremely useful in the diagnosis of this tumor because of its highly vascular nature.

Isotope liver scanning can confirm the presence of a mass in the liver, but is nondiagnostic. A small-size tumor in a cirrhotic liver may not be detected because of the irregular patchy uptake of the isotope. Gallium scanning can be helpful in differentiating cirrhosis from hepatocellular carcinoma. Gallium is not taken up by cirrhotic defects in the liver, but hepatocellular carcinoma is enhanced with gallium. In 30% of patients with hepatocellular carcinoma, however, the tumor may not concentrate the gallium.

Ultrasonography can differentiate between solid and cystic hepatic masses but does not necessarily distinguish between hepatocellular carcinoma and other solid tumors.

A definitive diagnosis can be achieved by liver biopsy. The risk of bleeding is rare, but it is greater than seen in non-neoplastic conditions. A liver biopsy can be directed by laparoscopy, ultrasonography, or even by computed tomography.

PRINCIPLES OF THERAPY

The surgical treatment depends on the stage of disease present at the time of diagnosis. At present a surgical resection with a partial hepatectomy offers the only chance of long-term cure. The major problem is that because the disease has an insidious onset, at the time of diagnosis the disease may be too widespread for a curative resection. With newer imaging techniques the extent of tumor involvement and operability can be determined with more accuracy. Tumors are considered resectable if there is no spread from one lobe of the liver to another and no evidence of any extrahepatic metastases. Because the liver can regenerate, 90% of the liver can be removed with recovery of good liver function.

Chemotherapy has a low response rate irrespective of the agents used. Intra-arterial infusion has been used and, in conjunction with radiotherapy, has yielded better results than chemotherapy alone.

Hepatic transplantation has also had unsatisfactory results. As this becomes a more standard surgical procedure, this approach may yield better results.

Surgical statistics might improve with earlier intervention in the course of the disease when hepatocellular carcinoma may be localized to a segment of the liver. Eradication of the disease is unlikely unless the large proportion of carriers of HBV can be reduced. Prevention of vertical transmission (mother to child) of HBV with hepatitis B vaccine in areas of high incidence of hepatocellular carcinoma may be helpful in eliminating one factor. In developed Western countries horizontal transmission is the common mode of transmission of HBV. Control strategies would therefore be directed at high-risk groups such as homosexuals. The cost of HBV vaccine and the relatively small supply may prohibit its use worldwide.

At present, early diagnosis, possibly through mass screening using alpha-fetoprotein measurement and x-ray studies in areas of high risk, may help make earlier diagnoses and lead to a better long-term prognosis. Hepatocellular carcinoma remains a tumor that is very difficult to treat.

REFERENCES

Arthur MJP, Hall AJ, Wright R: Hepatitis B, hepatocellular carcinoma, and strategies for prevention. *Lancet* 1984; 1:607–610. *A discussion of the approach to preventing vertical and horizontal transmission through mass vaccination.*

Beasley RP, Hwang LY: Hepatocellular carcinoma and hepatitis B virus. *Semin Liver Dis* 1984; 4:113–121. *An in-depth review of the association of HBV with hepatocellular carcinoma.*

Kew MC, Popper H: Relationship between hepatocellular carcinoma and cirrhosis. *Semin Liver Dis* 1984; 4:136–146. *A review and explanation of the relationship between hepatocellular carcinoma and cirrhosis.*

Oon CJ, Friedman MA: Primary hepatocellular carcinoma. *Cancer Chemother Pharmacol* 1982; 8:231–235. *A brief but succinct review of the recent treatment modalities as well as etiologic factors.*

64 PANCREATITIS

Christopher J. Barde, M.D.

Pancreatitis is an inflammation of the pancreas caused by the release of intrapancreatic enzymes. The initiating factors may be multiple. Acute pancreatitis is often but not always a limited process that on resolution leaves no functional impairment of the pancreas. This differs from chronic pancreatitis where exocrine or endocrine insufficiency, persistent pain, or histologic evidence of chronic inflammation exists. The definitions often overlap so that an acute attack is an individual inflammatory episode whether or not irreversible damage occurs. Clinically, acute pancreatitis causes abdominal pain associated with a rise in the serum level of amylase (or other pancreatic-specific enzymes) that returns to normal as the pain resolves.

CLINICAL SIGNS AND SYMPTOMS

An attack of pancreatitis usually begins as a dull ache in the epigastrium that reaches full intensity within an hour. This visceral pain radiates to the back in 50% of patients. Inflammation of the adjacent organs produces distention (70%) and nausea and vomiting (75%). The history may identify past illnesses, medications, trauma, a familial history, or symptoms that describe the initiating factor. The most common causes of acute pancreatitis are gallbladder disease and alcohol use. A more complete list is in Table 64–1. Much of the symptom complex may revolve around the underlying disease (i.e., peptic ulcer disease).

The patients appear ill and often are in the knees-up position to reduce peritoneal irritation. Hypotension and tachycardia secondary to volume depletion are present over half the cases. Tachypnea may be a sign of adult respiratory distress syndrome or acidosis. Fever is present in 60% to 80% early in the course,

but may herald an abscess if present after the first week. The abdomen may be distended with hypoactive or absent bowel sounds suggesting an ileus. Tenderness, frequently with rebound, is found over the epigastric or periumbilical regions. The presence of right upper-quadrant pain may suggest concomitant biliary disease. A palpable periumbilical mass may be a pseudocyst. A palpable periumbilical mass in acute pancreatitis may represent phlegmon though a patient with prior episodes of pancreatitis a pseudocyst must be considered. Ecchymosis on the flanks (Grey Turner's sign) or the periumbilical area (Cullen's sign) suggests hemorrhagic pancreatitis. The systemic findings of fat necrosis, tetany, or encephalopathy are rare. It is important to look for evidence of the initiating factor (i.e., the stigmata of liver disease, including jaundice and the xanthomas of lipid disorders, and trauma).

The majority of patients improve after 2 to 7 days. The 15% to 25% of patients with severe pancreatitis have a mortality rate of 16% to 100% depending on the risk factors that are present. Eleven risk factors (Table 64–2) allow prediction of which patients may have a severe course. The mortality rates correlate with the number of risk factors and are smaller for younger patients or those with prior episodes

---

TABLE 64–1.
Causes of Acute Pancreatitis

Cholelithiasis
Alcohol abuse
Idiopathic and/or hereditary
Trauma, postoperative
Drugs (azathioprine, thiazides, furosemide)
Hyperlipoproteinemia (types I, IV, V)
Hypercalcemia
Peptic ulcer
Pancreatic cancer
Miscellaneous: Viral infections, ischemia

TABLE 64–2.
Risk Factors in Acute Pancreatitis

PRESENT AT ADMISSION	PRESENT DURING FIRST 48 HOURS
Age over 55 years	Hematocrit decreases over 10%
WBC >16,000 cells/ml	BUN level increases more than 5 mg/dL
Blood glucose > 300 mg/dL	Serum calcium level < 8 mg/L
LDH >350 IU/L	Base deficit > 4 mEq/L
SGOT >250 SF units%	PaO_2 < 60 mm Hg
	Estimated fluid sequestration > 6 L

of pancreatitis. The higher-risk patients also have a higher morbidity rate. Up to 70% may have hypoxemia with some developing adult respiratory distress syndrome. Of concern is that up to 15% to 50% of the patients with severe pancreatitis will develop pseudocysts or pancreatic abscesses. If the initiating factor persists, recurrent attacks are likely. Those with repeated attacks or severe complications are more likely to develop chronic pancreatitis. In severe cases of chronic pancreatitis, there may be exocrine insufficiency (manifested by steatorrhea), endocrine insufficiency (hyperglycemia requiring insulin), and chronic pain.

PATHOPHYSIOLOGY

The pancreas produces large volumes of proteases for digestion. To protect the pancreas from autodigestion, the enzymes are stored in zymogen granule membranes until secreted and are inactive until the pancreatic juices reach the duodenum. The pancreas also produces trypsin inhibitor, which is present in pancreatic tissue and juice. In addition, the pancreas is perfused by blood containing $alpha_1$-antitrypsin and $beta_2$-macroglobulin, both antiproteolytic molecules.

Exactly how the protective mechanisms fail in pancreatitis is not known, but trypsinogen is converted to trypsin and the proteolytic cascade is activated. This premature activation of enzymes begins a process of autodigestion that results in mild edema to severe hemorrhagic necrosis. Trypsin activates phospholipase A and elastase which cause parenchymal and adipose tissue necrosis and dissolution of the elastic fibers in the blood vessels. Bradykinin is released causing vasodilation, increased vascular permeability, and pain. These effects are greater if the natural inhibitors $alpha_1$-antitrypsin and aprotinin are overwhelmed.

The tissue necrosis and kinin activity lead to edema and fluid sequestration in the peritoneal cavity resulting in hypovolemia. Calcium coming in contact with areas of fat necrosis may cause saponification and hypocalcemia. The hyperglycemia frequently seen is from an increased release of glucagon, not from insulin deficiency. Hypoxemia may be secondary to microthrombi from subclinical disseminated intravascular coagulation.

CLINICAL–PATHOLOGIC CORRELATIONS

The clinical manifestations of acute pancreatitis may occur in any organ system of the body. The major areas of concern are the cardiovascular, pulmonary, and gastrointestinal systems along with metabolic disorders such as hypoxemia, acidosis, and hyperglycemia. Table 64–3 shows the pathologic mechanisms behind these processes.

DIFFERENTIAL DIAGNOSIS

The symptoms and findings of the physical examination may be consistent with peptic ulcer disease, especially those involving the posterior aspect of the stomach or duodenum. The pain of cholelithiasis or cholangitis is usually in the right upper quadrant, but may appear as epigastric pain associated with nausea, vomiting, and fever. An amylase determination and an ultrasound or a hepatobiliary scan are useful in differentiating pancreatitis from cholecystitis. Patients with bowel perforation or infarction may present with an elevated serum amylase level and pain. The finding of free air on the x-ray film or a clinical suspicion of a bowel infarct are helpful. Patients with diabetic ketoacidosis often present with abdominal pain

TABLE 64–3.
Clinical–Pathologic Correlations for Pancreatitis

CLINICAL FINDINGS	MECHANISM	IDENTIFYING MEASUREMENTS OR PROCEDURES
Hypovolemia/shock	Fluid sequestration or hemorrhage	Vital signs Central venous pressure (Swan-Ganz monitor)
Hypocalcemia	Saponification Precipitation Decreased PTH response	Serum calcium Serum albumin
Hypoxemia	Atelectasis Pneumonitis Aspiration Adult respiratory distress syndrome	Arterial blood gases
Hyperglycemia	Insulin resistance Glucagon increases	Serum glucose Urine glucose
Acidosis	Lactate production Renal insufficiency Respiratory failure	Arterial blood gases Electrolytes
Hyperkalemia	Acidosis Renal insufficiency Tissue necrosis	Electrolytes
Ileus	Local inflammation Medications Hypokalemia	Abdominal examination Abdominal plain x-ray film
Gastrointestinal bleeding	Gastritis Peptic ulcer Varices Bowel infarction	Endoscopy
Atelectasis	Elevated diaphragm Poor excursion Supine position	Chest examination Chest x-ray film
Adult respiratory distress syndrome	Disseminated intravascular coagulation Pulmonary thrombi Hyperlipidemia Kinins	Swan-Ganz monitor Chest x-ray film Arterial blood gases
Pleural effusion	Activated pancreatic enzymes Diaphragmatic lymphatics	Chest examination Chest x-ray film Thoracentesis

and hyperamylasemia but without pancreatitis. This amylase is salivary amylase, so measurement of the serum levels of either lipase or isoamylase will distinguish this from pancreatitis.

DIAGNOSIS

An elevated serum amylase level associated with abdominal pain suggests pancreatitis. Hyperamylasemia is not specific for pancreatitis because the salivary glands, lungs, fallopian tubes, and certain tumors also secrete amylase. Amylase from these organs is an isoenzyme, salivary amylase, which is distinct from pancreatic amylase. Serum levels of amylase may also be elevated in renal failure or macroamylasemia (in which amylase is bound to a serum protein) because of ineffective glomerular filtration. A normal urinary level of amylase or lipase or identification of the isoenzyme can differentiate macroamylasemia from pancreatitis. The assays for amylase, lipase, trypsinogen (radioimmunoassay), and isoamylase (radioimmunoassay) have similar sensitivities and specificities (Table 64–4). Until the latter three assays are automated, the serum amylase will remain the most important test because of its ease of use in the laboratory.

Radiology has become useful in diagnosing severe pancreatitis and its complications. The

TABLE 64–4.
Assays in Acute Pancreatitis

ASSAY	SENSITIVITY (%)	SPECIFICITY (%)
Amylase	95	89
Lipase	86	99
Trypsinogen	95	86
Isoamylase	92	85

plain films of the abdomen, though, cannot be used to diagnose acute pancreatitis. The most frequent finding is an ileus. Findings of a sentinal loop or colon-cutoff sign in the splenic flexure may raise a suspicion of pancreatitis. Air in the biliary tract can be seen if a gallstone has recently been passed or if a duodenal ulcer has eroded into the common bile duct. It is of major importance to rule out air under the diaphragm that can be seen with a free perforation. Patients with repeated attacks may develop chronic pancreatitis with evidence of calcium deposits on the x-ray films. Ultrasound scans and computed tomography are relatively insensitive in diagnosing mild pancreatitis, missing the diagnosis in one-third of the cases. They are equally sensitive, however, for detecting complications in severe pancreatitis, although in up to 38% of the patients, the ultrasound scan provides incomplete information because of bowel gas.

PRINCIPLES OF THERAPY

The treatment of pancreatitis is the treatment of its complications and the prevention of further

pancreatic ischemia or renal failure. The hypotension resulting from loss of fluid into the abdominal cavity must be corrected. This often requires 4 to 10 L of intravenous fluids over 24 hours. In patients with a history of congestive heart failure, a Swan-Ganz monitor to measure pulmonary wedge pressures may be required. Neither nasogastric suction nor cimetidine alters the course of pancreatitis. Nasogastric suction is used for patients with an ileus to relieve the distention and prevent aspiration. Cimetidine is used to treat concomitant peptic ulcer disease or to prevent stress ulcerations in patients at risk. Monitoring for complications is crucial if treatment is to be instituted. An initial arterial blood gas measurement and a chest x-ray film should be made for all patients, repeated as necessary, and ventilatory support should be given as needed. Peritoneal dialysis has been attempted, but has not been found effective in controlled studies. Surgical treatment is reserved for patients with the complications of pseudocyst, abscess, hemorrhagic necrosis, or gallstone pancreatitis. Surgery for a pseudocyst is usually postponed for 6 weeks to allow maturing of the cyst wall so that the cyst can be drained by suturing to an adjacent viscus such as stomach, duodenum, or small bowel. A pancreatic abscess, on the other hand, needs prompt drainage because antibiotic therapy alone is not effective. Debate persists over the timing of biliary surgery in gallstone pancreatitis. Surgery done within the first 2 weeks has a low morbidity rate as long as the electrolyte status and fluid status have been corrected. Waiting 6 weeks reduces the edema, but attacks may recur during the waiting period.

REFERENCES

Dutta SK, Douglass W, Smalls UA et al: Prevalence and nature of hyperamylasemia in acute alcoholism. *Dig Dis Sci* 1981; 26:136–141. *A study showing that not all amylase elevations are of pancreatic origin.*

Geokas MC, Baltaxe HA, Banks PA et al: Acute pancreatitis. *Ann Intern Med* 1985; 103:86–100. *A review of the pathophysiology, diagnosis, and treatment, with extensive references.*

Loiudice TA, Lang J, Mehta H et al: Treatment of acute alcoholic pancreatitis: The roles of cimetidine and nasogastric suction. *Am J Gastroenterol* 1984; 79:553–558. *A well-referenced discussion of studies of the same topic.*

Ranson JHC: Acute pancreatitis: Pathogenesis, outcome and treatment. *Clin Gastroenterol* 1984; 13:843–863. *A good review of treatment with a surgical point of view.*

Soergel KH: Acute pancreatitis, in Sleisenger M, Fordtran JS (eds): *Gastrointestinal Disease.* Philadelphia, WB Saunders Co, 1983, pp 1462–1485. *A good general discussion of all aspects of pancreatitis.*

Steinberg WM, Goldstein SS, Davis ND et al: Diagnostic assays in acute pancreatitis. *Ann Intern Med* 1985; 102:576–580. *A comparison of the amylase, isoamylase, lipase, and trypsinogen assays.*

ADULT DIARRHEAL ILLNESSES

Clyde T. Miyaki, M.D.
Christopher J. Barde, M.D.

Diarrhea is an increase in stool frequency (more than three per day), liquidity, and total weight (more than 200 gm per day). A high-fiber diet may increase the stool weight without necessarily causing diarrhea. An important concept is that small-volume diarrhea due to disease of the lower colon or rectum may cause frequent defecation of blood or mucus without a large volume. The difference between acute and chronic diarrhea is duration, chronic diarrhea being longer than 2 weeks in length.

CLINICAL SIGNS AND SYMPTOMS

A detailed history will provide clues to the cause of the diarrhea. Information should be obtained about the onset, frequency, volume, consistency, color, odor, and associated findings of flatulence, blood, mucus, or fat droplets. The pattern of diarrhea is important. Nocturnal diarrhea usually signifies a pathologic process. Functional diarrhea seldom awakens the patient at night. Postprandial diarrhea may indicate altered motility or malabsorption.

In acute diarrhea, inquiry into recent drug ingestion such as antibiotics or antacids, food ingestion, recent travel, exposure to other infectious people, and sexual preference is important. Also information about systemic symptoms may lead to the cause of the acute diarrhea.

Determining the cause of chronic diarrhea is more involved, and the cause may remain a mystery even after an extensive work-up. General information about the duration (months vs. years), weight loss, fever, and malaise will indicate the degree of debilitation. The presence of rectal bleeding indicates a serious invasive or inflammatory process such as inflammatory bowel disease, amebiasis, or neoplasm. Information about prior operations such as gastrectomy or vagotomy, radiation, allergies, and familial illness should be sought. Dietary habits (especially fad diets) and drug intake (laxatives) should be investigated. Diarrhea may be an initial feature of certain systemic diseases such as diabetes mellitus, collagen vascular disease, or hyperthyroidism.

The physical examination provides few clues to the cause of diarrhea. The most important assessment is to determine the need for immediate medical therapy. Postural blood pressures, pulse rate, respiration, and skin turgor will indicate the state of hydration and the need for rapid fluid resuscitation. Other important signs are abdominal distension, peritonitis, or ileus. These may signify an impending abdominal catastrophe from perforation, or from a toxic megacolon resulting from amebiasis, shigellosis, or inflammatory bowel disease. Other less ominous signs which can be noted on examination and which may help differentiate the cause of the diarrhea are listed in Table 65–1.

The natural histories of diarrheal diseases are varied, and the clinical courses will depend on the causes. The cause of acute diarrhea is unknown in most cases, but is presumed to be viral (Norwalk or Rota). The viral illness is self-limited, lasting less than 48 hours, although the Rota virus may last up to 8 days. Most patients will use over-the-counter medications and not seek medical attention. Dehydration in very young or elderly persons may require hospitalization.

Most bacterial diarrheas are also self-limited and spontaneously resolve without specific therapy. Patients seek medical attention for prolonged diarrhea, rectal bleeding, fever, or increased symptomatic complaints. *Campylo-*

TABLE 65–1.
Physical Findings in Diarrhea

ORGAN	PHYSICAL FINDING	CAUSE OF DIARRHEA
Skin	Rose spot	*Salmonella typhosa*
	Pyoderma gangrenosum	Inflammatory bowel disease
	Dermatitis herpetiformis	Celiac sprue
	Purpura	Malabsorption, Schönlein-Henoch purpura
	Flushing	Carcinoid syndrome, vasoactive intestinal polypeptide
	Pigmentation	Addison's disease, Whipple's disease, sprue
Eyes	Exophthalmus	Hyperthyroidism
	Uveitis	Inflammatory bowel disease
Mouth	Pigmentation	Peutz-Jeghers syndrome
	Macroglossia	Amyloidosis
	Goiter	Hyperthyroidism
	Lymphadenopathy	Neoplasm, tuberculosis, Whipple's disease
Lung		Cystic fibrosis, tuberculosis
Abdomen	Surgical scar	Dumping syndrome, blind-loop syndrome, ileal resection
	Mass	Crohn's disease, carcinoma, amebiasis, diverticulitis
	Bruit	Vascular insufficiency
	Hepatomegaly	Cirrhosis, malignancy
Rectum	Mass	Neoplasm
	Stricture, fissure	Inflammatory bowel disease
Extremities	Arthritis	Inflammatory bowel disease, *Shigella* infection, *Yersinia* infection, Whipple's disease, collagen vascular disease
	Clubbing	Sprue, cystic fibrosis, ulcerative colitis
	Edema	Intestinal lymphangiectasia, sprue, inflammatory process
	Neuropathy	Diabetes mellitus, amyloidosis
	Postural hypotension	Addison's disease, diabetes mellitus
	Fever	Inflammatory bowel disease, tuberculosis, amebiasis, Whipple's disease, lymphoma, bacterial infection

bacter is the most common pathogen, occurring in up to 50% of cases of bacterial diarrheas. The diarrhea lasts up to 6 days, but has been known to last weeks and has a 25% relapse rate. This, plus the fact that 50% of patients have bloody diarrhea, may lead to a confusion of *Camplyobacter* enteritis with inflammatory bowel disease.

Salmonella gastroenteritis resolves in 4 days, although *Salmonella* colitis, present in up to 90% of hospitalized patients, may persist for 1 to 2 weeks and is associated with rectal bleeding. The incidence of chronic carriers is only 3 per 1000, but may be higher in the elderly or in those with biliary disease. *Salmonella*, like other gram-negative organisms, may invade several organs. Patients at high-risk for this complication are those with lymphoproliferative disease, prosthetic devices, valvular heart disease, hemolytic anemia, or advanced age.

Shigella causes 20% of bacterial diarrheas, which last up to 7 days. *Shigella* enteritis is usually self-limited, but antibiotics effectively shorten the duration. Mucosal invasion and bloody diarrhea cause confusion between *Shigella* enteritis with ulcerative colitis. The mortality rates for *Shigella* enteritis in the United States are less than 1%, but in developing countries may reach 32%. Although becoming a carrier and perforation are rare occurrences, 16% of patients with *Shigella* enteritis and with HLA-B27 will develop arthritis or Reiter's syndrome.

Yersinia infection is a rare disease in adults and may be first seen as ileitis or mesenteric adenitis. Bacteremia may rarely occur in immunocompromised hosts with a resulting high mortality rate despite antibiotic therapy.

Travelers' diarrhea may represent a number of bacterial or protozoan infections. Up to 60%

of travelers to Mexico may be affected, with toxigenic *Escherichia coli* being the agent in 40% to 70% of the cases. The episode lasts only 4 days, but if it persists, a search for other agents is imperative. Bacterial "food poisonings" result from enterotoxins that may be produced by *Staphylococcus*, *Clostridium perfringens*, *Bacillus cereus*, or *Vibrio parahaemolyticus*. The diseases caused by these organisms have an explosive onset but are so short-lived that they require no specific treatment.

Diarrhea produced by the exotoxin of *Clostridium difficile*, secondary to antibiotic therapy, has a 30% mortality rate in untreated cases. This cytotoxic agent produces a pseudomembranous colitis. Between 2% and 3% of normal adults carry *C. difficile* in fecal flora; 20% in those recently receiving antibiotics carry it.

The parasites *Giardia lamblia* and *Entamoeba histolytica* may cause acute, chronic, or intermittent diarrhea. *Giardia* is endemic in several geographic areas and is acquired through contaminated water or direct contact. Most patients are asymptomatic, but if the condition is untreated, it may produce malabsorption with low levels of vitamin B_{12} and folate, disaccharidase deficiency, and steatorrhea resulting in weight loss. *E. histolytica* is present in 5% of the population. While most people are asymptomatic, they do not spontaneously clear the infection and may become acutely ill. They develop chronic diarrhea or an acute colitis similar to ulcerative colitis or to dysentery. Bleeding or perforation may account for the 3% mortality rate. Amebic liver abscesses occur in 1% of patients with intestinal amebiasis.

The natural history of diarrhea varies according to the cause. Some resolve spontaneously (such as irritable bowel syndrome or 10% of ulcerative colitis cases). Lactose intolerance and celiac sprue will become asymptomatic as long as specific diets are maintained. Certain other patients with diarrhea will have persistent problems if the condition is not treated but may be cured with medication (i.e., patients with hyperthyroidism, bacterial overgrowth, or infestations).

Diseases such as amebiasis or inflammatory bowel syndrome may be chronic or form strictures requiring surgical treatment. Of special concern is the incidence of malignancy in certain cases of chronic diarrheas besides hormone-secreting tumors. Celiac sprue is associated with lymphomas (less than 10% of celiac sprue cases); long-standing ulcerative colitis and polyps are associated with adenocarcinoma.

PATHOPHYSIOLOGY

Under normal conditions, approximately 10 L of fluid reach the proximal duodenum each day. Two L of this fluid are ingested, with the rest coming from digestive secretions. The small bowel absorbs 8 L of fluid a day, so that only about 2 L enter the colon. The colon then actively absorbs the remaining fluid allowing only 100 ml of feces to be excreted per day. The absorption capacity of the colon is about 5 L per day. The final stool composition has about 30 mEq/L of sodium, 75 mEq/L of potassium, 10 mEq/L of chloride, 30 mEq/L of bicarbonate, HCO_3, and nonabsorbable solutes, giving an osmolarity of 400 mOsm/kg.

When absorptive capacities are exceeded, diarrhea develops. The four pathophysiologic mechanisms responsible for diarrheal illnesses are (1) osmotic changes, (2) secretory changes, (3) mucosal damage, and (4) altered motility. In the clinical setting, more than one mechanism may be responsible for the diarrhea.

Osmotic diarrhea occurs when poorly or nonabsorbable solutes are ingested and cause excessive retention of fluid in the intestine. The characteristics of osmotic diarrhea are: (1) stool osmolarity is greater than twice the sum of the stool sodium and potassium concentrations, (2) stool output ceases or decreases during fasting, and (3) stool sodium concentration is low (less than 45 mEq/L). Magnesium salts contained in laxatives or antacids are the most common agents causing osmotic diarrhea. An osmotic diarrhea may also occur in patients with lactose intolerance when milk is ingested. The unabsorbed carbohydrate enters the colon where bacterial fermentation produces short-chain fatty acids, hydrogen, carbon dioxide, and methane gases. These cause a rapid transit in the colon resulting in diarrhea and abdominal distention. Osmotic diarrhea causes no macroscopic or microscopic changes unless there is a submucosal infiltrative disease disrupting the intestinal absorption of nutrients.

Such is the case in lymphoma and amyloidosis, which interfere with small bowel recovery of carbohydrates. Enzymatic defects in the mucosal brush border can be measured in disaccharidase deficiencies.

Secretory diarrhea arises from enhanced active or passive ion secretion without gross mucosal injury. Secretory diarrhea characteristically shows: (1) a stool osmolarity close to plasma osmolarity, (2) stool output greater than 500 ml per day during fasting, (3) a high concentration of stool sodium (90 mEq/L), and (4) no osmolar gap. Secretory diarrhea can be caused by bacterial toxins, bile acids, hormones, laxative abuse, and fatty acids. Bacterial toxins such as from *Vibrio cholerae* or enterotoxigenic *E. coli* bind to specific cell-membrane receptors, which activates adenylate cyclase to form cAMP (or cGMP). This reduces the uptake of sodium chloride and the active secretion of chloride and bicarbonate. There is no evidence of microscopic mucosal damage.

Gastrointestinal hormones produced by certain tumors cause a secretory diarrhea by several mechanisms. A gastrinoma produces excessive gastrin causing an increase in gastric acid output and large volumes of pancreatic fluid containing bicarbonate to neutralize the acid. Pancreatic non-beta islet cell tumors cause a diarrhea by increasing production of cAMP through the secretion of hormones like vasoactive intestinal polypeptide (VIP). This is like the potent secretagogue activity of laxatives, which also increase intracellular cAMP. The secretory effect of bile salts on the colon is poorly understood, but in these cases there is usually no distal ileum subsequent to surgical removal or a diseased distal ileum, resulting in a large amount of bile salts being introduced into the colon.

Mucosal destruction is the third mechanism causing diarrhea. The diarrhea is usually not of a large volume and may be associated with impairment of absorption or exudation of leukocytes, red blood cells, or protein. Disease processes associated with this type of diarrhea include inflammatory bowel disease (IBD) or bacterial or protozoan invasion of the mucosa. Macroscopically, IBD may produce transmural disease or ulceration with a friable or cobblestone mucosa. There may be skip lesions involving both the small and large bowel. Microscopically, IBD can be suspected if granulomas or microabscesses are found. Amebiasis may produce a funnel-shaped ulceration in the sigmoid colon, however, ileal disease or hepatic abscess may also occur. Amebiasis can also be diagnosed by finding the cyst invading the mucosa. Microscopically, ischemic or radiation enteritis shows thrombosis of the submucosal arterioles in addition to nonspecific colitis.

Altered intestinal motility is the fourth mechanism producing diarrhea. This occurs with (1) rapid transit, (2) slow transit, or (3) rapid colonic emptying. Rapid transit occurs with hyperthyroidism, in which the overall metabolic activity is increased, or with gastric resection, in which the normal myoelectrical activity is disrupted with the ingested meal entering the small bowel rapidly. This causes an osmotic compensation by the small bowel and rapid evacuation into the colon, producing

TABLE 65–2.
Clinical–Pathologic Correlations for Diarrhea

CLINICAL FINDINGS	PATHOLOGIC FINDINGS	
	PATHOLOGIC MECHANISM	DISEASE
Dehydration	Increased secretion	Zollinger-Ellison syndrome, vasoactive intestinal polypeptide-secreting tumor
	Decreased reabsorption	Radiation enteritis, short-bowel syndrome
Fever	Infection	Bacterial, viral, parasitic
	Inflammation	Crohn's disease, ulcerative colitis
Cramping	Anatomical narrowing	Crohn's disease, tumor, amebiasis
	Spasm	Irritable bowel syndrome
	Rapid transit	Irritable bowel syndrome, large-volume diarrhea
Bleeding	Mucosal destruction	Tumor, infection, vasculitis, inflammatory bowel disease
Nausea, vomiting	Toxin	*Bacillus cereus*

TABLE 65–3.
Diagnostic Tests for Inflammatory Bowel Disease and Infectious Diarrhea

	WBCS IN FECES	SIGMOID EXAMINATION	BASIS FOR DIAGNOSIS
INFLAMMATORY BOWEL DISEASE			
Ulcerative	Present	Colitis (ulcerations, erosions, or friability of the mucosa)	Biopsy rules out other causes
Crohn's disease	Present	Colitis, but may be normal	Colon and small bowel examination
INFECTIOUS DIARRHEA			
Shigella	Present	Colitis	Stool culture
Campylobacter	Present	Mild to severe colitis	Stool culture
Clostridium difficile	May or may not be present	Pseudomembrane Colitis distal to beyond sigmoid in 15% of cases	Toxin assay
Salmonella	May or may not be present	Mild colitis	Stool culture
Entamoeba histolytica	Absent	"Punched-out" ulcers	Stool examination, mucosal biopsy, assay

diarrhea. Drugs such as quinidine cause a rapid transit by an unknown mechanism. Slow-transit diarrhea, seen in diabetes mellitus or blind-loop syndrome, decreases peristalsis, resulting in bacterial overgrowth in the normally sterile small bowel. This results in bacterial breakdown of carbohydrates, producing fatty acids that enter the colon resulting in an osmotic effect that produces diarrhea. Finally, rapid colonic emptying with an abnormal myoelectric pattern is seen in irritable bowel syndrome. This type of diarrhea is not associated with any macroscopic or microscopic pathologic changes.

CLINICAL–PATHOLOGIC CORRELATIONS

The correlation between clinical findings and the pathologic mechanisms behind them are listed in Table 65–2. Diseases that illustrate the mechanism are also listed.

DIFFERENTIAL DIAGNOSIS

The main concern in acute, severe diarrhea (i.e., fever, bloody stools, abdominal pain) is to distinguish inflammatory bowel disease from the other causes of acute colitis. The former is often treated with corticosteroids, which would be devastating to use in cases of infectious colitis. The main diagnostic points of each are listed in Table 65–3. The causes of chronic diarrhea are listed according to the pathogenic mechanism in Table 65–4.

DIAGNOSIS

In any case of diarrhea, after a complete history and physical examination are completed, a stool culture for bacteria, including an examination for ova and parasites, should be done. An examination for stool leukocytes will indicate if mucosal invasion or inflammation has occurred. If the results of all of these examinations are negative, no further work-up is usually indicated for an acute diarrhea, and the diarrhea is assumed to be of viral origin. If there are leukocytes in the stool or if the diarrhea persists, a proctosigmoidoscopy with a mucosal biopsy should be done. Further evaluation of chronic diarrhea with a complete blood count, an erythrocyte sedimentation rate, biochemical studies of the blood, thyroid function tests, and malabsorption screening tests should be done. The other specific radiologic, biochemical, and endoscopic examinations are done depending on the specific indications obtained from the history, physical examination, and laboratory tests (Table 65–5).

TABLE 65–4.
Causes of Chronic Diarrhea

OSMOTIC	SECRETORY	MUCOSAL INJURY	MOTILITY DISORDER

Drugs
Enzyme deficiency
Surgical:
  Gastroenterostomy,
  intestinal resection
Malabsorption: *Giardia*
  infection, celiac sprue,
  amyloidosis, lymphoma,
  Whipple's disease
	Bile salts; ileal resection or
	  disease (Crohn's)
	Fatty acid steatorrhea:
	  Pancreatic insufficiency,
	  bacterial overgrowth
	Hormonal: Carcinoid
	  syndrome, Zollinger-
	  Ellison syndrome,
	  medullary carcinoma of
	  thyroid, VIPoma
	Drugs: laxative
		Inflammatory bowel
		  disease
		Tumor: Polyp or cancer
		Ischemic: Vascular
		  insufficiency or
		  radiation-induced
		  ischemia
		Invasive organism:
		  Entamoeba histolytica
			Rapid transit:
			  Hyperthyroidism,
			  irritable bowel
			  syndrome,
			  postgastrectomy
			  syndrome, carcinoid
			  syndrome, Addison's
			  disease

TABLE 65–5.
Diagnostic Tests for Diarrhea

TESTS	DISEASE CAUSING A POSITIVE RESULT
Stool culture	Infections of *Salmonella, Shigella, Campylobacter, Yersinia*
Stool examination for ova and parasite	*Giardia* (60% of time), *Entamoeba histolytica*, and *Cryptospordia*
Stool WBC count	Infections of *Shigella, Salmonella, Campylobacter*, invasive *Escherichia coli, Yersinia, Clostridium difficile, Vibrio parahaemolyticus*, and *Entamoeba histolytica;* inflammatory bowel disease
Stool occult blood	Infections of *Shigella, Salmonella*, and *Campylobacter;* inflammatory bowel disease; tumor; ischemic colitis
Serum thyroxine (T_4) and Triiodothyronine (T_3) T_3 resin uptake (RT_3U)	Hyperthyroidism
Plasma levels of D-xylose	Disaccharidase deficiency, *Giardia* infection, Crohn's disease, blind-loop syndrome, celiac sprue, Whipple's disease, lymphoma
72-hour fecal fat	Pancreatic insufficiency, *Giardia* infection
SPECIFIC TESTS	
Clostridium difficile toxin	Pseudomembranous colitis
Cortisol, plasma	Addison's disease
5-HIAA, plasma	Carcinoid syndrome
Stool NaOH	Laxative abuse
Folate, vitamin B_{12} levels	Malabsorption, bacterial overgrowth
Gastrin, vasoactive intestinal polypeptide	Hormone-secreting tumors

PRINCIPLES OF THERAPY

The first requirement in therapy is to assess the patient's hydration status. Often fluid can be replaced orally with a glucose and electrolyte solution. If this is not feasible, intravenous hydration should be started. The levels of electrolytes should be corrected at the same time. Vitamin and mineral deficiencies should be corrected. For infectious diarrhea, few cases require treatment with antibiotics before the culture results are known. Some infectious agents are sensitive to antibiotics, but treatment does not alter the course of the disease. For other diseases, treatment with antibiotics in the acute phase may increase the carrier rate.

There are too many causes of chronic diarrhea to discuss therapy for each specific one. There are a number of concepts of treatment into which most cases will fall. The removal of offending agents can be useful in laxative abuse, and in drug-induced or food-related diarrheas. In cases of bile-induced diarrhea, a resin agent like cholestyramine is used. Enzyme replacement in lactase or pancreatic deficiency is beneficial. Anatomical causes, like tumors, strictures, or enterofistulas should be surgically removed. Abnomal bowel flora, as in pseudomembranous colitis or bacterial overgrowth, can be changed by antibiotic therapy.

Antidiarrheal agents will decrease transit time. Absorption can be increased by agents like clonidine, loperamide, or by the elemental diets. Finally, the use of vitamins (folic acid), if the origin is partly nutritional, will restore normal mucosal function. Difficult cases or cases of unknown cause may require empirical treatment with one of the described approaches.

REFERENCES

Blaser MJ, Berkowitz ID, LaForce FM et al: Campylobacter enteritis: Clinical and epidemiologic features. Ann Intern Med 1979; 91:179–185. A review of a large series of patients with good descriptions of their clinical manifestations.

Krejs GJ, Fordtran JS: Diarrhea, in Sleisenger M, Fordtran JS (eds): Gastrointestinal Disease. Philadelphia, WB Saunders Co, 1983, pp 257–280. An extensive review of the pathophysiology and evaluation of diarrhea, with numerous references.

Read NW, Krejs GJ, Read MG et al: Chronic diarrhea of unknown origin. Gastroenterology 1980; 78:264–271. A presentation of a large series of referred patients and eventual identification of the causes of their diarrhea.

Satterwhite TK, DuPont HL: Infectious diarrhea in office practice. Med Clin North Am 1983; 67:203–220. A concise review of the initial steps in evaluating diarrhea.

Tucker H, Schuster MM: Irritable bowel syndrome: Newer pathophysiologic concepts. Adv Intern Med 1982; 27:183–204. A presentation of the physiologic basis of IBD.

66   INFLAMMATORY BOWEL DISEASE

N. Gopalswamy, M.D.

Although there are many conditions that cause inflammatory changes in the large and small bowels, the term "inflammatory bowel disease" usually refers to ulcerative colitis and granulomatous ileitis or ileocolitis, commonly known as Crohn's disease, of unknown causes. The incidence of both diseases is 6 to 10 per 100,000 population, and their prevalence is 60 to 80 per 100,000. Both disorders affect adults between the ages of 20 and 40 years predominantly, and occasionally appear in the fifth or sixth decade. Inflammatory bowel disease is classified according to the extent of bowel involvement (Table 66–1). Inflammatory bowel disease in children, adolescents, and pregnant women is not discussed here (see Berk, 1985; "Inflammatory Bowel," 1984; Janowitz, 1985; Michener, Farmer, and Mortimer, 1979).

CLINICAL SIGNS AND SYMPTOMS

Rectal bleeding with increased frequency of bowel movements is common in ulcerative colitis. Diarrhea, abdominal pain, recurrent perianal abscesses, and fistulas are typical initial

TABLE 66–1.
Classification of Inflammatory Bowel Disease

ULCERATIVE COLITIS	CROHN'S DISEASE
Ulcerative proctitis	Regional ileitis and/or jejunitis (30%–40%)
Proctosigmoiditis or left-sided colitis	Granulomatous ileocolitis (45%–50%)
Universal (diffuse)	Granulomatous colitis (15%–20%)
	Crohn's disease of the upper gastrointestinal tract (5%–10%)
Segmental colitis (rare)	

TABLE 66–2.
Similarities and Differences between Ulcerative Colitis and Crohn's Disease

CLINICAL FEATURES	ULCERATIVE COLITIS	CROHN'S DISEASE
Rectal bleeding	>90%	<50%
Diarrhea	10%–30%	>70%
Abdominal mass	<1%	30%
Perianal abscesses, sinuses, and fistulas	2%	30%
Bowel perforation (free)	2%–3%	<1%
Toxic megacolon	5%–10%	<5%
Arthritis	10%	25%
Pyoderma gangrenosum	<5%	1%
Erythema nodosum	5%	15%
Pericholangitis/sclerosing cholangitis	30%	20%–30%
Renal stones	<5%	10%
Stomatitis, iritis, thrombophlebitis	10%	10%
Cancer of colon	Definite increase (5%)	Questionable increase
RADIOLOGIC, ENDOSCOPIC, AND PATHOLOGIC FINDINGS		
Rectal involvement	Almost 100%	<50% (looks grossly normal)
Ulcers	Superficial, multiple Irregular	Solitary ulcers in the rectum Linear, serpiginous and apthoid ulcers Collar-button ulcers
Crypt abscess, pseudopolyps, diminished goblet cells	>70%	<40%
Lymphoid aggregates and noncaseating granuloma	<10%	60%–70%
Extent of disease	Mucosal and continuous	Transmural and discontinuous with "skip lesions"
Ileal involvement	Nonspecific with mild inflammation and dilatation (backwash ileitis)	Ulcers, fissures, and stenosis
TREATMENT		
General	Supportive and symptomatic	Supportive, symptomatic
Definitive (drugs)	Sulfasalazine and corticosteroids	Sulfasalazine, corticosteroids, metronidazole

symptoms in Crohn's disease (Table 66–2). Fever, weight loss, arthritis, skin lesions, and occasionally massive gastrointestinal bleeding occur in both diseases.

The results of the physical examination are normal in early stages of the disease, except for evidence of fresh blood on rectal examination in ulcerative colitis and tenderness in the lower quadrants of the abdomen in Crohn's disease. Postural hypotension, tachycardia, fever, abdominal distention, palpable abdominal mass, and anemia occur in the later stages. Weight loss and evidence of malnutrition are frequent in Crohn's disease but occur only in severe ulcerative colitis.

Depending on the number of bowel movements and on the presence or absence of systemic signs and symptoms, ulcerative colitis can be classified clinically as mild, moderate, or severe. Four or fewer bowel movements in the absence of systemic symptoms are classified as mild, and eight or more bowel movements with fever, weight loss, or tachycardia are classified as severe.

The activity of Crohn's disease can be assessed by observing the general well-being of the patient, the number of stools per day, anemia, abdominal pain, abdominal mass, loss of body weight, the need for drugs to control diarrhea, and the presence or absence of complications. The Crohn's Disease Activity Index can be computed from these, with a score of less than 150 indicating inactive disease and greater than 150 indicating active disease.

Because corticosteroids were found to be beneficial in treating ulcerative colitis, a true natural history of untreated ulcerative colitis is not available. According to data from double-blind, placebo-controlled studies in both the United States and Europe, the mortality of Crohn's disease is relatively low. Spontaneous remission occurs in 25% to 30% of untreated patients, with 75% of these patients remaining in remission for 1 year. With longer follow-up, this figure diminishes.

The prognosis for diffuse ulcerative colitis is worse than that of idiopathic proctitis or left-sided ulcerative colitis, both regarding the mortality rate and the number of patients needing surgery. About 50% to 80% of patients with moderate or severe Crohn's disease need surgical treatment over a period of 10 to 20 years. Both diseases have remissions and exacerbations. Prophylactic treatment can prevent the recurrence of ulcerative colitis.

Intestinal and extraintestinal complications occur in both diseases (Tables 66–3 and 66–4).

PATHOPHYSIOLOGY

The etiology of both diseases is unknown. Chronic bacterial, fungal, or viral infections and autoimmune disorders have been cited as causes of inflammatory bowel disease. Ulcerative colitis is usually a mucosal disease of the colon with minimal nonspecific inflammatory changes of the terminal ileum. Crohn's disease is a transmural disease affecting all layers of the bowel wall and, in most cases, affecting both small and large bowel. In severe ulcerative colitis, the entire colon wall is thinned and the colon is dilated, which can lead to toxic megacolon or even free perforation of the colon. In both diseases, there may be extraintestinal involvement of joints, skin, eyes, mouth, liver, and kidneys (Table 66–4).

CLINICAL–PATHOLOGIC CORRELATIONS

The clinical—pathologic correlations for inflammatory bowel disease are presented in Table 66–5. Anemia is common in both

TABLE 66–3.
Intestinal Complications of Inflammatory Bowel Disease

ULCERATIVE COLITIS	CROHN'S DISEASE
Toxic megacolon (5%–10%)	Fistulas (50%)
Perforation of colon	Intestinal obstruction (20%)
Cancer of the colon (5%) (25% to 40% of patients with universal colitis of more than 20 years' duration)	Toxic megacolon (<5%)
	Cancer of the small bowel

TABLE 66–4.
Extraintestinal Manifestations

SYSTEM INVOLVED	FREQUENCY (% OF CASES)	
	ULCERATIVE COLITIS	CROHN'S DISEASE
Skin	Pyoderma gangrenosum	Erythema nodosum
Mouth		
Aphthous ulceration	4	4
Eyes		
Uveitis and iritis	4	5–10
Joints		
Spondylitis	<5	15–20
Peripheral arthritis	10	20
Liver		
Fatty	30–40	30–40
Pericholangitis	30	20
Sclerosing cholangitis	30	20–30
Cirrhosis	Rare	<1
Renal stones	Uric acid stones (after colectomy)	Oxalate stones 10–15
Gallstones	Rare	10–15
Thromboembolism with increased platelets and increased coagulant activity	Occurs	Occurs
Amyloidosis	Rare	1

diseases and is often related to blood loss from the diseased mucosa. In Crohn's disease, it is also related to the vitamin-B_{12} deficiency caused by dysfunction of the terminal ileum and to bacterial overgrowth. Folate deficiency may be related to lack of intake, reduced absorption with sulphasalazine therapy, and also to extensive jejunal involvement in Crohn's disease.

Diarrhea results from multiple factors such as mucosal inflammation, an excessive loss of bile salts, a diminished absorptive surface, and bacterial overgrowth due to internal fistulas. Intestinal obstruction and fistulas result from the transmural nature of the disease.

With steatorrhea and high oxalate in the diet, absorption of oxalate increases, leading to renal stones and resultant complications. Because of the ileal involvement and the excessive loss of bile salts, the bile acid pool is diminished, which leads to formation of gallstones.

Arthritis, both spinal and peripheral, skin lesions, uveitis, iritis, and aphthous stomatitis are common complications of inflammatory bowel disease. Their severity parallels that of the colitis or Crohn's disease, and they subside when the underlying disease is treated.

Fatty change in the liver is attributable to malnutrition and the use of corticosteroids. There is no good explanation for the rest of the liver abnormalities occurring as complications (Table 66–4). Osteoporosis and an increased incidence of peptic ulcer and thromboembolic disease occur in inflammatory bowel disease. With on-going chronic inflammation, amyloidosis can occur in Crohn's disease.

DIFFERENTIAL DIAGNOSIS

Although it is usually easy to differentiate ulcerative colitis from Crohn's disease, the diagnosis is extremely difficult in 20% of the cases. Either surgery or long-term follow-up is helpful in making the exact diagnosis, in such cases (Table 66–2).

DIARRHEA DUE TO INFECTIVE CAUSES

A history of travel, use of broad-spectrum antibiotics, examination of the stools for evidence of parasites or bacteria on culture or serologic tests help to establish the etiologic diagnosis of *Salmonella*, *Shigella*, *Campylobacter*, amebiasis, and occasionally *Yersinia* infections (Table 66–6).

TABLE 66–5.
Clinical–Pathologic Correlations for Inflammatory Bowel Disease

| | | PATHOLOGIC FINDINGS | |
CLINICAL FINDINGS	MACROSCOPIC	MICROSCOPIC
ULCERATIVE COLITIS		
Bleeding, diarrhea	Erythematous friable mucosa with superficial ulcerations	Breaks in epithelium Loss of architecture of the crypts Crypt abscesses Inflammatory cells in the lamina propria
Asymptomatic or bleeding	Shortened colon with loss of normal vascular network Granular mucosa Polypoid masses	Chronic inflammatory cell infiltrate Submucosal fibrosis
Weight loss, bleeding	Narrowed lumen of colon with abnormal-looking mucosa	Infiltrating carcinoma
Fever	Dilated colon with thin walls	Flattened mucosa with chronic inflammatory cells
Toxic condition	Many polypoid lesions	
Abdominal distention and tenderness		
Constipation or diminishing diarrhea		
CROHN'S DISEASE		
Diarrhea	Normal or erythematous mucosa, with solitary ulcers, linear ulcers, and "cobblestone" appearance	Noncaseating granuloma
Occult bleeding		Chronic inflammatory cells with aggregates of lymphocytes
Abdominal pain, distention, and mass	Narrow lumen, thickened bowel wall with "skip" areas	Inflammation from mucosa to serosa Fibrosis
Diarrhea	Abnormal connection between loops of bowel, or bowel and other organs (vagina, bladder, or skin)	Abnormal tract between the viscera lined by chronic and acute inflammatory cells
Weight loss		
Hematuria		
Dyspareunia		
Many draining lesions in the perianal area, with discomfort	Many abnormal openings in the perianal area, draining serosanguinous, purulent, or feculent matter, with indurated areas around them	Chronic inflammatory cells with necrotic debris or many polymorphonucleocytes

IRRITABLE BOWEL SYNDROME

Irritable bowel syndrome is a diagnosis by exclusion. A long history of alternating constipation and diarrhea, with no evidence of systemic signs and an absence of gastrointestinal bleeding or weight loss, coupled with normal investigations are helpful in making the diagnosis.

APPENDICITIS

Acute onset of periumbilical cramps, followed by severe pain in the right lower quadrant, and absence of diarrhea favor a diagnosis of appendicitis.

TABLE 66–6.
Differential Diagnosis

ULCERATIVE COLITIS	CROHN'S DISEASE
Bacterial infections	Bacterial infections
Salmonella	*Yersinia*
Shigella	*Campylobacter*
Clostridium difficile	Tuberculosis
Campylobacter	
Parasitic	Parasitic
Amebiasis	Giardiasis
Other	Other
Ischemic colitis	Appendicitis
Diverticulitis	Eosinophilic gastroenteritis
Radiation colitis	Peptic ulcer
	Irritable bowel syndrome

DIVERTICULITIS

In elderly patients, complaints of pain in the left lower quandrant and the presence of diverticuli on barium enema or sigmoidoscopy point to this diagnosis.

ISCHEMIC COLITIS

A history of coronary artery disease, resection of an abdominal aortic aneurysm in elderly persons with diarrhea and rectal bleeding and with characteristic involvement of the proximal descending colon near the splenic flexure, and rectosigmoid junction with intervening normal mucosa establish the diagnosis.

RADIATION-INDUCED COLITIS

Diarrhea or bleeding within weeks to years after abdominal radiation is helpful in diagnosing radiation colitis. Radiation may also cause enteritis resembling Crohn's disease.

TUBERCULOSIS

A positive skin test to tuberculin, involvement of the ileocecal area on barium enema, and caseating granuloma on biopsy favor the diagnosis of tuberculous enteritis.

PEPTIC ULCER DISEASE AND ESOPHAGITIS

Endoscopy and biopsy usually establish a diagnosis of peptic ulcer or esophagitis. Even if this procedure is performed, Crohn's disease can occasionally be misdiagnosed as peptic ulcer, and the correct diagnosis can be made retrospectively from histologic examination of the involved parts after surgery.

DIAGNOSIS

MILD TO MODERATELY SEVERE DISEASE

It is imperative to rule out the curable causes such as bacterial or parasitic infection before establishing the diagnosis of inflammatory bowel disease. Proctoscopic examination may show a friable mucosa with superficial ulcerations in ulcerative colitis, whereas the mucosa of the rectum may be normal on gross appearance or can show solitary ulcers or nonspecific inflammatory changes in Crohn's disease. Flexible sigmoidoscopy would delineate the extent of the disease in cases of less severe ulcerative colitis.

Barium enema should *not* be done in the active phases of ulcerative colitis and should be done only when the disease is under control with treatment. The rectum is invariably involved in ulcerative colitis, and radiologic findings consist of continuous lesions, superficial ulcerations, and pseudopolyps of the diseased segments of colon.

Barium examination of the small bowel is mandatory in all cases of suspected Crohn's disease. The ileum is involved in most cases and may show ulceration, spasm, stenosis, and fistulas.

SEVERE DISEASE

A flat plate of the abdomen showing a dilated transverse colon with filling defects establishes the diagnosis of toxic megacolon. An upper gastrointestinal series or barium enema can show fistulous communication between the loops of small bowel, the small bowel and colon, or the bowel and adjacent organs, such as the bladder or vagina, or between the bowel and skin.

Blood tests may show evidence of anemia, hypoalbuminemia, dehydration, and liver involvement. Special tests including slit-lamp examination of the eye, ultrasound examination of the abdomen, an intravenous pyelogram, liver biopsy, and endoscopic retrograde pancreatocholangiogram are helpful in diagnosing complications due to inflammatory bowel disease.

PRINCIPLES OF PREVENTION AND THERAPY

In mild to moderately active disease, a low-residue diet or elemental diet may be useful. In severe cases of either disease, total parenteral hyperalimentation is extremely helpful to improve nutrition, and occasionally has been claimed as a successful primary mode of therapy for healing fistulas in Crohn's disease.

Supportive treatment, such as correction of fluid and electrolyte imbalance, supplementation of vitamins and hematinics, and blood transfusions, is of vital importance. Symptomatic treatment, such as control of the diarrhea with diphenoxylate or codeine or morphine-like drugs, is needed in most cases but should be stopped promptly if toxic megacolon is suspected.

DEFINITIVE TREATMENT

Corticosteroids given systemically or topically in retention enemas are one of the mainstays of treatment. Sulfasalazine is very helpful in mild to moderately active ulcerative colitis and Crohn's disease and is broken down by the bacteria into sulfapyridine and 5-amino salicylic acid. The latter is not absorbed and is believed to be the active component of the drug. Azathioprine or 6-mercaptopurine is useful only to decrease the dose of corticosteroids in ulcerative colitis and is sometimes helpful in refractory cases of Crohn's disease. Oral sulfasalazine has been effective in preventing recurrent ulcerative colitis once the disease has been brought to remission by corticosteroids. It is not helpful as a prophylactic agent in Crohn's disease.

In cases of universal ulcerative colitis of more than 10 years' duration, an annual colonoscopy with multiple biopsies from different areas of the colon is recommended to detect dysplasia and predisposition to cancer of the colon. In patients with severe dysplasia or carcinoma in situ found on biopsy, proctocolectomy should be performed.

Proctocolectomy is indicated for cases of severe ulcerative colitis and of ulcerative colitis with either toxic megacolon or free perforation. It is curative for ulcerative colitis. Alternatives for patients with severe ulcerative colitis include continent ileostomy and sphincter-saving operations such as mucosal stripping of the rectum with ileoproctostomy. Conservative surgery with limited resection is the rule in Crohn's disease because the operation is not curative and also because the recurrence rate after surgery is higher than 50%.

REFERENCES

Allan RN: Long-term prognosis of Crohn's disease. *Current Med Lit Gastroenterol* 1984; 3(5):124–127. *Prognosis of the full spectrum of Crohn's disease from a British point of view.*

Berk JE (ed): *Bockus Gastroenterology* vol 4, ed 4. Philadelphia, WB Saunders Co, 1985, pp 2093–2362. *Excellent, up-to-date reference on inflammatory bowel disease.*

Farmer RG, Whelan G, Fazio VW: Long-term follow-up of patients with Crohn's disease—Relationship between the clinical pattern and prognosis. *Gastroenterology* 1985; 88:1818–1825. *A 13-year follow-up of 615 new patients with Crohn's disease in the Midwest.*

Greenstein AJ, Janowitz HD, Sachar DB: The extraintestinal complications of Crohn's disease and ulcerative colitis: A study of 700 patients. *Medicine* (Baltimore) 1976; 55(4):401–412. *Excellent account of the extraintestinal manifestations of inflammatory bowel disease.*

Janowitz HD: *Inflammatory Bowel Disease—A Personal View.* Field, Rich and Associates 1985, p 179.

Meyers S, Janowitz HD: Natural history of Crohn's disease—An analytical review of the placebo lesson. *Gastroenterology* 1984; 87:1189–1192. *Report of patient improvement on placebos.*

Michener WM, Farmer RG, Mortimer EA: Long-term prognosis of ulcerative colitis with onset in childhood or adolescence. *J Clin Gastroenterol* 1979; 1:301–305. *Follow-up of 336 Midwestern patients with ulcerative colitis.*

Ritchie JK, Power-Tuck J, Lennard-Jones JE: Clinical outcome of the first ten years of ulcerative colitis and proctitis. *Lancet* 1978; 1(1074)·1140–1143. *Follow-up of 203 British patients with ulcerative colitis.*

ACUTE APPENDICITIS

Dan W. Elliott, M.D.

Appendicitis is literally inflammation of the appendix attached to the cecum. This vestigial vermiform (worm-like) organ has no known function, and its removal produces no known consequences. The appendix is always present, has a lumen that normally contains loose fecal debris, and has a layered wall like that of the adjacent colon. No one can be certain as to how or why inflammation begins, but the most widely held belief is that it starts with obstruction of the lumen. In young people this may be due to lymphoid hyperplasia in the wall. In about 10% of cases of all ages, a stone-like fecalith (or appendicolith) is found. Secretions build pressure behind the blockade, producing edema in the wall and obliterating the microcirculation. Inflammation progresses to patchy necrosis. Bacteria normally contained within the colon invade and penetrate the wall. Cultures taken from the surface of the intact but acutely inflamed appendix usually grow two or three colonic species. Enormous quantities of bacteria are spilled into the abdomen after the appendix ruptures. Appendicitis occurs at all ages and almost equally between the sexes, except in the teens and twenties. Here at the peak age of occurrence, the incidence in males is greater than that in females by 3 to 2.

Appendicitis is a relatively acute process which progresses rapidly without treatment. In children the time from the first symptom to rupture averages 36 hours. In adults the process may take several days. It is important to determine, if possible, how long the patient has been ill when first seen.

In 10% of patients there may be a history of recurrent acute attacks that have resolved spontaneously. Later, an operation for some other cause may find a benign-appearing appendix with the lumen completely obliterated by scar tissue. Such a fibrosed appendix produces no symptoms, and chronic appendicitis does not occur. Recurrent acute appendicitis does occur, but once an attack begins the physician cannot assume that it may resolve spontaneously.

CLINICAL SIGNS AND SYMPTOMS

The history and physical findings depend very much on the stage of the disease in which the patient seeks help. The first symptom is pain of insidious onset. It may be either crampy or steady. It centers around the umbilicus in about 60% of patients. This location is typical of visceral pain arising in the stretch receptors of the appendiceal wall. Like all visceral pain, it is referred to the midline. It occurs at the level of the umbilicus because the appendix is innervated by thoracic segments 10 and 11. After the peritoneal surface is irritated, the pain "shifts" to the right lower quadrant. In 40% of patients the early visceral component is not felt and the pain first appears in the right lower quadrant. Shortly after the pain appears, anorexia is so universally present that its absence casts serious doubt on the diagnosis. Vomiting follows in only 50% of cases. There may be a brief history of diarrhea in 10% of patients. This represents irritability of the bowel because the stools are usually not liquid but frequent and scanty and do not relieve the pain. Vomiting and true liquid diarrhea occurring together suggest gastroenteritis rather than appendicitis.

Later on, pain in the right lower quadrant or pelvis becomes more generalized, and any jar of the abdomen hurts. The patient avoids walking and may resist any motion of the abdomen or legs, often preferring a fetal position. Anorexia persists and obstipation follows. In Table 67–1, symptoms are correlated with the stage of the disease, the physical findings, and the pathologic process.

TABLE 67–1.
Clinical–Pathologic Correlations for Acute Appendicitis

| | CLINICAL FINDINGS | | |
STAGE	SYMPTOMS	PHYSICAL FINDINGS	PATHOLOGIC FINDINGS
1. Earliest	Periumbilical pain, crampy or steady; urge to defecate; anorexia	Tenderness of the abdominal wall, well-localized over the appendix	Distention and edema of the appendiceal wall; plugging of the lumen with debris, a fecolith, or lymphoid hyperplasia
2. Early	Right lower quadrant abdominal pain; cramps; some vomiting; anorexia	Slight fever; tachycardia; abdominal distention; more tenderness in right lower quadrant with local rigidity	Distention; edema; fibrinous exudate; round cells through walls; patchy mucosal necrosis
3. Mature	Steady generalized lower abdominal pain, worse on any motion; occasional vomiting; anorexia	Low fever; tachycardia; dehydration; increasing distention; rigidity and rebound tenderness over appendix	Distention; edema; necrosis of appendiceal wall; microscopic perforation with pus around appendix
4. Ruptured	Steady generalized abdominal pain; bloating; guarding against motion; anorexia; vomiting in 50%	Fever; tachycardia; dehydration; distention; generalized tenderness and rigidity; rebound pain; referred rebound	Gross perforation; necrotic or missing wall; generalized pus; wide-spread fibrinopurulent peritonitis
5. Abscess	More localized right-sided abdominal pain; cramps; constipation; pain on motion; sweats; fever; vomiting in 50%	Low fever; tachycardia; tender firm mass in right lower quadrant or pelvic cul-de-sac; much less tender elsewhere	Thick exudate or fibrous wall binds together bowel and peritoneum around central pus; appendix is necrotic or missing; hole in cecum oozes stool

On physical examination, fever is usually absent early and becomes low grade later, not rising above 101°F until generalized abdominal sepsis appears. Tachycardia often precedes fever, but is not always present. In early appendicitis the most significant physical finding is tenderness sharply localized over the appendix, even when the pain is midline. This is most often at McBurney's point, which is one-third of the way from the iliac crest to the umbilicus. This location can vary because the appendix is attached to the cecum. The exact site of the tenderness will depend on how far the cecum descended in embryologic development. Sometimes the tenderness is so high it is hard to separate from the liver's edge. Sometimes it is so low that it cannot be defined by abdominal examination. In 30% of patients the cecum lies so inferiorly that the appendix hangs over the brim of the pelvis. Then sharp tenderness will be identified high on the right on vaginal and rectal examination, which must never be omitted. Bowel sounds are not of much help because there is localized paralytic ileus in the

nearby bowel. Early on, the bowel sounds may be obstructive above the ileus, and later are nearly silent after the ileus has become generalized.

As peritoneal reaction develops, the area of tenderness spreads and the examiner detects voluntary guarding. Hyperesthesia of the skin overlying the involved peritoneum has been noted. A little later, true involuntary rigidity of the abdominal wall develops, followed by rebound tenderness over the inflamed area. Rebound tenderness referred to the right lower quadrant from other quadrants, when present, provides the best possible localizing sign of peritoneal reaction. When the appendix lies very inferiorly or posteriorly, psoas and obturator signs may appear, but these are usually not found. When the appendix is encased within the peritoneal reflection attaching the cecum to the lateral abdominal wall, anterior abdominal findings are minimal. Tenderness may be most pronounced posteriorly in the flank. This makes retrocecal appendicitis notoriously difficult to diagnose.

Once generalized peritonitis has appeared, fever and tachycardia are expected. Abdominal distention appears. Tenderness and rigidity may extend to all four quadrants, but the most severe signs remain in the right lower quadrant, suggesting appendicitis as the underlying cause. If the peritonitis has spread more slowly, the patient's defenses may succeed in limiting the process to the right lower quadrant. As the abdominal wall grows less rigid elsewhere, a firm tender mass may become palpable. This suggests an appendiceal abscess. As a firm fibrous wall develops around the abscess, the more distant bowel resumes normal peristalsis and may even permit bowel movements. However, as the abscess wall contracts, it may capture and obstruct a knuckle of small bowel. Cramps, pain, vomiting, and obstipation reappear, and operation for bowel obstruction becomes mandatory.

If misdiagnosed or neglected, both peritonitis and appendiceal abscess will progress to systemic sepsis, bacteremia, septic shock, and death. If treated late or inadequately, metastatic abscesses can be expected. They may require multiple additional operations for drainage. These abscesses occur most frequently in the subhepatic or subphrenic spaces on the right, within the right lobe of the liver, or in the pelvic cul-de-sac. Pyelophlebitis of the portal vein is a rare but dramatic and deadly complication, producing gas in the portal vein visible on x-ray film, multiple hepatic abscesses, and thrombotic gangrene of intestinal segments.

DIFFERENTIAL DIAGNOSIS

A textbook devoted to the topic would be required to present all of the diseases to be ruled out in the differential diagnosis of acute appendicitis. However, it is possible to present the most frequent and important considerations in a consolidated list as in Table 67–2. A glance through this list should be convincing that a comprehensive history and physical examination are essential to make a diagnosis of acute appendicitis. The nasopharynx and lymph nodes of the neck are examined for infection leading to mesenteric adenitis. The lung bases are auscultated carefully for basilar pneumonia, and the chest x-ray film is never neglected, especially in children. The costovertebral angles are tapped for tenderness, and the urine sediment carefully examined for pus and red cells.

In young girls and women of childbearing age, a careful history of the menses is essential, together with a knowledge of sexual exposure. This may require a little time to get better acquainted with the patient. Perhaps the most difficult differential diagnosis lies between appendicitis and pelvic inflammatory disease, because both produce the same systemic signs of tachycardia, fever, and leukocytosis. The pelvic examination is crucial. Both appendicitis and salpingitis produce exquisite tenderness on the right, but salpingitis is usually bilateral with equal tenderness on the left. Moving the cervix produces much pain in pelvic inflammatory disease, but usually less pain in appendicitis.

In younger adults of both sexes, acute regional enteritis may have caused some prodromal diarrhea, but occasionally it does not. Both right-sided pyelonephritis and ureteral calculus may produce anterior abdominal pain. In tall thin individuals a distended gallbladder may descend to the right lower quadrant. In fat individuals, right lower quadrant tenderness may seem to extend to the costal margin. It may seem strange to see perforated duodenal ulcer and acute pancreatitis on this list. In both these diseases, exudate may drain downward in the right lumbar gutter or atop the colon, presenting the greatest tenderness just over the appendix.

In older individuals cancer becomes a serious concern, particularly cancer of the right colon, where surrounding inflammation may mimic appendicitis. Cancer is more common in the sigmoid, where colon obstruction may distend the cecum enough to cause right-sided pain and tenderness. The sigmoid colon may loop far to the right, where diverticulitis can mimic appendicitis. Mesenteric infarction often first appears as appendicitis because the longest branch of the mesenteric artery, the ileocolic branch, is often the first to be completely occluded. Necrosis begins in the terminal ileum or right colon and causes right lower quadrant pain and tenderness.

Table 67–3 lists some lesions that are almost never distinguished from appendicitis except at operation. The surgeon who operates on the appendix must be prepared to deal safely with any of these. Some may require a right colectomy in unprepared bowel.

TABLE 67–2.
Differential Diagnosis of Appendicitis:
More Common Lesions Classified by Patient Age and Sex

AGE GROUP	FREQUENT AND IMPORTANT LESIONS THAT MIMIC ACUTE APPENDICITIS	FINDINGS FAVORING DIAGNOSIS OF THIS LESION
INFANCY TO PUBERTY Both sexes	Mesenteric adenitis	Respiratory infection; cervical lymphadenitis
	Intussusception	Blood in stool; palpable mass
	Constipation	Relieved by bowel movement induced by suppository or low enema
	Pneumonia in right, middle, or lower lobe	Rales; rhonchi at right base; chest x-ray film findings
	Gastroenteritis, toxic or viral	Simultaneous vomiting and diarrhea
	Urinary infection	Pus in urine
	Allergic purpura	Dependent purpuric rash
PUBERTY TO 40 YEARS Female patients	*All of the above plus:*	
	Mittelschmerz	Midway between menses; no leukocytosis
	Ectopic pregnancy, right-sided	Missed menstrual period; mass in adnexa
	Twisted ovarian cyst, right side	Adnexal mass; positive pelvic ultrasound study
	Endometriosis	Cyclic pain with menses
	Salpingitis; pelvic inflammatory disease	Adnexal tender masses or bilateral tenderness
PREGNANT WOMEN		
	Right-sided hydronephrosis; pyelonephritis	Flank tenderness; pus in urine
PUBERTY TO 50 YEARS Both sexes	*All of the childhood lesions plus:*	
	Regional enteritis, acute	Chronic cramps, persistent diarrhea
	Right renal calculus	Blood in urine
	Pyelonephritis	Pus in urine
	Acute cholecystitis	Tenderness inseparable from liver edge
	Small-bowel obstruction	Hernias, prior abdominal surgery
	Perforated peptic ulcer draining in right gutter	Ulcer history; antacid use
	Acute pancreatitis	Alcohol abuse; gallstones
50 YEARS AND OLDER	*All of young adult lesions plus:*	
	Cancer of right colon	Nontender mass; anemia
	Sigmoid diverticulitis, colon looping to the right	History of diverticulitis; change in bowel habit
	Colonic obstruction	Distention; diffuse pain
	Mesenteric infarction	Atrial fibrillation; vascular disease
	Expanding aneurysm	Pulsatile mass

DIAGNOSIS

The physician must have sufficient confidence to base the diagnosis of acute appendicitis on the history and physical findings alone. The only positive finding in early appendicitis may be tenderness localized to the appendix. The laboratory tests and x-ray films provide insensitive and nonspecific help at best. The most helpful laboratory determination is the WBC count and differential, but both will be entirely normal in 10% of cases. However, the WBC count becomes elevated earlier and more uniformly in appendicitis than fever. A WBC

TABLE 67–3.
Lesions That Can Be Distinguished From Appendicitis Only At Operation

Diverticulitis of cecum
Perforated right colon from cancer or foreign body
Infarction of omentum
Infarcted appendix epiploica
Meckel's diverticulum
Right salpingo-ovarian abscess
Acute regional enteritis of the ileum or cecum

count over 10,000/mm^3 will be found in 90% of patients, whereas fewer than 10% of normal people have such elevations except during pregnancy, when the upper limit of normal is 12,000/mm^3. The differential count will show more than 75% neutrophils in 78% of patients with appendicitis. Either the total WBC count or the percent of neutrophils will be elevated in 96% of patients. Anemia shown by the complete blood count raises the question of a systemic disease and in older individuals of cancer.

A urinalysis should be essentially normal in appendicitis, but a few white cells or a few red cells per high-power field should not detract from the diagnosis. These are presumably due to irritation of the nearby ureter. More than 25 WBCs per high-power field in the centrifuged sediment suggests urinary tract disease or the need for a catheterized specimen, particularly in the female. Erythrocyte sedimentation rates will be quite high in acute salpingitis and not so high in appendicitis. Rapid pregnancy tests can be helpful in suspected tubal pregnancy.

X-ray films of the chest and abdomen without ingested barium for contrast provide little that is specific to appendicitis but are especially useful in children and older patients. Abdominal films should always be obtained with the patient in both supine and upright positions to show air–fluid levels. In a series of 100 children with acute appendicitis, such films were normal in only 18%. A right lower-quadrant ileus pattern was present in 30%, generalized ileus in 41%, and an obstructive pattern in 10%. There was a soft-tissue density in the right lower quadrant in 48%. Calcified fecoliths in the presence of abdominal pain clearly indicated appendicitis, but were present in only 22% (Fig 67–1). In older patients, x-ray films of the chest show underlying pulmonary and cardiac disease. X-ray films of the abdomen in the supine and upright positions are useful to show the absence of free air, bowel obstruction, and abscesses elsewhere. The films may confirm the paralytic ileus pattern most common in appendicitis.

Barium enema in the unprepared colon has become the most specific investigation available and has caused no complications. Findings indicative of appendicitis are (1) persistent nonvisualization or partial visualization of the appendix, (2) pressure defects in the cecum or ileum, or (3) mucosal changes in these structures (Fig 67–2). Nonvisualization of the appendix alone cannot be taken as evidence of appendicitis because this will be found in 10% of normal people. If the appendix is easily and completely filled with barium, appendicitis is very unlikely. Nevertheless, barium enema has had a false-negative rate of at least 7% or more.

When the suspicion of acute appendicitis is high, but there remains some doubt, a short period of active observation is in order without analgesics. The best diagnostic test is repeated physical examinations by the same examiner. In a series of 353 children up to 13 years of age, observation for up to 8 hours caused no ap-

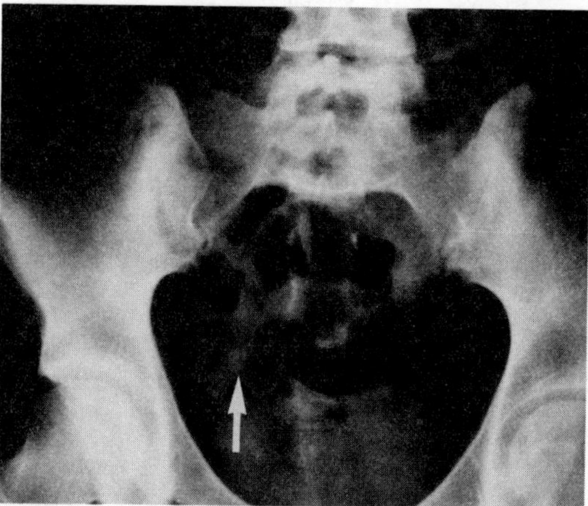

FIG 67–1.
A plain x-ray film of the abdomen showing a fecalith in the appendix with "egg-shell" layers of calcium (arrow). In the presence of abdominal pain, this strongly indicates appendicitis.

parent harm. In two-thirds of these patients, the pain subsided spontaneously or another cause was identified. In adults, observation may continue to 12 or even 18 hours, but if the diagnosis then remains in doubt, a barium enema is indicated without laxatives or any preparation.

PRINCIPLES OF THERAPY

When the history and physical findings, CBC, urinalysis, and plain x-ray films all point to acute appendicitis, an appendectomy should be performed within 2 to 5 hours. This permits fitting the operation easily into a busy schedule. The surgeon can make good use of a short delay to prepare the patient for a safe anesthesia. Intravenous fluids for full hydration are always helpful. High fevers can be lowered temporarily. The stomachs of little children and elderly persons should be emptied with a nasogastric tube to prevent vomiting at the induction of anesthesia. Any needed tests or therapy for coincident disease can be accomplished. Prophylactic intravenous antibiotics are indicated before operation. They should never be given until a clear decision to operate is reached because they are capable of masking the diagnostic signs that will confirm the need for surgery, but they cannot cure the lesion.

Appendectomy in the properly prepared patient is a very safe operation with an overall mortality rate of less than 0.8% in one large series. Therefore, it may be safer to operate than to assume the risks of rupture by delaying for a more certain diagnosis. However, if appendectomies are done quickly without careful thought, many normal appendices will be removed unnecessarily. If there is too much indecision and delay for tests, too many appendices will be perforated, with many complications and some deaths. A series of 1000 cases suggests that the right balance is struck when 80% of operations find appendicitis, and no more than 20% of these find perforation. The greatest dangers lie in children younger than 10 years of age, in whom the perforation rate is around 38%, and in patients over 65 years of age, in whom the perforation rate may be as high as

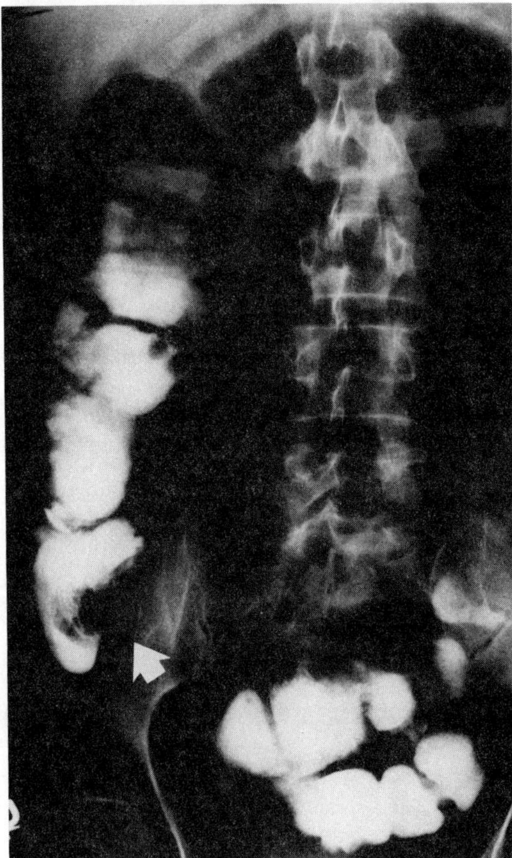

FIG 67–2.
A barium enema of the colon without any prior cleansing laxatives or enemas showing a definite filling defect in the cecum (*arrow*); the appendix cannot be visualized. This combination indicates appendicitis.

64%. Undue delay in these cases can almost always be recognized in retrospect. In patients over 70 years of age, such delay leads to many complications, and the mortality rate rises to 15%.

In patients with an established generalized peritonitis when first seen, it is too late to operate safely or to prevent peritonitis. These patients may be treated with intravenous fluids, high doses of intravenous antibiotics, and nasogastric suction until the process subsides. A delayed, or interval, appendectomy should always be performed before an exacerbation recurs.

REFERENCES

Bakhda RK, McNair MM: Useful radiological signs in acute appendicitis in children. *Clin Radiol 1977; 28:193–196. Subtle but useful help in interpreting plain abdominal x-ray films of children with appendicitis.*

Brewer RJ, Golden GT, Hitch DC, Rudolf LE, Wagensteen SL: Abdominal pain, an analysis of 1,000 consecutive cases in a university hospital emergency room. *Am J Surg 1976; 131:219–223. A careful analysis of the symptoms and signs differentiating appendicitis from other common complaints.*

Jones PF: Active observation in management of acute abdominal pain in childhood. *Br J Med 1976; 2:551–553. The usefulness and safety of a short period of observation in children with appendicitis are carefully documented.*

Lewis FR, Holcroft JW, Boey J, Dunphy JE: Appendicitis, a critical review of diagnosis and treatment in 1,000 cases. *Arch Surg 1975; 110:667–684. A very large retrospective series shows what can be accomplished by, and some of the pitfalls of operation in appendicitis.*

Raftery AT: The value of the leukocyte count in the diagnosis of acute appendicitis. *Br J Surg 1976; 163:143–144. Good documentation of the role of the WBC count and differential in the diagnosis of appendicitis.*

Rajagopalan AE, Mason JH, Kennedy M, Pawlikowski J: The value of the barium enema in the diagnosis of acute appendicitis. *Arch Surg 1977; 112: 531–533. A good exposition of the safety and usefulness and some limitations of barium enema in diagnosis.*

Storer EH. Appendix, in Schwartz SI, Shires GT, Spencer FC, Storer EH (eds): *Principles of Surgery*, ed 4. New York, McGraw-Hill Book Co, 1984, pp 1245–1256. *An excellent comprehensive description of appendicitis, including historic background, differential diagnosis, and details of operative treatment with good illustrations.*

68 DIVERTICULOSIS COLI

Dan W. Elliott, M.D.

Diverticula of the colon are thin-walled outpouchings of colonic mucosa. Their walls do not contain any of the muscularis that gives the colon wall its strength. This feature indicates they are acquired rather than congenital diverticula. They are rarely found before the age of 30 years, but their incidence steadily rises with age. In the United States about 60% of the population have multiple diverticula by the age of 80 years. In contrast, African natives who eat much indigestible fiber such as bran have almost no diverticula. These observations have been thought to imply that a low-fiber or constipating diet causes diverticulosis.

Diverticula develop most commonly in the narrowest part of the colon, the descending and sigmoid loop, where pressures are highest. They almost never occur in the rectum and are much less common in the right and transverse colon. They are most likely to begin at points where the muscular wall is penetrated by blood vessels, which presumably cause weak points. Many diverticula push out along these vessels between the layers of the mesentery. Many also occur in appendices epiploicae on the antemesenteric border. In patients with diverticulosis coli, manometric studies have shown that intraluminal pressures are unusually high. The smooth muscle bundles between diverticula are hypertrophic. At surgery the sigmoid colon with diverticula feels thick-walled and dense. However, multiple uncomplicated diverticula produce no symptoms, and patients are often unaware of their existence (Fig 68–1).

Diverticulitis is inflammation in the wall of a diverticulum. It may begin with the plugging of a single diverticulum, but edema will spread and occlude other nearby diverticula. The result is acute inflammation involving most of the circumference of the bowel and extending along its length for 8 cm to 10 cm or more. This is most likely to occur in the sigmoid or descending colon. Microscopically there are intramural microabscesses, and some may extend into the mesentery, which becomes thickened and edematous. This acute process can resolve completely with antibiotic treatment and occasionally without treatment. Sometimes it leaves behind a heavily fibrotic segment narrowing or occluding the lumen, but usually the fibrosis is mild and colon function returns to normal. Subsequent attacks occur in only about one-third of the patients, but once a second or third attack occurs many more usually follow. Chronic diverticulitis may follow between attacks, causing bowel irritability, cramps, excessive flatus, and diarrhea alternating with constipation. These symptoms may wax and wane between bouts of acute inflammation or occasionally subside completely.

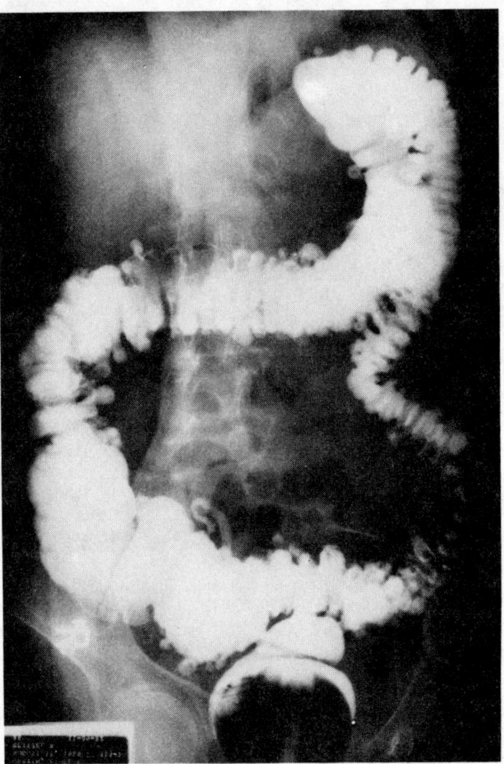

FIG 68–1.
Barium enema shows extensive involvement of the colon with diverticulosis coli in an elderly patient.

SYMPTOMS AND SIGNS OF ACUTE DIVERTICULITIS

Pain, the predominant symptom of acute diverticulitis is located directly over the involved bowel, usually in the left lower quadrant. There may be cramps and constipation or the passage of scanty liquid stool, but almost no gross blood. Anorexia is usual, but nausea and vomiting occur late and only in the more severe attacks.

The physical findings include low-grade fever, well-localized tenderness, and sometimes a tender, palpable and movable mass. Because the sigmoid colon may lie in the pelvis and swing far to the right, acute diverticulitis may mimic appendicitis. In women the vaginal and rectal examination may suggest a left tubo-ovarian abscess. If the condition is sufficiently severe, the physical signs of a localized peritonitis may appear, with rigidity and rebound tenderness directly over the involved bowel.

Treatment in this early acute stage employs primarily intravenous fluids and antibiotics, analgesics, and withholding all food and liquids by mouth. All laxatives and enemas should be avoided. Although the diagnosis can be readily confirmed by a barium enema, this should be delayed until the attack is subsiding because it can cause a major exacerbation or perforation and peritonitis. The typical findings on barium enema are of saw-toothed mucosal deformity and narrowing. Sometimes the barium will track outside the colon showing the site of a walled-off perforation (Fig 68–2). Sigmoidoscopy is indicated primarily to rule out such other diseases as colon cancer and granulomatous or ischemic colitis. The involved segment can rarely be visualized, but spasm, rigidity, angulation, and tenderness will be found as the instrument approaches. Leukocytosis is expected and can provide a useful guide to the efficacy of therapy. The clinicopathologic correlations of this process and

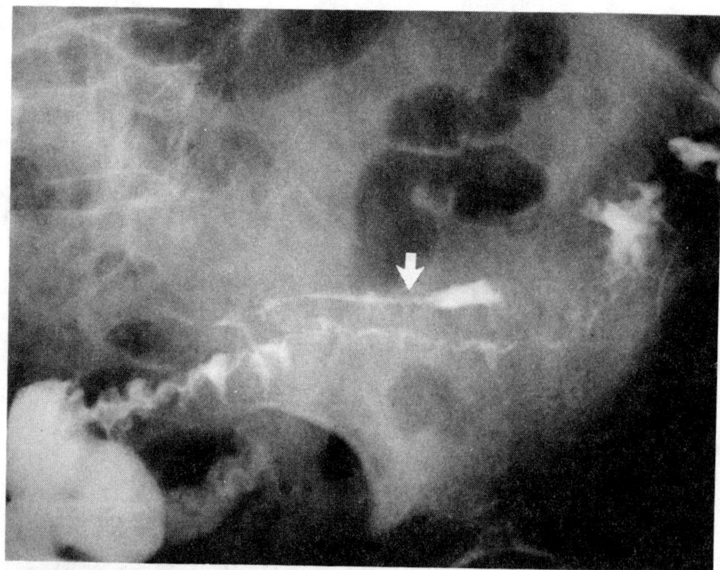

FIG 68–2.
Barium enema shows a segment of sigmoid colon with the spiking edges of acute diverticulitis and a walled-off fistula tracking along the wall of the colon (arrow).

the major complications of diverticular disease are listed in Table 68–1.

COMPLICATIONS OF ACUTE DIVERTICULITIS

In more severe and persistent attacks, a gross pericolic abscess may form in the lumbar gutter lateral to the colon or in its mesentery or in the pelvic cul-de-sac. Occasionally, a loop of small bowel is caught and obstructed by the abscess. In such cases abdominal distention and vomiting appear. Flat and upright plain x-ray films of the abdomen will show small bowel obstruction and the need for surgical relief. Very rarely the segmental inflammation obstructs the colon completely for gas as well as fluid passage. Complete colon obstruction is also an indication for surgical intervention.

FREE PERFORATION INTO THE ABDOMEN

A single acutely inflamed diverticulum can perforate freely into the peritoneal cavity. This is accompanied by relatively more intense pain, which usually starts insidiously in the left lower quadrant, but rapidly spreads and be-

comes generalized over the lower abdomen. The physical findings are those of peritonitis with widespread rigidity, tenderness, and rebound tenderness, followed by distention, tachycardia, and fever. Leukocytosis is rapid and more intense than in localized disease. An elevated hematocrit may reflect the rapid onset of dehydration as interstitial fluid pours into the area of injury. Flat and upright x-ray films of the abdomen usually show free air under the diaphragm, showing how rapidly the peritonitis can spread from the lower to upper quadrants. Intravenous fluids and antibiotics are essential. If the patient is in good health and the initial response to treatment is quite favorable, such an attack can occasionally be controlled with nonoperative measures. Close monitoring of the patient is essential so that prompt operation can be undertaken if improvement falters. More often, an emergency operation is required to stop the steady leak of bacteria and feces (Fig 68–3).

FISTULA FORMATION

Adjacent structures can become involved when a walled-off abscess forms outside the bowel. The abscess may be propagated by fecal ma-

TABLE 68–1.
Clinical–Pathologic Correlations for Diverticulosis Coli

CLINICAL FINDINGS	PATHOLOGIC FINDINGS
1. No symptoms—normal bowel function	1. Diverticulosis coli without inflammation
2. Left lower quadrant pain, cramps, obstipation, low fever, tender mass	2. Acute diverticulitis of the sigmoid colon

3. a. Anorexia, vomiting, abdominal distention
   b. Fever, leukocytosis, palpable mass
	3. Complications of acute diverticulitis:
	   a. obstruction of large or small bowel
	   b. intra-abdominal abscess

4. Spreading peritonitis, fever, leukocytosis, free air on upright x-ray film of abdomen	4. Free perforation of a diverticulum

5. a. Flatus in the urine, recurrent bladder infection
   b. Flatus from vagina or abscess opening, painful feculent drainage
	5. a. Colovesical fistula
	
	   b. Colovaginal fistula
	      Colocutaneous fistula

6. No pain; syncope, cramps with frequent passage of clots and black or bright red blood	6. Hemorrhage from the colon, usually but not always from a diverticulum

terial forced through a diverticular perforation in the wall of the colon. Such an abscess can erode its way into the dome of the bladder. This usually occurs in men whereas erosion of the uterus or vagina may also occur in women. When the abscess perforates into the bladder, it discharges its pus and the acute inflammation is temporarily improved. However, a fistula from colon to bladder is formed. This continues to feed fecal material into the bladder because of the higher pressures in the colon. Urine rarely moves in the opposite direction. Chronic and recurrent urinary tract infections result. Similarly, a fistula into the vagina or uterus produces uncontrollable, irritating, and painful fecal drainage.

The symptoms of diverticulitis that precede fistula formation can be sufficiently mild or vague so that the patient ignores them. However, a startling and instantly recognizable symptom is pathognomonic of the fistula: the passage of flatus in the urinary stream or from the vagina. Such an event always calls for careful investigation. The presence of the fistula can usually be confirmed by barium enema, and this helps to determine the nature and extent of the colonic disease. Cystoscopy should usually be performed not only becuase the orifice of the fistula can be seen, but also to assure that the bladder is otherwise healthy. The upper urinary tract should be visualized by intravenous pyelography. While the vast majority of such fistulas are caused by diverticulitis, sigmoidoscopy is also indicated to rule out

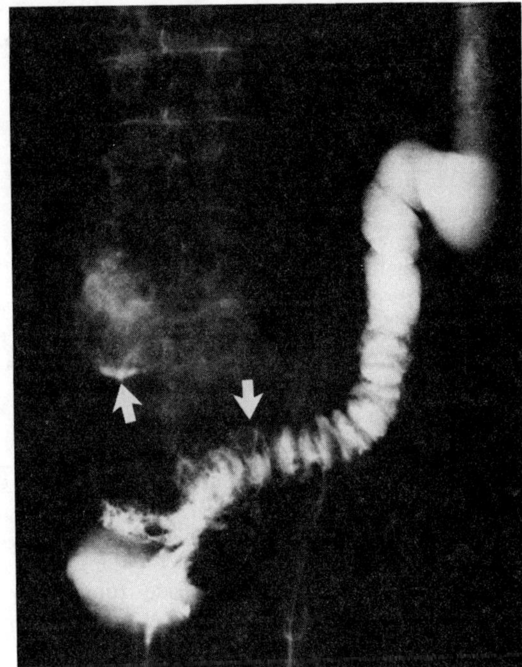

FIG 68–3.
Barium enema shows sigmoid diverticulitis (arrow) and a puddle of barium outside the bowel (arrow), indicating a free perforation of the colon into the abdomen.

Crohn's granulomatous colitis or an occasional occult carcinoma. It is unlikely that the colonic orifice of the fistula can be identified, and identification is not essential. Because these fistulas do not spontaneously close, an operation is needed. The inflammation around these fistulas makes them easy to identify at surgery. Resection of the involved segment of colon will be required, together with repair of the involved viscus.

A pericolic abscess can also appear at the skin surface in the left flank or left groin where it may mimic an incarcerated hernia. In the perineum the process resembles a perianal abscess, but the internal source lies much higher. Pain, redness, and bulging may necessitate incision and drainage, but this leaves behind a colocutaneous fistula. This usually requires resection of the underlying diverticular disease for control of the fistula. Oddly enough, such fistulas almost never develop between loops of bowel in diverticulitis. An enterocolic fistula suggests granulomatous colitis.

HEMORRHAGE FROM THE COLON

Major hemorrhage can occur from one or two nutrient arteries in a single diverticulum. Unlike all the other complications of diverticulosis, inflammation is minimal at the bleeding site. If surgery is needed to stop the bleeding, there are no gross changes in the bowel to guide the surgeon to the point of hemorrhage. Management of rapid rectal bleeding can therefore present a most difficult and life-threatening challenge, especially when it occurs in a patient past 70 years of age or with other complicating diseases, as it usually does.

Because there is no significant diverticulitis, there are almost no preceding symptoms. The onset is heralded by an urge to defecate, and the toilet bowl will be filled with bright red blood, currant-jelly clots, or blackened blood, followed quickly by faintness or syncope from blood loss. Such bleeding may arise from any point in the rectum, colon, or small bowel as high as the duodenum. However, blood from the upper small bowel that is still red and undigested in the rectum must be flowing very rapidly. Therefore, as a rule of thumb, if the patient is not in shock, the blood is coming from a point below the stomach and duodenum. In the older patient the most likely source is a single bleeding diverticulum, usually one of many lining the colon.

Resuscitation is begun and blood is transfused before diagnostic studies are undertaken. Coagulopathy should be ruled out by the

best screening tests available. Sigmoidoscopy should be performed to rule out a low-lying lesion such as an enormous hemorrhoid, ulcer, cancer, or acute ulcerative colitis. When the blood is seen to be coming from beyond the instrument, the next step in former years was a barium enema. Some thought the barium would plug the eroded diverticulum and stop the bleeding. When this idea was examined objectively, however, it was proved untrue. Bleeding does stop spontaneously, only to recur a few hours later. Although a barium enema will confirm diverticulosis, it fails to identify the bleeding point and interferes with more useful studies.

The next step in diagnosis is a nuclear scan with technetium or labeled red cells. The labeled red cell scan is more sensitive to slower rates of bleeding, but either scan will show increased activity where blood is pooling, provided the bleeding has not stopped. These scans are more likely to pinpoint pooling of blood than a selective mesenteric angiogram. If bleeding has stopped, colonoscopy can be performed after rapid preparation with an oral bowel-cleansing solution (GoLYTELY). The bleeding point may be identified precisely or even coagulated with this instrument.

When active bleeding makes adequate preparation for colonoscopy impossible, a selective mesenteric angiogram may show a blush of contrast at the bleeding point. If so, injection of vasopressin directly into the involved artery through the angiographic catheter may stop the hemorrhage. The angiogram may also identify angiodysplasia, a pathologic coil of small arteries and veins in the submucosa. There may be early filling of a dilated vein as in an arteriovenous fistula, or occasionally late filling of the vein. Mucosal erosions of these vessels can produce a major hemorrhage. This is probably the second most frequent cause of bleeding in older people.

When the surgeon must operate without any guide to the bleeding source, he or she is likely to find diverticulosis and a colon filled with blood. With no grossly identifiable pathologic changes, the safest operation is a total colectomy, removing distal ileum and all of the colon down to the rectum. Anything less risks disastrous recurrent hemorrhage a few days after surgery. The distal ileum can be anastomosed to the rectum to avoid a colostomy, but the penalty is frequent diarrheal stools. If the relative position of the bleeding source is known, that portion of the colon can be safely resected and the colon reanastomosed, preserving normal bowel function.

PRINCIPLES OF THERAPY

In addition to surgery for uncontrolled hemorrhage, emergency operations are needed for treating complete colon obstruction, secondary small-bowel obstruction, free perforation of the colon with spreading peritonitis, and large abscesses that are uncontrolled by antibiotics. Because the colon is unprepared and filled with stool, these operations are very hazardous and frequently complicated by wound infections and sepsis. In former years as many as three operative stages would be required: (1) a colostomy to divert the fecal stream, together with lysis of adhesions and drainage; (2) after the acute process subsided, local resection of the diseased bowel and anastomosis; and then (3) closure of the colostomy. More recently surgeons have learned that it is safer to remove the diseased segment at the initial operation, bringing the proximal bowel to the surface as a colostomy, and closing the distal end leading to the rectum. This is the Hartmann procedure, named for the French surgeon who devised it for perforated colon cancer (Fig 68–4). Later, after the infection has subsided, the two ends can be reanastomosed much more safely, eliminating the colostomy. The distal end may be brought to the surface as a mucous fistula, or if not long enough, it may be closed and fixed to the sacrum. Because very potent antibiotics have become available, surgeons have resected the diseased colon and reanastomosed it in a single procedure with acceptable results in highly selected low-risk patients. The danger of

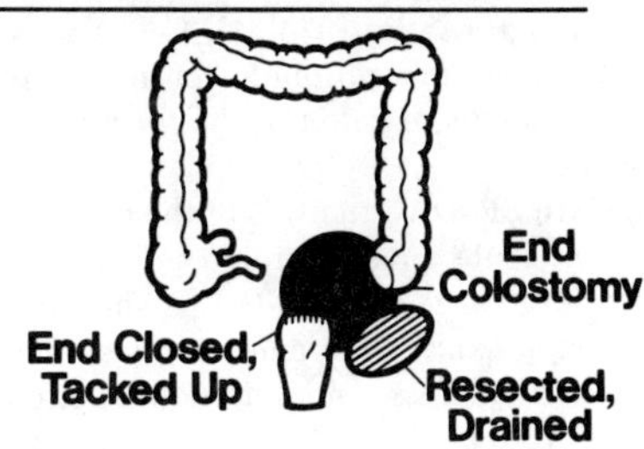

FIG 68–4.
Diagrammatic representation of a Hartmann resection of the sigmoid colon for perforated diverticulitis, with the location of the abscess indicated by the gray oval. The end of the descending colon is brought outside as a colostomy. The distal rectum is closed.

a leak is very great, however, from an anastomosis performed in these circumstances, and for most patients the Hartmann resection and colostomy are the safest at present.

The hazards of emergency surgery can be avoided in operations for fistulas because the inflammation is much more localized and the bowel can be cleansed and prepared with oral antibiotics. This is also true of elective colon resections for chronic or recurrent diverticulitis. Proper preparation can reduce the hazard of septic complications from more than 50% to less than 4% and make elective operation very safe. The medical treatment of chronic and recurrent diverticulitis with oral antibiotics, antispasmodics, and analgesics is usually effective temporarily, but recurrence of symptoms in an irregular and unpredictable pattern is the rule. A true test of a physician's best judgment is deciding when to advise a patient to undergo a safe resection for chronic or recurrent diverticulitis before more serious complications ensue.

REFERENCES

Boulos PB, Cowin AP, Karamanolis DG, Clark CG: Diverticula, neoplasia, or both? Early detection of carcinoma in sigmoid diverticular disease. *Ann Surg* 1985; 202(5):607–609. *A report of a study showing that patients with diverticulitis investigated by modern colonoscopy were found to have cancer in 6.6% of cases and adenomatous polyps in 27.6%, but the interpretation of the barium enema was inaccurate in 43%.*

Drapanas T, Pennington DG, Kappelman M, Lindsey ES: Emergency subtotal colectomy: Preferred approach to management of massively bleeding diverticular disease. *Ann Surg* 1073; 177(5): 519–526. *A classic well-documented article describing the rationale for subtotal colectomy in older patients with massive colonic bleeding.*

Laimon H: Hartmann resection for acute diverticulitis. *Rev Surg* 1974(31); 1–6. *A presentation of the history and rationale for resecting the diseased segments of colon at the initial emergency operation.*

Letwin ER: Diverticulitis of the colon: Clinical review of acute presentations and management. *Am J Surg* 1982; 143:579–581. *A short account of recent experience with emergency surgery for perforation, abscess, and colon obstruction due to diverticulitis.*

Painter NS, Truelove SC, Ardran GM, Tuckey M: Segmentation and the localization of intraluminal pressures in the human colon, with special reference to the pathogenesis of colonic diverticula. *Gastroenterology* 1965; 49(2):169–177. *A well-documented account of the physiologic abnormalities in diverticulosis coli.*

Rodkey GV, Welch CE: Changing patterns in the surgical treatment of diverticular disease. *Ann Surg* 1984; 200(4):466–478. *A comprehensive survey of the treatment of diverticulitis over a very long period of time, showing the risks of emergency surgery and the relative safety of elective resection.*

Storer EH, Goldberg SM, Nivatvongs S: Diverticular disease, in Schwartz SI, Shires GT, Spencer FC, Storer EH (eds): *Principles of Surgery*, ed 4. New York, McGraw-Hill Book Co, 1984, pp 1185–1190. *This brief but comprehensive textbook discussion of diverticular disease of the colon provides more details of treatment and surgery.*

Zollinger RW: The prognosis in diverticulitis of the colon. *Arch Surg* 1968; 97:418–422. *One of the very few well-documented long-term follow-up studies showing what may be expected after a single attack of diverticulitis.*

69 PERIANAL DISEASES

J. H. Wittoesch, M.D., M.S.

BASIC ANATOMICAL CONSIDERATIONS

The anal canal is of ectodermal origin. It is lined with stratified epithelium, a modified skin without such appendages as hair follicles and sweat glands. The blood supply comes from the inferior hemorrhoidal artery, a branch of the internal pudendal artery. The venous return goes through the inferior hemorrhoidal veins into the portal system. The anal lymphatic plexus drains toward the inguinal and internal iliac nodes. The nerve supply is somatic and thus very sensitive to painful stimuli.

The rectum is of endodermal origin and lined with glandular mucosa. Blood is supplied by the middle hemorrhoidal artery, a branch of the internal iliac artery, and the superior hemorrhoidal artery, which is the caudal branch of the inferior mesenteric artery. The venous drainage is through the inferior hemorrhoidal veins to the portal system. These veins have no valves. The lymphatics drain to the inferior mesenteric and aortic nodes. The nerve supply is sympathetic and parasympathetic. The sympathetic fibers stem from the inferior mesenteric plexus and the hypogastric nerve originating with three roots from the 2nd, 3rd, and 4th lumbar sympathetic ganglia. The sympathetic supply is derived from the 2nd, 3rd, and 4th sacral nerves.

The anal canal and the lowermost portion of the rectum are surrounded by a powerful sphincter mechanism, consisting of internal and external sphincters, levator ani, and longitudinal fibers which reduce the anal opening to a longitudinal slit.

The anal canal and rectum are joined by the mucocutaneous junction, or pectinate line, where the anal papillae and the anal glands are situated. These play a great part in anal pathologic changes. Surrounding the anal verge are normal skin appendages such as hair follicles, sweat glands, and a number of apocrine glands.

ANORECTAL EXAMINATION

Most patients with anorectal problems will complain of piles or hemorrhoids. It is important to take a thorough history of bowel habits, bleeding, pain, and itching. With the patient in a left lateral Sims' position or preferably in the knee–chest position on a proctologic table, the anal area should be inspected. A gentle digital examination is done. After palpation of the perianal structures, a sigmoidoscopic examination of the rectum and lower sigmoid should be done. A rigid sigmoidoscope will give more accurate results in this area, but if not available an anoscope must do. If examination further into the bowel is necessary, a sigmoidoscopy to 60 cm should be done with a flexible sigmoidoscope after proper preparation of the bowel. During the examination every step should be explained to the patient. This is referred to as vocal anesthesia and will relax the patient. One thing must be remembered: sedation will not replace gentleness.

HEMORRHOIDS

The hemorrhoidal plexus are situated under the anoderm and under the mucosa of the lowermost portion of the rectum. They constitute a corpus cavernosum of the anus and help accomplish tight closure after defecation. From the plexus, "internal and external" hemorrhoids develop. A hemorrhoid is not a varicose vein, but it is rather a vascular tumor. The vessels are increased in number and in size. In approximately 5% of cases, arteries are involved, which explains heavy hemorrhoidal bleeding. The chief cause of hemorrhoids is chronic, low-grade infection of the anal crypts causing increased vascularization. Straining,

chronic constipation, pregnancy, and anything increasing the intra-abdominal pressure will aggravate the preexisting condition. Hemorrhoids in the beginning states are asymptomatic and do not require any treatment other than basic anal hygiene.

External hemorrhoids are covered with skin and do not bleed unless thrombosed, with a break in the skin. Internal hemorrhoids, covered by mucosa, will bleed if irritated. Thrombosis is rare and not painful. A heavy pressure feeling is present. We distinguish four states:

1st degree: Asymptomatic; some bleeding

2nd degree: Protrusion with spontaneous post-defecation reduction

3rd degree: Protrusion after defecation or straining; manual reduction necessary

4th degree: fixed protrusion; cannot be reduced

The higher the degree, the more complicating features such as fissures, ulcers, and bleeding will be present and determine the therapeutic course.

TREATMENT

The treatment corresponds to the stage of the disease.

1st degree: Conservative; general anal hygiene

2nd degree: Conservative; anal hygiene, possible Blaisdell ligation treatment, if bleeding present

3rd degree: Anal hygiene; Blaisdell ligation (rubber band excision)

4th degree: Hemorrhoidectomy

The clamp and cautery operation and cryotherapy methods have been abandoned. Laser surgery does not offer any advantages. Injection therapy carries the risk of anaphylactic reactions and foreign body granuloma formation.

BASIC ANAL HYGIENE

Basic anal hygiene consists of the following:

1. Sitzbath, one to three times daily
2. Avoid toilet paper, soap.
3. Cleanse with witch hazel and cotton or commercial witch hazel pads.

4. Create a bulky stool by increasing fiber in the diet; give bulk-forming agents.
5. In case of painful irritation, an acid mantle cream with 1% hydrocortisone can be prescribed. For temporary use a topical anesthetic may be added. Do not order ointments because of their macerating effect.

The use of doughnut cushions is contraindicated because it increases the internal pressure on the anal ring. Suppositories are without any value for the treatment of anal conditions. If drainage is present, a dry piece of cotton should be placed in the rima ani.

FISSURE IN ANO

A fissure is one of the most painful anal conditions, often requiring surgical treatment. Most frequently, fissures are found in the posterior midline, less often in the anterior midline. Because of the angulation and fixation of the anal canal, these are the stress points. A fissure starts as a split in the anoderm, which eventually gets infected. Repeated tearing and healing lead to scarring in the base of the split with loss of elasticity. Due to the chronic infection, the adjacent papilla will hypertrophy, while at the anal verge the skin will thicken and form a fibrotic tag known as a sentinel pile. A chronic fissure is an anal ulcer.

Bowel movements are painful, associated with a tearing sensation. The pain lasts for 2 to 3 hours after defecation. Some bright red bleeding may be present. Constipation develops because of the fear of defecation. Patients often take laxatives to keep the stool soft. This may increase the pain due to the chemical irritation of semiliquid alkaline stools. Even when the acute pain subsides, there is a subthreshold pain that keeps the patient on edge.

Diagnosis can be made by external inspection, palpation, and gentle anoscopic examination. Usually the classic triad, sentinel pile, anal ulcer, and hypertrophied papilla will be present.

Treatment consists of basic anal hygiene and application of an anesthetic cortisone cream. Oral pain medication may be given to relieve the anal spasm. If there is no satisfactory improvement within 2 to 3 weeks of conservative treatment, surgical intervention should be considered. Fissurectomy and hemorrhoidectomy are the method of choice. If the general condition of the patient prohibits radical surgery, left lateral subcutaneous sphincterotomy or the Lord procedure (forceful dilatation of the anus under anesthesia) may be substituted.

THROMBOSED HEMORRHOIDS

Thrombosis of an external hemorrhoidal vein occurs after a sudden increase in venous pressure (e.g., straining with bowel movements, coughing, sneezing, childbirth, and emergency braking). Edema develops around the thrombosed vessel causing intense pain. Swelling of variable size will be seen. Gradually the edema will subside. Often the clot will penetrate the skin and spontaneously evacuate with considerable bleeding.

In the acute phase, instant relief can be accomplished by surgical evacuation of the clot under local anesthesia. This can be done if one or two major clots are present. If half or more of the anal circumference is involved, the thrombosis should be treated conservatively. A thrombosed prolapsed internal hemorrhoid should never by incised because of the resulting uncontrollable bleeding.

Conservative treatment consists of basic anal hygiene and use of anesthetic creams. Oral enzymes often will decrease swelling.

ANORECTAL ABSCESS

An abscess usually is the result of an infected crypt. Sometimes the infection penetrates the muscle and spreads into the pararectal spaces. The microorganisms most frequently involved are *Escherichia coli*, *Proteus vulgaris*, staphylococci, streptococci, and bacteroides. Anaerobic organisms are occasionally present. Abscesses are classified according to their location. Most frequent is the perianal abscess located under the anal skin and lower rectal mucosa. If it penetrates the muscular layers, we speak of an ischiorectal abscess. If found above the levator muscle, it is called a supralevator abscess, a rare occurrence. Abscesses in the posterior rectal space are hard to diagnose in the beginning. They are difficult to palpate, yet cause great discomfort because of the pressure buildup in this limited space. In rare occasions a foreign body, usually a swallowed toothpick or chicken bone, may penetrate the rectal wall just above the mucocutaneous juncture and cause an ischiorectal abscess. Care should be exercised in exploring abscess cavities so the examining finger is not injured.

In the beginning there is dull aching. As the infection progresses toward the surface, swelling, redness, and localized pain will occur. As soon as this takes place, surgical intervention is indicated. Antibiotics have no place in nondraining abscesses because with these drugs the infection will subside, and nonresponsive organisms will continue to spread the infection. Small abscesses can be drained in the office. If generalized toxic symptoms are present, incision and drainage should be done under anesthesia in the operating room. If the internal opening is found, primary fistulectomy can be done. Otherwise the patient should be informed that a fistula will develop which will need surgical removal later. Ninety percent of true anorectal abscesses will recur eventually. After incision and drainage, antibiotics are given to speed up healing and fistula formation. The patient should be instructed in anal hygiene for proper postoperative care.

Perianal hidradenitis suppurativa, a chronic infection of perianal apocrine glands, can mimic an abscess. Furuncles (folliculitis), infected comedones, and sebaceous cysts often have the appearance of an abscess. If the abscess is located anteriorly, bartholinitis in a woman or a urethroperineal abscess in a male must be ruled out. A thorough history and careful examination will help to arrive at the proper diagnosis.

FISTULA IN ANO

A fistula is a connection between a hollow organ and the outside. The anal fistula usually leads from a crypt through the former abscess cavity to the perianal area. According to their course, we distinguish among subcutaneous, intramuscular, submuscular, and submucosal fistulas. In general, one fistula develops, but if not surgically treated, several tracts will develop. If this complex fistula traverses the sphincter in more than one place, surgical repair will have to be staged to maintain sphincter function. Multitract fistulas are often seen in patients suffering from inflammatory bowel disease. Abscesses in the posterior space often will spread around the anus and appear as a horseshoe fistula with two anterior openings. An abscess in the anterior quadrant, if not treated promptly may drain spontaneously into the vagina, thus causing the dreaded rectovaginal fistula.

The diagnosis is obtained by palpating the track and watching for exit of pus from the internal opening, and then by passing of a probe through the fistulous tract. If this cannot be done gently, examination under anesthesia should be done followed by the appropriate surgical treatment. Goodsalls' rule will be helpful in determining the origin of the fistula. He pointed out that fistulas curve toward the posterior midline when the opening is situated posterior to an imaginary line passing through the anal opening. If the opening is anterior to the line, the origin is found in the regional crypt, hence the tract is straight to the anus.

The differential diagnosis of a fistula includes the same conditions as mentioned with anal abscess. A low opening of a pilonidal sinus may have the appearance of a posterior fistula.

The treatment of a fistula in ano is definitely surgical. All anal crypts should be removed during surgery to prevent further abscess formation. As in all anorectal operations, proper postoperative care is of utmost importance. If the sphincter is severed in one place only, satisfactory function will return.

PRURITUS ANI

Anal itch is a most distressing affliction. Etiologic factors include skin diseases such as psoriasis, seborrhea, and eczema. Fungal infections play a part, as do certain neoplasms (Bowen's disease, extramammary Paget's disease). Early diabetes should be considered. Parasitic infestations will cause itching, such as that often seen with pinworms (*Enterobius vermicularis*). The main cause is iatrogenic. The frequent, often unnecessary use of antibiotics will change the normal intestinal flora resulting in diarrhea. The pH of the perianal skin is acid. The highly alkaline contents of the small bowel are concentrated by absorption and acidified by bacterial action in the colon. Liquid stools are extremely irritating to the anal skin. Most digestive enzymes are still active and contribute to the irritation. Their deactivation takes place in an acid environment. The patient, feeling unclean, will use lots of soap to clean the area (all soaps are alkaline) and will resort to all kinds of over-the-counter preparations, especially local anesthetics (such as benzocaines). This may create formidable cross allergies.

The anoderm and perianal skin thickens, and lichenification of the skin is found. Usually excoriations are present.

The treatment consists of restoring the normal flora and clearing up the skin irritation. The patient is placed on the basic anal hygiene regimen and warned not to use anything except what is prescribed. Large doses of of *Lactobacillus acidophilus* (or *L. bulgaricus*) preparations are given, reinforced with buttermilk and yogurt. The intake of citrus juice and coffee is diminished. Mycostatin is prescribed to reduce fungal overgrowth. Oral antipruritics and antihistaminics should be given at night to keep the patient from traumatizing the area during sleep. The patient must be instructed to continue to practice reasonable anal hygiene so the condition does not recur.

ANAL EROTICISM

An increasing number of anorectal lesions are seen these days because of the current use of the anal opening for sexual gratification.

A rather common occurrence is condylomata accuminata (venereal warts), which often are caused by anal intercourse, especially if the lowermost rectum is involved. The causative agent is the human papilloma virus. If not treated promptly, these warts will grow into large cauliflower-like masses which bleed easily and are rather malodorous. If they are small, treatment with podophyllin resin can be attempted. If they are large, surgical treatment is indicated. Electrocoagulation or laser coagulation and vaporization are the treatments of choice. Cryotherapy is another frequently used method. Steroid creams should never be ordered to relieve the itching because they are about the best fertilizer for condylomata. Histologic study is mandatory because malignant de-

generation can occur, especially in the presence of the herpes virus.

Syphilis will occur in the area as an indurated painless ulcer or in the later stages as condylomata lata, flat broad-based lesions. Serologic and dark-field examinations will be diagnostic. Gonococcal proctitis causes severe pain. Drainage, skin irritation, mucosal redness, and cryptitis are the main symptoms. A smear and culture of the secretions should be made. Other sexually transmitted infections include hepatitis B, amebiasis, lymphogranuloma venereum, herpes genitalis, and shigellosis.

If a sexually transmitted disease is found, it may be well to include the HIV antibody test in the work-up to protect the medical personnel as well as the patient. An inspection should be made for anorectal trauma and the presence of foreign bodies.

PROCTITIS

Proctitis is an inflammatory condition of the rectal mucosa, causing bleeding and discharge of mucus. We distinguish several types.

Chronic ulcerative proctitis is a chronic ulcerative colitis limited to the rectum showing the typical granular mucosa with microulcerations. In Crohn's proctitis, larger ulcers are found. The treatment is that for inflammatory bowel disease with topical steroids added.

Campylobacter proctitis is mostly due to anal intercourse and resembles chronic ulcerative proctitis.

Ischemic proctitis is of similar, only duskier appearance.

Factitial proctitis is a side-effect of radiation treatment of adjacent organs. In the beginning the mucosa is very edematous with much bleeding. Gradually the swelling subsides, and the mucosa becomes atrophic.

The diagnosis of proctitis is made by history, inspection, tissue culture, and, if necessary, biopsy.

ANAL MALIGNANCIES

Malignant tumors of the anal canal and verge are seen infrequently. They always should be considered in making a diagnosis. The most common is the squamous cell epithelioma.

Small lesions have a wartlike appearance. Larger lesions will infiltrate and ulcerate. Cloacogenic carcinoma arises from the anal glands. Basal cell epithelioma of the anus is a rare lesion and resembles the rodent ulcer found in other parts of the body. The basiloid small cell carcinoma often mimics a basal cell epithelioma and carries a very poor prognosis. Bowen's disease is an intraepidermal carcinoma and appears as a reddish plaque. Ex-

tramammary Paget's disease is of similar appearance. Malignant melanoma of the anus has a poor prognosis because of early spread; only half of these tumors are pigmented.

The treatment for anal malignancies is surgical, the extent depending on the biopsy results, identification of the tumor, and its size, infiltration, and grade. X-ray therapy (Papillon) and chemotherapy may be valuable adjuvants.

REFERENCES

Buie LA: *Practical Proctology.* Springfield, Ill, Charles C Thomas Publisher, 1960. *Good standard text on clinical proctology.*

Goligher J: *Surgery of Anus, Rectum, and Colon.* London, Balliere Tindal, 1984. *Valuable background on full spectrum of colorectal problems.*

Jackman R, Beahrs O: *Tumors of the Large Bowel.* Philadelphia, WB Saunders Co, 1968. *Classification of colorectal tumors.*

Wittoesch JH, Woolner LB, Jackman RJ: Basal cell epithelioma and basiloid lesions of the anus. *Surg Gynecol Obstet* 1957; 104:75–80. *Anal malignancies.*

70 COLORECTAL CARCINOMA

Robert P. Turk, M.D.

In the United States cancer of the colon and rectum ranks second after cancer of the lung in incidence of new cases and in death rate. In 1984 an estimated 125,000 new cases were diagnosed, and 57,000 people died of the disease. The incidence increases with age beginning at age 40 years. About 50% of the carcinomas of the colon occur in the rectosigmoid area. The other 50% occur in the right colon (25%) followed by the descending colon and transverse colon. Both synchronous and metachronous lesions occur in less than 5% of cases.

Ninety-five percent of malignant tumors of the colon and rectum are adenocarcinomas. The other malignant neoplasms in these areas are lymphoma, leiomyosarcoma, and rectal carcinoids.

CLINICAL SIGNS AND SYMPTOMS

Adenocarcinoma of the colon and rectum may take a number of years to attain a size sufficient to cause symptoms. The only way the diagnosis can be made during this asymptomatic phase is during routine examination. There is evidence to suggest that patients diagnosed during this phase of their disease have a much better survival rate. In patients undergoing routine screening examinations and, when indicated, polypectomy, the incidence of colorectal carcinoma is considerably less than once projected.

The symptoms of advanced carcinoma of the colon and rectum depend on the location of the tumor, but cachexia is found with advanced carcinoma in all three areas (the right colon, left colon, and rectum). Because the right colon has the greatest bowel diameter and transports a liquid fecal stream and because tumors in this area grow in a fungating manner and tend to bleed, patients with these tumors usually present with a history of easy tiring and weakness, which is secondary to their anemia. The patient may also complain of postprandial dyspepsia or right lower-quadrant pain.

Tumors of the left colon tend to encircle the bowel. This, coupled with a narrower bowel lumen here and the semisolid fecal stream, leads to the symptoms of change in bowel habit with increasing constipation, abdominal distention, decrease in caliber of the stool, and occasionally rectal bleeding.

The most common symptom of rectal carcinoma is bleeding with bowel movements. The bleeding is usually painless and can be of varying amounts. The patient may also complain of a sensation of incomplete emptying of the rectum.

The only physical examination that can detect early carcinoma of the rectum is the rectal examination. Approximately 30% of colorectal carcinomas are within the reach of the examining finger. They tend to be hard and may be oval with a central depression, or flat. There may be blood on the examining finger.

All the other physical findings of colorectal carcinoma are found only in far-advanced disease. Cachexia is a systemic manifestation. On abdominal examination there may be a palpable mass. The liver may be enlarged by metastatic tumor. If there is accompanying portal obstruction, the patient may also have ascites or distended veins on the abdominal wall. Supraclavicular and groin nodes may be enlarged. On rectal examination, peritoneal metastases in the rectovesical or rectouterine pouch may feel like a hard shelf or a completely immobile pelvis.

A number of conditions are associated with a high risk of developing colon cancer (see Table 70–1).

The adenoma-carcinoma sequence has been well established. Most colonic polyps are non-neoplastic, but 20% to 30% are of the adenomatous type, which may become malignant. About 95% of all colon cancers slowly develop from neoplastic polyps. The interval between the appearance of the polyp and development of cancer may be as long as 15 years. Therefore, screening techniques for early detection and removal of colon polyps should be highly effective in the prevention of colon cancer.

Untreated carcinoma of the colon and rectum spreads by a number of methods including direct extension, lymphatic, hematogenous, intraluminal, perineural, and gravitational metastasis. The adenocarcinoma invades the submucosa and penetrates the muscular layers of the bowel and serosa. The tumor also grows circumferentially to form a constricting lesion and can produce obstruction of the bowel. When the tumor grows through the bowel wall, it may extend into contiguous structures such as the abdominal wall, the omentum, the mesentery, the kidneys, ureters, or vagina or any of the intra-abdominal organs. After invading the intramural lymphatics, the tumor may spread to the regional lymph nodes. When the tumor invades the colonic veins, it is carried to the portal venous system to the liver to produce hepatic metastases. The lumbar and vertebral venous emboli can lead to metastases in the lung. Tumor cells may be shed into the peritoneal cavity and become implanted throughout the peritoneum to produce a generalized carcinomatosis. They may also seed the ovary. In some instances, the tumor may produce a bowel perforation. A large tumor may bleed severely. The necrotic tumor may also serve as a portal of entry for nontraumatic clostridial myonecrosis.

CLINICAL–PATHOLOGIC CORRELATIONS

Because of the passage of the fecal stream, both benign and malignant colonic mucosal lesions tend to bleed in amounts sufficient to identify on a fecal occult blood test. Other clinical symptoms usually correlate with the size and location of the tumor and its involvement in contiguous structures or from the metastases from the primary location (see Table 70–2).

TABLE 70–1.
Colon Cancer Risk Factors

HIGH RISK	LOW RISK
Familial polyposis	Less than 40 years of age
Inflammatory bowel disease	No family history of colon carcinoma for two or
Familial colon cancer	more generations
Nonfamilial adenomatous polyps	Low-fat, high-bulk diet
Multiple cancers	
Previous ureterosigmoidostomy	
High-fat, low-bulk diet	
Previous colon cancer	

TABLE 70–2.
Clinical–Pathologic Correlations for Colorectal Carcinoma

CLINICAL FINDINGS	PATHOLOGIC FINDINGS
Easy tiring, malaise, anemia, and rectal bleeding	Anemia; tumor is friable and/or ulcerated, resulting in blood mixed with stool or gross blood.
Pain	
Periumbilical pain	Cecum is midgut derivative; ileocecal dysfunction causes autonomic system to refer pain to mid-abdomen.
Right lower quadrant pain and mass	Tumor grows larger, irritating parietoperitoneum; pain localizes to area of tumor.
Lower abdominal pain	Distal colon is hindgut derivative; encircling carcinoma may produce infraumbilical cramping pain.
Change in bowel habits	
Alternating constipation/diarrhea	Partial obstruction of distal colon; solid waste may not pass lumen easily, but liquid portion does.
Decrease in caliber of stool	In rectosigmoid annular carcinoma, "pencil-thin" stools are produced.
Constipation and obstipation	Progressive constriction of bowel lumen prevents passage of fecal stream.
Abdominal mass	Tumor grown to palpable size; metastasis to another organ (liver or ovaries), which becomes palpable.
Supraclavicular nodes	Tumor emboli may traverse cisterna chyli to thoracic duct to supraclavicular region.
Ascites	Metastatic involvement of liver with portal obstruction

DIFFERENTIAL DIAGNOSIS

Even after colorectal carcinoma grows to the point where it produces gastrointestinal symptoms, approximately one-fourth of these patients will have their symptoms mistakenly attributed to some benign condition.

The symptoms of a right colon carcinoma may be mistaken for appendicitis, biliary disease, peptic ulcer, ameboma, Crohn's disease, or ulcerative colitis. The anemia accompanying this tumor may be thought to be a primary hematologic disorder. Rectal bleeding from the left colon and colorectal lesions may be attributed to hemorrhoids, if they are present. Sigmoidoscopic examination should be done on all patients with rectal bleeding.

Probably the most difficult benign disease to differentiate from left colon cancer is diverticulitis. The patient may present with a tender mass, rectal bleeding, or intestinal obstruction which, with an incompetent ileocecal valve, may look like a small-bowel obstruction. Endoscopic and barium studies are often helpful in making the correct diagnosis.

Occasionally the patient with a pelvic mass may have a primary lesion of the colon that has metastasized to the ovary.

DIAGNOSIS

A summary of the diagnosis of colorectal cancer is in Table 70–3. No laboratory examinations are specific for colorectal carcinoma, but a CBC, urinalysis, liver function tests, fecal occult blood, and carcinoembryonic antigen (CEA) level may be helpful. The blood count may reveal the chronic blood loss of a right colon lesion; the leukocyte count may help in differentiating the carcinoma from an inflammatory lesion; the urinalysis may point to genitourinary involvement; and abnormal liver function tests may be a clue to metastatic disease.

Testing for fecal occult blood is a simple, inexpensive screening test for colorectal cancer. The test is based on detection of the peroxidase activity of blood. Ten to twenty percent of patients with positive tests for occult blood prove to have colon cancer when further studies are performed. Another 15% to 25% of patients are found to have adenomas greater than 5 mm in diameter. Most cancers in these patients are early, well-localized lesions, and survival rates after resection are reported to be 85%. The major problem in using fecal occult blood testing is the false-positive results produced by foods with high peroxidase levels. These include red meat, ascorbic acid, vitamin supplements, horseradish, cucumbers, carrots, cauliflower, and raw fresh fruit and vegetables (except oranges and strawberries). If an appropriate diet is followed for 3 days prior to testing, there are less than 10% false-positive reactions. With dietary noncompliance, the false-positive rate may be as high as 85%.

Carcinoembryonic antigen is a cell membrane glycoprotein found in many tissues including colon carcinoma. Its presence is not specific enough to diagnose colon cancer and, therefore, is not useful in screening. However, it is useful in monitoring the condition of patients who have had surgery for colorectal

TABLE 70–3.
Diagnosis of Colorectal Cancer

| | FINDINGS IN VARIOUS LOCATIONS | | |
	RIGHT COLON	LEFT COLON	RECTUM
SYMPTOMS	Unexplained weakness Dyspepsia Right-sided discomfort	Change in bowel habits Change in stool caliber Increasing constipation Lower abdominal cramping pain	Painless rectal bleeding Sensation of incomplete rectal emptying
SIGNS: *Early stage*	Occult blood in stools		Blood on rectal examination
Late stage	Palpable abdominal mass Palpable liver "Fixed pelvis" on rectal examination Ascites Supraclavicular nodes Cachexia	Palpable abdominal mass Palpable liver "Fixed pelvis" Ascites Supraclavicular nodes Cachexia	Palpable rectal mass Enlarged groin nodes Cachexia
LABORATORY STUDIES	Microcytic hypochromic anemia	Not helpful	Not helpful
BARIUM ENEMA	Fungating lesion in cecum	"Apple core" lesion	Not helpful
PROCEDURES	Colonoscopy	Colonoscopy	Sigmoidoscopy or colonoscopy

cancer. If the CEA level was normal preoperatively or fell to normal postoperatively, a progressive elevation in the postoperative follow-up period would suggest a recurrence. If the CEA level was elevated preoperatively and failed to return to normal level postoperatively, the patient has a poor prognosis.

The barium enema is helpful in diagnosing cancer in all areas of the colon except the rectum. It can demonstrate a fungating growth in the cecum or an "apple core" lesion in other areas of the bowel. The nondistensible "apple core" is produced by an encircling carcinoma that has destroyed the normal mucosal pattern. A chest x-ray film is used to rule out pulmonary metastasis.

The sequencing of procedures for establishing a diagnosis of colorectal cancer, particularly in the established high-risk group, would begin with rectal examination and a test for fecal occult blood. Anoscopy may find rectal lesions, but a sigmoidoscope is required to examine the colorectal area. With the rigid sigmoidoscope the distal 25 cm of bowel can be seen, whereas with the flexible sigmoidoscope, which comes in 36-cm or 60-cm lengths, greater distances can be seen. A barium enema is less expensive but is also less accurate than colonoscopy. However, a double-contrast barium enema (i.e., insufflating the colon previously coated with barium) can detect small lesions. The caveat of no barium enema for 1 to 2 weeks after endoscopic biopsy must be observed to prevent barium peritonitis. With the colonoscope one can directly see all of the colon, collect biopsies or cytologic brushings, and find synchronous lesions in the more proximal colon. The cost-effective sequencing of these examinations would be digital rectal examination, sigmoidoscopy, barium enema (including double-contrast barium enema), and colonoscopy.

PRINCIPLES OF THERAPY

The treatment of colorectal carcinoma is primarily surgical. The operations are done for various reasons (e.g., cure, staging, and palliation). Staging involves not only the histopathologic classification but also evidence of regional or distant metastasis (Table 70–4). The palliative operations prevent bowel obstruction and bleeding.

The operative principle is to respect the tumor and its lymphatic drainage, first exploring the abdomen for metastasis, then ligating the vascular supply (to prevent tumor embolization), and tying the intestinal lumen on both sides of the cancer with umbilical tape (to prevent seeding of exfoliated cells). The tumor is then mobilized and removed.

The extent of resection depends on the location of the cancer. Usually right, left, or transverse colectomies are done for tumors in those locations and low anterior resection for rectosigmoid lesions. Although the stapling devices now allow anastomoses to be created very low in the pelvis, lesions below 8 cm from the anal verge and rectal carcinomas are treated with abdominoperineal resection with end colostomy.

Colon carcinoma is basically treated surgically because effective chemotherapy is lacking. Cancer of the rectum can also be treated with x-ray or electrocoagulation if the tumor cannot be resected or is in a poor-risk patient.

TABLE 70–4.
Survival Rates for Various Stages of Colorectal Carcinoma

STAGE	DEFINITION	5-YEAR SURVIVAL RATE(% OF PATIENTS)
A	Limited to bowel wall	80
B	Penetrates through the serosa into pericolic fat	45
C	Regional nodal metastases	25
D	Distant metastases	10

REFERENCES

Beart RW Jr, O'Connel MJ: Postoperative follow-up of patients with carcinoma of the colon. *Mayo Clin Proc* 1983; 58(6):361–363. *Carcinoembryonic antigen is most sensitive in detecting recurrence, but in 95% of the cases, tumors were unresectable.*

Burkitt DP: Etiology and prevention of colorectal cancer. *Hosp Pract* 1984; 19(2):67–77. *Environmental factors play a role in the etiology of colorectal cancer, and the major factor is dietary.*

Ferguson E Jr: Operations of choice for cancer of the colon and rectum: An overview. *Am Surg* 1984; 50(3):121–127. *Diagrammatic illustration of the extent of colon and mesenteric resections recommended for tumors in various locations of the large bowel.*

Gastrointestinal Tumor Study Group: Adjuvant therapy for colon cancer—Results of a prospectively randomized trial. *N Engl J Med* 1984; 310(12):737–743. *Describes a study not supporting the use of chemotherapy with 5-fluorouracil as adjuvant treatment for patients at high risk for recurrent colon cancer.*

Goligher J et al: *Surgery of the Anus, Rectum, and Colon,* ed 5. Philadelphia, WB Saunders Co, 1983. *Best recent text reference.*

Nostraint TT, Wilson JA: How good is screening for colorectal cancer? *Postgrad Med* 1983; 73(6): 131–139. *Discusses the effectiveness of tests for fecal occult blood and endoscopy in the early detection of colorectal cancer.*

Pitluk H, Poticha S: Carcinoma of the colon and rectum in patients less than 40 years of age. *Surg Gynecol Obstet* 1983; 157:335–337. *Report that poor survival in this group seemed related to delay in diagnosis and to the histologic grade of the tumors.*

Webb WA, McDaniel L, Jones L et al: Experience with 1,000 colonscopic polypectomies. *Ann Surg* 1985; 201:626–632. *Discusses the polyp-cancer sequence and describes finding in polyps greater than 2 cm in diameter as well as preventing cancer by removing polyps that are smaller in size.*

Unger SW, Wanebo HJ: Colonoscopy: An essential monitoring technique after resection of colorectal cancer. *Am J Surg* 1983; 145:71–76. *Presents a protocol for follow-up of patients who have been operated on for colorectal cancer.*

71   COMMON HERNIAS

Margaret M. Dunn, M.D.

Hernias are abnormal defects through which other structures may protrude. Hernias of the abdominal wall are common clinical problems. The peritoneum, omentum, bowel, as well as properitoneal fat and the bladder can all protrude through fascial defects, beyond the usual confines of the abdominal wall. The types of abdominal wall hernias are listed in Table 71–1.

In the groin, inguinal hernias are those with defects immediately above the inguinal liga-

TABLE 71–1.
Differential Diagnosis for Common Hernias

Groin
Inguinal
indirect
direct
Femoral
Abdominal wall
Umbilical
Incisional
Epigastric

ment. In indirect inguinal hernias the peritoneum and its contents protrude through an enlarged internal ring into the inguinal canal. In direct inguinal hernias, the defect is in the attenuated floor of the inguinal canal medial to the internal ring and inferior epigastric artery and inferior to the border of the rectus sheath (i.e., Hesselbach's triangle). Femoral hernias are found below the inguinal ligament, medial to the femoral vessels, and protrude through the femoral canal. Groin hernias are present in about 5% of the adult male population.

Ventral hernias or hernias of the anterior abdominal wall include umbilical hernias and incisional hernias. Less common ventral abdominal wall defects include epigastric and spigelian hernias. Epigastric hernias represent defects of the linea alba between the xiphoid and umbilicus. The spigelian line along which those defects occur is the lateral border of the rectus sheath or the linea semilunaris. When the contents of a hernia can be returned to the abdomen, the hernia is said to be reducible. When the contents cannot be returned, the hernia is irreducible, or incarcerated. A strangulated hernia implies compromise of the blood supply of the hernia contents.

CLINICAL SIGNS AND SYMPTOMS

The most common initial complaints will be of pain or the presence of a mass. In the uncomplicated hernia, discomfort should differ from that secondary to other musculoskeletal problems in that it should be relieved by assumption of the supine position. Acute incarceration or strangulation will have constant pain referable to the hernia as well as abdominal pain, nausea, and vomiting.

A physical examination is usually diagnostic. The findings may be limited in the obese patient or in the patient with multiple abdominal scars. Examination of the patient in the erect position combined with a Valsalva maneuver may be necessary to demonstrate a defect. It is difficult and pointless to attempt to differentiate indirect and direct inguinal hernias on physical examination because in most cases recommendations for treatment and initial operative approach are the same for both. In the acutely incarcerated or strangulated hernia, a tender, unyielding mass will be found.

Bowel sounds are not specific for incarcerated bowel and can be occasionally heard in the normal groin of a thin individual.

Strangulation is not necessarily preceded by the presence of chronic symptoms, but may be heralded by the development of increasing difficulty in reduction of a hernia. A hernia can produce simple mechanical obstruction and should be sought in every case of small-bowel obstruction. Epigastric hernias, because of the normal position of the small intestine within the infracolic compartment, are less likely to entrap the small intestine than those lower on the abdominal wall. Hernias with large fascial deficits are also less likely to incarcerate bowel. The large intestine is rarely obstructed within hernias, though the sigmoid colon is often contained in large left-sided inguinal hernias. Direct inguinal hernias often may contain bladder, but these rarely incarcerate.

Over a period of years the contents of the abdominal cavity may gradually fill a hernia until the "right of domain" is lost. In ventral hernias, the skin overlying such giant hernias can become ulcerated and can rupture producing evisceration. Ulceration and rupture of the attenuated overlying skin can also occur in cirrhotic patients with ascites and umbilical hernias.

PATHOPHYSIOLOGY

A variety of congenital, mechanical, and possibly biochemical factors can contribute to the development of hernia. Factors contributing to a chronic increase in intra-abdominal pressure such as chronic cough, constipation, prostatism, and obesity have long been felt to contribute to hernia development. Occupational activities such as heavy lifting produce symptoms largely in cases of preexisting defects.

In the groin, hernias are far more common in men than women. The necessary passage of the testes through the abdominal wall as well as persistent patency of the processus vaginalis contribute to development of groin hernias in men. Approximately 20% of adult men have a patent processus vaginalis, a figure far in excess of the incidence of indirect inguinal hernias in the adult male population. Obviously other factors play an important role in the development of indirect inguinal hernia, and these hernias are best not thought of as strictly "congenital" hernias. Umbilical hernias are associated with failure of obliteration of the allantois as well as with ascites and pregnancy. The most controllable factors contributing to the development of incisional hernias are the location of the incision, the technique of closure, and wound sepsis.

Some investigators have identified a relationship between smoking and hernia. Both an increased incidence of hernias as well as increased serum proteolytic activity have been found in smokers. The development of abdominal aortic aneurysms has also been linked with that of inguinal hernias. Either increased collagen lysis or abnormal collagen synthesis could explain these findings.

DIFFERENTIAL DIAGNOSIS

The diagnosis of hernia is generally only in question in those patients where the physical examination is limited by obesity or other factors. However, a patient may have a history of long-standing discrete reproducible pain typical of hernia without a demonstrable mass. Young women with indirect inguinal hernias, as well as those patients with intraparietal spigelian hernias (i.e., where a properitoneal defect produces herniation deep to the external oblique and anterior rectus sheath) may present a history of recurrent pain without a mass apparent on examination.

Except in these exceptional circumstances, other causes of groin and scrotal pain such as ureteral obstruction, epididymitis, testicular torsion, and groin muscle injury should be differentiated by the absence of a reducible mass. Occasionally other groin masses may be difficult to distinguish from an incarcerated femoral hernia. A hydrocele may be confused with an incarcerated inguinal hernia extending into the scrotum.

In the case of a long-standing inguinal hernia, it is important to ascertain why the patient is presenting at this time. Constipation of recent onset secondary to colon cancer can worsen the symptoms of an inguinal hernia from increased intra-abdominal pressure. Similarly worsening prostatism or ascites may produce increased symptoms referable to a long-standing hernia and lead the patient to seek medical attention. Symptoms of large bowel or bladder-outlet obstruction should be investigated prior to elective herniorrhaphy.

Herniography, or demonstration of a patent processus vaginalis with intraperitoneal radiopaque or radionuclear contrast agents, is occasionally useful in evaluating the asymptomatic, contralateral groin in the pediatric patient with an inguinal hernia. In ambulatory peritoneal-dialysis patients, herniography has been used to differentiate scrotal swelling produced by extraperitoneal extravasation of peritoneal fluid from an indirect inguinal hernia.

CLINICAL–PATHOLOGIC CORRELATIONS

A review of the usual initial symptoms and signs and the probable underlying mechanical causes is given in Table 71–2.

PRINCIPLES OF THERAPY

All groin hernias should be repaired except for the large chronic hernia in the patient who is an extremely poor surgical risk. The majority of groin hernia repairs can be performed under lo-

TABLE 71–2.
Clinical–Pathologic Correlations for Common Hernias

CLINICAL FINDINGS	PATHOLOGIC FINDINGS
Discomfort	Distention or inflammation of parietal or visceral peritoneum or properitoneal fat entrapment
Mass	Properitoneal fat, omentum, bowel, bladder
Obstruction	Mechanical impingement of bowel lumen
Strangulation	Mechanical impingement of bowel mesentery impairs venous return
	Distention from closed-loop obstruction impairs arterial inflow
	Pressure necrosis from edge of hernial defect

cal or regional anesthesia so that serious underlying medical conditions are not strict contraindications to repair. Umbilical hernias may be observed in patients under 4 years of age, but otherwise should be repaired. In cirrhotic patients with ascites, vigorous efforts to control ascites should be made prior to elective repair. Peritoneovenous shunting should be considered in cases in which medical therapy fails to control the ascites.

Repair may be deferred in certain cases of incisional and recurrent hernias. Large fascial defects and recurrent hernias may require the use of prosthetic materials such as polypropylene mesh. The incidence of recurrence in inguinal herniorrhaphy is often reported as less than 5%, but is probably closer to 10%.

REFERENCES

Berliner SD: An approach to groin hernia. *Surg Clin North Am* 1984; 64:197–213. *A nicely written current personal series.*

Cannon DJ, Read RC: Metastatic emphysema. A mechanism for acquiring inguinal herniation. *Ann Surg* 1981; 194:270–278. *A controversial and stimulating paper on smoking as a systemic cause of groin herniation.*

Donahue PE, Nyhus LM: Surgical repair of groin and ventral hernia: The rationale and strategy of treatment. *Adv Surg* 1981; 15:93–121. *An excellent short treatment of the basic anatomy and standard repairs.*

Dunphy JE, Botsford TW: Examination of the inguinal and femoral regions and the male external genitalia—The differential diagnosis of hernia, in *Physical Examination of the Surgical Patient*, ed 4. Philadelphia, WB Saunders Co, 1975. *An illustrated discussion of the physical exam of the groin and possible findings.*

Nyhus LM, Condon RE: *Hernia*, ed 2. Philadelphia, JB Lippincott Co, 1978. *The standard reference work on this topic.*

Ponka JL: *Hernias of the Abdominal Wall.* Philadelphia, WB Saunders Co, 1980. *An extensive treatment of the subject by a single author.*

part VI

Hematologic Disorders

COAGULATION DISORDERS

Barrett H. Bolton, M.D.

Maintenance of the fluidity of blood, limitation of blood loss from damaged blood vessels, and repair to reestablish vascular integrity are essential conditions for human life. The balance between fluidity and the generation of clots to stop blood loss after vascular injury is delicate and amazingly efficient under most circumstances. Excessive or inappropriate clot production leads to ischemia, infarction, and the necrosis of tissue. Deficiencies in the substances needed to stop bleeding and produce clots lead to blood loss, hematomas, and ultimately to tissue damage, scarring, and occasionally death. Damage to a sufficiently large blood vessel may exceed the ability of even a perfectly functioning coagulation system to occlude the vascular defect, necessitating pressure occlusion, ligature, or operative repair to stop blood loss.

REVIEW OF NORMAL BLEEDING AND CLOTTING

Events following blood vessel damage can be grouped into four phases: (1) tissue or vascular, (2) platelet, (3) coagulation and, (4) fibrinolytic. These phases often overlap or proceed together at different rates. Included in the vascular phase are the immediate retraction of the cut ends of blood vessels, slowing of blood loss through constriction of the vascular lumen by its muscular layers, exposure of the blood to collagen fibers and tissue juice, and tissue swelling with resulting occlusive pressure on the injured vessel. The platelet phase depends on adequate numbers and function of platelets and involves the aggregation of platelets, their adherence to the defect in the blood vessel wall, production of a fragile temporary platelet plug, which slows or stops the flow of blood

further and activates the coagulation system. The coagulation phase consists of a series of plasma enzymatic reactions, which successively activate clotting factors ultimately generating a fibrin-mesh clot which stabilizes and occludes the blood vessel lumen. This clot eventually retracts and dissolves in the fourth and final phase of the process, the fibrinolytic phase, which is necessary to permit new blood, nutrients, fibroblasts, and phagocytic cells to be brought to the area for the repair of the damage and to restore the integrity and lumen of the injured blood vessel.

CLINICAL SIGNS AND SYMPTOMS

Bleeding and coagulation disorders become manifest when a patient bleeds excessively following an injury involving damage to blood vessels. Minor cuts such as scratches, nicks from shaving, laceration, and abrasion or more serious hemostatic challenges such as the loss of teeth, severe trauma, and surgical procedures may lead to continued active bleeding.

Coagulation deficiencies can be classified into congenital or acquired. Although most patients with congenital coagulation defects are discovered during childhood, some congenital deficiencies such as very mild hemophilia and von Willebrand's disease may not become apparent until late adolescence or adult life following a major surgical or obstetric challenge. Acquired abnormalities occur predominantly in adults with liver diseases, because most of the coagulation proteins are made in the liver, or with neoplastic diseases or their treatment.

Neonatal bleeding from vitamin K deficiency (hemorrhagic disease of the newborn) will often appear as bloody gastric regurgitation. Hemophilia may be suspected when undue bleeding is noted at circumcision. Epistaxis, easy bruising, hematomas and hemarthroses following falls, and bleeding from the loss of deciduous teeth may also be initial symptoms of congenital, inherited clotting-factor deficiencies such as the hemophilias. Acquired coagulation disorders may appear as major gastrointestinal (GI), genitourinary (GU), or surgical bleeding in patients who at an earlier age were apparently able to form adequate clots.

Some differences may be noted in the symptoms of bleeding from platelet disorders and coagulation defects. Platelet abnormalities commonly appear as small petechial skin hemorrhages or blood blisters in mucous membranes or as prolonged bleeding from skin cuts. Coagulation-protein defects more often result in continued GI or GU bleeding or in unduly large or persistent hematomas or hemarthroses.

Patients with tissue or vascular defects such as scurvy may develop nose bleeds, gum bleeding, perifollicular hemorrhages, and large hematomas in the skin. Patients with excessive fibrinolysis will have recurrent delayed bleeding and difficulty healing a deep hematoma.

Excessive utilization of coagulation factors or platelets by the body such as in a consumptive coagulopathy can also lead to bleeding. Finally, coagulation can take place in inappropriate amount, time, and tissue leading to thrombosis and infarctions.

Fibrinolysis can lead to normal healing but also to recurrent unsatisfiable demands on the coagulation system such as in patients with hemophilia who have healing wounds. Lack of fibrinolysis may delay healing in areas with large hematomas.

Each type of hemorrhagic disease has a different natural history. Patients with congenital coagulation defects have bruising and hematoma and hemarthrosis formation, often leading to ankylosis of a joint with limitation of motion and disability. The severity of the deficiency determines the frequency of the bleeding episodes and the need for repeated replacement coagulant therapy. Hemophiliacs whose level of factor VIII is less than 1% may require monthly, weekly, or even more frequent replacement with factor VIII concentrate. Hemophiliacs whose level of factor VIII is more than 5% may have fewer episodes and less severe bleeding. Repeated administration of blood products exposes patients to blood-borne viral infections such as hepatitis (A, B, or non-A

non-B) or to the virus associated with the acquired immunodeficiency syndrome (AIDS). Since the availability of concentrates of coagulation factors such as factor VIII, factor IX, and cryoprecipitate for von Willebrand's disease or low-fibrinogen syndromes, the danger of circulatory overload, which was of concern when only fresh plasma or fresh frozen plasma was available, has decreased considerably. In the past, few hemophiliac children survived to reproductive age, but with the easy availability of the concentrates now sponsored in the United States by the government, many more hemophiliacs are achieving adulthood, and many are quite functional.

Acquired coagulation defects, appearing most often in adulthood and frequently as a result of liver disease, result in bleeding that is commonly life threatening. If the liver disease is transient such as in hepatitis A, the risk may not be great or last long. In patients with cirrhosis or alcoholic liver disease, which is among the top six causes of death in adults, gastrointestinal hemorrhage worsened by multiple coagulation defects is second only to hepatic metabolic failure as the cause of death.

Immune platelet disorders may spontaneously remit or, more often, will improve with therapy, but will sometimes be chronic. The thrombocytopenia of alcoholic patients caused by multiple mechanisms often becomes chronic. Thrombocytopenia due to drugs may be permanent, such as in aplastic anemia due to chloramphenicol or phenylbutazone, or transient, such as with quinidine therapy. Tumors metastatic to the bone marrow may result in a thrombocytopenia that is often unresponsive to treatment. Bleeding that results from a low platelet count is a common cause of death in patients with leukemia because of the disease or sometimes its treatment. Most infectious processes leading to thrombocytopenia or disseminated intravascular coagulation are associated with sepsis and improve with an eradication of the infection. Platelet transfusions under most circumstances are short-lived solutions to a low platelet count. The prognosis of thrombocytopenia depends largely on its reversibility and the disease causing it.

Coagulation disorders are generally serious problems. A good long-term outlook is usually associated with transient drug-induced, infectious, or obstetric causes.

PATHOPHYSIOLOGY

(See Tables 72–1 through 72–6.) Although all organs can be affected by a coagulation disorder, the skin, mucous membranes of the oropharynx, nose, mouth, and the GI and GU tracts are the sites most often affected with bleeding leading to significant blood loss. With anemia and sufficient blood loss may come the secondary manifestations of weakness, tiredness, fatigue, and the symptoms of dizziness, and orthostatic hypotension if the blood loss is great enough.

In congenital coagulation-factor defects, the muscles and joints are often the site of bleeding. In all bleeding disorders, the central nervous system is an uncommon but dreaded and sometimes lethal site of bleeding. Bleeding damages the tissues by direct pressure, hematoma formation, and the repeated necessity for clot resorption and repair, sometimes producing scarring.

Congenital coagulation disorders are attributed to a genetic defect leading to the production of biochemically defective coagulation proteins, which are, therefore, deficient in function or in amount because of a decreased rate of synthesis. Except for hemophilia A and B and von Willebrand's disease, congenital coagulation factor deficiency is rare.

Acquired coagulation-factor deficiencies are most commonly associated with liver disease because the liver is the site of synthesis of most coagulation proteins with the notable exception of factor VIII and its variants: coagulation factor VIII, antigenic factor VIII, von Willebrand's factor VIII. Protein malnutrition may contribute to factor deficiency directly if it is severe enough or indirectly by contributing to liver damage. Vitamin K deficiency can lead directly to deficiency of the vitamin K-dependent factors II, VII, IX, and X. Vitamin K deficiency can be produced by a congenital lack (hemorrhagic disease of the newborn), dietary deficiency, disruption of the normal intestinal flora that synthesize and contribute to the supply of vitamin K, diseases such as obstructive jaundice (vitamin K as a fat-soluble vitamin requires bile for proper absorption), medications such as cholestyramine, laxatives that interfere with vitamin K absorption, and some antibiotics that interfere with its production. Coumarin anticoagulants prevent the conversion of the precursors of factors II, VII, IX, and X into functional coagulation proteins.

Tissue abnormalities may be the result of protein malnutrition or a vitamin deficiency such as scurvy in which the vitamin C deficiency results in a defective formation of collagen. In amyloidosis, abnormal gamma globulins are deposited in tissues and form complexes with factor X. This disease may appear to be a tissue abnormality with relatively normal in vitro coagulation test values.

TABLE 72–1.
Pathogenesis of Vascular Tissue-Phase Defects

DEFICIENCIES	
Vitamin C (Scurvy)	Defective production of collagen and mucopolysaccharides leads to skin,
Proteins	gum, and joint bleeding.
DISEASES	
Collagen disease, vasculitides	Vascular inflammation and necrosis leads to bleeding into tissues from
Allergic purpura	damaged vessels.
Amyloidosis	Amyloid infiltration damages blood vessels increasing fragility, or amyloid may complex with factor X leading to its deficiency.
Senile purpuras	Degeneration of collagen fiber and intercellular bridges leads to failure to limit spreading of subcutaneous hematomas.
DRUGS	
Corticosteroids	Inhibit collagen with consequent failure to limit extension of subcutaneous hematomas
HEREDITARY	
Rendu-Osler-Weber disease	Bleeding from the telangiectases of hereditary hemorrhagic telangiectasia because of thinning of blood vessel walls
Marfan's syndrome	Deficient mesenchymal support of vascular and perivascular tissues leads to
Ehlers-Danlos syndrome	an increase in bleeding tendency.

TABLE 72–2.
Pathogenesis of Coagulation Factor Deficiencies

Liver disease	May result in deficiencies of factors I, II, V, VII, IX, X, and XIII from decreased synthesis of these coagulation proteins and other proteins
Congenital defects	Factors VIII and IX are sex-linked recessive inherited qualitative or quantitative deficiencies of these factors, giving rise to hemophilia A and hemophilia B, respectively. Von Willebrand's disease is an autosomally recessive inherited defect of factor VIII production and defective platelet function. Factors II, V, VII, X, and XI deficiencies are rare autosomal recessive conditions with decreased quantities of these factors.
Vitamin K deficiency or vitamin K antagonist	Incomplete synthesis of the vitamin K-dependent factors II, VII, IX, and X result in these coagulation proteins being incompletely formed and functionally useless.
Disseminated intravascular coagulation or consumptive coagulopathy	By the intravascular utilization of coagulation proteins at inappropriate times and places, induced by the circulation of activated coagulation factors or thrombogenic substances, all coagulation proteins and platelets are consumed at rates exceeding the ability of the liver, vascular endothelium, or bone marrow to replace them.
Inhibitors of coagulation factors	As polypeptide proteins, most coagulation factors may become antigenic leading to the generation of corresponding antibodies following their administration. Some hemophiliacs will thus develop antibodies to factor VIII. In some immunologic diseases patients may rarely produce immunologic inhibitors, particularly of factors VIII and IX. Patients with inhibitors will be found to have "circulating anticoagulants."

Platelet disorders are qualitative or quantitative. With a qualitative platelet defect, the platelets fail to form an adequate platelet plug, usually because of a defective platelet membrane or inadequate platelet contents, such as in platelet storage pool disease or Bernard-Soulier disease. These are diagnosed by appropriate platelet aggregometric, retention, or adherence studies. Much more common than the congenital diseases is the acquired platelet function deficiency from the loss of thromboxane A2 caused by cyclooxygenase inhibitors including aspirin, most nonsteroidal anti-inflammatory drugs, and, to lesser degrees, many commonly used medications such as some antihistamines and antibiotics.

Quantitative platelet disorders may be caused by a tumor replacing the bone marrow causing a decrease in normal megakaryocytic elements and in platelet production. Many drugs such as chloramphenicol and phenylbutazone may also lead to thrombocytopenia by damaging the megakaryocytes specifically or the bone marrow cells generally. Some drugs such as quinidine may lead to an immunologic destruction of platelets. Some drugs, by interfering with folic acid absorption (estrogens) or metabolism (methotrexate), may lead to folic acid deficiency and thrombocytopenia. Hy-persequestration of platelets may lead to thrombocytopenia by an increased destruction or storage of platelets in the spleen.

In the disorders characterized by excessive clotting, a common pathologic mechanism is the release into the circulation of thrombogenic substances such as lipids, proteins, or lipoproteins from such diverse tissues or fluids as the brain, amniotic fluid, placental juice, the pancreas, or some malignant tumors. Endotoxins or exotoxins from various bacteria may also activate clotting factors. Quantities of activated coagulation factors generated in excess of their local need from the production of a clot in an area of trauma may lead to clots in distant blood vessels. Increases in the amounts of normal coagulation factors may be produced by estrogens (factor VIII) and by pregnancy (fibrinogen) and are thought to have some influence on the increased likelihood of venous thrombotic or thromboembolic disease associated with these conditions or substances.

PRINCIPLES OF THERAPY

The treatment of bleeding disorders depends on the nature of the defect. When the disorder is due to a deficiency for which a concentrate

TABLE 72–3.
Pathogenesis of Quantitative Platelet Disorders

CONGENITAL	
Passively acquired immunologic disorders	Antibodies from mother are transmitted to fetus leading to immunologic platelet destruction.
Leukemia	Rare congenital leukemia decreases megakaryocytes and platelets by myelopoietic replacement with leukemic cells.
Fanconi's anemia	Hereditary form of pancytopenia of uncertain pathogenesis
ACQUIRED	
Leukemia	Myelopoietic replacement with leukemic cells; toxicity of treatment or intercurrent septic processes often cause thrombocytopenia
Deficiencies Folic acid	Dietary deficiency such as in alcoholics. Increased metabolic requirements such as hemolytic anemias, interference with absorption such as with phenytoin or estrogen treatment, or metabolic interference such as with methotrexate may lead to decreased production and induration of megakaryocytes and platelets.
Vitamin B_{12}	Lack of intrinsic factor in stomach or disease of the terminal ileum leads to malabsorption of vitamin B_{12} which often leads to thrombocytopenia.
BONE MARROW REPLACEMENT	Leukemias, lymphomas, multiple myeloma, and metastatic solid tumors in the bone marrow may mechanically crowd out normal marrow elements by overgrowth or toxic suppression.
BONE MARROW FAILURE	
Aplastic anemia Paroxysmal nocturnal hemoglobinuria Idiopathic disorders Toxins Drugs	Decrease in stem cell pool, suppression of marrow by immune cells, metabolic damage to proliferation and maturation of marrow cells by drugs (chloramphenicol, phenylbutazone, and many others), toxins (such as benzene, alcohol), suppressants (thiazide, estrogens), radiation damage, and some viral, infectious, idiopathic, or unrecognized mechanisms will lead to varying degrees of thrombocytopenia.
PERIPHERAL DESTRUCTION	
Infections	Decrease in survival of platelets leading to thrombocytopenia seen with some viral, bacterial, or rickettsial infections, (especially in septic patients) may be due to direct toxicity of microbial toxins to immunologic damage, or disseminated intravascular coagulation.
Drugs	Many drugs agglutinate or lyse platelets by several proposed mechanisms, including haptenic binding to platelet membranes, and drug antibody reactions with platelets as "innocent bystanders." Antibodies may be to platelet constituents, and may fix complement.
Immunologic disorders	Idiopathic thrombocytopenic purpura is a relatively common cause of platelet destruction thought to be immunologically mediated and often follows infections, especially viral. Thrombotic thrombocytopenic purpura causes aggregation of platelets in an unknown manner probably through a substance in plasma.

TABLE 72–4.
Pathogenesis of Qualitative Platelet Deficiencies

CONGENITAL	
Platelet storage pool deficiencies	Diminished platelet ATP and ADP and serotonin lead to defective platelet aggregation.
Von Willebrand's disease Thrombasthenia Bernard-Soulier disease	The congenital qualitative platelet disorders are characterized by hereditary platelet membrane defects in function leading to defective aggregation and platelet plug formation.
ACQUIRED	
Drug-induced deficiencies	Acquired qualitative platelet disorders are regularly induced by aspirin or other prostaglandin-inhibiting drugs such as most nonsteroidal anti-inflammatory drugs, dipyridamole, and many other cyclooxygenase-inhibiting drugs.
Disease-induced deficiencies	Diseases such as myeloproliferative disorders, anemia, multiple myeloma, and liver disease may result in functionally defective platelets.

TABLE 72–5.
Pathogenesis of Fibrinolytic Disease

Liver disease	Activated fibrinolytic enzymes are normally metabolized in the liver. Patients with severe liver disease may have a prolonged and increased fibrinolysis.
Tumor	Some tumors may elaborate fibrinolytic enzymes or activate the normal fibrinolytic system excessively, leading to pathologic fibrinolysis.

TABLE 72–6.
Pathogenesis of Hypercoagulability

Increased coagulation factor levels	Pregnancy is accompanied by increases in fibrinogen and factor VIII; estrogens increase factor VIII and von Willebrand's factor, with associated increased risk of thrombotic disease.
Decreased circulation	Bedrest, heart failure, and immobilization all slow venous blood flow and increase the risk of venous thrombosis.
Increased risk factors	Stress, cigarette smoking, blood group A, increased estrogen levels, hyperlipidemia, cancer, diabetes, and decrease of antithrombin III are all risk factors for increased incidence of thromboembolic disease.
Atherosclerosis	Arterial plaques and narrowing lead to increased risk of thrombosis, embolism, ischemia, and infarction in many organs and sites.

of the deficient factor or cell is available, replacement is relatively straight forward. In thrombocytopenia, platelet transfusion may be effective in stopping bleeding and is often used in patients with platelet counts (under 30,000) that are sufficiently low to constitute a risk of spontaneous bleeding. If the thrombocytopenia is brief (days to a few weeks), transfusion may be of considerable value but if the thrombocytopenia is chronic or anticipated to be prolonged, platelets will usually be transfused only to stop actual bleeding because the transfusion of platelets other than those from type-specific compatible donors generally leads to antibody production and decreasing amounts of improvement in the platelet count with successive transfusions. Factor replacements for fibrinogen, factors II, VII, VIII, IX, and X are feasible with currently available concentrates. Multiple factor defects such as in liver disease are more difficult to treat because they may require plasma, fresh plasma, or fresh frozen plasma with its relatively large volume to provide the missing factors. Factor V deficiency, for which no appropriate concentrate is available, is an example of a defect, common in liver disease, for which fresh or fresh frozen plasma is necessary.

Inhibition of a late recrudescence of bleeding such as following dental extraction, which is common in hemophilia, may be minimized by an inhibition of fibrinolysis such as with epsilon-aminocaproic acid (EACA).

Correction of a deficiency of vitamin K-dependent factors induced by vitamin K deficiency or oral anticoagulant treatment with a coumarin derivative is successful with vitamin K administration if liver function is intact or, in urgent circumstances, with blood, plasma, or prothrombin complex (factor IX concentrate).

In uncharacterized or complex urgent bleeding problems, combination therapy with platelets and fresh frozen plasma is often used to cover a maximum of the possible deficiencies.

REFERENCES

Bennett JS: Blood coagulation and coagulation tests. *Med Clin North Am* 1984; 68:557–576. *A good concise review of coagulation and its disorders.*

Coleman RW, Hirsh J, Marder VF, Salzman EW (eds): *Hemeostasis and Thrombosis: Basic Principles and Clinical Practice.* Philadelphia, JB Lippincott Co, 1982. *An excellent multi-author text and reference source that is understandable and clinically satisfactory.*

Fischbach DP, Fagdahs RP: *Coagulation: The Essen-*

tials. Baltimore, Williams & Wilkins Co, 1981. *A basic graphic introduction to the complexities of blood coagulation that is directed at students and nonhematologists; easy to read and understand.*

Sirridge M: Laboratory evaluation of the bleeding patient. *Clin Med* 1984; 4:285–301. *A good review of coagulation tests, with description of the tests and the differential diagnosis.*

Williams WJ, Beutler E, Ersler AJ, Lichtman MA: *Hematology,* ed 3. New York, McGraw-Hill Book Co, 1983. *A multi-author text in general hematology with excellent, lucid chapters on platelets and thrombocytopenias as well as on coagulation defects.*

73   IRON DEFICIENCY ANEMIA

Jaime Pacheco, M.D.
Michael A. Baumann, M.D.

Iron is essential for hemoglobin synthesis and is also present in myoglobin, cytochromes, flavoproteins, and in other enzymes as a cofactor. Iron deficiency is the most common cause of anemia, but the cause of iron deficiency varies with age, sex, geographic, and cultural factors. Iron deficiency anemia is most often caused by chronic blood loss. Occasionally it is caused by malabsorption of iron or in infants by dietary insufficiency. The most common causes of iron deficiency are listed in Table 73–1.

CLINICAL SIGNS AND SYMPTOMS

The initial complaints of most patients are related to the severity of the anemia and do not indicate the cause of the iron deficiency. Fewer than 25% of the patients have symptoms and signs related to the primary illness responsible for the blood loss. Dyspnea on exertion, tachycardia, lightheadedness, and fatigue are related to the severity of the anemia. As body tissues are depleted of iron, the patient develops atrophy in several epithelial tissues. Signs and symptoms of gastrointestinal tract mucous membrane involvement are angular stomatitis and burning, redness, and atrophy of the tongue. Dysphagia is an uncommon complaint related to the development of hypopharyngeal web (Plummer-Vinson syndrome). The hair thins and becomes brittle. Easy splitting of nails is common, and spooning of the nails, or koilonychia, occurs in more advanced cases. Dyspnea, weakness, and fatigue are sometimes out of proportion to the degree of anemia and are perhaps related to depletion of enzyme iron. Splenomegaly may be present.

Up to 50% of patients have the symptom known as pica, a behavioral disorder characterized by compulsive eating of one particular item. Of these, about half eat ice (pagophagia); others eat dirt or clay (geophagia), starch (amylophagia), or other substances. Pica disappears with iron treatment and returns with the same or a different pica when iron deficiency recurs.

The medical history should include queries about prescribed or self-administered drugs because agents such as indomethacin, corticosteroids, and aspirin may cause gastrointestinal bleeding. Inapparent blood loss due to chronic use of aspirin or products containing aspirin (more than 260 preparations with acetylsalicylic acid are on the market) can reach 9 ml of blood a day.

TABLE 73–1.
Causes of Iron Deficiency

NUTRITIONAL CAUSES

Unsupplemented milk diet

INCREASED IRON REQUIREMENTS

Growth
  Infancy
  Pregnancy

MALABSORPTION

Postgastrectomy
Celiac disease

BLOOD LOSS

Gastritis
  Stress
  Alcoholism
  Drugs
Chronic use of aspirin
Peptic ulcer
Hiatal hernia
Inflammatory bowel disease
Gastrointestinal cancer
Hookworm parasitism
Hereditary telangiectasia
Benign tumors of GI tract
Hemorrhoids
Pulmonary hemosiderosis
Genitourinary bleeding
Hemosiderinuria
Paroxysmal nocturnal hemoglobinuria

Iron stores can be depleted by periodic blood donation or by frequent blood samples for laboratory studies. The average blood loss from phlebotomy for diagnostic purposes in hospitalized patients is 15 ml a day. Chronic epistaxis (hereditary telangiectasia) and hemorrhoids are frequently overlooked causes of iron deficiency. Documenting causes of blood loss in anemic patients is facilitated by a detailed history of changes in patterns of bowel movements, changes in stool color, or the presence of blood in the stool. To evaluate occult gastrointestinal (GI) bleeding, a rectal exam must always be performed to avoid falling prey to Sir William Osler's aphorism: "The chief function of the consultant is to make a rectal examination that you have omitted."

Untreated iron deficiency leads to a progressively reduced red cell mass. A hyperdynamic pulse and tachycardia protect temporarily from tissue hypoxia, but eventually the patient develops dyspnea and other signs of high output cardiac failure. Brisk blood loss results in signs of hypovolemia.

PATHOPHYSIOLOGY

A normal Western diet supplies more iron than is required to maintain normal iron metabolism. Because the daily iron loss by desquamation of skin and mucous membranes is only 1 mg a day, and because the body recycles iron from dead red cells, almost the only way an adult can become iron deficient is by bleeding.

Dietary iron is absorbed in the duodenum and proximal jejunum in the form of heme (of animal origin) or ferrous iron. While absorption is facilitated by gastric acid, which keeps iron soluble, phytates and other nonfood substances (pica) may interfere with iron absorption. Normally only 10% of dietary iron is absorbed, but absorption may increase fivefold in an iron-deficient state. In many gastrectomy patients, malabsorption of iron from the diet develops because of rapid transit, lack of gastric acid, and less surface contact with the mucosa of the proximal jejunum.

The absorbed iron is bound and transported by transferrin, a beta globulin, to the normoblasts of the marrow and to the reticuloendothelial system. Normally transferrin is 30% saturated with iron. In patients with uncomplicated iron deficiency, the production of transferrin increases as the level of serum iron decreases. Iron is stored as an intracellular iron protein complex called ferritin. Minute amounts of ferritin can be measured in the serum, and serum values reflect total body iron stores.

Nutritional iron deficiency is the most common cause of anemia in children under 3 years of age who are maintained on a milk diet without iron-fortified foods. In women of child-bearing age, the combination of blood loss through menses and the increased demand for iron during the second and third trimesters of pregnancy often results in iron deficiency. Iron deficiency in men and postmenopausal women always indicates blood loss until proven otherwise.

CLINICAL–PATHOLOGIC CORRELATIONS

Iron deficiency in the hematopoietic tissue results first in anemia followed by microcytosis and hypochromia as heme synthesis is further impaired. Lack of iron in nonhematopoietic tissues leads to depletion of cytochromes, reduced myoglobin concentration in skeletal and heart muscle, and decreased amounts of many enzymes that contain iron. Manifestations of these deficiencies are found in several epithelial tissues. The clinical–pathologic correlations are summarized in Table 73–2.

DIFFERENTIAL DIAGNOSIS

Iron deficiency must be differentiated from other microcytic hypochromic anemias. Red cell indices and morphology may be similar in thalassemia trait and some patients with anemia of chronic illness.

Serum iron levels are low in patients with iron deficiency and with anemia of chronic illness. The serum level of transferrin (iron-binding capacity, IBC) is elevated in two-thirds of the patients with iron deficiency, and normal or low in the remaining third. The IBC is usually low in anemia of chronic illness.

Transferrin saturation [(Iron × 100)/IBC] may be below 16% in both conditions. The values of serum iron levels, IBC, and transferrin saturation do not allow differentiation between iron deficiency and anemia of chronic illness. Ferritin, which better reflects iron stores, is low in iron deficiency and elevated in the anemia of chronic illness in which iron is poorly utilized. Usual values of serum iron levels, IBC, and serum ferritin in several conditions are illustrated in Figure 73–1.

Thalassemia trait occurs in 5% of American blacks and in people of Mediterranean origin. The diagnosis of β-thalassemia trait is established by hemoglobin electrophoresis and quantitation of HbA_2. The diagnosis of α-thalassemia trait is usually made by excluding other causes of hypochromic microcytic anemia. (See Table 73–3 for the differential diagnosis of iron deficiency and thalassemia trait.) A correct diagnosis is critical because iron therapy in anemias other than iron deficiency can be toxic and does not correct the anemia.

TABLE 73–2.
Clinical–Pathologic Correlations for Iron Deficiency

CLINICAL FINDINGS	PATHOLOGIC FINDINGS
HEMATOLOGIC EFFECTS	
Pallor, dyspnea, fatigue, tachycardia	Hypochromic, microcytic anemia due to reduced hemoglobin synthesis
NONHEMATOLOGIC EFFECTS	
Glossitis, stomatitis, koilonychia, brittle hair	Tissue iron deficiency
Sideropenic dysphagia (Plummer-Vinson syndrome)	Web formation in the hypopharynx due to inflammation
Pica	Mechanism unknown
Fatigue, dyspnea	Depletion of iron enzyme

TABLE 73–3.
Differential Diagnosis

PARAMETER	IRON DEFICIENCY	THALASSEMIA TRAIT BETA	THALASSEMIA TRAIT ALPHA
Red cell count	Low	High	High
Reticulocyte count	Low	Normal or elevated	Normal or elevated
Serum iron level	Low	Normal	Normal
Serum ferritin level	Low	Normal	Normal
Hemoglobin A_2 level	Normal or low	Elevated	Normal
Hemoglobin F level	Normal	Normal or elevated	Normal

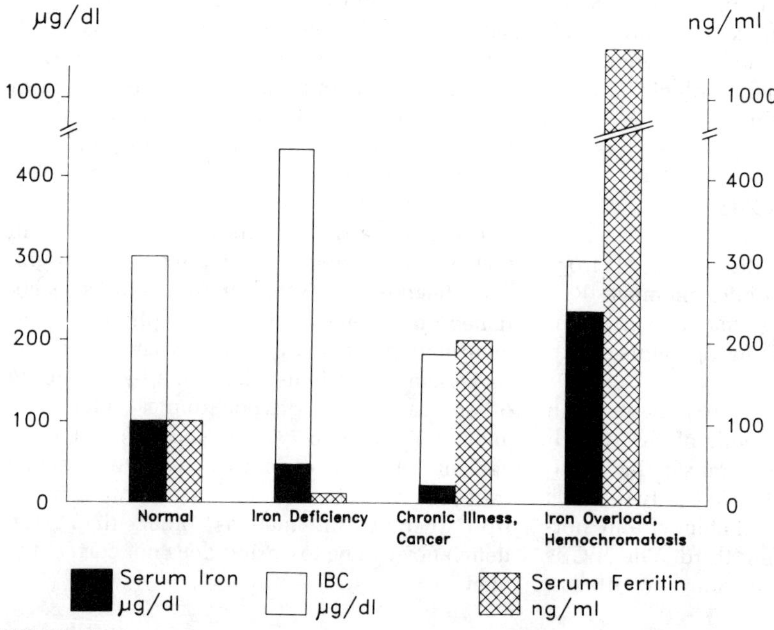

FIG 73–1.
Correlation among serum iron, IBC, and ferritin in several conditions.

DIAGNOSIS

Early in the evolution of iron deficiency, red cell morphology is normal. The first sign of the disease is some degree of anisocytosis with occasional microcytes and a normal hemoglobin content and normal red cell indices. Later the red cells become microcytic (low mean corpuscular volume) and finally hypochromic (low mean corpuscular hemoglobin concentration). Thrombocytosis is a common finding in bleeding patients. Occult blood loss should be considered in patients with unexplained thrombocytosis.

In uncomplicated iron deficiency, the serum iron level is low and the IBC is elevated. Many patients have low IBC values, and those values overlap with those found in patients with anemia of chronic illness. Serum ferritin is perhaps the best indicator of stored iron, and its level is low in iron deficiency. In the interpretation of this measurement, we must remember that several conditions raise its value, including chronic liver disease and hepatitis (release of ferritin from hepatocytes), active Hodgkin's disease, carcinomas, and leukemia (increased synthesis). Thus, a normal serum ferritin level associated with one of these disorders does not exclude iron deficiency.

When the previous tests are inconclusive, a bone marrow aspiration may be needed to evaluate iron stores.

PRINCIPLES OF PREVENTION AND THERAPY

Men, postmenopausal women, and infants require 1 mg of iron a day. Menstruating women require twice that amount. Women in the third trimester of pregnancy need up to 6 mg a day. To absorb these amounts, the amounts of dietary iron should be ten times the figures given.

Iron deficiency is best treated with inexpensive oral iron preparations such as ferrous sulfate or ferrous gluconate. Taking the iron before meals facilitates absorption. To replenish stores, iron therapy should be maintained 12 months beyond the time required to restore normal hemoglobin. Patients with chronic blood loss (hereditary telangiectasia or ulcerative colitis) may require parenteral iron.

REFERENCES

Aisen P: Current concepts in iron metabolism, in Jacobs A (ed): *Clinics in Hematology: Disorders of Iron Metabolism*. Philadelphia, WB Saunders Co, 1982, pp 241–486. *Current multi-author review of the topic.*

Bean WB (ed): *Sir William Ostler Aphorisms*, collected by Robert Bennett Bean. Springfield, IL, Charles C Thomas, 1968.

Crosby WH: Pica: A compulsion caused by iron deficiency. *Br J Haematol* 1976; 34:341–342. *Reviews a common symptom.*

Fairbanks VF, Beutler E: Chapter 33, Iron metabolism; Chapter 49, Iron deficiency, in Williams WJ, Beutler E, Erslev AJ, Lichtman MA (eds): *Hematology*. New York, McGraw-Hill Book Co, 1983, pp 300–310, 466–489. *An up-to-date textbook review.*

Jacobs A, Path FRC, Worwood M: Ferritin in serum. *N Engl J Med* 1975; 292:951–956. *Discusses the metabolism and clinical use of serum ferritin.*

Leonards JR, Levy G, Niemczura R: Gastrointestinal blood loss during prolonged aspirin administration. *N Engl J Med* 1973; 289:1020–1022. *Describes a frequently underestimated cause of blood loss.*

Rowley PT: The diagnosis of beta-thalassemia trait. *Am J Hematol* 1976; 1:129–137. *Reviews several screening methods.*

74   HEMOLYTIC ANEMIAS

Jaime Pacheco, M.D.
Michael A. Baumann, M.D.

The normal life span of an erythrocyte is 120 days. Conditions in which RBC survival is shortened are termed *hemolytic anemias*. A number of different pathophysiologic events are known to result in an early demise of RBCs.

CLINICAL SIGNS AND SYMPTOMS

Fatigue, dyspnea on exertion, and weakness are general symptoms of anemia and are related to the degree of reduction of the red cell mass. Patients with hereditary chronic hemolytic anemia may give a family history of frequent gallbladder surgery, jaundice, or splenectomy. Attention to race and origin will lead to consideration of certain syndromes: sickle cell anemia, hemoglobin (Hb) C in blacks, glucose-6-phosphatase dehydrogenase (G-6-PD) deficiency in blacks and individuals of Mediterranean extraction. The incidence of sickle cell gene among American blacks is 8% and of the HbC trait is 3%. A family history of hemolytic anemia involving members of different sexes and several generations suggests an autosomal dominant inheritance, as in hereditary spherocytosis. In other patients the mechanism of inheritance is a sex-linked pattern, as in G-6-PD deficiency. A detailed history of drug use is essential because certain drugs may result in hemolysis in previously normal individuals (methyldopa) or may precipitate hemolysis in G-6-PD deficient patients (sulfas, quinidine). Additional symptoms may be present depending on the underlying defect, such as painful crises in sickle cell disease, arthritis and serositis in SLE, and lymphadenopathy in lymphoproliferative diseases.

Patients with acute intravascular hemolysis present with abdominal and back pain, dark urine (hemoglobinuria), apprehension, fever, chills, and, in the more severe cases, shock and oliguria.

Mild jaundice is a very common finding in hemolytic anemia, but severe jaundice should arouse suspicion of complicating cholelithiasis or liver disease. Splenomegaly is a constant feature of hereditary spherocytosis and thalassemia. In sickle cell anemia, splenomegaly is found during childhood only, because recurrent thromboses and infarctions eventually result in splenic atrophy. Persistent splenomegaly also occurs in HbSC disease or with homozygous HbC. Some degree of cyanosis is seen in cases of M hemoglobins and hemoglobins with low affinity for oxygen. In hemolytic anemia related to drug exposure or to transfusion mismatch, signs of sudden intravascular hemolysis including hemoglobinuria, back pain, hypotension, oliguria, and acute renal failure may develop.

Patients with severe congenital hemolytic anemia (sickle cell anemia, thalassemia major) may develop prominent maxillary bones, "towering" of the skull, and other bony deformities from the expansion of the bone marrow caused by chronic erythroid hyperplasia. Chronic leg ulcers due to local hypoxia, stasis, and secondary infection are seen in patients with thalassemia major, sickle cell anemia, and hereditary spherocytosis.

Patients with hemolytic anemias and sickle cell anemia may rapidly become ill, requiring hospitalization and transfusions for the aplastic crises resulting from bone marrow suppression by viral infection or folate depletion.

PATHOPHYSIOLOGY

The mechanisms responsible for early death of RBCs can be divided into two categories, intrinsic abnormalities of the red cells and extrinsic mechanisms, and into subcategories, as presented in Table 74–1.

ABNORMALITIES OF THE RED CELL MEMBRANE

In hereditary spherocytosis, the microspherocytes are unable to deform because of a reduced surface area, and they become trapped in the narrow splenic sinusoids and are eventually destroyed. Splenectomy cures the hemolysis, although the primary defect remains. The defective membrane of the RBC allows a faster rate of sodium and water entry into the cells, which demands an accelerated glycolytic catabolism for the function of the sodium–potassium pump. In hereditary elliptocytosis, the primary defect is in spectrin, a membrane protein. Patients with this disease have few symptoms and only a few require splenectomy.

In alcoholic liver disease, the serum hyperlipidemia results in the accumulation of cholesterol and phospholipids in the red cell membrane. This results in membrane redundancy giving the morphologic appearance of a "target" cell. In more severe liver disease a much greater accumulation of cholesterol in the membrane results in "spur cells" with thorny, rigid, nondeformable membranes. These patients have severe hemolytic anemia, and the prognosis is poor because of the severity of the underlying liver disease. Splenectomy is associated with significant morbidity and mortality and is seldom recommended. Transient acquired stomatocytosis associated with alcoholism is a self-limited hemolytic anemia that resolves with abstention from alcohol. Hypersplenism secondary to portal hypertension may complicate any of the hemolytic syndromes due to alcoholic liver disease.

Paroxysmal nocturnal hemoglobinuria is an acquired stem-cell disorder resulting commonly in pancytopenia and rarely in acute nonlymphocytic leukemia. The patients have episodic or chronic intravascular hemolysis due to an abnormal membrane sensitivity to complement. There is also an acetylcholinesterase deficiency in the red cell membrane.

TABLE 74–1.
Pathophysiologic Classification of Hemolytic Anemias

I. Intrinsic abnormalities of the RBCs	
A. Membrane abnormalities	
1. Hereditary:	Hereditary spherocytosis
	Hereditary elliptocytosis
	Hereditary stomatocytosis
	Acanthocytosis
2. Acquired:	Paroxysmal nocturnal hemoglobinuria
	Hemolytic anemias of alcoholism
B. Enzyme deficiencies:	Glucose-6-phosphatase dehydrogenase deficiency
	Pyruvate kinase deficiency
	Other enzyme deficiencies
C. Globin abnormalities	
1. Amino acid substitutions in the globin chains:	Hb S
	Hb C
	Unstable hemoglobins
	Hbs. with low oxygen affinity
2. Abnormal globin synthesis:	Thalassemia syndromes
II. Extrinsic mechanisms	
A. Mechanical hemolysis:	March hemoglobinuria
	Prosthetic valves
	Microangiopathic anemias (thrombotic thrombocytopenic purpura, disseminated intravascular coagulation, hemolytic uremic syndrome, malignant hypertension)
B. Physical or chemical toxins	
C. Infections (protozoan, bacterial)	
D. Immune hemolysis:	Warm- and cold-reactive antibodies
	Drugs
	Alloimmune hemolysis of the newborn
	Incompatible blood
E. Hypersplenism	

ENZYME DEFICIENCIES (METABOLIC ABNORMALITIES)

A variety of enzymatic deficiencies or abnormalities result in hemolytic anemias. The most common among these are discussed here.

Of the more than 150 variants of G-6-PD, the most common are the "A-" type, which predisposes to hemolytic anemia and is present in 10% of American blacks, and the "Mediterranean" type, with an incidence of 15% in the eastern Mediterranean countries. Some variants of G-6-PD function more efficiently than others. In some cases, the deficiency is quantitative. Because G-6-PD deficiency is inherited as a sex-linked recessive trait, clinical illness is much more common in male patients. G-6-PD functions in the aerobic hexose-monophosphate shunt (pentose phosphate pathway) to reduce NADP to NADPH (which augments intracellular antioxidant activity). Hemolysis may be precipitated in these patients by infections, diabetic ketoacidosis, or exposure to oxidant chemicals and drugs (primaquine, sulfamethoxazole, nitrofurantoin, nalidixic acid, naphthalene, phenylhydrazine). Denatured hemoglobin precipitates within the cell (Heinz bodies) resulting in reduced deformability of the RBC and consequent extravascular hemolysis. In the more severe cases hemolysis may be intravascular. Patients of Mediterranean extraction may develop sudden and severe intravascular hemolysis precipitated by exposure to pollen or ingestion of fava beans.

Pyruvate kinase deficiency is the most common enzyme deficiency of the Embden-Meyerhof pathway of anaerobic glycolysis. The transmission is autosomal recessive, and patients have a moderate degree of hemolytic anemia with splenomegaly.

GLOBIN ABNORMALITIES (AMINO ACID SUBSTITUTIONS)

Over 400 hemoglobin variants have been described resulting from amino acid substitutions in globin chains. The more important hemoglobinopathies are due to the substitution of valine or lysine for glutamic acid in the sixth position of the beta globin chain, resulting in Hb S or C, respectively. Patients with sickle cell anemia (homozygous for Hb S) become symptomatic under circumstances that cause deoxygenation of hemoglobin. Deoxygenated Hb S aggregates and persistent or recurrent deoxygenation will result in irreversible distortion of the RBC membrane. The severity of the anemia and symptoms are related to the proportion of irreversibly sickled cells. The heterozygous state, or sickle cell trait (Hb AS), is asymptomatic except for episodes of hematuria and of impaired ability to concentrate urine.

Patients homozygous for Hb C have a mild, chronic hemolytic anemia. The heterozygous state (Hb AC) is asymptomatic.

Other less common substitutions may result in variable hemoglobin instability, expressed clinically as hemolytic anemia of variable severity. In these patients, oxidant drugs may precipitate hemolysis. Certain substitutions reduce hemoglobin affinity for oxygen, resulting in chronic cyanosis.

ABNORMAL GLOBIN SYNTHESIS (THALASSEMIA SYNDROMES)

A molecule of hemoglobin is comprised of heme and four globin chains (two alpha and two beta). In normal persons, synthesis of the globin chain is directed by four genes for the alpha chains and two genes for the beta chains. Deletion of one or more of these genes results in an imbalance of globin chain production. The severity of the defect depends on the number of genes affected. The chains produced in excess (Hb H [β_4] and Hb Bart [γ_4]) precipitate, resulting in intramedullary and splenic hemolysis. The thalassemias are named according to the globin chain whose synthesis is diminished.

Ineffective erythropoiesis and hypochromic anemia are constant features. In patients with the more severe syndromes such as thalassemia major, a chronic erythroid hyperplasia with ex-

pansion of the marrow and even extramedullary hematopoiesis develop.

MECHANICAL HEMOLYSIS

Among the extrinsic mechanisms leading to hemolytic anemia, trauma to erythrocytes can cause the intravascular hemolysis sometimes associated with thrombocytopenia. When this type of hemolytic anemia becomes chronic, the constant hemosiderinuria leads to development of iron deficiency. Red cell fragmentation is seen with some valve prostheses, arteritis, disseminated intravascular coagulation, thrombotic thrombocytopenic purpura, and march hemoglobinuria.

IMMUNE HEMOLYSIS

Immune hemolysis is initiated by the deposition of immunoglobulin on RBC membranes. This usually occurs at 37°C (warm reacting), but some antibodies (primarily IgM) bond to RBCs only at temperatures below 37°C, and thus are called "cold reacting." Complement fixation may follow antibody binding, after which the antibody may or may not remain in the RBC membrane. Red cell destruction occurs primarily in the splenic reticuloendothelial system and is thought to be related to the binding of the RBC associated IgG or C3b to specific surface receptors on macrophages. The RBCs may then be phagocytized, or may have the immunoglobulin "pitted" from the membrane resulting in loss of surface area, forming spherocytes, which are subsequently entrapped and destroyed in the splenic sinusoids. Less commonly, intravascular hemolysis may result from primary complement-mediated lysis.

Immune hemolysis either is associated with a number of lymphoproliferative disorders, autoimmune, and infectious diseases or is idiopathic. Drugs may also induce immune hemolysis either by inducing production of anti-RBC antibodies (methyldopa), by the "drug absorption" mechanism in which the drug acts as a hapten bound to the RBC membrane (penicillin), or by an "innocent bystander" mechanism resulting from the deposition of drug–drug antibody complexes on RBC membranes, which induces the attachment of complement to the RBC and then lysis (sulfa drugs, quinidine).

HYPERSPLENISM

Hypersplenism is a state characterized by splenomegaly, cytopenia of one or more of the blood elements, and reactive hyperplasia in the bone marrow. The blood cells become sequestered in the splenic sinusoids where they are destroyed by the augmented phagocytic function of this organ. The most common cause of hypersplenism is chronic liver disease; less common causes are many primary hematologic diseases and infections.

CLINICAL–PATHOLOGIC CORRELATIONS

The clinical manifestations of hemolytic anemias result from the reduction of the RBC mass, the metabolic stress created by increased RBC turnover, the compensatory efforts of the bone marrow, and several syndromes associated with some hemolytic illness. A summary of the important clinical–pathologic correlations appears in Table 74–2.

DIFFERENTIAL DIAGNOSIS

Anemia and reticulocytosis due to blood loss may simulate hemolytic anemia if blood loss is occult (e.g., bleeding into soft tissues or in the retroperitoneal space). Myoglobinuria is occasionally mistaken for intravascular hemolysis and hemoglobinuria. The history of muscle injury, lack of free hemoglobin in plasma, and specific testing for myoglobin in urine will clarify the diagnosis. Hemolysis is readily distinguished from hypoproliferative anemia by careful search for evidence of early RBC destruction and compensatory erythroid hyperplasia. Such evidence is obtained by a careful history and physical examination, review of peripheral blood smears for morphologic clues, a reticulocyte count, and if necessary an examination of the bone marrow.

DIAGNOSIS

The laboratory diagnosis of hemolytic anemia involves tests to document the destruction of RBCs and the compensatory increased production of RBCs by the marrow. A combination of some of these tests will confirm the clinical impression of hemolysis. Then specific diagnostic studies will reveal the mechanism of hemolysis (e.g., Ham test, G-G-PD, hemoglobin electrophoresis).

Increased catabolism of heme may be reflected in increased values of serum bilirubin, and lactate dehydrogenase, released by the hemolyzed RBCs. Haptoglobin binds free hemoglobin. In hemolysis the level of free haptoglobin will be very low or absent. In patients with intravascular hemolysis, unbound hemoglobin will give the plasma a pink color. As hemoglobin breaks down, it becomes bound to hemopexin and albumin, and the plasma will take on a brown color due to the presence of methemalbumin. Determination of RBC survival with ^{51}Cr to document the short life span

TABLE 74–2.
Clinical–Pathologic Correlations for Hemolytic Anemias

CLINICAL FINDINGS	PATHOLOGIC FINDINGS
Pallor, weakness, tachycardia	Decreased RBC mass
Tower-shaped skull, bony deformities	Chronic expanded erythropoiesis
Jaundice, gallstones	Elevated level of unconjugated bilirubin due to chronic hemolysis
Hypersplenism (single cytopenia or cytopenias)	Splenomegaly due to extravascular hemolysis
Acute back and abdominal pain, chills, fever, oliguria	Acute intravascular hemolysis
Aplastic crises	Folate depletion and/or marrow suppression by viral infection
Iron deficiency	Chronic hemosiderinuria
Megaloblastic anemia	Higher demand of folate due to increased erythropoiesis

of the RBCs is very seldom necessary. Increased RBC production is easily documented by erythroid hyperplasia in the bone marrow and by polychromasia and macrocytosis in the peripheral blood due to the increased number of reticulocytes. The reticulocyte count corrected for the number of RBCs or hematocrit is an excellent index of marrow ability to respond to the destruction of RBCs. Table 74–3 lists the diagnostic tests for hemolysis.

To specifically classify a hemolytic disease, one should start with a careful examination of the peripheral blood smear, looking for the morphologic features of the different hemolytic anemias, and then do some of the specific diagnostic tests. Table 74–4 lists these specific tests and the conditions for which they are indicated.

PRINCIPLES OF PREVENTION AND THERAPY

Hemoglobinopathies are preventable diseases. Prevention can be achieved to some degree by proper education of patients, their families, and the population at risk.

In patients with G-6-PD deficiency, hemolysis precipitated by drugs can be prevented by explaining to the patients which drugs to avoid and which ones are safe. Some patients with unstable hemoglobins also have to avoid oxidant drugs.

Bone deformities, hypersplenism, and most of the symptoms of thalassemia major are suppressed by starting the patient early in life on a chronic program of RBC transfusion. An adverse effect of this treatment is induction of the syndrome of iron overload, a lethal disease in itself. This iatrogenic complication may be delayed by simultaneous chelation of iron as part of the regimen.

Sickle cell crises are treated with hydration, analgesics, and oxygen. Severe cases require exchange transfusion.

Splenectomy will correct the anemia of hereditary spherocytosis (HS) and prevent gallstones and other complications of the disease. In patients with significant hypersplenism, splenectomy can be considered in selected pa-

---

TABLE 74–3.
Laboratory Diagnosis of Hemolytic Anemia

TEST	FINDING
RBC PRODUCTION	
Peripheral blood smears	Polychromasia, macrocytosis
	Reticulocytosis
Corrected reticulocyte count =	
Pt. reticulocyte count × Pt's Hct/Normal Hct	
Bone marrow studies	Erythroid hyperplasia
	Reduced or reversed myeloid-to-erythroid
	(M:E) ratio (normal 3:1)
Iron (^{59}Fe) turnover study	Increased turnover
X-ray films of skull	Skull "hair on end" trabeculation, expansion of
	medullary cavity in other bones
RBC DESTRUCTION	
Hemoglobin level and hematocrit	Low
Unconjugated bilirubin value in serum	High
Urobilogen level in urine and feces	High
Gallstones	Present
Lactic dehydrogenase level in serum	High
Haptoglobin level in serum	Low
Intravascular hemolysis:	
Hemoglobinemia in plasma	Present
Hemoglobinuria in urine	Present
Hemosiderinuria in urine	Present
Methemalbumin in plasma	Present
Haptoglobin level in serum	Low
Hemopexin level in serum	Low
RBC (^{51}Cr) life-span study	Decreased life span
Liver/spleen scan	Splenomegaly

TABLE 74–4.
Specific Diagnostic Tests Used in Classifying Hemolytic Anemias

TEST	CLASSIFICATION
Morphologic studies to diagnose	
Reticulocytes and microspherocytes	Hereditary spherocytosis
	Hemolytic anemia (autoimmune)
Howell-Jolly bodies	Hemolysis
	After splenectomy
Hypochromic cells (decrease Hb synthesis)	Thalassemia
Target cells	Hb C, Hb E
	Liver disease
	After splenectomy
Sickle cells	Hb S
Schistocytes	Mechanical destruction
	Microangiopathic anemia
Stomatocytes	Hereditary stomatocytosis, acquired in alcoholics
Acanthocytes	Abetalipoproteinemia
	Severe liver disease
Crenated cells	Pyruvate kinase deficiency
	Uremia
Heinz bodies	Unstable hemoglobins
	G-6-PD deficiency
Osmotic fragility of RBCs	Hereditary spherocytosis
Low levels of enzyme	G-6-PD
	Pyruvate kinase deficiency
	Other enzyme deficiencies
Positive sickling test	Hb SS, Hb AS, Hb SC, Hb C Harlem, and Hb S Travis
Hemoglobin electrophoresis	
Characteristic quantitation of Hbs	Disorders of Hb synthesis (thalassemia)
Mobility of different Hbs	Amino acid substitutions (Hb S, Hb C, etc.)
Sucrose hemolysis test	Paroxysmal nocturnal hemoglobinuria screening test
Acid hemolysis (Ham) test	Paroxysmal nocturnal hemoglobinuria diagnostic test
Heat and isopropanol denaturation test	Unstable hemoglobins
Direct and indirect Coombs' tests	Immune hemolysis

tients. For patients with hemolytic anemias due to mechanical, toxic, or infectious causes, removal of the underlying cause is the only reasonable approach. Immune hemolysis, if severe, is treated with corticosteroids while the underlying cause is addressed. In refractory idiopathic cases of immune hemolysis particularly, splenectomy is occasionally necessary. Because expanded erythropoiesis increases the need for folic acid, patients with chronic hemolytic anemias should take folic acid.

REFERENCES

Cooper RA: Abnormalities of cell membrane fluidity in the pathogenesis of disease. *N Engl J Med* 1977; 297:371–377. *Composition of the red cell membrane in several conditions.*

Crosby WH: Splenectomy in hematologic disorders. *N Engl J Med* 1972; 286:1252–1254. *Causes and treatment of hypersplenism.*

Nienhuis AW (moderator): Thalassemia major: Molecular and clinical aspects. *Ann Intern Med* 1979; 91:883–897. *Molecular analysis of the disease and recent advances in therapy.*

Prankerd TAJ, Bellingham AJ (ed): Hemolytic anemias. *Clin Haematology* 1975; 4:3–260. *Comprehensive review of this topic.*

Swisher SN (ed): Immune hemolytic anemias. *Semin Hematol* 1976; 13:251–253. *Excellent review of immune-mediated hemolysis.*

Valentine WN, Tanaka KR, Paglia DE: Hemolytic anemias and erythrocyte enzymopathies. *Ann Intern Med* 1985; 103:245–257. *Current review of the more important enzymopathies.*

Weed RI: Hereditary spherocytosis, a review. *Arch Intern Med* 1975; 135:1316–1323. *Physiopathology of HS.*

Wintrobe MM (ed): *Clinical Hematology.* Philadelphia, Lea & Febiger, 1981, pp 734–754. *Textbook review of the manifestations and diagnostic tests of hemolytic anemias.*

75   MEGALOBLASTIC ANEMIA

Jaime Pacheco, M.D.
Michael A. Baumann, M.D.

Vitamin B_{12} and folic acid are essential for DNA synthesis. Deficiency of either results in maturational abnormalities in rapidly proliferating tissues such as bone marrow and the mucosa of the gastrointestinal tract. Because RNA synthesis remains relatively unimpaired, cytoplastic maturation occurs normally while nuclear maturation lags behind (nuclear: cytoplasmic asynchrony), resulting in early cell death and the typical morphologic changes described as "megaloblastic." Although the adult nervous system is not a proliferative tissue, vitamin B_{12} appears to be essential for normal nervous system integrity. Prolongd B_{12} deficiency may lead to demyelination of certain anatomical areas of the spinal cord, resulting in a classic neurologic syndrome. Table 75–1 gives the etiology of B_{12} and folate deficiencies.

CLINICAL SIGNS AND SYMPTOMS

True pernicious anemia (PA) is a disease of the elderly. The median age of patients at presentation is 68 years, with few cases in whites under 40 years of age. Although PA occurs less often in blacks than in whites, 30% of blacks so afflicted are under 40 years of age. Deficiency of vitamin B_{12} due to causes other than PA occurs when the body stores of the vitamin are

depleted over a period of years following cessation of B_{12} absorption.

Regardless of cause, vitamin B_{12} deficiency is often first seen as complaints of fatigue, breathlessness, or weakness. Because anemia develops insidiously, the patient may adapt to severe anemia with few symptoms. Diarrhea or soreness of the tongue reflects damage to the mucosa of the gastrointestinal tract. Paresthesia, unstable gait, or irritability may reflect early neurologic damage.

Folate deficiency is much more common than B_{12} deficiency and usually results from a poor diet. Malnourishment and weight loss are the rule, and alcoholism is common. Up to 40% of patients admitted to hospitals with problems related to alcohol have folate deficiency. In addition to folate depletion, these patients often have iron deficiency anemia due to chronic blood loss, hemolysis, due to portal hypertension with hypersplenism, and direct marrow toxicity of alcohol.

Pallor with a yellow tint to the skin and sclera are due to anemia in combination with hyperbilirubinemia. More than 50% of patients with pernicious anemia have inflammation of the buccal mucosa. A smooth, red tongue is characteristic. A broad gait and abnormal vibratory and positional perceptions are early signs of demyelination of the dorsal columns of the

TABLE 75–1.
Etiology of Megaloblastic Anemias

B_{12} DEFICIENCY	FOLATE DEFICIENCY	OTHER
Inadequate intake (strict vegetarians)	Poor diet (alcoholism)	Inhibitors of purine and pyrimidine metabolism
Pernicious anemia (primary lack of IF)	Hyperalimentation	5-Fluorouracil
Gastrectomy (secondary lack of IF)	Defective absorption	6-Mercaptopurine
	Celiac sprue	6-Thioguanine
Selective malabsorption of B_{12} with proteinuria (Imerslund syndrome)	Whipple's disease	Azathioprine
	Scleroderma	Cytosine arabinoside
	Defective absorption due to drugs	Hydroxyurea
Defective absorption of B_{12}	Dilantin	Inherited metabolic defects
Regional enteritis	Isoniazid	Orotic aciduria
Tuberculosis of the ileum	Cycloserine	
Celiac disease	Phenobarbital	
Sprue	Oral contraceptives	
Consumption of B_{12}	Increased requirements	
By intestinal bacteria	Hemolytic anemia	
Scleroderma	Pregnancy	
Blind loop syndrome	Folic acid antagonists	
Fish tapeworm parasitization	Methotrexate	
Malabsorption due to drugs	Pentamidine	
Colchicine	Triampterene	
Neomycin	Trimethoprim	
PAS		

spinal cord. Patients with more advanced neurologic involvement have ataxia, hyperreflexia, clonus, and a positive Babinski's sign.

Folate deficiency does not have specific physical findings, but because many of these patients are generally malnourished, weight loss and signs of avitaminosis, such as perifollicular petechiae, peripheral neuropathy, and angular stomatitis, are common.

If untreated, deficiency of either vitamin may lead to profound cytopenias of all three blood cell lines, resulting in cardiovascular compromise, bleeding, and severe infection. Some patients with pernicious anemia have only hematologic signs of disease without neurologic involvement, and others have symptoms and signs of progressive neurologic syndrome without megaloblastic anemia. The most common evolution is anemia with some neurologic involvement. Progression of neurologic damage may result in severe loss of proprioception, spastic ataxia, and psychosis known as "megaloblastic madness." Although there are no apparent neurologic manifestations of folate deficiency per se, glove-stocking peripheral neuropathy due to thiamine deficiency is common.

PATHOPHYSIOLOGY

The common pathophysiologic effect of B_{12} and folate deficiency is impairment of DNA synthesis resulting in failure of nuclear maturation and early cell death ("ineffective hematopoiesis"). The bone marrow is hypercellular, but cell death occurs before maturity (intramedullary hemolysis), resulting in an inappropriately low reticulocyte count for the degree of anemia and in erythroid hyperplasia in the bone marrow. All rapidly proliferating tissues are affected, with the mucosa of the GI tract being affected somewhat less severely than the bone marrow.

Deficiency of vitamin B_{12} usually results from impaired absorption. Normal B_{12} absorption requires "intrinsic factor" (IF), produced by gastric parietal cells, to bind dietary B_{12}, the "extrinsic factor." Together they reach the terminal ileum where absorption takes place. Specific receptors in the microvilli receive the IF–B_{12} complex, and the vitamin enters the cell in the presence of Ca^{++}, Mg^{++} and a neutral pH. Damage to or surgical removal of the stomach or terminal ileum impairs absorption. Less commonly, anatomical or physiologic derangement of intestinal function may permit bacterial overgrowth of organisms that compete for dietary B_{12}. Other less common causes are included in Table 75–1.

The syndrome known as pernicious anemia results when gastric parietal cells fail to secrete IF. Achlorhydria also occurs because the parietal cells also cease to produce hydrochloric acid.

The mechanism of parietal cell failure is not completely understood, but some evidence suggests that autoimmune damage is a contributing factor. Serum autoantibodies to parietal cell cytoplasm are found in 90% of patients with PA, and anti-IF antibodies are present in about 50%. These antibodies, however, may be formed as the result of parietal cell injury and may not be the cause of that injury. Many PA patients have serum thyroid autoantibodies, and many patients with Hashimoto's thyroiditis or Graves' disease have anti-parietal cell antibodies.

Though the mechanism of neurologic damage in B_{12} deficiency is not clear, there is some evidence that lack of the B_{12} coenzyme in the metabolic pathway of propionate results in depressed synthesis of the normal fatty acids needed in myelin. This results in methylmalonic acid being present in the blood, cerebrospinal fluid, and urine. Thus quantitation of the methylmalonic acid in the urine is a tool for diagnosing PA.

Although body stores of B_{12} may last for 5 to 6 years after dietary absorption ceases, stores of folate are generally adequate for only a few weeks. Reduction of dietary folate intake is the most common cause of folate deficiency. Dietary folate occurs primarily as a conjugated polyglutamate, which must be degraded by an intestinal enzyme called conjugase before absorption can occur in the proximal small intestine. Diseases that affect the mucosa of the small intestine or drugs such as diphenylhydantoin that inhibit the activity of conjugase may cause clinical folate deficiency secondary to malabsorption (Table 75–1).

CLINICAL–PATHOLOGIC CORRELATIONS

The clinical manifestation of vitamin B_{12} or folate deficiency are the result of impaired DNA synthesis in rapidly proliferating tissues such as the bone marrow and the mucosa of the GI tract. Neurologic symptoms, expressed pathologically as subacute combined degeneration, result only from B_{12} deficiency. The important clinical–pathologic correlations are summarized in Table 75–2.

DIFFERENTIAL DIAGNOSIS

Megaloblastic anemia should be included in the differential diagnosis of a macrocytic anemia, defined by a mean corpuscular volume (MCV) greater than 100 μm^3 (Table 75–3). Examination of the peripheral smear, a reticulocyte count, and a careful history and physical examination will narrow the choices. Patients with severe macrocytosis (MCV > 125 μm^3) al-

TABLE 75–2.
Clinical–Pathologic Correlations in Megaloblastic Anemias

CLINICAL FINDINGS	PATHOLOGIC FINDINGS
Lemon-yellow hue, pallor	Intramedullary hymolytic anemia
Weight loss	Anorexia in pernicious anemia
	Malnutrition in folate deficiency
Red, smooth tongue	Megaloblastosis of the GI tract
Diarrhea	
Abnormal proprioception and vibratory sensation	Degeneration of dorsal columns of the spinal cord
Romberg's sign	
Clonus hyperreflexia	Degeneration of corticospinal tracts
Positive Babinski's sign	
Somnolence, impaired memory	Cerebral degeneration
Psychosis	

TABLE 75–3.
Causes of Macrocytic Indices

Alcoholism without folate deficiency
Liver disease
Reticulocytosis
Megaloblastic anemias
Aplastic anemia
Refractory (myelodysplastic) anemia
Hypothyroidism

most always have megaloblastic anemia. Patients with MCVs between 100 and 115 μm^3 may also have megaloblastic anemia, but other conditions associated with macrocytosis such as those listed in Table 75–3 must be considered. Alcoholism is probably the most common cause of macrocytosis even in the absence of folate or B_{12} deficiency. When PA and thalassemia coexist, macrocytosis may be minimal, making the diagnosis of PA difficult.

DIAGNOSIS

Peripheral blood and bone marrow examinations are essential for the diagnosis of megaloblastic anemia. The peripheral blood smear typically reveals the presence of macro-ovalocytes and hypersegmentation (five or more lobes) of polymorphonuclear leukocytes. Hypersegmentation is quantitated by counting the number of nuclear lobes in 100 neutrophils and dividing by 100. The average number is normally less than 3.42 lobes per cell. In advanced cases, leukopenia or thrombocytopenia may be present. The serum lactate dehydrogenase and unconjugated bilirubin levels are elevated because of intramedullary hemolysis. The values of both tend to be higher in B_{12} deficiency than in folate deficiency.

Examination of bone marrow reveals hypercellularity with a reduced myeloid-to-erythroid (M:E) ratio. Morphologic changes are most striking in the erythroid series with delayed nuclear maturation and the presence of megaloblasts. "Giant" band forms and metamyelocytes may be present in the myeloid series.

Once the diagnosis of megaloblastic anemia is established, serum B_{12} and folate levels are measured to determine the cause (Table 75–4). The finding of a low serum B_{12} level should be followed by a Schilling test when the diagnosis

of pernicious anemia is a possibility. One μg of radiolabeled B_{12} is given by mouth, and a 24-hour urine collection is begun. One milligram of unlabeled B_{12} is given intramuscularly to saturate serum binding sites and thus facilitate excretion of absorbed tagged B_{12}. Patients who malabsorb B_{12} excrete less than 7% of the radiolabeled vitamin in the urine. The test is repeated some days later, this time with a mixture of hog-IF and radiolabeled B_{12}. If B_{12} levels in the urine become normal, the cause of malabsorption is IF deficiency, as occurs in cases of true pernicious anemia or gastrectomy. If B_{12} levels remain low, another cause for malabsorption must be considered (Table 75–1).

The serum folate level is a reflection of the recent nutritional status of the patient and is not necessarily an accurate indication of tissue folate stores. Tissue stores are better estimated by measurement of the red blood cell folate level. Thus, an alcoholic patient with macrocytosis and a low serum folate level is not necessarily suffering from megaloblastosis. Careful review of blood cell morphology and measurement of the red blood cell folate level help to clarify the diagnosis.

PRINCIPLES OF PREVENTION AND TREATMENT

The recommended daily allowance of B_{12} is 5 μg of which 1 μg is absorbed. Liver, seafood, meat, milk, and eggs are rich in B_{12}. Patients with pernicious anemia become deficient in B_{12} on a normal diet because their lack of IF prevents absorption at the terminal ileum. These patients are treated with daily intramuscular injections of vitamin B_{12} for at least 2 weeks to prevent further neurologic damage and to start replenishment of body stores; then monthly injections are given for life. Only about 30 μg of B_{12} can be retained from injections of B_{12}. Patients and their relatives must be informed that discontinuing treatment leads to relapse. Patients who stop treatment develop macrocytosis in about 4 years if their stores have been completely replenished, and anemia in 6 years, as do total gastrectomy patients who do not receive intramuscular vitamin B_{12}.

The recommended daily allowance of folic acid is 0.4 mg. Lemons, melons, and bananas

TABLE 75–4.
Differential Diagnosis of Vitamin B$_{12}$ and Folate Deficiencies

DIAGNOSTIC POINT	VITAMIN B$_{12}$ DEFICIENCY*	FOLATE DEFICIENCY†
Dietary history	Normal diet	Malnutrition
	Little weight loss	Alcoholism
Neurologic signs	Ataxia	May have alcoholic peripheral neuropathy
	Impaired proprioception	
Gastric analysis	Achlorhydria	Normal
Serum folate level	Normal	
	Elevated in 1/3 of patients	< 3 µg/ml
Serum B$_{12}$ level	< 100 pg/ml	Normal
		100–200 µg/ml in 1/3 of patients
Schilling test	Abnormal	Normal

* Normal range of serum vitamin B$_{12}$ concentration: 200–900 pg/ml.
† Normal range of serum folate concentration: 5–19 µg/ml.

are rich in folate, as are spinach, lettuce, broccoli, and asparagus. Other good sources are liver, kidney, and mushrooms. Patients with folate deficiency are treated with oral folic acid, but it is equally important to evaluate the patient's diet and the sociopsychologic circumstances that led to malnutrition or alcoholism. Because of the high prevalence of folate deficiency among alcoholics, prevention could be accomplished by fortifying wine with folic acid. Neither the folic acid nor the wine seems to lose quality by being mixed.

REFERENCES

Beck WS: The megaloblastic anemias, in Williams WJ, Beutler E, Erlev AJ, Lichtman MA (eds): *Hematology.* Minneapolis, McGraw-Hill Book Co, 1983, pp 434–465. *An up-to-date textbook review.*

Carmel R, Johnson CS: Racial patterns in pernicious anemia. *N Engl J Med* 1978; 298:647–650. *Early age at onset and higher prevalence of IF antibodies in blacks.*

Frenkel EP: Abnormal fatty acid metabolism in peripheral nerves of patients with pernicious anemia. *J Clin Invest* 1973; 52:1237–1245. *Physiopathology of neurologic involvement.*

Green R, Kuhl W, Jacobson R et al: Masking of macrocytosis by alpha-thalassemia in blacks with pernicious anemia. *N Engl J Med* 1982; 307:1322–1325. *Thalassemias are prevalent in blacks. Black patients with PA may have a normal MCV.*

Holfbrand AV (ed): Megaloblastic anemia. *Clin Haematol* 1976; 5:471–769. *Recent comprehensive review.*

Kannitz JD, Lindenbaum J: The bioavailability of folic acid added to wine. *Ann Intern Med* 1977; 87:542–545. *Prevention of folate deficiency in alcoholism.*

Kass L: William B. Castle and intrinsic factor. *Ann Intern Med* 1978; 89:983–991. *Excellent chronicle of a fascinating chapter in the history of medicine.*

McPhedran P, Barnes MG, Weinstein JS et al: Interpretation of electronically determined macrocytosis. *Ann Intern Med* 1973; 78:677–683. *Degree of macrocytosis correlated with several conditions.*

Savage D, Lindenbaum J: Relapses after interruption of cyanocobalamin therapy in patients with pernicious anemia. *Am J Med* 1983; 74:765–772. *Recurrence of PA after discontinuation of treatment.*

MYELOPROLIFERATIVE DISEASES

Michael A. Baumann, M.D.
Jaime Pacheco, M.D.

The myeloproliferative disorders are a clinically heterogeneous group of disorders that result from the clonal proliferation of abnormal pluripotent bone marrow stem cells. The clinical manifestations result from the presence of too many or too few cells of one or more hematopoietic cell lines in the peripheral blood and from abnormal hematopoietic cell function or tissue infiltration. There is a tendency for the disorders to overlap or interconvert, and the development of acute leukemia is a common terminal event. Four clinical syndromes are recognized: polycythemia vera (PV), chronic myelogenous leukemia (CML), myelofibrosis with myeloid metaplasia (MMM), and essential thrombocythemia (ET).

CLINICAL SIGNS AND SYMPTOMS

The onset of myeloproliferative disorders is insidious, and it is not unusual for the diagnosis to be first entertained after finding splenomegaly or an abnormal complete blood count (CBC) during the evaluation of an unrelated problem. Clinical symptoms in PV result primarily from circulatory disturbances caused by increased red cell mass and include headache, dizziness, visual disturbances, angina, hemorrhage, and thrombosis or thromboembolism. Abdominal fullness may be a symptom of any of the disorders as a result of splenomegaly. Fatigue or lack of exercise tolerance are common complaints. Pruritis is an occasional symptom, particularly after a warm bath or shower, and is probably related to histamine release from an expanded basophil population. Gout or uric acid stones may develop. Patients having significant thrombocytosis are prone to hemorrhage or thrombosis. Infiltration of the skin or

destructive bone lesions may occur in CML patients and indicate aggressive illness.

At physical examination, plethora with engorgement of the mucous membranes is found in PV patients and in those CML patients with erythrocytosis. The retinal veins may be engorged. Splenomegaly is present in 50% to 75% of patients and is an especially valuable finding for limiting the differential diagnosis of PV. Hepatomegaly is found in 30% to 50% of patients. Lymphadenopathy is uncommon but is occasionally seen in CML patients during the transition to acute leukemia. Pallor is present commensurate with anemia in patients with CML, MMM, and ET. Signs of hypermetabolism may be present and include fever, weight loss, sweating, and gouty arthritis. Skin or soft tissue lesions (chloroma) may be found in a minority of CML patients in whom the disease appears to have an aggressive course. Petechiae and ecchymoses are common in advanced disease states and are related to thrombocytopenia, dysfunctional platelets, or paradoxical bleeding in patients having severe thrombocytosis ($> 1 \times 10^6/\mu l$).

POLYCYTHEMIA VERA

Without treatment, life threatening episodes of major hemorrhage or thrombosis may occur and account for 40% of deaths in PV patients. Mesenteric vein, renal vein, or hepatic vein thromboses are not unusual. Fifteen percent of patients enter a "spent" phase and may develop anemia, marrow fibrosis, and extramedullary hematopoiesis indistinguishable from MMM. Progressive enlargement of the spleen and liver may result in disabling mechanical difficulty or an aggravation of cytopenias by splenic sequestration. Fifteen percent of patients will develop acute leukemia as a terminal event. Although this is clearly treatment-related in most cases, we believe that it is likely a part of the natural history of the disease in a small percentage because a higher-than-expected incidence of acute leukemia has been reported in patients treated only by phlebotomy. The median survival time after diagnosis is 8 to 10 years.

CHRONIC MYELOGENOUS LEUKEMIA

In all untreated patients with CML, acute leukemia will eventually develop if death does not first occur due to intercurrent illness. This transition to acute leukemia appears to be a random event and may happen from weeks to years after the diagnosis of CML. Before the development of frank acute leukemia, many patients experience a brief "accelerated phase" during which systemic symptoms of fatigue, fever, and weight loss become more severe and hepatosplenomegaly becomes more marked. Leukocytosis may become extreme with increasing immaturity, and marked basophilia, severe anemia, and thrombocytopenia may supervene. Death occurs soon after acute transformation occurs and is due chiefly to infection or hemorrhage. The mean survival time after diagnosis of CML is about 3 years.

MYELOFIBROSIS WITH MYELOID METAPLASIA

Without treatment, 80% of newly diagnosed, asymptomatic MMM patients will remain stable for 5 years. The early morbidity of the disease most commonly results from anemia and progressive splenomegaly. Later, progressive failure of the bone marrow interacts to a variable degree with hypersplenism to cause pancytopenia. Acute leukemia develops in 25% of patients. Hemorrhage or infection causes death in 40% of all MMM patients. Cardiovascular complications cause death of most of the remainder.

ESSENTIAL THROMBOCYTHEMIA

Bleeding and thrombosis, both arterial and venous, are the major clinical problems of untreated ET and are aggravated by preexistent degenerative vascular disease in older patients. Eighty percent of treated patients survive 1 year, and 50% survive 5 years.

PATHOPHYSIOLOGY

Myeloproliferative disorders result from the clonal proliferation of an abnormal hematopoietic stem cell. The stem cell involved has been shown to be pluripotent for all three marrow cell lines by such evidence as finding the same chromosomal abnormality (Ph[1]) in all three cell lines in CML and by finding only a single isoenzyme of glucose-6-phosphate dehydrogenase (G-6-PD) in all three marrow cell lines of female G-6-PD heterozygotes with CML, PV, MMM, and ET. There is similar evidence that the stem cell involved in CML is common to the B-lymphoid and the hematopoietic cell lines. This explains the clinical observation that 20% of the acute leukemias developing in CML patients are lymphoblastic by morphologic, immunochemical, and cell-surface marker criteria. These patients have a somewhat improved prognosis because they may respond to relatively nontoxic regimens effective in treating de novo acute lymphocytic leukemia. Interestingly, patients with MMM who have an abnormal karyotype in hematopoietic cell lines have a normal karyotype in marrow fibroblasts, and female G-6-PD heterozygotes with only one isoenzyme in hematopoietic cells are G-6-PD mosaics in marrow fibroblasts. These findings suggest that the marrow fibrosis in MMM is reactive to the myeloproliferation. The recent characterization of a potent fibroblast growth factor elaborated by normal platelets and megakaryocytes supports this idea.

The cause of myeloproliferative disorders is completely unknown, although CML has been associated with exposure to ionizing radiation. The mechanism of the apparent growth advantage of the abnormal clone is also unclear, but may relate to a higher growth fraction (percentage of cells capable of self-renewal) in the abnormal clone or to feedback inhibition of normal hematopoiesis by a humoral substance produced by the autonomously proliferating clone.

CLINICAL–PATHOLOGIC CORRELATIONS

Clinical manifestations in myeloproliferative disorders are the result of too many or too few circulating blood cell elements, dysfunction of abnormal blood cell elements, and tissue infiltration by hematopoietic cells. A summary of the major clinical–pathologic correlations appears in Table 76–1.

DIFFERENTIAL DIAGNOSIS

POLYCYTHEMIA VERA

The chief problem in diagnosing PV is separating PV from secondary forms of erythrocytosis. The most helpful finding on physical examination is palpable splenomegaly, but this will be absent in 25% of cases. Leukocytosis, thrombocytosis, or basophilia suggest PV. Additional important differential features are included in Table 76–2. The rare patient with an abnormal high O_2-affinity hemoglobin may be discerned by measurement of the P_{50} oxygen-hemoglobin dissociation curve. Hepatomas or hypernephromas may occasionally cause erythrocytosis by elaboration of an erythropoietin-like substance.

CHRONIC MYELOGENOUS LEUKEMIA

Careful examination of peripheral blood and bone marrow samples usually permits easy diagnosis, although, because of some morphologic overlap, differentiation from other myelo-

TABLE 76–1.
Clinical–Pathologic Correlations in Myeloproliferative Disorders

CLINICAL FINDINGS	PATHOLOGIC FINDINGS
Plethora, ruddy cyanosis	Erythrocytosis due to autonomous erythropoiesis
Deep venous or intra-abdominal thrombosis, peripheral vascular ischemia, stroke, angina, congestive heart failure	Impairment of circulation due to increased viscosity (Hct $\geq$ 50%) or to thrombosis (increased number of functionally abnormal platelets)
Epistaxis, ecchymosis, GI bleeding, poor hemostasis	Increased number of functionally abnormal platelets (paradoxical bleeding)
Splenomegaly	Extramedullary hematopoiesis or hypertrophy of splenic reticulum
Hyperuricemia, gout, urate stones	High marrow cell turnover with increased nucleic acid breakdown
Pruritis	Histamine release from expanded basophil pool
Anemia, thrombocytopenia, leukopenia	Hypersplenism and bone marrow stem cell depletion (MMM); conversion to acute leukemia
"Tear-drop" RBCs (MMM)	Apparently due to RBC damage in spleen. Removal of spleen reduces number of teardrop RBCs.

TABLE 76–2.
Differential Diagnosis of Polycythemia

LABORATORY STUDY	POLYCYTHEMIA VERA	SECONDARY POLYCYTHEMIA	SPURIOUS POLYCYTHEMIA
Red cell mass	Increased	Increased	Normal
Splenomegaly	Present (in 75% of patients)	Absent	Absent
Arterial O_2 saturation	Normal	Decreased or normal	Normal
Leukocytosis or thrombocytosis	Present	Absent	Absent
Basophil count	Increased	Normal	Normal
Serum B_{12} level and B_{12}-binding capacity	Increased	Normal	Normal
Leukocyte alkaline phosphatase level	Increased	Normal	Normal
Marrow cellularity	Panhyperplasia	Erythroid hyperplasia	Normal
Serum erythropoietin level	Low	High	Normal

TABLE 76–3.
Laboratory Findings in Myeloproliferative Disorders

LABORATORY STUDY	PV	CML	MMM	ET
CBC	Erythrocytosis. May have thrombocytosis (50%),* leukocytosis (66%), basophilia (66%)	Leukocytosis with left shift. May have thrombocytosis (33%) or polycythemia basophilia	Anemia (66%), thrombocytopenia (33%), thrombocytosis (33%), leukopenia (15%), leukocytosis with left shift (30%), teardrop RBCs, nucleated RBCs	Thrombocytosis ($> 1 \times 10^6/\mu l$), giant platelets, platelet aggregates, megakaryocyte fragments, anemia due to blood loss (50%), may have leukocytosis
LAP	Increased (70%)	Low	May be increased	Usually normal
Bone marrow	Hypercellular—Three line increase. Reticulin increased (20%)	Hypercellular Myeloid: Erythroid cell ratio increased. Left shift without maturation arrest	Hypocellular (80%), hypercellular (10%), increased reticulin, fibrosis	Hypercellular, marked megakaryocytic hyperplasia, platelet aggregates. May have increased reticulin
Marrow karyotype	Abnormal (26%) Aneuploidy is most common abnormality	Ph[1] (translocation of long arm of chromosome 22 to short arm of 9) (90%)	May be normal. Most common abnormality is trisomy or monosomy of C group.	Majority normal

* Percents are percentages of patients with this finding.

proliferative disorders is occasionally difficult. "Leukemoid" reactions, sometimes seen in severe infection or with neoplasms, can be distinguished by the lack of peripheral blood immaturity beyond an occasional metamyelocyte, the absence of splenomegaly, a normal or high leukocyte alkaline phosphatase (LAP) score, and the absence of the Ph^1 chromosome.

MYELOFIBROSIS WITH MYELOID METAPLASIA

Red blood cell morphology and the degree of marrow fibrosis help in differentiating MMM from CML. The Ph^1 chromosome is absent in MMM. Bone marrow involvement by metastatic carcinoma, by tuberculosis, or by fungal infection may result in a "leukoerythroblastic" peripheral blood picture suggestive of MMM, but examination of adequate bone marrow aspirate and biopsy specimens should be diagnostic.

ESSENTIAL THROMBOCYTHEMIA

Careful examination of peripheral blood and bone marrow samples permits separation of ET from other myeloproliferative disorders (Table 76–3). It is vital that ET be distinguished from secondary thrombocytosis due to iron deficiency, to inflammation, or to carcinoma because platelet counts even greater than $1 \times 10^6/\mu l$ are not usually associated with complications in secondary thrombocytosis. Most patients with secondary thrombocytosis will have platelet counts of less than $1 \times 10^6/\mu l$. The bleeding time and the results of in vitro platelet aggregation studies should be normal in secondary thrombocytosis.

DIAGNOSIS

The peripheral blood and bone marrow findings in the myeloproliferative disorders are summarized in Table 76–3. Hyperuricemia is present in 40% to 60% of patients. Serum vitamin B_{12} levels and B_{12}-binding capacity are increased in many patients with PV and CML.

This results from an increased granulocyte turnover with release of granulocyte transcobalamins I and III, which function as B_{12} carriers. In patients with significant thrombocytosis, "pseudohyperkalemia" may result from release of platelet potassium during clotting. Measurement of the red cell mass and plasma volume will establish whether true polycythemia exists, but will not differentiate PV from secondary erythrocytosis. Measurement of serum erythropoietin levels is fraught with technical difficulty, but values should be low in PV because the erythrocytosis is autonomous.

PRINCIPLES OF THERAPY

Curative therapy does not exist at this time for myeloproliferative disorders with the possible exception of a subgroup of CML patients who may be cured by allogeneic marrow transplantation. In those cases, the best results are in young patients who are still in the chronic phase of the disease. For patients with other myeloproliferative disorders or for CML patients who are not transplantation candidates, treatment is palliative. Patients with PV who have hematocrits above 50% are best treated by periodic phlebotomy. If significant thrombocytosis exists or if phlebotomies are required very frequently, P^{32} may be given. Acute leukemia is a serious complication of treatment and appears to be more frequent with alkylating agents than with P^{32}. Extreme leukocytosis or thrombocytosis in any of the disorders may be treated with alkylating agents or hydroxyurea. Severe cytopenias in MMM may improve following splenectomy if the marrow reserve is adequate.

Although morbidity may be prevented by treatment of myeloproliferative disorders, it is not clear that survival is prolonged. The treatment of acute leukemia developing from a myeloproliferative disorder is very discouraging. Patients with CML in lymphoblastic transformation often respond to treatment, but the responses are usually quite brief.

REFERENCES

Berk PD, Goldberg JD, Silverstein MN et al: Raised incidence of acute leukemia in polycythemia vera associated with chlorambucil therapy. *N Engl J Med* 1981; 304:441–447. *A discussion of the leukemogenic potential of treatment of myeloproliferative disorders.*

Golde DW (moderator): Polycythemia: Mechanisms and management. *Ann Intern Med* 1981; 95:71–87. *Discussion of PV and secondary polycythemia including concepts of pathophysiology and therapeutic principles.*

Goldman JM, Lu DH: New approaches in chronic granulocytic leukemia—Origin, prognosis and treatment. *Semin Hematol* 1982; 14:241–256. *Excellent recent review of CML.*

Jabaily J, Iland HJ, Lazlo et al: Neurologic manifestations of essential thrombocythemia. *Ann Intern Med* 1983; 99:513–518. *Excellent recent clinical review of ET.*

Quesenberry P, Levitt L: Hematopoietic stem cells. *N Engl J Med* 1979; 301:755–760, 819–823, 868–877. *Concise review of hematopoietic stem cells in health and disease.*

Thomas ED: Marrow transplantation for malignant diseases. *J Clin Oncol* 1983; 1:517–531. *Recent overview of progress in marrow transplantation including discussion of recent results in CML.*

Varki A, Lottenberg R, Griffith R, Reinhard E: The syndrome of idiopathic myelofibrosis. A clinicopathologic review with emphasis on the prognostic variables predicting survival. *Medicine* 1983; 62:353–371. *Best recent review of MMM including analysis of prognostic variables in 56 cases.*

77 ACUTE NONLYMPHOCYTIC LEUKEMIA

Michael A. Baumann, M.D.
Jaime Pacheco, M.D.

Acute nonlymphocytic leukemia (ANLL) is a malignant disease of hematopoietic precursor cells and is characterized by replacement of the bone marrow with primitive blast cells and by reduction of normal marrow myeloid, erythroid, and megakaryocytic elements. Severe neutropenia, anemia, and thrombocytopenia result and are responsible for the majority of the clinical manifestations. Blast cells may remain largely confined to the marrow or may be present in peripheral blood or other tissues to various degrees.

CLINICAL SIGNS AND SYMPTOMS

ANLL occurs in all age groups, but the median age range of patients at diagnosis is 62 to 64 years. Patients usually complain of one or more of the symptoms and signs listed in Table 77–1. Early symptoms are usually due to reduction of normal hematologic elements and include fatigue, poor exercise tolerance, dypsnea, palpitations, bleeding into the skin or mucous membranes, and fever and chills with or without symptoms or signs of localized infection. Later symptoms and signs are related to the mechanical and metabolic effects of the increasing tumor cell burden. As many as 25% of patients may have a history of myelodysplasia ("preleukemia") lasting months or years.

The usual physical findings are summarized in Table 77–1. The signs related to peripheral cytopenias predominate, while the signs resulting from tissue infiltration (lymphadenopathy, hepatosplenomegaly, and skin or gingival lesions) occur in less than 25% of patients.

The clinical signs and symptoms may

TABLE 77–1.
Occurrence of Symptoms and Signs in ANLL

SYMPTOM	FREQUENCY (% OF ANLL PATIENTS)	SIGN	FREQUENCY (% OF ANLL PATIENTS)
Fatigue, weakness	80	Pallor	50
Bleeding into skin or mucous membranes	65	Tachycardia	35
Fever/chills	30	Petechiae, ecchymosis	65
Anorexia	20	Weight loss	20
Abdominal fullness	15	Bone tenderness	20
Bone pain	20	Lymphadenopathy	10
Headache	2	Splenomegaly	25
Nausea/vomiting	2	Hepatomegaly	10
Lethargy	2	Gingival hypertrophy	<10
		Skin infiltrates	<10
		Cranial nerve dysfunction	< 2

develop insidiously over a period of weeks to months, or may develop within days. Once diagnosed, untreated patients survive about 8 weeks. Hemorrhage and infection are equally important principal causes of death. Less common complications include cerebral or pulmonary vascular leukostasis when the circulating blast cell count exceeds 150,000/μl, congestive heart failure due to severe anemia, and uric acid nephropathy as a result of increased nucleic acid metabolism due to increased cell "turnover."

PATHOPHYSIOLOGY

ANLL results from the clonal proliferation of an abnormal hematopoietic stem cell. The level of the stem cell involved probably varies from case to case, but a cell pluripotent for all three marrow cell lines is probably involved in many cases (Fig 77–1). Evidence for this has accumulated from morphologic and functional study of myeloid, erythroid, and megakaryocytic cell lines, and more definitively, from karyotypic analysis or glucose-6-phosphodehydrogenase (G-6-PD) marker study of the marrow cell lines of ANLL patients. The morphologic expression of the disease depends on the level of the stem cell affected and the amount of differentiation occurring in the progeny of the abnormal clone. Thus, several variants of ANLL are recognized and are associated with certain clinical features (Table 77–2).

Sensitive techniques can identify karyotypic abnormalities in virtually all ANLL patients, and many patients appear to have coexisting marrow populations of normal and abnormal karyotypes. The abnormal clone becomes dominant not because the cells "divide more quickly" but because the growth fraction, or the percentage of cells capable of self-renewal, is greater in the abnormal population. Suppressed proliferation of normal bone marrow stem cells results. This may be due largely to a "crowding out" effect, or, as in vitro studies have suggested, may be produced by a humoral regulatory factor elaborated by the abnormal clone and capable of suppressing normal hematopoiesis.

Although successful treatment usually results in the return of normal polyclonal hematopoiesis of cells having normal morphology, function, and karyotype, cases have been described in which remission hematopoiesis has been shown to be clonal. Such observations suggest that the development of ANLL may be a multistep process in some cases, with the ascendency of a "preleukemic" clone preceding the development of frank ANLL or even obvious dyshematopoiesis.

The cause of ANLL is unknown. Environmental factors such as radiation or exposure to chemicals such as benzene or alkylating agents are implicated in some cases. Environmental factors may interact with a genetic susceptibility, most obvious in certain congenital disorders like Down's syndrome. RNA viruses are known causes of ANLL in some mammals, but direct evidence does not currently exist for a viral cause of human ANLL. The recent characterization of cellular "oncogenes" provides im-

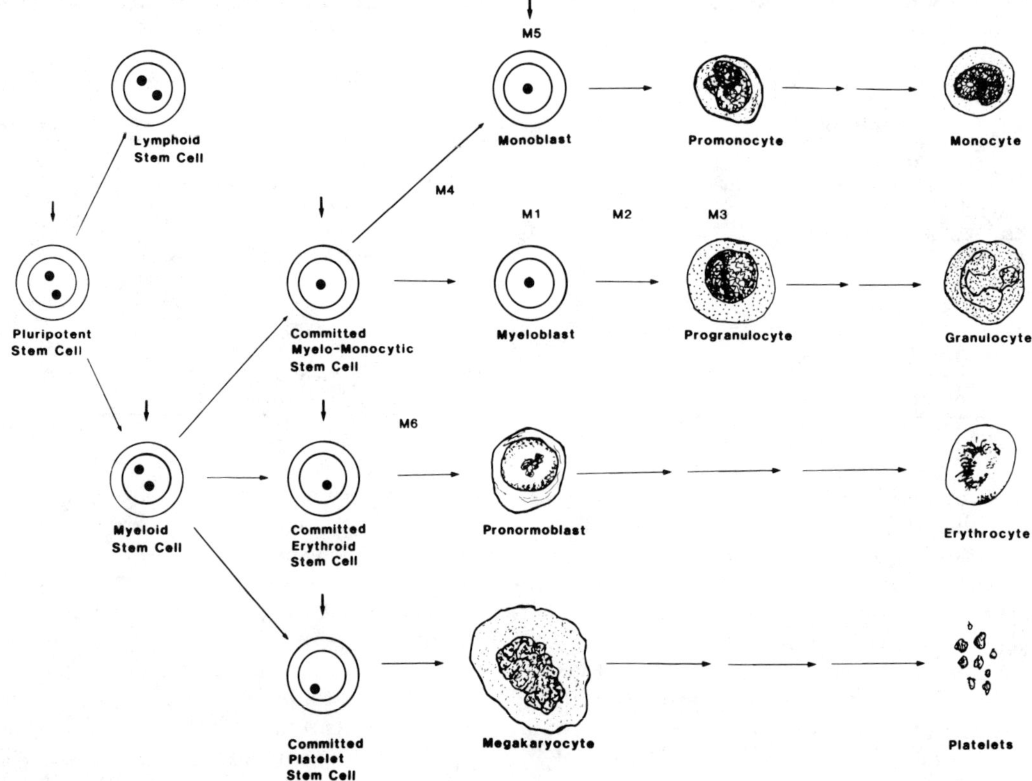

FIG 77–1.
Possible "hit points" for the leukemic transformation of hematopoietic stem cells in ANLL.

portant insight into the mechanism of malignant transformation through the observation that such genetic material may be involved in chromosomal translocations associated with ANLL and other malignancies.

CLINICAL–PATHOLOGIC CORRELATIONS

The clinical features of ANLL result from the reduction of normal hematopoietic elements and the mechanical and metabolic effects of tumor burden. A summary of the major clinical–pathologic correlations is shown in Table 77–3.

DIFFERENTIAL DIAGNOSIS

The diagnosis of acute leukemia is rarely a problem. Confusion with other clinical entities is unlikely if appropriate studies of peripheral blood and bone marrow are done. The major problem lies in distinguishing ANLL from acute lymphocytic leukemia (ALL), and this is often difficult based on morphology alone. The key differentiating features are summarized in Table 77–4. It is occasionally difficult to differentiate ANLL from a more "smoldering" myelodysplastic syndrome. The presence of 30% blast cells in the bone marrow is arbitrarily diagnostic of acute leukemia, but in equivocal cases in short period of observation may be necessary to assess the tempo at which the disease is developing.

DIAGNOSIS

LABORATORY TESTS AND PROCEDURES

About 90% of patients have anemia and thrombocytopenia. About 20% of patients have no or very few circulating blast cells, and another 20% have greater than 15,000 blast cells/μl. Hy-

TABLE 77–2.
French–American–British (FAB) Classification of ANLL

FAB CLASS	COMMON NAME	MORPHOLOGY	HISTOCHEMICAL REACTIONS AND SPECIAL STUDIES	SPECIAL CLINICAL FEATURES
M1	Acute myelocytic leukemia without differentiation	Myeloblasts predominate; distinct nucleoli; few granules	MP*	———
M2	Acute myelocytic leukemia with differentiation	Myeloblasts and promyelocytes predominate; further maturation abnormal	MP	———
M3	Acute promyelocytic leukemia	Promyelocytes predominate; hypergranular	MP	DIC common
M4	Acute myelomonocytic leukemia	Myelocytic and monocytic maturation evident; may be peripheral monocytosis	MP NSE*	Gingival hyperplasia or skin infiltrates
M5a	Acute monocytic leukemia with differentiation	Promonocytes predominate; large, cerebriform nuclei	NSE	Gingival hyperplasia or skin infiltrates
M5b	Acute monoblastic leukemia without differentiation	Undifferentiated blast cells	NSE	
M6	Erythroleukemia	Bizzare, multinucleated megaloblastoid erythroblasts; myeloblasts also present	MP (myeloblasts) PAS* (erythroblasts)	
M7	Acute megakaryoblastic leukemia	Polymorphic, undifferentiated blasts, may have cytoplasmic budding	Electron microscopy for platelet peroxidase; Platelet-associated cell surface markers	Myelofibrosis

* MP = myeloperoxidase, NSE = nonspecific esterase, PAS = periodic acid-Schiff.

TABLE 77–3.
Clinical–Pathologic Correlations in ANLL

CLINICAL FINDINGS	PATHOLOGIC FINDINGS
Fatigue, weakness, pallor, tachycardia	Anemia due to mechanical or humoral suppression of normal erythropoiesis by the leukemic clone
Bleeding into skin, mucous membranes, GI tract, and GU tract	Thrombocytopenia due to mechanical or humoral suppression or normal thrombopoiesis
	Hypofibrinogenemia and clotting factor depletion (DIC) due to release of procoagulants from leukemia cells (M3 variant)
Fever/chills, pneumonia, perirectal abscess, other soft-tissue infection, pharyngitis	Neutropenia due to mechanical or humoral suppression of normal myelopoiesis
Gingival hyperplasia, skin lesions	Leukemic infiltration (M4 and M5 variants)
Bone pain and tenderness	Intramedullary expansion of leukemia
Anorexia, abdominal fullness	Infiltration of abdominal viscera
Headache, nausea/vomiting, cranial nerve dysfunction, lethargy	Meningeal leukemia
	Leukostasis (blast cell count greater than 150,000/μl)

TABLE 77–4.
Differentiation of ANLL from ALL

LEUKOCYTE FEATURES	ANLL	ALL
Auer bodies	10% of patients	0% of patients
Myeloperoxidase	+	−
Sudan black	+	−
Nonspecific esterase	+	−
Myeloid cell-surface antigens	+	−
Lymphoid cell-surface antigens	−	+
TdT (terminal deoxyribonucleotidyl transferase)	< 5% of patients	+
Periodic acid-Schiff	± (may contain fine granules)	+ (large granules or blocks)

peruricemia is present in 36% of cases. Laboratory evidence of disseminated intravascular coagulation (prolonged prothrombin time [PT] and partial thromboplastin time [PTT], depressed serum levels of fibrinogen, and elevated serum levels of fibrin degradation products) is present in 5% of cases, most commonly in cases of the M3 variant.

Examination of bone marrow samples establishes the diagnosis. Stained preparations of bone marrow aspirate are essential for assessing the morphologic, cytochemical, and immunocytochemical characteristics of the leukemic cells. A core biopsy sample is useful for assessing marrow cellularity. In cases where marrow is not aspirable, the core biopsy sample may be used for cytochemical and immunocytochemical analysis.

PRINCIPLES OF THERAPY

Vigorous supportive care is essential for a favorable outcome and includes transfusion of red cells and platelets, treatment of a documented or suspected infection with synergistic broad-spectrum antibiotics, attention to adequate hydration, and correction of hyperuricemia with allopurinol. Patients having laboratory evidence of disseminated intravascular coagulopathy (DIC) or M3 morphology (Table 77–2) are treated with heparin and replacement of coagulation factors as needed. Intensive combination chemotherapy is capable of inducing remission in more than 70% of patients, but initially aggravates the cytopenias.

Following the induction of remission, patients who are under 45 years of age and have an HLA-matched sibling (about 10% of patients) should be considered for allogeneic bone marrow transplantation following high-dose chemotherapy and total-body radiation. About 50% of the patients who receive transplants will be alive and free of leukemia 5 years after treatment, compared with 10% to 20% of the patients who are treated with chemotherapy alone. However, the patients who receive transplants are at higher risk of dying during the first 6 months after treatment because of the transplant-related problems of infection, interstitial pneumonitis, and graft-versus-host disease.

REFERENCES

Appelbaum FR, Dahlberg J, Thomas ED et al: Bone marrow transplantation or chemotherapy after remission induction for adults with acute nonlymphoblastic leukemia. *Ann Intern Med* 1984; 101:581–588. *A recent comparison of modern postremission therapies.*

Foon KA, Gale RP: Controversies in the therapy of acute myelogenous leukemia. *Am J Med* 1982; 72:963–979. *A review of therapeutic options, supportive measures, and prognostic factors.*

Henderson ES: Acute myelogenous leukemia, in Williams WJ, Beutler E, Erslev AJ, Lichtman MA (eds): *Hematology.* New York, McGraw-Hill Book Co, 1983, pp 239–253. *A good, up-to-date general overview.*

Quesenberry P, Levitt L: Hematopoietic stem cells. *N Engl J Med* 1979; 301:755–760, 819–823, 868–877. *Concise review of human hematopoietic stem cells in health and disease.*

78 CHRONIC LYMPHOCYTIC LEUKEMIA

Russell A. Jones, M.D.

Chronic lymphocytic leukemia is a disorder characterized by the accumulation of small lymphocytes in blood, bone marrow, and other tissues. It is almost always a disease of B-lymphocytes as shown by the presence of monoclonal Ig on the cell surface of the involved cells. The disease occurs most commonly in the elderly and may be present in an asymptomatic state for years prior to diagnosis.

CLINICAL SIGNS AND SYMPTOMS

The signs and symptoms noted in the early states of chronic lymphocytic leukemia are outlined in Table 78–1. In early states, the disease is frequently asymptomatic and is detected by routine blood cell counts with white cell differential count. Other less common initial complaints relate to infection such as herpes zoster and pneumonia or worsening of some preexisting medical condition (e.g., chronic obstructive pulmonary disease, angina) usually due to anemia.

As chronic lymphocytic leukemia progresses, the sizes of lymph nodes, spleen, and liver steadily increase. Progressive involvement of the bone marrow results ultimately in pancytopenia. Skin lesions such as leukemia cutis may be seen as may herpes zoster for which the chronic lymphocytic leukemia patient is markedly susceptible. Exaggerated reactions to bee

TABLE 78–1.
Frequency of Symptoms and Signs of Chronic Lymphocytic Leukemia at Diagnosis

SYMPTOM	FREQUENCY (% OF PATIENTS)	SIGN	FREQUENCY (% OF PATIENTS)
No symptoms	25	No signs	25
Vague fatigue, malaise	60	Enlarged lymph nodes	70
Masses (nodes, spleen) noted	40	Enlarged spleen	60
Infection	25	Enlarged liver	50

stings and bug bites may also be seen. Death is usually due to infection or to coexisting medical problems.

PATHOLOGIC MECHANISMS

The pathogenetic mechanisms at work in chronic lymphocytic leukemia are best considered in three categories: the chronic lymphocytic leukemia cell, organ dysfunction due to infiltration by the cells, and the immune protein changes that accompany the disease.

CELL BIOLOGY OF CHRONIC LYMPHOCYTIC LEUKEMIA

The abnormal cell is almost always a B-lymphocyte. There is, in CLL, an increased production of long-lived and short-lived lymphocytes as well as a prolonged survival of the long-lived lymphocytes. Dameshek (1967) described CLL as "an accumulative disease of immunologically incompetent lymphocytes." There is a decrease in the response of these cells to certain substances, called mitogens, demonstrating a lack of normal lymphocyte function (especially B-lymphocyte function). There is also a decrease in gammaglobulin production.

ORGAN DYSFUNCTION

As these lymphocytes accumulate, tissues become filled with them. Lymphocytosis of the blood and marrow progressively develops. This is followed or accompanied by diffuse infiltration of the lymph nodes with small lymphocytes. The spleen, liver, and other tissues such as skin, pleura, and nerves become involved. Usually, organ dysfunction is limited, despite the presence of these cells. For example, the results of liver function tests are characteristi-

cally normal or only slightly abnormal despite hepatomegaly. However, problems, unfortunately, do arise as indicated in Figure 78–1 and Table 78–2.

BIOCHEMICAL CHANGES

Hypogammaglobulinemia is a characteristic development in chronic lymphocytic leukemia. Even more common is an impaired antibody response to antigenic challenge. The IgM level is reduced most severely. All this makes the chronic lymphocytic leukemia patient especially susceptible to certain infections (primarily bacterial). Herpes zoster is also very common in chronic lymphocytic leukemia. Agranulocytosis (especially after treatment) and a possible decrease in cell-mediated immunity also predispose the chronic lymphocytic leukemia patient to infection. Immunosuppressive (corticosteroid) therapy is a definite risk factor for infection.

Monoclonal gammopathies may be observed. Usually these are IgM and at times IgG or IgA. Some of these promote hyperviscosity. Others are rheumatoid (anti-IgG) factor or cryoglobulins.

For some reason, autoantibodies may develop in 20% or more of chronic lymphocytic leukemia patients. Usually these are directed as red cell membrane antigens and are IgG. The "direct" Coombs' test reveals IgG on the red cell membranes. Hemolysis is noted less often (5% of the cases). Autoimmune thrombocytopenia is also noted in chronic lymphocytic leukemia from time to time and is usually demonstrated in the patient by thrombocytopenia resolving after a brief course of corticosteriods. It is always difficult to exclude thrombocytopenia due to marrow replacement or hypersplenism in these patients. They also may coexist.

The clinical features of CLL are correlated

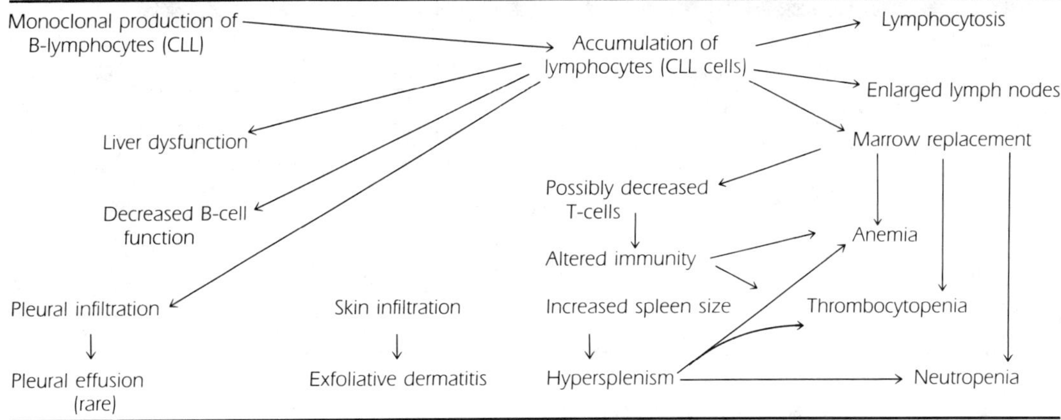

FIG 78–1.
Pathophysiologic correlations in CLL. CLL results when a monoclonal accumulation of certain lymphocytes (CLL cells) causes lymphocytosis of peripheral blood and marrow. Marrow replacement, enlarged lymph nodes and spleen, and infiltration of various organs eventually develop.

with the pathologic aspects in Table 78–3. The interrelationship is further demonstrated in Figure 78–1.

DIFFERENTIAL DIAGNOSIS

The presence in an elderly or middle-aged patient of an elevated absolute lymphocyte count above 15,000 cells/ml (the % lymphocytes in white cell differential count times the white cell count), usually with lymphadenopathy, splenomegaly, and mild nonspecific malaise often leads quickly to the diagnosis of chronic lymphocytic leukemia. It is important to examine the peripheral smear, looking for the characteristic small lymphocytes with scanty cytoplasm, fragmented (smudge) cells, and absent nuclear "immaturity."

The presence of large atypical-looking lymphocytes with cleaved nuclei and prominent nucleoli in the blood smear are more characteristic of lymphosarcoma cell leukemia. The patient with lymphosarcoma cell leukemia has more prominent lymph node enlargements (masses) and a far worse prognosis. A lymph node biopsy is necessary for an accurate diagnosis of this type of lymphoma. In these cases, the lymph node biopsy specimen usually reveals malignant lymphoma of the small cleaved-cell type (follicular) despite the fact that the cells are larger than chronic lymphocytic leukemia cells in the peripheral blood

TABLE 78–2.
Organ Dysfunction in Chronic Lymphocytic Leukemia

Marrow dysfunction
  Anemia
  Thrombocytopenia
  Neutropenia
Lymph nodes
  Local pressure (e.g., on airway)
  Cosmetic deformity
Hypersplenism
Mild hepatic dysfunction
Pleural effusion
Exfoliative dermatitis due to skin infiltration
Very rare
  Chronic lymphocytic leukemia meningitis
  Gastrointestinal involvement
  Significant lung parenchymal involvement
  Epidural mass

smear. Lymphosarcoma cell leukemia is much less common than chronic lymphocytic leukemia.

Acute lymphoblastic leukemia may be confused with chronic lymphocytic leukemia because this acute leukemia may occur in adults although it usually occurs in children. Lymphadenopathy and splenomegaly are features of both diseases as are anemia, thrombocytopenia, and infections. However, acute lymphoblastic leukemia is characterized by lymphoblasts, not "mature" lymphocytes, in the peripheral blood smear. Lymphoblasts have large, immature nuclei with delicate chromatin and one or two

TABLE 78–3.
Clinical–Pathologic Correlations in CLL

CLINICAL FINDINGS	PATHOLOGIC FINDINGS
Anemia, neutropenia, thrombocytopenia	Bone marrow replacement, hypersplenism, therapy-induced hypoplasia of marrow, autoantibodies
Enlarged lymph nodes	Replacement of lymph nodes by CLL cells in diffuse pattern
Infections	Hypogammaglobulinemia, altered lymphocyte function, neutropenia
Miscellaneous (enlarged liver, spleen), pleural effusion, dermatitis	Infiltration of organ by CLL cells

TABLE 78–4.
Differential Diagnosis of Chronic
Lymphocytic Leukemia

Lymphosarcoma cell leukemia
Acute lymphoblastic leukemia
Prolymphocytic leukemia
Hairy cell leukemia
T-cell chronic lymphocytic leukemia
Waldenström's macroglobulinemia
Benign lymphocytosis
Sézary syndrome

nucleoli. The cytoplasm is scanty, and no Auer bodies (=AML) are seen. These cells are present in peripheral blood, lymph nodes, marrow, and spleen and may be differentiated from the abnormal cells in lymphosarcoma cell leukemia and in chronic lymphocytic leukemia.

Prolymphocytic leukemia is characterized by very high counts of white blood cells, mainly large lymphocytes with condensed nuclear chromatin and a single, large, vesicular nucleolus. Lymphadenopathy is not prominent, but massive splenomegaly is regularly seen. Evidence of increased mitotic activity is unusual in tissue sections despite the nuclear immaturity. This disease has a poor prognosis and is resistant to treatments used for chronic lymphocytic leukemia. More aggressive treatment is at times beneficial, so distinguishing it from chronic lymphocytic leukemia is important.

Hairy cell leukemia (leukemic reticuloendotheliosis) is characterized by splenomegaly, pancytopenia, and infections, but usually no lymphadenopathy. The abnormal cells are much larger than chronic lymphocytic leukemia cells and have characteristic fine filamentous projections of cytoplasm ("hairs"). These cells are tartrate-resistant, and in contrast to the cells of chronic lymphocytic leukemia and lymphoma, are acid-phosphatase positive. Treatment options include splenectomy, corticosteroids, and interferon. Cytotoxic chemotherapy has a more limited role and may be detrimental.

Waldenström's macroglobulinemia is usually distinct from chronic lymphocytic leukemia. Waldenström's macroglobulinemia is usually characterized by marrow lymphoplasmacytosis, elevated levels of monoclonal IgM, an enlarged spleen, and evidence of hyperviscosity. A mild lymphocytosis may be present. Conversely, typical chronic lymphocytic leukemia may be associated with an IgM monoclonal protein (chronic lymphocytic leukemia with macroglobulinemia). Thus, the distinctions between the two diseases may be blurred. They are both diseases of monoclonal overproduction by B cells and, in a way, are the same disease manifested differently, as could be said for all the B-cell disorders (such as chronic lymphocytic leukemia, nodular lymphoma, myeloma, Waldenström's macroglobulinemia, hairy cell leukemia).

T-cell chronic lymphocytic leukemia is an extremely rare disease and is mentioned here just to emphasize that point. It may involve the skin and the central nervous system. A new variety has been noted in Japan. Sézary syndrome is erythroderma with T-lymphocytosis at times evolving into lymphoma. It seems to be a malignant disorder of helper T-cells.

Benign lymphocytosis is extremely unusual, but "lymphocytic leukemoid reactions" are described in the older literature, for example, with tuberculosis and carcinomas. Lymphocytosis with pertussis is seen in childhood whereas chronic lymphocytic leukemia is virtually unheard of in patients younger than 40 years.

The differential diagnosis of chronic lymphocytic leukemia can be found in Table 78–4.

DIAGNOSIS

Almost always the diagnosis is made by noting an elevated white blood cell count with increased number of lymphocytes. Lymph nodes are filled with the same abnormal cells in a diffuse manner and may mimic diffuse, well-differentiated lymphocytic lymphoma. Bone marrow examination is usually done but is seldom required for the diagnosis. Diseases which may mimic B-cell CLL include T-cell CLL, lymphosarcoma cell leukemia, hairy cell leukemia, and prolymphocytic leukemia.

Routine blood chemistry values are usually normal with the notable exception of a low globulin level in 20% to 40% of patients. Some patients have a monoclonal gammopathy (frequently IgM).

As the disease progresses, anemia and thrombocytopenia ultimately develop due to bone marrow replacement by leukemic cells and, at times, hypersplenism. They may be seen earlier in the disease than otherwise if an autoimmune red cell or platelet destruction is occurring (autoimmune hemolytic anemia, autoimmune thrombocytopenia). Autoimmune hemolytic anemia is characterized by a positive reaction to a "direct" Coombs' antiglobulin test, reticulocytosis, microspherocytosis, and marrow erythroid hyperplasia.

Lymph node enlargement, spleen enlargement, anemia, thrombocytopenia, and possibly extreme lymphocytosis are of prognostic significance in patients with CLL. A staging system based on these was developed by Rai and co-workers in 1975 (Rai et al., 1975) (see Table 78–5) and has been modified by others to reflect the number of lymphoid sites involved and the degree of lymphocytosis.

In general, these various systems simply reflect the degree of lymphocyte mass and will be used more and more to direct the timing and aggressiveness of treatment. The rapidity of change from one stage to another also influences therapy.

PRINCIPLES OF TREATMENT

There are similarities between the treatment of chronic lymphocytic leukemia and follicular lymphoma. No treatment is given to the asymptomatic patient or the patient with minimal symptoms, stable disease, and in a favorable state.

Patients with symptoms such as weight loss, painful adenopathy, or painful splenomegaly

---

TABLE 78–5.
Rai Staging of Chronic Lymphocytic Leukemia*

SURVIVAL (MONTHS)	STAGE	DESCRIPTION
150+	0	Marrow (> 40%) and peripheral lymphocytosis (> 15,000 cells/ml)
100	I	Lymphocytosis (M, B) (+) LN increased
70	II	(+) Enlarged liver or spleen (with or without enlarged lymph nodes)
20	III	(+) Anemia (excluding AHA) (with or without enlarged lymph nodes, H, S)
20	IV	(+) Thrombocytopenia

* Adapted from Rai KR, Sawitsky A, Cronkite EP, Chanana AD, Levy RN, Pasternak BS: Clinical staging of chronic lymphocytic leukemia. *Blood* 1975; 46:225; Baccarani M, Cand M, Gobbi M, Lauria F, Tura S: Staging of chronic lymphocytic leukemia. *Blood* 1982; **59**:1191–1196.
M = marrow.
B = blood (peripheral blood).
AHA = autoimmune hemolytic anemia.
H = liver.
S = spleen.

are usually treated as are those with rapidly enlarging masses. Autoimmune cytopenias are treated with corticosteroids. Bone marrow replacement with pancytopenia is treated with corticosteroids and cytotoxic drugs (alkylating agents) with treatment started when early compromise is evident but before the marrow is totally packed with malignant cells. Chlorambucil is the alkylating agent usually used, but cyclophosphamide is also used and is less apt to lower the number of platelets. Corticosteroids are used for as short a time as possible (4 weeks or less) because of their complications (infections, compression fractures, and cataracts) except in cases of bone marrow failure. In those cases, corticosteroids are often used longer than would be desirable otherwise because of the difficulty in using only cytotoxic drugs, which have neutropenic and thrombocytopenic side-effects, in cases of bone marrow failure. Corticosteroid therapy lacks these adverse effects. The aim is to use corticosteroids first, and then gradually shift to the cytotoxic drugs.

With therapy, the condition generally improves, but some things do not. Lymphocytosis improves in 75% of patients, whereas lymph nodes decrease in size in 50%, and the spleen decreases in 25%. Usually the hypogammaglobulinemia gets worse, if anything. There may be a gradual improvement in white cell counts. Intermittent infections develop, which are treated as indicated by type of infection. One curious but important factor is the capacity of corticosteroid therapy to often elevate the lymphocyte count even higher in some patients with CLL. This is contrary to a slight reduction of peripheral lymphocytes with corticosteroids in normal subjects.

Combination chemotherapy, including therapy following very aggressive protocols, and total body irradiation are under study for certain stages of chronic lymphocytic leukemia (those with an extremely poor prognosis).

REFERENCES

Boggs DR, Sofferman SA, Wintrobe MM, Cartwright GE: Factors influencing the duration of survival of patients with chronic lymphocytic leukemia. *Am J Med* 1966; 40:243–244. *This classic paper reviews the clinical findings and analyzes the prognostic variables in chronic lymphocytic leukemia.*

Dameshek W: Chronic lymphocytic leukemia—An accumulative disease of immunologically incompetent lymphocytes. *Blood* 1967; 29:566–584. *Another classic paper in which Dr. Dameshek sets out his hypothesis as stated and reviews lymphocyte function as understood at that time.*

Galton DAG, MacLennan ICM: Clinical patterns in B-lymphoid malignancy. *Clin Haematol* 1982; 11:561–587. *A summary of the clonality concept of lymphoproliferative malignancies as well as the humoral immunity problems seen in these diseases (including CLL).*

Rai KR, Sawitsky A, Cronkite EP, Chanana AD, Levy RN, Pasternak BS: Clinical staging of chronic lymphocytic leukemia. *Blood* 1975; 46:219–234. *"Rai staging" has become routine practice in chronic lymphocytic leukemia because the stage has prognostic and therapeutic significance.*

Rozman C, Montserrat E, Finin E et al: Prognosis of chronic lymphocytic leukemia: A multivariate survival analysis of 150 cases. *Blood* 1982; 59:1001–1005. Rai staging was amplified by the addition of the number of lymphoid sites in other work and by attention to the degree of lymphocytosis in this work.*

Sweet DL Jr, Golomb HM, Ultmann JE: Chronic lymphocytic leukemia and its relationship to other lymphoproliferative disorders. *Clin Haematol* 1977; 6:141–157. *Chronic lymphocytic leukemia is compared to and contrasted with Waldenström's macroglobulinemia, hairy cell leukemia, PLL, MM, and other "lymphoproliferative" states on morphologic, immunologic, and clinical grounds.*

Sweet DL Jr, Golomb HM, Ultmann JE: The clinical features of CLL. *Clin Haematol* 1977; 6:185–202. *An excellent pathophysiologic analysis of the clinical features of chronic lymphocytic leukemia as well as an overview of immune phenomena, second malignancies, and therapy in relation to pathophysiology are presented here. The best reference for pathophysiologic descriptions.*

Wiltshaw E: Chemotherapy in chronic lymphocytic leukemia. *Clin Haematol* 1977; 6:223–235. *An overview of chronic lymphocytic leukemia treatment, including present practice and future prospects, is presented.*

79 NON-HODGKIN'S LYMPHOMA

Michael A. Baumann, M.D.
Jaime Pacheco, M.D.

The non-Hodgkin's lymphomas (NHL) are solid cancers of the immune system. Because the immune system comprises a number of cell populations of differing functions and stages of activation, the clinical behavior of non-Hodgkin's lymphoma varies greatly from case to case. Over the past few decades, a number of classification systems have been developed in an attempt to delineate prognostic subgroups of non-Hodgkin's lymphoma. All of these systems have prognostic utility and have facilitated the development and comparison of therapeutic strategies. However, the common use of several differing classification schemes led to a great deal of confusion. An attempted codification of the most useful features of the various systems resulted in the recent, proposed International Working Formulation of Non-Hodgkin's Lymphoma (Table 79–1). An in-depth discussion of the various entities recognized is beyond the scope of this chapter, but general comments will be made about the major prognostic groupings (low, intermediate, and high grade).

CLINICAL SIGNS AND SYMPTOMS

The clinical manifestations of non-Hodgkin's lymphoma are related to the mechanical effects of tumor mass, the metabolic effects of tumor burden, and the impairment of immune system function that results from (or may permit) malignant lymphoproliferation. A summary of the common symptoms and signs of NHL appears in Table 79–2.

The natural history of these diseases varies greatly. Low-grade lymphomas may be indolent and may cause few or no clinical problems for 8 to 10 years or more. High-grade lymphomas are among the most malignant of neoplasms and are fatal within weeks to months if un-

TABLE 79–1.
The International Working Formulation of Non-Hodgkin's Lymphoma

LOW GRADE

A. Small lymphocytic consistent with chronic lymphocytic leukemia
B. Follicular
Predominantly small cleaved cell
   Diffuse areas
   Sclerosis
C. Follicular
Mixed, small cleaved and large cell
   Diffuse areas
   Sclerosis

INTERMEDIATE GRADE

D. Follicular
Predominantly large cell
   Diffuse areas
   Sclerosis
E. Diffuse
Small cleaved cell
   Sclerosis
F. Diffuse
Mixed, small and large cell
   Sclerosis
   Epithelioid cell component
G. Diffuse
Large cell
   Cleaved cell
   Noncleaved cell
   Sclerosis

HIGH GRADE

H. Large cell, immunoblastic
   Plasmacytoid
   Clear cell
   Polymorphous
   Epithelioid cell component
I. Lymphoblastic
   Convoluted cell
   Nonconvoluted cell
J. Small noncleaved cell
   Burkitt's
   Follicular

TABLE 79–2.
Common Symptoms and Signs in Non-Hodgkin's Lymphoma*

SYMPTOM	FREQUENCY (% OF PATIENTS)	SIGN	FREQUENCY (% OF PATIENTS)
Painless adenopathy	66	Lymphadenopathy	75
Painful adenopathy	8	Splenomegaly	30
Anorexia	25	Weight loss	20
Decreased exercise tolerance	25	Hepatomegaly	15
Fever	20	Abdominal mass	15
Night sweats	20	Pallor	10
Abdominal fullness/pain	10	Skin lesions	5
Back pain	10	Superior vena cava syndrome	2
Fatigue	8		
Dysphagia	5		
Cough	4		
Bone pain	4		
Pruritis	2		

* Data from Lester EP, Ultmann JE: Non-Hodgkin's lymphoma, in Williams WJ, Beutler E, Erslev AJ, Lichtman MA: *Hematology.* New York, McGraw-Hill Book Co, 1983, pp 1035–1056, and from personal experience.

treated. Morbidity and mortality result from interference with normal organ function, either as a result of obstruction by enlarged lymph nodes or by direct tumor infiltration. In addition, death may result from infection in the setting of the immunosuppression often associated with malignant lymphoma. Both humoral and cell-mediated immunity may be impaired, and resultant infections may be opportunistic and unusual.

PATHOPHYSIOLOGY

Clinical malignant lymphoma results from a monoclonal proliferation of lymphocytes. The structure and function of the immune system are complex, and so expression of disease is diverse and depends on the lineage of the cell line involved and the level of differentiation achieved by the abnormal clone. Our current concepts of lymphocyte maturation and functional diversity have resulted from correlation of normal and malignant lymphocyte morphology, in vitro culture studies, analysis of cell-surface antigenic determinants, and the recognition of specific genetic rearrangements that occur early in lymphoid maturation. A hypothetical scheme of lymphoid development correlated with corresponding non-Hodgkin's lymphoma subtypes is shown in Figure 79–1. Although 85% of lymphocytes in normal subjects are T-cells, most non-Hodgkin's lymphomas are of B-cell derivation. The reasons for this are unknown.

The cause of monoclonal lymphoproliferation is unknown. The risk of developing lymphoma is greatly increased in patients having congenital or acquired immunodeficiency syndromes or iatrogenic immunosuppression (as with renal transplants). This suggests that lymphoma may be due in some instances to a failure of normal immunoregulatory mechanisms to limit the lymphoproliferative response to antigenic stimulation. A strong association exists between Epstein-Barr viral infection and African Burkitt's lymphoma, and between HTLV-I infection and human adult T-cell leukemia/lymphoma. Survivors of the atomic bomb in Japan are also at a somewhat increased risk of developing non-Hodgkin's lymphoma.

When high-resolution techniques are employed, most non-Hodgkin's lymphoma patients are found to have an abnormal karyotype in the tumor cells. The recent characterization of cellular oncogenes is providing important insight into the relation between karyotypic abnormality and malignant growth. Involvement of such oncogenes in chromosomal translocations [e.g., t(8;14) in Burkitt's lymphoma] may lead to oncogene activation or release from inhibition, resulting in unregulated cell proliferation.

Lymphomas proliferate and disseminate preferentially in the lymphatic system, presumably because of favorable local conditions for lymphocyte-derived cells. Hematogenous metastases do occur (extranodal lymphoma) and are more common in intermediate- and high-

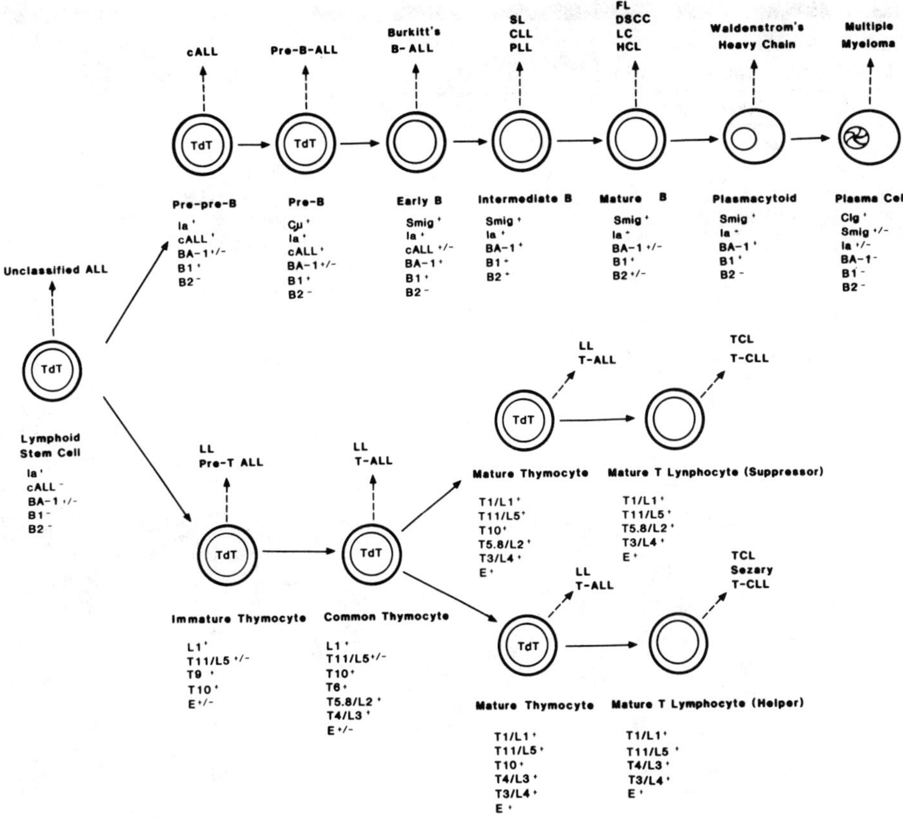

FIG 79–1.
Hypothetical correlation of malignant lymphoma cell-surface phenotype with normal lymphocyte development and maturation. [Modified from Foon KA, Schroff RW, Gale RP: Surface markers on leukemia and lymphoma cells: Recent advances. *Blood* 1982; 60:10. Used by permission.]

grade lymphomas. Central nervous system involvement is uncommon and is most frequently seen in patients with bone marrow involvement. An unusually high incidence of primary CNS large cell lymphoma occurs with immunosuppression after renal transplantation.

Recent long-term studies of low-grade lymphomas suggest that up to two-thirds of patients may eventually have a "transformation" to a higher grade. This may have important implications for subsequent therapy.

CLINICAL–PATHOLOGIC CORRELATIONS

The clinical manifestations of the non-Hodgkin's lymphomas result primarily from the mechanical and metabolic effects of tumor burden. In addition, impairment of immune responses occurs and may be aggravated by treatment, resulting in susceptibility to opportunistic infection. A summary of the important clinical–pathologic correlations appears in Table 79–3.

DIFFERENTIAL DIAGNOSIS

Lymph node enlargement due to malignant lymphoproliferation must be differentiated from reactive lymphadenopathy or other neoplastic illness. Serologic studies may aid in establishing a presumptive diagnosis of infectious mononucleosis, cytomegalovirus infection, or toxoplasmosis. Careful review of a chest roentgenograph or skin testing may suggest the possibility of tuberculosis or histoplasmosis. Persistence of unexplained adenopathy in an adult for longer than 6 weeks is an indication for biopsy. Patients with persistent cervical adenopathy should have a careful examination of the upper aero-digestive tract,

TABLE 79–3.
Clinical–Pathologic Correlations for Non-Hodgkin's Lymphoma

CLINICAL FINDINGS	PATHOLOGIC FINDINGS
Lymphadenopathy/splenomegaly	Expansion of malignant clone in favorable milieu of lymph node and spleen
Extranodal mass lesions	Hematogenous metastases
Fever/night sweats/weight loss	Hypermetabolism related to malignant clonal expansion by uncertain mechanism
Abdominal fullness/pain	Splenomegaly/hepatomegaly, mesenteric nodal involvement, extranodal GI tract involvement
Back pain	Retroperitoneal node enlargement, vertebral body lesions
Anemia/leukopenia/thrombocytopenia	Bone marrow involvement, hypersplenism, autoimmune hemolytic anemia (1.7% of patients)/ thrombocytopenia (1%) resulting from immunoregulatory abnormalities
Dysphagia	Waldeyer's ring adenopathy
Cough, superior vena cava syndrome	Mediastinal adenopathy, lymphangitic parenchymal spread
Opportunistic infection, dissemination of herpes zoster	Impaired cell-mediated and/or humoral immunity, possibly due in part to immunoregulatory reaction to abnormal lymphoproliferation (activation of suppressor cells); immunosuppression due to therapy

including indirect laryngoscopy, to exclude a primary head and neck carcinoma.

The major problems of pathologic diagnosis relate to accurate subclassification of non-Hodgkin's lymphoma. This requires considerable expertise, and often necessitates submission of tissue samples to highly trained and experienced "referee" pathologists. Confusion occasionally arises over whether lymphoproliferation is reactive (benign) or malignant. In such situations, immunologic analysis of lymphocyte cell-surface markers can aid in establishing whether a monoclonal (malignant) proliferation exists. The presence of surface immunoglobulin of uniform heavy and light chain class is strong presumptive evidence for monoclonal B-cell proliferation. Monoclonality cannot be proven by cell-surface analysis of T-cell tumors. Recently developed techniques, allowing the study of gene rearrangements in DNA segments coding for immunoglobulin production (B-cell) or T-cell receptor proteins (T-cell), provide more definitive evidence for monoclonality. Unfortunately, these studies are not widely available.

Anaplastic carcinomas or sarcomas are also occasionally mistaken for lymphomas. Analysis of cell-surface markers, special histochemical staining, or electron microscopy may be necessary to make the distinction.

DIAGNOSIS

The diagnosis of non-Hodgkin's lymphoma requires biopsy of an involved lymph node. Because classification of these diseases (which predicts prognosis) is dependent on morphologic assessment of lymph node architecture, biopsy of other involved tissues is suboptimal for accurate diagnosis.

Following diagnosis, the extent of disease, or stage, must be determined in order to plan therapy rationally. Staging criteria outlined in Table 79–4 are analogous to a scheme originally developed during studies of Hodgkin's disease. A staging evaluation may include a number of the following studies:

1. Complete history and physical examination
2. Complete blood count and serum chemistry studies, including measurement of alkaline phosphatase, uric acid and creatinine levels, and liver function studies
3. Chest roentgenogram
4. Computed tomography of chest and abdomen

TABLE 79–4.
Staging of Non-Hodgkin's Lymphoma

Stage I:	Involvement of a single lymph node region
I$_E$:	Involvement of a single extralymphatic organ or site
Stage II:	Involvement of two or more lymph node regions on the same side of the diaphragm
II$_E$:	Plus localized involvement of an extralymphatic organ or site
Stage III:	Involvement of lymph node regions on both sides of the diaphragm
III$_E$:	Plus localized involvement of an extralymphatic organ or site
III$_S$:	Involvement of the spleen
III$_{SE}$:	Both III$_E$ and III$_S$
Stage IV:	Diffuse or disseminated involvement of one or more extralymphatic organs with or without associated lymph node involvement

Note: The presence of symptoms (unexplained fever, sweats, more than 10% loss of body weight) is indicated by the suffix letter B; the absence of symptoms is indicated by the suffix letter A.

5. Bipedal lymphangiogram
6. Bilateral bone marrow aspiration and biopsy
7. Selected studies (radionuclide bone scan, plain bone films, intravenous pyelogram) depending on clinical symptoms or abnormal screening studies
8. Staging laparotomy

The extent of the staging evaluation depends on the effect of a positive finding on subsequent therapy. For example, because more than 80% of non-Hodgkin's lymphoma patients are found to have at least stage III disease by less aggressive studies, staging laparotomy is seldom indicated.

PRINCIPLES OF THERAPY

The treatment of NHL is guided by knowledge of the histopathologic type and the extent of disease (stage). For most histopathologic types, localized disease (stages I and II) may be treated for cure by radiotherapy. Paradoxically, the low-grade lymphomas are least likely to be localized initially. Because even disseminated low-grade lymphomas may be indolent, therapy may not be necessary until symptoms appear, often years after the diagnosis is established. Symptomatic, disseminated low-grade lymphoma may be effectively palliated with low- or moderate-dose chemotherapy. Attempts to cure these patients through the use of aggressive high-dose chemotherapy have been disappointing because relapse is usual. In contrast, advanced intermediate- and high-grade lymphomas may apparently be cured in up to 50% of patients following aggressive combination chemotherapy. For the remaining 50% who either relapse or fail to achieve a complete remission, the prognosis is poor, although transient second responses may occur after retreatment.

REFERENCES

Fisher RI, DeVita VT, Hubbard SM et al: Diffuse aggressive lymphomas: Increased survival after alternating flexible sequences of ProMACE and MOPP chemotherapy. *Ann Intern Med* 1983; 98:304–3049. *A summary of recent work at the National Cancer Institute suggesting the potential curability of a significant proportion of intermediate- and high-grade lymphomas after intensive therapy.*

Foon KA, Schroff RW, Gale RP: Surface markers on leukemia and lymphoma cells: Recent advances. *Blood* 1982; 60:1–19. *A discussion of recent studies of cell-surface phenotype in non-Hodgkin's lymphoma with hypothetical correlation to normal lymphoid maturation.*

Greene MH: Clinical and environmental predisposing factors, in Berard CW (moderator): A multidisciplinary approach to non-Hodgkin's lymphomas. *Ann Intern Med* 1981; 94:218–235. *A concise discussion of epidemiologic considerations in non-Hodgkin's lymphoma.*

Hait WN, Farber L, Cadman E: Non-Hodgkin's lymphoma for the non-oncologist. *JAMA* 1985; 253: 1431–1435. *A discussion of the interrelationships between the various classification systems with emphasis on the Working Formulation proposal.*

Horning SJ, Rosenberg SA: The natural history of initially untreated low-grade non-Hodgkin's lymphomas. *N Engl J Med* 1984; 311:1471–1475. *An analysis of the results of deferral of therapy for selected patients with low-grade lymphomas, including a discussion of histologic transformation.*

Lester EP, Ultmann JE: Non-Hodgkin's lymphoma, in Williams WJ, Beutler E, Erslev AJ, Lichtman MA: *Hematology.* New York, McGraw-Hill Book Co, 1983, pp 1035–1056. *A recent, comprehensive overview of the non-Hodgkin's lymphomas.*

Waldman TA (moderator): Molecular genetic analysis of human lymphoid neoplasms. *Ann Intern Med* 1985; 102:497–510. *An explanation of recent studies of molecular-level occurrences during early lymphoid development and the relation of cellular oncogenes to malignant proliferation.*

80   HODGKIN'S DISEASE

Russell A. Jones, M.D.

Hodgkin's disease is a malignant condition of unknown cause primarily of lymph nodes and potentially involving multiple sites (such as the liver, lung, spleen, and bone marrow). The characteristic Reed-Sternberg cell is uniformly present but not pathognomonic. Recent studies suggest that Hodgkin's disease begins as a malignant change in interdigitating reticulum cells. Defects in cellular (T-lymphocyte-mediated) immunity, which may have to do with susceptibility to the disease, are seen early in Hodgkin's disease.

CLINICAL SIGNS AND SYMPTOMS

In Hodgkin's disease, the usual patient is asymptomatic. However, various symptoms may be present including fever, weight loss, night sweats, itching, fatigue, and painful adenopathy. In late Hodgkin's disease with failure of therapy, these symptoms are regularly encountered (especially weight loss, fever, and fatigue). An unusual symptom unique to Hodgkin's disease is alcohol-induced pain in areas of nodal involvement.

The physical findings may include lymphad-enopathy (usually present at diagnosis), and hepatosplenomegaly. Jaundice is usually a very late development in Hodgkin's disease. Most patients present with painless, rubbery nodes in the neck, axillary, or iliac-inguinal-femoral regions. Unlike non-Hodgkin's lymphoma, popliteal and epitrochlear lymph nodes are usually not affected.

Late in the disease, multiple problems may develop (Table 80–1). Physical findings may therefore be diverse including jaundice, weakness, sensory loss, pallor, petechiae, organomegaly, ascites, pleural effusion, evidence of infection, and cachexia.

Untreated Hodgkin's disease is uniformly fatal with an average survival of about 1 year from diagnosis for all cases considered together. Important prognostic variables are outlined in Table 80–2.

The outlook and treatment of Hodgkin's disease depends on the "stage." The most commonly used staging classification, a modification of the Ann Arbor modification of the Rye staging system, is outlined in Table 80–3.

Modern treatment has resulted in as many as 86% of all patients being free of disease at 5 years. Even patients with extensive disease may have cure rates of 50% to 60%.

TABLE 80–1.

Complications in Advanced Hodgkin's Disease

1. Jaundice (such as from liver involvement, biliary obstruction due to enlarged nodes)
2. Anergy, immunosuppression, opportunistic infections
3. Hematologic abnormalities
   a. Anemia (decreased production, plus or minus marrow involvement, hypersplenism, rarely significant hemolysis)
   b. Lymphocytopenia (lymphocytosis usually means a wrong diagnosis)
   c. Eosinophilia, monocytosis
4. Spinal cord compression
5. Ivory vertebrae, sclerosis of bones
6. Serous effusions (pleural, pericardial, ascitic)
7. Miscellaneous
   a. Nephrosis
   b. Marrow aplasia
   c. Multifocal leukoencephalopathy

TABLE 80–2.

Prognostic Variables in Hodgkin's Disease

1. Histologic subtype
   a. Lymphocyte predominant (LP) has best prognosis (rare).
   b. Nodular sclerosis (NS) has better prognosis.
   c. Mixed cellularity (MC) has intermediate prognosis.
   d. Lymphocyte depletion (LD) has worse prognosis.
2. Clinical stage
   a. Better prognosis with lower stage
   b. B symptoms equal worse prognosis.
3. Immune competence—better prognosis with preservation of cellular immune mechanisms
4. Better for female patients than for male patients—more nodular sclerosis in females
5. Older age has worse prognosis.
6. Modern treatment has resulted in improved prognosis for all stages of Hodgkin's disease.

TABLE 80–3.

Staging System for Hodgkin's Disease

Stage I:	Involvement of a single lymph node region
I_E:	Single extralymphatic site
Stage II:	Involvement of two or more lymph node regions on the same side of the diaphragm
II_E:	Plus single contiguous extralymphatic site
Stage III:	Involvement of lymph node regions (spleen or lymph node) on both sides of the diaphragm
III_S:	Spleen involved
III_1:	High abdominal nodes only (splenic hilar, celiac porta hepatis nodes)
III_2:	Low abdominal nodes (para-aortic, iliac, mesenteric, or inguinal nodes) with or without spleen or upper abdominal lymph node involvement
Stage IV:	Diffuse or disseminated involvement of one or more extralymphatic organs or tissues (with or without lymph node involvement)

Note: The presence of symptoms (unexplained fever, sweats, more than 10% loss of body weight) is indicated by the suffix letter B; the absence is indicated by the suffix letter A.

DIAGNOSIS

The diagnosis of Hodgkin's disease rests on the light microscopic examination of involved tissue preferably not of inguinal nodes but of cervical, supraclavicular, or axillary nodes.

The presence of the characteristic Reed-Sternberg cell is required for the diagnosis of Hodgkin's disease. Most of the cells present in involved lymph nodes are benign, reactive cells such as eosinophils, lymphocytes, and plasma cells. A variable number of Reed-Sternberg cells are found. Sometimes they are rare, for example, in the lymphocyte predominant subtype. Nodular-sclerosing Hodgkin's disease, characterized by "lacunar cells" and collagen bands, is the most common subtype, whereas lymphocyte predominant and lymphocyte depletion are uncommon. Table 80–4 details the pathologic changes and relative frequencies of the subtypes.

The hematologic manifestations of Hodgkin's disease are outlined in Table 80–1. Early in the disease, however, these tests are normal. Late in the disease, elevated erythrocyte sedimentation rates and serum copper levels have been noted in many patients.

The results of liver function tests such as measurement of alkaline phosphatase, SGOT, and bilirubin may be abnormal even in the absence of hepatic involvement. When the results are abnormal, however, a liver biopsy may be needed prior to therapy if the presence of proven liver involvement would change the planned therapy.

Staging follows diagnosis. Clinical staging (CS) is based on the history, physical examination, chest x-ray film, and the procedures in Table 80–5 up to biopsy. Pathologic staging (PS) includes exploratory laparotomy and splenectomy. Twenty-five percent of patients appear to be CS IV, but over twice that percentage are PS IV, demonstrating the limits of clinical staging in Hodgkin's disease.

Computed tomography (CT scan) of the abdomen is of major use in detecting disease high in the abdomen, whereas the bipedal lymphangiogram is most useful in evaluating the lower abdominal lymph nodes and detecting abnormalities in small lymph nodes. Mesenteric and splenic hilar nodes are not seen in the lymphangiogram, and neither test is diagnostic of Hodgkin's disease specifically. Laparotomy is used to determine the presence or absence of Hodgkin's disease in the abdomen in cases where the therapy would change if Hodgkin's disease is found. Other indications for laparotomy such as removal of the spleen in order to reduce the risks of chemotherapy and the incidence of radiation nephritis, are unproven and possibly erroneous.

TABLE 80–4.

Histopathologic Classification of Hodgkin's Disease*

| CLASSIFYING TERM | | | RELATIVE FREQUENCY |
JACKSON AND PARKER	RYE, 1965	DISTINCTIVE FEATURES	(% OF CASES)
Paragranuloma	Lymphocyte predominance	Abundant stroma of mature lymphocytes and/or histiocytes; no necrosis; Reed-Sternberg cells may be sparse.	10–15
	Nodular sclerosis	Nodules of lymphoid tissue partially or completely separated by bands of doubly refractile collagen of variable width; atypical Reed-Sternberg cells in clear spaces ("lacunae") in the lymphoid nodules	30–70
Granuloma	Mixed cellularity	Usually numerous Reed-Sternberg cells and atypical mononuclear cells with a pleomorphic admixture of plasma cells, eosinophils, lymphocytes, and fibroblasts; foci of necrosis commonly seen	20–40
Sarcoma	Lymphocyte depletion	Reed-Sternberg and malignant mononuclear cells usually, though not always, numerous; marked paucity of lymphocytes; diffuse fibrosis and necrosis may be present.	5–15

* From Rosenberg, SA: Hodgkin's disease, in Holland J, Frei E (eds): *Cancer Medicine*. Philadelphia, Lea & Febiger, 1982. Reproduced with permission.

TABLE 80–5.
Recommended Procedures to Classify Disease Stage

A. Required evaluation procedures
  1. Adequate surgical biopsy specimen, reviewed by a hematopathologist
  2. Detailed history of fever, sweating, pruritus, and weight loss
  3. Complete physical examination with attention to lymphadenopathy, Waldeyer's rings, and liver, spleen, and bone tenderness
  4. Laboratory studies
    a. Complete blood count, platelet count, erythrocyte sedimentation rate, serum alkaline phosphatase level
    b. Evaluation of renal function and liver function
  5. Radiologic studies
    a. Chest radiograph (posteroanterior and lateral views)
    b. Computerized tomographic (CT) scan of abdomen
    c. Bilateral lower-extremity lymphangiogram
  6. Bone marrow biopsy, by needle or open-surgical technique
B. Required evaluation procedures under certain conditions
  1. Whole-chest tomography or CT scan of thorax for suspected intrathoracic disease
  2. IVP, ultrasound, or inferior vena cavagram for equivocal lymphangiogram or abdominal CT scan
  3. Skeletal radiographic survey for areas of bone pain or tenderness
  4. Liver biopsy, by percutaneous needle or open-surgical technique for suspected liver involvement
  5. Laparoscopy
  6. Exploratory laparotomy and splenectomy, if management decisions will depend on the identification of abdominal disease
C. Useful ancillary procedures
  1. Whole-body gallium 67 tomographic scanning
  2. Liver and spleen scan
  3. Bone scan
  4. Estimate of patient's delayed hypersensitivity

The differential diagnosis of Hodgkin's disease is that of lymphadenopathy. Infectious mononucleosis, toxoplasmosis, metastatic carcinoma, and other malignancies of the reticuloendothelial system (NHL) may be confused histologically with Hodgkin's disease as may collagen diseases such as rheumatoid arthritis, polymyositis, or systemic lupus erythematosis. Careful examination of lymph node samples by light microscopy by an experienced hematopathologist should resolve these uncertainties, however. Frequently an involved lymph node resides beside other histologically uninvolved lymph nodes (perhaps also enlarged by a benign process, reactive hyperplasia). Therefore, it is important to remove the most suspicious of the enlarged lymph nodes.

The condition most commonly misdiagnosed as Hodgkin's disease in one study was non-Hodgkin's lymphoma, but other (rare) conditions also were encountered including Lennert's lymphoma and angioimmunoblastic lymphadenopathy. The key problems in differentiating these conditions can be solved by re-examination of the tissue histologically with the light microscope.

PATHOPHYSIOLOGY AND CLINICAL CORRELATIONS

The involved cell (Reed-Sternberg cell) may be a dendritic interdigitating reticulum cell that resides primarily in the thymic-dependent portions of lymphoid tissue. Perhaps in response to a viral agent or other factors, this cell undergoes malignant transformation to the Reed-Sternberg cell. Because this cell is somehow involved in cellular immunity (e.g., antigen processing), a defect in cellular immunity is common early in the disease. Most of the cells present in the diseased lymphoid tissue are inflammatory cells (eosinophils, neutrophils, lymphocytes). Hodgkin's disease tends to spread "in contiguity" from one area to another as opposed to non-Hodgkin's lymphoma where "skip areas" are more common. The spleen has a central role in Hodgkin's disease; involvement of the retroperitoneal nodes or the liver in the absence of splenic disease is unusual. The spleen lacks afferent lymphatics so it must be seeded by hematologic spread of malignant cells or other factors (perhaps a virus) early in the disease in certain situations.

Defects in cellular immunity, such as absent delayed skin-test reactivity (anergy), are common in Hodgkin's disease. Opportunistic infections (herpes zoster and cytomegalovirus infection, tuberculosis, *Pneumocystis carinii* pneumonia, and fungal infections such as candidiasis and cryptococcal meningitis) may be seen. Graft-versus-host disease after blood component therapy may occur but is rare.

Fever is at times due to infection, but commonly is present in Hodgkin's disease without obvious infection. Night sweats result when the elevated temperature drops toward normal. The exact cause of fever in Hodgkin's disease is unclear but may be due to necrosis within large, diseased lymph nodes or other organs with release of pyrogens into the circulation. Similar mechanisms may explain itching (histamine or Kinin release) and weight loss (intermediary unknown). Vascular invasion by the malignant cells has also been mentioned as a cause of fever in Hodgkin's disease. The cause of alcohol-induced pain (in areas of enlarged lymph nodes) is unknown.

Anemia, granulocytopenia, and thrombocytopenia (pancytopenia) are usually present late in the disease. When present they are frequently due to therapy but can be due to bone marrow involvement by the disease, hypersplenism (uncommon) and immune destruction (rare).

Jaundice in Hodgkin's disease is usually due to hepatic involvement by Hodgkin's disease and is usually a very late development. Other causes of jaundice include biliary duct obstruction by enlarged lymph nodes in the porta hepatis, viral hepatitis, and idiopathic cholestasis. Noncaseating granulomas with or without abnormal liver function are found in Hodgkin's disease and are reversible without treatment directed to the liver.

The common clinical features of Hodgkin's disease are correlated with pathologic features in Table 80–6. The pathophysiologic aspects are further demonstrated in Figure 80–1.

PRINCIPLES OF THERAPY

Extended field radiation for cure has been the mainstay of treatment for more localized disease (stages I, II, and IIIA). "B" symptoms (fever, weight loss, or night sweats) most often signal more advanced disease (IIB, IIIB, IVB). Stage IIIA patients receive either very aggressive radiation therapy or chemotherapy (sometimes with radiation to the sites of involvement). The combination of aggressive chemotherapy and total nodal radiation therapy is avoided if possible because of early hematologic toxicity and late sequelae (secondary malignancies, especially acute leukemia). Patients with low abdominal nodal (stage III_2A) disease, large mediastinal masses (mass-to-chest ratio $\geq$ 0.35), and extensive spleen involvement (five or more splenic nodules) are thought by some to need chemotherapy at times with radiation therapy to sites of bulk disease. The best way to combine the two modalities (radiation therapy and chemotherapy) is uncertain and under study.

Palliative therapy is of value in Hodgkin's disease but should obviously be reserved for patients failing all attempts at cure or unable to tolerate aggressive therapy (such as extremely

TABLE 80–6.
Clinical–Pathologic Correlations in Hodgkin's Disease

COMMON CLINICAL FINDINGS	PATHOLOGIC FINDINGS
Asymptomatic patient	Lymphocyte predominant and nodular sclerosis subtypes, low stage
Symptoms of fever, night sweats, and weight loss	Bulky masses, necrosis; mixed cellularity and lymphocyte depletion subtypes
Young patient, typically female, with a mediastinal mass	Nodular sclerosis subtype
Elderly, symptomatic patient with a large retroperitoneal mass	Lymphocyte deletion subtype, advanced stage
Anemia, pancytopenia	Marrow involvement, therapy-related marrow hypoplasia, enlarged spleen (hypersplenism, not common)

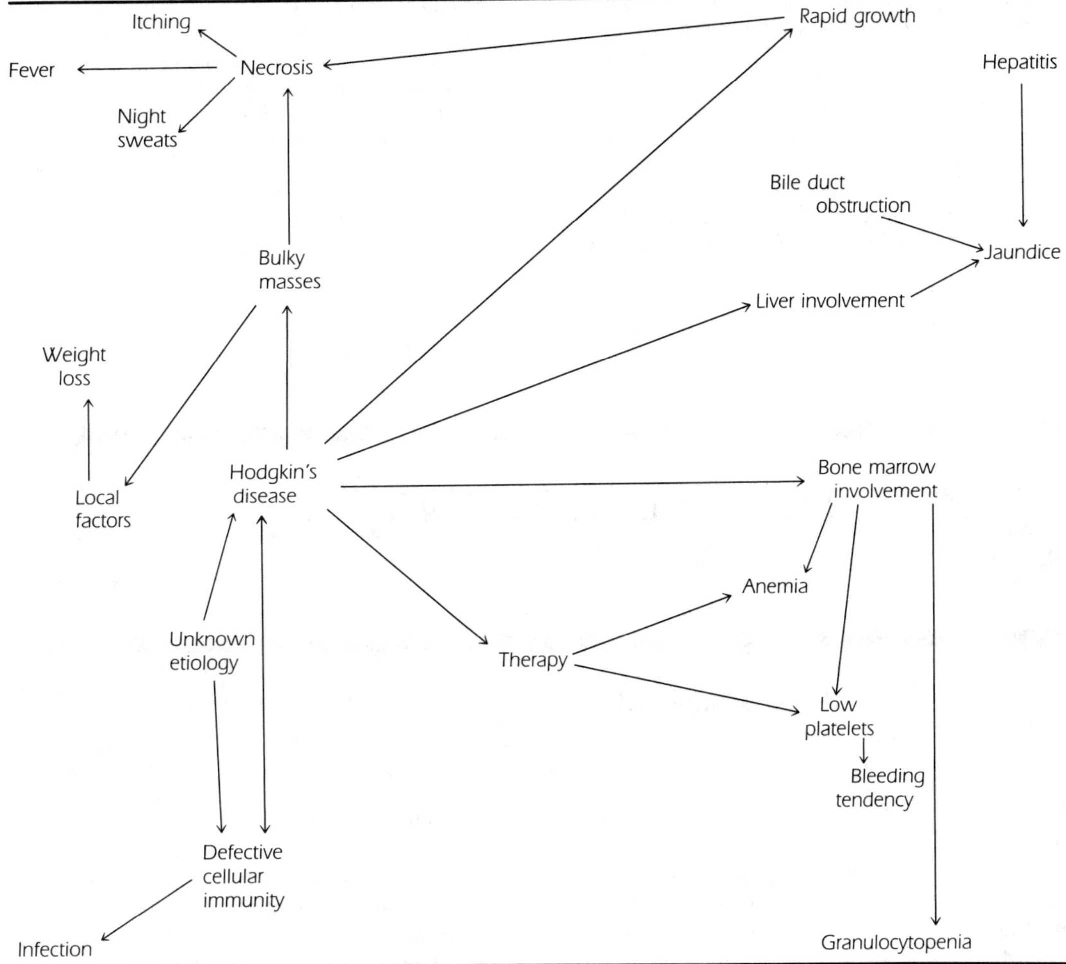

FIG 80–1.
Clinical–pathologic correlations in Hodgkin's disease.

old patients). Even with stage IVB disease, 40% to 60% of patients may have prolonged complete remissions following aggressive chemotherapy. After extensive treatment, relapsing or unresponsive (to chemotherapy) patients may be aided by local radiation to bothersome areas, by corticosteroids (especially helpful to decrease the constitutional symptoms but increases risks of infection) and, at times, by single-agent cytotoxic chemotherapy.

REFERENCES

Coltmann CA (ed): Hodgkin's disease. *Semin Oncol* 1980; 7:91–220. *Introductory remarks and twelve papers dealing with epidemiology, pathology, immunology, staging, treatment, and complications of treatment of Hodgkin's disease.*

Desfornes JF: Hodgkin's disease. *N Engl J Med* 1979; 301:1212–1222. *A review of pathology, epidemiology, genetic factors, immune defects, and management of Hodgkin's disease.*

Kaplan HS: Hodgkin's disease. Cambridge, Harvard

University Press, 1980. *This is the best recent and most complete review of all aspects of Hodgkin's disease.*

Kaplan HS: Hodgkin's disease: Biology, treatment, prognosis. *Blood* 1981; 57:813–822. *This paper focuses on the biology of the malignant cell, the mode of spread of Hodgkin's disease, and the nature of the immunologic defect, treatment, and prognosis of Hodgkin's disease.*

Proceedings of the symposium on contemporary issues in Hodgkin's disease: Biology, staging, and treatment. *Cancer Treat Rep* 1982; 66:601–1055. *An extensive review of developments in Hodgkin's disease (48 papers) with special emphasis on treatment as related to the stage and on the cell of origin of Hodgkin's disease.*

Rosenberg, SA: Hodgkin's disease, in Holland J, Frei E (eds): *Cancer Medicine.* Philadelphia, Lea & Febiger, 1982. *An excellent and concise review of the management of the patient with Hodgkin's disease.*

81 MULTIPLE MYELOMA

Jae C. Chang, M.D.

Multiple myeloma is a relatively common hematologic malignancy characterized by a neoplastic proliferation of plasma cells in the bone marrow and in most instances production by the plasma cells of a monoclonal immunoglobulin or one of its constituent polypeptide chains. Although the disease may begin as a solitary myeloma of bone or soft tissue, it is usually disseminated in the marrow at the time of diagnosis.

CLINICAL SIGNS AND SYMPTOMS

The clinically apparent stage of multiple myeloma is commonly preceded by an asymptomatic period of variable duration. The typical patient usually complains initially of low back pain. The age range of peak incidence is between 50 and 60 years, and both sexes are equally affected.

In the early symptomatic stage of the disease, the common symptoms and signs are related to the infiltration of the bone marrow by neoplastic plasma cells and the subsequent destruction of the bones. These symptoms and signs include weakness, weight loss, anorexia, bone pain, and pallor. As the disease progresses, they become more pronounced.

In the end stage of the disease, the patient becomes debilitated and cachectic as happens with other advanced neoplastic diseases. Intractable bone pain due to progressive bone destruction is often a prominent symptom. Increasing hypercalcemia may produce mental confusion, somnolence, and eventually coma.

There are no characteristic physical findings specific for multiple myeloma. Bone tenderness, especially in the sternum and lumbosacral vertebral bodies, may be present. If anemia is severe, conjuctival pallor can be easily detected. Lymphadenopathy, hepatomegaly, and splenomegaly are uncommon.

Untreated multiple myeloma progresses gradually. Although the initial, asymptomatic state may continue for several months to more than 1 year after the diagnosis, the disease, once symptoms appear, advances rapidly. In untreated patients life expectancy from time of diagnosis is approximately 1.5 years. Over 50%

of patients respond to multidrug chemotherapy. In this group median survival approaches 4 years. Regardless of treatment (whether the patient is treated or not), the terminal stage is manifested by bone marrow failure, destructive bone disease, and renal failure. Death in myeloma is usually caused by serious infections such as bacterial pneumonia and sepsis, which are related in part to decreased production of normal immunoglobulins and immunosuppression from chemotherapy.

PATHOPHYSIOLOGY

The pathophysiologic changes of abnormal plasma cell proliferation and production of abnormal immunoglobulin are hematopoietic suppression, bone destruction, renal disease, hypogammaglobulinemia, and monoclonal gammopathy.

The hallmark of multiple myeloma is infiltration of the marrow by abnormal plasma cells, which in this disease make up more than 20% of the nucleated marrow cells. Bone marrow aspiration samples almost always show typical changes: increased number of plasma cells, often with abnormal morphology; reduction of normal erythroid and granulocytic precursors, and megakaryocytes. As infiltration by the plasma cells progresses, normal hematopoiesis becomes impaired and deficiencies in the formed elements in the peripheral blood occur. Anemia, which is normochromic and normocytic, is common and is an early hematologic change. Neutropenia and thrombocytopenia also eventually develop in the later stages of the disease. Diffuse or localized osteolytic bone destruction occurs around areas of excessive plasma cell growth and produces bone pain as well as bone tenderness.

Plasma cell infiltrates or tumors may develop at extramedullary sites such as the oropharynx, skin, and spinal cord, but these manifestations are clinically uncommon.

Renal disease with progressive renal failure is common in multiple myeloma patients. Hypercalcemia resulting from bone destruction, deposition of "myeloma" protein in the renal tubules, development of amyloidosis, and hyperuricemia, may contribute to the renal failure.

The neoplastic plasma cells usually secrete one of the immunoglobulins, IgG, IgA, IgD, IgE, or one of their constituent polypeptide chains. Therefore, a monoclonal spike is present in the electrophoretic pattern of either the serum or urine proteins except in the rare cases of nonsecretory multiple myeloma. Immunoelectrophoresis identifies the monoclonal immunoglobulin class and usually shows a reduced amount of normal immunoglobulins. A variety of clinical syndromes may result from an accumulation of abnormal proteins in the blood.

CLINICAL–PATHOLOGIC CORRELATIONS

The clinical features of multiple myeloma reflect the result of (1) infiltration of the bone marrow and other organs by neoplastic plasma cells, and (2) production of a monoclonal immunoglobulin. A summary of the major clinical–pathologic correlations is shown in Table 81–1.

DIFFERENTIAL DIAGNOSIS

The diagnosis of multiple myeloma is not difficult when the patient presents with osteolytic bone lesions, a marked increase in plasma cells in the bone marrow, and a monoclonal spike in the electrophoretic patterns of serum or urine proteins. Each of these manifestations may occur in other diseases. Osteolytic bone lesions may be seen in non-Hodgkin's lymphoma (especially histiocytic lymphoma), metastatic cancer, and hyperparathyroidism.

Marrow plasmacytosis may be present in patients with acute and chronic liver disease, Hodgkin's disease, amyloidosis, granulomatous diseases, and certain chronic infections but not usually to the degree seen in myeloma. In these, however, the patients usually have a broad-based, heterogenous, polyclonal gammopathy as shown by serum protein electrophoresis. Monoclonal gammopathy is sometimes seen in diseases other than multiple myeloma, and the differential diagnosis of monoclonal gammopathy is summarized in Table 81–2.

The excretion of a monoclonal protein in urine usually supports the diagnosis of multiple myeloma, but such protein has also been re-

TABLE 81–1.
Clinical–Pathologic Correlations of Multiple Myeloma

CLINICAL FINDINGS	PATHOLOGIC FINDINGS
Anemia Leukopenia Thrombocytopenia Plasma cells in the blood Leukoerythroblastosis	Plasma cell infiltration into the bone marrow
Osteoporosis Osteolytic bone lesions Hypercalcemia	Plasma cell invasion of the bone
Hepatomegaly and splenomegaly Neuropathy and encephalopathy Myelomatous meningitis Lymphadenopathy	Plasma cell infiltration into the tissue or organ
Hyperuricemia	Increased plasma cell turnover rate
Hyperviscosity syndrome Increased sedimentation rate Rouleau formation of red cells Abnormal clotting Amyloidosis Nephrotic syndrome Adult Fanconi's syndrome Renal tubular dysfunction	Monoclonal protein in serum and urine
Increased susceptibility to infection	Hypogammaglobulinemia

ported to be present in benign idiopathic Bence Jones proteinuria, amyloidosis, and Waldenström's macroglobulinemia. Nonsecretory multiple myeloma can be easily distinguished from hypogammaglobulinemia because in multiple myeloma there is plasmacytosis in the marrow and osteolytic bone lesions also may be found.

DIAGNOSIS

The laboratory diagnosis of multiple myeloma is simple. Serum and urine protein electrophoreses are essential first tests (Fig 81–1). A monoclonal spike in the serum or urine suggests a neoplastic proliferation of plasma cells. The next important test is immunoelectrophoresis on the sample of serum or urine which shows a monoclonal spike. The presence of monoclonal IgG, IgA, IgD, IgE, or its constituent polypeptide chain suggests multiple myeloma. If only a light chain is produced by the abnormal plasma cells, the serum protein electrophoresis shows hypogammaglobulinemia, but the urine electrophoresis reveals a

monoclonal spike because the light chains are excreted in the urine. The percentages of multiple myeloma cases manifesting the various immunoglobulin classes are shown in Table 81–3.

The excretion of more than 60 mg of a monoclonal light chain per 24 hours in the urine or a level of monoclonal protein greater than 2 gm/dl in the serum is suggestive of the diagnosis of multiple myeloma. Unlike benign monoclonal gammopathy, multiple myeloma is characterized by a progressively increasing concentration of the monoclonal protein as measured by periodic serum protein electrophoreses.

Anemia may be an initial clinical manifestation calling for an investigation of multiple myeloma. Blood smears often show rouleau formation of red cells if significant amounts of monoclonal protein are present.

Bone marrow aspiration and biopsy are also essential because plasma cells, either mature or immature, are increased to more than 20% of the nucleated marrow cells. Because marrow infiltration by plasma cells is sometimes sporadic, failure to demonstrate plasmacytosis

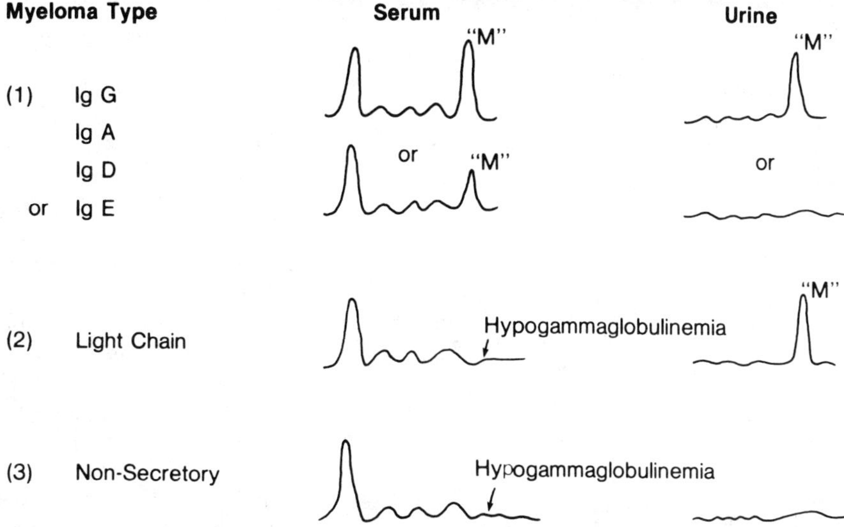

FIG 81–1.
Electrophoretic patterns of serum and urine proteins in multiple myeloma.

TABLE 81–2.
Differential Diagnosis of Monoclonal Gammopathy

DISEASE	CLINICAL–PATHOLOGIC FEATURES
Benign monoclonal gammopathy	"M" protein in serum < 1.5 gm%, stable for years Marrow plasma cells $< 15\%$ Lack of cytopenias Lack of bone destruction Absence of Bence Jones protein
Solitary myeloma	Small "M" spike in serum or urine Marrow plasma cells $< 15\%$ A tumor localized in bone or tissue
Macroglobulinemia	IgM as "M" spike in serum Lymphoid cells in the marrow Lack of bone destruction
Heavy chain disease	"M" spike of one of the heavy chains in serum Lymphadenopathy Splenomegaly
Amyloidosis	Small "M" spike in urine "M" spike as light chain Amyloidosis in tissue biopsy
Skin diseases	Small "M" spike in serum Seen with Papular mucinosis Pyoderma gangrenosum
Lymphoproliferative disorders	Small "M" spike in serum Seen with Chronic lymphocytic leukemia Non-Hodgkin's lymphoma

TABLE 81–3.
Occurrence of Immunoglobulin Classes in Cases of
Multiple Myeloma*

TYPES OF PROTEINS†	PERCENT OF CASES
IgG	50–60
IgA	20–25
IgD	about 1
IgE	<0.01
Light chains only	15–20
Biclonal	0.5–1

* Data from Oken MM: Multiple myeloma. *Med Clin North Am* 1984; 68:757–787; Bergsagel DE: Plasma cell myeloma, in Williams WJ et al (eds): Hematology. New York, McGraw-Hill Book Co, 1983, pp 1078–1104; and personal experience.

† Nonsecretory multiple myeloma occurs in < 1% of cases.

should not preclude the diagnosis of multiple myeloma. To avoid this situation, bone marrow biopsies are recommended in addition to bone marrow aspiration. In immunochemical studies using immunofluorescent staining of bone marrow aspiration samples, the neoplastic plasma cells labeled with a monoclonal protein may be demonstrated.

A bone survey is an important diagnostic test because virtually all patients have either generalized osteoporosis or osteolytic "punched-out" lesions of the axial skeleton (skull, ribs, vertebral bodies, and pelvis) and of the proximal extremities that contain hematopoietically active marrow. The bone lesions are almost always osteolytic without osteoblastic changes. In the early, asymptomatic stage, bone lesions may not be readily appreciated. In the advanced stage, pathologic fractures are frequent, and hypercalcemia is a common complication.

PRINCIPLES OF THERAPY

Important objectives in the management are to relieve symptoms such as fatigue and pain and to prevent complications such as hypercalcemia, pathologic fracture of bones, renal failure, and infections. All patients should be encouraged to remain ambulatory in order to retard demineralization of bones and prevent hypercalcemia. Fluid intake and nutrition must be adequate. Pain can be controlled with analgesics, and anemia should be corrected with blood transfusion.

More definitive treatment is chemotherapy using alkylating agents and adrenal corticosteroids. In the early stage of the disease a number of patients respond well to chemotherapy and enjoy an improved quality of life. Combination chemotherapy of L-phenylalanine mustard and prednisone can achieve response in about 50% of the patients. Other agents such as carmustine, cyclophosphamide, and vincristine also have been found to be effective in combination with adrenal corticosteroids. Remission is accompanied by a reduction of the level of monoclonal protein, which seems to be fairly proportional to the reduction in number of plasma cells. When chemotherapy is effective, the improvement of clinical symptoms may be dramatic, and an objective response such as correction of anemia is often observed.

The response to chemotherapy is usually partial, and the duration of remission is generally limited to about a year or two due to the development of resistance to chemotherapeutic agents. When the disease becomes progressive on one regimen, it tends to be refractory to other regimens, as well. A few patients occasionally achieve complete remission, and these patients seem to have a genuine extension of life span. A distressing observation is the development of acute nonlymphocytic leukemia in some patients with a prolonged remission, especially after treatment with L-phenylalanine mustard. A leukemogenic effect of L-phenylalanine mustard has been suggested.

Severe back pain may be treated with radiation therapy and a back brace. Laminectomy is the treatment of choice for spinal cord compression and should be followed by radiation. Impending fracture or pathologic fracture of long bones should be managed with an intramedullary rod and then with radiation therapy.

Hypercalcemia can be prevented with adequate fluid intake and ambulation and can be treated with hydration, diuretics, adrenal corticosteroids, phosphates, and, if refractory, mithramycin. Hyperuricemia should be prevented and treated with allopurinol.

REFERENCES

Bergsagel DE: Treatment of plasma cell myeloma. *Ann Rev Med* 1979; 30:431–443. *An excellent discussion of the pathophysiologic basis for the chemotherapeutic treatment of multiple myeloma.*

Bergsagel DE: Plasma cell myeloma, in Williams WJ et al (eds): *Hematology.* New York, McGraw-Hill Book Co, 1983, pp 1078–1104. *A recent up-to-date review of multiple myeloma.*

Durie BGM: Staging and kinetics of multiple myeloma. *Clin Haematol* 1982; 11:3–18. *A concise presentation of a proposed staging system of multiple myeloma and of survival data in tables and graphs.*

Kyle RA: Multiple myeloma. Review of 869 cases. *Mayo Clin Proc* 1975; 50:29–40. *A detailed analysis and description of clinical manifestations of multiple myeloma.*

Kyle RA: Monoclonal gammopathy of undetermined significance. Natural history in 241 cases. *Am J Med* 1978; 64:814–826. *An excellent discussion of the significance of monoclonal gammopathy and the natural history of the abnormality.*

Oken MM: Multiple myeloma. *Med Clin North Am* 1984; 68:757–787. *An excellent review of the current understanding of multiple myeloma.*

Endocrine and Metabolic Disorders

82 DIABETES INSIPIDUS

Barry A. Warner, D.O.
James V. Hennessey, M.D.

Diabetes insipidus is a disorder characterized by excessive urination (polyuria). When caused by a complete or partial defect in pituitary synthesis and/or secretion of antidiuretic hormone (ADH, vasopressin), it is termed central diabetes insipidus (vasopressin-sensitive). When it is caused by insensitivity of the renal collecting tubule to the water-permeability modulating effect of ADH, it is termed nephrogenic diabetes insipidus (vasopressin-insensitivity). In either case, there is a failure of the antidiuretic response to water depletion. The most common causes of central diabetes insipidus are neoplasia, trauma, and idiopathic disease (Table 82–1), while most nephrogenic diabetes insipidus is drug-induced (Table 82–2).

CLINICAL SIGNS AND SYMPTOMS

Patients with diabetes insipidus present with polyuria ranging from 2.5 to 40 L/day (normal values are about 1.5 L/day). Unless thirst sensation is also impaired, diabetes insipidus patients will match their voluminous urinary losses with an equivalent intake, thus generating concomitant polydipsia. Although few other symptoms are commonly associated with the disorder, symptoms may be discovered which relate to an underlying disease causing the diabetes insipidus (Tables 82–1 and 82–2). When thirst is impaired or when fluids are unavailable, urine fluid losses can result in life-threatening dehydration. Physical examination may reveal dry mucous membranes, poor skin turgor, reflex tachycardia, decreased intraocular pressure, either supine or orthostatic hypotension, lethargy, weakness, confusion, and occasionally coma. Polyuria may also lead to bladder distention with decreased tone, which may produce associated hydroureter and hydronephrosis.

TABLE 82–1.
Etiology of Central (Vasopressin-Sensitive) Diabetes Insipidus

Idiopathic (30%)*
Neoplastic disease (30%)
  Craniopharyngioma
  Suprasellar cysts
  Metastatic carcinoma
  Leukemia
  Hypothalamic hamartoma
  Lymphoma
  Pinealoma
  Other primary brain tumors
Posttraumatic (30%)
  Postneurosurgical
  Postpartum
  Post-head injury
Autoimmune†
  Antibodies to ADH-synthesizing neurons
  Antibodies to circulating ADH
Cerebral vascular disease†
  Sheehan's syndrome (postpartum necrosis)
  Vasculitis
  Aneurysms
  Sickle cell anemia
Congenital intracranial structural defects†
  Septo-optic dysplasia
  Microcephaly
  Hydrocephaly
Granulomatous disease†
  Histiocytosis X
  Sarcoidosis
  Syphilis
  Tuberculosis
  Wegener's granulomatosis
Hereditary disease†
  Autosomal dominant
  X-linked recessive
  Autosomal recessive
Infection†
  Viral (mumps, encephalitis)
  Bacterial (rheumatic fever)
  Fungal (cryptococcal meningitis)
  Postvaccination
  Guillain-Barré syndrome

* The percents are percentages of all cases of diabetes insipidus.
† These causes together account for about 10% of the cases of diabetes insipidus.

TABLE 82–2.
Etiology of Nephrogenic (Vasopressin-Insensitive) Diabetes Insipidus

Dietary
  Decreased protein intake
  Decreased salt intake
  Primary polydipsia
Electrolytes
  Hypercalcemia
  Hyperphosphaturia
  Hypocalemia
Hereditary
  Sex-linked dominant
Pharmacologic (Most Common)
  Aminoglycosides
  Amphotericin B
  Barbiturates
  Colchicine
  Iodinated contrast agents
  Isophosphamide
  Lithium
  Loop diuretics
  Methicillin
  Methoxyflurane
  Osmotic diuretics
  Propoxyphene
  Saline infusion
  Sulfonylureas
  Tetracyclines
  Vinca alkaloids
Renal disease
  Acute renal failure (diuretic phase)
  Analgesic nephropathy
  Gout
  Hydronephrosis
  Interstitial nephritis
  Medullary cystic disease
  Polycystic kidney disease
  Postobstructive uropathy
  Postrenal transplant
  Pyelonephritis
  Radiation nephritis
  Renal tubular acidosis
Systemic diseases
  Addison's disease
  Amyloidosis
  Cirrhosis
  Diabetes mellitus
  Fanconi's syndrome
  Hypercatabolism (malignancy)
  Hypertension
  Multiple myeloma
  Primary hyperaldosteronism
  Sarcoidosis
  Sickle cell anemia
  Sjögren's syndrome

Diabetes insipidus is transient in some traumatic conditions, especially after neurosurgical procedures in the area of the hypothalamus, pituitary and pituitary stalk, where as many as one-third of the patients develop diabetes insipidus. Permanent diabetes insipidus persists in less than 5% of these patients. In other cases, the degree of polyuria may not be perceived as abnormal, especially if onset occurred in early childhood. When fluid intake matches urine output, the untreated disorder has little consequence other than the associated polyuria and polydipsia.

PATHOPHYSIOLOGY

Homeostatic water balance is rigidly maintained within a plasma osmolar range of 280 to 295 mOsm/kg of water. The osmolality is kept within the range through a feedback system in which water loss stimulates both thirst and ADH release. Appropriate interplay of these mechanisms depends on (1) the integrity of osmoreceptors (sensors of plasma osmolality), (2) an intact supraopticoneurohypophyseal tract (hypothalamic cell bodies that produce ADH with extended axons terminating in the posterior pituitary), (3) a functional hypothalamic thirst center, (4) responsive renal collecting tubules (site of water reabsorption via cyclic AMP-dependent ADH action), and (5) an adequate renal medullary osmotic gradient. Central diabetes insipidus patients have an abnormality of one or more of the first three components, whereas nephrogenic diabetes insipidus patients have a collecting tubule defect or, as frequently seen in patients with primary polydipsia, a renal medullary gradient defect.

Systemic water loss normally results in increased plasma osmolality, which stimulates ADH release and thirst to return plasma osmolality to normal. ADH causes the collecting tubules to reabsorb free water, while thirst leads to increased water intake. With some individual variation, ADH secretion is completely suppressed at a plasma osmolality less than or equal to 280 mOsm/kg of water, which allows maximum water diuresis (the lowest urine osmolarity). Peak antidiuretic effect and maximum urine osmolality are reached at an osmolality of 295 to 300 mOsm/kg of water, which is also the range in which thirst stimulation occurs.

In the diabetes insipidus patient, thirst is the only available mechanism to maintain water homeostasis. With a lack of or an insensitivity to ADH, the kidney is unable to maintain antidiuresis, thus constant fluid losses must be matched by an equal fluid intake. This response can effectively modulate the system only as long as there is free access to fluids and even then, in more severe cases, the serum osmolality may be slightly elevated, due to the patient's inability to drink enough fluid. Lack of fluid results in an unabated rise in plasma osmolarity in the face of unchecked diuresis.

In some nephrogenic diabetes insipidus patients, a specific impairment of the collecting tubules makes the cells unresponsive to ADH's cyclic AMP-mediated alteration of the luminal surface to favor water reabsorption. In other nephrogenic diabetes insipidus patients, diminished medullary hyperosmolarity renders the kidney ineffective in concentrating the urine. This concentrating function is highly dependent on the interstitial tonicity gradient of the medulla even in the presence of maximal ADH activity. In a third group of nephrogenic diabetes insipidus patients with polyuria, a renal or extrarenal disease alters renal blood flow or urine flow rates, thus impeding effective urine concentration.

CLINICAL–PATHOLOGIC CORRELATIONS

The polyuria, polydipsia, and hypertonic dehydration of diabetes insipidus are a direct result of either vasopressin deficiency or renal refractoriness to vasopressin (Fig 82–1).

DIFFERENTIAL DIAGNOSIS

The differential diagnosis of major nonosmotic polyuric states is limited to central diabetes insipidus, nephrogenic diabetes insipidus, and psychogenic or primary polydipsia. The latter involves an abnormal thirst mechanism, in which ingestion of large quantities of fluid can result in moderate hypotonicity, overhydration, vasopressin suppression, urine dilution, renal osmotic gradient diminution, and polyuria. Because basal measurements of plasma and urine osmolarity cannot adequately distinguish

among the three polyuric states, dynamic dehydration testing or hypertonic saline infusion testing or both are necessary.

The principle of dehydration testing is to increase plasma osmolality enough to stimulate maximal endogenous vasopressin-mediated antidiuresis. This produces maximum urine hypertonicity such that additional exogenous vasopressin administration causes no further increase in urine concentration. Normally, after dehydration alone there is a modest increase in plasma osmolarity, which results in a signficant increase in urine osmolarity. In normal subjects, the administration of exogenous vasopressin at that point produces little change in the osmolality of an already concentrated urine.

This test is conducted in two phases. First, all oral intake is withheld under supervision, and urine volume and osmolality and body weight are measured at 60-minute intervals. The end-points of this phase are either a 3% to 5% reduction of body weight or a plateau of urine osmolality in three consecutive samples. Second, 5 units of aqueous vasopressin are administered intramuscularly, while urine volume and osmolality and body weight are monitored for 2 or 3 more hours. Responses in the various polyuric states are listed in Table 82–3. The results of even properly performed dehydration tests may be equivocal in up to 21% of polyuric patients.

Alternatively, hypertonic saline infusion can exogenously induce a hypertonic state. When the patient is hypertonic, the discrimination of this test is optimized by using direct vasopressin measurement, as well as plasma and urine osmolality. Primary polydipsic patients have ADH levels appropriate for their urine osmolality, while nephrogenic diabetes insipidus patients have increased ADH levels in the face of low urine osmolality. This test is critically dependent on a reliable ADH assay, which is not commonly available (Table 82–3).

PRINCIPLES OF THERAPY

CENTRAL DIABETES INSIPIDUS

When the thirst mechanism is intact, treatment for central diabetes insipidus is necessary only to alleviate the inconvenience of polyuria and polydipsia. Replacement therapy with a vaso-

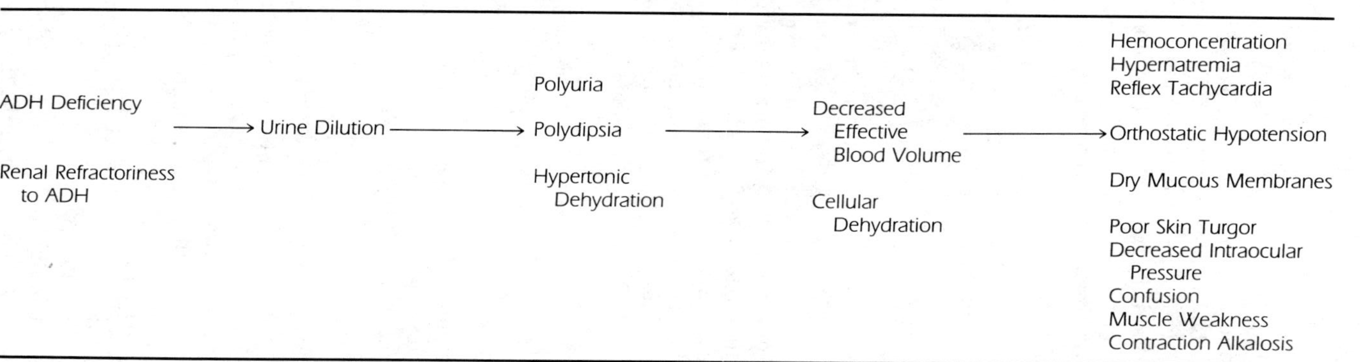

FIG 82–1.
Clinical–pathologic correlations of diabetes insipidus.

TABLE 82–3.
Differential Diagnosis

| | DEHYDRATION TEST | | | HYPERTONIC SALINE INFUSION TEST | | |
| | POSTDEHYDRATION | | POSTVASOPRESSIN | | | |
CONDITION	PLASMA OSMOLARITY (mOsm/kg)	URINE OSMOLARITY (mOsm/kg)	URINE OSMOLARITY (mOsm/kg)	PLASMA ADH (Pmol/L)	PLASMA OSMOLARITY (mOsm/kg)	URINE OSMOLARITY (mOsm/kg)
Normal	280–295	> 750	> 750*	> 4	> 300	> 750
Complete central diabetes insipidus	> 295	< 300	> 750†	< 4	> 300	< 300
Partial central diabetes insipidus	280–295	< 750	< 750‡	< 4	> 300	< 750
Nephrogenic diabetes insipidus	> 295	< 300	< 300*	> 4	> 300	< 300
Primary polydipsia	280–295	< 750	< 750§	> 4	> 300	> 750

* Not changed from postdehydration value.
† > 50% increase over postdehydration value.
‡ > 10% increase over postdehydration value.
§ < 10% increase over postdehydration value.

pressin analogue will effectively decrease urine output. If the thirst mechanism is disrupted, matching urinary output to oral intake is critical. Adding roughly 500 ml/24 hours for insensible losses to the amount of urine output is required to avoid life-threatening dehydration in patients unable to compensate with spontaneous oral fluid intake. Vasopressin analogues will also decrease polyuria.

In partial central diabetes insipidus, several agents can potentiate the renal response to vasopressin; other drugs can simulate a tubular ADH effect or stimulate endogenous ADH release. Single-agent or combination therapy has potential therapeutic benefit in selected cases.

NEPHROGENIC DIABETES INSIPIDUS

Nephrogenic diabetes insipidus is best treated by ensuring adequate fluid intake, salt restriction, and administration of a diuretic agent that reduces polyuria by sodium depletion and volume contraction, thus enhancing proximal water reabsorption. Prostaglandin synthetase inhibitors may serve as adjunctive therapy by causing water and sodium retention. In an occasional patient, there will be a partial sensitivity to vasopressin, so ADH may be used for therapy, even though endogenous ADH production is not impaired.

REFERENCES

Anderson O, Jacobsen BB: The renin-aldosterone system in nephrogenic diabetes insipidus and the influence of hydrochlorothiazide and indomethacin. *Acta Paediatr Scand* 1983; 72:717–720. *Mechanistic discussion of treatment rationale in nephrogenic diabetes insipidus.*

Baylis PH, Gill GV: The investigation of polyuria. *Clin Endocrinol Metab* 1984; 13:295–310. *Succinct review of neurohypophyseal physiology and testing procedures for the work-up of central diabetes insipidus.*

Culpepper RM, Herbert SC, Andriaoi TE: The posterior pituitary and water metabolism, in Williams RH (ed): *Textbook of Endocrinology.* Philadelphia, WB Saunders Co, 1985, pp 614–652. *General reference text for clinical endocrinology.*

Jamison RL, Maffly RH: The urinary concentrating mechanism. *N Engl J Med* 1976; 295:1059–1067. *Classic review on all aspects of the countercurrent mechanism.*

Moses AM, Schienman SJ, Oppenheim A: Marked hypotonic polyuria resulting from nephrogenic diabetes insipidus with partial sensitivity to vasopression. *J Clin Endocrinol Metab* 1984; 59:1044–1049. *Describes partial renal resistance to ADH; updates the nomenclature.*

Robertson GL: The regulation of vasopressin function in health and disease. *Recent Prog Horm Res* 1977; 33:333–385. *The single most complete discussion of ADH by a true pioneer in the field.*

Singer I, Forest JN Jr: Drug-induced states of nephrogenic diabetes insipidus. *Kidney Int* 1976; 10:82–95. *A general review of nephrogenic diabetes insipidus.*

<h1 style="font-size:3em; margin-right:0.5em;">83</h1>
<h1>Hyperthyroidism</h1>

H. Verdain Barnes, M.D.

Hyperthyroidism is a clinical syndrome resulting from excess circulating unbound (free) thyroxine (T_4) and/or triiodothyronine (T_3). Excess thyroid hormone has significant effects on the integument, nervous, muscle, skeletal, cardiovascular, reticuloendothelial, hematopoietic, gastrointestinal, and reproductive systems. Overt effects on these systems may or may not be clinically apparent or prominent. There are at least nine identifiable types of thyrotoxicosis (Table 83–1). The most common form in the United States is toxic diffuse goiter (Graves' disease), which accounts for about 90% of cases.

CLINICAL SIGNS AND SYMPTOMS

The typical patient complains of several of the signs and symptoms listed in Table 83–2. The onset is usually insidious with continuous progression over several months. In a few patients, however, the disease seemingly has an abrupt onset. A rare patient will present with a sudden marked exaggeration of the adrenergic manifestations of the disease termed thyroid storm, which is usually associated with major trauma, sepsis, and extraordinary psychosocial stress, discontinuation of an antithyroid drug or iodine therapy, or the effects of surgical or radioactive iodine treatment of uncontrolled disease.

The early course of thyrotoxicosis typically includes a history of increased nervousness, hyperhydrosis, palpitations, heat intolerance, and fatigue. In some cases, however, single organ system symptoms or signs will predominate (Table 83–3). Some patients, particularly those over 50 years of age, may have no striking features of hypermetabolism or present with unexplained weight loss, tachycardia, or atrial fibrillation. Some display a remarkable lack of signs and symptoms (apathetic hyperthyroidism).

On physical examination, the typical patient has a resting tachycardia, wide pulse pressure, thyroid enlargement, fine tremor of the outstretched fingers, stare, smooth warm skin, and hyperhydrosis. For those who have toxic diffuse goiter (Graves'), a thrill and/or bruit is often detected over the thyroid, and the eye manifestations of an infiltrative ophthalmopathy may appear (Table 83–3). A rare patient will have localized myxedema, most commonly seen in the anterolateral pretibial area. Later in the disease course there is often increasing bilateral proximal limb-girdle muscle weakness.

In untreated toxic diffuse goiter, spontaneous remission is thought to occur after months or years. Those patients who have hyperthyroidism due to symptomatic or silent acute nonsuppurative thyroiditis or toxic chronic lymphocytic thyroiditis (Hashitoxicosis) will usually have a spontaneous resolution of their hyperthyroidism in 2 to 6 months. The long-term prognosis for the former condition is usually a return to normal thyroid function, although some may become hypothyroid, while the prognosis for the latter is that most will in time become hypothyroid. Patients with iodine induced hyperthyroidism usually return to a normal thyrometabolic status after excess iodine intake is stopped; however the long-term prognosis is variable. The other types of hyperthyroidism probably do not remit except in the rare patient who hemorrhages into a solitary toxic adenoma or a thyroid-stimulating hormone (TSH)-producing pituitary adenoma. Patients with long-standing untreated thyrotoxicosis may progress to high-output congestive heart failure, persistent atrial fibrillation, profound muscle weakness, or psychosis.

TABLE 83–1.

Types of Hyperthyroidism Classified by Pathophysiologic Mechanism(s)

TYPE	PATHOLOGIC MECHANISM(S)
Toxic diffuse goiter (TDG) (Graves' disease)	Autoimmune: IgG human thyroid-stimulating immunoglobulin (TSI)
Toxic nodular goiter (TNG)	
Uninodular	Autonomous functioning adenoma(s)
Multinodular	Etiology unknown probably heterogenous; potential mechanisms include thyroid growth-stimulating immunoglobulin (TGI) and/or marine cycle changes
Chronic lymphocytic thyroiditis with thyrotoxicosis (Hashitoxicosis)	Probably autoimmune
Acute nonsuppurative thyroiditis (ANST) (subacute thyroiditis)	
Symptomatic	Probably postviral inflammation
Silent	Probably autoimmune
Toxic thyroid carcinoma (TTC)	Autonomous functioning follicular thyroid carcinoma (usually with widespread metastasis)
Struma ovarii (SO)	Ovarian dermoid cyst with autonomous functioning thyroid tissue in a cystic teratoma
Iodine-provoked hyperthyroidism (jodbasedow)	Excess iodine in presence of autonomously functioning thyroid parenchyma or adenoma(s)
Paraneoplastic hyperthyroidism (PH)	
Excess TSH	Autonomous functioning TSH-producing pituitary adenoma
Excess TSH-like substance	Hydatidiform mole, choriocarcinoma or embryonal cell, carcinoma of the testes producing excess molar thyrotropin
Excess exogenous thyroid hormone (EETH)	
Factitia	Chronic ingestion of excess T_4 and/or T_3
Medicamentosa	

TABLE 83–2.

Occurrence of Selected Symptoms and Signs of Hyperthyroidism*

SYMPTOM	FREQUENCY (% OF PATIENTS)	SIGN	FREQUENCY (% OF PATIENTS)
Nervousness	98	Thyroid enlargement	97
Hyperhydrosis	90	Smooth skin	94
Palpitations	88	Fine tremor of fingers	94
Fatigue	85	Hyperhydrosis	90
Weight loss	84	Wide pulse pressure	80
Heat intolerance	81	Stare	80
Tachycardia	80	Thyroid bruit or thrill	78
Weakness	72	Infiltrative ophthalmopathy[†]	60
Dyspnea	70	Atrial fibrillation	12
Increased appetite	61	Hepatomegaly or splenomegaly	6
Eye complaints		Gynecomastia	6
Stare	56	Pretibial myxedema[†]	1
Proptosis[†]	30		
Hyperdefecation			
Without diarrhea	28		
With diarrhea	20		
Anorexia	10		
Weight gain	3		

* From Werner SC, Ingbar SH (eds): *The Thyroid: A Fundamental and Clinical Text.* New York, Harper & Row, 1978, and a personal series ($N = 380$).

[†] Seen in autoimmune cases of toxic diffuse goiter or toxic chronic lymphocytic thyroiditis.

TABLE 83–3.
Hyperthyroidism First Seen as Single Organ System Manifestations

ORGAN SYSTEM	MANIFESTATIONS
Eyes	Stare
	Infiltrative ophthalmopathy
	Periorbital edema
	Excess lacrimation
	Chemosis
	Proptosis
	Ophthalmoplegia (extraocular)
	Optic nerve involvement (retro-orbital neuritis, papilledema, papillitis)
Cardiac	Arrythmia (first-degree heart block, atrial fibrillation), angina and/or congestive heart failure (high output)
Skeletal muscle	Easy muscle fatigue
	Weakness, wasting (temporal and/or proximal)
	Periodic paralysis
Gastrointestinal	Abdominal cramping
	Pernicious hyperdefecation or diarrhea
	Pernicious vomiting
	Malabsorption
Genital or breast	Infertility
	Spontaneous abortion
	Oligomenorrhea or amenorrhea
	Gynecomastia
	Testicular atrophy
Psychologic	Chronic anxiety
	Hyperactivity
	Apathy
	Psychosis
Skin	Onycholysis
	Myxedema circumscripta
	Vitiligo
	Hyperpigmentation
	Alopecia areata
	Pruritis

PATHOPHYSIOLOGY

Maintaining normal thyroid homeostasis requires: (1) an adequate number of functioning thyroid cells, (2) an adequate amount of circulating and intrathyroidal iodine, (3) a normally functioning thyroid autoregulatory system, (4) an intact hypothalamic-pituitary-thyroid negative feedback system, (5) effective intracellular control of the deiodination of T_4 to T_3, and (6) an adequate number of nuclear receptors for thyroid hormone in those cells responsive to thyroid hormone. The principal control mechanism for circulating free T_4 and T_3 levels is the hypothalamic-pituitary-thyroid negative feedback system. Both T_4 and T_3 are probably needed for this system to function normally, although T_3 within the thyrotrophs appears to be the primary regulator.

Normally about 80% of the circulating T_3 comes from the deiodination of T_4 in the cytosol of the liver and kidney cells. In the target organ cells, T_3 is bound to a specific nuclear receptor that initiates the unique hormone action of the cell. A logical, but as yet unproven, intracellular sequence includes the alteration by T_3 of nuclear DNA transcription followed by an increase in RNA formation leading to the synthesis of a specific protein by which thyroid hormone regulates the metabolic activity of the cells in responsive organ systems.

Thyroid hormone increases: (1) heat production by stimulating the sodium pump of plasma membranes; (2) oxygen consumption; (3) carbohydrate, fat, and protein metabolism; (4) cardiac output; and (5) neuron irritability. Excess thyroid hormone accentuates these effects in varying degrees.

TABLE 83–4.
Typical Macroscopic and Microscopic Features of the Thyroid in Hyperthyroidism

TYPE OF HYPERTHYROIDISM	MACROSCOPIC FEATURES	MICROSCOPIC FEATURES
Toxic diffuse goiter	Enlarged thyroid, firm, red-brown, smooth (occasionally lobular without district nodules), nongelatinous tissue	Small follicles, hyperplastic columnar epithelium with papillary projections into the follicle lumen, scant colloid, various degrees of aggregated lymphocytes and plasma cells
Toxic nodular goiter Uninodular	Distinct encapsulated nodule	Fibrous capsule, normal follicle size, hyperplastic columnar epithelium and normal amounts of colloid
Multinodular	Enlarged, nodular thyroid; red-tan granular tissue in the nodules or between colloid-filled nodules	Glandular tissue (in or between the nodules) with some follicles showing hyperplasia of columnar epithelial cells, papillae with small follicles enclosed in their struma and/or increased amounts of colloid
Toxic chronic lymphocytic thyroiditis	Enlarged thyroid; pale, firm tissue	Diffuse lymphocyte infiltration with germinal centers, some destruction of epithelial cells, degeneration and fragmentation of the follicle basement membrane, some cells with oxyphilic cytoplasm (Askanazy cells) and hyperplasia, and plasma cell accumulation
Acute nonsuppurative thyroiditis	Enlarged thyroid; pale, hard tissue	Patchy involvement with various degrees of mononuclear cell infiltration with disrupted epithelium and partial or complete loss of colloid, central core of the colloid surrounded by multinucleated giant cells with or without granuloma formation
Toxic thyroid carcinoma	Variable size nodule(s), usually encapsulated, stone-hard, gray-pink, granular tissue	Variable with areas resembling normal tissue except for smaller follicles and diminished amounts of colloid to areas with solid sheets of cells containing mitotic forms, invasion of blood vessels and/or adjacent parenchyma
Excess exogenous thyroid hormone	Usually small, firm thyroid	Usually atrophic normal tissue

The major gross and microscopic findings of the thyroid in the various types of hyperthyroidism are shown in Table 83–4.

CLINICAL–PATHOLOGIC CORRELATIONS

The clinical features of hyperthyroidism result from: (1) the underlying pathology, (2) an overstimulation of responsive cells by the excess hormone, and (3) a summation of the cellular effects of thyroid hormone and catecholamines. The primary clinical–pathologic correlations are shown in Table 83–5.

DIFFERENTIAL DIAGNOSIS

The differential diagnosis of hyperthyroidism is shown in Table 83–1. The differential diagnosis for the most common nonthyroid diseases that may mimic thyrotoxicosis clinically, especially if the initial manifestations are seen mainly in a single system, are shown in Table 83–6. The most common of these is acute and/or chronic anxiety.

DIAGNOSIS

The laboratory diagnosis of hyperthyroidism is usually simple, requiring only determinations of the total serum T_4 (TT_4) and/or the total serum T_3 (TT_3) level and an estimate of the serum's thyroxine-binding capacity. The TT_4 and TT_3 levels can be precisely measured by specific radioimmunoassays; the thyroxine-binding capacity can be indirectly determined by measuring the T_3 resin uptake which estimates the number of available binding sites on TBG or directly by measuring the serum level of thyroxine-binding globulin (TBG).

Although the amount of unbound (free) T_4 and T_3 in the serum is far less than 1% of the total amount of the hormone, it is advantageous to quantitate or estimate the level of "free" hormone. Because the "free" fraction is controlled by mass law equilibrium for bound and unbound hormone, a measurement can be made by equilibrium dialysis or more economically estimated mathematically by the equation: TT_4 or TT_3 concentration times the T_3 resin uptake

(T_3RU). The product is a free T_4 or T_3 index (FT_4I or FT_3I).

In typical cases of hyperthyroidism, the TT_4 and TT_3 levels, RT_3U, FT_4I, and FT_3I are elevated. By using the FT_4I or FT_3I, most of the changes that can occur in TBG concentration are resolved, thus usually eliminating the potential for erroneous clinical judgments based on TT_4, TT_3, or T_3RU measurements alone if there are significant changes in the binding or level of TBG such as with oral contraceptives.

An occasional patient will have "T_3 toxicosis," in which case the TT_4 level, T_3RU, and FT_4I are normal, while the TT_3 level and FT_3I are substantially elevated. Levels of TT_3, however, can also be elevated in persons without hyperthyroidism, including those with iodine deficiency, chronic lymphocytic thyroiditis, disorders that increase the serum concentration of TBG and those who have had radioiodine therapy for thyrotoxicosis. Consequently, it is necessary to demonstrate autonomous thyroid gland function to firmly establish the diagnosis.

Thyroid gland autonomy can be assessed by the T_3-suppression test or thyrotropin-releasing hormone (TRH) stimulation test. When the hypothalamic-pituitary-thyroid negative feedback system is intact, the 24-hour radioactive iodine uptake (RAIU) is suppressed by 50% or more after 1 week of exogenous T_3 administration (50 µg twice daily). If the thyroid is functioning autonomously, the RAIU is not normally suppressed. Normally with TRH stimulation, the serum TSH level increases by at least threefold to fivefold over baseline at 30 or 60 minutes after injecting 500 µg of TRH and with autonomous function TRH stimulates little or no increase in the TSH level. Autonomous function is seen in toxic diffuse goiter (Graves'), toxic nodule(s), toxic thyroid carcinoma, and iodine-induced hyperthyroidism.

The routine RAIU measurement is now less useful in the United States as a diagnostic test for hyperthyroidism than in the past because of the increased iodine intake. However, the RAIU is usually elevated in toxic diffuse goiter, paraneoplastic hyperthyroidism, and toxic thyroid carcinoma. It may be elevated or normal in toxic nodule(s) and toxic chronic lymphocytic thyroiditis (Hashitoxicosis). Thyroid uptake is low in acute nonsuppurative thyroiditis, excess exogenous thyroid hormone ingestion, struma ovarii, and occasionally in toxic chronic lymphocytic thyroiditis.

TABLE 83–5.
Clinical–Pathologic Correlations in Hyperthyroidism*

CLINICAL FINDINGS	PATOLOGY	PATHOLOGIC FINDINGS
Increased appetite	Hypermetabolism†	Increased basal metabolism rate
Weight loss	Increased oxygen consumption	Increased lipolysis and fat metabolism
Hypocholesterolemia	change in oxidative	Increased utilization of carbohydrates
Heat tolerance	phosphorylation (uncoupling)	Increased synthesis and degradation of
Weakness	Stimulation of the plasma membrane	proteins
Fatigue	sodium pump	
Increased skin temperature		
	Increased adrenergic activity	
Tachycardia	(Summation of thyroid hormone and	Increased adrenergic stimulation
Palpitations	catecholamine effects)	Increased cardiac output
Hyperdefecation		Increased gastrointestinal motility
Nervousness		Increased alveolar ventilation
Hyperkinesis		
Dyspnea		
Stare		
Connective tissue	Proptosis	
proliferation	Infiltrative ophthalmopathy‡	Increased bulk extraocular muscles and
	Increased mucopolysaccharides in	fat
	collagen ground substance	Increased connective tissue
	Increased water retention	Localized myxedema‡
	Probable immune response:	
	lymphocyte and plasma cell	
	infiltration	

* From Werner SC, Ingbar SH (eds): *The Thyroid: A Fundamental and Clinical Text.* New York, Harper & Row, 1978.
† Current hypothesis.
‡ Commonly found in toxic diffuse goiter but not other types of hyperthyroidism.

In toxic diffuse goiter, an antibody that stimulates human thyroid hormone production is measurable in at least 90% of patients. In toxic chronic lymphocytic thyroiditis, high titers of antithyroglobulin and/or antimicrosomal antibodies are typically present, whereas in toxic diffuse goiter low titers are common and in acute nonsuppurative thyroiditis low titers occasionally occur. The serum TSH level is elevated when the patient has hyperthyroidism due to a TSH-secreting pituitary adenoma. Those patients with paraneoplastic hyperthyroidism due to molar thyrotropin, which appears to be chemically/structurally identical to human chorionic gonadotropin (HCG), have markedly elevated levels of circulating HCG.

The laboratory diagnosis of hyperthyroidism can be misleading. In the presence of acute nonthyroid illness, some inherited diseases of the liver, and with certain drug treatments, where an elevated TT_4 level or normal FT_3I may not rule out the diagnosis. In the euthyroid sick (acute nonthyroid illness) syndrome, the FT_4I may be elevated and the TT_3 level and FT_3I decreased due to changes in TBG-binding capacity, relatively rapid decreases in liver production of thyroid-binding prealbumin (TBPA), and a decrease in the peripheral conversion of T_4 to T_3 by monodeiodination resulting from a decreased concentration or activity of the enzyme 5' deiodinase. This decreased enzyme activity results in increased circulating levels of reverse T_3 $(3, 3', 5'T_3)$.

In patients with alcoholic cirrhosis there are also changes in the production and binding capacity of the thyroid-binding proteins (TBG, TBPA, and albumin), which may result in an increased FT_4I. With acute viral hepatitis, chronic active hepatitis, and primary biliary cirrhosis, an increased TT_4 level is common due to increased TBG binding. In the patients with primary biliary cirrhosis, the FT_4I is usually normal but may be elevated without thyrotoxicosis being present. The inherited diseases associated with hyperthyroxinemia without thyrotoxicosis include excess thyroid-binding globulin, familial dysalbuminemic hyperthyroxinemia, prealbumin-associated hyperthyroxinemia, and generalized thyroid-hormone resistance syndromes. In the resistance syndromes the TT_4 and TT_3 and FT_4I are commonly elevated.

TABLE 83–6.
Disorders That May Mimic Hyperthyroidism or the Ophthalmopathy of Toxic Diffuse Goiter

HYPERTHYROIDISM	OPHTHALMOPATHY
Anxiety	Pituitary adenoma
Acute	Cushing's disease
Chronic	Acromegaly
Pheochromocytoma	Retro-orbital tumors or infection
Pregnancy	Lymphoma
Malignancy	Histiocytosis
	Pseudotumor
	Cirrhosis
	Superior mediastinal obstruction
	Mechanical ventilation
	Carotid sinus thrombosis
	Trichinosis
	Nephrotic syndrome
	Myasthenia gravis

The drugs that may produce: (1) elevated TT_4, TT_3, FT_4I, and FT_3I values include some of the iodides; (2) an elevated TT_4 and FT_4I values include iopanoic acid, ipodate, and amiodarone; and (3) an elevated TT_4 and occasionally TT_3 levels with a normal FT_4I include estrogens, methadone, heroin, perphenazine, and clofibrate. These drug-induced changes are due to actions on thyroid hormone biosynthesis, alterations in the deiodination of T_4 to T_3, and increased production and concentrations of TBG, respectively.

Finally, in some patients with acute nonthyroid disease and in some with certain liver diseases, thyrotoxicosis may be masked by normal or low levels of TT_4 and/or TT_3 with an elevated T_3RU and FT_4I. When the routine thyroid function studies are equivocal, the clinical picture is unclear or the patient appears to be euthyroid, a TRH-stimulation test will usually resolve the dilemma.

PRINCIPLES OF THERAPY

The primary goal of therapy is to lower the level of circulating thyroid hormone. In toxic diffuse goiter and toxic nodular goiter, this can be accomplished by administering a thioamide that blocks the synthesis of thyroid hormone (blocks organification and coupling) or by ablative treatment with radioactive iodine or surgery. Surgical or radioiodine treatment is usually preferred for toxic nodular goiter. Ablative treatment is usually not considered for toxic chronic lymphocytic thyroiditis or acute nonsuppurative thyroiditis because of their natural histories.

The secondary goal of therapy is to control clinically disabling adrenergic manifestations of the disease. This can be accomplished by beta-adrenergic blockade or the depletion of norepinephrine from the adrenergic nerve terminals.

The long-term prognosis for adequately treated patients with hyperthyroidism is good except for those with thyroid storm, toxic thyroid carcinoma, and malignant struma ovarii.

REFERENCES

Hamilton CR, Maloof F: Unusual types of hyperthyroidism. *Medicine* 1973; 52:195–215. *A well-referenced discussion.*

Larsen PR, Sliva JE, Kaplan MM: Relationships between circulating and intracellular thyroid hormones: Physiologic and clinical implications. *Endocrine Reviews* 1981; 2:87–102. *A provocative description of thyroid hormone effects and interactions.*

Werner SC, Ingbar SH (eds): *The Thyroid: A Fundamental and Clinical Text.* New York, Harper & Row, 1978. *The best detailed presentation of the clinical spectrum of hyperthyroidism.*

Woolf PD: Transient painless thyroiditis with hyperthyroidism: A variant of lymphocytic thyroiditis? *Endocrine Reviews* 1980; 1:411–420. *A detailed discussion of this variant of hyperthyroidism.*

84   HYPOTHYROIDISM

Richard A. Serbin, M.D.

Hypothyroidism is a deficiency of circulating unbound (free) thyroxine T_4 or triiodothyronine T_3 or both. The deficiency leads to diminished metabolism in virtually all tissues. The incidence of hypothyroidism is high following radioactive iodine therapy or subtotal thyroidectomy.

CLINICAL SIGNS AND SYMPTOMS

Early to late manifestations of hypothyroidism vary in severity. No symptoms are usually present until the process is well advanced. Symptoms, when present, are often nonspecific and nondiagnostic, and individual symptoms are less helpful than the constellation of symptoms. Frequent symptoms (typically elicited only by direct questioning) include cold intolerance, constipation, dry skin, and thin brittle hair. Mentation is usually not significantly impaired, but some patients demonstrate intellectual impairment varying from subtle memory deficits to coma. The physical findings can also be nonspecific with many also seen in some euthyroid patients. For example, dry skin, pallor, puffy facies, and loss of eyebrows are not unusual in the euthyroid elderly patient. A hoarse voice, sluggish reflexes, bradycardia, a thick tongue, and hypothermia, however, are more suggestive of hypothyroidism (Table 84–1).

The natural history of hypothyroidism is not well-delineated because treatment is usually begun when the diagnosis is made. Clinical experience, however, suggests that in some patients mild hypothyroidism may not be progressive. On the other hand, hypothyroidism occurring after ablative therapy (with radioactive iodine or subtotal thyroidectomy) may be rapid in onset and severe in presentation with pronounced myalgia and weakness.

PATHOPHYSIOLOGY

All major organ systems are involved in hypothyroidism. The direct effects of thyroid hormone deficiency can be directly attributed to the lack of metabolic stimulation by the active hormone and include decreased oxygen consumption in most, but not all, tissues, decreased new protein synthesis, tissue infiltration with a characteristic mucopolysaccharide, decreased thermogenesis, and decreased metabolic clearance of drugs. The indirect effects include increased atherosclerosis, which is at least in part attributable to increased levels of serum lipids. This may increase the incidence or accelerate coronary atherosclerosis, although not necessarily angina. Pleural and pericardial effusions of protein-rich fluid occur in up to half of hypothyroid patients.

DIFFERENTIAL DIAGNOSIS

Many of the manifestations of hypothyroidism are found often enough in normal patients that routine thyroid function studies are recommended to detect subclinical or atypical cases in elderly patients.

Patients with pernicious anemia and azotemia may appear clinically to be hypothyroid, but this can usually be differentiated by appropriate laboratory studies such as measurement of T_4 levels, T_3 resin uptake (T_3RU), free thyroid hormone index (FTI), and thyroid-stimulating hormone (TSH) levels. One must be cautious in interpreting the results of these tests in patients with a nonthyroid illness (euthyroid sick syndrome).

DIAGNOSIS

Hypothyroidism can be diagnosed in most patients by a combination of a low T_4 level and an elevated TSH level. Total (free plus bound)

TABLE 84–1.
Signs and Symptoms of Hypothyroidism*

SIGNS AND SYMPTOMS	INCIDENCE (% OF CASES)
Weakness	99
Dry skin	97
Coarse skin	97
Lethargy	91
Slow speech	91
Edema of eyelids	90
Sensation of cold	89
Decreased sweating	89
Cold skin	83
Thick tongue	82
Edema of face	79
Coarseness of hair	76
Pallor of skin	67
Memory impairment	66
Constipation	61
Gain in weight	59
Loss of hair	57
Pallor of lips	57
Dyspnea	55
Peripheral edema	55
Hoarseness or aphonia	52
Anorexia	45
Nervousness	35
Menorrhagia	32
Palpitation	31
Deafness	30
Precordial pain	25

* From Means JH: *The Thyroid and Its Diseases*, ed 2. Philadelphia, JB Lippincott Co, 1948, p 233.

T_4 values should be corrected for thyroid-binding globulin (TBG) concentration by measuring a T_3RU, which then allows a free thyroxine index (FT_4I) to be calculated. The FT_4I and T_4 level have a high degree of correlation. Total T_3 levels are not reliable in the diagnosis of hypothyroidism.

A list of conditions causing problems in evaluation follows (Table 84–2).

EUTHYROID SICK SYNDROME

A significant proportion of patients with nonthyroid disease have a low total T_4 concentration, but are euthyroid. The FT_4I and free T_4 levels, however, are usually normal. A normal TSH level in these patients usually clarifies the patient's thyrometabolic status. Occasionally the results are equivocal, and a thyrotropin-releasing hormone (TRH) stimulation test may be needed to clarify the patient's status.

TABLE 84–2.

Classification of Hypothyroidism

Thyroprivic
  Postablative hypothyroidism
  Primary idiopathic hypothyroidism
  Sporadic athyrotic cretinism (thyroid asplasia or dysplasia)
Trophoprivic
  Sheehan's syndrome
  Infiltrative disorders of pituitary or hypothalamus
Goitrous
  Hashimoto's thyroiditis
  Endemic iodine deficiency
  Antithyroid agents (para-aminosalicylic acid, phenylbutazone, resorcinol, lithium, cruciferous plants,
    cassava)
  Iodide goiter and hypothyroidism
  Heritable defects in hormone biosynthesis and action
  Peripheral resistance to thyroid hormone (may also be nogoitrous)

PITUITARY INSUFFICIENCY

Hypothyroidism of a mild degree may be present in patients with other manifestations of hypopituitarism. Occasionally, however, the hypothyroidism is clinically blatant and the predominant initial manifestation seen clinically. The key difference between pituitary insufficiency and primary hypothyroidism is a normal or low TSH value in hypothyroidism. Prolactin measurement is important in cases of pituitary insufficiency because prolactinomas may appear as hypothyroidism, especially in men. Clinical evaluation of the hypothalamic-pituitary axis in cases of suspected hypothyroidism is complex and beyond the scope of this chapter.

Long-standing hypothyroidism may lead to an enlarged pituitary and a decreased responsiveness to TRH stimulation, although in most patients a response will differentiate secondary from primary hypothyroidism. A brisk TSH response to TRH suggests normal pituitary function indicating either hypothalamic or primary hypothyroidism. When an abnormally low TSH response is seen, repeated TRH testing is required to confirm the diagnosis of secondary hypothyroidism.

TRANSIENT HYPOTHYROIDISM

In subacute thyroiditis (acute nonsuppurative thyroiditis), patients usually present with a painfully enlarged thyroid. As destruction of the follicles occurs, the hyperthyroxinemia may result in symptoms of hyperthyroidism. These symptoms may be followed by transient hypothyroidism during the process of thyroid follicle regeneration. Clinically this is usually relatively mild and does not require treatment. The diagnosis of this form of thyroiditis is usually suspected by the clinical picture. Elevation of the erythrocyte sedimentation rate, fine needle aspiration biopsy, a positive gallium scan, and elevated serum thyroglobulin level may be of considerable diagnostic help.

THYROID BLOCKING ANTIBODIES

Occasionally patients who later develop Graves' disease have a history of hypothyroidism. It is postulated that antibodies blocking the TSH receptor may have previously been present. This is rare and need not be considered at the time of the initial evaluation for hypothyroidism.

TRANSIENT ELEVATION OF TSH FOLLOWING THE DISCONTINUATION OF THYROID REPLACEMENT

Occasionally it is desirable or necessary to stop thyroid replacement. Following discontinuation, the thyroid hormone level will drop and the TSH level will rise. Elevated TSH levels may be seen before the thyroid responds with enough hormone synthesis and release to suppress TSH secretion. This response may take 6 or more weeks. Consequently, if testing occurs too early, an elevated TSH level and a low normal thyroid hormone level may give misleading results.

SUBCLINICAL HYPOTHYROIDISM

An elevated TSH level and normal T_4 level may occur early in destructive or ablative settings such as chronic lymphocytic thyroiditis or radioiodine therapy. In most cases thyroid function is progressively lost, and replacement hormone therapy or close surveillance or both are needed.

MYXEDEMA COMA

Myxedema coma is an unusual and severe manifestation which has a high mortality rate. It requires prompt and aggressive therapy if the process is to be reversed. The diagnosis is made on clinical grounds and confirmed by appropriate laboratory tests on specimens obtained before institution of thyroid hormone therapy.

Myxedema coma occurs most often in the elderly and is usually associated with hypothermia, bradycardia, and hypotension. The patient's physical appearance is usually suggestive, but not pathognomonic. The history, if obtainable, may reveal prior thyroid ablation therapy or give clues to other disease states (e.g., infection, myocardial infarction, or stroke) which are almost always present.

Once a presumptive diagnosis is made, supportive therapy should be prompt. A major factor is hypoventilation, which usually requires a respirator to correct the hypercarbia and hypoxia. Corticosteroids should be given promptly because most patients have some degree of functional adrenal insufficiency.

Intravenous L-T_4 thyroxine or L-T_3 triiodothyronine should be given initially. If an intravenous preparation is not available, administration can be by nasogastric tube. Severe hyponatremia may be present and require hypertonic saline therapy. Hypoglycemia is also a potential problem.

The prognosis depends largely on the precipitating disease, particularly if it is coronary ar-

tery disease. Coronary events following the institution of replacement therapy appear to be common and are associated with a high mortality. Beta-adrenergic blockers may be beneficial in preventing tachyarrhythmias.

Vigilance is essential so that early therapy for such complications as hypostatic pneumonia, decubitus ulcer, and impaction can be instituted. Prevention of myxedema coma is more effective than treatment, which argues for routine thyroid screening in older patients.

PRINCIPLES OF THERAPY

Except in myxedema coma, thyroid replacement should be started only after laboratory confirmation of the diagnosis. Requirements for thyroid hormone are to a degree age-dependent and decrease with age (Fig 84–1). Occasionally patients who have long-standing or severe hypothyroidism will not show a prompt decrease in TSH levels even with relatively high doses of L-thyroxine (T_4). Doses can be initially titrated from the total T_4 values with the goal of attempting to maintain levels in the normal range and the final dose adjustment being based on the TSH level. Patients who have high total T_4 values may have total T_3 values in the normal range, which is also acceptable. In patients with symptomatic coronary artery disease, therapy may be difficult. Fatal coronary events can occur, and extreme caution must be used.

Triiodothyronine in microgram doses given incrementally may be useful initially because of its relatively short half-life (18 to 36 hours). Calcium-channel or beta-adrenergic blockers may be useful in managing angina during replacement therapy.

In patients needing coronary bypass surgery, in whom it has been impossible to replace the thyroid hormone, surgery can be accomplished with no apparent increase in surgical morbidity or mortality if beta-adrenergic blockade is instituted. Slowly progressive thyroid hormone replacement then may be instituted after the operation.

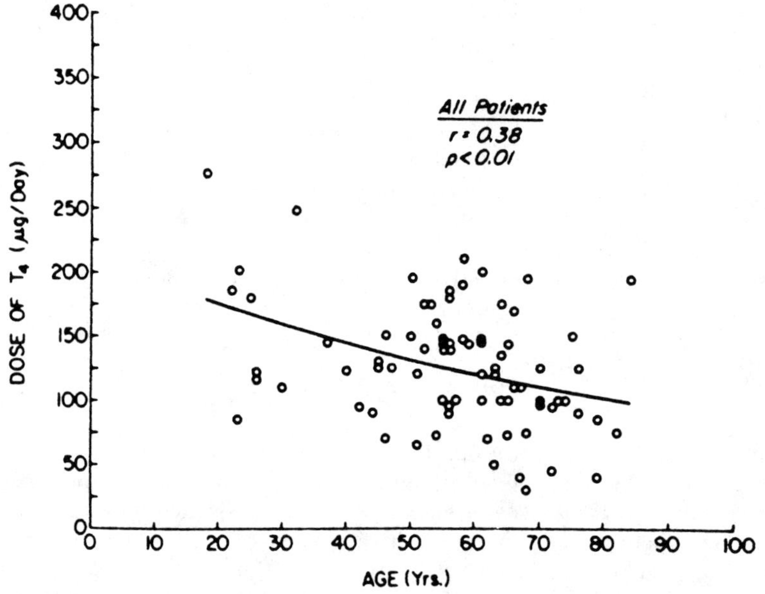

FIG 84–1.

Relationship of daily maintenance dose of levothyroxine to age in male and female patients with hypothyroidism. Maintenance dose is that required to lower the serum TSH concentration into the normal range. (From Sawin C, Herman T, Molitch ME et al: Aging in the Thyroid: Decreased requirement for thyroid hormone in older hypothyroid patients. *Am J Med* 1983; 75:206–209. Used by permission.)

REFERENCES

Bacci V, Schussler GC, Kaplan TB: The relationship between serum triiodothyronine and thyrotropin during system illness. *J Clin Endocrinol Metab* 1982; 54:1229–1235. *A discussion of the physiologic profile in this setting.*

Becker C: Hypothyroidism and atherosclerotic heart disease. *Endocrine Reviews* 1985; 6:432–440. *An up-to-date review.*

Kaptein EM, Grieb DA, Spencer CA et al: Thyroxine metabolism in the low thyroxine state of medical nonthyroidal illnesses. *J Clin Endocrinol Metab* 1981; 53:764–771. *A study of the euthyroid sick syndrome.*

Madeddu G, Casu AR, Costanza C et al: Serum thyroglobulin levels in the diagnosis and follow-up of subacute painful thyroiditis. *Arch Intern Med* 1985; 145:243–247. *The use of serum Tg in diagnosis.*

Sanders LR, Moreno AJ, Pitman DL et al: Painless giant cell thyroiditis diagnosed by fine needle aspiration and association with intense thyroidal uptake of gallium. *Am J Med* 1986; 80:971–975. *Describes the use of gallium in diagnosis.*

Sawin C, Herman I, Molitch ME et al: Aging in the thyroid: Decreased requirement for thyroid hormone in older hypothyroid patients. *Am J Med* 1983; 75:206–209. *Good review of the aging thyroid.*

Steinberg AD: Myxedema and coronary artery disease. A comparative autopsy study. *Ann Intern Med* 1968; 68:338–344. *Good study of descriptive pathology.*

85 THYROIDITIS

James V. Hennessey, M.D.
Barry A. Warner, D.O.

Thyroid inflammatory processes can be grouped clinically, pathologically, or etiologically (Tables 85–1 and 85–2). Acute bacterial infections are rare. Viral-initiated and immunologically mediated subacute forms of thyroiditis are more commonly encountered. Chronic lymphocytic conditions, resulting in hypothyroidism (e.g., Hashimoto's thyroiditis), represent the most common form of this heterogenous group of conditions.

CLINICAL SIGNS AND SYMPTOMS

Patients with thyroiditis commonly seek medical attention for the symptoms of hyperthyroidism, hypothyroidism, or for the presence of a goiter. In thyroiditis, the thyroid is usually firm and may be significantly greater than normal size, depending on the cause. Local pain and compression symptoms, as well as systemic manifestations, usually help distinguish among the various types of thyroiditis. The history and physical findings depend on the cause of the disease and on the thyrometabolic state of the patient.

Acute suppurative thyroiditis (AST) is a deep-seated bacterial infection often associated with septicemia. If it is untreated, local spread of the infection into adjacent deep structures of the neck may occur, and an advanced systemic infection may lead to death.

Typically, subacute (painful) thyroiditis (SubT) and a painless form of thyroiditis, often associated with the immediate postpartum period, are characterized by four clinical phases of thyroid function as outlined in Figure 85–1. Pain, an elevated erythrocyte sedi-

TABLE 85–1.
Types of Thyroiditis and Underlying Causes of Pathologic Changes

TYPE	CAUSE
ACUTE THYROIDITIS	
Acute suppurative thyroiditis	Gram-positive bacteria, fungi
Radiation thyroiditis	Iodine 131
Traumatic thyroiditis	Trauma
SUBACUTE THYROIDITIS	
De Quervain's (painful) thyroiditis	Viral and possibly autoimmune
Silent (painless) thyroiditis	Probably autoimmune
CHRONIC THYROIDITIS	
Lymphocytic (Hashimoto's) thyroiditis	Autoimmune
Riedel's thyroiditis	Unknown
Tuberculous thyroiditis	*Mycobacterium tuberculosis*
Syphilitic thyroiditis	*Treponema pallidum*
Echinococcal thyroiditis	*Echinococcus*
INFILTRATIVE THYROID DISEASE	
Amyloidosis	Unknown
Sarcoidosis	Unknown

TABLE 85–2.
Typical Macroscopic and Microscopic Features of the Thyroid in Thyroiditis

TYPE OF THYROIDITIS	MACROSCOPIC FEATURES	MICROSCOPIC FEATURES
Acute suppurative	Enlarged with abscess formation	Isolated or "diffuse focal" polymorphonuclear and lymphocytic involvement with suppuration, necrosis, hemorrhage, and thrombophlebitis in local veins. Progresses to fibrosis.
Radiation	Enlarged, nodular	Epithelial swelling and necrosis. Disruption of follicular architecture. Edema and leukocytic infiltration progresses to irregular hyaline fibrosis of interstitial thyroid tissues and vessel walls.
Trauma	Enlarged, inflamed, firm	Mild follicular destruction. Mild fibrosis with infrequent lymph follicles and abundant interstitial plasma cells.
Subacute (de Quervain's)	Enlarged, pale, hard	Patchy involvement with varying stages of development. Mononuclear cell infiltration with disrupted epithelium and partial or complete loss of colloid. Some lesions have a central core of colloid surrounded by multinucleate giant cells with or without granuloma formation.
Chronic	Enlarged, pale, firm	Diffuse lymphocyte infiltration and germinal centers formation. Some destruction of epithelial cells with degeneration and fragmentation of follicle basement membranes. Some oxyphilic cytoplasm (Askanazy cells). Hyperplasia and plasma cell accumulation
Riedel's	Enlarged, asymmetric, stony hard, adherent to surrounding tissue	Dense fibrosis with scattered solitary follicular cells and occasional acini with small amounts of colloid

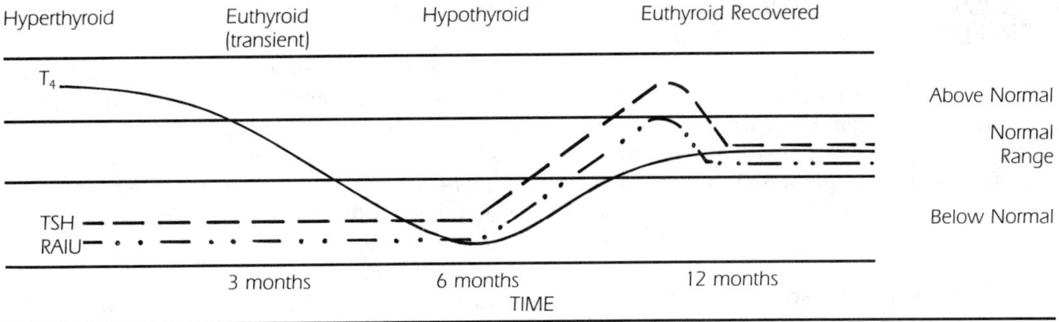

FIG 85–1.
Variation of the clinical parameters of thyroxine level, serum TSH, and 24-hour radioactive iodine uptake (RAIU) and their relationship to time during the course of subacute thyroiditis.

mentation rate (ESR), and hyperthyroidism with a low radioactive iodine uptake (RAIU) lasting for 1 to 3 months are characteristic initial findings. A transient euthyroid phase follows, usually with gradual abatement of the pain, but with persistence of the elevated ESR and suppression of radioactive iodine uptake. The thyroid status subsequently reaches a nadir during the time of tissue recovery, and finally an intact and functional gland returns to normal function in more than 95% of cases.

Chronic lymphocytic thyroiditis (CLT) (Hashimoto's thyroiditis) appears to be autoimmune initiated and perpetuated. It affects women 10 to 20 times more often than men. Lymphocyte- mediated processes result in high titers of circulating antimicrosomal or antithyroglobulin antibodies or both along with lymphocytic infiltration of the thyroid gland, characterized by germinal center formation and fibrosis (Table 85–2). The insidious failure of the thyroid gland to generate thyroid hormone leads to primary hypothyroidism and a thyroid-stimulating hormone (TSH)-stimulated diffuse enlargement of the gland, resulting in a firm, somewhat lobulated goiter.

PATHOPHYSIOLOGY

The pathologic changes associated with the various types of thyroiditis are listed in Table 85–1. AST is often caused by common gram-positive organisms or fungi entering the thyroid through the circulation, fistulas, or direct trauma. SubT (de Quervain's thyroiditis) is probably a viral disease and has been documented to be associated with mumps, in-

fluenza, and adenovirus. A strong association with certain HLA types has been reported, giving insight into the genetic predisposition and the basis of the immunologic mediation. Histologically, disruption of thyroid follicles by polymorphonuclear leukocytes or lymphocytes and the presence of characteristic giant cells proceeds to microabscess formation and fibrosis (Table 85–2). The disruption of follicular cells is the basis for the low radioactive iodine uptake seen during the inflammatory phases of this condition (Fig 85–1.)

To understand the pathophysiologic process in autoimmune thyroiditis, one must understand why autoimmune disease does not occur in normal individuals. Random mutations of lymphocytic clones that are self-reactive ("forbidden") is a normal occurrence. These "forbidden" clones are suppressed by specific clones of "suppressor" T-lymphocytes, resulting in tolerance and thus prevention of autoimmune disease. Lymphocytic (Hashimoto's) thyroiditis can be viewed as a genetically predisposed defect of the specific "suppressor" T-lymphocytes (see Strakosch et al., 1982). This defect allows "forbidden" clones to proliferate and autoreact as "helper" T-lymphocytes against normal thyroid cell membranes and to induce autoreactive B-lymphocytes with subsequent antibody production. Thyroid cell destruction results from the cell-mediated T-lymphocyte activity combined with humoral antibody production by B-lymphocytes. This immunologic attack damages the follicular cells. Iodine organification defects cause a decreased production of thyroxine (T₄) and consequent unchecked TSH hyperstimulation.

CLINICAL–PATHOLOGIC CORRELATIONS

Table 85–2 describes the macroscopic and microscopic pathologic changes in the various forms of thyroiditis. Figures 85–1 and 85–2 illustrate the clinical–pathologic correlations in SubT.

DIFFERENTIAL DIAGNOSIS

The differential diagnosis of thyroiditis falls into two main categories: goitrous conditions and thyrotoxic conditions that have a low RAIU. These are considered in Tables 85–3 and 85–4. The features that most easily distinguish the various forms of thyroiditis from one another and from toxic diffuse goiter (Graves' disease) are listed in Table 85–5. Ultimate differentiation among the goitrous conditions may necessitate histologic confirmation.

DIAGNOSIS

Thyroid function tests including measurement of the serum T_4 level, the T_3 resin uptake, and the serum level of TSH are usually adequate to define the metabolic state of the patient with thyroiditis. Specific diagnosis relies on tests that reflect inflammation and the presence or absence of thyroid autoantibodies (Table 85–5). Antithyroglobulin or antimicrosomal antibodies or both are elevated in almost all cases of CLT. As indicators of inflammation, the ESR and leukocyte counts are often useful in diagnosing acute suppurative and subacute thyroiditis. Measurement of RAIU can be helpful in separating the thyrotoxicosis of thyroiditis from the much more common diffuse toxic goiter in which uptake values are increased. The RAIU in thyroiditis is usually suppressed to less than 8% at 24 hours.

Thyroid scanning provides little useful information. Specimens from a needle-aspiration

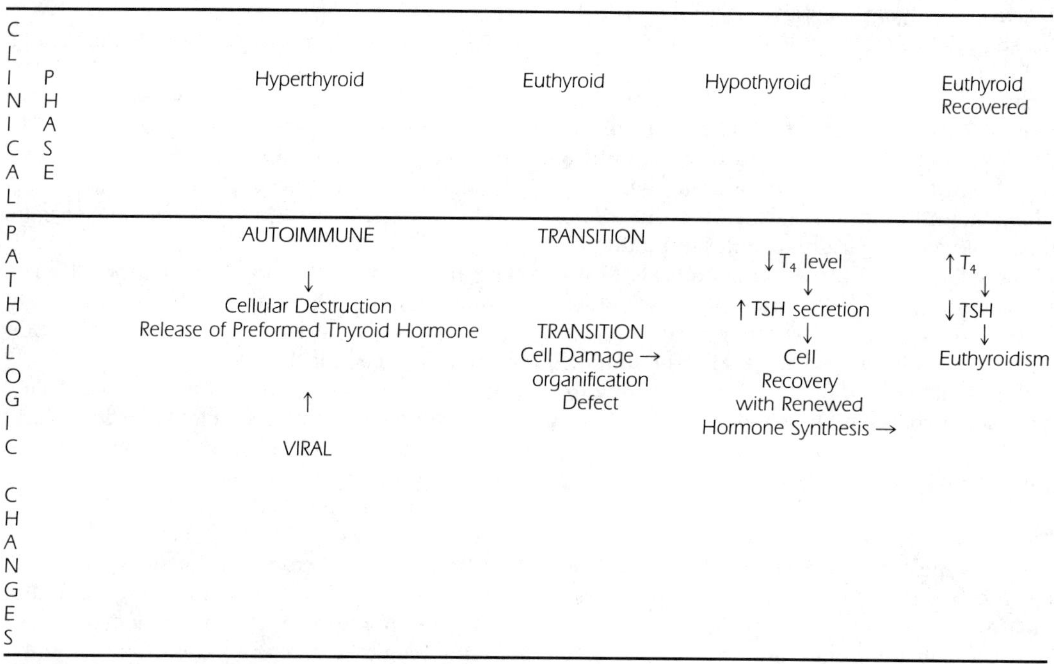

FIG 85–2.
Clinical–pathologic correlations in subacute thyroiditis.

biopsy, although rarely necessary, may be useful to distinguish thyroiditis from malignancy and to define infiltrative conditions. These key features are listed in Table 85–5.

PRINCIPLES OF TREATMENT

The therapeutic approach to the patient with thyroiditis depends on the specific pathologic changes. AST requires appropriate antibiotic therapy, in addition to surgical intervention for abscess drainage or for fistula excision. SubT requires only symptomatic therapy because it usually resolves spontaneously. The pain of SubT usually responds well to salicylates. Resistant cases may require glucocorticoid treatment for 2 to 3 weeks. Propranolol is useful in treating the symptoms attributed to hyperthyroxinemia, and short-term administration of levothyroxine may be required for significant symptoms observed during the hypothyroid period.

Patients with CLT may have little prospect of regaining normal thyroid function and consequently benefit from levothyroxine therapy titrated to reduce the TSH value into the normal range to avoid significant clinical or biochemical signs of overreplacement (thyrotoxicosis medicamentosa).

Surgical intervention for symptomatic relief of goiter associated with dysphagia, stridor, or hoarseness may be indicated when the thyroid in CLT is unresponsive to thyroid hormone therapy. The rarely encountered Riedel's struma, however, commonly requires surgical removal to relieve the compression symptoms caused by extensive fibrosis.

TABLE 85–3.
Differential Diagnosis of Common Goitrous Conditions

GOITROUS CONDITION	THYROID STATE
Simple diffuse goiter	Euthyroid
Nodular goiter	Euthyroid
Cancerous goiter	Euthyroid
Riedel's thyroiditis	Euthyroid/hypothyroid
Acute suppurative thyroiditis	Euthyroid
Hashimoto's thyroiditis	Hypothyroid
Subacute thyroiditis	Hyperthyroid/hypothyroid
Graves' disease	Hyperthyroid
Lymphoma	Euthyroid

TABLE 85–4.
Differential Diagnosis of Thyrotoxicosis with Decreased RAI Uptake

TYPE OF THYROTOXICOSIS	GOITER	IODINE LEVEL	THYROGLOBULIN LEVEL	24 HOUR RAIU	SED RATE	CLINICAL FINDING
Subacute thyroiditis (painful, painless)	+	Nℓ	High	< 8%	High	Fever, leukocytosis
Iodine-induced thyrotoxicosis (jodbasedow)	+	High	High	Low	Var	Often MNG* by history
Exogenous iodine ingestion in Graves' disease	+	High	High	Low	Var	Infiltrative eye disease
Exogenous thyroid hormone ingestion (thyrotoxicosis facticia)	θ	Nℓ	Low	Low	Nℓ	Typically medical personnel
Ectopic thyroid tissue	θ	Nℓ	High	Ectopic	Nℓ	Consider lingual goiter
Struma ovarii	θ	Nℓ	High	Pelvis	Nℓ	Pelvic mass
Functioning metastasis from thyroid malignancy	θ	Nℓ	High	Ectopic	Nℓ	History of thyroid carcinoma frequent

* MNG = multinodular goiter.

TABLE 85–5.
Differential Diagnosis of Major Thyroid Diseases as Gauged by Typical Findings

	HASHIMOTO'S THYROIDITIS	DE QUERVAIN'S THYROIDITIS	SILENT THYROIDITIS	ACUTE SUPPURATIVE THYROIDITIS	RIEDEL'S THYROIDITIS	GRAVES' DISEASE
GOITER						
Type	Diffuse	Diffuse	Diffuse	Focal	Diffuse	Diffuse
Consistency	Firm	Firm	Firm	Fluctuant	Hard	Spongy
Pain on palpation	No	Yes	No	Yes	No	No
Local compressive symptoms*	No	No	No	No	Yes	No
Associated lymphadenopathy	No	No	No	Yes	No	No
THYROID STATE						
Hyperthyroid	No	Yes (early)	Yes (early)	No	No	Yes
Hypothyroid	Yes	Yes (late)	Yes (late)	No	No	No
24-HOUR RADIOACTIVE IODINE						
UPTAKE (Nℓ = 10%–25%)	Variable	Low (< 8%)	Low (< 8%)	Normal	Low	Elevated (> 30%)
SYSTEMIC SYMPTOMS						
Acute onset	No	Yes	Yes	Yes	No	No
Fever	No	Variable	No	Yes	No	Variable
Prodromal syndrome	No	Yes	No	No	No	No
ESR elevated	No	Yes	Variable	Yes	No	Yes
Leukocytosis	No	Yes	No	Yes	No	No
ASSOCIATED FINDINGS						
Sex ratio of incidence F > M	Yes	Yes	Yes	No	Yes	Yes
Known significant autoantibody titers	Yes	No	No	No	+/−	Yes
HLA haplotype-associated	B8, DR5	Bw35	DR4	No	No	B8, DR3 (Caucasians); Bw46 (Chinese); Bw35 (Japanese)
Associated with other autoimmune disease	Yes	No	No	No	No	Yes
PRIMARY TREATMENT						
Medical	Yes	Yes	Yes	Yes	No	Yes
Surgical	No	No	No	Yes	Yes	Yes

* Dysphagia, dyspnea, hoarseness.

REFERENCES

Hamburger JI: The various presentations of thyroiditis. *Ann Intern Med* 1986; 104:219–224. *Brief recent review from voluminous clinical experience.*

Hay ID: Thyroiditis: A clinical update. *Mayo Clin Proc* 1985; 60:836–843. *Review of experience with thyroiditis at the Mayo Clinic.*

Hayashi Y, Tamai H, Fukata S et al: A long-term clinical, immunologic, and histologic follow-up study of patients with goitrous chronic lymphocytic thyroiditis. *J Clin Endocrinol Metab* 1985; 61(6): 1172–1178. *Most up-to-date discussion of the natural course of treated and untreated disease.*

Ingbar SH: The thyroid gland, in Williams RH (ed): *Textbook of Endocrinology.* Philadelphia, WB Saunders Co, 1985, pp 682–815. *The standard reference textbook for general clinical endocrinology.*

Nikolai TF, Coombs GJ, McKenzie AK: Lymphocytic thyroiditis with spontaneously resolving hyperthyroidism and subacute thyroiditis. Long-term follow-up. *Arch Intern Med* 1981; 141:1455–1458. *A 15-year follow-up study on the natural history of subacute thyroiditis.*

Strakosch CR, Wenzel BE, Row VV, Volpe R: Immunology of autoimmune thyroid diseases. *N Engl J Med* 1982; 307(24):1499–1507. *Understandable review of the complexities of thyroid immunology from one of the world's premier laboratories in that area.*

Volpe R: Pathogenesis of autoimmune thyroid disease, in Werner SC, Ingbar SH (eds): *The Thyroid: A Fundamental and Clinical Text,* ed 5. Philadelphia, JB Lippincott, 1986, pp 747–767. *Widely accepted to be the best of only a few complete books on the thyroid.*

Volpe R, Row VV, Ezrin C: Circulating viral and thyroid antibodies in subacute thyroiditis. *J Clin Endocrinol Metab* 1967; 27:1275–1284. *One of many studies by Volpe's group outlining the pathophysiology of subacute thyroiditis.*

Woolf PD: Transient painless thyroiditis with hyperthyroidism: A variant of lymphocytic thyroiditis? *Endocrinol Rev* 1980; 1(4):411–420. *Clinical cyclicity of thyroiditis discussed with data from many studies.*

86 ADRENAL CRISIS

James W. Agna, M.D.

Adrenal crisis is an overwhelming, life-endangering disorder due to a deficiency of adrenal corticosteroids. It occurs in patients with primary adrenal insufficiency from disease of the adrenal cortex or in patients with secondary adrenal insufficiency from lack of adrenocorticotrophic hormone (ACTH) due to disease or dysfunction of the hypothalamus or the pituitary gland. Patients stressed by trauma, surgery, or sepsis whose hypothalamic-pituitary-adrenal axis is incapable of producing adequate amounts of adrenal corticosteroids are prone to adrenal crisis. In primary and secondary insufficiency most signs and symptoms are attributable to a lack of glucocorticoids (cortisol). The renin-angiotensin system instead of ACTH controls production of mineralocorticoids (aldosterone). Therefore, a lack of mineralocorticoids does not occur in secondary insufficiency but accounts for the signs and symptoms related to alterations in sodium, potassium, and hydrogen ion concentration in primary insufficiency.

CLINICAL SIGNS AND SYMPTOMS

Patients with adrenal crisis frequently have weakness, confusion, anorexia, nausea, vomiting, and abdominal or flank pain. They are hypotensive, often have fever, and have evidence of dehydration. If untreated, shock and vascular collapse develop rapidly. The signs and symptoms of acute adrenal insufficiency are listed in Table 86–1. Probably the most common cause of acute adrenal insufficiency is secondary to the therapeutic use of corticosteroids in the millions of patients with allergic, neoplastic, and autoimmune diseases. Exogenous steroids taken for prolonged periods suppress ACTH release resulting in adrenal cortical atrophy. Thus a large population is at risk for secondary insufficiency and adrenal crisis. The insufficiency may persist for a year or more after steroid intake is discontinued.

Adrenal crisis occurs also in patients with known or unrecognized chronic primary adrenal insufficiency. Hyperpigmentation of the skin and mucous membranes is a sign that often alerts the clinician to a predisposing chronic insufficiency. The signs and symptoms and their relative frequency in chronic primary insufficiency are listed in Table 86–2. Because a significant number of patients with primary adrenal cortical insufficiency have an autoimmune disease with associated manifestations of gonadal failure, hypoparathyroidism, hypothyroidism, hyperthyroidism, Hashimoto's thyroiditis, diabetes mellitus, vitiligo, or pernicious anemia, evidence of these disorders in the history or physical examination may be helpful in establishing the diagnosis of adrenal crisis. Likewise a history of tuberculosis,

TABLE 86–1.
Signs and Symptoms of Acute Adrenal Insufficiency

Weakness
Fever
Hypotension
Hypoglycemia
Tachycardia
Anorexia, nausea, vomiting
Abdominal or flank pain
Confusion, coma
Hyponatremia, hyperkalemia, hypovolemia*

* More likely in primary insufficiency.

trauma, infection, anticoagulant therapy, and other clinical states listed in Table 86–3 may lead to early recognition of primary or secondary adrenal crisis.

Often clinical clues are not readily apparent, leading to a delay in recognition of the crisis. This circumstance occurs frequently in the emergency department, the recovery room, or the intensive care unit. When a patient has fever, nausea, vomiting, confusion, and hypotension disproportionate for the initial clinical problem, adrenal crisis should be considered as a possible cause of the clinical deterioration of the patient.

PATHOPHYSIOLOGY

Secondary adrenocortical insufficiency is due to disease or dysfunction of the hypothalamus or pituitary resulting in ACTH deficiency, adrenal atrophy, and decreased cortisol secretion. The suppression of ACTH by glucocorticoid therapy is the most common cause of secondary insufficiency. Destructive infiltrative diseases of the hypothalamic-pituitary region (neoplasms, infections, granulomas) may cause secondary (ACTH) insufficiency. These pathologic processes are often also associated with decreased secretion of growth hormone, gonadotropin, and thyrotropin (panhypopituitarism). ACTH deficiency from hemorrhage or from infarction due to hypotension or hypoxia will lead to similar manifestations. Postpartum ACTH deficiency is referred to as Sheehan's syndrome. A rare syndrome is isolated ACTH deficiency.

With ACTH deficiency, cortisol secretion is decreased, but aldosterone secretion is normal because aldosterone production in the zona glomerulosa is controlled by the renin-angiotensin system and not by ACTH. Therefore, in secondary adrenal insufficiency hyperkalemia and acidosis are not characteristic. Hypoglycemia is often profound and the overriding clinical manifestation. The lack of cortisol in secondary insufficiency may cause a mild hyponatremia from renal loss of sodium and retention of water, the latter from enhancement of the effect of antidiuretic hormone due to cortisol deficiency. Because of a lack of ACTH and β-lipotropin, which shares a common precursor with ACTH, patients with secondary insufficiency do not have hyperpigmentation.

Primary adrenocortical insufficiency occurs when there is a loss of function of more than 90% of both adrenal cortices. Prior to the acute manifestations, there is usually a gradual destruction of the adrenals with clinical manifestations of chronic insufficiency (Table 86–2). The production of both glucocorticoids (cortisol) and mineralocorticoids (aldosterone) is affected. The hormonal secretion may be adequate for normal activities, but the stress of surgery, trauma, or infection results in adrenal crisis. Destruction of the adrenals by hemorrhage or infarction causes adrenal insufficiency abruptly. Although a number of conditions are associated with adrenal hemorrhage, most patients with adrenal hemorrhage at autopsy did not before death have evidence to document or suggest the presence of acute adrenocortical insufficiency during their terminal illness.

Cortisol deficiency results in impaired gluconeogenesis, glycogen depletion, impaired fat mobilization and utilization, and hypoglycemia. There is an impaired response to catecholamines, decreased cardiac output, hypotension, and an impaired ability to excrete "free water." These disorders are common to both primary and secondary adrenal insufficiency. A concomitant aldosterone deficiency in primary adrenal disease results in the inability to conserve sodium and to secrete potassium and hydrogen ions by the kidney. Hyponatremia, hyperkalemia, and acidosis ensue. The disorder of sodium metabolism causes hypovolemia, hypotension, postural syncope, and shock. Impaired secretion of hydrogen and potassium ions leads to acidosis and hyperkalemia and may result in cardiac arrest.

CLINICAL–PATHOLOGIC CORRELATIONS

Some clinical-pathologic correlations are listed in Table 86–4. Major factors accounting for the clinical manifestations of adrenal insufficiency and adrenal crisis are deficiencies of cortisol or aldosterone production or both.

DIFFERENTIAL DIAGNOSIS

Cases of shock due to sepsis, trauma, drug overdose, myocardial infarction, massive gastroenteric bleeding, or hypoglycemia may

TABLE 86–2.

Occurrence of Signs and Symptoms of Chronic Primary Adrenal Insufficiency

IN ABOUT 90% OF PATIENTS
Weakness
Anorexia
Weight loss
Hyperpigmentation
Hypotension
Electrolyte derangement
IN ABOUT 50% OF PATIENTS
Gastrointestinal symptoms
Hypoglycemia
IN ABOUT 25% OF PATIENTS
Associated disorders (thyroid, parathyroid, ovarian, pancreatic)
IN LESS THAN 20% OF PATIENTS
Salt craving
Postural symptoms
Vitiligo

TABLE 86–3.

Classification of Adrenocortical Insufficiency According to Cause

SECONDARY INSUFFICIENCY (ACTH DEFICIENCY)
Hypothalamic-pituitary disorders
Acute
Hemorrhage or infarction
Trauma
Hypotension
Infection
Atherosclerosis
Chronic
Glucocorticoid therapy
Tumor (pituitary or suprasellar)
Infiltrative and granulomatoris diseases
Aneurysm
Isolated ACTH deficiency (rare)
PRIMARY INSUFFICIENCY (ACTH EXCESS)
Adrenal cortical diseases
Acute
Hemorrhage or infarction
Trauma
Sepsis
Coagulopathy (anticoagulant therapy)
Adrenal vein thrombosis
Chronic
Autoimmune disease
Infection (tuberculous, fungous)
Infiltrative (granuloma, neoplasm)
Congenital adrenal hyperplasia (enzyme defect)
Cytotoxic agents

TABLE 86—4.
Clinical—Pathologic Correlations of Adrenal Crisis

CLINICAL FINDINGS	PATHOLOGIC FINDINGS	
	CORTISOL DEFICIENCY	ALDOSTERONE DEFICIENCY
Fever	+	−
Hypoglycemia	+	−
Anorexia	+	−
Nausea, vomiting	+	−
Abdominal pain	+	−
Hypotension, shock	+	+
Apathy, confusion, coma	+	+
Weakness	+	+
Hyponatremia	+	+
Hypovolemia	−	+
Postural syncope	−	+
Acidosis	−	+
Hyperkalemia	−	+

simulate or be associated with adrenal insufficiency. These conditions predispose to accelerated utilization of corticosteroids with subsequent feedback stimulation of ACTH, causing intensive adrenocortical stimulation. Focal and diffuse hemorrhages of the adrenal cortex have been found in stressed patients, some with adrenal insufficiency, but others with elevated plasma cortisol levels. When the clinical condition is confusing and adrenal crisis is suspected, cortisol therapy has been instituted in critical states until a more accurate assessment of adrenocortical function can be determined. If the patient has a history of weakness, anorexia, weight loss, and hyperpigmentation, the differential diagnosis includes chronic illnesses such as malabsorption, cirrhosis, chronic renal disease, anorexia nervosa, hemochromatosis, malnutrition, dermatomyositis, acanthosis nigricans, the use of certain drugs and heavy metal poisoning.

DIAGNOSIS

In adrenocortical insufficiency, abnormal results of several laboratory tests may be suggestive but are not diagnostic of the disorder (see Table 86–5). Significant hypoglycemia is common to both primary and secondary adrenocortical insufficiency, whereas electrolyte derangements, especially hyperkalemia and acidosis, are more commonly observed in primary adrenal insufficiency. However, if the patient's disease develops suddenly as a result of hemorrhage or infarction, or if the patient is on maintenance therapy for known adrenal insufficiency and has become acutely stressed, many of these suggestive laboratory values will be normal. Hypercalcemia due to decreased cortisol levels and impaired renal perfusion is a rare but dramatic manifestation of adrenocortical insufficiency.

Basal plasma and urine concentrations of corticosteroids are not diagnostic because various degrees of adrenocortical insufficiency may exist. Furthermore, the plasma cortisol level with its wide normal range may not exclude the diagnosis of acute adrenocortical insufficiency. High levels of plasma cortisol under stress make the diagnosis of adrenocortical insufficiency less likely, however.

Specific assessment of adrenocortical reserve and delineation of primary from secondary adrenocortical insufficiency involve the assessment of plasma and urine cortisol concentration after rapid and prolonged ACTH stimulation tests and measurement of plasma ACTH concentration (see Table 86–5). In patients with known adrenocortical insufficiency, these tests are not required, but for suspected cases they are imperative. A normal plasma cortisol response to a rapid ACTH stimulation test (30 to 60 minutes) rules out primary adrenocortical insufficiency, but it does not exclude the possibility of decreased ACTH reserve or secondary

TABLE 86–5.
Laboratory Tests in the Diagnosis of Adrenocortical Insufficiency

I ABNORMAL CONDITIONS THAT SUPPORT THE DIAGNOSIS

Hypoglycemia
Hyponatremia
Hyperkalemia
Acidosis
Azotemia
Eosinophilia
Lymphocytosis
Hypercalcemia

II ABNORMAL VALUES THAT SUGGEST THE DIAGNOSIS

Laboratory Finding	Diagnosis
Low plasma cortisol and high plasma ACTH levels	Primary insufficiency
Low plasma cortisol and normal or low plasma ACTH levels	Secondary insufficiency

III DIAGNOSTIC TESTS THAT CONFIRM THE DIAGNOSIS

Diagnostic Test	Subnormal Response	Normal Response
Rapid (30–60 min) ACTH stimulation test	Primary or secondary insufficiency	Excludes primary but not secondary insufficiency
Prolonged (3 day) ACTH stimulation test	Primary insufficiency	Possible secondary insufficiency
Metyrapone or insulin-induced hypoglycemia test	Secondary insufficiency	Excludes secondary insufficiency

insufficiency. During the period of diagnostic testing, the patient is treated with appropriate fluid replacement and dexamethasone, which does not interfere with the diagnostic testing. Prolonged infusion of ACTH (3 days) resulting in increased cortisol concentration excludes the diagnosis of primary adrenocortical insufficiency; lack of a response to ACTH establishes the diagnosis. At the time of initial assessment, an elevated plasma ACTH is indicative of primary adrenocortical insufficiency, whereas a normal or low level is indicative of secondary adrenocortical insufficiency. Further evaluation of ACTH reserve may be determined by metyrapone or insulin-induced hypoglycemia tests.

PRINCIPLES OF PREVENTION AND THERAPY

Recognition of the need for supplementary glucocorticoids during periods of stress for patients on treatment for adrenal insufficiency will prevent adrenal crisis. This is especially important in patients with known compromised adrenal reserve who are undergoing surgery or who have severe infections. The treatment of acute adrenocortical insufficiency includes intravenous hydrocortisone, saline, and glucose, careful monitoring, correction of precipitating factors, and general supportive measures. In most cases the use of potent mineralocorticoids is not necessary.

REFERENCES

Bondy PK: Adrenocortical insufficiency, in Wilson JD, Foster DW (eds): *Williams Textbook of Endocrinology,* ed 7. Philadelphia, WB Saunders Co, 1985, pp 851–858. *A succinct discussion of the subject in seventh edition of a standard textbook.*

Crigler JF Jr, Gang DL: Case records of the Massachusetts General Hospital. *N Engl Med* 1985; 312:976–983. *Case presentation and excellent discussion of adrenal crisis with emphasis on autoimmune processes involving adrenal as well as other endocrine glands.*

Leshin M: Acute adrenal insufficiency: Recognition, management, and prevention. *Urol Clin North Am* 1982; 9:229–235. *Excellent review of adrenal crisis with important discussion of prevention.*

Nerup J: Addison's disease—clinical studies. A report

of 108 cases. *Acta Endocrino (Copenh)* 1974; 76:127–141. *Emphasizes the "idiopathic" etiology, the frequency of signs and symptoms, and the associated autoimmune diseases.*

Passmore JM Jr: Adrenal cortex, in Geelhoed GW, Chernow B (eds): *Endocrine Aspects of Acute Illness.* New York, Churchill Livingstone, 1985, pp 97–134. *Thorough current review of adrenal crisis with extensive references.*

Shapiro M, Zalewski S, Steiner Z et al: Adrenal insufficiency in a general hospital over a 14 year period. *Isr J Med Sci* 1984; 20:381–387. *Representative spectrum of causes of primary and secondary insufficiency.*

Xarli VP, Steele AA, David PJ, Buescher ES, Rios CN, Garcia-Bunuel R: Adrenal hemorrhage in the adult. *Medicine* 1978; 57:211–221. *Thorough review with emphasis on low incidence of adrenal insufficiency with adrenal hemorrhage.*

87 DIABETES MELLITUS

Stephen D. McDonald, M.D.

Diabetes mellitus, a disease first described over 3400 years ago in Egypt, is the most commonly seen endocrine disorder in the United States. It is currently considered to be a heterogeneous group of metabolic disorders that have in common the presence of hyperglycemia which usually results from an absolute or relative lack of insulin. The presence of hyperglycemia chronically over a number of years may lead to degenerative conditions of the vascular and nervous systems.

A classification of diabetes mellitus has been developed by the National Diabetes Data Group of the National Institutes of Health (Table 87–1). Two major types of diabetes mellitus are now recognized: type I, insulin-dependent diabetes mellitus (IDDM), and type II, noninsulin-dependent diabetes mellitus (NIDDM).

Type I disease is characterized by a severe lack of insulin and a tendency to develop life-threatening ketoacidosis. Patients with this disorder are dependent on exogenous insulin to prevent death. This type of diabetes was formerly called juvenile-onset diabetes and accounts for approximately 10% to 15% of all cases. It is now known that this type of diabetes may occur at any age, but it usually has an abrupt onset of signs and symptoms before age 40 years.

Type II diabetes mellitus is characterized by a less severe insulin deficiency, and indeed some patients may have hyperinsulinemia. This type of diabetes was formerly known as maturity or adult-onset. It is generally diagnosed in patients over the age of 40 years but may occur at any age. This type of diabetes accounts for 85% to 90% of the diabetes in the United States and is associated with obesity in 60% to 80% of the patients. Patients with type II diabetes are not dependent on insulin for survival, although it may be required to control the symptoms of hyperglycemia that persist despite other forms of therapy.

Hyperglycemia may occur in association with other medical conditions or syndromes. These are classified as "other types of diabetes mellitus" (Table 87–1).

Alterations of glucose homeostasis that do not meet the criteria established for the diagnosis of diabetes mellitus should not be designated as diabetes, but rather classified according to the criteria for impaired glucose

TABLE 87–1.
Classification of Diabetes Mellitus and Impaired Glucose Tolerance*

CURRENT TERMS	FORMER TERMS (NO LONGER RECOMMENDED)
1. *Diabetes mellitus*	
a. *Type I*	Juvenile-onset diabetes
Insulin-dependent (IDDM)	
b. *Type II*	Adult-onset diabetes
Noninsulin-dependent (NIDDM)	
c. *Other types of diabetes mellitus*	Secondary diabetes
2. *Impaired glucose tolerance*	Chemical diabetes
	Borderline diabetes
	Subclinical diabetes
3. *Gestational diabetes mellitus*	
4. *Previous abnormality of glucose tolerance*	Subclinical diabetes

* Adapted from National Diabetes Data Group: Classification and diagnosis of diabetes mellitus and other classes of glucose intolerance. *Diabetes* 1979; 28:1042–1043.

tolerance. Hyperglycemia that begins or is discovered during pregnancy is appropriately classified as "gestational diabetes mellitus." Patients who have a normal glucose tolerance but a history of transient diabetes mellitus or impaired glucose tolerance are categorized as having "previous abnormality of glucose tolerance."

CLINICAL SIGNS AND SYMPTOMS

Patients with type I diabetes mellitus often present with an abrupt onset of polyuria, polydypsia, and polyphagia ("the poly's"). Patients with severe insulin deficiency may present in ketoacidosis. Other symptoms include weight loss, fatigue, unexplained infection, and dehydration. Patients with type II diabetes often are asymptomatic, in which case the disease is usually diagnosed by identifying hyperglycemia on routine blood testing. Other patients with type II disease may present with symptoms of hyperglycemia similar to those found in type I diabetes. Occasionally type II diabetes remains undiagnosed for years until a vascular or nervous system complication prompts the physician to look for hyperglycemia.

Early in the course of diabetes mellitus, the typical patient has few, if any, physical findings of hyperglycemia. Patients with type I diabetes may present with one or more of the acute manifestations of diabetic ketoacidosis: decreased level of consciousness, rapid deep respirations, fruity odor to the breath, abdominal tenderness, and dehydration. With a profound depletion of extracellular fluid, the patient may have dry mucous membranes and postural hypotension.

Late in the course of diabetes, patients may have numerous physical findings associated with complications of the disease (e.g., atherosclerosis, retinopathy, and neurologic deficits), particularly numbness and loss of vibratory sensation in the lower extremities.

NATURAL HISTORY

The early descriptions of diabetes mellitus dramatically depict the acute demise of patients who lacked insulin and died during the acute metabolic crisis of ketoacidosis. Others who presented with polyuria and polydypsia were treated with a diet regimen and most lived no longer than 1 to 2 years. With the discovery and beginning clinical use of insulin in 1921, there has been a dramatic decrease in the number of deaths from ketoacidosis. However, the use of insulin has not prevented the chronic complications of hyperglycemia. Those diabetic patients living 10 to 15 years after diagnosis have been plagued with the chronic complications of diabetes mellitus, particularly complications of the cardiovascular and renal systems, and microvascular retinopathy.

The chronic complications are similar in type I and type II disease. They are generally seen when the disease has been present for more than 10 or 15 years. Diabetic retinopathy is the leading cause of new onset blindness in the United States, with diabetic patients being 25 times more susceptible to blindness. Renal failure is 15 times more common in diabetic patients, myocardial infarctions 5 times more common, and peripheral vascular disease 20 times more common than in the nondiabetics. Patients with diabetes generally die of renal failure, cardiovascular complications, or infection related to peripheral vascular complications.

PATHOPHYSIOLOGY

Both type I and type II diabetes mellitus are characterized by a lack of insulin effect, in the former case because of absolute insulin deficiency and in the latter because of a relative resistance to the effect of insulin. Insulin has numerous physiologic effects. In adipose tissue it promotes glucose utilization and lipogenesis. It inhibits lipolysis resulting in lower plasma levels of glucose, triglycerides, and free fatty acids. In muscle, insulin inhibits proteolysis and promotes glucose utilization leading to increased levels of glycogen. In the liver insulin promotes glycogenesis and inhibits gluconeogenesis and glycogenolysis. These effects contribute to decreased plasma levels of glucose and the preservation of tissue and liver glycogen stores. Glucose use by muscle requires more circulating insulin than does the inhibition of lipolysis and proteolysis. This explains why patients with moderate insulin deficits have hyperglycemia whereas those with absolute insulin deficiency develop marked lipolysis and ketoacidosis. Glucagon is also an important hormone in the development of diabetes and in particular ketoacidosis.

Glucagon and insulin in nondiabetic patients have a reciprocal relationship. Glucagon is suppressed by small increases in insulin concentration, and insulin secretion is stimulated by increases in glucagon concentrations.

When tissues need glucose, the insulin level falls and the glucagon level rises, promoting glycogen breakdown in the liver and an increase in free fatty acid and ketone levels in the blood. During glucose intake, insulin secretion is stimulated thus suppressing glucagon secretion and enhancing glycogenesis in the liver and lipogenesis in the adipose tissue.

Type I diabetes is considered to result from destruction of the beta cells of the pancreatic islets. This appears to be an autoimmune phenomenon that develops in susceptible individuals. The susceptibility to islet cell destruction appears to be determined by the histocompatibility allelic genes found on chromosome six. Patients who express the high-risk HLA alleles DR3 and DR4 have the highest risk of type I diabetes, more than 20 times the risk of those without these alleles.

Type II diabetes generally does not involve a primary islet-cell destruction. There is now, however, evidence for abnormal islet cell function and in addition there is convincing evidence that patients with type II have a resistance to the glucoregulatory effects of insulin in these patients. This is most prominent in the obese patient with type II diabetes. Insulin's effect is mediated by specific insulin receptors on the cell membrane. Some patients with type II diabetes have decreased numbers of insulin receptors. Other type II patients who have not been found to have decreased numbers of receptors are considered to have postreceptor defects in insulin action.

CLINICAL–PATHOLOGIC CORRELATIONS

The acute features of diabetes, hyperglycemia, and ketoacidosis are the result of insulin deficiency. The hallmark of long-standing diabetes is the presence of microvascular changes. This involves the capillaries throughout the body but predominantly the vasculature of the eye and kidney. Atherosclerotic vascular lesions of the large vessels are more prominent in the diabetic and are a major cause of the morbidity and mortality from coronary and peripheral artery disease.

The pathogenetic mechanisms of chronic diabetic complications are not entirely clear. The causes of the various complications may be different. Three major mechanisms have been suggested: (1) the glycosylation of proteins leading to structural and functional changes throughout the body; (2) the polyol metabolic pathway in which glucose is reduced by aldose reductase to sorbitol, which, when present in the retina, kidney, and nerve cells, may cause damage; (3) the hemodynamic hypothesis, which suggests that blood flow is increased early in the course of type I diabetes, causing increased hydrostatic pressure in the capillary beds, leading to damage of the vascular endothelial proteins. All three mechanisms may be important in the overall development of the chronic complications in diabetes.

DIFFERENTIAL DIAGNOSIS

Diabetes mellitus is the most likely cause of fasting hyperglycemia. Certain other conditions, however, may lead to frank hyperglycemia or impaired glucose tolerance (Tables 87–2 and 87–3). The diagnosis of diabetes mellitus in a patient who has symptoms of hyperglycemia is easily confirmed by finding fasting hyperglycemia. A plasma glucose level during fasting that is greater than 140 mg/dl on two separate occasions is sufficient for the diagnosis of diabetes mellitus. The accepted criteria for the diagnosis of diabetes are listed in Table 87–4.

For defining milder forms of glucose intoler-

TABLE 87–2.
Possible Causes Other Than Diabetes Mellitus of Hyperglycemia or Impaired Glucose Tolerance*

BROAD CATEGORY	SPECIFIC EXAMPLE
Pancreatic disease	Cystic fibrosis
	Chronic pancreatitis
	Hemochromatosis
Endocrine conditions	Cushing's syndrome
	Acromegaly
	Pheochromocytoma
	Hyperthyroidism
	Glucagonoma
Drugs	Alcohol
	Thiazide diuretics
	Estrogens
	Glucocorticoids
Miscellaneous conditions	Pregnancy
	Malnutrition
	Liver disease
	Renal failure

* Adapted from National Diabetes Data Group: Classification and diagnosis of diabetes mellitus and other classes of glucose intolerance. *Diabetes* 1979; 28:1045–1046.

TABLE 87–3.
Pathophysiologic Mechanisms in Diabetes Mellitus and Hyperglycemic States

CLINICAL CONDITION	PATHOLOGIC MECHANISMS
Type I diabetes mellitus	Autoimmune: associated HLA DR3, DR4 alleles; insulin antibodies; absolute insulin deficiency
Type II diabetes mellitus	Relative resistance to insulin action; decreased insulin receptors; postreceptor defects
Endocrine diseases	
Cushing's syndrome, acromegaly	Excess counterregulatory hormones perhaps related to insulin resistance
Hyperthyroidism	Unknown
Pheochromocytoma	Catecholamine-induced glycogenolysis
Aldosteronism	Hypokalemia inhibits insulin secretion.
Glucagonoma	Excess glucagon suppresses insulin secretion.
Acanthosis nigricans	Insulin-receptor deficiency; insulin-receptor antibody
Pancreatic disease	Loss, destruction, or removal of pancreatic islets leading to insulin deficiency
Cystic fibrosis	
Hemochromatosis	
Pancreatitis	
Pancreatectomy	
Medications	
Glucocorticoids	Increase gluconeogenesis
Thiazide diuretics	Potassium depletion inhibits insulin secretion.
Sympathomimetic agents	Increase glycogenolysis
Oral contraceptives	Unknown; probably causes peripheral resistance to insulin action

TABLE 87–4.

Criteria for the Diagnosis of Diabetes Mellitus and Impaired Glucose Tolerance in Nonpregnant Adults*

| | VENOUS PLASMA GLUCOSE CONCENTRATION (mg/dl)[†] | | |
DIAGNOSIS	FASTING	OGTT[‡](2 HR)	OGTT (1/2, 1, OR 1-1/2 HR)
Normal	< 115	< 140	< 200
Diabetes	≥ 140 or	≥ 200	≥ 200
Impaired glucose tolerance	< 140	140–200	≥ 200

* Adapted from National Diabetes Data Group: Classification and diagnosis of diabetes mellitus and other classes of glucose tolerance. *Diabetes* 1979; 28:1049.

[†] Values that do not fit into the defined categories would be considered non-diagnostic.

[‡] Oral glucose tolerance test.

ance, the oral glucose tolerance test has been widely used. Because of the wide variety of conditions affecting glucose tolerance, this test, to be useful, must be done according to an established protocol in otherwise healthy individuals. Glucose tolerance testing to diagnose diabetes mellitus is not recommended in patients who have fasting hyperglycemia, are acutely ill, or are hospitalized for other illness. Patients taking medications such as diuretics, beta-adrenergic blockers, phenytoin, glucocorticoids, or estrogens should not have a glucose tolerance test because these drugs interfere with the test results. For the test, the patient is given a 75-gm glucose load after an 8-hour fast preceded by at least 3 days of an unrestricted diet. Blood glucose levels are then determined every 30 minutes for the 2 hours after administration of the glucose. Patients who do not specifically meet the established National Diabetes Data Group criteria (Table 87–4) should not be classified as having diabetes mellitus. Glycohemoglobin levels are generally not considered to be useful in the diagnosis of diabetes mellitus but are useful in the management of those who have been determined to have the disease.

PRINCIPLES OF PREVENTION AND THERAPY

The goal of diabetic treatment is to help the patient remain symptom free, to achieve a near-normal metabolic state including a normal or near-normal fasting plasma glucose, and to prevent the chronic complications of the disease. Long-term control of blood glucose levels may delay or prevent the development of complications, although this has not been rigorously proven. Evidence that close control reverses complications is lacking. It is reasonable, however, to attempt to normalize blood glucose levels.

The mainstays of diabetes therapy are diet, exercise, insulin, and oral sulfonylurea hypoglycemic agents. In type I diabetics who are insulin deficient, insulin must be used to maintain life. The goal is to balance the dietary caloric intake with the level of insulin and physical activity. Insulin is given in an effort to mimic the normal secretion of insulin in response to meals. Because most type I diabetic patients are not overweight, adequate calories must be maintained to prevent weight loss. In the type I diabetics, great care should be taken to prevent hypoglycemia with appropriate insulin adjustments and the proper timing of meals and snacks. In the type II, or non-insulin dependent, diabetes, proper dietary measures and consistent exercise to achieve an "ideal" body weight are generally the management of choice, using the oral hypoglycemic agents and insulin as adjunctive measures. If the patient is taking oral hypoglycemics, care should be taken to ensure that he or she does not develop refractory hypoglycemia.

Appropriate diabetes education is the cornerstone of effective long-term management of all types of diabetes. Active involvement of the patient is necessary to ensure that the unique aspects of the individual's type of diabetes and life-style are addressed and managed. In the past, diabetic patients have adjusted their insulin dosage on the basis of urine glucose testing. However, because of the wide fluctuations in values, frequent changes in renal function, and poor accuracy, this measurement is not as beneficial as the use of home blood glucose monitoring. This technique uses a small paper strip impregnated with glucose oxidase and a coloring agent. The patient places capillary blood from a finger stick on the paper strip to determine relatively accurately, visually or with a small machine, his or her actual level of blood glucose. This can be done, if needed, several times throughout the day. This technique provides excellent information for physician and patient in the management of the disease.

Long-term control can now be assessed by laboratory determinations of hemoglobin A1c, a hemoglobin fraction which has been irreversibly glycosylated. The concentration of this glycosylated hemoglobin reflects the average glucose concentration over the previous 6 to 10 weeks, thus giving the physician and patient a better idea of overall control rather than an isolated blood glucose value.

In addition to the ongoing management for glycemic control, the patient and physician must be alert to developing complications. This necessitates a multidisciplinary approach including the primary care physician, an ophthalmologist, a dietitian, a nephrologist if necessary to handle renal complications, a podiatrist to help with foot problems, and occasionally a psychiatrist to handle the dramatic psychosocial issues involved in diabetes. Associated medical conditions such as hypertension and hyperlipidemia require control because they appear to worsen or accelerate the development of the chronic complications. The overall management of diabetes mellitus, to accomplish the goal of near-euglycemia, is a lifelong endeavor requiring a diligent patient and a compassionate, knowledgeable physician.

REFERENCES

American Diabetes Association: *The Physician's Guide to Type II Diabetes (NIDDM) Diagnosis and Treatment.* New York, American Diabetes Association, 1984. *A handy reference guide to the evaluation and management of the most common form of diabetes.*

Davidson JK: *Clinical Diabetes Mellitus: A Problem-Oriented Approach.* New York, Thieme, Inc, 1986. *A comprehensive clinical reference text which is well indexed and provides details of diabetes organizations and aids for clinical care of diabetic patients.*

Eisenbarth GS: Type I diabetes mellitus: A chronic autoimmune disease. *N Engl J Med* 1986; 314:1360–1368. *A recent review of the dramatic advances in the genetics of diabetes mellitus.*

Marble, A et al (eds): *Joslin's Diabetes Mellitus,* ed 12. Philadelphia, Lea & Febiger, 1985. *A comprehensive reference text on all aspects of diabetes mellitus; well-referenced and detailed.*

National Diabetes Data Group: Classification and diagnosis of diabetes mellitus and other classes of glucose intolerance. *Diabetes* 1979; 28:1039–1057. *The basis for the current classification of diabetes mellitus and the proper use of the oral glucose tolerance test.*

Unger RH, Foster D: Diabetes mellitus, in Wilson JD, Foster DW (eds): *Williams Textbook of Endocrinology,* ed 7. Philadephia, WB Saunders Co, 1985, pp 1018–1080. *A detailed chapter on diabetes mellitus in a standard endocrine text with an excellent discussion of genetics and physiology.*

FASTING HYPOGLYCEMIA

Barry A. Warner, D.O.
James V. Hennessey, M.D.

Hypoglycemia is a clinical syndrome in which low levels of blood glucose are associated with symptoms that abate after ingesting glucose. This sequence has been labeled "Whipple's triad." Semantic confusion exists when symptoms are present in the absence of a low glucose level, or when a low glucose level is present without symptoms. Further, confusion arises because the definition of abnormally low glucose levels is sex-dependent. Glucose values less than 50 mg/dL in men who have fasted for 72 hours are more than two standard deviations below the mean. Women's levels, on the other hand, can fall to as low as 30 mg/dl in 24 hours without being more than two standard deviations below the mean. These values are true blood glucose measurements; plasma and serum values are about 15% higher. Fasting hypoglycemia occurs in the postabsorptive state, whereas reactive hypoglycemia occurs in the postprandial period.

CLINICAL SIGNS AND SYMPTOMS

The symptoms of hypoglycemia can be classified as adrenergic (excess sympathetic discharge) and neuroglycopenic (cerebral dysfunction) (Table 88–1). A host of other signs and symptoms may be associated with the disease underlying the hypoglycemia.

In untreated fasting hypoglycemia, the brain's nutrient requirements cannot be met. Brain damage, coma, and eventually death ensue.

PATHOPHYSIOLOGY

The restoration of euglycemia following antecedent hypoglycemia depends on the neural and hormonal factors that alter glucose production and utilization. Normally, this recovery is heralded by an initial rise in glucagon levels with later peaks in epinephrine, growth hormone, cortisol, and norepinephrine levels. These hormone responses result in a marked increase in glucose production, but only a small decrease in glucose utilization. The net effect is normalization of the blood glucose level. Conversely, fasting hypoglycemia is prompted by a decrease in glucose production, an increase in glucose utilization, or both (Table 88–2). The exact alterations in gluconeogenesis and glycogenolysis in most hypoglycemic states are unclear but are probably multifactoral.

Decreased glucose production is exemplified by alcohol-induced hypoglycemia. The oxidation of alcohol proceeds via NAD-dependent steps, thus consuming NAD which is necessary for gluconeogenesis. Because alcohol does not impair glycogenolysis, hypoglycemia occurs when glycogen stores are depleted.

Hormone deficiency as a cause of hypoglycemia is rare in the absence of diabetes mellitus. This is secondary to the redundant counterregulation produced by the interplay of thyroid hormone, glucagon, catecholamines, and cortisol.

During the postabsorptive state, a relative or absolute increase in either endogenous or exogenous insulin necessarily leads to hypoglycemia because glucose utilization in that state is accelerated and glucose production through the breakdown of glycogen and gluconeogenesis is decreased.

CLINICAL–PATHOLOGIC CORELATIONS

The normal response to fasting is outlined in Figure 88–1. If glucose production is inadequate or glucose utilization is excessive, hypoglycemia results. Catecholamine discharge leads to adrenergic symptoms, while an inadequate supply of nutrient to the brain results in neuroglycopenic symptoms (Table 88–1). The type of symptom depends in part on the rate at which the glucose level falls. Adrenergic symptoms predominate during precipitous falls, and neuroglycopenic symptoms predominate during gradual falls or prolonged hypoglycemia.

DIFFERENTIAL DIAGNOSIS

The differential diagnosis is listed in Table 88–2. The history, physical examination, and routine blood studies effectively rule out many of these possibilities. Other cases require one or more diagnostic tests (Table 88–3) to make a diagnosis.

TABLE 88–1.
Classification of Symptoms of Hypoglycemia

ADRENERGIC SYMPTOMS	NEUROGLYCOPENIC SYMPTOMS
Anxiety	Visual disturbances
Diaphoresis	Dysarthria
Tachycardia	Headaches
Palpitations	Confusion
Hunger	Amnesia
Tremors	Stupor
Irritability	Coma
Flushing	Lethargy
Piloerection	Seizures
Hypertension	Incoordination
Faintness	Focal neurologic deficits
Nausea	Weakness
Vomiting	Affective disorders
Oral and acral paresthesias	Hypothermia
	Nightmares
	Vertigo

TABLE 88–2.
Pathophysiology Related to Differential Diagnosis

DECREASED GLUCOSE PRODUCTION	INCREASED GLUCOSE UTILIZATION	DECREASED PRODUCTION AND INCREASED UTILIZATION
Starvation	Excessive exercise	Insulin excess
Cachexia	Growth hormone deficiency	Insulinoma
Hepatic failure	Pregnancy	Beta-cell hyperplasia
Congestive heart failure		Nesidioblastosis
Hormonal deficiency		Antibody-mediated
Thyroid hormones		Autoimmune hypoglycemia
Glucagon		D-penicillamine
Catecholamines		Insulin-secreting
Cortisol		nonendocrine tumors
Drugs		Uremia
Ethanol		Sepsis
Beta-blocking agents		Insulin-like-substance secreting
Salicylates		nonendocrine tumors
Akee fruit (hypoglycin)		Cancer
Thionamides		Drugs
Sulfonamides		Insulin
PABA		Biguanides
Pentamidine		Sulfonylureas
Chloramphenicol		EDTA
Oxytetracycline		
Phenylbutazone		
Manganese		
Propoxyphene		
Coumadin derivatives		
MAO inhibitors		
Anabolic steroids		
Disopyramide		
Acetaminophen		
Colchicine		
Quinine		
Phenothiazines		

0 to 24 Hours	1 to 3 Days	More Than 3 Days
Decreased Blood Glucose Levels (2° to Glucose Consumption) ↓ Increased Counterregulatory Hormone Levels (Increased Catabolism → Adrenergic Symptoms) ↓ Decreased Insulin Level (Decreased Anabolism) ↓ Increased Hepatic Glycogenolysis ↓ Maintain Blood Glucose Level (If CNS has inadequate supplies, neuroglycopenic symptoms follow.)	Hepatic Glycogen Stores Depleted ↓ Gluconeogenesis ↓ Maintain Blood Glucose Levels (If CNS has inadequate supplies, neuroglycopenic symptoms follow.)	Lipolysis ↓ Free Fatty Acid Substrate to Liver ↓ Keto-genesis ↓ Decreased Need for Gluconeogenesis (Muscle-protein Preservation) ↓ Maintain Blood Glucose Levels (If CNS has inadequate supplies, neuroglycopenic symptoms follow.)

FIG 88–1.
Clinical–pathologic correlations for fasting hypoglycemia.

TABLE 88–3.
Diagnostic Tests

TEST	ABNORMAL RESULT	CONDITION WHERE MOST APPLICABLE
72-hour fast	Immunoreactive insulin (IRI) not suppressed when blood glucose levels low	Hyperinsulinism
Fasting immunoreactive insulin-to-glucose ratio	> 0.3	Hyperinsulinism
Amended ratio of Turner (immunoreactive insulin ÷ 100/glucose − 30)	> 50	Hyperinsulinism
Proinsulin-to-insulin ratio	> 0.25–0.35	Endogenous hyper-insulinism (EH)
Fish-insulin suppression	Immunoreactive insulin levels not suppressed	EH
C-peptide suppression	C-peptide levels not suppressed	EH
Provocative tests Tolbutamide Leucine Glucagon Calcium	Exaggerated release of immuno-reactive insulin	EH
Dextrose infusion via biostator	Increasing amounts of dextrose required per time to maintain preset blood glucose level	EH
C-peptide measurement with immunoreactive insulin measurement	Increased immunoreactive insulin level with suppressed C-peptide level Increased immunoreactive insulin level with increased C-peptide level	Factitious hyper-insulinism (FH) Antibody-mediated hypoglycemia (AH); EH; sulfonylurea ingestion
Species-specific immuno-reactive insulin	Increased levels of bovine or porcine immunoreactive insulin	FH
Insulin antibodies	Present	FH or AH
Drug measurements	Drugs present in plasma or urine	Sulfonylurea ingestion
Glycosylated hemoglobin	Less than normal	Hyperinsulinism
Insulin-induced hypoglycemia	Decreased cortisol, decreased GH, decreased epinephrine	Counterregulatory hormone deficiency
Argenine infusion	Decreased GH, decreased glucagon	Counterregulatory hormone deficiency
HCG or subunits	Increased	Malignant insulinoma
Ultrasonography/computed tomography/arteriography	Tumor visualization	Tumor localization
Pancreatic venous sampling for immunoreactive insulin	Increased immunoreactive insulin at some locations	Tumor localization
Measurement of calcitonin, calcium, catecholamines, prolactin, ACTH, gastrin	Increased	Multiple endocrine neoplasia

DIAGNOSIS

Fasting hypoglycemia is considered to be present if after a 24-hour fast, the fasting plasma glucose value is less than 50 mg/dL in men or less than 40 mg/dL in women. The presence of Whipple's triad adds credence to the diagnosis on clinical grounds. If hypoglycemia is strongly suspected but the glucose level is not below the stated value, fasting is continued for 72 hours, with blood glucose, immunoreactive insulin, and C-peptide levels measured periodically or at any time symptoms appear. Symptoms may be induced in asymptomatic patients by having them exercise during the last 2 hours of a 72-hour fast. Failure to document hypoglycemia after a 72-hour fast virtually eliminates a diagnosis of fasting hypoglycemia.

Demonstration of Whipple's triad during a 72-hour fast with documentation of hyperinsulinemia by an abnormal insulin-to-glucose ratio and elevated proinsulin or C-peptide level (Table 88–2) in the absence of a detectable sulfonylurea level and insulin antibodies is virtually diagnostic of endogenous hyperinsulinism associated with beta islet-cell hyperactivity (insulinoma). When hormone deficiency syndromes and the obvious contributions of drugs can be ruled out, the remaining diagnoses listed in Table 88–2 can usually be readily differentiated.

Artifactual hypoglycemia is a diagnostic consideration in the presence of leukocytosis because leukocytes metabolize glucose. Failure to measure plasma glucose immediately may result in a spuriously low value. Such findings have been reported in patients with leukocyte counts of 55,000 and greater. This is a rare occurrence.

Hypoglycorrhachia (low CSF glucose levels) may be diagnostically helpful because CSF glucose levels remain low for several hours after plasma glucose has returned to normal. The CSF level may be of diagnostic value in unusual cases where the glucose level nadir is elusive.

PRINCIPLES OF PREVENTION AND THERAPY

Acute hypoglycemia is treated with an intravenous administration of a 50% solution of glucose, which serves as a diagnostic and therapeutic trial by aborting a hypoglycemic episode. Alternatively, glucagon administration will induce rapid glycogenolysis, which elevates the blood glucose level. However, patients without glycogen stores or with hepatic failure may not respond to glucagon.

Therapy of chronic hypoglycemia is directed toward the underlying disorder. In most cases, correction of that disorder or removal of an offending agent results in euglycemia. When the cause of insulin excess is a discrete lesion such as an insulinoma or an insulin-secreting, non-endocrine tumor, surgical removal is appropriate. When a malignant metastatic insulinoma or diffuse histologic changes (nesidioblastosis) is the source of excess insulin production, inhibitors of insulin secretion are generally necessary, along with cytotoxic therapy. Alternatively, artificial pancreata in the form of closed-loop devices (devices where a glucose sensor is coupled to an insulin infusion device) to infuse insulin and glucose have been successful as a research technique.

In fasting hypoglycemia, anticipatory preventive measures other than decreasing the duration of fasting are not helpful.

REFERENCES

Cryer PE: Glucose homeostasis and hypoglycemia, in Wilson JD, Foster DW (eds): *Williams Textbook of Endocrinology*, ed 7. Philadelphia, WB Saunders Co, 1985, pp 999–1017. *The standard reference textbook for general clinical endocrinology.*

Fajans SS, Floyd JC Jr: Fasting hypoglycemia in adults. *N Engl J Med* 1976; 294:766–772. *Most comprehensive review on the topic.*

Gerich J, Cryer P, Rizza R: Hormonal mechanisms in acute glucose counterregulation: The relative roles of glucagon, epinephrine, norepinephrine, growth hormone, and cortisol. *Metabolism* 1980; 29(11): 1164–1175. *Elegant yet simple description of glucose counterregulatory mechanisms.*

Merimee TJ, Tyson JE: Stabilization of plasma glucose during fasting. Normal variations in two separate studies. *N Engl J Med* 1974; 291: 1275–1278. *The basis for normal ranges of blood glucose levels in fasting subjects.*

Nelson RL: Hypoglycemia: Fact or fiction? *Mayo Clin Proc* 1985; 60:844–850. *Well-referenced recent review.*

Osei K, O'Dorisio TM: Malignant insulinoma: Effects of a somatostatin analog (compound 201–995) on serum glucose, growth, and gastroenteropancreatic hormones. *Ann Intern Med* 1985; 103(2): 223–225. *State-of-the-art discussion of the inhibition of insulin secretion.*

Seltzer HS: Drug-induced hypoglycemia—A review based on 473 cases. *Diabetes* 1972; 21(9):955–966. *The most comprehensive look at drug-induced hypoglycemia.*

89 HYPERNATREMIA

Joseph Premanandan, M.D.

Hypernatremia results from the excess loss of free water from the body. A patient with a serum sodium concentration greater than 147 mEq/L, is considered to be hypernatremic. Symptoms and signs of hypernatremia occur when the serum sodium level is above 150 mEq/L, and death may occur when the serum sodium level is above 160 mEq/L. Excess loss of free water has significant clinical impact, mostly on the central nervous system, and the clinical manifestations of hypernatremia depend on the underlying cause of the hypernatremia (Table 89–1).

CLINICAL SIGNS AND SYMPTOMS

Patients with hypernatremia develop clinical manifestations that depend on the severity of hypernatremia (Table 89–1). The common signs and symptoms are thirst, weakness, and other neurologic signs.

The physical findings depend on the underlying cause of the hypernatremia. If the hypernatremia is associated with hypovolemia or intravascular volume depletion (also called the state of dehydration), the patient will have all the signs and symptoms of a volume-depleted state such as postural hypotension, loss of skin texture and turgor (not a reliable sign in elderly patients), sunken eyeballs, loss of sweating in the axilla, decreased urine output, and tachycardia. At this point it should be understood that hypovolemia refers to decrease in both intra- and extravascular volume. If the hypernatremia is due to hypervolemic situations such as can result from administration of excess sodium bicarbonate during cardiac arrest or for lactic acidosis, or if hypernatremia occurs during hemodialysis, the patient will gain weight and manifest edema of the legs and presacral region and a gallop rhythm. It should be again noted that hypervolemia means an increase in both intra- and extravascular volume. Normovolemic patients with hypernatremia may not have any symptoms, except for the patient with diabetes insipidus (central or nephrogenic) who will have intense thirst and polyuria. In these patients, the signs of hypernatremia will develop to the point of death if the patient becomes comatose due to some other unrelated CNS or metabolic causes like head trauma and if their associated medical illness like diabetes insipidus goes unrecognized. These patients, too, may have clinical manifestations of the underlying disease that is causing

TABLE 89–1.
Clinical–Pathologic Correlations for Hypernatremia

CLINICAL FINDINGS	PATHOLOGIC FINDINGS
Severe thirst	Intracellular dehydration
Headache	Shrinkage of the cerebral hemisphere
Nausea, vomiting	
Disorientation	
Convulsions, coma	(In severe hypernatremia, the intracellular compartment is
Intracerebral hemorrhage	hypotonic in relation to the hypertonic extracellular
Cerebrovascular accident	compartment, so free water moves out of the cell, producing
	cellular dehydration.)

the central or nephrogenic diabetes insipidus like pituitary or hypothalamic tumors, sarcoidosis, or hypercalcemia.

The natural course of hypernatremia depends on the degree of hypernatremia, the rapidity with which it develops, and the underlying cause. Severely hypernatremic patients, if left untreated, will develop seizures and coma or may die of intracerebral hemorrhage, especially if the serum sodium level is above 160 mEq/L.

The laboratory diagnosis of hypernatremia is made by the measurement of serum sodium levels. When the serum sodium level is above 147 mEq/L, the patient may be considered to be hypernatremic. The serum sodium level is not, however, the true measurement of total body sodium. It only gives the ratio between total body sodium and total body water.

$$\text{Serum Sodium} = \frac{\text{Total Body Sodium}}{\text{Total Body Water}}$$

If the denominator, total body water, is decreased, the outcome would be hypernatremia. So hypernatremia for all practical purposes means less free water or a ratio of salt to water that is greater than normal. If the serum sodium level is significantly high, one needs both to calculate and to measure directly the serum osmolality. The serum osmolality may be calculated by using the following formula:

$$2 \times \text{Na} + \frac{\text{Blood Glucose}}{18} + \frac{\text{BUN}}{2.8}$$

If the hypernatremic patient is found to be normovolemic with a low urine osmolality, and variable spot urine sodium values, then conditions like central or nephrogenic diabetes insipidus or compulsive water drinking should be considered. (The different causes of central or nephrogenic diabetes insipidus are discussed in the chapter on diabetes insipidus.) level will be less than 20 mEq/L because of the coexisting hypovolemic condition.

If the hypernatremic patient is found to be normovolemic with a low urine osmolality, and variable spot urine sodium values, then conditions like central or nephrogenic diabetes insipidus or compulsive water drinking should be considered. (The different causes of central

or nephrogenic diabetes insipidus are discussed in the chapter on diabetes insipidus.)

If the hypernatremic person is clinically hypervolemic and if his or her serum osmolality is high and the spot urine sodium values are high, one should consider situations like excess sodium bicarbonate administration during cardiac resuscitation or for treatment of metabolic acidosis, excess saline administration during dialysis to be the possible causes.

DIFFERENTIAL DIAGNOSIS

The differential diagnosis of hypernatremia is given in Table 89–2. In addition passing mention needs to be made about essential hypernatremia in which the hypothalamic secretion of ADH in response to osmotic stimuli is blunted because of an underlying pathologic condition of the hypothalamus. Most hypernatremic situations are associated with a loss of free water in the urine relative to the sodium salt excretion. In psychogenic polydipsia and central or nephrogenic diabetes insipidus, the concentrating ability of the kidney is lost because of either insufficient ADH release or ineffective ADH.

PATHOPHYSIOLOGY

The pathophysiology of different types of hypernatremia depends on the underlying cause. In hypernatremia associated with hypovolemia (a state of dehydration, a hyperosmolar state), the end result is hypertonic serum due to an excessive urinary loss of free water as a consequence of the osmotic diuretic effect of excessive glucose, mannitol, or urea excretion, which in turn is a consequence of postobstructive diuresis or prolonged tube feeding. The pathophysiology of different types of diabetes insipidus associated with normal or high serum sodium levels in a normovolemic patient are discussed in the chapter on diabetes insipidus.

In compulsive water drinking, the excessive intake of free water results in excessive free water excretion. Chronic ingestion of excess free water will result in loss of renal medullary tonicity, disrupting the counter-current mechanism, which results in loss of concentrating

TABLE 89–2.
Differential Diagnosis of Hypernatremia

ASSOCIATED WITH HYPOVOLEMIA (DEHYDRATION)	ASSOCIATED WITH NORMOVOLEMIC SITUATIONS	ASSOCIATED WITH HYPERVOLEMIC SITUATIONS
Hyperosmolar state	Central diabetes insipidus	$NaHCO_3$ excess
Tube feeding	Nephrogenic diabetes insipidus	Excess saline administration
Hot temperature	Psychogenic polydipsia	Hypertonic saline administration
Gastroenteritis	Febrile state	
Peritoneal dialysis		
Excess mannitol		
Postobstructive diuresis		

ability of the kidney, all of which present a picture similar to nephrogenic diabetes insipidus. The diagnosis of psychogenic polydipsia or compulsive water drinking is difficult to make because these patients' underlying psychiatric problems and psychopharmacologic medications will induce inappropriate ADH secretion in addition to their habit of compulsive water drinking. Lastly, hypernatremia due to hypervolemia is due to excess salt in the body relative to the free water in the body, which results in hypertonic serum.

CLINICAL–PATHOLOGIC CORRELATIONS

The clinical features of severe hypernatremia are mainly due to cell shrinkage, or intracellular dehydration, especially of the cerebral hemispheres when the patient's extracellular fluid is hypertonic compared to the intracellular tonicity. In this situation, the free water moves from the intracellular compartment into the extracellular area resulting in intracellular dehydration. Because of the sudden shrinkage of the cerebral hemispheres, from the tentorium in a severe hyperosmolar state, areas of intracerebral hemorrhage may be seen in extreme situations.

PRINCIPLES OF THERAPY

The primary goal of therapy in hypernatremia should be directed toward removing the underlying cause; for example, through adequate correction of intravascular volume depletion, timely treatment of hypervolemic situations with diuretic agents or dialysis, appropriate management of central or nephrogenic diabetes insipidus, and treating compulsive water drinking disorder with water restriction and psychotherapy. The correction of a coexisting volume-depleted state deserves the top priority in such a situation and can be effectively done by giving an appropriate amount of isotonic saline. After appropriate treatment of the volume-depleted state, persisting hypernatremia may be treated with dextrose in water or preferably with dextrose in a 0.2 N saline solution.

REFERENCES

Feig PU: Hypernatremia and hypertonic syndromes. Med Clin North Am 1981; 65:271–289. *Review of the definition, pathophysiology, differential diagnosis, and treatment of hypernatremia and hyperosmolar syndromes.*

Jamison RL, Oliver RE: Disorders of urinary concentration and dilution. *Am J Med* 1982; 72:308–322. *A good review of the different pathophysiologic mechanisms responsible for urinary concentration and dilution.*

Narins RG, Jones ER, Stom MC, Rudnick MR et al: Diagnostic strategies in disorders of fluid, electrolyte and acid base homeostasis. *Am J Med* 1982; 72:496–503. *The reader will appreciate the diagnostic strategies that are required for patients with hypernatremia.*

Singer I: Differential diagnosis of polyuria and diabetes insipidus. *Med Clin North Am* 1981; 65:303–320. *The differential diagnosis and routine work-up of patients with polyuria are presented.*

Singer I: *Inappropriate Antidiuretic Hormone Secretion and Related Syndromes. Clinical Update in Nephrology,* vol 1. New Canaan, Nassau Publications, 1984, pp 2–12. *The reader will note the different mechanisms (both physiologic and pathologic that operate in disorders of urinary concentration and dilution.*

Weitzman R., Kleeman CR: Water metabolism and the neurophysiological hormones, in Maxwell MH, Kleeman DR (eds): *Clinical Disorders of Fluid and Electrolyte Metabolism.* New York, McGraw-Hill Book Co, 1980, pp 531–633. *Basic principles of urinary concentration and dilution and different pathophysiologic mechanisms responsible for disorders of urinary concentration and dilution are reviewed.*

90 HYPONATREMIA

Joseph Premanandan, M.D.

Hyponatremia is a clinical syndrome resulting from an excess of total body water in relation to total body sodium irrespective of the underlying cause, the only possible exception being spurious hyponatremia which will be discussed later. Excess body water has significant clinical effect mainly on the central nervous system and on the musculoskeletal system, and the clinical manifestations depend on the underlying cause of hyponatremia.

CLINICAL SIGNS AND SYMPTOMS

Symptoms and signs develop in the hyponatremic patient, depending on the severity of the hyponatremia and the rapidity with which hyponatremia develops (Table 90–1.) It is very unusual for a patient to manifest signs and symptoms of hyponatremia unless the serum sodium concentration is below 115 mEq/L. Chronic, persistent hyponatremia, if unrecognized and untreated, may result in demyelination of the central nervous system. The acute manifestations of hyponatremia include anorexia, vomiting, seizures, lethargy, and coma.

The physical findings depend on the underlying cause of the hyponatremia. If the hyponatremia is due to hypovolemia, the patient will have postural hypotension, loss of skin texture and turgor (not a reliable sign in elderly patients), sunken eyeballs, loss of sweating in the axilla, decreased urine output, and tachycardia. It should be noted here that hypovolemia refers to decrease in both intra- and extravascular volume. If the hyponatremia is due to hypervolemic situations like congestive heart failure, the patient will have a daily gain in weight, edema of the legs and presacral region, an elevated jugular venous pulse, and a gallop rhythm. One has to keep in mind that hypervolemia may mean an increase in extravascular volume only. For example, in conditions like hepatic cirrhosis or nephrotic syndrome there is intravascular volume depletion and a corresponding increment of interstitial fluid volume

TABLE 90–1.
Signs and Symptoms of Hyponatremia

CLINICAL FINDINGS	PATHOLOGIC FINDINGS
GASTROINTESTINAL	
Anorexia, nausea	Cellular edema
Vomiting	Cerebral edema (In severe hyponatremia the intracellular compartment
MUSCULOSKELETAL	is hypertonic in relation to the relatively dilute intravascular area, so
Weakness	free water moves into the cell from the extracellular area, producing
Cramps	the cellular edema.)
NEUROPSYCHIATRIC	
Lethargy, apathy	
Disorientation	
Personality changes	
Organic psychosis	
Abnormal sensorium	
Seizures	
Depressed tendon reflexes	
Pseudobulbar palsy	
Cheyne-Stokes respiration	
Hypothermia	
Coma	

due to decreased intravascular oncotic pressure as a result of either increased urinary loss or decreased hepatic synthesis of albumin. Usually the clinical signs and symptoms of hepatic cirrhosis or the nephrotic syndrome will be obvious if they are the underlying causes of hyponatremia. On the other hand, normovolemic patients with hyponatremia may not manifest any acute symptoms unless the hyponatremia is very severe, but they may have symptoms and signs of underlying disorders, like disease processes and drugs that produce the syndrome of inappropriate antidiuretic hormone (ADH) production (SIADH), hypothyroidism, glucocorticoid deficiency, psychogenic polydipsia, reset osmostat, and chronic hypokalemia.

The natural course of hyponatremia depends on the degree of hyponatremia, the rapidity with which it develops, and the underlying cause. Severely hyponatremic patients, if left untreated, will develop seizures, coma and may ultimately die.

PATHOPHYSIOLOGY

The pathophysiologic mechanisms of different types of hyponatremia are best appreciated through a familiarity with ADH, its mode of action, and the site, mode, and regulation of its secretion. ADH is secreted in the supraoptic and paraventricular nuclei of the hypothalamus and is ultimately stored in the posterior pituitary gland. Many stimuli including physical stress, emotions, drugs, and nicotine are responsible for increased secretion of ADH. Among them the most important factors that augment or inhibit the secretion of ADH are the intravascular volume and the tonicity or the osmolality of the serum. Hypertonic or hyperosmolar serum, which deviates 1% to 2% from normal, increases and hypotonic serum decreases ADH secretion. Volume changes of about 10% alter ADH secretion. Hypovolemia stimulates and hypervolemia inhibits ADH secretion. When the hypothalamus is confronted by a volume stimulus and a tonicity stimulus at the same time, the volume stimulus receives the top priority. For example, volume depletion of 10% or greater augments the secretion of ADH from the hypothalamus irrespective of what the serum osmolality is. Once ADH is released, it acts on the collecting tubule of the nephron and promotes antidiuresis. The mechanism by which antidiuresis is achieved by ADH is shown in Figure 90–1. The effective osmotic force in the body is executed by the sodium because it is primarily confined to the extracellular fluid.

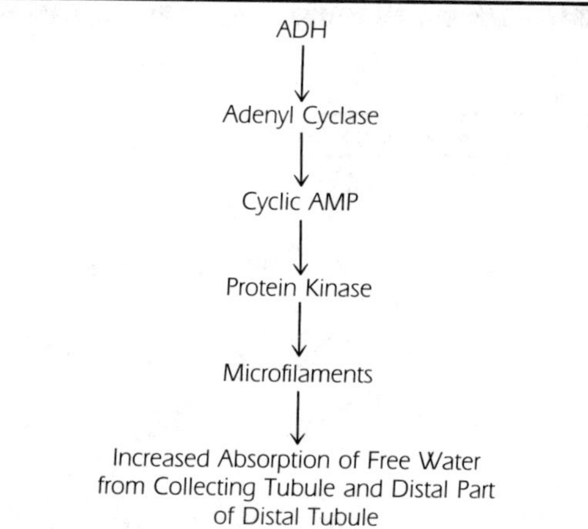

FIG 90–1.
Mechanism of antidiuresis produced by antidiuretic hormone (ADH).

CLINICAL–PATHOLOGIC CORRELATIONS

The clinical features of severe hyponatremia are mainly due to the edema or swelling of the cells, especially of cells of the central nervous system. When the patient's extracellular fluid is dilute and hypotonic compared to the intracellular tonicity, then the free water moves from the extracellular compartment into the intracellular compartment and thus promotes cellular swelling or edema especially of CNS.

DIAGNOSIS

The laboratory diagnosis of hyponatremia is made by the measurement of serum sodium levels. When the patient's serum sodium level is less than 135 mEq/L, then he or she may be considered to be hyponatremic. The serum sodium level is not, however, a measurement of total body sodium. The serum sodium level only reflects the ratio between total body sodium and total body water.

$$\text{Serum Sodium} = \frac{\text{Total Body Sodium}}{\text{Total Body Water}}$$

If the denominator, total body water, is increased, low serum sodium levels or hyponatremia will result.

True hyponatremia (as opposed to spurious hyponatremia, which occurs in hyperlipidemic and dysproteinemic states) usually means an increase in intravascular or total body water. If the serum sodium level is significantly low, the serum osmolality must be calculated by using the following formula:

$$2 \times \text{Na} + \frac{\text{Blood Sugar}}{18} + \frac{\text{BUN}}{2.8}$$

It is also always necessary to measure the serum osmolality directly.

If a patient is hyponatremic and asymptomatic and if his or her measured serum osmolality is normal, than we should consider possible causes like hyperlipidemia or dysproteinemic states such as multiple myeloma. This situation is called spurious hyponatremia, which necessitates further studies like lipoprotein electrophoresis and serum protein electrophoresis. If the measured osmolality is high in a hyponatremic patient, then conditions like severe hyperglycemia or administration of excess mannitol should be given serious consideration.

After these possibilities are ruled out, true hyponatremia in which the measured osmolality is less than 270 mOsm with coexisting low serum sodium levels can be associated with hypovolemic, hypervolemic, and normovolemic situations. If the patient is hyponatremic and if his random urine sodium level is below 20 mEq/L, then the possible causes are intravascular volume depletion, congestive heart failure, hypoalbuminemic states like nephrotic syndrome, cirrhosis of liver, and malnutrition, and conditions in which there is fluid loss into a third space such as acute pancreatitis. Further investigation should be directed depending on the above considerations. If the patient is hyponatremic but if his or her spot urine sodium level is above 20 mEq/L, one should consider situations like diuretic abuse, salt-losing renal abnormalities, Addison's disease, or chronic or acute renal failure. Administration of diuretics should, however, be avoided before measuring the spot urine sodium levels because diuretics will disrupt the spot urine sodium value.

If a patient is normovolemic, if his or her serum sodium level osmolality is low, and if the spot urine sodium level is more than 40 mEq/L, then one should consider measurement of the urine osmolality and the serum uric acid levels.

TABLE 90–2.
Differential Diagnosis of Hyponatremia

TRUE HYPONATREMIA	PSEUDOHYPONATREMIA	TRANSIENT HYPONATREMIA

Hypovolemia
Hypervolemia
Normal volume
  SIADH
  Hypothyroidism
  Glucocorticoid deficiency
  Psychogenic polydipsia
  Reset osmostat
  Chronic hypokalemia
	Hyperlipidemia
	Hyperproteinemia
	Marked hyperglycemia
		Severe hyperglycemia
		Excess mannitol administration

TABLE 90–3.
Differential Diagnosis of Hyponatremia Associated with Hypovolemia

RENAL LOSSES OF SODIUM (SPOT URINE Na $>$ 20 mEq/L) CONCENTRATION	EXTRARENAL LOSSES OF SODIUM (SPOT URINE Na $<$ 10 mEq/L) CONCENTRATION
Excessive use of diuretic agents Addison's disease Salt-losing nephritis Partial obstructive uropathy Renal tubular acidosis with bicarbonaturia Hypercalcemia Use of diuretic agents	Sweating Gastrointestinal loss (vomiting, diarrhea) Third space loss (pancreatitis, peritonitis, burns)

If the patient's urine osmolality is inappropriately higher than the serum osmolality and if the serum uric acid level is low, the probable cause is SIADH or another clinical situation that mimics SIADH, like hypothyroidism, isolated glucocorticoid deficiency, reset osmostat, chronic hypokalemia, or certain drugs. Further investigations should then be continued depending on the patient's history and clinical findings which may include searches for an occult malignancy, a connective tissue disorder, a chronic illness like tuberculosis, a metabolic disorder like porphyria and studies such as chest x-ray films, thyroid function tests, ACTH stimulation test, and electrolyte measurements.

If the patient is clinically normovolemic and is hyponatremic, has low urine osmolality (urine osmolality being lower than the serum osmolality), and variable spot urine sodium values, then psychogenic polydipsia or compulsive water drinking is a probable cause.

TABLE 90–4.
Differential Diagnosis of Hyponatremia Associated with Hypervolemia

CONDITIONS WITH SPOT URINE Na CONCENTRATION $Na^+ <$ 10 mEq/L	CONDITIONS WITH SPOT URINE Na CONCENTRATION $Na^+ >$ 20 mEq/L
Congestive heart failure Nephrotic syndrome Cirrhosis of liver	Acute renal failure Chronic renal failure

DIFFERENTIAL DIAGNOSIS

The differential diagnosis of hyponatremia is given in Table 90–2. The differential diagnosis of hyponatremia associated with hypovolemic and hypervolemic situations is given in Tables 90–3 and 90–4. True hyponatremia is invariably associated with the kidney's inability to dilute the urine. Hyponatremia is not a diagnosis by itself, but is the end result of an underlying problem that needs to be carefully studied. The different causes of SIADH are given in Table 90–5.

TABLE 90–5.
Causes of Syndrome of Inappropriate ADH Secretion (SIADH)

I.	CNS Disorders Encephalitis, meningitis, brain tumors, brain abscess, head trauma, stroke, subarachnoid or subdural hemorrhage, psychosis, Guillain-Barré syndrome
II.	Systemic diseases Systemic lupus erythematosis Acute intermittent porphyria
III.	Drugs A. *Release of Endogenous Vasopressin*—Nicotine, clofibrate, vincristine, cyclophosphamide, carbamozepine, morphine, barbiturate, amitriptyline, isoproterenol, chlorpropamide, diuretics B. *Enhancement of Tubular Action of ADH*—Indomethacin, chlorpropamide, acetaminophen C. *Antidiuretic Effect on Renal Tubule*—Vasopressin, oxytocin, acetaminophen, diuretics
IV.	Tumors Bronchogenic, Hodgkin's disease, lymphoma, thymoma, adenocarcinoma of pancreas, duodenum, ureter
V.	Miscellaneous Pneumonia, tuberculosis of lung

PRINCIPLES OF THERAPY

The primary goal of therapy should be directed toward treatment of the underlying cause, namely through correction of the hypovolemia or adequate and appropriate treatment of hypervolemic and normovolemic situations that are responsible for the onset of hyponatremia. Severe, life-threatening hyponatremia should be treated with hypertonic solutions. Chronic hyponatremia should be treated with agents that nullify the action of ADH on its target site, namely the collecting tubule and the distal part of the distal tubule of the nephrons. One should use hypertonic saline with caution in asymptomatic patients with serum sodium levels above 120 mEq/L. In situations like reset osmostat associated with occult malignancy or chronic illness where there is loss of intracellular idiogenic osmoles the cell and its contents become rather vulnerable, especially cells of the cerebral cortex. The administration of hypertonic saline to those patients will result in significant intracellular dehydration, with deleterious clinical consequences. Mild to moderate hyponatremia not associated with hypovolemic conditions can be treated effectively with water restriction alone.

REFERENCES

Goldberg M: Hyponatremia. *Med Clinc North Am* 1981; 65:251–269. *The reader will find definition, pathophysiology, differential diagnosis, and treatment of hyponatremia.*

Jamison RL, Oliver RE: Disorders of urinary concentration and dilution. *Am J Med* 1982; 72: 308–322. *A good review of the different pathophysiologic mechanisms responsible for urinary concentration and dilution.*

Narins, RG et al: Diagnostic strategies in disorders of fluid, electrolyte and acid base homeostasis. *Am J Med* 1982; 72:496–503. *A review of diagnostic and therapeutic strategies required for assessment and treatment of hyponatremia.*

Singer I: *Inappropriate Antidiuretic Hormone Secretion and Related Syndromes. Clinical Update in Nephrology,* vol 1. New Canaan, Nassau Publications, 1984, pp 2–12. *Physiologic and pathophysiologic mechanisms that are operating to enhance the secretion of ADH are presented.*

Weitzman R, Kleeman CR: Water metabolism and the neurophysiological hormones, in Maxwell MH, Kleeman CR (eds): *Clinical Disorders of Fluid and Electrolyte Metabolism.* New York, McGraw-Hill Book Co, 1980, pp 531–633. *Basic principles of urinary concentration and dilution and their alteration in diseases are reviewed.*

91

HYPERKALEMIA AND HYPOKALEMIA

Daniel Simon, M.D.

Potassium (K^+) is the predominant intracellular cation and is necessary for proper function of almost all cells. The high intracellular K^+ concentration is required for maintenance of cell volume as well as acid–base balance, optimal carbohydrate and protein metabolism, and activation of several enzyme systems. The ratio of intracellular-to-extracellular K^+ concentrations has an important role in regulating neuromuscular and cardiac excitability.

CLINICIAL SIGNS AND SYMPTOMS AND CLINICAL–PATHOLOGIC CORRELATIONS

While the disease process responsible for hypokalemia or hyperkalemia will appear with its own signs and symptoms, the manifestations of an abnormal serum K^+ concentration will be related to the degree of severity, rapidity of development, and to the change in intracellular-to-extracellular concentration ratio. The manifestations will also be modulated by calcium, sodium, magnesium, and hydrogen ion concentrations. Although in normal subjects serum K^+ is rarely greater than 5.0 mEq/L, hyperkalemia is defined as a serum K^+ concentration greater than 5.5 mEq/L, and symptoms are rarely noted until the concentration is greater than 6.0 mEq/L. While hypokalemia is usually defined as a serum K^+ concentration less than 3.5 mEq/L, symptoms are rarely noted until the concentration is less than 3.0 mEq/L. The most obvious manifestations of an abnormal serum K^+ concentration will be related to neural transmission alterations because the ratio of intracellular-to-extracellular K^+ concentrations is the most important determiner of the resting membrane potential. This ratio is more likely to be altered by acute than by chronic changes in K^+ balance and serum K^+ concentration. Metabolic abnormalities secondary to alterations in cellular function are also seen. Although hyperkalemia occurs less frequently than hypokalemia, its consequences are likely to be much more immediately severe.

HYPERKALEMIA

The clinical signs and symptoms of patients with hyperkalemia are usually predominately those of the underlying disease state until the point that severe potentially life-threatening consequences of hyperkalemia supervene (Table 91–1).

Neuromuscular and cardiac alterations due to hyperkalemia are most threatening. Initially the cardiac alterations may be manifest simply by peaking of the precordial T waves on the electrocardiogram (ECG) when the serum K^+ concentration is greater than 6 mEq/L. With progressive elevations in the serum K^+ concentration, a series of ECG changes occur that only poorly correlate with the serum K^+ level. Ventricular arrhythmias or cardiac arrest can occur at any point in this progression and occur more commonly than in hypokalemia. The progression from a peaked T wave to decreased amplitude of the P waves with prolonged PR intervals leads to atrial asystole. Widening of the QRS complex is a medical emergency and can progress at any moment to fuse with the T wave to produce the classic sine wave of hyperkalemia associated with terminal ventricular fibrillation and asystole.

Muscle weakness due to hyperkalemia is not generally seen until the serum K^+ concentration is greater than 7 mEq/L. The weakness is generally ascending and can lead to quadriplegia often with paresthesias and muscle cramps. Respiratory depression may occur, as can confusion, but cranial nerves are usually spared. Gastrointestinal symptoms include nausea,

TABLE 91–1.
Clinical-Pathologic Correlations of Hyperkalemia

CLINICAL FINDINGS	PATHOLOGIC FINDINGS
Neuromuscular	Reduced resting transmembrane potential (E_M) = partial depolarization
Paresthesias	
Muscle cramps	
Muscle weakness	$E_M = -61 \, Log \dfrac{K \text{ intracellular}}{K \text{ extracellular}}$
Respiratory insufficiency	
	Unchanged threshold potential (E_T)
Cardiac	
Conduction disturbances	Increased excitability of conducting tissue (initially)
Atrial arrhythmias	
Ventricular arrhythmias	Decreased rate and amplitude of depolarization (reduced Na^+ entry)
Smooth muscle	Accelerated repolarization (increased K^+ permeability)
Nausea	
Vomiting	Eventual progressive inexcitability of conducting tissue
Abdominal pain	
Ileus	
Metabolic acidosis	Transcellular redistribution of K^+ and hydrogen ion
	Decreased proximal tubule bicarbonate reabsorption
Lethal events	
Paralysis	
Respiratory arrest	Depolarization block when $E_M \geq E_T$
Asystole	

vomiting, ileus, and abdominal pain. Metabolic acidosis of a mild to moderate degree may also be present.

HYPOKALEMIA

The hypokalemic patient may present with complaints of weakness, constipation, polyuria, and polydipsia. Neuromuscular and cardiovascular alterations have the greatest clinical significance (Table 91–2). Both striated and smooth muscle may be involved. The hypokalemia may be manifested as muscle weakness (proximal greater than distal) progressing to paralysis, often associated with diminished deep tendon reflexes and can be associated with hypoventilation leading to respiratory arrest. Vomiting due to gastric atony, constipation with intestinal ileus, or urinary retention because of diminished bladder motility may be noted. Necrosis of muscle (rhabdomyolysis), when secondary to hypokalemia, is not generally seen until the serum K^+ concentration is less than 2.5 mEq/L and is reflected in elevated serum creatine phosphokinase or aldolase activity. This rarely involves cardiac muscle, is more common in skeletal muscle following ex-

ercise, is associated with muscle cramps or myalgias, and can cause myoglobinuria complicated by acute renal failure. Occasional hypokalemic patients complain of paresthesias with a "restless leg syndrome" or exhibit tetanic spasms. Rarely patients have been described as presenting with neuropsychiatric disturbances manifested as depression or encephalopathy.

The most obvious cardiac effects are the ECG alterations initially manifest as flattening of T waves and the development of prominent U waves. This may give rise to the mistaken impression of the presence of a prolonged QT interval, which in reality is a QU interval. P waves may become peaked, ST segments depressed, and amplitude and duration of the QRS complex increased. Utlimately atrial and ventricular ectopic beats develop, which presage the development of paroxysmal atrial tachycardia (often with atrioventricular block), atrioventricular dissociation, Mobitz type 1 atrioventricular block, ventricular tachycardia, and ventricular fibrillation. These arrhythmias are aggravated by the presence of digitalis glycosides, and patients receiving these preparations may suffer fatal arrhythmias with a rela-

TABLE 91–2.
Clinical–Pathologic Correlations of Hypokalemia

CLINICAL FINDINGS	PATHOLOGIC FINDINGS
Neuromuscular	*Initially*
Muscle cramps	
Restless legs	Increased resting transmembrane potential (E_M) =
Muscle weakness	hyperpolarization
Respiratory insufficiency	
Decreased deep tendon reflexes	Decreased excitability of conducting tissue
Rhabdomyolysis	
Paralysis	Increased velocity of conduction
Respiratory arrest	
	Subsequently
Cardiac	
Conduction abnormalities	Decreased E_M = partial depolarization (reduced K^+
Atrial arrhythmias	permeability)
Ventricular fibrillation	Decreased velocity of repolarization (reduced K^+
	permeability)
	Prolonged relative refractory time increases risk of
	arrhythmias.
Smooth muscle	
Nausea	
Vomiting	
Gastric atony	
Constipation	
Ileus	
Urinary retention	
Metabolic abnormalities	
Impaired glucose tolerance	Decreased insulin release
	Increased hepatic gluconeogenesis
Polyuria	Vasopressin-resistant urinary concentrating defect
Polydipsia	
Metabolic alkalosis	Renal tubular chloride wasting
Hyponatremia	Transcellular redistribution of K^+ and Na^+
Renal failure	Proximal tubular vacuolization
	Interstitial fibrosis
Hepatic encephalopathy	Increased renal ammoniagenesis from glutamine

tively modest K^+ deficiency. Rare patients have been reported to have congestive heart failure resulting from hypokalemia.

The renal and metabolic manifestations of hypokalemia are generally not as obviously symptomatic with the exception of the precipitation of hepatic encephalopathy in patients with borderline liver function and worsened glucose intolerance in patients with non-insulin-dependent diabetes mellitus. Hypokalemia may cause a mild, usually reversible decline in the glomerular filtration rate (GFR) and renal blood flow. Polyuria and polydipsia are seldom severe and are associated with an impairment of maximal urinary concentration that is not corrected by the administration of antidiuretic hormone (nephrogenic diabetes insipidus). Severe K^+ depletion may be associated with a tendency for sodium retention, edema formation, and modest hyponatremia, and a sodium chloride-resistant metabolic alkalosis.

PATHOPHYSIOLOGY OF POTASSIUM DISORDERS

The total body K^+ has been estimated in humans by the methods of isotope dilution (^{42}K or ^{43}K) and total body counting of the naturally occurring isotope ^{40}K. A higher total body K^+ (56 mEq/kg body weight in men, 43 mEq/kg in women) is found with the latter technique than with the former (46 mEq/kg in men, 32 mEq/kg in women). This is because the isotope dilution method only measures exchangeable K^+. With either technique, though, men appear to have about 33% more K^+ per kilogram of body weight than women, presumably because of greater muscle mass and less fat. Adipose tissue contains only 9 mEq K^+ per kilogram. In addition, K^+ content per kilogram of body weight decreases with age, based on a relative decline in muscle mass and increase in fat.

While total body K^+ is estimated to be about 50 mEq/kg, only 2% is extracellular at a concentration of 3.8 to 5.0 mEq/L and 98% is intracellular at a concentration of 150 mEq/L. Most K^+ in the body is contained in the muscle and viscera.

In order to maintain K^+ balance, the typical daily intake of 50 mEq to 100 mEq must be excreted. In addition, to maintain a normal extracellular fluid (ECF) concentration, K^+ distribution between the intracellular and extracellular fluid spaces must be regulated. The concentration difference of K^+ and sodium (Na^+) between ECF and intracellular fluid (ICF) would rapidly dissipate if an energy-dependent cation transport system failed to maintain the K^+ concentration higher and Na^+ concentration lower in the ICF than in the ECF. The essential component of this transport system is the Na^+–K^+ ATPase enzyme system located in the cell membrane of mammalian cells. The K^+ concentration modulates the activity of the cation pump such that high ECF K^+ concentrations increase the activity of the pump and increase the rate of uptake of K^+ by cells.

In general, acute metabolic or respiratory acidosis results in an increase in plasma K^+ levels, whereas acute respiratory or metabolic alkalosis results in a decrease in plasma K^+ levels because of transcellular K^+ redistribution. It had generally been assumed that the transcellular alteration in K^+ distribution was related to hydrogen ions shifting into or out of cells in exchange for K^+ and Na^+ in an effort to correct ECF pH. However, more recent information indicates that changes in ECF bicarbonate concentrations, independent of pH changes, can influence transcellular K^+ movement such that a decreased ECF bicarbonate concentration will result in bicarbonate redistributing into the ECF from ICF along with K^+. Chronic acid–base disorders may also influence K^+ distribution superimposed on alterations in total body K^+ resulting from changes in renal K^+ excretion.

Insulin administration has been shown to decrease plasma K^+ levels, and KCl infusions have been shown to acutely increase plasma insulin levels in animals and humans. In addition, when insulin secretion is inhibited, there is a small abrupt rise in plasma K^+ concentrations, and the ability to dispose of an exogenous K^+ load is markedly impaired. The alteration in plasma K^+ levels attributable to insulin appears to be due to cellular uptake predominately in muscle, liver, and fat. The mechanism is unclear, but evidence demonstrates that it is independent of glucose uptake.

Catecholamines play a complex role in transcellular K^+ distribution. The acute infusion of epinephrine results in a biphasic response in which there is a brief increase in the plasma K^+ level followed by a sustained decrease. The initial response results from the hepatic release of K^+, whereas the sustained decline appears to be due to cellular uptake of K^+ mediated by $beta_2$ receptors. The uptake is reversed by the nonselective beta-adrenergic blocking agent propranolol, but it is not influenced by the $beta_1$ selective adrenergic blocking agent metoprolol.

Mineralocorticoids such as aldosterone primarily regulate plasma K^+ concentrations by increasing K^+ secretion by the transporting epithelia of the renal distal tubule, colon, and salivary glands. Potassium is one of the major regulators of aldosterone production and in selected situations such as in anephric humans may be predominant. Chronic aldosteronism may create a buffer capacity for acute loads of K^+ by depleting muscle K^+ which will be replenished by transcellular redistribution of K^+ before hyperkalemia can occur from any given K^+ load.

Renal excretion of K^+ is the predominant regulator of K^+ balance in health, accounting for 90% of dietary intake. Plasma K^+ is freely filtered at the glomerulus, but reabsorption in the proximal tubule and loop of Henle results in only 10% of the filtered K^+ reaching the distal tubule. Subsequently, further reabsorption or K^+ secretion can occur depending on physiologic conditions including total body K^+ balance. Potassium secretion is increased by chronic or acute loads of K^+, by mineralocorticoids, by acute metabolic or respiratory alkalosis, by chronic metabolic acidosis, and by conditions that increase the rate of delivery of solute (especially of poorly reabsorbed anions) and fluid to distal nephron sites. Potassium secretion is inhibited by chronic K^+ depletion, mineralocorticoid deficiency, acute metabolic or respiratory acidosis, and by conditions that decrease the rate of delivery of solute and fluid to distal nephron sites.

Fecal excretion of K^+ in health accounts for 10% to 15% of dietary intake. The usual 5 mEq to 15 mEq of stool K^+ may triple in patients with severe renal failure. Generally K^+ is absorbed in the small intestine, and fecal K^+ excretion is determined by colonic secretion. Mineralocorticoids appear to enhance colonic K^+ secretion, and stool K^+ losses become potentially important in conditions characterized by increased aldosterone production, especially if fecal water or mucus losses are concomitantly increased.

Exocrine glands normally do not play a role in K^+ homeostasis because sweat volume is low. Because of a Na^+-K^+ exchange mechanism in sweat glands that is stimulated by aldosterone, sweat K^+ concentration is greater than plasma K^+ concentration. Under conditions of excercise or heat stress, K^+ depletion can occur.

DIFFERENTIAL DIAGNOSIS AND DIAGNOSIS

The differential diagnosis of hyperkalemia and hypokalemia is shown in Tables 91–3 and 91–4. Generally the history and physical examination will suggest the specific cause. Where the cause is not immediately apparent, measurements of urinary pH, K^+, Na^+, chloride, or aldosterone levels and of plasma renin levels will be most rewarding if collected prior to institution of therapy. In clinical situations where a 24-hour urine collection prior to therapy is not practical, a spot urine will be nearly as accurate. A diagnostic approach to the patient with hyperkalemia or hypokalemia is shown in Figures 91–1 and 91–2.

Aside from the occasional patient with pseudohyperkalemia, diagnostic confusion most commonly occurs when the patient provides an inaccurate history or deliberately misleads the physician. This will occur in hyperkalemic patients ingesting excessive quantities of K^+-rich substances or medications that impair renal tu-

bular K^+ secretion. In hypokalemic patients, various combinations of surreptitious emesis, diuretic or laxative abuse may result in the erroneous diagnosis of Bartter's syndrome. On occasion these patients will maintain denial of suspected abuse, and screening urine for the presence of diuretics or senna, a sigmoidoscopy searching for melanosis coli, or other tests searching for cathartic or emetic drug abuse may prove necessary before psychiatric referral. The persistently hypokalemic patient who fails to respond to apparently large doses of K^+ replacement may be noncompliant. In general 24-hour urine collection should contain 90% of the prescribed K^+ intake. If it contains less, the patient is either not taking the dose prescribed or has extrarenal losses. Finally any condition that leads to loss of upper gastrointestinal fluids can lead to K^+ depletion and hypokalemia. The major site of K^+ loss, however, is urinary because the K^+ concentration of gastric, biliary, pancreatic, and small intestinal secretions is rarely greater than 10 mEq/L. The metabolic alkalosis that develops from gastric fluid losses leads to transcellular redistribution of K^+ intracellularly while increased distal tubular delivery of bicarbonate with associated secondary aldosteronism (because of volume depletion) leads to renal K^+ wasting.

PRINCIPLES OF PREVENTION AND THERAPY

Prevention of hyperkalemia requires identification of those patients at risk for this problem and institution of measures to minimize the occurrence. Those with acute oliguric renal failure or advanced chronic renal failure invariably require dietary K^+ restriction (2–3 gm daily). Under most circumstances this, in association with regular dialysis therapy, will maintain the serum K^+ concentration within acceptable limits. Occasional patients require the regular intake of a K^+-binding resin (sodium polystyrene sulfonate) to maintain control of K^+ levels because of dietary noncompliance, catabolic states, or gastrointestinal bleeding. Patients with lesser degrees of renal failure, diabetic patients with marginal reserve for maintaining K^+ balance, and occasional patients with a normal GFR and a high K^+ intake may become frankly hyperkalemic when

TABLE 91–3.
Differential Diagnosis of Hyperkalemia

CAUSE	CLINICAL CLUES
Facitious hyperkalemia	Absence of expected ECG changes and symptoms
In vivo release	Prolonged tourniquet
In vitro release	
Hemolyzed specimen	Difficulty obtaining blood specimen, pink specimen
Thrombocytosis	Platelet count > 500,000/mm^3
Leukocytosis	White blood cell count > 100,000/mm^3
Transcellular redistribution	
Acidosis	Clinical setting
Drug induced	Known exposure
Depolarized muscle from a paralytic agent	Succinylcholine
Arginine hydrochloride	
Digitalis glycoside overdose	
Nonselective beta-adrenergic blocking agent	
Hyperglycemia	Glucose infusion with insulin and aldosterone deficiency
Hyperkalemic periodic paralysis	Recurrent attacks of weakness with myotonia, often familial
Excessive K$^+$ intake	Often associated with impaired renal excretion
Exogenous	
Dietary	High intake of K$^+$ salt substitute, high K$^+$ diet, pica (clay)
Medicinal	K$^+$ preparations (PO or IV), rapid transfusion of aged blood
Endogenous	
Hemolysis	Clinical setting
Bleeding	Gastrointestinal bleeding, hematoma
Tissue necrosis	Ischemia or crush injury
Tumor cell lysis	Chemotherapy or radiation therapy with brisk response
Catabolic states	Clinical setting
Impaired renal excretion	
Physiologic rate limitation	Inadequate tubular flow rate and delivery of Na$^+$
Acute renal failure	Negligible GFR and oliguria
Chronic renal failure	GFR < 15–20 ml/min
Primary renal tubular K$^+$ secretory defect	Known associated disease
Obstructive uropathy	
Systemic lupus erythematosus	
Amyloidosis	
Sickle cell nephropathy	
Renal transplant	
Congenital	
Pseudohypoaldosteronism	Infant with failure to thrive, salt wasting, metabolic acidosis, elevated plasma aldosterone and renin levels
Pseudohypoaldosteronism type II	Older children and adults often hypertensive with low plasma renin level and without salt wasting
Inhibited tubular secretion	Known exposure
K$^+$-sparing diuretics	Spironolactone, triamterene, or amiloride
Digitalis glycoside overdose	
Mineralocorticoid-deficient states	
Addison's disease	Usually dehydrated, hypotensive, acidemic and hyperpigmented
Hyporeninemic hypoaldosteronism	Diabetes mellitus ± greater than mild renal insufficiency
Drug-induced hypoaldosteronism	Intake of PGE$_2$-inhibiting nonsteroidal anti-inflammatory drug, angiotensin-converting enzyme inhibitor, or heparin
Enzyme defects in mineralocorticoid metabolism	
21-hydroxylase deficiency	Virilization and salt wasting; increased urinary 17-ketosteroids and pregnanetriol levels
3-beta hydroxy dehydrogenase	Ambiguous genitalia, salt wasting
20-hydroxylase deficiency	Survival beyond infancy uncommon

TABLE 91–4.
Differential Diagnosis of Hypokalemia

CAUSE	CLINICAL CLUES
Inadequate K$^+$ intake	Malnourished (tea and toast diet, alcoholism, anorexia nervosa)
Gastrointestinal binding of K$^+$	Ingestion of cation-binding resin, pica (clay low in K$^+$ content)
Transcellular redistribution	
Alkalemia	Clinical setting
Insulin	Exogenous or secreted in response to glucose infusion
Vitamin B$_{12}$ or folic acid	With reticulocytosis after treatment of megaloblastic anemia
Beta-adrenergic agonist	Salbutamol, terbutaline
Hypokalemic periodic paralysis	Recurrent attacks, often familial, occasional hyperthyroidism
Barium intoxication (soluble salts)	Associated hypertension, vomiting, and diarrhea
Excessive loss from integument	Extensive burns or excessive sweating, usually with a renal contribution
Gastrointestinal losses	
Gastric losses	Metabolic alkalosis with emesis, gastric suction, or gastrocolic fistula
Small bowel losses	Metabolic acidosis, cholera, pancreatic nonbeta islet cell tumor, bile fistula, long or obstructed ureteroileostomy
Large bowel losses	Villous adenoma of colon or rectum, inflammatory bowel disease, ureterosigmoidostomy, laxative or enema abuse
Renal losses	
Drug-induced losses	
Diuretic agents	All except K$^+$-sparing diuretics
Penicillins	High doses, especially with secondary aldosteronism
Amphotericin B	Often with associated distal renal tubular acidosis
Secondary to gastrointestinal losses	Chloride depletion with secondary aldosteronism
Diabetic ketoacidosis	Salt wasting secondary to glycosuria and ketouria
Renal tubular disorders	
Renal tubular acidosis (proximal or distal)	Hereditary or acquired, hyperchloremic metabolic acidosis
Fanconi's syndrome	
Nephrocalcinosis	
Polyuric tubular dysfunction	Postobstructive diuresis, diuretic phase of acute tubular necrosis, or postrenal transplantation
Bartter's syndrome	Metabolic alkalosis, salt wasting, normotension, increased plasma aldosterone and renin levels
Magnesium deficiency	Hypomagnesemia
Familial	Renal magnesium wasting associated with K$^+$ wasting
Acquired	Drug-induced renal magnesium wasting (gentamicin, cisplatin, diuretic agents), diabetic ketoacidosis, aldosteronism, malabsorption, alcoholism
Leukemia with lysozymuria	Often complicated by drugs that may cause renal K$^+$ wasting
K$^+$-wasting nephropathy	Rare cases of pyelonephritis, interstitial nephritis
Excessive mineralocorticoid activity	Usually associated with hypertension
Hyperreninemic	
Accelerated or malignant hypertension	
Renovascular hypertension	
Renin-secreting tumors	Hemangiopericytomas of the kidney, rarely hypernephromas and Wilms' tumors
Oral contraceptives	
Adrenocortical dysfunction	
Primary aldosteronism	Several forms aside from a single adenoma
Cushing's syndrome	Adrenal neoplasm; pituitary, ectopic, or exogenous ACTH
Congenital adrenal hyperplasia	11-beta or 17-alpha hydroxylase deficiency (rare)
Pseudoaldosteronism	Familial (Liddle's syndrome)
Medicamentosa	Exogenous mineralocorticoids, glycyrrhizin (in licorice and chewing tobacco)

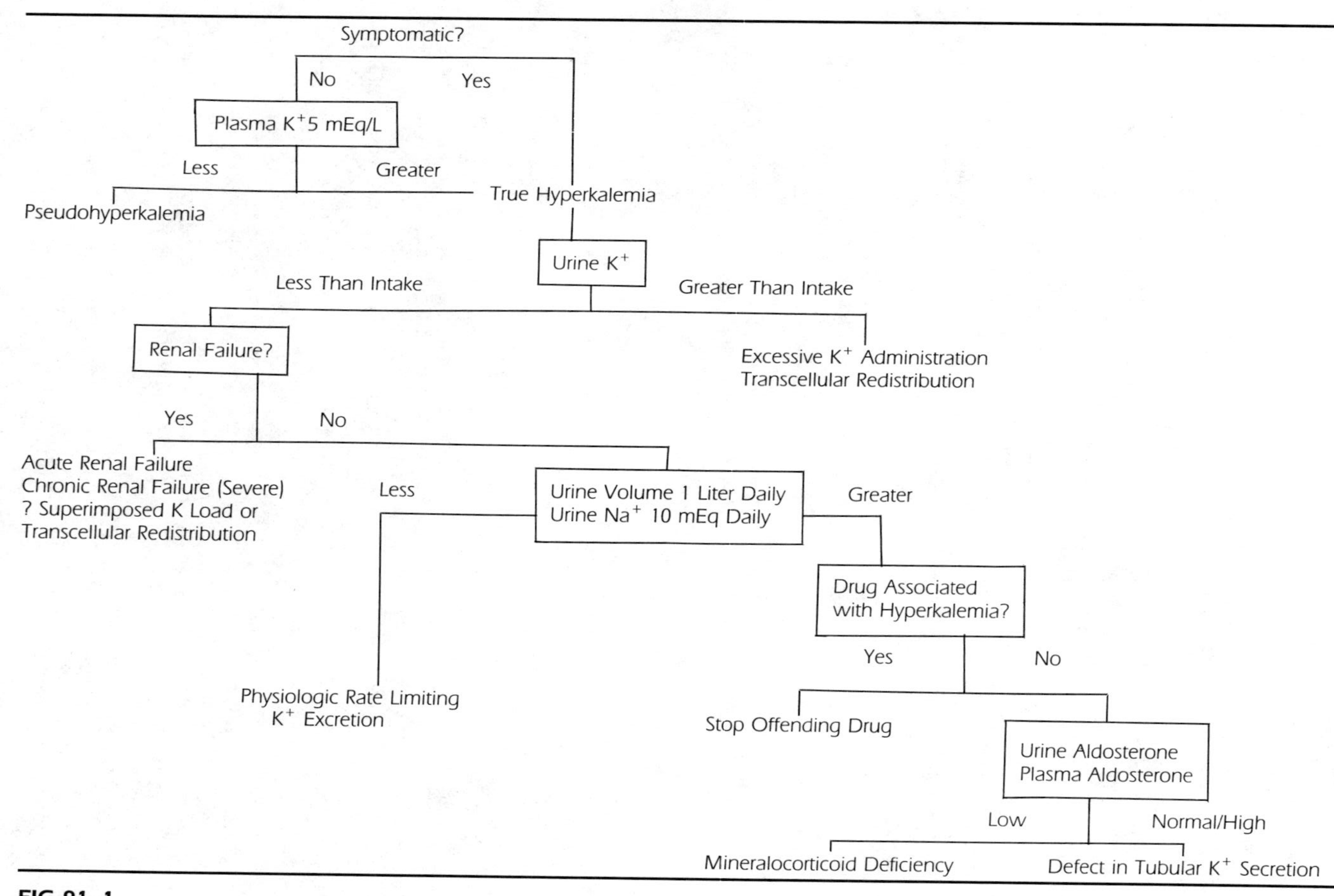

FIG 91–1.
Diagnostic approach to hyperkalemia.

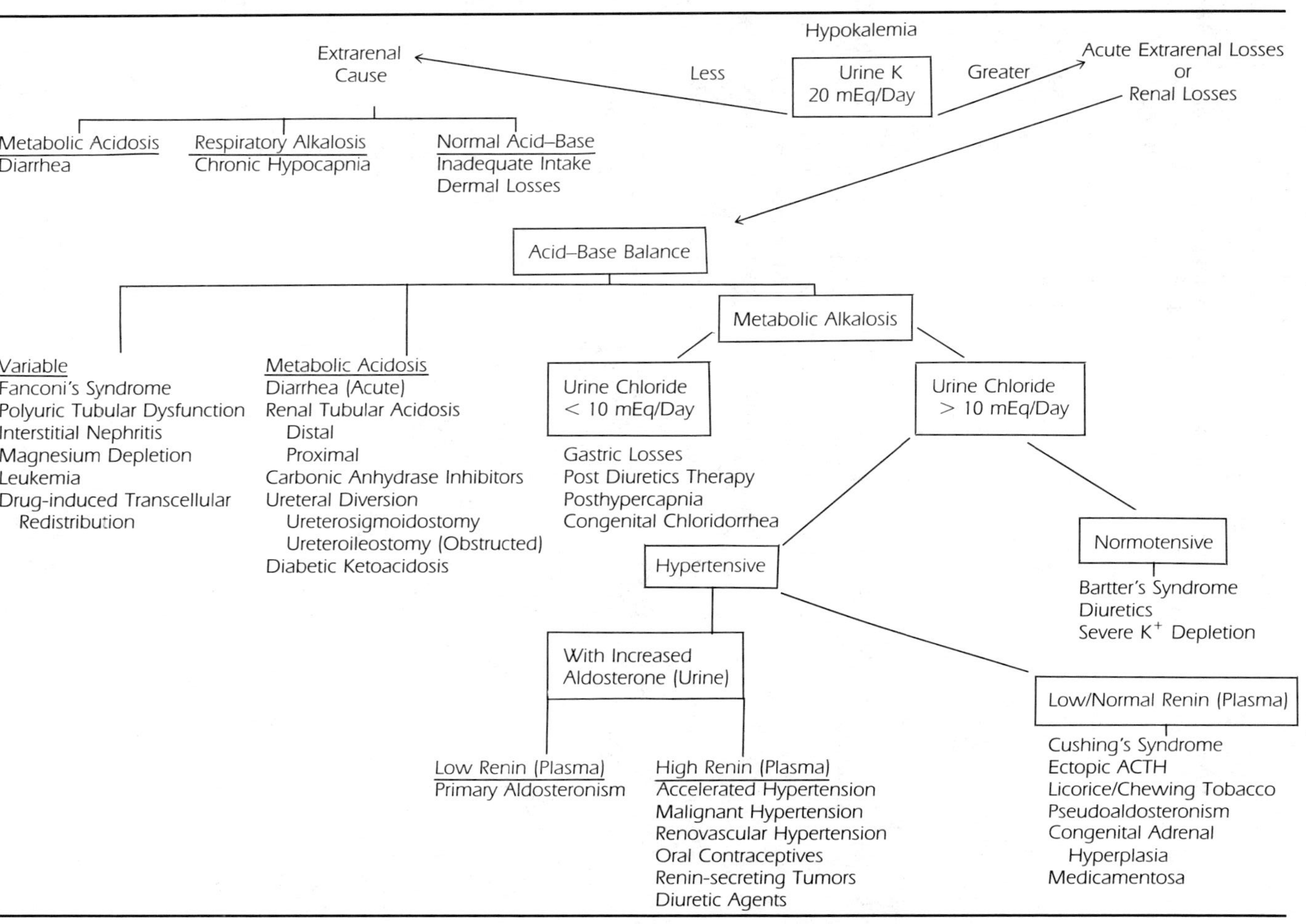

FIG 91–2.

Diagnostic approach to hypokalemia.

treated with K^+-sparing diuretics, nonsteroidal anti-inflammatory drugs with the capacity to inhibit prostaglandin E_2 synthesis, or an angiotensin-converting enzyme inhibitor. These agents are best avoided in these patients, or close monitoring for the development of hyperkalemia will be required. Because of alterations in transcellular K^+ distribution, nonselective beta-adrenergic blocking agents should also be used cautiously in patients at risk for hyperkalemia. It would seem prudent to favor selective beta$_1$-adrenergic blocking agents in this situation because cellular K^+ uptake appears to be mediated by beta$_2$-adrenergic activity.

Although hypokalemia is more frequently encountered clinically, it rarely is severe. Many patients receiving diuretic therapy for essential hypertension will have mild degrees of hypokalemia (serum K^+ concentrations of 3.0 to 3.5 mEq/L). The desirability of K^+ supplements for this group of patients is vigorously debated. There are risks of hyperkalemia with K^+ supplements or K^+-sparing diuretic agents. The benefits generally outweigh the risks in those patients with edema or known heart or liver disease and in those receiving digitalis or glucocorticoids. The risks are often greater in patients with diabetes mellitus or renal insufficiency and in those receiving drugs known to impair normal K^+ homeostasis. In hospitalized patients in the Boston Collaborative Drug Surveillance Program, 31% of patients received KCl for prevention and treatment of hypokalemia. Hyperkalemia developed in 3.6% of those treated and was described as life threatening in 0.4% and fatal in 0.1%.

The therapy of hyperkalemia will depend on the severity of the elevation, the rapidity of its development, and the specific cause. The presence of cardiac or neuromuscular manifestations of hyperkalemia is a medical emergency and requires immediate and aggressive therapy, as does any patient with an acute rise in serum K^+ levels to greater than 6 mEq/L. Therapy is aimed at antagonizing the membrane effects of hyperkalemia, redistributing K^+ from the ECF to the ICF, enhancing K^+ removal from the body, and specifically treating the cause of hyperkalemia when possible (see Table 91–5). In general, calcium gluconate is a temporizing measure employed to prevent a lethal cardiac arrhythmia or respiratory arrest until measures that will redistribute K^+ intracellularly and re-

move K^+ can have their desired effect. The need for dialysis will be determined by the patient's renal function, the severity of the hyperkalemia, and the presence of a remediable condition. The diabetic patient with a serum K^+ concentration of 6.5 and moderate renal failure who was taking supplemental K^+ and a drug known to impair renal K^+ excretion can usually be managed without dialysis. In contrast, a catabolic patient with acute renal failure will undoubtedly require dialysis in addition to the medical measures described. Once the acute situation has stabilized, it is necessary to attempt to identify the specific cause of the hyperkalemia. If no specific therapy is available, the patient will require dietary K^+ restriction with avoidance of salt substitutes high in K^+, control of metabolic acidosis if present (with sodium bicarbonate, sodium citrate, or calcium carbonate), adequate dietary fluids so that urine volume is at least 1 liter daily, and avoidance of any drug with the potential to interfere with K^+ excretion or cause K^+ transcellular redistribution to the ECF. Under some circumstances chronic administration of diuretic agents to enhance renal K^+ excretion or of a cation-exchange resin to promote fecal K^+ excretion may be necessary.

Most hypokalemic patients can usually be treated with oral K^+ supplements. Dietary K^+ is not generally more than 100 mEq daily unless the diet is very high in fruits. The choice of anion to accompany the K^+ depends on the underlying acid–base disturbance. Only those patients with a metabolic acidosis should be given an alkalizing salt (acetate, bicarbonate, citrate, or gluconate), while the majority should receive KCl. Patients with concomitant phosphate depletion can be given K^+ phosphate to provide part of the K^+ supplement. Of the KCl preparations, the liquid preparations are more rapidly absorbed than tablets. For chronic administration, KCl in one of several timed-release formats has better compliance. Intravenous administration should be reserved for hospitalized patients unable or unwilling to take K^+ orally or by nasogastric tube and for those with severe hypokalemia until stabilized. The dose required should be roughly estimated from the serum K^+ concentration.

Estimation of the total K^+ deficit in any individual patient is difficult, especially when a concomitant acid–base disturbance is present.

TABLE 91–5.
Therapy of Hyperkalemia

MODALITY	ONSET OF ACTION	DURATION OF EFFECT	MECHANISM	COMMENTS
Calcium gluconate	Immediate	30–60 min	Membrane antagonism	Increased E_T Increased sodium channels Faster conduction Enhanced digitalis toxicity
Sodium bicarbonate	10–30 min	2 hr	Transcellular redistribution	Decreases ionized calcium level Risk of sodium overload
Glucose and insulin	15–30 min	During infusion	Transcellular redistribution	Risk of hypoglycemia Risk of hyperglycemia
Cation-exchange resin (sodium polystyrene sulfonate)	1–2 hr	4–6 hr	Excretion (fecal)	May cause vomiting, fecal impaction, sodium overload
Kaliuretic diuretic agent	Onset of diuresis	Hours	Excretion (renal)	Requires renal function
Hemodialysis	Immediate	During dialysis	Removal	Risk delay in treatment
Peritoneal dialysis	Gradual	During dialysis	Removal and transcellular redistribution	K^+ removal < 5 mEq/hr

As a guideline, a decrease in serum K^+ concentration from 4 to 3 mEq/L in a 70-kilogram man represents a 100 mEq to 200 mEq deficit of K^+ and each additional decrease of 1 mEq/L will reflect an additional 200 mEq to 400 mEq deficit of K^+. Acid–base changes alter plasma K^+ levels acutely and as a rule of thumb there is an inverse change in serum K^+ of 0.6 mEq/L for each 0.1 unit decrease in arterial blood pH.

When replenishing K^+, consideration must also be given to continuing K^+ losses, the current serum K^+ concentration, the chronicity of the problem, accompanying medical problems, and the complication induced by hypokalemia. Generally K^+ can be given orally in a dose of 20 mEq every 2 hours to 50 mEq every 4 hours to the patient who has normal renal function, insignificant ongoing losses or transcellular redistribution, an absence of severe acidosis and no life-threatening hypokalemic manifestations with a serum K over 2 mEq/L. Modifications to greater or lesser doses should be anticipated if any of the above conditions exist, and, in any event, repeated measurements of serum K will be necessary after each 60 mEq to 100 mEq have been administered. It is unusual to require more than 200 mEq of K^+ daily although patients with severe renal K^+ wasting may need 200 mEq to 400 mEq daily. It should be recalled that K must be redistributed intracellularly from the low concentration and low capacity ECF space. If K^+ is provided intravenously, continuous EKG monitoring will be required if the rate exceeds 10 mEq/hour although normal subjects given KCl at 0.75 mEq/kg over 2 hours will increase serum K^+ by less than 0.8 mEq/L. *Rarely,* rapid intravenous administration of K^+ is required for *life-threatening* cardiac arrhythmias or paralysis *with serum K^+ of less than 2 mEq/L.* When these very unusual situations are associated with ongoing losses, K^+ may be given at rates exceeding 40 mEq/hour for brief periods while the EKG is continuously monitored and the serum K^+ is determined hourly. The rate of administration should be markedly slowed once the serum K^+ increases to approximately 2.5 mEq/L or sooner if there is EKG evidence of toxicity. These rates cannot be considered safe and require extreme caution. During rapid repletion the altered ratio of intracellular to extracellular K^+ may be manifest by increased neural or cardiac excitability especially if the patient has concomitant hypocalcemia and/or hypomagnesemia. Deficiencies of these divalent cations should be corrected if present. Once the emergent condition is under control, the remainder of the required K^+ replacement should be attempted orally.

REFERENCES

Giebisch G, Mainic G, Berliner RW: Renal transport and control of potassium excretion, in Brenner BM, Rector FC (eds): *The Kidney.* Philadelphia, WB Saunders Co, 1985, pp 177–205. *An extensively referenced authoritative monograph on renal potassium metabolism.*

Kaplan NM, Carnegie A, Raskin P, Heller JA, Simmons M: Potassium supplementation in hypertensive patients with diuretic-induced hypokalemia. *N Engl J Med* 1985; 312:746–749.

Kassirer JP, Harrington JT: Fending off the potassium pushers (editorial). *N Engl Med* 1985; 312:785–787. *The above references highlight some of the debate concerning routine potassium supplementation of patients receiving diuretics for hypertension.*

Katz LD, Defronzo RA: Hyperkalemia, in Glassock RJ (ed): *Current Therapy in Nephrology and Hypertension 1984–1985.* Philadelphia, BC Decker, 1984, pp 13–20. *A discussion of the current classification and treatment of hyperkalemia.*

Levy AS, Harrington JT: Hypokalemia, in Glassock RJ (ed): *Current Therapy in Nephrology and Hypertension 1984–1985.* Philadelphia, BC Decker, 1984, pp 20–25. *A discussion of the current classification and treatment of hypokalemia.*

Nardone DA, McDonald WJ, Girard DE: Mechanisms in hypokalemia: Clinical correlation. *Medicine* 1978; 57:435–446. *A discussion of the physiology relevant to the development of hypokalemia.*

Sebastian A, Hernandez RE, Schambelan M: Disorders of renal handling of potassium, in Brenner BM, Rector FC (eds): *The Kidney.* Philadelphia, WB Saunders Co, 1985, pp 519–550. *The most current clinical review of potassium disorders, extensively referenced by authors who have done much to describe the clinical syndrome of hyporeninemic hypoaldosteronism.*

92

HYPERMAGNESEMIA AND HYPOMAGNESEMIA

James W. Agna, M.D.

Patients with abnormal concentrations of serum magnesium may or may not have symptoms or signs. Furthermore, an altered concentration does not necessarily reflect an abnormal total body content of magnesium. The serum magnesium concentration normally is maintained in a narrow range from 1.5 to 2.0 mEq/L. Clinically significant problems do not usually occur unless the serum magnesium concentration is below 1.0 mEq/L or above 4.0 mEq/L. When these abnormal levels are obtained, significant symptoms and signs may ensue involving principally the neuromuscular and cardiovascular systems. Alterations of serum magnesium concentration are not disease entities but biochemical abnormalities and occur in a variety of clinical disorders.

CLINICAL SIGNS AND SYMPTOMS

Hypomagnesemia and magnesium deficiency occur in clinical states in which there is decreased intake, decreased intestinal absorption, excessive losses of body fluids, or excessive urinary losses of magnesium. Conditions associated with hypomagnesemia are listed in Table 92–1. Signs and symptoms of hypomagnesemia are related principally to the neuromuscular, cardiovascular, and gastrointestinal systems. In acute magnesium deficiency, neuromuscular irritability as evidenced by positive Chvostek's and Trousseau's signs may evolve rapidly into frank tetany. On the other hand, in chronic magnesium deficiency, muscle tremors, fasciculations, wasting, and weakness may occur; the patient may complain of anorexia, nausea, and dysphagia. Cardiac arrhythmias are an important, serious clinical manifestation of magnesium deficiency. Premature ventricular contractions, ventricular tachycardia, and ventricular fibrillation have been reported. The common signs and symptoms of hypomagnesemia are listed in Table 92–2.

Hypermagnesemia usually requires an increased intake of the ion and abnormal renal

---

TABLE 92–1.
Clinical Settings for Hypomagnesemia

DECREASED INTAKE
Starvation
Prolonged intravenous therapy
Prolonged nasogastric suction

GASTROINTESTINAL DISORDERS
Malabsorption syndromes
Prolonged diarrhea
Short bowel syndrome
Bowel and biliary fistulas
Cirrhosis
Pancreatitis

RENAL MAGNESIUM WASTING
Renal diseases
Diuretic phase of acute tubular necrosis
Chronic glomerulonephritis and pyelonephritis
Obstructive nephropathy
Renal tubular acidosis
Postrenal transplant
Osmotic diuresis
Glucose (diabetic ketoacidosis)
Mannitol
Alcohol ingestion
Hypercalciuria
Aldosteronism
Bartter's syndrome
Syndrome of inappropriate ADH secretion
Diuretic therapy
Amphotericin toxicity
Aminoglycoside therapy
Cisplatin therapy
Cardiac glycoside therapy

ENDOCRINE AND METABOLIC
Parathyroid disease
Thyroid disease
Hungry bone syndrome
Phosphate deficiency
Protein-calorie malnutrition
Excessive lactation

function. However, it may occur in patients with normal renal function who have an excessive intake of magnesium from compounds used for diagnostic or therapeutic reasons. The conditions associated with hypermagnesemia are listed in Table 92–3. The symptoms and signs of hypermagnesemia are correlated to some degree with the plasma concentration and range from hypoactive tendon reflexes, hypotension, nausea, vomiting, and urinary retention at lower levels of hypermagnesemia to somnolence, paralysis, respiratory depression, and asystole at higher levels. The symptoms and signs related to the serum magnesium concentrations are listed in Table 92–4.

PATHOPHYSIOLOGY

The adult human contains approximately 2000 mEq of magnesium, which makes it the fourth most abundant cation in the body. It is a major intracellular cation, ranking second in amount to potassium. About half the total body magnesium is contained in bone, the remainder being distributed in muscle and other tissue. A small but vitally important pool of magnesium is in the serum where the concentration ranges from 1.5 to 2.0 mEq/L as measured by the atomic absorption method of analysis; other colorimetric methods give similar but possibly less accurate values. A third of plasma magnesium is bound to protein; the remainder is diffusible except for a small percentage bound to phosphates and other anions. Normally we ingest from green vegetables, grains, and meat 25 mEq of magnesium per day and absorb one-third of the intake from the gastrointestinal tract. Excretion and regulation of magnesium concentration is principally through the kidney. Renal handling of magnesium is by glomerular filtration and tubular reabsorption.

The major factors controlling magnesium excretion are the glomerular filtration rate, filtered load, extracellular fluid volume, hypermagnesemia, hypomagnesemia, phosphate depletion, hyperkalemia, and parathyroid hormone (PTH). Therefore, altered intake, gastrointestinal function, and renal function are keys to the production of hypomagnesemia or hypermagnesemia.

Magnesium functions as a cofactor or metalloenzyme for enzymes or enzyme systems, especially where phosphate is a substrate. The enzymes include the phosphatases and others concerned in the reactions involving adenosine triphosphate (ATP). Thus magnesium is involved in oxidative phosphorylation, nerve conduction, muscle contraction, membrane transport, and nucleic acid synthesis. Magnesium is required by the enzyme adenyl cyclase for the conversion of ATP to cyclic adenosine monophosphate (cAMP), the generally accepted mediator of the peripheral action of PTH. The maintenance of cell transmembrane ratios of potassium to sodium and

---

TABLE 92–2.
Signs and Symptoms of Hypomagnesemia

GASTROINTESTINAL SYSTEM

Anorexia
Nausea
Dysphagia

CARDIOVASCULAR SYSTEM

Prolonged PR and QT intervals and flat broad T waves
Premature ventricular contractions
Severe ventricular dysrhythmias

NEUROMUSCULAR SYSTEM

Muscle twitching and tremor
Muscle weakness
Chvostek's sign
Paresthesia
Carpopedal spasm
Hyperreflexia
Vertigo
Ataxia
Nystagmus
Tetany
Seizures
Athetoid movements

MENTAL EFFECTS

Lethargy
Confusion
Delirium

TABLE 92–3.
Clinical Settings for Hypermagnesemia

Acute renal failure
Chronic renal failure
Toxemia therapy (mothers and infants)
Administration of magnesium-containing compounds*
  Orally (antacids, cathartics)
  Parenterally
  Irrigation

* Especially in patients with impaired renal function.

magnesium to calcium are important for cell excitation and intracellular metabolism. Excitable tissues including heart muscle depend on electrochemical potential differences across cell membranes for impulse generation and propagation. These electrical impulses initiate neuromuscular activity. The cell membrane ATPases, which are magnesium dependent, regulate the egress and ingress of potassium, sodium, and calcium. In fact, magnesium has been termed "nature's physiologic calcium blocker." Therefore, the effect of magnesium on CA^{++} ATPase and NA^{+}-K^{+}-ATPase probably accounts for a number of the signs and symptoms of magnesium deficiency or excess. Competition between calcium and magnesium for common receptor sites is thought to play a major role in the effects observed particularly in the nervous system.

CLINICAL–PATHOLOGIC CORRELATIONS

Hypomagnesemia and hypermagnesemia affect basic cell function. The significant manifestations clinically involve principally the neuromuscular and cardiovascular systems. Somewhat paradoxically very low and very high magnesium concentrations both inhibit parathyroid gland function. Some of the clinical–pathologic correlations of hypomagnesemia and hypermagnesemia are listed in Tables 92–5 and 92–6.

DIFFERENTIAL DIAGNOSIS

Differential diagnostic considerations in hypomagnesemia include delirium tremens, hypocalcemia, and toxic substances causing neuromuscular irritability. In delirium tremens, the neuromuscular irritability may be due to both alcohol and magnesium deficiency. The tetany from hypocalcemia is indistinguishable from the tetany of hypomagnesemia, and in a significant number of patients with tetany, the serum concentrations of both ions are abnormally low.

Cases of symptomatic hypermagnesemia may be confused with cases of myopathies, polyneuropathies, and myasthenia gravis. In the latter condition, weakness and respiratory de-

TABLE 92–4.
Signs and Symptoms of Hypermagnesemia Correlated with Plasma Levels

SERUM LEVEL OF MAGNESIUM (mEq/L)	SIGN OR SYMPTOM
4–9	Hypotension
	Nausea and vomiting
	Urinary retention
	Bradycardia
	Cutaneous flushing
5–10	EKG changes
	Increased PR, QRS, and QT intervals
	Decreased P wave voltage
	Variable T wave peaking
	Heart block at high concentrations
	Hyporeflexia
	CNS depression
9–10	Respiratory depression
	Coma
15	Asystolic arrest

pression may occur, but in contrast to hypermagnesemia, the reflexes are spared. Those patients with hypermagnesemia who manifest hypotension and cardiac conduction problems must be distinguished from patients who have heart disease or digitalis intoxication. Measurement of the serum magnesium concentration is crucial in differentiating these conditions.

DIAGNOSIS

The diagnosis of hypomagnesemia or hypermagnesemia can be suspected from the history and physical examination, but it is confirmed by obtaining abnormal serum concentration values. The abnormal values, usually indicative of a deficiency or an excess of magnesium, do not always indicate abnormalities in the total body content. Tissue analysis for magnesium has not proved to be a practical procedure, and blood cell analysis for magnesium is not an accurate method for estimating total body stores.

Characteristic of other electrolyte abnormalities, abnormalities in serum magnesium concentration are not usually an isolated event but are associated with other abnormalities. Hypokalemia, hypocalcemia, hypophosphatemia, and hyponatremia appear to be good predictors of coexisting hypomagnesemia. As reported in

TABLE 92–5.
Clinical–Pathologic Correlations of Hypomagnesemia

CLINICAL FINDINGS	PATHOLOGIC FINDINGS
NEUROMUSCULAR SYSTEM	
Muscle weaknesses Muscle twitching Dysphagia Hyperreflexia Tremor Tetany Seizures	Electromyographic changes of myopathic-like potentials in animals. Facilitation of acetylcholine release at motor endplate or any cholinergic synapse because magnesium not available to inhibit calcium
CARDIOVASCULAR SYSTEM	
Premature ventricular contractions Ventricular tachycardia and fibrillation Refractory hypokalemia	Diminished activation of Mg^{++}-dependent membrane Na^{+}-K^{+} ATPase resulting in cell loss of K^{+} and cell gain of Na^{+}. Diminished activation of Mg-dependent Ca^{++} ATPase resulting in increased calcium entry into myocardial cells. Catecholamine stimulation of heart because magnesium not available to suppress catecholamine release
PARATHYROID FUNCTION	
Refractory hypocalcemia and tetany	Inhibition of synthesis or release of PTH and inhibition of end-organ responsiveness

a recent study, hypomagnesemia occurred in 42% of patients with hypokalemia, 22% of patients with hypocalcemia, 29% of patients with hypophosphatemia, and 27% of patients with hyponatremia (Whang et al., 1984). A coexisting potassium or calcium deficiency may be more easily corrected if the magnesium deficiency is addressed initially. Certain cases of hypocalcemia are refractory to treatment unless the magnesium deficiency is corrected.

PRINCIPLES OF PREVENTION AND THERAPY

Prevention of hypomagnesemia is predicated on recognizing the predisposing clinical settings, for example, patients on gastric suction or prolonged intravenous therapy or in other clinical states listed in Table 92–1. In treatment of hypomagnesemia and hypermagnesemia, attention to the basic disorder causing the deficiency or excess is paramount. Hypomagnesemia is treated with magnesium salts. Mild deficiencies may be ameliorated with oral intake of magnesium. However, most patients with symptomatic magnesium deficiency require intramuscular or preferably intravenous infusions of magnesium salts. Total body deficits of magnesium may be several hundred mEq but need not be restored quickly. In fact, because magnesium equilibrates slowly with the intracellular compartment, it is desirable to replenish the stores over several days with appropriate monitoring of other electrolyte derangements and urinary output. Rapid infusion of magnesium could result in abnormally high levels affecting vital body functions. Commonly associated hypokalemia and hypocalcemia will become more easily corrected once the magnesium deficiency is corrected. If renal function is impaired, frequent measurement of the serum magnesium concentration is indicated.

The prevention of hypermagnesemia is associated with the judicious use of magnesium-containing antacids and laxatives, careful monitoring of patients receiving magnesium for the toxemia of pregnancy, and the cautious replacement of magnesium in deficiency states. In the treatment of hypermagnesemia, the first steps are discontinuing magnesium ingestion or administration and addressing the clinical problems related to hydration and renal function. Calcium given intravenously acts as an antidote to counteract life-threatening signs

TABLE 92–6.
Clinical–Pathologic Correlations of Hypermagnesemia

CLINICAL FINDINGS	PATHOLOGIC FINDINGS
NEUROMUSCULAR SYSTEM	
Hyporeflexia	Impaired nerve conduction
Respiratory depression	Paralysis of voluntary muscles
Paralysis	Neuromuscular blockade by suppressing release of acetylcholine
Somnolence coma	CNS depression
CARDIOVASCULAR SYSTEM	
Hypotension and bradycardia	Depressant effect on vascular smooth muscle and sympathetic nervous system (possibly by blocking calcium)
Asystolic arrest	Depressed myocardial contractility through interaction with calcium, potassium, and sodium
PARATHYROID FUNCTION	
Hypocalcemia	Inhibition of PTH secretion

and symptoms of excess magnesium. However, if there is persistence of the hypermagnesemia, peritoneal dialysis or hemodialysis may be required to effectively and rapidly lower the plasma concentration of magnesium to a safe level.

REFERENCES

Cronin RE, Knochel JP. Magnesium deficiency. *Annu Rev Med* 1983; 28:509–533. *Excellent recent review of the subject.*

Dirks JH: The kidney and magnesium regulation. *Kidney Int* 1983; 23:771–777. *Good review of the role of the kidney in magnesium metabolism.*

Fassler CAA, Rodriguez M, Badesch DB, Stone WJ, Marini JJ: Magnesium toxicity as a cause of hypotension and hypoventilation. Occurrence in patients with normal renal function. *Arch Intern Med* 1985; 145:1604–1606. *Brief review of magnesium toxicity with detailed list of magnesium-containing compounds.*

Flink EB, Stutzman FL, Anderson AR, Konig T, Fraser R: Magnesium deficiency after prolonged fluid administration and after chronic alcoholism complicated by delirium tremens. *J Lab Clin Med* 1954; 43:169–183. *A paper written at mid-century that heightened clinical awareness of major causes of magnesium deficiency.*

Hirschfelder AD, Hawry VG: Clinical manifestations of high and low plasma magnesium. *JAMA* 1934; 102:1138–1141. *A landmark article written 50 years ago containing numerous clinical observations.*

Iseri LT, Freed J, Bures AR: Magnesium deficiency and cardiac disorders. *Am J Med* 1975; 58: 831–846. *An important paper linking magnesium deficiency with serious cardiac arrhythmias.*

Iseri LT, French JH: Magnesium: Nature's physiological calcium blocker. (Editorial) *Am Heart J* 1984; 108:188–193. *A succinct discussion of magnesium–calcium interaction.*

Mordes JP, Wacker WEC: Excess magnesium. *Pharmacol Rev* 1978; 24:273–300. *A comprehensive review of the causes and effects of excess magnesium.*

Wacker WEC: *Magnesium and man.* Commonwealth Fund Book. Cambridge, Harvard University Press, 1980. *A definitive monograph on normal and abnormal metabolism of magnesium.*

Whang R, Tjien OO, Aikawa JK, Watanabe A, Vanatta J, Fryer A, Markanich M: Predictors of clinical hypomagnesemia, hypokalemia, hypophosphatemia, hyponatremia, and hypocalcemia. *Arch Intern Med* 1984; 144:1794–1796. *Underscores the high incidence of multiple electrolyte derangements.*

93

HYPERCALCEMIA AND HYPOCALCEMIA

James W. Agna, M.D.

Bone contains 99% of the total body calcium. The 1% present in the extracellular fluid and the soft tissue cells, though small in quantity, plays a vital role in cellular function. Under normal conditions the serum calcium concentration is maintained within relatively narrow limits. The ionized fraction is critical to optimal cell function. Although many patients with an abnormal serum calcium concentration have no related symptoms, the detection of this abnormality is important because in most instances the altered calcium concentration is indicative of a significant disease. Rapid changes in calcium concentration, as well as chronically low and high levels, can result in dramatic and life-threatening conditions ranging from tetany and convulsions with low levels to coma and cardiac arrest with high levels. Although there is some variation based on analytic methods, the normal range for serum calcium is 9 to 10.5 mg/dL. Therefore, hypocalcemia is definable as a serum calcium level of less than 9 mg/dL and hypercalcemia as a level greater than 10.5 mg/dL.

CLINICAL SIGNS AND SYMPTOMS

Hypocalcemia causes neuromuscular, cardiac, mental, dermal, and ocular abnormalities. A common and characteristic finding is neuromuscular irritability which may be expressed as tetany. The patient may experience paresthesias, muscle spasms, and cramps. Carpopedal spasm occurs frequently. The most common cause of tetany seen in an emergency department is hyperventilation, which is not associated with an actual decrease in total serum calcium, but a fall in the concentration of ionized calcium resulting from the increased protein–calcium binding induced by the respiratory alkalosis. Hypocalcemic tetany, on the other hand, does not usually occur until the serum calcium level drops below 7.0 mg/dL. Occasionally tetany is subclinical and may be identified by producing a twitch or grimace from tapping over the facial nerve (Chvostek's sign) or by inflating a blood pressure cuff to greater than the systolic pressure for 3 minutes to produce carpal spasm (Trousseau's sign). Table 93–1 lists the signs and symptoms of hypocalcemia. The more acute and dramatic manifestations of hypocalcemia involve the neuromuscular and cardiovascular system, whereas sustained hypocalcemia may be associated with intellectual impairment, movement disorders, ocular manifestations, and ectodermal disorders.

Hypercalcemia affects many body systems including the cardiovascular, gastroenteric, genitourinary, and neuromuscular systems. Psychiatric manifestations may include depression and psychosis. Metastatic calcification in one or more tissues of the body may be present. Often the patient has polyuria and polydipsia from an impaired ability of the kidney to concentrate. Renal calculi may be the initial symptom. If the hypercalcemia is rapidly progressive, stupor, coma, heart block, and cardiac arrest may develop. A serum calcium concentration in excess of 15 mg/dL is a true medical emergency. Occasionally, if the plasma calcium rise is unusually rapid, vital functions may be threatened when the calcium level is between 12 and 15 mg/dL. The signs and symptoms of hypercalcemia are listed in Table 93–2.

PATHOPHYSIOLOGY

The maintenance of a normal extracellular calcium concentration is under the control of parathyroid hormone (PTH), vitamin D, and probably calcitonin. In response to a fall in the

TABLE 93–1.
Signs and Symptoms of Hypocalcemia

ACUTE HYPOCALCEMIA	CHRONIC HYPOCALCEMIA
Paresthesias	Depression
Chvostek's sign*	Hallucinations
Trousseau's sign	Psychosis
Muscle spasm	Mental retardation
Carpopedal spasm	Weakness and myopathy
Anxiety	Dry skin
Seizures	Eczema
Laryngeal stridor	Brittle nails
Bronchospasm	Moniliasis (polyendocrine deficiency)
Apnea	Dental changes
Hypotension	Cataracts
Arrhythmias	Basal ganglia calcification
Heart failure	Movement disorders
Papilledema	

* Approximately 15% of normals have this sign.

TABLE 93–2.
Signs and Symptoms of Hypercalcemia*

Gastrointestinal—Nausea, vomiting, abdominal pain, constipation, pancreatitis, peptic ulcer
Neurologic—Fatigue, weakness, hypotonia, hyporeflexia, confusion, stupor, coma
Psychiatric—Impaired memory, apathy, hallucinations, depression, psychosis
Genitourinary—Polyuria, renal calculi, nephrocalcinosis, renal failure
Cardiovascular—Hypertension, arrhythmias, short QT interval, heart block
Skeletal—Fractures, deformities, bone pain
Metastatic calcification—Joints, cornea (band keratopathy), vessels, soft tissue

* Pancreatitis, peptic ulcer, calculi, and skeletal changes are primarily associated with hyperparathyroidism.

ionized serum calcium concentration, PTH acts to restore calcium to a normal level by increasing bone resorption and renal tubular calcium reabsorption and by increasing the intestinal calcium absorption through augmentation of the synthesis of 1,25-dihydroxy/vitamin D $(1,25\text{-}(OH)_2D)$ by the kidney. The effects of PTH are mediated through its interaction on a membrane-bound receptor, the adenylate cyclase complex, resulting in an increase in intracellular cyclic AMP. Cyclic AMP recovered in the urine, nephrogenous cyclic AMP, can serve as an index of PTH activity. Parathyroid hormone also causes an increase in the renal reabsorption of magnesium, as well as a phosphaturia and a bicarbonaturia. Vitamin D stimulates the absorption of calcium from the gut, decreases its renal excretion, and enhances calcium resorption from bone. Vitamin D is produced nonenzymatically by the exposure of the skin to ultraviolet light, or is ingested in food.

In the body, vitamin D is initially hydroxylated in the liver to 25-hydroxy-cholecalciferol $(25\text{-}(OH)D)$. It is further hydroxylated to a more active form, by the kidney under the influence of PTH, 1,25-dihydroxycholecalciferol $(1, 25\text{-}(OH)_2D)$. Calcitonin secretion is stimulated by a rise in the concentration of ionized calcium in the serum. Calcitonin decreases calcium resorption from bone and increases calcium excretion by the kidney. In contrast to that of PTH and vitamin D, the role of calcitonin in calcium homeostasis is not well defined.

Of an average daily intake of 800 mg to 900 mg of calcium, approximately 30% to 35% is absorbed from the small bowel. Approximately 150 mg to 200 mg of calcium are normally excreted each day in the urine. Calcium is also lost through the gastroenteric secretions. The serum calcium concentration, kept in a narrow range (9 to 10.5 mg/dL) contains three components: approximately 45% as a protein-bound fraction; 10% as a complexed nonionized fraction in the form of salts of phosphate, sulfate, and citrate; and approximately 40% as the most important, physiologically active, ionized fraction. Spuriously high or low values of total serum calcium, not reflecting changes in ionized calcium levels, may occur with correspondingly elevated or decreased serum protein concentrations. The ionized component is also influenced by body pH, the higher the pH the lower the ionized calcium.

Of the 1200 gm of calcium in the adult human body, the 1% outside of bone in the extracellular fluid and soft tissues is critical for normal cardiac contraction, cardiac conduction, blood coagulation, nerve conduction, muscle contraction, hormone secretion, and enzyme activation. The transmembrane flux of calcium ions is intertwined with the transfer of other ions including potassium, sodium, chloride, phosphate, and magnesium. Calcium movement is regulated by a voltage-dependent and a phosphorylation-dependent gate. The movement of calcium, potassium, sodium, and chloride is controlled by specific channels, and the harmonious relationship of these ions is crucial to cell function. The role of magnesium is especially important because the magnesium-dependent cell membrane ATPases regulate the egress and ingress of potassium, sodium, and calcium.

The causes of hypocalcemia are listed in Table 93–3. The major causes are impaired PTH metabolism, vitamin D deficiency, impairment of calcium function through chelation or chemical combination, and hypomagnesemia. Hypomagnesemia decreases PTH secretion and diminishes PTH end-organ responsiveness to PTH.

The causes of hypercalcemia are listed in Table 93–4. Hypercalcemia may result from increased bone resorption, increased gut absorption, or decreased renal excretion of calcium. Primary hyperparathyroidism and malignancy are the most common serious causes of hypercalcemia, the former because of excess PTH and the latter because of increased bone resorption from tumor secretion of osteoclastic ac-

TABLE 93–3.
Causes of Hypocalcemia

A lack or defect in PTH synthesis, release, or end-organ responsiveness
  Hypoparathyroidism
  Pseudohypoparathyroidism
  Hypomagnesemia
  Neonatal hypocalcemia
  Pancreatitis
Disturbance in vitamin D metabolism from decreased intake, decreased 25-(OH)D production, accelerated 25-(OH)D catabolism, decreased 1,25-(OH)$_2$D production, or end-organ resistance to 1,25-(OH)$_2$D
  Dietary deficiency
  Malabsorption
  Liver disease
  Anticonvulsant therapy
  Renal failure
  Resistant rickets
Drugs and compounds affecting bone resorption, increasing calcium excretion, and chelating or chemically combining calcium
  Mithramycin
  Calcitonin
  Citrate
  Colchicine
  Protamine
  Ethylene glycol
  Loop diuretics
  EDTA
Miscellaneous
  "Hungry bone" syndrome
  Malignancies with increased osteoblastic activity
  Hyperphosphatemia

TABLE 93–4.
Causes of Hypercalcemia

CAUSES	PATHOGENETIC MECHANISMS
Malignancies	Secretion of PTH-like substance
	Metastases (resorption)
	Osteoclast activating factor
	Prostaglandins
Primary hyperparathyroidism	PTH secretion
Tertiary hyperparathyroidism	PTH secretion
Hypervitaminosis D	Vitamin D
Sarcoidosis	Vitamin D
Thiazide therapy	Decreased renal calcium excretion
	Increased bone resorption
Milk-alkali syndrome	Increased calcium intake
	Decreased renal calcium excretion
Hypervitaminosis A	Increased bone resorption
Immobilization	Relative increase in bone resorption
Familial hypocalciuric hypercalcemia	Decreased renal calcium excretion
Adrenal insufficiency	Decreased renal calcium excretion
	Relative vitamin D increase (cortisol lack)
Hyperthyroidism	Increased bone resorption
Lithium	PTH secretion
Postrenal transplantation	PTH secretion
Recovery from acute renal failure	Mobilization of tissue calcium
	PTH secretion
Acromegaly	Possible increased PTH or vitamin D levels
Pheochromocytoma	Increased bone resorption directly from catecholamines or indirectly through their effect on PTH

tivating factor, prostaglandins, PTH-like substances or by the production of vitamin D-like sterols. A malignancy with bone metastases may, independent of the aforementioned factors, also produce hypercalcemia by bone breakdown. Solid tumors producing prostaglandins and neoplasms of lymphoid origin producing osteoclastic activating factor may cause hypercalcemia. PTH-like substances are produced by carcinomas of the lung, genitourinary tract, and gastrointestional tract, as well as by lymphomas, leukemias, and melanomas. Hypervitaminosis D due to excess ingestion or associated with granulomatous diseases such as sarcoidosis account for a significant number of hypercalcemia cases. Excess ingestion of milk and alkali is a rare cause of hypercalcemia compared to several decades ago. Probably the most common cause of mild hypercalcemia occurs in patients who take a thiazide, which causes a decrease in renal calcium excretion. These patients are usually asymptomatic but should be investigated for a cause other than the thiazide itself because a significant number have been found to have primary hyper-

parathyroidism that was unmasked by the thiazide.

CLINICAL–PATHOLOGIC CORRELATIONS

Hypocalcemia decreases the excitation threshold of nerves and muscles and may result in tetany and seizures. Hypercalcemia increases the threshold for brain and muscle excitation and may result in weakness, lethargy, and eventually coma. The clinical–pathologic correlations of these abnormal states are listed in Table 93–5.

DIFFERENTIAL DIAGNOSIS

The differential diagnosis of hypocalcemia includes disorders of magnesium metabolism. Hypomagnesemia may impair PTH release and function. Parathyroid insufficiency, lack of vitamin D, and drug therapy causing calcium binding or a decrease in the vitamin D level

TABLE 93–5.
Clinical–Pathologic Correlations for Hypocalcemia and Hypercalcemia

CLINICAL FINDINGS	PATHOLOGIC FINDINGS
HYPOCALCEMIA	
Paresthesias	Decreased threshold of neuromuscular excitation:
Chvostek's sign	Frequent repetitive discharges on EMG
Trousseau's sign	Convulsive effects on EEG
Carpopedal spasm	
Laryngeal stridor	
Seizures	
Prolongation of QT interval on ECG	Prolongation of phase 2 of the transmembrane
Arrhythmias	action potential of myocardial cells
Hypotension	Lack of calcium binding to troponin causing
Depressed ventricular function and potential	inhibition of myosin–actin interaction resulting
heart failure	in muscle relaxation in the myocardium and
	vascular smooth muscle
HYPERCALCEMIA	
Weakness	Increased threshold of neuromuscular excitation
Hypotonia	
Hyporeflexia	
Confusion	
Stupor	
Coma	
Short QT interval on ECG	Decreased duration of phase 2 of the
Prolongation of PR interval; higher degrees of	transmembrane action potential of myocardial
atrioventricular block	cells
Ventricular tachyarrhythmias	Calcium binding of troponin causing
	augmentation of myosin–actin interaction
Hypertension	resulting in muscle contraction in the
	myocardium and vascular smooth muscle
Polydipsia	Impaired renal concentration
Polyuria	Nephrocalcinosis
Dehydration	
Renal failure	

should be considered. The disorders included in the differential diagnosis of hypocalcemia are listed in Table 93–3.

Hypercalcemic patients with primary hyperparathyroidism may have hypertension, weakness, renal colic, epigastric pain, peptic ulcer, pancreatitis, polyuria, arthralgias, or bone pain. There may be a family history of hyperparathyroidism or the patient may have a history of multiple endocrine neoplasia (MEN syndrome) involving the pituitary gland, pancreas, thyroid (medullary carcinoma), and adrenal medulla (pheochromocytoma). Familial hypocalciuric hypercalcemia should be considered in the differential diagnosis of hypercalcemia. The presence of a malignancy should also alert the clinician to the possibility of hypercalcemia. Excessive ingestion of vitamin D, vitamin A, milk, alkali, and calcium supplements should likewise alert the clinician to the possibility of hypercalcemia. Rarely the initial manifestation of adrenal cortical insufficiency is hypercalcemia due to the impaired renal excretion of calcium plus a relative excess of vitamin D. Other conditions in the differential diagnosis of hypercalcemia are listed in Table 93–4 along with the proposed mechanisms producing the elevated calcium.

DIAGNOSIS

Alterations in serum calcium concentration may be detected through routine laboratory testing or be strongly indicated from the history or physical examination. Having established the abnormality inadvertently or by design, it is incumbent upon the physician to determine the underlying cause.

With the advent of reliable methods to measure PTH, vitamin D, and nephrogenic cAMP, many alterations in calcium metabolism previously diagnosed by more indirect evidence are more quickly and accurately assessed. This is especially true for parathyroid disease. Nonetheless, a thorough history and physical examination often makes the diagnosis obvious. Alteration in plasma protein concentration can result in a spuriously high or low total plasma calcium concentration with the ionized fraction being normal. This situation occurs most frequently with hypoalbuminemia.

In hypocalcemia a family history of rickets, hypoparathyroidism, or pseudohypoparathyroidism should be sought. Also a history of the ingestion of certain medications (Table 93–3), poor dietary intake, malabsorption, or a gastrectomy may lead to hypocalcemia. Skeletal abnormalities and ectodermal changes noted on the physical examination are important clues. Low calcium, high phosphate, and low PTH values suggest hypoparathyroidism. A low serum magnesium concentration may be the major factor explaining a patient's hypocalcemia particularly in the alcoholic. Determining the levels of vitamin D metabolites (25-(OH)D and 1,25-(OH)$_2$D) may delineate the various forms of vitamin D deficiency. The response of serum calcium, urinary phosphate, and nephrogenic cAMP levels to the administration of PTH will usually differentiate hypoparathyroidism from pseudohypoparathyroidism.

In hypercalcemia, a positive family history may suggest the possibility of primary hyperparathyroidism, familial hypocalciuric hypercalcemia, or one of the MEN syndromes. Rapid-onset hypercalcemia suggests a malignancy, excessive calcium ingestion, or vitamin D intoxication. The physical examination may point to an obvious cause (e.g., malignancy or sarcoidosis). Elevated plasma levels of PTH and 1,25-(OH)$_2$D and elevated urinary levels of nephrogenic cAMP assist in establishing a diagnosis of hyperparathyroidism. Nephrogenic cAMP concentrations may be high in a malignancy with or without ectopic PTH production. The plasma concentration of 1,25-(OH)$_2$D is high in sarcoidosis, normal in the hypercalcemia of malignancy, and normal or high in primary hyperparathyroidism. In vitamin D intoxication, the 25-(OH)D level is elevated. In general, plasma levels of PTH are suppressed in

hypercalcemic conditions other than hyperparathyroidism and neoplasms producing a PTH-like molecule.

The urine calcium level is low in familial hypocalciuric hypercalcemia, high in primary hyperparathyroidism, and very high in nonparathyroid hypercalcemia. In primary hyperparathyroidism, the serum phosphate level is usually low, and a mild hyperchloremic acidosis may be present. Glucocorticoids suppress serum calcium levels in vitamin D intoxication, sarcoidosis, and some malignancies but not in primary hyperparathyroidism. Other diagnostic tests which have been used include computed tomography (CT scan), ultrasound and radionucleotide studies, serial PTH sampling from the neck or chest through a venous catheter, and arteriography for the preoperative localization of parathyroid neoplasia.

PRINCIPLES OF PREVENTION AND TREATMENT

It is important to recognize that hypomagnesemia, unless corrected, may make hypocalcemia refractory to treatment. Anticipation of potential hypocalcemia in patients with gastrointestinal diseases associated with malabsorption may avert significant hypocalcemia. Patients who take anticonvulsant drugs may develop hypocalcemia and require vitamin D supplementation. Acute symptomatic hypocalcemia requires emergency treatment with intravenous calcium to prevent tetany and seizures. The calcium is usually administered in the form of a 10% solution of calcium gluconate. Long-term calcium deficiency requires oral calcium supplements as well as vitamin D. The type of vitamin D chosen is determined to some degree by the nature of the disease causing the hypocalcemia and its duration of action. Cost factors are an additional consideration.

In hypercalcemia, attention should be directed toward ameliorating or correcting the cause (e.g., parathyroidectomy for hyperparathyroidism and chemotherapy or surgery for a malignancy). The discontinuance of calcium or vitamin D ingestion is obviously indicated in cases of excess ingestion. When the serum calcium concentration approaches or exceeds 15 mg/dL the problem is considered an emergency requiring rehydration with large amounts of saline and the use of furosemide for calcium diuresis. Careful attention to electrolyte balance is important under these conditions to prevent concomitant deficiencies in potassium and magnesium. Calcitonin acts within a few hours, has minimal toxicity, and may be used in the acute management of hypercalcemia. Mithramycin, which interferes with osteoclastic activity, is effective and acts within 12 to 24 hours. Its toxic effects, however, must be monitored closely. For long-range management of persistent hypercalcemia, glucocorticoids are efficacious in hypervitaminosis D, sarcoidosis, and certain malignancies. Glucocorticoids are not recommended for hyperparathyroidism. Glucocorticoids inhibit vitamin D secretion as well as the bone resorption stimulated by osteoclastic activating factor and prostaglandin. Prostaglandin synthetase inhibitors such as indomethacin may be helpful in the hypercalcemia of prostaglandin producing malignancy. Diphosphonates can be employed in the long-term management of hypercalcemia because they inhibit osteoclastic bone resorption through their effect on PTH secretion. Other treatment modalities include oral phosphate and more recently cisplatin. Phosphate given intravenously is potentially hazardous because it may result in widespread deposition of calcium phosphate, so-called metastatic calcification, and is, therefore, not recommended for the rapid lowering of serum calcium.

REFERENCES

Agus ZS, Goldfarb S: Calcium metabolism: Normal and abnormal, in Arieff AI, DeFronzo RA (eds): *Fluid, Electrolyte, and Acid Base Disorders*, 2 vols. New York, Churchill Livingstone, 1985, Vol 1, pp 511–573. *Thorough review; fine discussion of differential diagnoses; extensive references.*

Agus ZS, Wasserstein A, Goldfarb S: Disorders of calcium and magnesium homeostasis. *Am J Med* 1982; 72:473–488. *A concise review of factors maintaining serum calcium concentration.*

Conner FB, Rosen BL, Blaustein MP, Applefeld MM, Doyle LA: Hypocalcemia precipitating congestive heart failure. *N Engl J Med* 1982; 307:869–872. *An unusual manifestation of hypocalcemia with a good discussion of calcium–digoxin interaction.*

Fisch C: Electrolytes and the heart, in Hurst JW (ed): *The Heart*, ed 6. New York, McGraw-Hill Book Co, 1986, pp 1473–1476. *Excellent discussion of calcium and the transmembrane action potential.*

Jacobson H, Knochel JP: Calcium and magnesium, renal handling and disorders of metabolism, in Brenner BM, Rector FC Jr (eds): *The Kidney*, ed 3. Philadelphia, WB Saunders Co, 1986, pp 567–584. *A complete review with focus on renal pathophysiology.*

Marx SJ, Stock JL, Attie MF et al: Familial hypocalciuric hypercalcemia: Recognition among patients referred after unsuccessful parathyroid exploration. *Ann Intern Med* 1980; 92:351–356. *Increased awareness of this disorder might reduce the incidence of parathyroid explorations.*

Mundy GR, Cove DH, Fisken R: Primary hyperparathyroidism: Changes in the pattern of clinical presentation. *Lancet* 1980; 1:1317–1320. *Discussion of the high incidence in elderly women with hypercalcemic crisis being an initial manifestation.*

Zaloga GP, Chernow B: Calcium metabolism, in Geelhoed GW, Chernow B (eds): *Endocrine Aspects of Acute Illness*. New York, Churchill Livingstone, 1985, pp 169–204. *Another fine general review, but particularly valuable for the discussion of cellular physiology.*

94

HYPOPHOSPHATEMIA

Mohammad G. Saklayen, M.D.

Phosphate, an integral constituent of all tissues, is critical to many physiologic functions. Although most of the phosphate in the body is intracellular and cannot be readily measured, the serum level of phosphate provides an indirect estimate of total body phosphate. The lower limits of normal are 2.8 mg/dL in adults and 4.0 mg/dL in children. A serum phosphate level of less than 1.0 mg/dL is considered severe and may be associated with catastrophic complications. Tables 94–1 and 94–2 list causes of severe and moderate hypophosphatemia, respectively. Although many conditions can cause hypophosphatemia, chronic alcoholism accounts for more than 70% of all severe cases in the United States. Depletion of body phosphate can cause a host of clinical syndromes.

CLINICAL SIGNS AND SYMPTOMS

Clinical manifestations of hypophosphatemia depend on the magnitude and rapidity of phosphate depletion. Thus, a serum phosphate level of 1.5 mg/dL in a chronic alcoholic patient may be associated with mild muscle weakness only, while further lowering of the serum phosphate level (to 0.5 mg/dL or less) as a result of glucose infusion in the same patient may be associated with confusion, coma, or acute respiratory failure. Most of the clinical manifestations listed in Table 94–3 are associated with acute severe hypophosphatemia.

Although the exact incidence of the different clinical expressions of low phosphate levels has never been studied in a comprehensive way, the available literature indicates that muscular weakness, reduced ventilatory capacity with or without acute respiratory failure, platelet and leukocyte dysfunctions, confusion, coma (metabolic encephalopathy), rhabdomyo-

lysis, and sepsis are relatively common complications of severe hypophosphatemia. Rhabdomyolysis is especially common in chronic alcoholic patients. Alcoholic myopathy apparently plays a synergistic role in the genesis of rhabdomyolysis in acute hypophosphatemia.

Myoglobinuria following rhabdomyolysis often causes acute tubular necrosis of the kidneys. Hemolytic anemia, Guillain-Barré syndrome, ataxia, and ballismus are relatively rare complications of acute hypophosphatemia.

Chronic hypophosphatemia, as occurs in vitamin D deficiency or renal tubular disorders, usually affects only the musculoskeletal system. Osteomalacia or rickets with or without associated muscle weakness is the usual sequela in these conditions.

Because most patients with acute hypophosphatemia have chronic alcoholism, the stigmata of chronic alcoholism are usually present on physical examination. Other physical findings may include irritability, confusion or coma, nystagmus or ptosis, tachypnea with shallow respiration, and signs of sepsis. The muscles are usually weak, and reflexes are usually depressed.

Mild to moderate hypophosphatemia in a chronically debilitated patient usually resolves with adequate dietary phosphate. Merely stopping the precipitating event, namely glucose infusion, antacid therapy, or hyperventilation, usually allows serum phosphate levels to return to normal. In chronic alcoholic patients, good meals containing dairy products and the cessation of drinking often bring phosphate levels to normal. However, severe hypophosphatemia may not resolve spontaneously and may result in death if untreated or unrecognized.

Chronic hypophosphatemia from primary hyperparathyroidism, Fanconi's syndrome, or

TABLE 94–1.
Causes of Severe Hypophosphatemia (PO_4 Level < 1.0 mg/dl)

Chronic alcoholism
  Especially in hospitalized patients receiving glucose infusion
Diabetic ketoacidosis
  Recovery phase
Hyperalimentation/hypertonic glucose infusion
  When phosphate is not added to the solution
Intensive antacid therapy
  Given every 1 or 2 hours for 1 or 2 days
Severe acute respiratory alkalosis
  When PCO_2 is less than 20 mm Hg
"Nutritional recovery syndrome"
  Overzealous feeding of simple carbohydrates to patients who have protein-calorie malnutrition
Severe burns
  Recovery phase
Hereditary fructose intolerance
  When affected children ingest fructose

TABLE 94–2.
Causes of Moderate Hypophosphatemia (PO_4 Level = 1 to 2.5 mg/dl)

Glucose infusion
Hyperparathyroidism
Diuresis
Gram-negative sepsis
Malabsorption
Hypomagnesemia
Vitamin D deficiency
Vitamin D-resistant rickets
Pregnancy
Renal tubular defects (Fanconi's syndrome)
Vomiting/nasogastric suction
Fructose ingestion
Epinephrine administration
Androgen therapy
Recovery from hypothermia
Items listed in Table 94–1

other renal tubular disorders usually never resolves unless renal failure superimposes.

PATHOPHYSIOLOGY

Table 94–4 lists mechanisms involved in the development of hypophosphatemia. In chronic alcoholic patients, several mechanisms act together. In the prehospital phase, there is underlying phosphate depletion due to inadequate intake, poor absorption, and renal wasting of phosphate. In the hospital phase, acute hypophosphatemia is usually precipitated by glucose infusion, respiratory alkalosis due to liver disease or alcohol withdrawal, and increased catecholamine secretion.

Hypophosphatemia affects most systems of the body, mostly at the biochemical level. Two fundamental abnormalities seen are a decreased adenosine triphosphate (ATP) content of all the cells and a decreased 2,3-diphosphoglycerate (2,3-DPG) content of red cells. The P_{50}, which is the oxygen tension at which hemoglobin is 50% saturated, drops from normal (about 27 mm Hg) to about 16 mm Hg. The resting muscle membrane potential decreases. The intracellular sodium and calcium content of muscles increases. The ability of platelets to aggregate and the chemotactic and bactericidal activity of leukocytes decrease. A mild elevation of serum creatine phosphokinase (CPK) level is much more common than is frank rhabdomyolysis and hemolysis of the red cells.

A gross examination of tissues reveals little change. A microscopic examination of muscle tissue often shows intracellular edema. The platelet count may be low, and the platelets may be large. In long-standing phosphate depletion from vitamin D deficiency or renal tubular disorders, the usual sequela is osteomalacia or rickets. Examination of the bone will reveal defective mineralization with wide osteoid seams.

CLINICAL–PATHOLOGIC CORRELATIONS

Two fundamental biochemical abnormalities are thought to underlie the different clinical manifestations of hypophosphatemia: (1) depletion of the intracellular ATP content of all tissues, and (2) depletion of the 2,3-DPG content of red cells.

A decreased level of cellular inorganic phosphate activates the enzyme adenosine monophosphate deaminase and leads to a rapid irreversible production of inosine 5'-monophosphate. This depletes the intracellular ATP content. The production of new ATP is also impaired because inorganic phosphate is a cofactor in converting several intermediate metabolites in the glycolytic process.

An ATP deficiency impairs all energy-requiring metabolic processes (Table 94–5). Decreased levels of 2,3-DPG in the red cells increases hemoglobin's affinity for oxygen. This impairs tissue oxygenation and adds to the effect of low ATP levels in the cells. Phosphate deficiency may also alter the cell membrane and the sodium/calcium exchange system in the cell membrane.

DIFFERENTIAL DIAGNOSIS

Because phosphate depletion affects many systems of the body, hypophosphatemia must be considered in the differential diagnosis of many conditions (Table 94–3). It should be entertained as a possible cause of confusion, coma, seizure, sepsis, or respiratory failure developing in patients with a history of chronic alcoholism or in other high-risk groups (Table 94–1). Hypophosphatemia should also be considered in the etiologic diagnosis of rhabdomyolysis, unexplained hemolysis, and osteomalacia. Severe somatic muscle weakness is common in cases of hypophosphatemia. Hypokalemia can mimic hypophosphatemia and often coexists with it. In chronic alcoholic patients, subdural hematoma, meningitis, or alcohol withdrawal can mimic the metabolic encephalopathy seen with hypophosphatemia and can coexist in the same patient. Hypophosphatemia should be considered in patients with unexplained acute cardiomyopathy and in patients who cannot easily be weaned off mechanical ventilation.

TABLE 94–3.
Signs and Symptoms of Hypophosphatemia

NERVOUS SYSTEM
Paresthesia
Decreased attention span
Confusion/delirium
Seizure
Coma
Nystagmus
Ballismus/ataxia
Guillain-Barré syndrome
EEG abnormality

MUSCLE (SOMATIC) SYSTEM
Generalized muscle weakness
Rhabdomyolysis
Increased serum levels of creatine phosphokinase (CPK)
EMG abnormalities

HEMATOLOGIC SYSTEM
Impaired leukocyte function
Thrombocytopenia
Thrombocytopathy (platelet dysfunction)
Hemolysis

RESPIRATORY SYSTEM
Reduced diaphragmatic contractility
Tachypnea
Decreased vital capacity
Acute respiratory failure

GASTROINTESTINAL SYSTEM
Anorexia
Dysphagia

ENDOCRINE SYSTEM
Insulin resistance
Increased 1,25-dihydroxy viatmin D_3

CARDIAC SYSTEM
Cardiomyopathy
Congestive heart failure

RENAL SYSTEM
Myoglobinuria
Acute renal failure
Hypercalciuria
Nephrolithiasis

SKELETAL SYSTEM
Osteomalacia/rickets
Growth retardation
Bone pain
Pseudofractures

TABLE 94–4.
Pathogenesis of Hypophosphatemia

MECHANISM	EXAMPLES OF CAUSES
Reduced dietary phosphate	Chronic alcoholism
	Starvation
Reduced absorption of phosphate from gut	Phosphate-binding antacids
	Malabsorption
	Vomiting/nasogastric suction
Increased loss in urine	Fanconi's syndrome
	Hyperparathyroidism
	Vitamin D deficiency
	Hypomagnesemia
	Chronic alcoholism
	Glycosuria (as in diabetic ketoacidosis)
Intracellular shift	Glucose infusion
	Respiratory alkalosis
	Fructose ingestion/infusion
	Epinephrine infusion or release of epinephrine from adrenal glands

DIAGNOSIS

The diagnosis of hypophosphatemia is not difficult if it is clinically suspected and requires only determination of serum phosphate levels. More often than not, it is discovered on routine blood chemistries of hospitalized patients. The serum phosphate level should be measured in all patients at high risk for developing severe hypophosphatemia (Table 94–1). Once low levels are found, the cause can be established by following the simple leads shown in Table 94–6.

PRINCIPLES OF PREVENTION AND THERAPY

The potential hazards of hypophosphatemia can be avoided by paying proper attention to the possibility of the condition in situations known to induce it, and correcting it promptly when serum readings confirm suspicions.

In parenteral hyperalimentation, prevention rather than correction is the rule, simply by adding phosphate to the hyperalimentation solution, unless a contraindication like chronic renal failure exists. It is common practice to administer phosphate to all patients treated for diabetic ketoacidosis. However, recent studies indicate that not all such patients need phosphate. The small percentage of patients with low serum levels of phosphate when first seen, despite a coexisting metabolic acidosis, are the ones who tend to develop a life-threatening hypophosphatemia as treatment with fluid and insulin proceeds. Phosphate should be included in the treatment regimen of this subgroup. In chronic alcoholic patients, serum phosphate levels should be measured before starting any intravenous glucose infusion.

Phosphate deficiency can generally be corrected by oral medications. The available preparations are mostly phosphate salts of sodium or potassium. Milk is a readily available and very good source of phosphate. Diarrhea is the most common side-effect of oral phosphate therapy.

A few days of oral phosphate replacement is usually sufficient, except in renal phosphate wasting in which long-term phosphate therapy with or without added vitamin D is necessary to prevent osteomalacia.

Parenteral replacement of phosphate should be reserved for patients with severe complications of hypophosphatemia, like seizures or coma, and for those who cannot tolerate or absorb oral medication. Phosphate levels should be monitored frequently (at least every 8 hours) in these situations. Iatrogenic hyperphosphatemia due to excessive phosphate administration can cause hypocalcemia or visceral deposition of calcium phosphate crystals or both.

TABLE 94–5.
Clinical–Pathologic Correlations of Hypophosphatemia

CLINICAL FINDINGS	PATHOLOGIC FINDINGS	
	BIOCHEMICAL ABNORMALITY	AFFECTED TISSUE
		Muscle
Muscle weakness	Reduced intracellular ATP content (less energy available for all functions)	Decreased transcellular membrane potential
Guillain-Barré syndrome		
Reduced ventilatory capacity		
Acute respiratory failure	Alteration in cell membrane	Increased intracellular levels of Na^+ and Ca^{++}
Rhabdomyolysis (may lead to acute renal failure)		Decreased muscle contractility
Cardiomyopathy with congestive heart failure		
		Leukocytes
Increased incidence and severity of infection	Reduced intracellular ATP content (less energy available for all functions)	Decreased chemotactic, phagocytic, and bactericidal activity
Sepsis	Alteration in cell membrane	
		Platelets
Increased tendency to bleed, especially in gut and into skin	Reduced intracellular ATP content (less energy available for all functions)	Decreased aggregate ability
	Alteration in cell membrane	Decreased numbers
		Red cell
Hemolysis	Reduced 2–3 DPG in red cells	Increased fragility
	Reduced intracellular ATP content	Decreased oxygen-supplying capacity of Hgb (low P_{50}; O_2–Hb curve shifts left)
		Nervous system
Irritability	Reduced 2–3 DPG in red cells	Decreased oxygen availability (low P_{50}) in tissue dependent on oxidative glycolysis
Paresthesia	Reduced intracellular ATP content	
Confusion/obtundation		
Seizure/coma		
		Bone
Bone pain	Reduced ability for mineralization of osteoid in bone	Osteomalacia
Growth retardation		Rickets
Fractures		

TABLE 94–6.
Etiologic Diagnosis of Hypophosphatemia

Step 1.	Consider intracellular transfer of phosphate as cause of hypophosphatemia in the following clinical situations: Glucose or fructose infusion Hyperventilation causing respiratory alkalosis Recovery phase of diabetic ketoacidosis Recovery phase of rickets or osteomalacia Epinephrine administration
Step 2.	If none of the above is present, measure urinary phosphate level.
Step 3.	If urinary phosphate level is > 4 mg/dl, consider renal loss from Primary hyperparathyroidism Fanconi's syndrome Vitamin D-resistant rickets Diuresis
Step 4.	If urinary phosphate level is < 4 mg/dl, consider gastrointestinal loss from Phosphate-binding antacid Persistent vomiting or nasogastric suction Malabsorption Dietary phosphate deficiency

REFERENCES

Agus Z, Goldfarb S, Wasserstein A: Disorders of calcium and phosphate balance. Hypophosphatemia, in Brenner BM, Rector FC Jr (eds): *The Kidney*, ed 2. Philadelphia, WB Saunders Co, 1981, pp 990–1022. *Detailed discussion of causes, pathophysiology, and treatment of hypophosphatemia. Over 900 references cited.*

Aubier M, Murciano D, Lecocguic Y et al: Effect of hypophosphatemia on diaphragmatic contractility in patients with acute respiratory failure. *N Engl J Med* 1985; 313:420–424. *Recent, well-done study showing the effects of acute hypophosphatemia on ventilatory capacity.*

Juan D, Elrazak M: Hypophosphatemia in hospitalized patients. *JAMA* 1979; 242:163–164. *One of the few studies about the incidence of this disorder.*

Knochel JP: The pathophysiology and clinical characteristics of severe hypophosphatemia. *Arch Intern Med* 1977; 137:203–220. *In-depth review of the subject, emphasizing the pathogenic mechanism and clinical–pathologic correlation.*

Knochel JP: The clinical status of hypophosphatemia—an update. *N Engl J Med* 1985; 313(7):447–449. *Succinct editorial, updating information regarding the subject.*

Kreisberg RA: Phosphate deficiency and hypophosphatemia. *Hosp Pract* 1977; 12:121–128. *Another useful review on the subject with graphic representation of pathophysiology and clinical manifestation.*

part VIII

Renal and Reproductive Disorders

95 NEPHROLITHIASIS

Mohammad G. Saklayen, M.D.
Chetna Mital, M.D.

Kidney stones are abnormal concretions precipitated from urinary solutes in the kidneys, the pelvocaliceal system, and the ureter. Calcium oxalate or calcium phosphate is present in 80% to 90% of the stones. Other stones contain uric acid, magnesium ammonium phosphate (struvite), cystine, or xanthine and related compounds. Table 95–1 lists the frequency of occurrence of various stones. The annual incidence of nephrolithiasis, a condition characterized by the presence of kidney stones, in the United States is 1.6 per 1,000 population. Kidney stones are most common in young men.

CLINICAL SIGNS AND SYMPTOMS

Patients with kidney stones may present with characteristic renal colic, which often is excruciating at its peak and has a crescendo-decrescendo pattern beginning in the costovertebral angle and radiating to the groin. This pattern is frequently associated with a stone in the ureter. In other patients the initial feature is gross hematuria or microscopic hematuria with no associated pain, or gravel passed in the urine with minimal discomfort. When urinary tract infection is superimposed in cases of kidney stones, the patient may present with flank pain, fever, chill, and dysuria. In few asymptomatic patients, kidney stones are diagnosed by a radiographic examination done for unrelated reasons. In rare cases, patients with kidney stones present with unexplained renal failure (Table 95–2).

The results of a physical examination are unremarkable in most cases except for costovertebral angle tenderness.

Most cases of renal colic resolve spontaneously with passage of the stone, but a large stone causing urinary tract obstruction or stones associated with urinary tract infection, if untreated, can lead to renal failure or sepsis or both. Magnesium ammonium phosphate (struvite) stones are never passed in the urine and usually continue to grow, often destroying the involved kidney if untreated.

While 40% of the patients have no recurrence of stones, the other 60% have one or more recurrences within 2 or 3 years of the first episode. The highest rate of recurrence takes place in patients with calcium oxalate stones secondary to primary or secondary hyperoxaluria and hyperuricosuria.

PATHOPHYSIOLOGY

The formation of kidney stones involves the following factors:

1. Supersaturation of urine with certain solutes
2. Alteration of urine pH, changing ionic activities
3. Homogenous nucleation
4. Heterogenous nucleation
5. Inorganic and organic crystallization inhibitors
6. Epitaxy

Supersaturation is a physicochemical state that drives the solute from a liquid to a solid phase. An increased excretion of the solute in the urine, a decreased urine volume, or a

TABLE 95–1.
Frequency of Various Compositions of Renal Stones

TYPE	FREQUENCY (% OF STONES)
Calcium oxalate	70
Calcium phosphate	10
Magnesium ammonium phosphate	10
Uric acid	< 5
Cystine	< 1
Other (xanthine, hypoxanthine, triamterene)	< 1

TABLE 95–2.
Initial Manifestations of Kidney Stones

Renal colic
Gross or microscopic hematuria
Gravel passed in the urine
Urinary obstruction
Urinary tract infection
   Increased frequency, urgency, dysuria
   Fever and chills
Unexplained renal failure
Asymptomatic

change in urine pH can cause supersaturation of urine in respect to a particular solute and cause precipitation of crystals of that solute. Heterogenous nuclei, like dust particles or bacteria, facilitate crystallization by reducing the thermodynamic energy necessary for homogenous nucleation or for spontaneous formation of de novo crystals. On the other hand, the absence of crystallization inhibitors, such as pyrophosphate, citrate, and some peptides yet to be fully characterized, facilitates stone formation. Epitaxy, which refers to two crystals having similar atomic lattices (e.g., uric acid and calcium oxalate crystals), also facilitates stone formation. The importance of any one factor varies from one stone-forming disease to another.

The most common causes of calcium stones are idiopathic hypercalciuria, primary hyperparathyroidism, renal tubular acidosis, hyperoxaluria, and hyperuricosuria. Idiopathic hypercalciuria is the most common cause and is present in 30% to 40% of patients with calcium stones. Normal men usually excrete up to 300 mg of calcium in the urine per day, and normal women excrete up to 250 mg. Higher levels than these are defined as hypercalciuria, which is idiopathic when the serum calcium level is normal and other usual causes of normocalcemic hypercalciuria (such as sarcoidosis, Paget's disease, immobilization, a diet very high in calcium, or malignancy) are absent.

Idiopathic hypercalciuria occurs in 2% to 4% of otherwise normal adults. The fact that only 10% to 20% of people with this condition form kidney stones suggests that factors other than hypercalciuria also play a role in forming the stones. Excessive intestinal calcium absorption (absorptive hypercalciuria) occurs in most cases, while renal type hypercalciuria stemming from depressed reabsorption of calcium in the kidney tubules is the primary problem in others.

Primary hyperparathyroidism is caused by a adenoma in one of the parathyroid glands in 90% of cases or by hyperplasia of all four glands. Parathyroid hyperactivity mobilizes calcium from the bone. The resultant excessive excretion of calcium in the urine facilitates calcium stone formation. Both nephrocalcinosis and stones in the pelvocaliceal system can occur in primary hyperparathyroidism. Calcium phosphate stones are more common than calcium oxalate stones in this condition, and stones often recur and become bilateral. Of all those who form calcium stones, 5% have primary hyperparathyroidism.

Classic distal (type I) renal tubular acidosis is often associated with nephrocalcinosis and ureteral stones. Again, hypercalciuria is present secondary to mobilization of bone calcium due to persistent systemic acidosis. The alkaline urine and hypocitruria encountered in this condition also facilitate stone formation.

Primary hyperoxaluria results when oxalate synthesis is increased in two hereditary conditions, type I and type II hyperoxaluria, which are secondary to a deficiency of certain enzymes. Pyridoxine deficiency and high doses of ascorbic acid can also increase oxalate synthesis. Overabsorption of oxalate (secondary or enteral hyperoxaluria) is associated with gastrointestinal disorders such as Crohn's disease, celiac sprue, pancreatic insufficiency, and bypass surgery of the small intestine. Dietary fat malabsorption and steatorrhea are common to all these conditions. Dietary oxalate binds with calcium to form nonabsorbable calcium oxalate. In steatorrhea, however, calcium is bound to the abundant free fatty acids in the lumen leaving oxalate ions free to be absorbed, mainly in the colon.

Hyperuricosuria, the second most common metabolic abnormality in the formation of kidney stones, occurs in 26% of the patients with calcium stones. It is usually defined as a 24-hour urinary uric acid excretion greater than 700 mg in women and 800 mg in men and is caused either by excessive ingestion of purine-rich foods or by a metabolic abnormality leading to excessive synthesis of uric acid. Calcium oxalate stones are seen about four times more often than uric acid stones in patients with hyperuricosuria because (1) crystals of sodium urate or uric acid initiate calcium oxalate precipitation from a metastable solution (epitaxy), (2) a small urate crystal can lodge in a caliceal niche and become a heterogenous nucleus for a calcium oxalate stone, and (3) uric acid crystals may absorb certain urine crystal-growth inhibitors. Hypercalciuria coexists with hyperuricosuria in 10% of patients with calcium stones.

Uric acid stones develop in 20% of people with hyperuricosuria. The urine pH is critical in their pathogenesis. A rise of urine pH from 5 to 6 increases the solubility of uric acid sixfold. Below pH 6, supersaturation of urine with uric acid may occur even in normal subjects. Uric acid stones therefore occur only in persistently acidic urine. Reduced generation of ammonia in the renal tubules contributes to a low urine pH. Dehydration causes reduction in urine pH and higher urate concentration. High doses of uricosuric drugs like probenecid or aspirin can also facilitate uric acid stone formation.

Cystine stones are found in patients with cystinuria, an autosomal recessive disorder in which dibasic amino acids (ornithine, arginine, lysine, and cystine) are not reabsorbed in the proximal renal tubules. Cystine, the least soluble of the group, frequently precipitates in urine with a pH less than 7.4. Fewer than 1% of kidney stones are secondary to cystinuria.

Magnesium ammonium phosphate (also called struvite and triple phosphate) stones are formed when the urine is repeatedly infected with urea-splitting bacteria such as *Proteus* organisms. Bacterial urease hydrolyses urea, releasing free ammonia, which often elevates urine pH to 8 or 9, causing magnesium ammonium phosphate crystals to precipitate. Bacteria also form a nidus in the pelvocaliceal system and facilitate stone formation. Magnesium ammonium phosphate stones tend to grow continuously, branching and filling the whole renal collecting system, giving the stones a "staghorn" appearance.

CLINICAL–PATHOLOGIC CORRELATIONS

Different pathologic conditions lead to the formation of different kinds of kidney stones. Table 95–3 lists these basic pathologic abnormalities, associated clinical test abnormalities, and types of stones that result from such abnormalities.

DIFFERENTIAL DIAGNOSIS

The differential diagnosis of kidney stones is based on the initial signs and symptoms. Renal colic must be differentiated from other causes of acute abdomen. Because 90% of stones are radiopaque, an abdominal radiograph that shows no stones and the absence of microscopic hematuria virtually rules out a diagnosis of renal calculi. The differential diagnosis of asymptomatic microscopic or gross hematuria includes glomerulonephritis, tumors. infection, and trauma. Normal findings in an intravenous pyelogram excludes stones as a cause of hematuria. Similarly, normal findings in a urogram exclude stones as a cause of recurrent urinary tract infection or unexplained renal failure.

DIAGNOSIS

Most kidney stones are radiopaque. The findings in a standard abdominal x-ray film of the kidney-ureter-bladder area are diagnostic of 90% of kidney stones. Uric acid, xanthine, and hypoxanthine calculi are radiolucent and are seen as filling defects in intravenous pyelograms.

A urinalysis should be done to detect microscopic hematuria. The absence of hematuria usually precludes a diagnosis of kidney stones. A midstream "clean-catch" urine specimen for Gram's stain, culture, and sensitivity helps

TABLE 95–3.

Clinical–Pathologic Correlations of Nephrolithiasis

| | PATHOLOGIC FINDINGS | |
CLINICAL FINDINGS	CLINICAL TEST ABNORMALITY	TYPE OF KIDNEY STONES
Reduced reabsorption of calcium in renal tubules	Hypercalciuria, renal type Normal serum calcium level High serum PTH level	Calcium phosphate Calcium oxalate
Increased absorption of calcium from gastrointestinal tract	Hypercalciuria, absorptive type Normal serum calcium level Low/normal serum PTH level	Calcium phosphate Calcium oxalate
Increased production of PTH	Hypercalciuria High serum PTH level Hypercalcemia Increased urinary excretion of phosphate	Calcium phosphate Nephrocalcinosis Calcium oxalate
Defect of H^+ excretion in distal renal tubular acidosis	Hypocitruria Alkaline urine pH Increased urinary excretion of calcium and phosphate	Calcium phosphate Nephrocalcinosis
Primary hyperoxaluria (Increased production of oxalate)	Hyperoxaluria	Calcium oxalate
Secondary hyperoxaluria (Increased absorption of oxalate from gastrointestinal tract)	Hyperoxaluria	Calcium oxalate
Increased production of uric acid with or without hypercalciuria	Hyperuricosuria with or without hypercalciuria	Calcium phosphate Calcium oxalate
Increased production of uric acid Reduced generation of ammonia in renal tubules	Hyperuricosuria with acidic urine (pH <6)	Uric acid
Reduced reabsorption of dibasic amino acids in renal tubules	Cystinuria	Cystine
Urinary tract infection with urea-splitting organism (*Proteus* organisms)	Release of ammonia from urea Persistently alkaline urine (pH 8 to 9)	Magnesium ammonium phosphate (struvite)

TABLE 95–4.

Procedures for Evaluating Recurrent Kidney Stones

History and physical examination
Chemical analysis of stone
Abdominal x-ray films
Intravenous pyelogram
Urinalysis
Urine pH
Urine culture
Measurement of serum calcium, uric acid, creatinine, and phosphate levels
Measurement of 24-hour urinary excretion of creatinine, calcium, oxalate, uric acid, phosphate, citrate, and cystine
Chest x-ray film
Measurement of serum PTH level
Ammonium chloride loading test (in suspected renal tubular acidosis)
Nitroprusside screening test (in suspected cystinuria)

identify infection either as a cause or a sequela of kidney stones. All urine specimens should be strained, and any stone, however small, should be sent for chemical analysis, which directs further management.

An extensive metabolic work-up to find the underlying cause is expensive and time consuming. Those patients with two or more episodes of stones should have this done for etiologic diagnosis. Table 95–4 lists some useful tests that may need to be done for full evaluation of patients with recurrent stones. The exact sequence and number of tests to be done for any one patient should be based on the history and physical findings.

PRINCIPLES OF PREVENTION AND THERAPY

Table 95–5 summarizes the treatment of different types of kidney stones. The main aim of medical management is to prevent recurrence by correcting the underlying disorder. No known drug dissolves kidney stones. Surgical removal of stones is necessary if they do not

TABLE 95–5.
Management of Kidney Stones

TYPE	TREATMENT	EFFECT OF TREATMENT
Calcium stones		
Idiopathic hypercalciuria	Thiazides	Diuresis and contraction of extracellular fluid (ECF) volume increases reabsorption of calcium in proximal tubule
		Potentiates the action of PTH
Absorptive hypercalciuria	Orthophosphates	Decreases urinary calcium levels
		Increases urinary phosphate levels
		Increases level of urinary inhibitors in urine
Hyperuricosuria	Allopurinol	Decreases uric acid excretion by blocking uric acid synthesis
Hyperparathyroidism	Parathyroidectomy	Decreases urinary excretion of calcium
Primary hyperoxaluria	High doses of pyridoxine	Decreases oxalate formation
Secondary hyperoxaluria	Cholestyramine	Decreases absorption of oxalate from the gastrointestinal tract by binding it.
	Calcium gluconate	
	Low-fat diet	
Magnesium ammonium phosphate (struvite) stones		
	Surgical removal	
	Antibiotic therapy	Sterilizes the urine
Uric acid stones		
	Oral alkali	Increases urinary pH, which increases the solubility of uric acid in urine
	Allopurinol	Decreases urinary excretion of uric acid by blocking its synthesis
Cystine stones		
	Oral alkali	Increases urinary pH, which increases the solubility of cystine in urine
	D-Penicillamine	Reduces urinary excretion of cystine

pass spontaneously. Percutaneous lithotripsy and extracorporeal shock lithotripsy are recent developments in the area of surgical management.

Treatment for the prevention of recurrence is prolonged and requires patient compliance. Fluid intake at a level that ensures a urine volume of at least 2 L a day is advised. Patients with intestinal overabsorption of calcium should decrease consumption of dairy products. Patients that form uric acid stones should limit their purine intake to decrease the uric acid load.

In patients with calcium stones, specific management of systemic diseases such as hyperparathyroidism, distal renal tubular acidosis, and multiple myeloma eliminates the cause of the stones. In idiopathic hypercalciuria, thiazides and related diuretics are the mainstay of treatment and increase proximal tubular reabsorption of calcium, augment the action of PTH on the distal tubule, and conserve calcium. These effects in turn suppress the absorption of calcium from the gastrointestinal tract by decreasing the activity of 1,24-dihydroxy-vitamin D. Orthophosphates can be used to decrease hypercalciuria.

High doses of pyridoxine given to patients with primary hyperoxaluria decrease oxalate synthesis. In secondary (enteral) hyperoxaluria, a low-fat diet is advised, so that calcium may combine with oxalate to form a compound that is not absorbed. Calcium lactate or gluconate administration achieves the same result. Cholestyramine, an anion-exchange resin, can also be used to reduce oxalate absorption. Whenever possible, bowel continuity should be restored.

In patients with uric acid stones, urine pH above 6 is achieved by administering alkali orally and prevents the crystallization of uric acid. Allopurinol, a xanthine oxidase inhibitor, is used to decrease the synthesis of uric acid. Allopurinol is used for patients with hyperuricosuria and calcium stones.

In patients with cystine stones, alkalinizing the urine by giving alkali orally helps reduce cystine stone formation because the solubility of cystine is increased when the urine pH is over 7. D-Penicillamine can decrease the urinary excretion of cystine, but its toxicity should limit its use to patients with recurrent stones not responsive to other measures.

Magnesium ammonium phosphate stones are difficult to treat because even a small piece left in the kidney after treatment can act as a nidus for further stone formation. Appropriate antibiotic therapy sterilizes the urine. Acidifying the urine can help dissolve these crystals, but acidification is difficult to achieve because the bacteria produce ammonium ions. Half the patients are cured by surgically removing the stone and instituting appropriate antibiotic therapy. The other half have recurrences.

REFERENCES

Coe FL: *Nephrolithiasis: Pathogenesis and Treatment.* Chicago, Year Book Medical Publishers, 1978. *Detailed review of causes, pathogenesis, clinical manifestations, and treatment of kidney stones.*

Coe FL, Favus MJ: Disorders of stone formation, in Brenner BM, Rector FC Jr (eds): *The Kidney,* ed 3. Philadelphia, WB Saunders Co, 1986, pp 1403–1442. *In-depth review of all medical aspects of kidney stones, with 300 references.*

Gill WB: Urolithiasis update: Biophysical and radiologic advances enhance antistone therapy. *Am J Kidney Dis* 1981; 1(2):66–90. *Detailed discussion of pathogenetic mechanisms and principles of treating kidney stones.*

Health and Public Policy Committee, American College of Physicians: Lithotripsy. *Ann Intern Med* 1985; 103:626–629. *Succinct discussion of the new surgical treatment of renal stones, detailing the methods, safety, efficacy, and cost of the procedures, along with recommendations when to use.*

Lemann J Jr: Nephrolithiasis, in Massry SG, Glassock RJ (eds): *Textbook of Nephrology,* vol 2. Baltimore, Williams & Wilkins, 1983, pp 6266–6282. *Good chapter on the subject. Clinical orientation with emphasis on management of different kinds of kidney stones.*

Pak CYC, Britton F, Peterson R et al: Ambulatory evaluation of nephrolithiasis: Classification, clinical presentation and diagnostic criteria. *Am J Med* 1980; 69:19–30. *A detailed discussion of the out-*

patient protocol used for the etiologic diagnosis of nephrolithiasis.
Smith CL: When should the stone patient be evaluated? *Med Clin North Am* 1984; 68:455–459.

Author tries to answer one very important clinical question from available data in the literature and personal experience.

96 GLOMERULONEPHRITIS

Nicholas P. Christoff, M.D.

The term *glomerulonephritis* refers to an inflammatory injury to the capillary loops of the glomeruli of the kidney. Glomerulonephritis may be acute, with a relatively abrupt onset and a course measured in days to weeks. Subacute glomerulonephritis, or rapidly progressive glomerulonephritis (RPGN), progresses over weeks to months with little tendency to spontaneous improvement. The term *chronic glomerulonephritis* is used to describe glomerulonephritis with an insidious onset and a subclinical progression over years, often to advanced deterioration of renal function at the time of diagnosis. In chronic glomerulonephritis, it may be impossible to ascertain whether the initial renal injury was of a glomerular, tubulointerstitial, or vascular nature, or of another type.

Nephritic glomerular injury can be due to primary renal disorders or to multisystemic disease processes. This chapter will address primary renal disorders that commonly present as nephritic syndromes, including anti-glomerular basement membrane (anti-GBM) nephritis, poststreptococcal glomerulonephritis (PSGN), other postinfectious glomerulonephritides, IgG-IgA nephritis (Berger's disease), membranoproliferative glomerulonephritis (MPGN) (types I and II), and idiopathic (crescentic) glomerulonephritis. Not considered in detail will be glomerulonephritides due to noninfectious multisystemic disorders (such as systemic lupus erythematosus [SLE], Henoch-Schönlein purpura [HSP], essential mixed cryoglobulinemia, polyarteritis nodosa, Wegener's granulomatosis, hemolytic-uremic syndrome, and thrombotic thrombocytopenic purpura) and disorders that present primarily as nephrosis (including minimal change disease, membranous nephropathy, and focal sclerosis). Classification of the nephritic syndromes is shown in Table 96–1.

CLINICAL SIGNS AND SYMPTOMS

Nephritic glomerular injury is manifested by gross or microscopic hematuria, varying degrees of proteinuria (usually in the "nonnephrotic" range), reduced glomerular filtration rate (GFR) and azotemia, and the presence of RBC casts and other cellular elements in the urine. Secondary manifestations include varying degrees of oligoanuria, sodium and water retention, edema, hypertension, and circulatory overload. Uremic symptoms may also occur secondarily, including lethargy, somnolence, twitching, nausea, vomiting, abdominal pain, headache, seizures, and pruritus may also occur. Hematuria can be considered the hallmark of nephritic glomerular injury. The presence of hematuria, proteinuria, and RBC casts implies the potential for rapid deterioration of renal function.

TABLE 96–1.

Classification of Nephritic Syndromes

Acute and rapidly progressive (subacute) glomerulonephritides
  I. Anti-GBM antibody-mediated with/without pulmonary hemorrhage
  II. With glomerular immune deposits
    A. Poststreptococcal glomerulonephritis
    B. Other postinfectious glomerulonephritides (such as associated with subacute bacterial endocarditis "nephritis" shunt, and visceral abscesses)
    C. IgG-IgA nephritis (Berger's disease)
    D. Type I membranoproliferative glomerulonephritis
    E. Due to systemic disorders (such as systemic lupus erythematosus, HSP, and essential mixed cryoglobulinemia)
  III. Without glomerular immune deposits
    A. Type II membranoproliferative glomerulonephritis
    B. Idiopathic (crescentic) RPGN
    C. Due to vasculitides (polyarteritis nodosa; Wegener's granulomatosis; hemolytic-uretic syndrome/thrombotic-thrombocytopenic purpura)
Chronic glomerulonephritis

Poststreptococcal glomerulonephritis (PSGN) is considered the prototype of acute nephritic syndromes. Poststreptococcal glomerulonephritis occurs following infection with group A (beta-hemolytic) streptococci of nephritogenic M type, usually type 12 in the United States. It is primarily a disease of children between the ages of 3 and 12 years. It is rare in infancy and in those over 50 years. In the northern part of the United States, streptococcal pharyngitis is the most common antecedent event. Glomerulonephritis occurs in less than 5% of these patients, and the average latent period prior to the onset of nephritis is 10 days. Males are affected more than females, and outbreaks tend to occur in winter and spring. In the southern part of the United States, impetigo is a more common antecedent event. The incidence of associated glomerulonephritis is higher (25% to 50%), and the latent period is longer (average, 20 days). Again, males are more commonly affected. Outbreaks may be seen in summer and fall.

In poststreptococcal glomerulonephritis, there is typically an abrupt onset of hematuria (dark, "smoky," or "Coca-Cola" urine), with proteinuria, oligoanuria, and azotemia. There is malaise, nausea and vomiting, abdominal pain, periorbital and peripheral edema, and hypertension. There may be CNS manifestations including confusion, headaches, somnolence, encephalopathy, and seizures. Ninety percent of patients will recover completely, with the onset of spontaneous diuresis in 4 to 7 days. Twenty to fifty percent will continue to have abnormal proteinuria or hematuria, with a tendency to hypertension and some impairment of glomerular filtration rate. There may be slow progression of renal disease in these instances. The 5% who are oliguric longer than 9 days have a worse prognosis.

The nephritic syndrome may also appear as a sequel to a variety of other types of bacterial, viral, and parasitic infection. Glomerulonephritis is often associated with subacute bacterial endocarditis (SBE) and visceral abscesses, most commonly of the lung. Glomerulonephritis may present as the abrupt onset of acute renal failure with hematuria, proteinuria, and red blood cell casts in a patient with a pyogenic visceral abscess. In addition to the respiratory tract, other frequent locations of such infections are the abdomen or uterus. Patients with infected prostheses or vascular grafts in various locations may be similarly affected. Eradication of the infection may lead to recovery of renal function in 50% of such cases; however, mortality is high in this setting. Infection of ventriculoatrial shunts with *Staphylococcus albus* and various other organisms may give rise to glomerulonephritis associated with an SBE-like syndrome featuring malaise, fever, weight loss, and anemia (*shunt nephritis*). Other frequently seen infections that can give rise to glomerulonephritis include pneumococcal and *Klebsiella* pneumonias, *Staphylococcus aureus* or gram-negative sepsis, hepatitis B, cytomegalovirus, and Epstein-Barr virus. Glomerulonephritis can also be seen in association with

Mycoplasma infection, meningococcemia, secondary syphilis, leptospirosis, typhoid fever, mumps, coxsackieviruses, Rocky Mountain spotted fever, histoplasmosis, trichinosis, and toxoplasmosis. In the developing world, malaria is a common cause of glomerulonephritis.

IgG-IgA nephropathy (Berger's disease) represents 20% of acute glomerulonephritis in the United States, but is thought to be the most common cause of primary glomerular disease in Europe and Australia. It is considered a monosymptomatic form of Henoch-Schönlein purpura, lacking nonthrombocytopenic leukocytoclastic vasculitic purpura, abdominal pain, and arthralgias. It is two to three times more common in men than in women. It is rare in blacks. Eighty percent of cases appear in patients between the ages of 16 and 35 years. The classic presentation is with gross hematuria coincident with or following within 24 to 48 hours a viral upper respiratory infection (50% of cases), a flu-like illness (15%), a gastrointestinal (GI) syndrome (10%), or other infectious prodrome. Other symptoms may include fever, myalgias, dysuria, and loin pain. Some cases are identified during medical evaluation of a persistent asymptomatic hematuria or proteinuria. About 25% of patients will have an impaired glomerular filtration rate during active disease, but the serum creatinine is usually less than 3 mg/dl. Proteinuria is less than 1 gm per day. The gross hematuria usually lasts 2 to 6 days, but microscopic hematuria often persists between attacks. Half the patients have a single attack of gross hematuria; the rest have recurring episodes for many years, triggered by viral infections. Progression to renal failure may occur in 15% to 20% of the patients within 6 months. Progression to death or end-stage renal disease occurs in 50% of patients over a period of 20 years. This type of "synpharyngitic" nephritis is distinguished from poststreptococcal glomerulonephritis by the absence of a latent period.

The descriptive term "rapidly progressive glomerulonephritis" (RPGN) includes glomerular disorders characterized by rapid deterioration of renal function over weeks to months in association with extensive formation of fibrocellular crescents in many glomeruli. Approximately 20% of such cases are associated with anti-glomerular basement membrane (anti-GBM) antibodies. Anti-GBM nephritis in association with pulmonary hemorrhage is known as Goodpasture's syndrome. Pulmonary hemorrhage accompanies anti-GBM nephritis in about two-thirds of the cases. Goodpasture's syndrome is primarily a disease of young males, who are affected more often than females by a ratio of 6:1. Presenting manifestations include hemoptysis and pulmonary alveolar infiltrates on chest x-rays (CXR), with dyspnea and iron-deficiency anemia. There may be a history of a preceding flu-like illness or exposure to pulmonary toxins such as volatile hydrocarbons or cigarettes. Acute nephritis follows the onset of pulmonary symptoms by days to weeks. Half of the patients are azotemic at presentation. There may be arthralgias, fever, myalgias, abdominal pain, and hypertension, as well as uremic symptoms. Thirty percent die of pulmonary hemorrhage, and 80% require treatment for end-stage renal disease within 1 year. The survival rate now approaches 50%. Patients with anti-GBM nephritis without pulmonary hemorrhage are older, with a mean age of 50 years. In these cases, men and women are equally affected. The nephritis is otherwise similar to that seen in Goodpasture's syndrome. Recurrence of anti-GBM nephritis is seen in 10% to 30% of renal allografts. It is unknown whether bilateral nephrectomy reduces this recurrence rate.

About 40% of cases of (crescentic) RPGN are not associated with anti-GBM antibodies or significant glomerular immune deposits such as are seen in postinfectious glomerulonephritides, systemic lupus erythematosus, and IgG-IgA nephritis, and are classified as idiopathic. This is a disease of older patients, with a mean age at onset of 55 to 60 years. There is a slight male predominance. There is some tendency for such cases to appear in clusters. Many patients have a prodrome resembling a viral illness or vasculitis. Symptoms include myalgias, arthralgias, loin pain, abdominal pain, fever, malaise, and minor hemoptysis with fleeting pulmonary infiltrates on CXR. Patients may require dialysis at or shortly after presentation.

Membranoproliferative glomerulonephritis occurs mostly between the age of 5 and 30 years. Males and females are affected equally. There are only minor differences clinically between types I and II. Membranoproliferative glomerulonephritis appears in about 10% of renal biopsies. Twenty to thirty percent present with an acute nephritic syndrome (more common in type II). Thirty percent present with recurrent gross or microscopic hematuria. Fifty percent present with nephrotic syndrome. There is a history of antecedent upper respiratory infection in 50% of cases, sometimes in association with elevated antistreptolysin O (ASO) titers. Hypertension is found in one-third of patients and an impaired glomerular filtration rate in 25% to 50% at presentation. In type II disease, one-third of cases may progress to end-stage renal disease within 6 to 10 years. Progression is somewhat slower in type I disease. Only a few patients with either type I or type II disease will experience spontaneous remission. One-third will have persistent nephrotic syndrome with relatively stable renal function. One-third will have persistent hematuria and non-nephrotic range proteinuria. Poor prognostic signs include impaired glomerular filtration rate, gross hematuria, hypertension, and nephrosis on presentation.

PATHOPHYSIOLOGY

There are two generally accepted mechanisms of immunologic injury responsible for glomerulonephritis. The first is anti-GBM antibody deposition along the GBM, which appears as uninterrupted linear staining along the glomerular capillary walls by immunofluorescence staining. The second is the discontinuous, granular deposition of immunoglobulins and complement in various locations within the glomerulus leading to glomerular injury. Such deposits may occur primarily in the mesangium in IgG-IgA nephritis, Henock-Schönlein purpura (HSP), and systemic lupus erythematosus. Alternatively, the deposits may be found along the subendothelial surface of the capillary wall between the endothelial cells and the GBM, as in type I membranoproliferative glomerulonephritis or more severe forms of lupus nephritis. Finally, deposits may appear on the outer, subepithelial surface of the glomerular capillary wall as in membranous nephropathy or poststreptococcal glomerulonephritis ("subepithelial humps").

Mesangial and subendothelial granular immune complex deposits can result from either passive trapping of preformed immune complexes from the circulation, or local formation

due to glomerular localization of the antigens followed by antibody binding to the antigens. Subepithelial immune complex deposits, on the other hand, appear to form only on a local basis.

The type and severity of glomerular disease induced by immune deposits depends on the quantity, type, and location of the deposits (Table 96–2). Most glomerular antibody deposits contain IgG, which activates complement via the classical sequence. Such deposits occurring in mesangial and subendothelial sites are accessible to circulating inflammatory cells, which are recruited into the inflammatory response by chemotactic and immune adherence mechanisms. Polymorphonuclear leukocytes and macrophage effector cells damage the glomeruli by releasing proteolytic enzymes resulting in hematuria, proteinuria, and impaired glomerular filtration rate. IgA deposits activate complement primarily by the alternate pathway and engender a less vigorous inflammatory response. Immune deposits forming at subepithelial sites, as in membranous nephropathy, are not accessible to circulating inflammatory cells and thus give rise to a noninflammatory glomerular lesion, manifested clinically as the nephrotic syndrome rather than as acute nephritis. Nephrosis may also be induced by a direct membranolytic effect of complement activation leading to enhanced capillary wall permeability.

Impairment of the glomerular filtration rate in acute nephritic syndromes may be minimal or may progress to severe oliguria or anuria. Contributing factors include the adverse effects of immune injury on glomerular hemodynamics and structural integrity, formation of glomerular intracapillary thromboses, development of acute tubular necrosis due to glomerular ischemia, tubular obstruction by casts, and compression of glomerular tufts by proliferating cells or epithelial cell crescent formation. Return of the glomerular filtration rate to normal depends on cessation of the process initiating the injury and the extent of irreparable damage (necrosis, fibrosis, and sclerosis) occurring within the glomerulus.

Red blood cells apparently gain access to Bowman's space by passing through rents within the glomerular capillary walls, although such defects are not often observed histologically. The RBCs can potentially also enter the

TABLE 96–2.
Microscopic and Laboratory Features of Various Types of Glomerulonephritis

TYPE OF GLOMERULO NEPHRITIS	MICROSCOPIC FEATURES			LABORATORY FEATURES
	LIGHT MICROSCOPY	IMMUNE DEPOSITS	ELECTRON MICROSCOPY	
Anti-GBM*	Crescents; focal proliferative necrotizing glomerulonephritis	Continuous linear IgG deposition along GBM	Nonspecific	Anti-GBM antibodies; HLA-DRw2 antigens
Poststreptococcal glomerulonephritis	Diffuse proliferative glomerulonephritis; endothelial and mesangial hypercellularity and crescents	Coarsely granular IgG/C3 deposits along GBM	Electron-dense subepithelial "humps"	C3 levels depressed; ASO elevated; cryo/CIC present; C3NF.
Membranoproliferative glomerulonephritis type I	Diffuse proliferative glomerulonephritis; lobular glomeruli; "tram track" glomerular capillary wall on silver staining	Coarsely granular C3/IgG/IgM/C4/fibrin in peripheral capillary loops	Dense subendothelial and mesangial deposits; mesangial matrix interposition and capillary wall thickening	Markedly depressed C3 levels; CICs; cryo's; C3NF; B-cell alloantigen
Type II	Ribbon-like dense deposits in capillary walls; double linear pattern of capillary walls; crescents	Granular IgG deposits	Replacement of lamina densa of GBM with dark-staining material	Markedly depressed C3 levels; C3NF^{+++}
Idiopathic rapidly progressive glomerulonephritis	Extensive crescents; diffuse proliferative GN	Focal granular deposits of IgM and C3	"Gaps" in glomerular capillary walls; IgM and no immune deposits	Nondiagnostic
IgG-IgA	Focal/segmental proliferative GN; mesangial expansion and hypercellularity; crescents	Diffuse mesangial IgA deposits	Finely granular to homogeneous electron dense deposits	IgA CICs; HLA-Bw35 and Dr4

* Glomerular basement membrane.

urine via extravasation from the peritubular capillaries. Red blood cell casts form when red cells are present in the tubule lumen proximal to the site of Tamm-Horsfall protein secretion in the ascending limb of the loop of Henle and become incorporated into a matrix composed of polymerized Tamm-Horsfall proteins and filtered plasma proteins. Red blood cell casts are highly indicative of renal parenchymal disease.

Nephritic edema is the result of primary renal sodium retention which is typically seen in acute glomerulonephritis. The plasma oncotic pressure is normal, and progressive salt and water retention leads to circulatory congestion and pulmonary and peripheral edema. The renin-angiotensin-aldosterone axis is typically suppressed. This is in contradistinction to the secondary sodium retention seen in the nephrotic syndrome, where massive proteinuria leads to low plasma oncotic pressure, circulatory underfilling, low to normal blood pressure, and activation of the renin-angiotensin-aldosterone axis.

Although glomerular filtration rate is reduced in acute glomerulonephritis, renal sodium reabsorption is not. An adaptive increase in fractional excretion of sodium which should occur with expansion of the extracellular fluid (ECF) volume, tending to restore sodium balance, is not seen. The sodium reabsorption of acute glomerulonephritis cannot be explained by increased absolute or fractional reabsorption in the proximal tubule. Experimental evidence suggests that altered reabsorption of salt and water in distal nephron segments plays an important role. Sodium reabsorption in acute glomerulonephritis probably represents a decline in the glomerular filtration rate and decreased delivery of sodium to distal nephron segments coupled with a constant or increased fractional sodium reabsorption by these segments.

Although aldosterone is not increased in acute glomerulonephritis syndromes, it sometimes may not be appropriately suppressed. Plasma renin activity is usually significantly reduced. Another possible mechanism for sodium retention is suppression of an endogenous natriuretic substance. In acute glomerulonephritis, despite edema and expansion of the extracellular fluid volume, adaptive natriuresis does not occur until healing ensues. In chronic glomerulonephritis, adaptive natriuresis is commonly seen so that edema disappears and the ECF volume is only mildly expanded.

The hypertension of acute glomerulonephritis is usually mild to moderate and volume dependent, being due to the expanded ECF volume. In some forms of chronic glomerulonephritis (CGN), there may be a variably severe hyperreninemia, especially during ECF volume depletion, that may be associated with severe and refractory hypertension necessitating nephrectomy. The mechanism for such renin stimulation is unclear, but may involve reduced sodium delivery distally to the macula densa, or stimulation of the renin-producing cells of the afferent arterioles by glomerular capillary obstruction. Hypertension in acute glomerulonephritis is adaptive to the extent that glomerular hydraulic pressures and renal plasma flow are enhanced, thus tending to restore glomerular filtration rate to normal. For this reason, abrupt reduction of the systemic blood pressure may be associated with further deterioration of glomerular filtration rate.

Congestive heart failure in acute glomerulonephritis is due to hypertension (increased afterload), myocardial depression (which may be due to uremia, myocarditis, or coronary vasculitis), and ECF volume expansion (increased preload). Depressed cardiac output may further contribute to the kidney's impaired ability to increase fractional excretion of sodium as an adaptation to decreased glomerular filtration rate.

Proteinuria is invariably present in acute nephritic syndromes, but is usually in the "non-nephrotic" range, or less than 3.5 gm per day. The proteinuria is usually nonselective, containing serum globulins as well as albumin. The filtration of proteins across the glomerular capillary wall depends on (1) properties of the individual protein molecules (size, shape, deformability, ionic charge); (2) the protein concentration in plasma; (3) the structural and functional integrity and ionic charge of the glomerular capillary wall; and (4) the glomerular pressures and flows determining the rate of ultrafiltration. Thus, the proteinuria of acute nephritic syndromes is related to (1) a generalized increase in the permeability characteristics of the glomerular capillary wall; (2) altered glomerular hemodynamics; and (3) mechanical disruptions in the glomerular capillary wall structure.

Glomerular disorders may result in a defect in the size-selective barrier of the glomerular capillary wall. Increased permeability of the GBM based on size could result from various abnormalities of molecular organization of the hydrated GBM gel. Electron-microscopically demonstrated gaps in the glomerular capillary wall suggest increased protein permeability based on size considerations. Glomerular immune deposits may also act to alter the glomerular wall permeability to proteins. Focal loss of visceral epithelial cells may result in a local increase in water flux, which could result in increased transglomerular protein movement.

Alteration of the net negative charge of the GBM could lead to disruption of the charge-selective barrier to protein movement. The (anionic) sialic acid content of isolated GBM has been shown to be decreased in various experimental models of glomerulonephritis. Decreased sialoprotein content of epithelial cells has been found to correlate with the onset of proteinuria. Effacement of the epithelial cell foot processes, commonly seen in proteinuric states, may result from loss of negative charge in the interdigitating epithelial cell foot processes, preventing their normal separation. Focally distributed abnormalities of the slit-pore membrane or the GBM or both may result in discontinuous disturbances in capillary wall charge, transglomerular water flux, or "pore size." Thus, glomerular proteinuria can result from diffuse or generalized, or focal or segmental disturbances of the size- and/or charge-selective barriers to protein filtration.

CLINICAL–PATHOLOGIC CORRELATIONS

The clinical–pathologic correlations for glomerulonephritis are listed in Table 96–3.

DIFFERENTIAL DIAGNOSIS

In the differential diagnosis of acute nephritic syndromes, it is useful at the outset to ascertain the presence of a systemic disorder strongly associated with nephritis. A history of drug abuse or hepatitis B antigenemia might suggest polyarteritis nodosa. The presence of purulent rhinorrhea with active sinusitis, oral ulcerations, and bilateral nodular pulmonary infil-

TABLE 96–3.
Clinical–Pathologic Correlations for Glomerulonephritis

CLINICAL FINDINGS	PATHOLOGIC FINDINGS
Fatigue Weakness Malaise Nausea/vomiting	Manifestations of uremia
Headache Lethargy Confusion Somnolence Seizures	Central nervous system manifestations may be due to uremia, hypertension, or electrolyte disturbance
Hypertension Dyspnea Orthopnea Edema/anasarca	Due to ECF volume expansion
Hemoptysis	Seen in Goodpasture's syndrome
Loin pain Abdominal pain Hematuria	Due to active renal inflammation

trates should indicate renal involvement with Wegener's granulomatosis. Purpura, microangiopathic hemolytic anemia, and pulmonary infiltrates with hemoptysis would be expected features of a hypersensitivity vasculitis. The clinical syndrome of systemic lupus erythematosus should be recognizable by the usual criteria. Henoch-Schönlein purpura, or anaphylactoid purpura, features palpable purpura involving the lower extremities and buttocks, arthralgias of large joints (knees and ankles), GI involvement with abdominal pain and GI bleeding, and active nephritis. Raynaud's phenomenon with purpura and arthralgias could be a clue to essential mixed cryoglobulinemia. Hemolytic uremic syndrome and thrombotic thrombocytopenia purpura are characterized by fever, microangiopathic hemolytic anemia, thrombocytopenic purpura, and prominent neurologic manifestations that often cause death. The syndromes of subacute bacterial endocarditis and of chronic infection of a ventriculo-atrial (VA) shunt or other prosthesis as contributory to glomerulonephritis should be readily recognized. The presence of a lung abscess is readily ascertained, and a persistent focus of intra-abdominal infection can be considered in many postoperative settings. Poststreptococcal glomerulonephritis should be considered in a young patient with antecedent pharyngitis or impetigo and a suitable latent interval. Gross hematuria coincident with or following within 24 to 48 hours a viral upper respiratory infection suggests Berger's disease. Goodpasture's syndrome and anti-GBM nephritis should be suspected in a young male with hemoptysis and pulmonary infiltrates. Types I and II membrano-proliferative glomerulonephritis and idiopathic (crescentic) glomerulonephritis have no particular distinguishing clinical features.

DIAGNOSIS

The diagnosis of acute nephritic syndromes depends on clinical and laboratory features, and renal biopsy findings on light, immunofluorescence, and electron microscopy (Table 96–2).

The most specific laboratory finding in anti-GBM nephritis is the presence of serum antibodies to GBM. Such antibodies can be detected by an immunofluorescence test using normal human kidney tissue as substrate or by a commercially available radioimmunoassay. The former is 80% to 90% sensitive, and the latter is 95% sensitive. Complement levels are normal. Circulating immune complexes and cryoglobulins are absent. Fibrin degradation products may be elevated in serum. Antistreptolysin O (ASO) titers may be positive. The presence of HLA-DRw2 antigen confers a relative risk 15 to 34 times normal. Immunofluorescence microscopy is highly characteristic (Table 96–2). Light microscopy shows a diffuse proliferative necrotizing glomerulonephritis with fibrocellular crescents in more than half the glomeruli. Immunofluorescence microscopy shows continuous linear staining for IgG along the glomerular capillary wall.

In poststreptococcal glomerulonephritis the ASO titer is usually greater than 200 Todd units by 1 to 3 weeks and remains elevated for months. A rise may not be seen if antibiotics are given early in the course of infection. The ASO titers rise little or none in poststreptococcal glomerulonephritis associated with impetigo. The levels of antibodies to other streptococcal enzymes may be elevated as well. The streptozyme test utilizes five streptococcal antigens in a single assay. In impetigo-related glomerulonephritis, anti-hyaluronidase and anti-deoxyribonuclease-B antibodies are often present. Urine analysis shows proteinuria, RBCs, WBCs, and red blood cell casts. Ninety percent of patients with poststreptococcal glomerulonephritis have reduced total hemolytic complement or C3 during the first 2 weeks, with a return to normal within 3 weeks in 50%. Persistent or profound hypocomplementemia should suggest other disorders such as membranoproliferative glomerulonephritis, SBE, cryoimmunoglobulinemia, systemic lupus erythematosus, or occult visceral sepsis. Cryoglobulins and circulating immune complexes are often present. The levels of Clq and C4 are usually normal, suggesting complement activation by the alternate pathway. Fractional excretion of sodium is usually less than 0.5%. Table 96–2 shows characteristic microscopic features.

In Berger's disease, "synpharyngitic" gross hematuria may last 4 to 6 days. There may be persistent microscopic hematuria between attacks. Ten percent of patients may have nephrotic range proteinuria. Complement levels are normal. Cryoglobulins and rheumatoid factor are not found. Fifty percent of patients have elevated serum IgA levels, and circulating immune complexes containing IgA may be present. Skin biopsies from the volar surface of the forearm reveal dermal capillary deposits of IgA in 90% of patients with Berger's disease. There is an increased incidence of HLA-Bw35 and HLA-DR4 antigens in Berger's disease. Immunofluorescence microscopy shows immune deposits in the mesangial areas of all glomeruli with IgA as the predominant immunoglobulin.

In membranoproliferative glomerulonephritis, there is often marked and persistent hypocomplementemia. Seventy percent of patients have depressed C3 levels. In type I, the complement levels fluctuate, and both the classic (Clq and C4) and alternate pathway components are depressed at some time. Circulating immune complexes are present in 50% of cases; cryoglobulins may be present. Over 75% with type I MPGN have a particular B-cell alloantigen, suggesting a possible genetic susceptibility. Table 96–2 shows characteristic microscopic features.

Type II membranoproliferative glomerulonephritis features a more persistent and severe hypocomplementemia. Only alternate pathway complement components are depressed (C3). The C3 nephritic factor (C3NF), an IgG autoantibody to the C3 convertase of the alternate complement pathway, is present in 60% of patients with type II membranoproliferative glomerulonephritis (and in 20% with type I). It is a heat-stable factor capable of cleaving C3 in fresh normal plasma in the presence of magnesium EGTA. The levels of C3NF and C3 are unaffected by bilateral nephrectomy but have a tendency to normalize with time. Cryoglobulins may be present, although not as often as in type I disease. The HLA-B7 antigen may be positive in type II disease. Table 96–2 shows characteristic microscopic features.

PRINCIPLES OF PREVENTION AND TREATMENT

Various supportive measures can be taken in acute nephritis (Table 96–4). Restriction of sodium and water intake is helpful in managing edema, circulatory congestion, and hypertension. Dietary protein restriction may be useful in delaying the appearance of uremic symptoms. Dietary potassium restriction will

---

TABLE 96–4.
Management of Glomerulonephritis

GENERAL SUPPORTIVE MEASURES	
	Sodium and water restriction
	Protein restriction
	Potassium restriction
	Diuretics (not potassium-sparing diuretics)
	Antihypertensives
	Dialysis
SPECIFIC MEASURES	
Poststreptococcal glomerulonephritis	Usually no specific therapy needed
	?Plasma-exchange; pulse corticosteroids
Postinfectious glomerulonephritis	Appropriate management of infection
Berger's disease	No specific therapy
Anti-GBM nephritis	Prednisone and cyclophosphamide plasma exchange
Idiopathic (crescentic) glomerulonephritis	?Plasma exchange
	?Pulse corticosteroids
	?"Quadruple therapy" (dipyridamole, sulfinpyrazone, prednisone, cytotoxic drugs)
Membranoproliferative glomerulonephritis	?Continuous low doses of prednisone
	?"Quadruple therapy"

also be appropriate under most conditions when the glomerular filtration rate is severely reduced. Diuretics may be useful if the glomerular filtration rate is not too severely impaired, but potassium-sparing diuretics should be avoided. Appropriate antihypertensive therapy is essential. Dialysis therapy is indicated for severe circulatory congestion, uremic symptoms, electrolyte disturbances, and severe metabolic acidosis.

In poststreptococcal glomerulonephritis, recovery can be anticipated in most cases without specific therapy. Penicillin therapy does not alter the incidence or severity of poststreptococcal GN. Corticosteroids and cytotoxic agents have no proven role in the treatment of poststreptococcal glomerulonephritis and may prove harmful. In patients who have prolonged oliguria and extensive crescent formation, under certain circumstances plasma exchange or pulse corticosteroids can be considered for use, as in the management of idiopathic (crescentic) RPGN. Appropriate antibiotic therapy of streptococcal pharyngitis or impetigo is in order.

In glomerulonephritis associated with subacute bacterial endocarditis, renal function will often return to normal following successful antibiotic therapy. "Shunt nephritis" is appropriately managed with antibiotic therapy and removal of the infected shunt. In glomerulonephritis associated with visceral abscesses, eradication of the infection leads to recovery of renal function in 50% of cases, although overall mortality remains high.

There is no specific therapy for Berger's disease. Glomerular IgA deposition may recur in renal allografts, usually with no serious clinical consequences.

In anti-GBM nephritis there is little evidence that oral corticosteroids or immunosuppressives alone alter the course of the disease. Pulmonary hemorrhage may respond to high doses of prednisone or pulse methylprednisolone; however, pulse methylprednisolone does not benefit the renal lesion. Most institutions are now using vigorous plasma exchange (4 L/day) combined with prednisone and cyclophosphamide administration until anti-GBM antibody is no longer detectable or until disease progression halts. Survival in anti-GBM nephritis appears to be improved with plasma exchange therapy, but the response rate is low if the serum creatinine level is greater than 6

mg/dl. Allograft transplantation should be delayed until the anti-GBM antibody is undetectable. Spontaneous recovery is rare in anti-GBM nephritis.

In idiopathic (crescentic) glomerulonephritis without immune deposits, and with immune deposits in the absence of any clearly defined systemic illness (SLE, HSP, PSGN, and so forth), the response to therapy is similar. There is a paucity of data which would allow a truly rational choice of therapy. Modalities currently employed include plasma exchange, pulse methylprednisolone followed by oral corticosteroids, and "quadruple therapy" (dipyridamole, sulfin pyrazone, prednisone, and cytotoxic drugs). These modalities have not been shown in prospective trials to improve outcome, but are nonetheless considered by different authors to represent therapeutic advances. Response rates as high as 75% have been reported in small numbers of patients treated with pulse methylprednisolone followed by oral corticosteroids tapered over several months. Response, if any, usually occurs within 1 to 4 weeks. Long-term follow-up has been limited. Such a regimen is generally safe and could be considered a reasonable first approach. If no response is obtained, consideration can then be given to plasma exchange. Idiopathic (crescentic) RPGN rarely recurs in kidney allografts.

A variety of therapeutic modalities have been employed in an uncontrolled fashion in membranoproliferative glomerulonephritis types I and II. Generally, membranoproliferative glomerulonephritis is slowly progressive, with the outlook somewhat worse in type II than type I. The 10-year rate of progression to end-stage renal disease is about 50%. High doses of corticosteroids have not been shown to improve the prognosis. There is some suggestion of benefit with continuous low doses of prednisone. The benefit of "quadruple therapy" is uncertain. Generally, the results with corticosteroid and cytotoxic regimens have been unimpressive. There is no treatment program that is commonly accepted to be of long-term value.

Protein restriction may be beneficial in slowing the progression of various forms of chronic glomerulonephritis. Protein restriction has been shown to substantially modify experimentally induced glomerular hyperfiltration. Glomerular hyperfiltration occurs with a loss of functioning nephron mass via an adaptive increase in glomerular capillary plasma flow rates and transcapillary hydraulic pressure gradients in order to maximize glomerular filtration rate in the remaining nephrons. Glomerular hyperfiltration appears to result in increased capillary permeability to protein and structural glomerular damage when sustained above a certain level over time. The histologic manifestation of this process is focal glomerular sclerosis.

REFERENCES

Couser WG: Idiopathic rapidly progressive glomerulonephritis. *Am J Nephrol* 1982; 2:57. *Recent detailed review of idiopathic RPGN.*

Couser WG: Glomerular disorders, in Wyngarden JB, Smith LH (eds): *Textbook of Medicine*, ed 17. Philadelphia, WB Saunders Co, 1985, p 568. *Overview of primary and systemic glomerulopathies.*

Couser WG: Mechanisms of glomerular injury in immune-complex disease. *Kidney Int* 1985; 28: 569–583. *Reviews the mechanisms of immunologically mediated renal disease.*

Glassock RJ, Cohen AH, Adler S, Ward H: Primary glomerular disorders, in Brenner BM, Rector FC Jr (eds): *The Kidney*, ed 3. Philadelphia, WB Saunders Co, 1986, p 929. *Comprehensive discussion of the primary glomerulopathies.*

Glassock RJ, Cohen AH, Adler S, Ward H: Secondary glomerular disorders, in Brenner BM, Rector FC Jr (eds): *The Kidney*, ed 3. Philadelphia, WB Saunders Co, 1986, p 1014. *Comprehensive discussion of glomerulopathies due to systemic disorders.*

Madaio MP, Harrington JT: The diagnosis of acute glomerulonephritis. *N Engl J Med* 1983; 309 (21):1299–1302. *Emphasizes the utility of serum complement levels in the differential diagnosis of acute glomerulonephritis.*

Neugarten J, Baldwin DS: Glomerulonephritis in bacterial endocarditis. *Am J Med* 1984; 77:297–304. *Reviews the epidemiologic, laboratory, and clinical features of glomerulonephritis associated with bacterial endocarditis.*

97   NEPHROTIC SYNDROME

Robert T. Witty, M.D., Ph.D.

Nephrotic syndrome is one of the more common presentations of glomerular disease. The definition of nephrotic syndrome is arbitrary but is usually defined in an adult as a condition in which more than 3.5 gm of protein are excreted in the urine a day. This is associated with a decreased serum albumin level (less than 3 mg/dl), edema formation, lipidemia (increased serum cholesterol levels, Type II hyperlipoproteinemia) and lipiduria (oval fat bodies in the urine). Hypertension may or may not be a concomitant finding.

CLINICAL SIGNS AND SYMPTOMS

The typical patient with idiopathic nephrotic syndrome will present with edema formation. The severity of the edema depends on the serum albumin level which also depends on the amount of proteinuria. Peripheral edema can be a nuisance without being very disabling.

The amount of edema formed depends on the Starling forces in the capillary plus the amount of salt and water retained. In the periphery, the edema usually accumulates over the tibia and in the more severe cases in the thigh and flank. Periorbital and presacral edema can accumulate in patients overnight or in those patients who are bed bound. Occasionally salt and water retention can be severe and can lead to the accumulation of ascites, pericardial fluid, or pleural fluid.

Without affecting renal function, the nephrotic syndrome may increase the morbidity and mortality of a concomitant illness. For example, before the era of corticosteroids, a significant percentage of children with nephrotic syndrome would die from infectious or thrombotic complications.

Approximately one-third of all patients presenting with idiopathic nephrotic syndrome will initially present with a thrombotic complication, typically renal vein thrombosis and occasionally pulmonary emboli. Patients may also present initially with infectious complications such as pneumonia due ·to immunoglobulin deficiency. Patients who also have a systemic disease, for example, diabetes or systemic lupus erythematosus, may present initially with the signs and symptoms of the systemic disease.

At the time of diagnosis most patients with nephrotic syndrome will have good renal function but may still have constitutional symptoms such as malaise and increased fatigability. Patients who have long-term nephrotic syndrome may develop lipid disorders, atherosclerotic complications, and disturbances in vitamin D and calcium metabolism with subsequent bone disease.

The natural history of nephrotic syndrome is variable, depending on the underlying disease. Some patients may go on to end-stage renal disease within a few months, or they may continue to have nephrotic syndrome with good renal function for years. Some patients may develop infectious or thrombotic complications.

PATHOPHYSIOLOGY

Edema formation in nephrotic syndrome occurs when large amounts of protein are lost through the urine leading to a decreased serum level of albumin when the liver production of albumin cannot keep up with urinary losses. The low albumin level reduces the oncotic pressure of the plasma, and the Starling forces shift the fluid from the vascular compartment to the interstitium. The small decrease in intravascular volume stimulates the homeostatic mechanisms that increase salt and water retention. These mechanisms include baroreceptor activation, which increases antidiuretic hormone, and renin release, which then mediates aldosterone stimulation of the kidneys to retain salt and water. Intrarenal factors and other hormones may also play a role in sodium retention.

The proteinuria in nephrotic syndrome may be produced by many different types of glomerular damage. The basis for the increased glomerular selectivity for certain serum proteins is unclear but is probably related to the molecular size, configuration, and charge of the protein as well as to the structural changes in the glomerular basement membrane.

The amount of proteinuria in nephrotic syndrome is influenced by the plasma albumin concentration and the filtration rate. Commonly as renal function deteriorates, the amount of proteinuria also declines, sometimes even below the nephrotic range. There is a significant correlation between serum albumin and protein excretion rates. The liver attempts to keep up with the albumin loss in the urine by synthesizing more albumin. The stimulus to synthesize more albumin seems to be a low plasma oncotic pressure.

Albumin is the main plasma protein loss in the urine. It accounts for most of the protein in the urine of children who have lipoid nephrosis. However, in more severe glomerular diseases, heavier proteins are also lost in the urine; this proteinuria is said to be nonselective as opposed to the selective proteinuria of lipoid nephrosis. The selectivity in a case can be roughly gauged by immunoelectrophoresis of the urine. The plasma levels of proteins other than albumin may be altered in the nephrotic syndrome. The alpha and beta globulin levels are increased. The total gamma globulin level may be decreased from a decrease in the IgG level, but IgA, IgM, and IgE levels may be normal or increased. Some complement components such as Clq are lost in the urine.

Serum transferrin levels may be decreased, leading to a microcytic hypochromic anemia that is resistant to iron therapy. Serum ferritin levels, however, may be increased. Transcortin levels may be decreased, which can lead to a change in the proportion of bound cortisol. This can be important in patients with nephrotic syndrome who are treated with corticosteroids.

Thyroid-binding globulin deficiency can affect the measured levels of thyroid hormones, although clinically the patients are euthyroid.

Loss of cholecalciferol-binding globulin can result in a vitamin D-deficiency state in which levels of 25-hydroxycholecalciferol are decreased. Osteomalacia and hyperparathyroidism can develop when renal function is normal. The total serum calcium levels are usually decreased because of the marked decrease in serum albumin.

In conclusion, changes in a number of serum proteins may change the results of laboratory tests or, more importantly, the physiology.

In nephrotic syndrome, the primary lipid disorder is an increase in the serum cholesterol level or a type II hyperlipoproteinemia. High-density lipoproteins (HDL) levels may also be reduced. When the nephrotic syndrome is severe, triglyceride levels may also be increased. There is a significant inverse correlation between the serum cholesterol level and the serum albumin level and, therefore, with the oncotic pressure. As with the increased protein synthesis by the liver, the increased lipid synthesis seems to be related to the decrease in oncotic pressure because restoring the oncotic pressure to normal decreases the lipid synthesis to normal.

CLINICAL–PATHOLOGIC CORRELATIONS

The clinical–pathologic correlations for nephrotic syndrome are listed in Table 97–1.

In any given case, edema may not be important clinically, or it can be debilitating. Pedal edema can be treated with diuretics so that the patient will be more comfortable. In some cases, a small amount of edema may be desirable because this makes intravascular volume depletion less likely. Patients with low serum albumin levels and marginal intravascular volumes may have orthostatic hypotension.

Because of protein losses, maintenance of good nutrition can be a serious problem in nephrotic syndrome. Dietary protein of high biologic quality containing the essential amino acids plus histidine should be prescribed. Vitamin D supplements and iron may also be required. The degree of atherosclerotic risk in nephrotic syndrome is unclear. For that reason, and also because there are a lot of side-effects from lipid-lowering drugs, the cost-to-benefit ratio of these drugs must be carefully weighed. Diet and exercise are still standard therapy for

TABLE 97–1.
Clinical–Pathologic Correlations for Nephrotic Syndrome

CLINICAL FINDINGS	PATHOLOGIC FINDINGS	TREATMENT
Edema, ascites, pleural effusion, pericardial effusion	Proteinuria, decreased serum albumin level, salt and water retention	Diuretics
Weakness, dizziness, symptoms of renal failure	Reduced intravascular volume in severe nephrotic syndrome, acute renal failure	Dialysis
Weakness, poor nutrition, bone fractures	Protein loss, decreased vitamin D, osteomalacia, anemia	Protein of high biologic value, vitamin D, iron
Accelerated atherosclerosis	Increased serum cholesterol, type II hyperlipoproteinemia	Possible lipid-lowering agents
Symptoms of deep vein thrombosis, renal vein thrombosis, cerebrovascular disease	Hypercoagulable state	Anticoagulation, possible prophylactic anticoagulation
Short of breath, weakness, symptoms of bone disease	Renal tubular acidosis, Fanconi's syndrome	Alkalinizing agents
Weakness, malaise	Constitutional symptoms, anemia	Attempt to reverse nephrotic syndrome, possible steroids

preventing atherosclerotic complications. Patients with nephrotic syndrome may have significant morbidity and mortality from bacterial infections, especially pneumonia. This may be related to IgG deficiency.

Several important factors contribute to the hypercoagulable state (see Llach, 1985, for an excellent review of the hypercoagulable state) seen in nephrotic syndrome: (1) increased serum fibrinogen levels leading to an increased plasma viscosity, (2) a deficiency of antithrombin III, and (3) increased platelet aggregation. Renal vein thrombosis is a common occurrence, especially in patients with membranous glomerulonephritis. The incidence of deep vein thrombosis, especially of the extremities is 20% to 40%. Arterial thrombosis causing cerebrovascular ischemia also occurs. Anticoagulation for documented renal vein thrombosis is indicated, but whether prophylactic anticoagulation should be instituted for all patients with nephrotic syndrome is not clear.

Nephrotic syndrome may be associated with renal tubular dysfunction in some patients. This may be first seen as a full-fledged Fanconi's syndrome with phosphaturia, glycosuria, aminoaciduria, and a proximal renal tubular acidosis.

With severe nephrotic syndrome and marginal vascular volume, it is possible to develop acute renal failure although this is an unusual occurrance.

Patients with nephrotic syndrome may complain of the constitutional symptoms of decreased energy, decreased stamina, and malaise. These symptoms may be caused by anemia, nutritional problems, or blood pressure problems.

DIFFERENTIAL DIAGNOSIS

The differential diagnosis for nephrotic syndrome is listed in Table 97–2. The most common cause of nephrotic syndrome in the world is probably infections related to malaria. The most common cause of nephrotic syndrome in the United States is diabetes mellitus. The most common cause of idiopathic nephrotic syndrome (Table 97–3) in adults is membranous glomerulonephritis and in children is minimal change glomerulonephritis, previously known as lipoid nephrosis. These four conditions account for most cases of nephrotic syndrome. The other causes of nephrotic syndrome listed in Table 97–2 are less common.

DIAGNOSIS

Laboratory findings that support a diagnosis of a nephrotic syndrome in the adult include (1) proteinuria greater than 3.5 gm a day, (2) a serum albumin level usually less than 3 mg/dl, (3) a serum cholesterol level usually greater than 300 mg/dl, and (4) increased or decreased serum levels of other proteins depending on the severity of the renal disease and the molecular weight of the protein.

Radiology studies such as intravenous pyelography, renal scan, or ultrasound study usu-

---

TABLE 97–2.
Differential Diagnosis of Nephrotic Syndrome

I. Idiopathic nephrotic syndrome
II. Medications
    Gold, penicillamine, angiotensin captopril, converting enzyme inhibitors such as nonsteroidal anti-inflammatory agents most commonly feroprofen
III. Allergies
    Bee sting, snake venoms
IV. Collagen vascular disease, systemic lupus erythematosus, polyarteritis, Goodpasture's syndrome, Henoch-Schönlein purpura, sarcoid, amyloidosis
V. Infections
    Poststreptococcal glomerulonephritis, syphilis, malaria, viral infections (cytomegalovirus, hepatitis B), schistosomiasis
VI. Tumors
    Hodgkin's, myeloma, solid tumors
VII. Metabolic disease, hereditary disease, diabetes, Alport's syndrome

TABLE 97–3.
Pathologic and Clinical Characteristics of Conditions Causing Idiopathic Nephrotic Syndrome

CONDITION	RENAL PATHOLOGIC FEATURES	CLINICAL PRESENTATION	CORTICOSTEROID RESPONSIVENESS	PROGNOSIS
Minimal change glomerulonephritis	Fusion of foot processes on electron microscopy	Nephrotic syndrome	Yes	Good
Mesangial proliferative glomerulonephritis	Increased mesangial cellularity	Uncommon cause of nephrotic syndrome, occasional cause of nephritis	May respond if no sclerosing lesions are present	Fair
Focal sclerosing glomerulonephritis	Focal and segmental glomerulosclerosis	Nephrotic syndrome Occasionally nephritis	No	Poor; frequent progression to end-stage renal disease
Rapidly progressive glomerulonephritis	Cellular proliferation, crescent formation	Nephrotic or nephritic syndrome Renal failure	Bolus steroids may help	Poor
Membranoproliferative glomerulonephritis, Type I, type II*	Cellular proliferation, thickening of the basement membrane	Nephrotic or nephritic syndrome	No	Poor
Membranous glomerulonephritis	Thickening of basement membrane on light microscopy; subepithelial immune complex deposition; little cellular proliferation	Nephrotic syndrome	Often questionable Steroid trial for 8 weeks appropriate	Fair to good

* For more details, see Chapter 96.

ally do not add much information useful for a diagnosis of nephrotic syndrome. However, the kidney size may be useful, and kidney size and position and the presence of two kidneys must be confirmed before renal biopsy is undertaken.

The role of renal biopsy in the diagnosis and treatment of nephrotic syndrome is controversial. Nephrotic syndrome remains a strong indication for renal biopsy when the cause of the nephrotic syndrome is unclear, assuming that the kidney size is fairly normal. Some types of glomerulonephritis as shown in Table 97–3, for example, minimal change glomerulonephritis, are responsive to corticosteroids. Other types of glomerulonephritis, for example, membranoproliferative glomerulonephritis and focal sclerosing glomerulonephritis, are not responsive to corticosteroids. (The utility of doing a renal biopsy in all patients with nephrotic syndrome is reviewed in Kassirer, 1983.)

PRINCIPLES OF THERAPY

A diet with protein of high biologic value should be prescribed, and salt should be restricted. If renal function is decreased, restricted protein intake may be indicated.

Diuretics should be used cautiously to control the volume status of the patient. Combining a loop diuretic that acts on the loop of Henle with metolazone may have an additive effect. Occasionally in hospitalized patients who are severely hypoalbuminemic, intravenous (IV) infusions of albumin in combination with diuretics may mobilize edema fluid. Diuretics should be used cautiously when the serum albumin is very low because a relative

intravascular volume depletion may be easily produced.

The use of corticosteroids in idiopathic nephrotic syndrome can be valuable. The diseases usually considered to be responsive to corticosteroids are listed in Table 97–3. Some systemic diseases that cause nephrotic syndrome may also respond to corticosteroids. These include collagen vascular disease, especially systemic lupus erythematosus, polyarteritis, and Wegener's granulomatosis; sarcoidosis; and myeloma or a solid tumor. Occasionally if the patient with myeloma or a solid tumor causing nephrotic syndrome undergoes remission, the nephrotic syndrome will also resolve. Kassirer (1983) recently suggested that patients with idiopathic nephrotic syndrome should be treated empirically with corticosteroids without first doing a renal biopsy based on a controlled study that showed no differences in morbidity, mortality, and response of the renal disease to the two treatment regimens. If this approach is adopted, the single most important issue to remember is that the trial of steroids should be limited to a finite time such as 8 weeks, and if the patient does not respond by that time corticosteroid use should be discontinued.

The lesions usually considered to be responsive to corticosteroids are minimal change glomerulonephritis and occasionally cases of mesangial proliferative glomerulonephritis and membranous glomerulonephritis. It may be reasonable to treat all children with nephrotic syndrome empirically with corticosteroids because the overwhelming majority have lipoid nephrosis.

REFERENCES

Brenner BM, Rector FC Jr (eds): *The Kidney*, ed 3. Philadelphia, WB Saunders Co, 1986, p 929. *A comprehensive review of nephrotic syndrome.*

Kassirer J: Is renal biopsy necessary for optimal management of the idiopathic nephrotic syndrome? *Kidney Int* 1983; 24:561. *Renal biopsy can*

be considered as a research tool in nephrotic syndrome.

Llach F: Hypercoagulability, renal vein thrombosis, and other thrombotic complications of nephrotic syndrome. *Kidney Int* 1985; 28:429. *Thrombotic complications as a cause of significant morbidity in nephrotic syndrome.*

98 ACUTE RENAL FAILURE

Venkatachalam Muthiah, M.D.

Acute renal failure is a relatively common problem in clinical medicine. This form of renal failure may have many etiologies but is characterized by a relatively sudden onset of progressive retention of nitrogenous products such as urea and creatinine. There is usually, but not always, a decrease in the 24-hour urine production to less than 400 ml per day. Total anuria is rarely seen, and at times the urine volume can be normal or excessive. The outcome depends on the underlying cause, the presence, if any, of a systemic disease, the patient's age, and associated complications.

CLINICAL SIGNS AND SYMPTOMS

The onset of acute renal failure is sudden, and if the blood urea nitrogen (BUN) and serum creatinine levels rise rapidly to high levels, the patient may present with convulsions, hypertension, pulmonary edema, pericarditis, dehydration, acidosis, hyperkalemia, anorexia, vomiting, and weight loss. A prior or current history of systemic disease, renal disease or infection, fluid and electrolyte imbalance, surgery, trauma, drug use, exposure to nephrotoxins, anesthesia, or contrast agents should be sought.

It is important to evaluate prerenal and postrenal factors. Hydration and vascular volume should be assessed. The cardiac and circulatory status must be evaluated. A careful examination for flank tenderness, enlarged kidneys, distended bladder, and palpable enlarged prostate is essential, and when present these conditions suggest the possibility of acute renal failure. To exclude urethral obstruction, a Foley catheter should be temporarily inserted.

PATHOPHYSIOLOGY

Acute renal failure can follow prerenal, postrenal, and intrinsic renal pathology. Acute tubular necrosis (ATN), also known as vasomotor nephropathy, is one of the common intrinsic causes of acute renal failure which is characterized by necrosis of the glomerular tubular epithelial cells. Urine volume typically decreases rapidly (oliguric phase) to oliguria and rarely anuria (less than 100 ml per day). The serum creatinine and BUN levels rise. In some cases, however, these changes may occur despite the production of normal urine volume. ATN usually persists for 7 to 21 days but may be irreversible. Recovery is accompanied by an increasing urine volume (diuretic phase).

Prerenal azotemia is the result of a decrease in renal blood flow; effective renal perfusion pressure decreases; and vasoconstriction follows. There is an increase in tubular reabsorption of sodium and water. The BUN shows a disproportionate increase compared to creatinine. The patient becomes oliguric with a concentrated urine and a low urinary sodium level, which signifies intact tubular function. The BUN level will be high, and the creatinine level will be near normal. Correcting the underlying cause reverses the renal dysfunction. If not treated promptly, prerenal azotemia may result in the development of acute tubular necrosis.

Several conditions can decrease renal blood flow, for example, blood loss, vigorous diuretic therapy, gastrointestinal losses (vomiting or diarrhea), and interstitial fluid loss (burns, pancreatitis, peritonitis, and soft-tissue injury). Decreased cardiac output, as in congestive heart failure, cardiogenic shock, acute myocardial infarction, and pericardial effusion with or without tamponade, can also decrease renal flow. Peripheral pooling of blood with capillary bed vasodilatation in gram-negative sepsis, vasodilator drug therapy, anaphylaxis, and exogenous toxins can also reduce renal blood flow.

Liver disease such as acute fulminant hepatitis and cirrhosis can produce prerenal azotemia. If these patients are treated vigorously with diuresis, the hepatorenal syndrome may develop. This syndrome may also develop following massive gastrointestinal bleeding or overly aggressive paracentesis.

Postrenal azotemia can also follow postrenal obstruction, occurring from the pelvis of the kidney to the external uretheral meatus, either intrinsic or extrinsic to the lumen (Table 98–1). Bladder neck or external meatal obstruction is the most common in children. Ureteral obstruction due to nephrolithiasis, pelvic malignancy with paravertebral involvement, postoperative adhesions, and, rarely, fibrosis (retroperitoneal fibrosis due to methergiside therapy) is more frequent in middle-aged persons. Postrenal etiologies of acute renal failure should always be among the first causes considered. They are easily detected and corrected. Correcting the underlying problem will usually correct the abnormal renal function.

Intrinsic renal pathology may be due to changes in the vascular, glomerular, interstitial, or tubular elements or in all of these combined. If effective renal perfusion is decreased, ischemic tubular necrosis will occur. Renal tubules and the medulla receive the least amount of blood supply and hence oxygen despite the high workload of the tubular cells. Reduced perfusion significantly compromises renal function. Acute tubular necrosis is most frequently seen in patients who have undergone major surgery or have major trauma, sepsis, or toxemia.

Causes of intrinsic renal disease include exogenous and endogenous nephrotoxins, interstitial nephritis, papillary necrosis, other parenchymal and renal vascular disease. Exogenous nephrotoxins such as antibiotics are among the most common causes. High doses of aminoglycosides and cephalosporins can cause direct tubular damage. Amphotericin-B, usually prescribed in systemic fungal infection, can cause similar damage. Sulphonamides can cause crystalluria and associated acute renal failure. Chemotherapeutic agents can cause direct injury to the tubules or produce a secondary hyperuricemic nephropathy due to the necrosis of the tumor mass. Acute renal failure can follow the intravenous injection of contrast agents for procedures such as pyelography, cardiac catheterization, cerebral angiography and aortography. Predisposing factors are hypovolemia, preexisting renal impairment, diabetes mellitus, and multiple myeloma. Anesthetic agents (methoxyflurane), ethylene glycol (antifreeze), organic solvents (carbon tetrachloride), heavy metals (cisplatin, mercury, lead, cadmium, and gold), and radiation to the kidneys can also be nephrotoxic.

Endogenous nephrotoxins found in some systemic diseases, may cause acute renal failure by obstructing the renal tubules and ducts with epithelial debris of excretory products such as crystals. They can also cause tubular necrosis and interstitial inflammation. Important causes are myoglobinuria following rhabdomyolysis, and hemoglobinuria as seen after a posttransfusion reaction. Uric acid nephropathy can occur due to primary gout or drug-induced secondary hyperuricemia. Hypercalcemia which initially causes dehydration and prerenal azotemia may progress to hypercalciuric renal failure. Multiple myeloma (light- or heavy-chain disease) may result in a precipitation of Bence Jones protein in the distal nephrons where the urine is acidic.

Interstitial nephritis is often caused by a drug-induced hypersensitivity reaction which is associated with edema, cellular infiltration, and, not uncommonly, eosinophils in the urine. Here the onset of renal failure is usually slow, but it may be acute, severe, and irreversi-

---

TABLE 98–1.

Causes of Postrenal Obstruction

Blood Clots
Stones
Sloughed papillae
Fungus balls
Prostatic hypertrophy or malignancy
Neuropathy
Strictures
Phemosis
Malignancy
Retroperitoneal fibrosis
Inadvertent ligation

ble. Antibiotics such as the penicillins, cephalosporins, sulfonamides, and rifampin are well-known causes of interstitial nephritis. Other drugs such as diuretics, allopurinol, phenylbutazone, phenytoin, phenindione, and nonsteroidal anti-inflammatory drugs are also recognized causes.

Papillary necrosis usually follows acute pyelonephritis, obstructive uropathy, diabetes mellitus, and rarely sickle cell (trait or disease) nephropathy or tuberculosis. Back pain, flank tenderness, fever, oliguria, and gastrointestinal symptoms are common. Ischemia and infarction of the papillae along with cellular infiltration and inflammation of the cortex and the medulla are seen.

Renal parenchymal diseases such as post-streptococcal glomerulonephritis, systemic lupus erythematosis, Goodpasture's syndrome, and bacterial endocarditis can also cause acute renal failure. These syndromes are usually associated with the pathologic findings of rapidly progressive glomerulonephritis. This renal failure is almost invariably irreversible.

Vascular diseases such as renal artery occlusion (thrombotic or embolic) of a single functioning kidney, aortic dissection with renal involvement, vasculitis (polyarteritis, Wegener's granulomatosis) can cause acute renal failure. Malignant hypertension with its necrotizing arteritis can also cause renal failure. Acute cortical necrosis can occur in toxemia of pregnancy and septic abortion. Coagulopathies such as thrombotic thrombocytopenic purpura and hemolytic uremic syndrome can result in occlusion of the microcapillaries. Vascular diseases should be considered in all age groups with acute renal failure. Except for the hemolytic uremic syndrome, they are usually irreversible.

CLINICAL–PATHOLOGIC CORRELATIONS

Clinical findings do not correlate well with pathologic changes in the kidney. For example in pre- and postrenal diseases there is no microscopic histopathology. In intrinsic renal disease, micropuncture studies show significant cellular edema and debris, which, if prolonged, may produce necrosis.

DIFFERENTIAL DIAGNOSIS

With a thorough history and bedside examination, a presumptive diagnosis of acute renal failure can be made and the process can be ascribed to a prerenal, postrenal, or intrinsic mechanism. The urinalysis, biochemical and radiologic studies are useful to document and support the diagnosis. A flow sheet documenting the clinical events, fluid balance, daily blood chemistry values, and body weight is needed to assess the course of the disease.

DIAGNOSIS

The urine should be examined by the physician in every case of acute renal failure. The presence of proteinuria, detected with a dip stick or sulfosalicylic acid, suggests an underlying primary renal disease, such as glomerulonephritis. A positive hematest suggests the presence of red cells, hemoglobin, or myoglobin. In cases of myoglobinuria occurring with rhabdomyolysis, the supernatant of centrifuged urine is brownish-red due to the heme pigments, but the urine contains no red cells and the serum hemoglobin is negative. Staining the sediment will reveal myoglobin casts. Cellular casts, seen in acute tubular necrosis and, at times, in severe vasculitis are broad, reddish-brown, and granular. Coarse granular casts are seen in acute glomerulonephritis. Red cell casts are also seen in acute glomerular disease (Table 98–2).

The typical values for tubular function studies are listed in Table 98–3. In prerenal conditions such as prerenal azotemia, the urine osmolality and creatinine concentration are high due to the concentrated urine; the urinary sodium level is low, denoting intact tubular function. In renal and postrenal conditions such as acute tubular necrosis with tubular damage, however, the findings are opposite (i.e., the urine osmolality and creatinine level are low and the sodium level high) indicating damaged tubules that are unable to conserve sodium and water.

Fractional excretion is a useful diagnostic test to differentiate intrinsic renal disease from prerenal azotemia by quantitating the fraction of plasma sodium filtered at the glomerulus

TABLE 98–2.
Clinical Findings in Some Instrinsic Renal Pathologic Conditions That Cause Acute Renal Failure

DISORDER	URINE SEDIMENT	PROTEINURIA	FEna %	HYPERTENSION	MISCELLANEOUS FINDINGS
Glomerlonephritis	RBC.LIPD.OFB casts:RBC. pigmented.WBC.	2–4 +	<1	Unusual in RPGN* Common in AGN*	Nephrotic syndrome; signs of systemic disease
Vasculitis	Scant if pre-glomerular: RBC and RBC casts	2–4 +	V	Common	Multisystem disease; drug allergy; HAA- post-renal aneurysms
Interstitial nephritis	RBC.WBC.EOS- casts:RTE.WBC.	1–2 +	>3	Unusual pyelonephritis	Fever; rash; eosinophilia; drug allergy
Tubules (acute tubular necrosis)	RTE.casts:RTE. pigmented FGC.CGC.	1–2 +	>3	No	Hypotension; sepsis; nephrotoxins.

* RPGN = rapidly progressive glomerulonephritis; AGN = acute glomerulonephritis.

TABLE 98–3.
Tubular Function Values Differentiating Prerenal from Renal and Postrenal Changes

URINE STUDIES	PRERENAL CHANGES	RENAL/POSTRENAL CHANGES
Osmolality* (mOsm)	> 500	< 350
Sodium level† (mEq/L)	< 20	> 40
Fractional excretion‡ of sodium (%)	< 1	> 1.5

* Ten percent of prerenal patients have value < 350 mOsm; 10% of renal patients have value > 500 mOsm.

† Thirty-five percent of prerenal patients have 20–40 mEq/L, 30% of renal/postrenal patients have < 20 mEq/L.

$$\ddagger \ FEN_a = \frac{U_{Na}/P_{Na}}{U_{Cr}/P_{Cr}} \times 100\%$$

where U_{Na} = sodium level in urine and P_{Na} = sodium level in plasma; U_{Cr} = creatinine level in urine and P_{Cr} = creatinine level in plasma.

that escapes tubular reabsorption and thus excreted (Table 98–1). In obstructive uropathy, the indices are the same as acute tubular necrosis, but the urinary sediment findings differ. In acute renal failure resulting from acute glomerulonephritis, the urinary sodium level is low and there is proteinuria, casts in the urine, and red cells and granular casts in the sediment.

The urine volume is usually less than 200 ml per day in patients with obstructive uropathy, renal arterial occlusive disease, cresentic glomerulonephritis, and cortical necrosis. Fluctuations in the urine volume suggest obstructive uropathy.

The BUN-to-creatinine ratio is about 15:1 in normal subjects. In prerenal azotemia it is increased due to the preferential tubular reabsorption of urea compared to creatinine during decreased perfusion and urine flow. Rapid increases in the serum potassium, phosphorus, and creatinine levels suggest hypercatabolism, such as in rhabdomyolysis. Serum uric acid and calcium levels also change rapidly in hypercatabolic states. Serologic markers such as complement and antibodies should be checked in suspected cases of acute renal failure associated with acute glomerulonephritis or vasculitis.

Plain x-ray films of the abdomen may show the size and shape of the kidneys, ureters, and bladder, but tomograms are more accurate and, therefore, more useful. The kidneys are usually small in chronic renal failure compared to normal size or large in acute tubular necrosis.

Asymmetric kidneys suggest renal artery stenosis or a contracted kidney due to chronic pyelonephritis. Enlarged kidneys may be due to a hydronephrosis caused by obstruction or reflex nephropathy. There is no reason for an intravenous pyelogram in suspected cases of acute renal failure because the excreted contrast agent, as a toxin, may cause further damage to the tubules. It has been replaced by the sonogram, which can usually detect kidney enlargement, hydronephrosis, caliectasis, and stones more accurately. Sonography is a noninvasive, safe procedure. It can also be helpful in differentiating acute tubular necrosis from renal transplant rejection.

A radionuclide renal scan and renogram are useful in detecting perfusion and excretory defects. For example, technetium-labeled DPTA can detect altered renal blood flow and can assess renal perfusion as well as excretion. In acute tubular necrosis the ^{99m}Tc-DPTA is slowly and diffusely taken up to gradually show a dense mass. In primary parenchymal renal disease, the uptake is patchy or occasionally absent. Indications for the use of a radioactive hippurate renogram include the assessment of (1) symmetry of renal function in the presence of unilateral or bilateral renal disease, (2) patients with vascular hypertension, (3) urinary tract drainage, (4) the effect of urinary tract obstruction on renal function, and (5) the function of a transplanted kidney.

Cystoscopy and retrograde studies are performed if the suspicion of obstruction is high and to place a stent or a catheter to relieve an obstruction. Renal biopsy is indicated in cases of acute renal failure associated with systemic causes where the results will have an important therapeutic implication. For example, a biopsy is useful in acute renal failure due to systemic lupus erythematosis, Wegener's granulomatosis, Goodpasture's syndrome, and acute interstitial nephritis. Biopsy in acute tubular necrosis is indicated when there is no recovery of function over several weeks and irreversibility is a concern.

PRINCIPLES OF PREVENTION AND THERAPY

Patients with preexisting renal disease and those prone to develop prerenal azotemia should be identified. They should be adequately hydrated or, if indicated, given a diuretic that acts on the loop of Henle to potentially reduce the incidence of acute tubular necrosis. Prophylactic saluretic treatment will help to avoid nephrotoxicity when cytotoxic or nephrotoxic drugs are administered. Bicarbonate infusion may be of added benefit under those conditions. Saluretic therapy is useful in rhabdomyolysis or a hemolytic crisis due to a blood-transfusion reaction.

Nephrotoxic antibiotics such as aminoglycosides and nonsteroidal anti-inflammatory drugs should be avoided, if possible, in patients with reduced renal function. In cases where they must be given, the renal chemistry values should be monitored. The dosage of nephrotoxic drugs should be adjusted according to the renal function, and, if possible, the blood levels of the drug monitored. Osmotic therapy has been helpful in preventing complications in high-risk patients when given an hour or two before the onset of an anticipated renal injury.

Prompt investigation is necessary to diagnose and relieve obstructive uropathy in order to preserve renal function and prevent further renal deterioration. Simultaneous treatment of associated sepsis and urinary tract infection is important. Renal failure associated with obstruction and infection is a life-threatening problem. Fluid and electrolyte imbalance are common, particularly in partial obstruction of the urinary tract.

Volume depletion (dehydration) should be treated promptly. Fluid and electrolyte replacement should match the estimated deficit and the ongoing losses. Half of the estimated loss should be replaced over the first 24 hours. Fluid replacement should be monitored closely, and the patient should be examined frequently for signs or symptoms of hyper- or hypovolemia. Invasive monitoring, with central venous pressure and Swan-Ganz catheter, may be required in critically ill patients to avoid fluid overload.

The extracellular fluid volume, body weight, and fluid balance should be assessed daily, and fluid replacement should match the total output and insensible loss. If the patient is anuric and is in a euvolemic state, the daily fluid replacement should meet the daily measured loss and 10 ml/kg of body weight for the insensible loss. Sodium intake should be restricted to 2 gm/day for those who do not require dialysis. Hyponatremia is a good index of excessive fluid administration. In cases of septic shock, congestive heart failure, and hypoprotenemia, it may be necessary to accept anasarca in order to maintain the intravascular volume.

Hyperkalemia can become a serious problem within a few hours after the onset of acute renal failure. It is frequently seen in cases of rhabdomyolysis, burns, crush injury, auto accident trauma, and following major surgery. If the serum potassium level is high, immediate therapy should be instituted with drugs such as intravenous bicarbonate infusion, insulin and dextrose infusion, exchange resins orally or rectally, and dialysis.

Metabolic acidosis is a consequence of renal failure. Treatment with sodium bicarbonate is indicated when the arterial blood pH is less than 7.25 or the serum bicarbonate level is less than 12 mEq/L. Treatment should be given until the level reaches 16 mEq/L. Under such conditions, dialysis should be started as soon as possible.

Hyperphosphatemia occurs in all patients with renal failure due to the decreased renal clearance. It may be severe in cases of burns, muscle necrosis, and myolysis. Phosphate binders are given orally to bind the phosphate in the gut. Aluminum or calcium binders should be used instead of the magnesium derivatives to prevent magnesium intoxication.

Mild hypocalcemia is not uncommon, is not a major problem, and is usually asymptomatic. It can, however, become a major problem if the metabolic acidosis is corrected too rapidly. Rapid alkalinization can acutely worsen hypocalcemia and may precipitate tetany or seizures.

Hypermagnesemia is not a major problem in acute renal failure. Magnesium-containing antacids should not be given. Hyperuricemia occurs in acute renal failure due to the kidneys' inability to clear uric acid. It is usually not a problem.

The diet of patients with acute renal failure should be near normal with adequate calories and protein. These patients need 2000 calories to 3000 calories and 1 gm of protein per kg of body weight each day. Adequate nutrition prevents delayed wound healing and reduces the risk of infection. Nonessential drugs should be stopped, and essential drug administration should be kept to the minimum. Dosage of all the medicines requiring renal metabolism or excretion should be adjusted and reduced according to the renal function. When antibiotics are given, the nephrotoxic drugs should be avoided or given with caution in reduced doses based on renal function.

The indications for dialysis include hypervolemia, electrolyte imbalance, rapidly rising BUN and creatinine levels, congestive heart failure, pulmonary edema, hyperkalemia, acidosis, hyponatremia, asterixis, muscle twitching, jerks, somnolence, seizures, pericarditis, bleeding diathesis, or nausea and vomiting. The BUN level should be kept under 80 mgs%, and serum creatinine level should be kept under 8.0 mg/dl. Hemodialysis is chosen more often than peritoneal dialysis in the treatment of acute renal failure. Catheters can be inserted into the subclavian or femoral veins for temporary access.

Peritoneal dialysis is done by placing a temporary or permanent catheter (Tenchkoff catheter) in the abdominal cavity under local anesthesia. This modality is useful in those who have a low catabolic rate, are in circula-

tory collapse, or have an unstable cardiac condition. A recent abdominal operation precludes using this procedure. It is simple and has little risk. Peritoneal dialysis helps to remove the excess extracellular fluid without precipitating hypotensive episodes. It is very useful in patients who have suffered a recent episode of myocardial infarction or congestive heart failure.

Secondary infection is a frequent complication of acute renal failure. To avoid sepsis, indwelling catheters should be removed as soon as possible. Prophylactic antibiotic therapy should be avoided because such treatments predispose to secondary fungal and nosocomial infections. Antibiotic treatment should be specific and based on a bacterial culture and sensitivity study.

Gastrointestinal bleeding is a common complication following the onset of acute renal failure. Antacids may be given as prophylaxis, although magnesium-containing antacids should be avoided due to the reduced renal clearance of magnesium. If cimetidine is used, the dose must be reduced. Frequent dialysis appears to help prevent bleeding diathesis and platelet dysfunction.

If the patient has a strong history of drug-induced interstitial nephritis, corticosteroid therapy may reverse the damage. The dose of the steroid should be reduced rapidly as recovery progresses.

Recovery of renal function depends on several factors. The most important are the severity of the renal injury, the age of the patient, and the underlying renal disease. Acute renal failure following a coronary bypass, any other major surgery, trauma, or sepsis carries a high mortality and morbidity rate, about 40% to 80% respectively. Nonoliguric acute renal failure has the lowest morbidity and mortality. Sepsis, bleeding, hepatic decompensation, and congestive heart failure are also high-risk factors for increased mortality and morbidity.

REFERENCES

Berkseth RO, Kjellstrand CM: Radiologic contrast induced nephropathy. *Med Clin North Am* 1984; 68:351–370. *Comprehensive discussion of this complication.*

Brenner BM, Lazsarus JM: Nature of cellular insult in acute renal failure in *Acute Renal Failure*, Philadelphia, WB Saunders Co, 1983. *A discussion of the pathophysiology.*

Brenner BM, Rector FC Jr (eds): *The Kidney*, ed 3. Acute renal failure and pathogenesis of renal diseases, Philadelphia, WB Saunders Co., 1986. *An up-to-date discussion.*

Hamburger J, Crosnier J, Grunfeld JP: Acute renal failure; pathogenesis, diagnosis and treatment in *Advances in Nephrology*, Year Book Medical Publishers, 1981. *A well-referenced discussion of all aspects of the process.*

Massey SG, Glascock RJ (eds): *Textbook of Nephrology*, Management of uremic state, Baltimore, Williams & Wilkins, 1983, *An in-depth discussion of therapy.*

Shapiro JI, Schrier RW: General aspects of acute renal failure. Paper presented at the First National Acute Renal Failure Symposium. Pittsburgh, November 1984. *An overview.*

Welton A: Antibiotic pharmacokinetics and clinical application in renal insufficiency. *Med Clin North Am* 1982; 66:267–381. *Discusses the required antibiotic modifications in renal failure.*

99 CHRONIC RENAL FAILURE

H. Allan Feller, M.D.

Chronic renal failure implies a reduction in the number of functioning nephrons. The onset is usually insidious with progression over several months to years, but a few patients have an abrupt onset over a period of several weeks. As a result, by-products of protein and amino acid metabolism accumulate and anion-gap metabolic acidosis occurs secondary to retention of phosphates, sulfates, and other organic acids as well as a decrease in the translocation of total hydrogen ions into the tubular lumen. As function declines, early renal insufficiency is not symptomatic in a large number of individuals unless there are major changes in vascular volume or alterations of other metabolic or protein balance. Azotemia refers to an elevation in BUN without symptoms. Uremia refers to the symptoms, signs, and findings of advanced renal failure. Dependent on the geographic area of the world, 80 to 100 persons per million population each year will develop end-stage renal disease and become candidates for dialysis or transplantation. The normal glomerular filtration rate (GFR) is 100 to 120 ml/minute. Dialysis is necessary when the (GFR) falls below 5 ml/minute for the nondiabetic patient or below 10 ml/minute for the diabetic patient. The causes of renal failure are listed in Table 99–1.

CLINICAL SIGNS AND SYMPTOMS

As the GFR falls below 25 ml/minute, the symptoms of chronic renal failure occur with not all patients developing all symptoms. In fact many patients remain remarkably asymptomatic with the GFR in the 10-ml/minute range. During this period of declining function, a gradual ammoniacal or metallic taste develops along with mild anorexia and nausea. As function worsens, intermittent, sudden episodes of emesis and singultus plague the individual. If the person is a child, impaired growth and development can be observed. Fatigue is a progressive problem that worsens as the renal function declines. The physician may be informed about sleep disturbances in the form of insomnia or restlessness. At a GFR of 10 to 15 ml/minute, calf and other muscle cramps evolve along with fascicular twitching. The skin is noted to be sallow, and pruritus may lead to excoriations of the skin. Ecchymoses and capillary oozing from the gums and nose may rarely be the presenting clinical picture. The patient or the patient's relatives may note impaired mentation that interferes with employment or other activities. Hypertension is a frequent management problem at any phase of chronic renal

TABLE 99–1.
Causes of Chronic Renal Failure

CAUSES	PERCENTAGE OF PATIENTS (%)*
Diabetes mellitus	30
Nephrosclerosis	22
Glomerulonephritis	17
Polycystic kidney disease	6
Interstitial nephritis	6
Other	19
Obstruction	
Hereditary nephritis	
Collagen vascular disease	
Congenital abnormalities	
Nephrotoxins	
Multiple myeloma	
Amyloidosis	

* Ohio Valley Renal Disease Network, Annual Report, 1984.

failure. In addition uremia affects multiple other organ systems, some of which are depicted in Table 99–2. Although some forms of chronic renal failure may be retarded or decelerated by treatment, many cases are not preventable and are irreversible.

Some of the more severe complications of uremia are shown in Table 99–3. Salt and water imbalances can cause severe worsening of the renal insufficiency. A few conditions, such as polycystic kidneys, medullary cystic disease, and interstitial nephritis, may lead to salt and water loss, which results in volume contraction and diminished renal function because of inadequate renal perfusion. In other cases, gastrointestinal or diuretic-induced hypovolemia may worsen the renal insufficiency and require rehydration. The term salt-losing nephritis is used when sodium conservation is severely impaired. In general, however, the patient handles moderate sodium loads well until advanced renal failure when the capacity of the kidney to excrete sodium falls below intake. In this situation, volume overload and edema appear, dyspnea develops, and hypertension may worsen. Generally, potassium balance is well regulated until the GFR falls below 5 to 10 ml/minute. Certain drugs such as spironolactone, triamterene, and amiloride may cause life-threatening hyperkalemia. For this reason, these preparations should be avoided in patients with any degree of renal insufficiency. Acidosis also leads to hyperkalemia. For every 0.1 unit change in pH, there may be a recipro-

cal change in serum potassium concentration of about 0.6 mEq/L. Hyperkalemia in the absence of excessive intake of potassium, acidosis, or medications may be associated with hyporeninemic hypoaldosteronism with reduced serum levels of renin and aldosterone. This abnormality may be related to interstitial or microvascular damage leading to decreased renin and aldosterone production and hence defective tubular secretion of potassium. Frequently these patients have diabetes mellitus, interstitial nephritis, or nephrosclerosis. The hyperkalemia responds to treatment with fludrocortisone acetate or sometimes to potassium-wasting diuretics.

The hypertension may be related to volume expansion in most cases (85%–90%) or may be renin mediated in a small percentage (10%–15%). In either case poor control can result in a malignant phase that is associated with a rapid decline in renal function. In the past, bilateral nephrectomy was a common treatment, but modern antihypertensive therapy has almost obviated this type of surgery.

In some uremic patients uremic pericarditis occurs at a point in the progress of the disease when dialysis treatment is about to or has already begun. Uremic pericarditis may be very painful and can cause pleuritic substernal chest pain. In addition, it may be associated with fever. No underlying pathogenic mechanism has been incriminated. A friction rub is heard in at least 85% of the cases. The fibrinous and hemorrhagic effusion may produce tamponade,

Clinical–Pathologic Correlations of Chronic Renal Failure

CLINICAL FINDINGS	PATHOLOGIC FINDINGS
METABOLIC ABNORMALITIES	
Carbohydrates Glucose intolerance in > 50% of patients Lipids	Peripheral insulin antagonism at tissue level Decreased insulin binding
Type IV hyperlipoproteinemia	Increased synthesis or decreased removal of triglyceride Defective lipoprotein lipase, elevated VLDL and LDL, decreased HDL
Nutrition Failure to gain weight	Negative nitrogen balance Uremic plasma inhibitors of growth
ENDOCRINE ABNORMALITIES	
Thyroid Most patients euthyroid	T_4 level normal or decreased T_3 level decreased TSH level normal or increased
SEXUAL DYSFUNCTION	

Females
  Amenorrhea, infertility
  Decreased libido
	Plasma estradiol and progesterone levels normal
	FSH level normal or increased
	Prolactin levels increased
	Absence of increase in LH after estradiol stimulation

Males Gynecomastia, testicular atrophy, azospermia, impotence, decreased libido	Testosterone level low Leydig's cell dysfunction Prolactin level increased LH level increased in response to low testosterone level
PARATHYROID GLAND HYPERPLASIA AND DECLINING LEVELS OF ACTIVE VITAMIN D	

Osteodystrophy
  Bone pain
  Subperiosteal resorption
  Fractures
Metastatic calcification in eyes, arteries, lungs, heart, skeletal muscle, skin, and around joints
Osteosclerosis
	Kidneys unable to excrete phosphorus
	Kidneys unable to manufacture 1,25-$(OH)_2$-vitamin D, decreased calcium absorption by gut
	Increased levels of parathyroid hormone

HEMATOLOGIC DISORDERS	
Anemia—Normocytic, normochronic	Decreased erythropoietin production Shortened RBC survival Hemolysis Uremic inhibitors of RBC function Iron and folic acid deficiency
Qualitative platelet defects Prolonged bleeding time	Factor III deficiency Abnormal processing of Factor VIII and von Willebrand factor Capillary fragility
Hypersplenism	
NEUROLOGIC DISORDERS	
Peripheral neuropathy Restless leg syndrome Hypalgesia of toes and sometimes fingers Sleep disturbances Somnolence Seizures Coma Asterixis, myoclonus	Nerve conduction velocities diminished by unknown toxin causing nerve demyelination Other specific causes unknown

TABLE 99–3.
Life-Threatening Complications of Uremia

COMPLICATIONS	RESULT	TREATMENT
Hypovolemia	Postural hypotension Dehydration Tachycardia	Rehydrate to attain normovolemia
Hypervolemia	Dyspnea and rales Edema Cardiomegaly S$_3$ gallop	Control hypervolemia with diuretics and sodium restriction Digitalis administration
Hyperkalemia	Arrythmia and death	Administration of sodium bicarbonate, Glucose + insulin, calcium, potassium exchange resins Dialysis
Severe hypertension	Seizures Coma Death	Antihypertensive agents such as nitroprusside IV and volume reduction by diuretics or dialysis
Pericarditis with tamponade	Dyspnea Hypotension Paradoxical pulse Death	Nonsteroidal anti-inflammatory agents Intensive dialysis Pericardiocentesis with steroid irrigations Anterior pericardiectomy
Profound anemia HCT < 15%	Weakness Dyspnea Chest pain	Transfusion of packed cells Androgens
Severe metabolic acidosis	Kussmaul's breathing Hypotension	Alkalinization with sodium bicarbonate Dialysis

which is a true medical emergency. Coronary artery disease is a slowly progressive complication producing angina and myocardial infarction. Hyperlipoproteinemia may be linked to the arteriosclerotic heart disease, which is five times more common in the dialysis patient than the general population.

Renal osteodystrophy is a broad complex of skeletal abnormalities that results from disturbed calcium and phosphorus metabolism and consists of *osteitis fibrosa cystica, osteomalacia,* and *osteosclerosis.* Osteomalacia, or inadequate mineralization of bone, is generally associated with osteitis fibrosa cystica. The bone lesion in osteitis fibrosa cystica, due to secondary hyperparathyroidism, has increased numbers of osteoblasts and osteoclasts, increased layers of collagen, and fibrosis. The parathyroid hormone stimulates osteoclastic activity, resulting in the resorption of mineral and matrix along the trabecular surfaces of cortical bone. The parathyroid hormone is stimulated by hypocalcemia which results from an impaired renal conversion of 25-hydroxy-

vitamin D$_3$ to 1,25-dihydroxy-vitamin D$_3$ resulting in poor absorption of calcium from the gastrointestinal tract. Hyperphosphatemia, which occurs when advancing renal insufficiency prevents further phosphate excretion, and hypocalcemia result in an elevated level of parathyroid hormone, which is associated with skeletal changes (subperiosteal erosions), bone pain, and fractures. Changes in the bones are most frequently seen in roentgenograms of the hands, skull, and lateral clavicles. A peculiar proximal muscle myopathy, particularly of the lower extremities, may be disabling and lead to gait abnormalities. The exact pathogenesis of this myopathy remains unclear, but it may be related to the elevated parathyroid hormone levels.

Osteosclerosis, the result of bone redistribution and reformation, is frequently seen in roentgenograms as dense areas in the upper and lower margins of the vertebrae, producing the x-ray picture of the "rugger jersey spine." Acidosis adds to the dissolution of bone mineral buffers causing further osteomalacia.

When the product of the calcium and phosphorus concentrations exceeds 70 mg/dl, metastatic calcification can occur in the skin, arteries, sclera, joints, and occasionally the lungs and myocardial conduction system. Joint involvement may occur as a form of pseudogout, an acute monoarticular arthritis that more commonly affects the larger joints. Joint aspiration samples typically contain crystals of calcium pyrophosphate. Calcific periarthritis arises presumably from deposition of hydroxyapatite crystals in the periarticular tissues. Vascular calcifications may involve the intima of the aorta and large arteries or develop as medial calcification. Conjunctival calcifications are believed to be hydroxyapatite crystals beneath the epithelium.

Uremic neuropathy (Table 99—2) develops in patients when the GFR falls below 10 ml/minute. It cannot be distinguished from neuropathies associated with other metabolic diseases. It is usually a distal, symmetric, mixed polyneuropathy. Sensory manifestations occur first and may be followed by motor abnormalities in some patients. It may be progressive in spite of dialysis. Although the exact cause is unclear, it most probably is the result of one or multiple neurotoxins which cause axonal degeneration and segmental demyelination. Transplantation may lead to progressive improvement in nerve function but may take as long as a year. In some individuals with severe neuropathy at the time of renal transplantation, only partial amelioration can be expected.

DIFFERENTIAL DIAGNOSIS

The differentiation between acute and chronic renal failure is essential and sometimes difficult (Table 99–4). When the ratio of blood urea nitrogen (BUN) to serum creatinine level exceeds 10:1, the physician should consider a prerenal or extrarenal cause for this disparity (Table 99–5). In the case of decreased renal perfusion, the BUN is elevated because urea reabsorption depends on tubular urine flow. At a urine flow less than 2 ml/minute, the proportion of urea reabsorbed is increased. The rate of clearance of creatinine does not depend on urine flow.

DIAGNOSIS

It is mandatory to measure the BUN, creatinine, electrolytes, calcium, phosphorus, alkaline phosphatase, and hematocrit in the initial evaluation. A urinalysis can provide clues as to whether the process is acute, by virtue of the type of cells and casts in the sediment. Red blood cell casts are diagnostic of glomerulonephritis and therefore are of considerable diagnostic aid. The serum creatinine level provides a more precise measurement of renal function than does the BUN. The BUN is influenced by those factors reviewed in Table 99–5. However, small changes in serum creatinine are difficult to interpret. A more reliable and predictable measurement of GFR is the creatinine clearance based on a carefully timed urine collection, usually for 24 hours.

There are several other useful diagnostic maneuvers that may provide information. Renal ultrasound is a good noninvasive two-dimensional technique that provides accurate measurement of renal size and identification of hydronephrosis, masses, cysts, or obstructive uropathy. An abdominal "flat plate" (KUB—kidney, ureter, and bladder) x-ray may also reveal renal size or calculi but provides less anatomical data. Renal radionuclide imaging does

TABLE 99–4.
Differentiating Acute from Chronic Renal Failure

ACUTE	CHRONIC
Usually normal-sized kidneys	Small kidneys—KUB, ultrasound, or other x-ray techniques
No bone abnormalities	Renal osteodystrophy
Anemia uncommon	Anemia frequent
Recent evidence of normal renal function	History of progressive renal impairment
Sudden anuria or oliguria	Slow decline in urine output
Setting of sudden shock or trauma	

supply information about renal function in terms of isotope entry and clearance from each kidney. It also delivers an impression of renal size, or a disparity thereof, and whether obstruction is present. In a patient with any degree of moderate renal impairment, but especially in the diabetic patient, radiocontrast agents should be avoided because these may produce superimposed acute renal failure. In some cases, renal biopsy may be required to differentiate between acute and chronic renal failure. However, if the kidneys are abnormally small, the disease is not remediable, and biopsy is not indicated.

PRINCIPLES OF THERAPY

Treatment frequently is directed toward salt and water balance and prevention of hypervolemia and hypovolemia. Table 99–6 lists the conditions that should be considered when there is a decline in renal function. Diet should include 30 kcal/kg/day of high biologic grade protein. Recently the progression of the disease has been shown to be retarded with early restriction of protein intake to 0.6 gm/kg. Nitrogen-free amino acid analogue supplements are also of benefit but are not widely available nor very palatable. Dietary calcium needs are 1200 mg to 1500 mg per day. The anemia can frequently be improved with androgen administration. Administration of phosphorus binders such as oral aluminum hydroxide or calcium carbonate helps avoid the effects of secondary hyperparathyroidism. Normalization of the serum calcium with oral supplements of calcium and of the active form of vitamin D is also useful in reducing parathyroid hormone production. Occasionally the effects of renal osteodystrophy on the skeleton are so

TABLE 99–5.

Causes of a BUN-to-Creatinine Ratio of Greater than 10:1

GI bleeding with or without hypotension
Increased protein intake
Catabolic–anabolic states
   Infection—Catabolic event
   Steroid intake—Catabolic event
   Tetracycline intake—Anti-anabolic event
Decreased renal perfusion
   Dehydration
   Intravascular volume depletion
   Congestive heart failure

TABLE 99–6.

Reversible Factors Inducing Renal Function Deterioration

Decreased renal perfusion
   Volume depletion
   Congestive heart failure
   Shock
   Pericardial tamponade
Obstruction
Nephrotoxic drugs
Uncontrolled hypertension
Hypercalcemia
Hypokalemia prolonged
Hyperuricemia (> 15 mgm%)

calamitous that a subtotal parathyroidectomy is necessary. When absolutely required, nephrotoxic drugs may be used in reduced doses. Drugs that are primarily eliminated through renal mechanisms also require reduction of dosage and frequency of administration to avoid excessive accumulation in blood and tissue. When the GFR falls below 20 ml/minute, most patients require counseling and must make plans regarding dialysis and transplantation.

REFERENCES

Alfrey AC: Chronic renal failure: Manifestations and pathogenesis, in Schrier RW (ed): *Renal and Electrolyte Disorders*. Boston, Little, Brown & Co, 1976, pp 319–347. *Excellent discussion of pathophysiology of uremia.*

Brenner BM, Lazarus JM: Chronic renal failure, in Petersdorf R, Adams R, Braunwalt E, Isselbacher K, Wilson J (eds): *Harrison's Principles of Internal Medicine*, ed 9. New York, McGraw-Hill Book Co, 1980, pp 1299–1307. *In-depth coverage of some but not all aspects of renal failure.*

Coburn JW: Renal osteodystrophy. *Kidney Int* 1980; 17:677–693. *Clear presentation of renal osteodystrophy.*

Coburn JW: Renal osteodystrophy. *Adv Intern Med* 1984; 30:387–424. *Offers recent knowledge of renal osteodystrophy.*

Earle DP: Chronic renal insufficiency, in Earle DP, DelGreco FD, Levin ML, Quintanilla, AP (eds): *Manual of Clinical Nephrology.* Philadelphia, WB Saunders Co, 1982, pp 277–308. *Covers discussion of chronic renal insufficiency thoroughly.*

Klahr S, Buerkert J, Purkerson N: Role of dietary factors in the progression of chronic renal disease. *Kidney Int* 1983; 24:579–587. *Reasons for proper diet in retarding development of chronic renal failure.*

100 HYPERNEPHROMA

Gilbert L. Wergowske, M.D.

Renal cell carcinoma is a malignant tumor probably arising from the tubule cells of the kidney. Its appearance reminded premicroscopic anatomists of the adrenal gland, thus the name hypernephroma. Renal cell carcinoma comprises about 3% of malignancies in adults and is even less common in children. The tumor occurs in male patients twice as often as female and usually appears in the fifth to seventh decades of life. It is more common in urban dwellers, pipe and cigar smokers, male cigarette smokers exposed to cadmium, and after exposure to Thorotrast. Patients with polycystic kidney disease and von Hippel-Lindau disease have increased risk for renal cell carcinoma, and familial cases have been reported.

CLINICAL SIGNS AND SYMPTOMS

Because renal cell carcinoma is so protean in its manifestations, it has been called the internist's tumor. The "classic triad" of pain, hematuria, and flank mass appears in only 10% of cases and usually indicates advanced disease. Symptoms of metastatic disease are more frequent than pain and hematuria from the primary tumor. Weight loss, fever, night sweats, hypertension, and symptoms of hypercalcemia and paraneoplastic syndromes are common. The sudden appearance of a varicocele in a man over 50 years of age should raise suspicion.

Fever (18% of patients), hypertension (38%), cachexia (35%), and pallor may be present. A flank mass is present in about 25% of patients. Hepatosplenomegaly may indicate metastatic disease or an unexplained paraneoplastic syndrome of hepatic dysfunction, which is seen in 20% of patients. Weakness and mental status changes may be present as the result of hypercalcemia or neuromyopathy. In one case, acute delirium without a detectable cause was resolved with removal of the renal cell carcinoma. Extension of a tumor thrombus into the right atrium (in less than 10% of cases) may produce a heart murmur.

The prognosis for renal cell carcinoma depends primarily on the stage of disease at the time of diagnosis. Several staging systems are in use at present; their complexity prevents detailed discussion here. A simplified scheme for staging is presented in Table 100–1. Only 10% of untreated patients with distant metastases will survive 1 year. Between 25% and 30% of patients have distant metastases at the time of diagnosis. There are no studies of survival rates in patients with stage I disease (limited to the renal capsule) without intervention, but with

TABLE 100–1.
Staging and Prognosis of Renal Cell Carcinoma*

| | | SURVIVAL RATE WITH THERAPY† (% OF CASES) | |
| | | 2 YEARS | 5 YEARS |
STAGE	DESCRIPTION		
I	Tumor confined within renal capsule	100	60–82
II	Tumor invasion of perinephric fat but confined to Gerota's fascia	88	47–80
III	Involvement of regional lymph nodes and/or renal vein or vena cava‡	65	35–50
IV	Invasion of adjacent organs or distant metastasis	4–15	0

* Adapted from Siminovitch JMP, Montie JE, Straffon RA: Prognostic indicators in renal adenocarcinoma. *J Urol* 1983; 130: 20–23.
† Therapy varies with studies, but usually includes radical nephrectomy except in stage IV patients.
‡ Recent data suggest that renal vein and/or vena cava involvement implies a prognosis more like that of stage II than of stage III, especially when involvement is subdiaphragmatic.

surgical treatment the 5-year survival rate is 82%. Bilateral renal cell carcinoma does not have a worse prognosis unless the tumors are asynchronous.

PATHOPHYSIOLOGY

Renal cell carcinoma probably arises from proximal convoluted or distal collecting tubule cells. Metastases can be found throughout the body, but the most common sites are lung, liver, subcutaneous tissue, central nervous system, and bone.

The primary tumors vary greatly in size, gross appearance (though most are round), and the amount of hemorrhage and necrosis. Multiple cysts from resorption of necrotic areas appear among areas of yellow-brown soft tumor and fibrosis. Stippled or plaque-like areas of calcification may be present. A pseudocapsule of compressed fibrous tissue or renal parenchyma is common. The tumor may displace or invade the collecting system or Gerota's fascia or both, or extend into the renal vein as a thrombus, propagating as far as the right atrium. Local invasion of surrounding organs and muscles is fairly common for larger tumors.

Rounded or polygonal cells with abundant cytoplasm, called clear cells, are characteristic of renal cell carcinoma, although granular cells with eosinophilic cytoplasm and abundant mi-

tochondria sometimes predominate. Some tumors contain primarily spindle cells reminiscent of fibrosarcoma, a bad prognostic sign. Aneuploid and bizarre nuclear patterns also appear to worsen the prognosis. The cells may appear in sheets or trabecular arrangements, form alveoli, or, rarely, show papillary or tubular patterns.

Hematuria is present in 38% of patients with renal cell carcinoma. The erythrocyte sedimentation rate is elevated in 56%, often above 100 mm/hour. Either anemia (36%) or polycythemia (3.5%) may be present, but leukocyte and platelet counts remain normal. Liver transaminase and lactate dehydrogenase levels are abnormal in 14% of patients. The alkaline phosphatase level is elevated in 10% and, when accompanied by a prolonged prothrombin time and elevated haptoglobin levels, may indicate the hepatic dysfunction syndrome. Hypercalcemia complicates 5% of cases and usually does not respond to removal of the primary tumor. Renal cell carcinoma is responsible for about 30% of all amyloidosis associated with cancer. Amyloid protein (AA or AL type) may be seen with special stains in kidney, muscle, liver, and nerve tissue. The resulting nephropathy, neuropathy, or cardiomyopathy can be detected with appropriate paraclinical tests. Bence Jones proteinuria and an elevation of serum immunoglobulin levels have been reported in cases of renal cell carcinoma-associated amyloidosis. Renin levels may be elevated.

CLINICAL–PATHOLOGIC CORRELATIONS

Renal cell carcinoma is associated with many biologic derangements, few of which are well understood. A list of the common findings and possible explanations are given in Table 100–2. The diversity of metastatic sites precludes presenting an exhaustive list of the symptoms and signs in this chapter.

DIFFERENTIAL DIAGNOSIS

Combinations of pain, hematuria, and fever are seen with urinary tract infections, lithiasis, primary tumors other than renal cell carcinoma, and metastasis, but few of these conditions carry a worse prognosis. The other signs and symptoms listed above may represent almost any illness. The main problem of differential diagnosis in this cancer is not ruling out other

TABLE 100–2.
Clinical–Pathologic Correlations for Renal Cell Carcinoma*

CLINICAL FINDINGS	APPROXIMATE PREVALENCE (% OF CASES)	PATHOLOGIC FINDINGS
Pain (local)	41	Invasion of surrounding tissue or obstruction of urine flow
Hematuria	38	Invasion of blood vessels by tumor or necrosis of tumor
Flank mass	24	Large, palpable tumor mass
Varicocele	†	Obstruction of venous return
Weight loss	36	Common symptom for malignancy, related to parasitism of nutrients or decreased intake
Fever (night sweats)	18	Common symptom for malignancy, renal cell carcinoma is often associated with large areas of inflammation around the tumor
Hypertension	38	Possibly from increased renin production or segmental artery occlusion by tumor
Anemia	38	Bone marrow suppression, blood loss, hemolysis
Erythrocytosis	4	Increased production of erythropoietin by tumor
Increased erythrocyte sedimentation rate	56	Inflammation produced by tumor, immunoglobulin secretion
Hypercalcemia	6	Possible elaboration of PTH-like substance, bone metastasis
Abnormal liver function tests	14	Poorly understood, occurs with or without metastasis
Increased alkaline phosphatase level	10	Poorly understood, occurs with or without metastasis; may indicate bone metastasis
Hepatic dysfunction	20	Hepatosplenomegaly, prolonged prothrombin time, elevated alkaline phosphatase and haptoglobin levels; etiology unclear, occurs without metastasis; may be related to amyloidosis
Neuromyopathy	3	Probably from amyloidosis
Amyloidosis	2	Stimulation of plasmacytes by tumor (primary) or reaction to inflammation (secondary)

* Adapted from deKernion JB: Renal Tumors, in Walsh PC, Gittes RF, Perlmutter AD, Stamey TA (eds): *Campbell's Urology*, ed 5. Philadelphia, WB Saunders Co, 1986, p 1310; and Chisholm GD: Nephrogenic ridge tumors and their syndromes. *Ann NY Acad Sci* 1974; 230: 405.
† No published data.

diseases, but remembering to look for renal cell carcinoma.

DIAGNOSIS

The various laboratory abnormalities seen with renal cell carcinoma were discussed under Pathophysiology. No single test is pathognomonic, so the synthesis of data from the history, physical examination, and laboratory studies is crucial.

Infusion pyelography with nephrotomography usually is the primary diagnostic procedure. Ultrasound studies and percutaneous cyst puncture may improve the accuracy of the diagnosis in cystic lesions. The presence of blood in a cyst should prompt further investigation. Radionuclide scans have a limited role; uniform distribution of the isotope in the area of the suspected renal mass usually indicates absence of tumor.

Renal arteriography, long the final diagnostic step, is being replaced by computerized tomography (CT scan). A CT scan is superior in accuracy and cost-effectiveness and reveals smaller tumors, renal vein (91% accuracy) and vena cava (97%) involvement, perirenal extension (79%), nodal metastasis (87%), and invasion of adjacent organs (96%) not seen with arteriography. Magnetic resonance imaging may eventually supplant CT scanning as the procedure of choice. Ultrasound studies are reliable in detecting renal vein and vena cava involvement and produce fewer complications than inferior venacavography. Echocardiography reliably documents extension to the heart.

PRINCIPLES OF PREVENTION AND THERAPY

No preventive efforts have been shown to be effective. However, elimination of cigar and pipe smoking and caution about exposure to cadmium may reduce risks for renal cell carcinoma.

Surgery is the only effective treatment for primary renal cell carcinoma. Complete excision of the tumor and the involved adjacent organs is essential; radical nephrectomy is the procedure most often used. Partial excision does not improve survival. A regional lymphadenectomy is often also done. It certainly adds valuable information for staging, but its therapeutic value is not certain. Preoperative occlusion of the renal artery may be of value for large vascular tumors. Surgical treatment does not appear to improve survival if a distant metastasis is present. Regression of a metastasis after removal of the primary tumor has been reported with renal cell carcinoma, but remains rare. Palliative nephrectomy should be reserved for control of severe symptoms or hemorrhage or for a select group of otherwise healthy patients in whom a solitary metastasis can also be excised.

Radiotherapy may reduce the size of a large tumor preoperatively, but its only proven value is in palliative treatment of skeletal metastasis. Local palliation may be achieved with arterial implantation of radioactive "seeds."

Chemotherapy and hormonal manipulation have not been effective. Medroxyprogesterone may be of value when no other therapy is available.

Active specific immunotherapy, adoptive immunotherapy, and interferons have shown some promise in early studies but remain investigative treatments.

The course of the disease with treatment depends on the stage at time of diagnosis (Table 100–1). Involvement of the renal vein and inferior vena cava appears to convey a more favorable prognosis than the earlier staging systems indicated. This may be due to improvements in diagnostic and surgical technique.

REFERENCES

Dalakas MC, Fujihara S, Askansas V, Engel WK, Glenner GG: Nature of amyloid deposits in hypernephroma. Immunocytochemical studies in 2 cases associated with amyloid polyneuropathy. *Am J Pathol* 1984; 116:447–454. *A discussion of systemic amyloidosis in association with renal cell carcinoma.*

deKernion JB: Renal tumors, in Walsh PC, Gittes RF,

Perlmutter AD, Stamey TA (eds): *Campbell's Urology*, ed 5. Philadelphia, WB Saunders Co, 1986, pp 1305–1332. *A well-written textbook chapter discussing all features of the disease except the use of MRI in diagnosis.*

Ehman RL, Wesbey GE, Moon KL et al: Enhanced MRI of tumors utilizing a new nitroxyl spin label contrast agent. *Magnetic Resonance Imaging* 1985; 3:89–97. *Reports of enhanced tumor imaging with use of a paramagnetic contrast agent (human renal cell carcinoma transplanted to rats).*

Goldman A, Parmeswaran R, Kotler MN, Hartman J: Renal cell carcinoma and right atrial tumor diagnosed by echocardiography. *Am Heart J* 1985; 110:183–186. *A brief but impressive demonstration of the value of echocardiography with references to more exhaustive works.*

Lack EE, Cassady Jr, Sallan SE: Renal cell carcinoma in childhood and adolescence: A clinical and pathological study of 17 cases. *J Urol* 1985; 133:822–828. *A complete review of renal cell carcinoma in childhood.*

Marshall FP, Reitz BA, Diamond DA: A new technique for management of renal cell carcinoma involving the right atrium: Hypothermia and cardiac arrest. *J Urol* 1984; 131:103–107. *Describes a surgical technique for removing a tumor involving the right atrium.*

Patel NP, Lavengood RW: Renal cell carcinoma: Natural history and results of treatment. *J Urol* 1978; 119:722–726. *Presents survival data comparing simple and radical nephrectomy and the effects of radiation therapy.*

Schwerk WB, Schwerk WN, Rodeck G: Venous renal tumor extension: Prospective US evaluation. *Radiology* 1985; 156:491–495. *A prospective evaluation of ultrasound (US) for detection of venous tumor extension.*

Siminovitch JMP, Montie JE, Straffon RA: Prognostic indicators in renal adenocarcinoma. *J Urol* 1983; 130:20–23. *An understandable staging system for renal cell carcinoma with discussion of prognostic implications.*

101 PROSTATE CANCER

Barrett H. Bolton, M.D.

Cancer of the prostate is a malignant neoplastic disease of men causing major mortality and morbidity. It is the second most common cancer in men in developed countries. Its cause is unknown. Race is a predisposing factor, with a low incidence in Orientals and a high incidence in blacks. Prostate cancer is rare before age 40 years and is increasingly common in old age. Because it is androgen dependent, it is rare in eunuchs. Geography, heredity, and exposure to chemicals and infectious agents, particularly viruses, are thought to contribute to its development. In the United States, the annual incidence is about 69 per 100,000 men, and the annual mortality rate is about 20 per 100,000.

CLINICAL SIGNS AND SYMPTOMS

In early stages, cancer of the prostate may produce no symptoms. The initial symptoms may be caused by local prostatic infiltration leading to bladder neck obstruction and the symptoms of urinary retention including nocturia, frequency, difficulties in initiation of urination, and/or reduced caliber of the urinary stream.

Pain from the prostate may be perceived as arising in the pelvis, lower abdomen, or poorly defined areas of the lower back. Dysuria, hematuria, and urinary tract infections may indicate the presence of a prostatic tumor. Symptoms at early or late stages may be from metastases and may include bone pain, weight loss, lymphedema or lymphadenopathy, and symptoms of anemia or uremia.

The digital rectal examination of the prostate is still the most valuable method of detection. Induration, firmness-to-hardness, or the presence of one or more nodules within the prostate suggests cancer. Extension of the tumor beyond the prostate may make margins of the gland indistinct or the seminal vesicles firm and palpable or may lead to fixation to adjacent structures. Not all firm or nodular prostates contain tumor. The specificity of digital rectal examination varies considerably and improves with experience.

Large tumors can produce urinary obstruction with urinary retention, a distended bladder, and even hydronephrosis with palpable discomfort in the costovertebral angle areas. Direct extension beyond the prostate may lead to lymphedema of the legs or perineum, or to lymphadenopathy. Metastatic disease may produce bone pain with local tenderness, deformity, or pathologic fracture.

The natural history of untreated prostate cancer is enormously variable. Clinical stage A tumors are diagnosed only incidentally when prostatic tissue is examined microscopically after prostatic resection for obstruction. Half of men over age 65 years harbor an occult carcinoma of the prostate, which would be demonstrated if the prostate were examined micro-scopically in its entirety. This incidence rises with advancing age.

Of patients with focal occult prostate cancer, defined as three transurethral resection chips containing tumor, or $\leq$ 5%, only 2% die of the tumor, and 10% develop apparent metastases. Patients with distant metastases (stage D2) at the time of diagnosis have a mortality rate of 50% within 2-1/2 years and of 90% within 10 years.

Table 101–1 lists the approximate percentages of patients in various clinical stages, the staging criteria, and estimated 5-year survival rates. Tumor grade (degree of differentiation), patient age, concomitant disease, and, to some extent, treatment may influence the prognosis and natural history. The general results of surgery, radiation, hormonal therapy, and chemotherapy shown in Table 101–2 demonstrate the effect of treatment on the natural history of the disease.

PATHOPHYSIOLOGY

Most cancers of the prostate are adenocarcinomas and originate in the acinar structures in the periphery of the gland. Other pathologic types are less common.

While *stage* refers to the anatomical extent of the tumor, *grade* refers to malignant potential and prognosis on the basis of histologic pat-

TABLE 101–1.
Staging and Prognosis in Prostatic Cancer

STAGE	DEFINITION	STAGE OF TUMOR AT DIAGNOSIS (% OF ALL PATIENTS)	5-YEAR SURVIVAL (% OF PATIENTS) WITHIN STAGE
A1	Three or more chips on TURP	10	75
A2	Multifocal		
B1	Nodule, < 1.5 cm in diameter	15	60–70
B2	Intracapsular nodule, > 1.5 cm in diameter		
C1	< 6 cm extracapsular	40	35–45
C2	> 6 cm to seminal vesicle		
D1	Metastases to lymph nodes, rectum, bladder, pelvis	35	20%
D2	Distant metastases		
D3	Recurrence after hormonal treatment		

TABLE 101–2.
Effect of Treatment of Prostatic Cancer

TREATMENT	EFFECT
Radical prostatectomy	Some survival value in patients with stage A2 and B lesions, although some studies show little or no survival benefit
External x-ray	Some survival value in patients with stage A2, B, and C lesions
Interstitial radiation with external radiation	Stage A2, B, and C lesions respond better than to external x-ray alone.
Orchiectomy	Simple, probably safest hormonal manipulation
Estrogen	No survival benefit, although 80% of patients show response
Leuteinizing hormone releasing hormone (LH-RH) antagonists	Probably as good as orchiectomy. Less toxicity than estrogens. Promising
Chemotherapy	Many patients' symptoms improve. No definite survival benefit shown consistently

terns, differentiation, anaplasia, and cellular characteristics. The greater the architectural change from the normal linear pattern radiating from the urethra and the greater the degree of anaplasia of individual cells, the more malignant and aggressive the tumor. The tumor may invade perineural spaces (of uncertain significance), lymphatics (a poor prognostic sign), and striated muscle. Extension to the seminal vesicles, pelvic wall, or rectum may occur.

Histochemically, prostatic cancer cells lose their acid phosphatase content as they become more anaplastic.

Spread of tumors within the prostate may lead to urethral obstruction, bladder dilatation, and eventually hydroureter, hydronephrosis, and uremia, as well as urinary tract infection and sepsis. Locally the tumor may cause pain, perineal or pelvic discomfort, and sometimes constipation and other bowel symptoms from pressure on the rectum or anus.

Metastases from prostate cancer occur by lymphatic extension and hematogenous spread. Obturator, common iliac, inguinal, para-aortic, mediastinal, and supraclavicular nodes can be involved. Hematogenously spread tumor most often involves bone, especially cancellous bone in the lumbar spine, proximal femurs, pelvis, thoracic spine, ribs, sternum, skull, and humerus. A popular explanation for this distribution has been that the tumor was disseminated through the vertebral venous system (Batson's plexus). Many other tumors that metastasize to bone share this metastatic pattern. Prostatic metastases to bone are 90% osteoblastic, although many are mixed with some osteolytic features.

Visceral metastases most often involve lungs, liver, and adrenals. The fact that metastases occur more often in some tissues than in others such as skeletal muscle must represent histochemical factors in some tissues that provide a more fertile soil for the establishment and growth of metastatic cells or tumor emboli.

CLINICAL–PATHOLOGIC CORRELATIONS

The clinical–pathologic correlations for prostate cancer are listed in Table 101–3. The pain sometimes associated with local prostate cancer is from nerve infiltration or pressure, lymphatic blockage with edema, or direct invasion into adjacent structures and their nerve supply. Partial to complete obstruction of the urinary tract results in urinary frequency, urgency, or retention.

Urinary obstruction may lead to the uremic syndrome with confusion or depression, seizures, muscle fasciculations, heart failure, nausea, vomiting, diarrhea, hiccups, weakness, and anemia. Pain from bony metastases results from pressure exerted with growth, especially when the periosteum is stretched or because of destruction of bone with collapse of architecture or fracture. Considerable relief may be effected by relatively small decreases in tumor

TABLE 101–3.
Clinical–Pathologic Correlations for Prostate Cancer

CLINICAL FINDINGS	PATHOLOGIC FINDINGS
Pain (perineal, pelvic, low back)	Local infiltration into neural structures in prostate and adjacent tissues, seminal vesicles, bladder, and bowel
Pain (skeletal)	Metastatic osteoblastic lesions infiltrate or create pressure on periosteum, or destroy bone, leading to collapse or fracture
Uremic syndrome nausea, nausea, vomiting, lethargy, anorexia, muscle twitching, heart failure, hiccups	Obstruction of urinary tract from direct blockage or from edema at level of prostate and bladder, or from neurogenic bladder secondary to spine metastases and cord compression
Edema of legs, scrotum, and perineal area	Lymphatic blockage from extension of tumor or surrounding edema
Hypercalcemia with dehydration, lethargy, constipation, polyuria, and cardiac arrythmias	Bony metastases with destruction of bone, perhaps humoral secretion from tumor tissue
Weight loss	Hypermetabolism from tumor, humoral cachexia, producing secretion, anorexia from metabolic complications (uremia)

size or reduction in edema surrounding the tumor, perhaps because of the relative rigidity of bones and the substantial loss of pressure that occurs with small volume losses in hydraulic type mechanical systems.

DIFFERENTIAL DIAGNOSIS

The differential diagnosis includes pathologic processes causing pelvic pain, prostatic nodules, induration and fixation of prostatic and periprostatic tissues, and metastases to bone and other sites. These include benign prostatic hypertrophy: adenomas of the prostate, which are generally less firm and show no tumor on biopsy; abcesses, which are often softer, more tender, and contain no tumor on excision or drainage; other neoplasms originating in adjacent organs such as the bladder, seminal vesicles, and rectum; and tumors that may have spread to the peritoneal cavity and pelvis such as to the pancreas or stomach. Bony metastases from other tumors which present differential difficulty because of their osteoblastic nature include carcinoma of the stomach and carcinoid tumors of the lung. The osteoblastic, rather than osteolytic, character of the bony metastases may explain the infrequency of hypercalcemia.

If the prostatic metastases are atypical, that is, are not osteoblastic, the differentiation becomes more difficult because most tumors that metastasize regularly to bone (such as lung, breast, and cervix tumors), or start in bone (such as osteosarcomas, chondrosarcomas, and multiple myeloma) must be considered. It is important to recognize the possibility of prostatic origin of metastatic adenocarcinoma in bone biopsies because of the potentially helpful and relatively nontoxic treatments available for this disease.

DIAGNOSIS

The diagnosis of carcinoma of the prostate requires microscopic confirmation of neoplastic cells and tissue patterns. The serum acid phosphatase level is elevated in less than 60% of patients with metastatic disease and is not a good screening test, although it can be followed as a tumor marker to assist in assessing response to therapy or progress of disease. Elevated acid phosphatase levels are not specific for prostatic cancer because 10% of elevations may be due to prostatic examination or instrumentation, osteosarcoma, breast or pancreatic cancer, Gaucher's disease, and thrombocytopenia, in some patients, even with the newer radioimmunoassay methods for measuring acid phosphatases. Alkaline phosphatase levels are more likely to be increased in metastatic stages of prostate cancer, thus being somewhat more sensitive, but less specific because bony metastases from most tumors lead to its elevation.

X-ray films of the pelvis may show enlargement of the prostate, which can be more clearly outlined if the bladder is filled with radiopaque dye, as in cystograms or intravenous urograms. Metastatic lesions to bone are most often seen on x-ray films of the pelvis, hips, and spine, but any bone may be involved. Bone x-ray surveys seeking metastases have been used as staging procedures.

Bone scanning with technetium-labeled methylene diphosphonate is a more reliable method of detecting bony metastases and may disclose abnormal uptake suggesting metastases up to 6 months before x-ray film changes are visible. Bipedal lymphangiography can show abnormal lymph node architecture suggesting tumor involvement in the 50% to 60% of patients whose metastases are large enough for detection in this way. The inconvenience of the procedure and a false-positive rate of 10% have further limited the use of lymphangiography in staging prostatic cancer.

Computerized tomography (CT scans), helpful in ruling in but not ruling out metastases, is about 66% sensitive in detecting lymph node metastases when they are large enough and has a 10% false-positive rate. Transrectal or transurethral ultrasonography does not distinguish prostatitis from calculi and tumor, but has been used in staging and assessing the response to therapy. See Table 101–4 for test values.

PRINCIPLES OF PREVENTION AND THERAPY

Venereal diseases, particularly gonorrhea, are the only known likely risk factors for carcinoma of the prostate over which any possible control might be exerted.

The management of prostatic carcinoma is determined by the stage of the disease. Stage A disease carries such a good prognosis that observation alone is recommended. In stage A2 and stage B disease, radical prostatectomy is often curative and is likely to control local disease even if metastases appear later. External beam x-ray or interstitial radiation with iodine 125 or gold 198 each benefit many patients, used alone or in combination with each other. Some patients with stage C disease are treated with radical prostatectomy, although the mortality and morbidity of radical surgery are felt to outweigh potential advantages for most patients. Radiation therapy is often recommended for patients with stage C disease. Treatment of stage D metastatic disease is palliative. It is important to remember that palliation is the relief of symptoms. Thus the asymptomatic patient with stage D disease is usually not treated.

For patients with symptomatic disease or po-

TABLE 101–4.
Relative Value of Diagnostic Tests for Prostatic Cancer

TEST	SPECIFICITY (%)	SENSITIVITY
Total prostatectomy	100	100
TURP 100	50	
Needle biopsy	99	70–95
Rectal examination	50	80
Acid phosphatase level (biochemical)	94	56
Acid phosphatase level RIA	85	20
Acid phosphatase level SIEP	95	20
Alkaline phosphatase level	low	≤50
Bone survey (x-ray films)	50*	70†
Technetium scan	≤50	70†
Lymphangiogram	88	50
CT scan	70	50
Urine cytologic study	98	20–30

* Estimate.
† In patients with bone metastases.

tential symptomatic disease, such as major bony lesions in the spine or long bones in danger of pathologic fracture, local x-ray treatment is usually effective, but only to the area treated. Systemic treatment of metastatic prostate cancer starts with hormonal manipulation, the goal of which is to reduce or block the effect of androgens because an overwhelming majority of prostatic cancers are initially hormone dependent. Bilateral orchiectomy is the most reliable and ultimately the simplest and safest of all hormonal manipulations, with the fewest side-effects. Treatment with estrogens, most commonly diethylstilbesterol, can be dramatic and lastingly effective although controlled prospective studies show no net survival benefit. Newer treatments with luteinizing hormone releasing hormone (LH-RH)

agonists are similarly effective, have fewer serious side-effects, but have the inconvenience of parenteral administration. Antiandrogenic substances such as megestrol and flutamide also show therapeutic promise. All hormonal manipulations produce impotence in many patients, a source of concern and frequent noncompliance with therapy.

Patients whose symptoms and disease are not controlled or who relapse after initial control with hormonal manipulation are candidates for cytotoxic chemotherapy with single or multiple drugs whose beneficial effects are usually brief. Treatment is often measured in terms of stability or nonprogression of the disease, and benefits are often offset by the toxicity, expense, and inconvenience of therapy.

REFERENCES

Klein LA. Prostatic carcinoma. *N Engl J Med* 1979; 300:824–833. *A succinct medical progress review of incidence, diagnosis, staging, and treatment considerations.*

Murphy GP, Karr JP (eds): *Urology* 1981; 17(3 suppl):1–82 and 1981; 17(4 suppl):1–56. *Supplements to two successive issues of Urology in which papers on incidence, etiology, pathology, diagnosis, prognosis, and surgical, radiotherapeutic, endocrinologic, and chemotherapeutic approaches to treatment are collated.*

Perez CH, Fair WR, Ihde DC, Labrie F: Cancer of the prostate, in DeVita VT, Hellman S, Rosenberg SA (eds): *Cancer Principles and Practice of Oncology*, ed 2. Philadelphia, JB Lippincott Co, 1985, pp 929–964. *An excellent chapter covering most clinical aspects of current understanding and treatment of carcinoma of the prostate. Outstanding multiple-author oncology textbook.*

Sheldon CA, Williams RD, Fraley EE: Incidental carcinoma of the prostate: A review of the literature and critical reappraisal of classification. *J Urol* 1980; 124:626–631. *A critical discussion of the significance of focal tumors of the prostate, staging, prognostic features, and natural history.*

Torti FM, Carter SK: The chemotherapy of prostatic adenocarcinoma. *Ann Intern Med* 1980; 92: 681–689. *A discussion of medical treatment of prostatic cancer.*

Warner B, Worgul TJ, Drago J et al: Effect of very high dose D-leucine[6]-gonadotropin-releasing hormone proethylamide on the hypothalamic-pituitary testicular axis in patients with prostatic cancer. *J Clin Invest* 1983; 71:1842–1853. *Reports some results with newer attempts at endocrinologic manipulations in the treatment of metastatic prostatic cancer.*

102 BENIGN BREAST DISEASE

Margaret M. Dunn, M.D.

A wide variety of clinical entities other than malignancy can affect the female breast. Often the clinical focus is on the need to rule out the presence of carcinoma. Certain benign breast processes, particularly fibrocystic disease, can be highly symptomatic and difficult problems to treat, and thus deserve attention. Fibrocystic disease is the most common benign disease of the breast affecting American women and is found so often that in some cases the changes in the breast may not reflect a true pathologic entity.

SIGNS AND SYMPTOMS

The usual initial symptoms of breast disease are a mass, pain, or far less commonly, a nipple discharge. Both breast pain and breast masses may vary in a cyclic and constant relationship to the menstrual calendar. Engorgement, nodularity, and tenderness will typically worsen a few days prior to the menses. In fibrocystic disease bilateral involvement is usual, although unilateral symptoms may predominate. Typically, the symptoms of fibrocystic disease abate after menopause, but some women, particularly those being treated with hormone replacement, have persistent pain and nodularity past middle age. Fibroadenoma has its peak incidence in the third decade of life and cystosarcoma phylloides in the fifth, 10 years earlier than breast carcinoma. The older the patient, the greater the risk of malignancy. A history of trauma, recent breast feeding, or breast surgery should be sought, as well as reproductive, drug and medication, and family histories.

The physical examination will be limited in the obese, fibrous, or gravid breast. In the premenopausal patient, the optimal period for breast examination is 5 to 7 days after the onset of the menses. Occasionally, findings in the breast during another point in the cycle will resolve on reexamination. An unhurried examination increases accuracy. Moderate fibrous change may make it difficult to define the highly significant finding of a dominant mass. Symmetric nodularity is often felt in the fibrocystic breast, particularly in the upper outer quadrants and just above the inframammary fold.

Breast changes in fibrocystic disease may be localized or diffuse. The dominant smooth, firm, rubbery, sometimes lobulated, mass in a younger woman suggests a fibroadenoma, although a cyst should be ruled out by needle aspiration. The uncommon finding of a bulky discrete mass without skin invasion in the older patient is seen in cystosarcoma phylloides. Signs of malignancy such as skin fixation, new nipple retraction, peau d'orange, or lymphadenopathy should be sought.

Fat necrosis secondary to direct breast trauma, superficial thrombophlebitis of the breast (Mondor's disease), and mammary duct ectasia are all entities significant only because their initial features may include mass and skin retraction, suggesting malignancy. Where a discharge can be expressed, an attempt should be made to localize its origin to a single quadrant of the involved breast. Intraductal papillomas, which most often produce nipple discharge, are rarely palpable. Warmth, erythema, and induration, particularly in the lactating breast, point to infection. With an abscess, there may be no additional development of discrete swelling and fluctuance until quite late because of Cooper's ligaments.

PATHOPHYSIOLOGY

Fibroadenoma, intraductal papilloma, and fibrocystic disease are often felt to represent a spectrum of pathologic changes. From the microscopically dense fibrous whorls of fibroadenoma to the gross cystic changes of chronic cystic mastitis, fibrocystic mastopathy includes the pathologic diagnoses of sclerosing adenosis, ductal papillomatosis, and cystic hyperplasia. Often the form of this disease without dominant masses may simply be referred to as mastodynia. All these entities are felt to represent a change in the normal response of the breast to cyclic hormonal influences. Whether the underlying problem is largely an abnormally increased systemic estrogen effect or disturbed end-organ response is still not clear. Increased risk of malignancy is only associated with the minority of pathologic subtypes where hyperplasia atypia or carcinoma in situ is found.

Cystosarcoma phylloides was once felt to be the late outcome of untreated fibroadenomas, however, this tumor is now considered to arise *de novo*. It is a variant of fibroadenoma, usually of large size, with an unusually cellular stroma, and it occasionally metastasizes. However, nonaggressive malignancy has been found in large, long-standing tumors. Cystosarcoma is of fibroepithelial origin as is fibroadenoma and is not a sarcoma in either its pathologic features or behavior. These uncommon tumors can grow rapidly, producing skin ulceration, and can be quite imposing in appearance.

In the lactating breast, nipple trauma and stasis contribute to the development of infection. Predisposing factors often cannot be identified in nonlactating infections. *Staphylococcus aureus* is the most common bacterial agent.

CLINICAL–PATHOLOGIC CORRELATIONS

The clinical–pathologic correlations for benign breast disease are presented in Table 102–1.

DIAGNOSIS

The diagnostic steps for benign breast disease are shown in Figure 102–1. Mammography should largely be used for screening clinically uninvolved breast tissue for occult malignancy and rarely to confirm a clinical impression of benign disease. Both conventional x-ray techniques and xerography now deliver very low dosages, and each has relative advantages in different breast tissues. Sonography may distinguish cystic from solid lesions, as can aspiration.

Cytologic studies of tissue obtained by fine-needle aspiration are being applied to the evaluation of breast lesions on a limited basis. Tissue aspirated through a fine needle into a dry syringe is smeared on a slide, prepared, and evaluated by cytologic criteria. This technique may prove particularly useful in evaluating diffuse, bilateral breast disease because multiple sampling over a wide area may be performed. However, the accuracy of aspiration biopsy in the breast is not yet firmly established. Cytologic examination of nipple discharge or cyst fluid may be helpful.

Core needle biopsy, as with the Tru-cut needle, is generally only obtainable in cases of obvious malignancy. Open surgical biopsy re-

TABLE 102–1.
Clinical–Pathologic Correlations for Benign Breast Disease

	PATHOLOGIC FINDINGS	
CLINICAL FINDINGS	MICROSCOPIC FINDINGS	LESION
Ill-defined induration Diffuse nodularity	Increased fibrous stroma and/or dilatation of ducts and/or epithelial proliferation	Fibrocystic disease
Sanguinous discharge Small subareolar mass	Papillary lesion in dilated duct	Intraductal papilloma
Smooth, rubbery, discrete mass	Dense fibrous stroma compressing glandular elements	Fibroadenoma

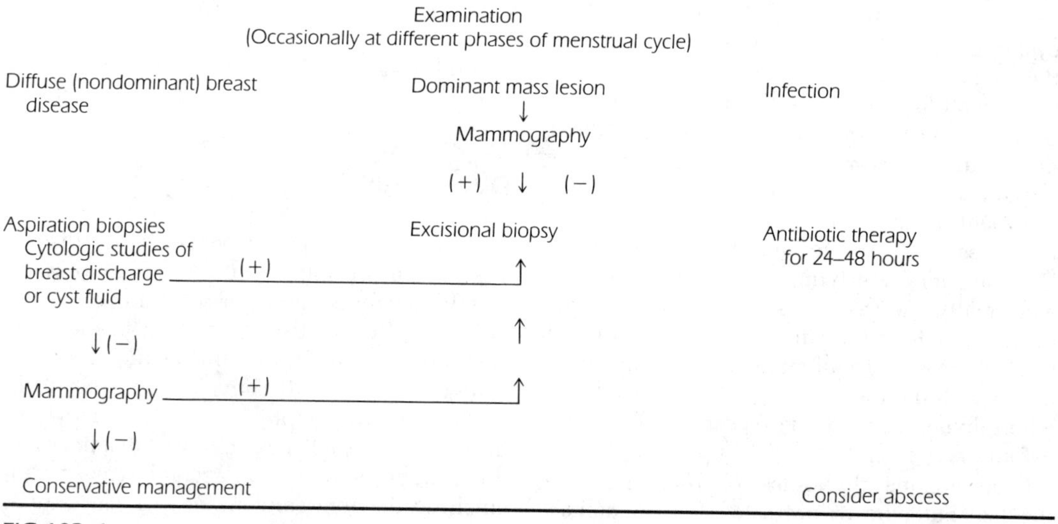

Examination
(Occasionally at different phases of menstrual cycle)

Diffuse (nondominant) breast disease	Dominant mass lesion	Infection
	↓ Mammography	
	(+) ↓ (−)	
Aspiration biopsies Cytologic studies of breast discharge or cyst fluid ——— (+) ———→	Excisional biopsy ↑	Antibiotic therapy for 24–48 hours
↓ (−)	↑	
Mammography ——— (+) ———→	↑	
↓ (−)		
Conservative management		Consider abscess

FIG 102–1.
Diagnostic steps for benign breast disease.

mains the standard for establishing a histologic diagnosis. Sclerosing adenosis, a form of fibrocystic disease, can be confused with carcinoma in frozen sections.

DIFFERENTIAL DIAGNOSIS

The differential diagnosis for benign breast disease is given in Table 102–2. The discrete firm rounded mass in the breast of a teenager has a high probability of being a fibroadenoma.

TABLE 102–2.
Differential Diagnosis for Benign Breast Disease

Fibrocystic disease
Benign tumors
  Fibroadenoma
  Cystosarcoma phylloides
  Intraductal papilloma
Infection
  Lactational mastitis
  Nonlactational mastitis
Inflammation
  Fat necrosis
  Mondor's disease
Malignancy
  Carcinoma
  Sarcoma

In the patient in her twenties, the possibility of cyst or malignancy must be excluded. There have been rare reports of medullary carcinoma mimicking fibroadenoma. In any patient over age 20 years with a dominant lesion. The possibility of carcinoma can only be excluded by pathologic diagnosis. The absence of mammographic evidence of malignancy does not eliminate the need for biopsy, because all carcinomas do not produce radiographic signs of malignancy. Unilateral bloody nipple discharge is most often associated with an intraductal papilloma, but can also be an initial sign in carcinoma. Bilateral serous discharge, on the other hand, will more likely be a symptom of a systemic endocrine disturbance. Infection can easily be recognized in the lactating breast. In the nonlactating breast, the uncommon entities of mammary duct ectasia, Mondor's disease (defined as subcutaneous vein phlebitis, involving breast veins from the epigastric region to the axilla and occurring in both men and women), recurrent subareolar abscesses, and inflammatory carcinoma can mimic infection. Because the breast is a specialized skin structure, conditions that affect the entire integument may manifest here. Skin lesions that may be confused with primary breast problems include epidermal inclusion cysts and nevi.

PRINCIPLES OF TREATMENT

Fibrocystic disease is often considered more significant for its ability to mask and mimic carcinoma than as a distinct clinical problem. In the highly symptomatic patient, many agents including vitamin E, thyroid hormone, diuretic agents, estrogen or progesterone or both, and anti-estrogens like tamoxifen have been tried without success. Initial reports suggesting that withdrawal of methylxanthines (e.g., in cola, coffee, and chocolate) leads to improvement in fibrocystic disease have not been supported by later evidence, although this is an innocuous and probably otherwise beneficial recommendation. Danazol, an androgen-related steroidal agent, has been useful in moderate to severe disease, but is not without troublesome side-effects such as muscle cramps, acne, oiliness of the skin, hot flashes, and occasionally, mild hirsutism.

Excision is the recommended therapy of all dominant masses. Even where a strong presumptive diagnosis of a benign tumor such as fibroadenoma can be made, carcinoma can only be definitely excluded with histologic examination. In most cases excisional breast biopsy can be performed under local anesthesia on an outpatient basis. If a mass is determined to be a cyst, an excisional biopsy may be deferred if the lesion completely resolves after needle aspiration.

Excision is also recommended for cystosarcoma phylloides. These lesions can be bulky enough to require simple mastectomy merely to accomplish excision. Because intraductal papillomas are often not palpable, but are located within 1 cm of the areola, the quarter of the breast whose palpation produced discharge is defined. Excision of the subaveolar ducts in the involved quarter of breast is the standard procedure.

Infection should initially be treated with antibiotics effective against S. aureus, in the absence of findings suggestive of a pus collection. Occasionally aspiration of suspicious areas with an 18-gauge needle will be helpful in defining the extent of infection. Failure to improve after a 24- to 48-hour trial of therapy points toward the presence of a breast abscess. Exploration and drainage of the breast is best accomplished under general anesthesia. Limited drainage secondary to inadequate anesthesia prolongs the septic process, produces increased scarring, and can result in a chronic breast abscess, which also may be confused with carcinoma.

REFERENCES

Dupont WD, Page DL: Risk factors for breast cancer in women with proliferative breast disease. *N Engl J Med* 1985; 312:146–151. *This large series examines subtypes of breast disease in terms of cancer risk.*

Haagensen CD: *Diseases of the Breast*, ed 3. Philadelphia, WB Saunders Co, 1986, p 1050. *The standard work on all breast problems.*

London RS, Sundaram GS, Goldstein PJ: Medical management of mammary dysplasia. *Obstet Gynecol* 1982; 59:519–523. *The best current review of all touted therapies.*

Love S, Gelman RS, Silen W: Fibrocystic "disease" of the breast—a nondisease? *N Engl J Med* 1982; 307:1010–1014. *A provocative discussion of the significance of this entity.*

Schwartz GF: Benign neoplasms and "inflammations" of the breast. *Clin Obstet Gynecol* 1982; 25:373–385. *Excellent overview of benign breast disorders.*

Townsend C: Breast lumps. *CIBA Clinical Symposia* 1980; 32(2):32. *Excellent illustrations of common lesions and basic breast examination.*

103 BREAST CANCER

Andrew B. Rittenberry, Jr., M.D.

Breast cancer is a very common malignancy affecting women in the United States. Each year, 90,000 to 100,000 new cases are discovered, and about 35,000 women die from breast carcinoma.

CLINICAL SIGNS AND SYMPTOMS

Breast cancer should always be suspected when evaluating patients with breast complaints. Any sign of breast disease can be produced by cancer. Eighty-five percent of breast cancers occur after age 45 years and 10% are in patients less than 40 years old. The incidence of new cases continues to increase in the elderly.

The most frequent initial complaints are listed in Table 103–1. A mass is not necessarily a prerequisite to diagnosis. Increasing numbers of patients without symptoms or signs are being referred from screening centers. These patients with so-called occult breast cancer have the best prognosis.

The medical history of all women should include the following information about their breasts: whether signs or symptoms are unilateral or bilateral, whether there is breast discomfort or pain and its relation to menses, and whether there are nipple or skin changes. In addition, information should be obtained about the menstrual history, particularly menarche and menopause; her age at the birth of first child; parity; history of lactation and its duration; trauma; exposure to x-rays or carcinogens; previous breast surgery, aspirations, or mammograms and the results; previous pelvic surgery especially for castration; use of birth control pills or hormones; and family history of breast cancer, particularly in close female relatives. The risks of breast carcinoma are listed in Table 103–2.

Late in the course of breast cancer, the patient may report breast pain, redness, or drainage. If skin ulceration has occurred, the symptoms may include bleeding and a foul odor. An axillary or supraclavicular mass may be reported. Patients who have disseminated disease commonly have associated constitutional symptoms such as weight loss, cough, shortness of breath, bone pain, pathologic fracture(s), ascites, or jaundice. Female patients with metastatic lesions from an undiagnosed primary site frequently have breast carcinoma.

Physical examination of the breast by a skilled examiner is accurate in detecting breast pathology 60% of the time. The breasts should be examined by inspection and a methodic palpation of the breast tissue with the patient upright and supine, first with the arms at the sides and then extended above the head both singly and together. Early changes in breast cancer are often subtle and may only consist of a crusty nipple as in Paget's disease, localized flattenings, or vague dimpling. Carcinoma is seldom palapable unless the mass is 1 cm or greater in diameter. The lesion is usually

---

TABLE 103–1.
Presenting Complaints in Breast Cancer*

	PERCENT OF CASES
Painless mass	66
Painful mass	11
Nipple discharge (usually bloody)	9
Edema	4
Nipple retraction	3
Nipple crusting	2
Erythema	1
Local swelling	1
Abscess	1
Other	2

* From Donegan WL, Spratt JS: *Cancer of the Breast, Major Problems in Clinical Surgery.* Philadelphia, WB Saunders Co, 1979, p 50.

TABLE 103–2.
Risk Factors of Breast Cancer*

RISK FACTOR	INCREASE IN RISK
Female sex	Yes
Age over 45 years	Yes
Family history	9.0 times
Bilateral premenopausal carcinoma in mother or sister	
Benign breast disease	2.5 times
Benign breast disease plus atypia	5.0 times
Previous carcinoma of breast	5.0 times; higher if first cancer occurs before 50 years of age and in an early stage
Previous carcinoma of endometrium	1.3 times
Nulliparous female	3.0 times
Late first parity (> 35 yr)	4.0 times
Protracted menstrual activity	1.3 times
Estrogen use	Uncertain
Birth control pill use	Uncertain
Obesity	2.0 times
High dietary fat	2.0 times
Wet cerumen	2.0 times
Mammographic parenchymal pattern—DY pattern	17.0 times
Abnormal thermogram	15.0 times
Drug use	
Reserpine, dextroamphetamine, methyldopa, phenothiazines	Uncertain
Immune incompetence	Uncertain
Thymic atrophy, chemotherapy, immunosuppressive drugs	

* From Leif, HP, Risk Factors in Breast Cancer, in *Breast CPC Communications*, 1980; 6(4):22.

discrete, hard, poorly defined, relatively immobile, and not tender. Axillary and supraclavicular areas should be carefully examined for lymph node enlargement. The findings usually indicating advanced local or regional disease include obvious dimpling of the skin, lesions greater than 5 cm in diameter, nipple inversion, and enlarged axillary nodes.

Inflammatory changes deserve special mention. Erythema, heat, and pain can represent infection, advanced local carcinoma, or the hallmarks of inflammatory carcinoma. The latter runs a rapidly fatal course and closely mimics infection, except that the white blood cell count is usually normal and there are typically massively enlarged axillary lymph nodes (greater than 80%).

Breast carcinoma often appears to begin as a single focus, but about 15% present with bilateral involvement or multiple primary tumors within the same breast. The upper outer quadrant is most frequently involved (40% of cases), followed by subareolar (30%), upper inner quadrant (15%), lower outer quadrant (10%), and lower inner quadrant (5%).

PATHOPHYSIOLOGY

Breast carcinoma most frequently arises from ductal epithelium and subsequently invades the surrounding parenchyma. A scirrhous histopathologic pattern accounts for 80% of breast lesions. About 30 doubling times and 5 years appear to be required for a breast carcinoma to progress from a single cell to a palpable mass 1 cm in size. Thus, a so-called early lesion may have been present for a substantial period of time, thus often allowing metastases to occur before the primary tumor is clinically evident. This in part explains the inadequacy of some extensive local-regional operations.

As the tumor increases in size and extends into the parenchyma along the ducts and fascial strands into the less resistant mammary fat, the associated scirrhous desmoplastic reaction tends to shorten Cooper's ligaments which leads to skin indentation. Obstruction of the dermal lymphatics usually results in edema. Local extension may reach the skin and result in ulceration, and/or additional adjacent sites of cutaneous involvement, the satellite nodules of advanced local disease.

Extension of breast cancer into the lymphatics is largely an embolic phenomenon, although it can occur by direct extension. The central group of axillary nodes is most commonly (47.5% of cases) the first and most extensively involved. About 30% of women have axillary metastases at the onset of symptoms. In general, the smaller the primary tumor and the shorter the duration of symptoms, the fewer axillary metastases. In very early breast cancer detected by mammography, less than 10% have axillary metastases. Involvement of axillary nodes is an important prognostic indicator.

Cancer cells may pass via the nodal chains, right lymphatic trunk, left thoracic duct, or directly into the circulation, all of which lead to systemic spread. About 95% of patients dying of breast cancer have distant metastases. The most frequent metastatic sites are listed in Table 103–3.

Lung metastases can be solitary, multinodular, or lymphangitic. The latter two are ominous and often lethal. Pleural involvement may lead to a pleural effusion.

Skeletal metastases are almost as frequent as pulmonary and pleural metastases. These may be osteolytic in which destruction of bony trabeculae occurs causing lesions which may cause bone pain, a pathologic fracture(s), and/or nerve root or spinal cord compression. Os-

teoblastic metastases occur in fewer than 10% of patients. In this type, the trabeculae coalesce to form thickened masses of new bone. Osseous metastases can occur by direct arterial-borne route or via the intercostal and vertebral veins to the lower vertebrae. The latter probably explains the more frequent involvement of these bones by breast cancer.

Liver metastases are less frequent but are important because they are particularly resistant to therapy. The lesions are usually widely distributed throughout the liver, and hepatic enlargement and jaundice are often lacking until late in the disease.

Between 5% and 10% of patients develop a primary tumor in the contralateral breast. The incidence of carcinoma in the contralateral breast is 17 times greater than breast cancer in the general population. A few patients have simultaneous primary tumors in both breasts. One particular histologic variant, lobular carcinoma, is bilateral in up to 40% of patients. The threat of carcinoma in the opposite breast is greatest in women with early lesions in the first breast permitting them to survive long enough to develop another lesion. These second tumors have roughly the same prognosis as the first.

Careful study reveals multicentricity in as many as 54% of breast cancer specimens, and studies of the opposite breast in cancer victims shows latent tumors 19 times more frequently than the reported incidence of clinical malignancy. This suggests that not all in situ or latent lesions progress to invasive cancers. There is strong evidence for heterogeneity among the tumors and among the patients.

Untreated breast carcinoma was extensively studied at the Middlesex Hospital in England in the last century. Of 250 cases, the range of survival was 30.2 months to 39.8 months from the onset of symptoms to death with a median survival of 2.7 years. Eighteen percent of the patients survived 5 years and 10.8% survived 10 years.

Currently the treatment of breast cancer can be effective. Presently, a patient with a clinically occult breast carcinoma has a 90% probability of a 10-year survival. For early lesions with a small primary tumor and uninvolved axillary nodes (stage A), disease-free survival for 10 years occurs in about 80% of cases.

TABLE 103–3.
Most Frequent Sites of Distant Metastases from Carcinoma of Breast as Determined at Autopsy*

SITE	PERCENT OF CASES
Lungs	77
Pleura	65
Liver	61
Bone	73
Mediastinal nodes	66
Skin and soft tissues	20

* Derived from Haagensen CD: Diseases of the Breast. Philadelphia, WB Saunders Co, 1971, p 426.

CLINICAL–PATHOLOGIC CORRELATIONS

Among the best known of the many classifications of the histopathology of breast carcinoma is that of Foote and Stewart (Rush, 1974, p 539):

1. Carcinoma of nipple (Paget's disease)
2. Carcinoma of ducts
   a. Infiltrating: Ductal (adenocarcinoma), medullary, papillary, comedo
   b. Noninfiltrating: Papillary, comedo
3. Carcinoma of lobules
   a. Noninfiltrating
   b. Infiltrating

The clinical–pathologic correlations of breast cancer are based on numerous studies, most of which are retrospective. These correlations are shown in Table 103–4. These studies have centered on the involvement of regional nodes, histologic grading, size of the primary tumor, histologic type, tumor margins, vascular invasion, inflammatory infiltrate, and lymph node involvement. The most important prognostic indicator is the status of the regional axillary lymph nodes. Survival falls off sharply if four or more nodes are involved. Up to 50% of patients have nodal metastases when first seen. Of those, up to 40% have four or more involved nodes. The 10-year survival rate for these patients is 40%. In those patients showing no nodal metastases, the 10-year survival rate approximates 75%, and the 20-year rate approximates 65%.

The size of the primary tumor is also important. As a rule, the larger the lesion, the higher the chance of axillary or distant metastases. Tumors larger than 6 cm are associated with a 70% incidence of nodal metastases and a 10-year survival rate of only 17%.

DIFFERENTIAL DIAGNOSIS

The differential diagnosis of breast cancer includes all forms of benign breast disease (see Chap 102).

TABLE 103–4.
Clinical–Pathologic Correlations for Breast Cancer*

CLINICAL FINDINGS	PATHOLOGIC FINDINGS
Lump: small, painless, hard	The smaller the cancer, the less chance of axillary metastasis; hardness is directly related to amount of connective tissue or inflammation present
Tumor attached to skin	Tumor growing just beneath skin
Discharge from nipple	If bloody, cancer has grown into a major duct; is Paget's disease or intraductal cancer
Prominent veins in region of tumor	Tumor blocking venous return
Edema; orange-skin appearance of skin (peau d'orange)	Tumor growing in subdermal and dermal lymphatics
Fixation to chest wall	Invasion of pectoral fascia and rarely of muscle
Satellite nodules	Extensive dermal and subdermal lymphatic involvement
Hard supraclavicular node	Usually a metastasis; can rule out benign lesions by biopsy
Enlarged contralateral axillary lymph nodes	Usually metastasis; can rule out benign lesions by aspiration or biopsy
Fixed masses in axilla	Tumor growing in nodes, breaking through capsule, and growing in loose fat
Edema of arm	Tumor blocking lymphatics and venous return
Horner's syndrome (miosis, enophthalmos, and narrowing of palpebral fissure)	Metastatic tumor pressing on or invading cervical sympathetic chain
Diffuse chest pain, dyspnea	Tumor involving pleura and probably lung
Girdle chest pains (lumbar or sciatic pains)	Possible metastasis to vertebrae or sacroiliac region
Marked weight loss	May mean distant metastasis, possibly to liver

* Derived from Ackerman LV, del Regato JA: *Cancer—Diagnosis, Treatment and Prognosis,* ed 4. St Louis, CV Mosby Co, 1970.

DIAGNOSIS

The history and physical examination will lead the examiner to an appropriate suspicion in 60% of cases. Because women who detect malignant lesions by their own monthly self-examination are much more likely to present with an earlier stage of the disease, self-examination should be strongly encouraged. Adjunctive methods of detection include mammography, needle aspiration, and ultrasound studies. There are currently no chemical markers available for the detection of breast cancer.

Biopsy is the only method of definitive diagnosis with a diagnostic accuracy of about 99%, but between 2% and 5% of frozen section examinations require permanent sectioning for clarification.

Once a diagnosis of breast carcinoma is made, the stage of the disease should be determined, and appropriate therapy selected. Staging systems are essential to accurately stratify patients into groups that can or cannot be cured. A variety of staging schemes are recognized. The most complete is the TNM International System for clinical and pathologic staging (Table 103–5).

The extent to which a patient should be studied prior to treatment varies. In general, extensive testing with x-ray or radionucleotide imaging techniques is unwarranted. In addition to taking tissue for histopathologic studies, it is important to preserve 1 gm of the tumor to measure estrogen and progesterone receptors. These receptors can be reliably measured and have proved valuable in managing patients who later manifest recurrent or metastatic disease. These measurements may also help predict who might respond to selected chemotherapy.

Paget's disease is a unique variant that first appears as an eczema of the nipple. It arises in the small ducts of the nipple and areola and secondarily invades the skin. Often a mass is not palpable. It is a favorable lesion because it usually is diagnosed early.

TABLE 103–5.

Clinical Staging of Breast Carcinoma

PRIMARY TUMOR (T)

T1   Tumor of 2 cm or less in its greatest dimension; skin not involved, or involved locally with Paget's disease

T2   Tumor over 2 cm in size or with skin attachment (dimpling of skin) or nipple retraction (in subareolar tumors); no pectoral muscle or chest wall attachment

T3   Tumor of any size with any of the following: skin infiltration, ulceration, peau d'orange, skin edema, pectoral muscle or chest wall attachment

REGIONAL LYMPH NODES (N)

N0   No clinically palpable axillary lymph node(s) (metastasis not suspected)

N1   Clinically palpable axillary lymph nodes that are not fixed (metastasis suspected)

N2   Clinically palpable homolateral axillary or infraclavicular lymph node or nodes that are fixed to one another or to other structures (metastasis suspected)

DISTANT METASTASIS (M)

M0   No distant metastasis

M1   Clinical and radiographic evidence of metastasis other than to homolateral axillary or infraclavicular lymph nodes

SUMMARY OF CLINICAL STAGING

Stage I   T1, N0, M0;
           T2, N0, M0;
Stage II   T1, N1, M0;
           T2, N1, M0 (includes all N1, M0 except for T3)
Stage III   T3, N0, M0;
           T3, N1, M0;
           T3, N2, M0;
           T1, N2, M0;
           T2, N2, M0;
           includes any combination of T1, T2, or T3 with N2 and M0
Stage IV   Any clinical stage of disease with distant metastasis (M1)

The adenocarcinoma, or scirrhous carcinoma, accounts for over 75% of all breast malignancies. Grossly, the lesion is stellate with serrated edges. On cut section, these lesions are gritty and hard, and yellow streaking is common. Microscopic features vary from well-differentiated to highly anaplastic types. There is a dense fibrous stroma. Electron microscopic studies suggest that the myoepithelial cells of the mammary duct are the point of origin of these highly malignant tumors.

The other types of ductal carcinoma are relatively rare. Five percent of ductal carcinomas assume the medullary pattern of a large, bulky tumor at least 4 cm in diameter. These lesions have a more favorable prognosis than scirrhous carcinoma.

Papillary carcinomas represent 1% or less of primary tumors. Like medullary and colloid carcinomas, they progress slowly, attain a large size, and metastasize late. They can be a cystic lesion, with bloody cyst fluid. Microscopically, this carcinoma is difficult to distinguish from a benign ductal papilloma—stromal invasion being the deciding feature. Improved cure rates are also seen with this tumor.

Comedo, or intraductal, carcinomas account for 3% to 5% of all breast cancers. The distinctive feature of this tumor is the intraductal component. Tumor cells desquamate and fill the ducts, giving rise to ductal casts of tumor, which are called comedos. These also tend to be large. The ducts may become infected giving the condition a prominent inflammatory component. Calcification may be prominent and suggest the diagnosis when seen on mammography.

The noninfiltrating ductal tumors, carcinoma in situ, account for a very small percentage of breast cancer and may be quite difficult to recognize.

Carcinomas of the mammary lobules (lobular carcinoma) arise in the acini or in the epithelium of the terminal ducts. They compromise 6% of all breast tumors. Grossly, this lesion is indistinguishable from ductal carcinoma. Microscopically, its appearance is characterized by cells arranged in linear clusters, a so-called Indian file configuration. Another appearance is that of a bull's eye or target board. Lobular carcinoma is probably the invasive counterpart of lobular carcinoma in situ. The two frequently coexist. It is generally agreed that lobular carcinoma in situ can and does progress over a period of time into invasive lobular carcinoma. Hallmarks of lobular lesions include multicentricity and bilaterality, with 88% showing the former and 35% to 39% the latter. The noninvasive form occurs more frequently in young, premenopausal women.

The only clinically significant sarcoma of the breast is the cystosarcoma phylloides—the malignant counterpart of the benign giant fibroadenoma. It is rare and seen primarily in older women. It may become extremely large.

Inflammatory carcinoma is a highly aggressive and lethal form of breast cancer characterized microscopically by tumor cells in the dermal lymphatics and clinically by erythema, heat, ulceration, and pain. Axillary metastases are usually present (in 80% of cases) and may be massive. Inflammatory carcinoma is nonoperable and is usually rapidly fatal.

PRINCIPLES OF PREVENTION AND THERAPY

Therapy for breast cancer is controversial. It can be divided into management of the primary breast lesion and its regional tissues and management of the recurrent or disseminated tumor.

The standard radical mastectomy (Halsted's operation), modified radical mastectomy, and total mastectomy are surgical procedures used in the United States, along with irradiation and/or axillary dissection, simple mastectomy, radiation therapy alone, and recently local excision of the breast tumor (tylectomy, lumpectomy, segmental mastectomy) with or without axillary dissection and with or without radiation therapy.

Primary treatment failures due to local recurrence or systemic dissemination require advanced therapy.

If a local recurrence is suspected, a biopsy should be taken. If confirmed, the patient should have a metastatic evaluation including bone, liver, and brain scans, as well as chest x-ray films, chemical hepatic profile, and a serum calcium level. Forty-five percent of patients will have demonstrable metastases.

Knowledge of the estrogen receptor status is critical in managing the patient with metastatic disease. Between 60% and 70% of patients with metastases from tumors with estrogen receptors can expect a response to hormone manipulation, and 80% of those with both estrogen- and progesterone-positive tumors will respond. For premenopausal patients who have solitary, nonvital, generally slow-growing metastases (in the soft tissues, skin, bone, nodular lung), castration is recommended and can be expected to produce tumor regression for an average of 9 months. Recent evidence suggests that the initiation of systemic multidrug chemotherapy in the pericastration period lengthens survival. In those with life-threatening metastases (in mul-

tiple sites, liver, lymphangitic lung, brain), systemic cytotoxic multidrug chemotherapy is used. In the postmenopausal patients with positive estrogen receptor status and non-life-threatening metastases, hormone therapy with Tamoxifen is the treatment of choice. Thirty percent of these patients can be expected to respond for as long as 2 years. About 20% of these patients with extensive metastases will respond with a complete remission of variable duration. Fewer than 5% of patients with tumors that show no estrogen receptors respond to chemotherapy.

REFERENCES

Donegan WL, Spratt JS: *Cancer of the Breast, Major Problems in Clinical Surgery.* Philadelphia, WB Saunders Co, 1979. *An up-to-date reference with detailed chapters on diagnosis and management and chapters on nursing care and emotional disturbances.*

Greenblatt RB: Benign breast disease. *Contemp Surg* 1981; 18:27–36. *A superb, succinct article by a leading authority in endocrinology. Emphasizes breast pathophysiology. Contains an excellent bibliography.*

Haagensen CD: *Diseases of the Breast,* ed 3. Philadelphia, WB Saunders Co, 1986. *A major reference text for breast disorders by one of the foremost authorities on the subject. Contains a classic chapter on the natural history of breast cancer.*

Haagensen CD et al: *Breast Carcinoma Risk and Detection.* Philadelphia, WB Saunders Co, 1981. *An assessment of the risk of developing breast cancer and an up-to-date evaluation of available diagnostic methods.*

Hintz BL et al: Primary irradiation for carcinoma of the breast. *Curr Probl Surg* 1981; 6:305–316. *A good review of historic practices and current radiation methods, with provident insight into alternatives to surgical treatment.*

Rush BF Jr: Breast, in Schwartz SI (ed): *Principles of Surgery.* New York, McGraw-Hill Book Co, 1974, pp 527–551. *A concise presentation of the anatomy and physiology of the breast and of both benign and malignant breast disorders that should be read by every student.*

Shehlin JS et al: Treatment of carcinoma of the breast. *Surg Gynecol Obstet* 1979; 149:911–922. *An excellent treatise of the current treatment, emphasizing history taking.*

Veronesi U et al: Comparing radical mastectomy with quadrantectomy, axillary dissection, and radiotherapy in patients with small cancers of the breast. *N Eng J Med* 1981; 305:6–11. *An important article providing insight into the controversial area of conservative treatment for minimal breast cancer.*

104 DYSMENORRHEA

Dennis D. Barber, M.D.

The word *dysmenorrhea* is derived from a Greek root meaning "difficult menstrual flow." A number of myths and misconceptions have long been associated with this condition. Although most women have some degree of discomfort and disruption of activity during normal menstrual flow, dysmenorrhea is more than a passing nuisance. An estimated 600 million working hours are lost annually because of unrelieved, incapacitating dysmenorrhea—the single greatest cause of lost time in the work force. About 52% of postpubescent girls are affected by dysmenorrhea, and about 10% of that group miss 1 to 3 days of school a month. Viewed from a national scale, dysmenorrhea is a large medical problem.

Multiple symptoms associated with menses affect some women more than others. It is important to differentiate symptoms related directly to menstruation from symptoms of poorly understood causes and related temporarily to menses. Psychological influences must also be carefully evaluated.

CLINICAL SIGNS AND SYMPTOMS

Only in those women in whom other pathologic change has been excluded and in whom the cramping discomfort coincides with the onset of flow and usually subsides within 48 to 72 hours, is the diagnosis of primary dysmenorrhea appropriate. Although associated pathologic changes may at times contribute to the total clinical picture, failure of medication that inhibits prostaglandin synthesis to provide relief should alert the physician to look for an additional cause.

In secondary dysmenorrhea, the onset of symptoms may coincide with surgical events or trauma such as delivery. The onset of pain several days prior to menstrual flow suggests endometriosis, particularly if tender nodularity is found in the pelvic structures prior to menses. Aggravation of pain by altered bowel function, or relief of pain upon bowel or bladder evacuation may suggest a functional or inflammatory component. Past pelvic inflammations may suggest chronic residuals of infection that may aggravate primary dysmenorrhea. Chronic pain throughout the cycle suggests a diagnosis other than primary dysmenorrhea.

Repeated observation of the patient with pain will identify psychosomatic or psychogenic components, which make judgment of the true degree of disability difficult. The longer the physician cares for the patient and evaluates the patient's environment, the better he or she can evaluate the disability and response to therapy. Secondary causes for dysmenorrhea require appropriate treatment.

In primary dysmenorrhea, which generally begins 6 to 12 months after menarche and is usually associated with ovulatory cycles, the menstrual pain is intrinsic and idiopathic and is not related to any identifiable gynecologic disorder. The pain usually begins a few hours before, or with the onset of, the menstrual flow. It usually occurs in the lower abdomen, may radiate to the back and upper thighs, and is colicky or "like labor pains." The cramps may occasionally be associated with nausea, vomiting, diarrhea, or pallor.

PATHOPHYSIOLOGY

Folk stories of many countries convey the idea of a menotoxin. In our era, Schich reported that the sweat of a menstrous women was toxic to plants. Macht and Davis noted the acetone extract of menstrual fluid could potentiate the adrenalin-induced contractions of the vas deferens in rats in vitro. These studies were confirmed by others. Embry then showed that the action of prostaglandin F_2 (PGF_2) was one of smooth muscle stimulation. Later studies confirmed the increased concentrations of prostaglandin activity in menstrual effluvia. Pickler postulated that this active substance affected smooth muscle elsewhere as well. Thus there is evidence for the idea that a substance released at the time of menses contains active agents that cause contractions of the myometrium, resulting in cramping or dysmenorrhea.

It now appears that phospholipids are present in the cell membrane, and that arachidonic acid is released by the action of phospholipase A_2, the precursor of prostaglandins. Cyclooxygenase catalyzes the biosynthesis of cyclic endoperoxides from arachidonic acid. The action of this enzyme can be inhibited by drugs such as aspirin, indomethacin, and nonsteroidal anti-inflammatory drugs (NSAIDs) such as ibuprofen and naproxin.

Dysmenorrheic women have a high concentration of PGF_2 in the endometrium and menstrual blood. The administration of PGF_2 causes increased uterine contractility and elevated intrauterine pressures. Treatment with prostaglandin synthetase inhibitors promotes relaxation of the uterine muscle and marked reduction of dysmenorrhea.

CLINICAL–PATHOLOGIC CORRELATIONS

The clinical–pathologic correlations for dysmenorrhea are presented in Table 104–1.

DIFFERENTIAL DIAGNOSIS

A careful history and physical examination must be performed to differentiate primary from secondary dysmenorrhea. A brief summary of the clinical characteristics of primary and secondary dysmenorrhea is presented in Table 104–2. Secondary dysmenorrhea is acquired or extrinsic. The pain usually begins several days before the menses or may be present at other times during the menstrual cycle. It usually occurs in women between 30 and 40 years of age. The pain is usually due to associated pelvic pathologic changes. Commonly

TABLE 104–1.
Clinical–Pathologic Correlations of Dysmenorrhea

CLINICAL FINDINGS	PATHOLOGIC FINDINGS
Cyclic pain related to the menses with increase in severity over 6 to 12 months; infertility	Endometriosis
Painful menses associated with pelvic pressure and an enlarged or irregular uterus	Leiomyomata
Pelvic pain with an associated history of fever, discharge or contact with an infected partner	Pelvic inflammatory disease
Increased prostaglandin syntheses	Pelvic cramping pain associated with the onset of menses; absence of known pelvic pathology.

TABLE 104–2.
Diagnosis—Clinical Characteristics of Primary and Secondary Dysmenorrhea

PAIN CHARACTERISTICS	PRIMARY DYSMENORRHEA	SECONDARY DYSMENORRHEA
Type	Cramping, wave-like	Dull, localizing
Onset	During or a few hours prior to onset of flow	May start before menses
Duration	Rarely lasts beyond 48 to 60 hours	May last longer than 72 hours
History	Usually starts 6 to 12 months after menses begin	First occurs in patients > 20 years of age

TABLE 104–3.
Treatment of Dysmenorrhea*

DEGREE OF PAIN	TREATMENT†
Mild	Education
	Reassurance
	Proprietary analgesics
Moderate	Oral contraceptive if not contraindicated
	Mefenamic acid
	Ibuprofen
	Naproxin sodium
Severe	Combined oral contraceptive plus non-steroidal anti-inflammatory drugs

* From Dawood MY, McGuire JL, Demers LM (eds): *Premenstrual Syndrome and Dysmenorrhea.* Baltimore-Munich, Urban and Schwarzenberg, 1985.
† If symptoms persist, laparoscopy should be considered to assess for other conditions such as endometriosis.

associated conditions include endometriosis, endometrial polyps, pelvic inflammatory disease, uterine leiomyoma (especially intramural or pedunculated), outflow obstruction due either to a congenital anomaly or to post-traumatic or postsurgical scarring, adenomyosis, and uterine malformation.

PRINCIPLES OF THERAPY

Because pain is subjective, assessment of its severity is difficult. In an effort to assess dysmenorrheal disability, Andersch and Milsom (1982) developed a scale to quantify pain. Likewise, observation of the patient and the degree of disability in her everyday working environment allows the physician to rate the pain with a reasonable degree of certainty. The treatment depends on the degree of pain (Table 104–3).

Providing accurate information may help dispel myths relating to dysmenorrhea. The physician should review the physiology of menstruation with young patients and answer their questions truthfully and in a straightforward manner.

Where there is significant discomfort or disability, use of nonsteroidal anti-inflammatory drugs (NSAIDs) that inhibit prostaglandin synthesis helps relieve symptoms in 80% to 90% of patients. Because symptoms relate to prostaglandin release, treatment prior to the onset of menstruation does not seem to increase relief. The NSAIDs should be taken regularly over the first 48 to 72 hours to suppress prostaglandin synthesis in dysmenorrhea. They should *not* be taken every 3 to 4 hours for pain.

In women where contraception is desired, oral contraceptives have proven to be beneficial. Because prostaglandin formation is greater in secretory endometrium, achieving anovulation by hormonal control reduces menstrual fluid volume and prostaglandin activity. For patients who get no relief, the combination of oral contraceptives and prostaglandin synthetase inhibitors may prove helpful.

Unless stenosis of the cervical canal during menstruation is evident, dilatation and curettage should only be done in cases of primary dysmenorrhea when laparoscopy or hysteroscopy is performed to rule out secondary dysmenorrhea. Dilatation and curettage should be resorted to only when other therapy fails.

REFERENCES

Aberlund M: Pathophysiology of dysmenorrhea. *Acta Obstet Gynecol Scand* 1979; 87(suppl):27–32. *Excellent summary of pathophysiology.*

Andersch B, Milsom J: An epidemiologic study of young women with dysmenorrhea. *Am J Obstet Gynecol* 1982; 144:655–660.

Dawood MY, McGuire JL, Demers LM (eds): *Premenstrual Syndrome and Dysmenorrhea.* Baltimore-Munich, Urban and Schwarzenberg, 1985. *Excellent text on this subject.*

Embry MP: Experimental results reproduced from Memoir Soc Endocr 1966; 14, 90.

Macht DI, Davis ME: Experimental Studies, old and new, on menstrual toxin. *J Comp Physical Psychol* 1934; 18:113.

Novak ER, Jones GS, Jones HW (eds). *Textbook of Gynecology*, ed 10. Baltimore, Williams & Wilkins, 1981, pp 817–829. *Good description of clinical symptomatology.*

Pickles VR: Prostaglandins and dysmenorrhea in historical survey. *Acta Obstet Gynecol Scand* 1979; 87(suppl):7–12. *Excellent review of early work on dysmenorrhea.*

Wellman EA, Collins WP, Clayton SG: Studies in the involvement of prostaglandins in uterine symptomology and pathology. *Br J Obstet Gynecol* 1976; 83:337–350. *Basic study on pathophysiology of dysmenorrhea.*

Wiquist N, Widholm O, Nillius S, Nilsson B (eds). *Acta Obstet Gynecol Scand* 1979; 87(suppl). *This whole supplement is devoted to dysmenorrhea.*

Yleborkala O, Dawood MY: New concepts in dysmenorrhea. *Am J Obstet Gynecol* 1978; 130: 833–847. *Excellent review article.*

105 AMENORRHEA

Jack S. Gruber, M.D.

Amenorrhea is a symptom of numerous pathophysiologic states including an array of potential diseases and disorders involving several organ systems, some including serious and life-endangering illnesses. Most patients with amenorrhea have relatively simple problems that can be easily managed by the patients' primary care physician. Our increased understanding of the pathophysiology common to both primary and secondary amenorrhea has made the classic distinction less important.

Concern should be raised to a clinical level if (1) by age 14 years menstruation has not begun and there is no growth or development of secondary sexual characteristics, (2) by age 16 years menstruation has not begun even if there is normal growth and development with the appearance of secondary sexual characteristics, and (3) the absence of menses in a previously menstruating woman for a time equal to at least three previous cycles, or 6 months of amenorrhea in a previously menstruating woman.

These are only general guidelines about when to initiate testing. The patient should be seen whenever her anxieties or, in the case of a teenage girl, those of her parents are brought to the physician's attention. Clinical evaluation of the patient is necessary so that the physician can effectively counsel the patient and her family about menstrual delay.

NORMAL MENSTRUAL FUNCTION

The basic principles underlying the physiology of menstrual function can be divided into four discrete compartments as follows: (1) disorders of the outflow tract or uterine target organ, (2) disorders of the ovary, (3) disorders of the anterior pituitary, and (4) disorders of the hypothalamus (Speroff, Glass, and Kase, 1983).

The presence or absence of menstrual flow is clearly demonstrated by the presence or absence of the visible external evidence of the menstrual discharge. Its presence demonstrates a patent outflow tract that connects the internal genital source of flow to the vaginal orifice. The presence of menstrual flow depends on the necessary existence and development of a functional endometrium. The endometrium must be stimulated by estrogen and regulated by progesterone in the proper sequence. The secretion of estrogen and progesterone originates in the ovary undergoing normal follical development, ovulation, and corpus luteum function. The ovarian cycle is controlled by gonadotropins, follicle-stimulating hormone (FSH), and luteinizing hormone (LH) from the anterior pituitary. The secretion of these depend on gonadotropin-releasing hormone (Gn-RH) being released at the proper pulse frequency. The feedback regulation of GnRH secretion is complex involving the ovarian steroid hormones, pituitary gonadotropins, and other neuroregulators.

EVALUATION OF AMENORRHEA

In addition to careful history of the patient, a family history should be taken. A careful physical examination should be made, and pregnancy should be ruled out. Psychological dysfunction or emotional stress should be noted. Problems with nutrition, growth, and development may be found.

The initial step in the evaluation of the amenorrheic patient includes a measurement of thyroid-stimulating hormone (TSH) and prolactin level, and a progestogen challenge test (Fig 105–1). A few patients presenting with amenorrhea or galactorrhea or both will have hypothyroidism that is not clinically apparent. It is not sufficient to do only the routine thyroid function tests because patients may be in a compensated state with normal thyroxine (T_4) levels achieved by increased secretion of thyroid-stimulating hormone (TSH).

The progestogen challenge test assesses the level of endogenous estrogen, responsiveness of the endometrium, and the patency of the outflow tract and requires a pure progestogen devoid of estrogen activity. Either injectable progesterone (200 mg) in oil or orally active medroxyprogesterone acetate (Provera) may be given, (10 mg daily) for 7 to 10 days. Estrogen-progestogen combinations, such as in birth control pills, are not appropriate because they do not exert a purely progestational effect. Within 2 to 7 days after the progestogen challenge test, the patient will either bleed or not bleed. If the patient bleeds, the diagnosis is anovulation because the test has demonstrated a patent outflow tract, an estrogen-primed endometrium, and follicles in the ovaries with at least basal FSH stimulation.

In the absence of galactorrhea, further testing is usually not needed for the patient with a normal prolactin level and a normal TSH level. All anovulatory patients require therapeutic management, which may vary according to the patient's complaint such as hirsutism, infertility, acne, or may require treatment to prevent the development of carcinoma of the endometrium.

If the progestogen challenge does not produce withdrawal bleeding, either the outflow tract is not patent or estrogen priming of the endometrium is inadequate. Next check compartment I by administering an estrogen. If an endometrium and patent outflow exist, when a progestogen challenge is administered after priming with estrogen then withdrawal bleeding will occur. Estrogen priming can be best accomplished with 2.5 mg of conjugated estrogens daily for 21 days. Medroxyprogesterone acetate (10 mg daily) is then added for the last 7 days. The patient with amenorrhea and a negative progestogen challenge test, when primed with estrogen and again challenged with a progestogen will either bleed or not bleed. If withdrawal bleeding does not occur, then a component of compartment I is defective. If withdrawal bleeding does occur, the endometrium and outflow tract have normal capabilities if properly stimulated by estrogen followed by a progestogen.

If withdrawal bleeding does not occur with a progestogen but does with a combination of estrogen followed by a progestogen, then the ovary is failing to provide adequate estrogen. The question is then does the ovary contain unstimulated follicles or is it devoid of follicles? Because the pituitary regularly monitors the activity of the ovaries and regulates folliculogenesis, testing of pituitary function is next. This can be done by measuring the serum levels FSH and LH by radioimmunoassay (Table 105–1).

This is best done during early folliculogenesis 6 to 7 days after stopping the administration of estrogen and progesterone for the progestogen challenge test to avoid the midcycle surge and to avoid the luteal phase when gonadotropin levels are low. This step is designed to determine whether the lack of estrogen is due to a lack of follicles or a lack of pituitary stimulation and therefore is due to a defect in the CNS-pituitary axis (compartments

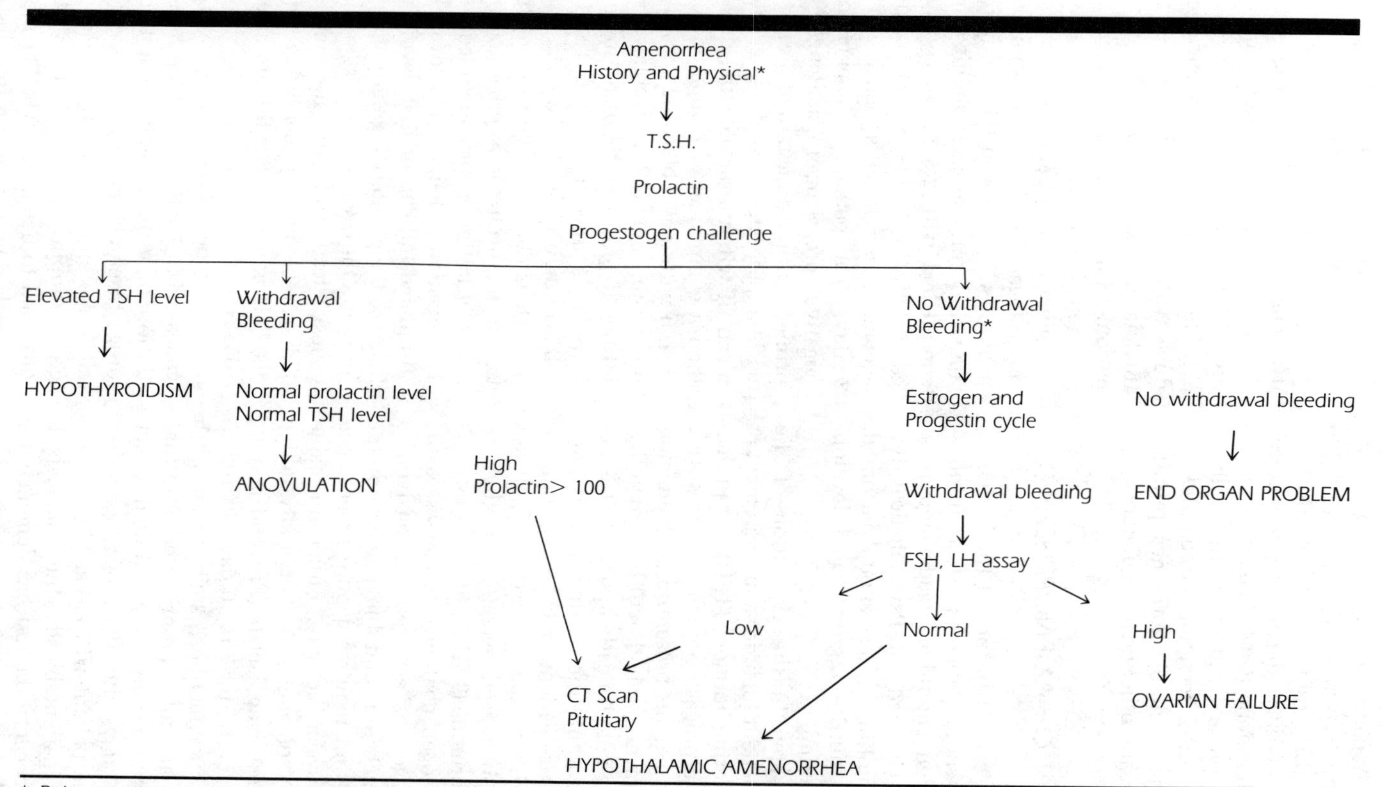

* Rule out pregnancy and anatomical abnormalities.

FIG 105–1.
Flow diagram for the evaluation of amenorrhea.

TABLE 105–1.
Gonadotropin Levels During Basal or Early Follicular Phase (Day 6 or 7 of the Menstrual Cycle)

CLINICAL STATE	SERUM FSH LEVEL	SERUM LH LEVEL
Normal young adult female	6–18 mIU/ml (range) 10 ± 2 mIU/ml (mean)	6–18 mIU/ml 10 ± 2 mIU/ml
Perimenopausal	18–30 mIU/ml	18–25 mIU/ml
Hypogonadotropic state (prepubertal hypothalamic, or pituitary dysfunction)	<6	<6
Hypergonadotropic state (postmenopausal, castrate, and ovarian failure)	>40	>25

III and IV). The serum gonadotropin level in the amenorrheic woman who does not have withdrawal bleeding with progestogen challenge will either be abnormally high, abnormally low, or in the low-normal range.

High gonadotropin levels almost always indicate ovarian failure, an ovary devoid of follicles. The exceptions include resistance or insensitive ovary syndrome in which follicles are resistant to gonadotropins, probably due to the lack of gonadotropin receptors (Speroff, Glass, and Kase, 1983). An ovarian biopsy would be needed to differentiate this from ovarian failure, but since pregnancy is still unobtainable, the pursuit is not recommended.

High levels may also be measured in conditions in which a single gonadotropin has been deficient since fetal development resulting in defective gametogenesis. The level of one gonadotropin may be high and the other undetectable.

Perimenopausal women may have low numbers of follicles and only relatively resistant follicles left; the response of the follicles may be limited until gonadotropins rise to a higher level and then call forth follicles again. During this time, postmenopausal levels of FSH may be followed by the return of folliculogenesis for a short time. This is differentiated by measuring both FSH and LH because it is associated with a high FSH but a normal LH.

A patient with a complete 17-hydroxylase deficiency in both the ovary and adrenal gland would have high gonadotropin levels and normal ovarian follicles. The patient would present with absent secondary sexual development because the sex steroids could not be produced.

The karyotype should be determined for patients under the age of 30 years who have ovarian failure diagnosed on the basis of elevated gonadotropin. The presence of a Y chromosome in the karyotype of a phenotypic female requires gonadectomy, because the presence of any testicular component within the gonad carries a 25% chance of neoplasia. In patients over the age of 30 years secondary amenorrhea with high gonadotropin levels is best labeled *premature menopause.*

Low-normal levels of gonadotropins sometimes occur in hypoestrogenic patients, that is, patients with no withdrawal bleeding after a progestogen challenge. The levels would be normal for the luteal phase followed by menstruation, but they are inadequate to initiate follicular growth and maintain estrogen levels high enough to proliferate the endometrium sufficiently to have withdrawal bleeding. The low-normal levels of FSH and LH in a patient with a negative progestogen challenge test are consistent with pituitary-CNS failure. Further evaluation is in order using the same tests as for patients with below-normal levels of gonadotropins.

When the gonadotropin levels are either abnormally low or in the low-to-normal range, whether the pituitary cells are underdriven, oversuppressed, or pushed aside must be determined. A space-occupying lesion of the sella turcica should be ruled out. The most modern computed tomography (CT) scan (capable of high-resolution 1-mm "cuts") is best able to evaluate the contents of the sella turcica as well as the suprasellar area. The scans can be enhanced by dye perfusion because many pituitary tumors are vascular.

Patients with amenorrhea and without galactorrhea who have reached this point in the work-up and have normal x-ray films of the sella turcica are diagnosed as having hypothalamic amenorrhea. The cause of the amenorrhea is suppression of the pulsatile Gn-RH secretion outside its critical range.

Endocrine testing does not discriminate between disorders of the hypothalamus and the anterior pituitary secretion (including Gn-RH stimulation, thyroid-releasing hormone (TRH) stimulation, and other tests to alter prolactin, growth hormone, and ACTH secretion). Tremendous variability in response is the rule. Patients with pituitary tumors may or may not respond. Amenorrhea can be classified according to compartments of dysfunction that correlate with specific organ systems enabling the clinician to further evaluate the specific disorder which led to the amenorrhea.

COMPARTMENT I: DISORDERS OF OUTFLOW TRACT OR UTERINE TARGET ORGAN

Asherman's syndrome is defined as secondary amenorrhea following destruction of the endometrium. This classically follows postpartum curettage and results in intrauterine adhesions which may partially or completely obliterate the endometrial cavity, the internal cervical os, or the cervical canal. Destruction of the endometrium can be caused by tuberculosis but this is rare in the United States. The diagnosis would be made by a hysterogram and confirmed and treated by hysteroscopic-directed lysis of the intrauterine adhesions. After dissection of the adhesions, a custom-made Silastic intrauterine balloon is placed to prevent the sides of the uterine cavity from adhering. The endometrium is encouraged to proliferate across defects by administering estrogens to prolong the proliferative phase.

MÜLLERIAN ANOMALIES

In primary amenorrheas, developmental anomalies should be ruled out. Cost-effective clinical practice is starting the evaluation with the first compartment. Inspection and palpation would thus rule in or out imperforate hymen, obliteration of the vaginal orifice, and segmental atresia of the vaginal canal. The cervix or the entire uterus may be absent. The uterus may be present but the cavity absent, or the endometrium may be congenitally absent.

Further evaluation should include radiologic studies. About one-third of the patients with müllerian anomalies have urinary tract abnormalities, and about 12% have skeletal anomalies, usually involving the spine. When the presence of an abnormal uterine structure is suspected from the physical examination, ultrasound studies can be used to confirm it. If a partial endometrial cavity is present, cyclic abdominal pain may occur. Removal of the müllerian remnants may be necessary if fibroid growth, hematometra, endometriosis, or symptomatic herniation into the inguinal canal occurs. Distal obstruction of the genital tract is the only condition that can be considered an emergency.

CONGENITAL ANDROGEN-INSENSITIVITY SYNDROME

Congenital androgen-insensitivity syndrome is the likely diagnosis when a blind canal is encountered and the uterus is absent. These patients appear normal at birth except for the possible presence of an inguinal hernia. The growth and development are normal. Puberty occurs with breast development but with absent or scant pubic and axillary hair. Although the individual is phenotypically female, the karyotype is XY, the gonad is a testis, and the hormones produced are androgens. There is no intracellular androgen-receptor protein in the cytosol, so no androgen effect of any type is visible. Transmission is by means of an X-linked recessive gene. Because the incidence of neoplasia is high, the gonads should be removed once full development is attained after puberty. The patient should then be placed on estrogen-replacement therapy.

COMPARTMENT II: DISORDERS OF GONAD

The characteristics of Turner's syndrome are short stature, webbed neck, "shield" chest, increased carrying angle at the elbow, and hypergonadotropic hypoestrogenic amenorrhea. Less common findings include renal anomalies and coarctation of the aorta. The karyotype should be determined for all patients with elevated gonadotropin levels. The presence of a pure syndrome (i.e., a single cell line with the 45, X chromosome) should be confirmed.

MOSAICISM

The presence of multiple cell lines of varying sex chromosome composition must be ruled out because the presence of a Y chromosome in the karyotype requires gonadectomy. The presence of any testicular component within the gonad increases the risk of neoplasia and may cause virilization at puberty. Even in the absense of a Y-containing cell line, XX mosaicism is expressed in a variety of ways, from complete gonadal dysgenesis to functional ovarian tissue with varying degrees of female development. Pregnancy and delivery may even occur before premature menopause occurs. Such patients are usually born with a normal amount of functional follicles, which undergo an acclerated atresia because of the lack of granulosa cell-supporting structure.

XY GONADAL DYSGENESIS

Patients with Swyer's syndrome have an XY karyotype but no gonads, so they develop a müllerian system. At the time of expected puberty, no spontaneous puberty occurs. Neoplasia of the gonadal streaks can occur at any age, so gonadectomy should be performed and estrogen therapy begun.

XX GONADAL AGENESIS

Although a female karotype and phenotype are present, puberty does not occur in XX gonadal agenesis. Such patients have hypergonadotropic hypogonadism and no propensity for neo plasms. *Premature ovarian failure* is probably a genetic disorder with either a reduced number of primordial follicles or an increased rate of atresia. When loss of follicles has been rapid, primary amenorrhea and a lack of sexual development are present. If loss of follicles takes place during puberty or later, secondary amenorrhea occurs. Accelerated atresia may be due to a genetic problem within the germ cells. Because the primordial follicle number corre-

lates with the fetal level of gonadotropins, there may have been a deficiency of the gonadotropin secretion during fetal life, or the fetus may have been exposed to an antigonadotropin.

COMPARTMENT III: DISORDERS OF PITUITARY FUNCTION

Growth of a benign tumor in the pituitary can cause pressure. The suspicion of pituitary tumor is increased if there are clinical signs either of acromegaly due to excessive secretion of growth hormone or of Cushing's disease due to excessive secretion of ACTH. Prolactin-secreting tumors seen in preadolescent and adolescent children may cause both primary amenorrhea and failure of growth and development. Prolactin-secreting adenomas are the most common pituitary tumors. Tumors less than 1 cm in diameter are called *microadenomas;* those greater than 1 cm are called *macroadenomas.*

A high prolactin level may be found in about one-third of women with amenorrhea. One-third of patients with high prolactin levels have galactorrhea. One-third of the women with galactorrhea have normal menses. As the prolactin level increases, the patient may progress sequentially from normal ovulation to an inadequate luteal phase to intermittent anovulation to total anovulation to complete amenorrhea. The amenorrhea associated with elevated prolactin levels appears to be due to prolactin inhibition of the pulsatile secretion of Gn-RH. Treatment that lowers the circulating levels of prolactin restores ovarian and menstrual function. This can be accomplished either by surgical removal or medical supression with bromocriptine. This drug is a dopamine agonist that binds to a dopamine receptor, thereby directly mimicking dopamine inhibition of pituitary prolactin secretion.

THE EMPTY SELLA SYNDROME

Instead of a tumor, a patient may have an abnormal sella turcica in which the sella diaphragm is incomplete from birth, allowing an extension of the subarachnoid space into the pituitary fossa. The pituitary gland is flattened, and the sella floor may be eroded by pressure from the cerebrospinal fluid. The empty sella syndrome may also occur secondary to surgery or radiotherapy and may arise because of tumor infarction. Enlargement of the sella turcica with a normal shape is more likely to be due to an empty sella than to a tumor. Because of possibility of a coexisting adenoma, the patient with an elevated prolactin level or galactorrhea should be surveyed annually to rule out tumor growth.

COMPARTMENT IV: DISORDERS OF HYPOTHALAMUS

Few tests are available to evaluate hypothalamic function in suspected cases of hypothalamic amenorrhea. Problems in this area are usually diagnosed by exclusion of pituitary lesions. Hypothalamic dysfunction may be associated with stress, weight loss, or excessive exercise. These patients have low or low-normal levels of gonadotropins and fail to have withdrawal bleeding following a progestogen challenge.

TABLE 105–2.
Diagnostic Characteristics of Anorexia Nervosa

1. Onset between ages 10 and 30 years
2. Weight loss of 25%, or weight 15% below normal for age and height
3. Special attitudes
   Denial
   Distorted body image
   Unusual hoarding or handling of food
4. At least one of the following:
   Lanugo
   Bradycardia
   Overactivity
   Episodes of overeating (bulimia)
   Vomiting, which may be self-induced
5. Amenorrhea
6. No known medical illness
7. No other psychiatric disorder
8. Other characteristics:
   Constipation
   Low blood pressure
   Hypercarotenemia
   Diabetes insipidus

ANOREXIA

A classic example of hypothalamic amenorrhea is that associated with weight loss. Amenorrhea in the patient who is chronically underweight or has lost weight rapidly is commonly due to a hypogonadotropic state. The patient may present in various ways, from the thin chronic dieter to the severely ill patient with the life-threatening attrition of anorexia nervosa. It occurs mainly in young middle- to upper-class girls under the age of 25 years in success-oriented families where high expectations are placed on the child.

The normal weight gain of puberty may be interpreted as excessive in a diet-conscious adolescent. The children are often high achievers, rigid, self-critical, and preoccupied with food. The patient provides much rationale for low-calorie foods. Diuretic and laxative abuse is common. The borderline anorexic patient frequently presents as a teenager who has a low body weight, amenorrhea, hyperactivity, excellent grades, and many extracurricular activities (Table 105–2).

The problems associated with anorexia represent dysfunction of the body mechanisms regulated by the hypothalamus: appetite, thirst and water conservation, temperature, sleep, autonomic balance, and endocrine secretion. Patients have low levels of FSH and LH. Cortisol levels are elevated due to a decreased clearance with normal production; prolactin levels are normal; the levels of TSH and T_4 are normal, but the T_3 level may be low. Many of the symptoms can be explained by relative hypothyroidism: constipation, cold intolerance, bradycardia, hypotension, dry skin, and low metabolic rates. With sufficient weight gain, all the metabolic changes revert to normal. Even though normal gonadotropin secretions may be restored with sufficient weight gain, 30% of patients remain amenorrhagic. Patients with anorexia nervosa have persistent low levels of gonadotropins similar to prepubertal children. Presentation of the dynamics of the problem to the patient may be all that is necessary, but many require continued supportive counseling and manipulative management such as calorie counting. If weight gain is slow, hormone replacement therapy may be used until some weight gain has been attained.

EXERCISE AND AMENORRHEA

Today women are active—running and competing in athletics or engaging in other forms of strenuous recreational exercise including dance and body building. The loss of a critical amount of body fat combined with stress results in hypothalamic suppression and a high incidence of menstrual irregularity and amenorrhea.

The onset and regularity of menstrual function necessitate maintaining a body weight above a critical level and therefore maintaining a critical amount of body fat. The competitive female athlete has about 50% less body fat than the noncompetitor. This change in body fat can occur with no discernible change in total body weight because fat is converted to lean muscle mass. The amenorrhea is due to hypothalamic dysfunction similar to that seen in anorexia nervosa.

HORMONE REPLACEMENT THERAPY

The patient who is hypoestrogenic and who is not a candidate for induction of ovulation should be placed on hormone replacement therapy. Young women with weight-loss amenorrhea, runner's amenorrhea, or hyperprolactinemic amenorrhea, lose bone density if left hypoestrogenic. These women may be taken off replacement therapy and reevaluated yearly. Once a decision to replace hormones has been made, it is reasonable to mimic the ovarian cycle with daily estrogen and cyclic progestogens. This can be done by using 1.25 mg of conjugated estrogens daily and adding 10 mg of medroxyprogesterone acetate 10 days each month. The dose of either may be reduced to half this amount if side-effects occur.

REFERENCES

Archer DF, Lattanzi DR, Moore EE, Harger JH, Herbert DH: Bromocriptine treatment of women with suspected pituitary prolactin-secreting microadenomas. *A J Obstet Gynecol* 1982; 143:620–625. *Classic paper on management of hyperprolactinemia associated with amenorrhea.*

Kase N: The neuroendocrinology of amenorrhea. *J Reprod Med* 1983; 28:251–255. *A good, easily understood review of the pathophysiologic basis of amenorrhea of hypothalamic origin.*

Killanski A, Neer RM, Beitins IZ, Ridgway EC, Zervas NT, McArthur JW: Decreased bone density in hyperprolactinemic women. *N Engl J Med* 1980; 303:1511–1514. *Classic paper on risk of bone loss associated with hyperprolactinemic amenorrhea.*

Speroff L, Glass R, Kase N: *Amenorrhea. Clinical Gynecologic Endocrinology and Infertility,* ed 3. Baltimore, Williams & Wilkins, 1983, pp 141–184. *The most practical and easily understood approach to the subject of amenorrhea.*

Speroff L, Levin RM, Haning RV Jr, Kase NG: A practical approach for the evaluation of women with abnormal polytomography or elevated prolactin levels. *Am J Obstet Gynecol* 1979; 135:896–906. *Detailed presentation of data on polytomography of sella tursica.*

Warren MP, Vande Wiele RH: Clinical and metabolic features of anorexia nervosa. *Am J Obstet Gynecol* 1973; 117:435–449. *Review of laboratory finding in series of patients with anorexia nervosa.*

106 PREGNANCY COMPLICATIONS

Richard J. Hildebrandt, M.D.

ABORTION

Abortion is the spontaneous or elective termination of pregnancy before viable extrauterine life is possible; the latter is usually defined by a mass of 500 gm and a length of 25 cm or 20 weeks of gestation. The incidence of spontaneous abortion is approximately 15% of all pregnancies.

A threatened abortion is defined as uterine bleeding with minimal pain and a closed uneffaced cervix. An inevitable abortion is usually associated with heavy bleeding, moderate to severe pain, and dilatation of the internal os. The term *missed abortion* applies to a conceptus that has expired in utero but has not been expelled from the uterus.

CLINICAL SIGNS AND SYMPTOMS

The patient usually gives a history of one or more missed menstrual periods and often has had a pregnancy test at home or in a physician's office. She reports vaginal spotting, a brownish discharge, or frank bleeding. Moderate to severe lower abdominal cramping occurs in the case of an inevitable abortion.

Examination may reveal brownish discharge, blood or clots in the vagina, an enlarged uterus, softening of the isthmus, and pulsations of the adnexa. A slightly enlarged ovary may be felt in one adnexa. With a threatened abortion, the uterus is usually not tender. With an inevitable abortion, the lower uterine segment is thin, the cervix may be dilated, and the uterus may be tender. A missed abortion may be suspected when, in absence of the above signs and symptoms, serial examinations fail to reveal any growth. Approximately 35% to 50% of threatened abortions will proceed to viability, although as many as 40% of these may end with premature delivery. Between 50% and 65% proceed to passage of tissue and then may be termed complete or incomplete abortions depending on whether or not the uterus is completely emptied.

PATHOPHYSIOLOGY

Death of the conceptus probably occurs in 50% to 80% of abortions. The most common cause is a chromosomal abnormality (35% to 50% of deaths). Most chromosomal abnormalities are the result of spontaneous mutation, but a small percentage are the result of one parent being the carrier of a balanced translocation. Other factors include defective implantation, maternal infections (toxoplasmosis, herpes simplex, cytomegalovirus, rubella, t-strain *Mycoplasma*, and *Listeria*), defective hormone production (inadequate corpus luteum), and ingestion of cytotoxic agents. Mid-trimester abortions may be associated with an incompetent cervix or a uterine anomaly such as a uterine septum or bicornuate uterus.

DIFFERENTIAL DIAGNOSIS

The primary conditions to be distinguished from abortion are ectopic pregnancy and hydatidiform mole. The signs and symptoms may be the same as for abortion, but, in addition, a patient with an ectopic pregnancy often presents with severe unilateral lower-abdominal pain. A molar pregnancy is commonly first seen later than most spontaneous abortions, and the symptoms usually occur in the late first or early second trimester. The uterus is often of inappropriate size for the duration of pregnancy.

DIAGNOSIS

Ultrasound and beta-human chorionic gonadotropin (BHCG) test titers are the laboratory cornerstones in diagnosis. A positive BHCG test

TABLE 106–1.
Clinical–Pathologic Correlations in Abortion

CLINICAL FINDINGS	PATHOLOGIC FINDINGS
Spotting or bleeding	Spontaneous first-trimester abortion a. Trophoblasts erode into maternal vessels.
Heavy bleeding usually with moderate to severe cramping	b. Hemorrhage into decidua basalis with necrotic changes in the adjacent tissues.
Increased bleeding and severe cramping with expulsion of products of conception	c. The ovum becomes detached with increasing hemorrhage in the decidua around the ovum.
	Spontaneous second-trimester abortion
Bleeding may sometimes be occult. Cramping is more apt to resemble labor.	The pathology is usually similar to that of abruptio placentae.

differentiates between bleeding due to abnormal menses and pregnancy. Serial BHCG titers are helpful in determining the duration and location of the pregnancy. A case of ectopic pregnancy or missed abortion may have titers that are low and/or falling for the calculated menstrual age. A case of hydatidiform mole may have high titers. Ultrasound studies should be able to detect an intrauterine gestational sac if the HCG titer is above 6500 units (about 6 weeks gestation). Fetal heart activity is usually detected by 7 to 8 weeks gestation and predicts a viable pregnancy outcome in over 90% of individuals. Absence of a gestational sac after 6 weeks may indicate an ectopic pregnancy or an incomplete abortion. If an adnexal mass is observed without an intrauterine sac, an ectopic pregnancy is highly probable. A hydatidiform mole gives a characteristic intrauterine "snow" pattern.

PRINCIPLES OF THERAPY

A threatened abortion requires no specific treatment. Bedrest has not been shown to be of benefit. The patient should be informed about the probabilities of the various outcomes and about the symptoms of an inevitable abortion. It should be emphasized that the patient was not herself at fault in determining the fate of her pregnancy.

An inevitable or incomplete abortion should be completed with due haste. Infusion of Ringer's lactate solution should be started through a large-bore intravenous (IV) tube because blood loss is often of magnitude sufficient to result in hypovolemia. A blood sample should be taken for a complete blood count (CBC) and differential as well as typing (for crossmatching and for Rh immune globulin administration). A suction curettage may be performed under paracervical block with a plastic cannula if the size of the uterus indicates that the conceptus is less than 8 weeks gestation. If the uterus is larger than 8-week size, the procedure is best performed in the operating room under general anesthesia. All tissue removed should be sent to the pathology department for diagnosis. Any signs of infection demand immediate treatment with antibiotics. Because most infections are mixed, with gram-positive and gram-negative aerobes and anaerobes, the spectrum of antibiotics should include a penicillinase-resistant penicillin or cephalosporin and an aminoglycoside.

Septic shock is rare since abortions were legalized in 1973. However, one occasionally sees a neglected incomplete abortion with severe infection. In this instance coagulation studies should be performed, and massive antibiotic therapy including parental chloramphenicol should be instituted. Large doses of glucocorticoids may be life saving. A central venous pressure (CVP) line or Swan-Ganz catheter should be inserted to take samples for determining fluid balance.

A mid-trimester abortion is sometimes associated with a retained placenta, and oxytocin stimulation may be necessary to effect delivery. If bleeding is excessive, curettage under general anesthesia may be necessary. The mid-trimester abortion should raise the concern of uterine pathology, and the patient ought to be informed that a hysterosalpingogram should be performed after two or three normal menstrual periods.

THIRD-TRIMESTER BLEEDING

Bleeding in the third trimester is most often associated with one of the two major causes, placenta previa and abruptio placentae. Each of these entities occurs in 0.5% to 1.0% of all pregnancies. Placenta previa is defined as the implantation of trophoblastic tissue on the lower uterine segment, obstructing the presenting part prior to or during labor. The entire internal cervical os is covered in a total placenta previa. Only a portion of the os is covered in a partial placenta previa.

Abruptio placentae is defined as the premature separation of a normally implanted placenta after 20 weeks of gestation. In the mild form, separation is minimal, involving less than 15% of the surface and less than 500 ml of blood is usually lost. In the severe form, more than 65% of the placental surface separates, and more than 1000 ml of blood is lost.

CLINICAL SIGNS AND SYMPTOMS

Painless vaginal bleeding is the usual initial symptom with a placenta previa and may be associated with a history of unusual exertion or recent coitus. However, it is not uncommon for the patient to awaken in a pool of blood. The presenting part is often elevated out of the pelvis and can be palpated above the symphysis. A placental souffle can sometimes be heard with the fetoscope low on the abdomen. The uterus is not tender or soft, although approximately 10% of patients may show some signs of abruption.

Abruptio placentae is first seen with various degrees of symptoms, depending on the severity of the separation. The bleeding is usually painful, and the uterus is tender and tense. The blood loss is almost always more than initially evident. The severe form is associated with maternal cardiovascular collapse, fetal death, and coagulopathy.

PATHOPHYSIOLOGY

Placenta previa is more common in multiparas and is thought to be due to previous scarring of the uterus from former implantations in the fundus, thus leaving the lower portion for subsequent nidation. An abruption is due to a decidual arterial vascular insult, resulting in hemorrhage into the decidual plate and subsequent separation of the placenta. Abruption is associated with hypertension, smoking, and multiparity, presumably because these conditions affect the vasculature.

DIFFERENTIAL DIAGNOSIS

Placenta previa should be distinguished from abruptio placentae, genital lacerations, cervical lesions, excessive show, bladder or rectal bleeding, and blood dyscrasias. In the diagnosis of abruptio placentae, one must also consider degenerating fibroids, placenta previa, twisted ovarian cyst, appendicitis, and any other acute adbominal condition.

DIAGNOSIS

Do not perform a bimanual vaginal examination until placenta previa is ruled out. Manipulation of the lower uterine segment can result in massive and sudden hemorrhage. Ultrasound is the most valuable tool aiding in the diagnosis of placenta previa and abruptio placentae. A full bladder is necessary to evaluate for placenta previa (this aids in visualizing the cervix). In placenta previa, the placental substance can be seen impinging on or covering the internal cervical os. In abruptio placentae, a sonolucent area can sometimes be seen between the placenta and the uterine wall. However, the absence of such findings does not rule out an abruption. If ultrasound is not available, a "double set-up" examination must be performed if bleeding is significant and delivery therefore indicated. The patient is taken to the operating room after blood has been crossmatched and the cardiovascular system stabilized. With the entire delivery team prepared for an immediate cesarean birth, the patient is examined internally to palpate the granular, sometimes gritty, placental tissue impinging on the internal cervical os.

PRINCIPLES OF THERAPY

Placenta previa rarely produces profuse hemorrhage with the first episode of bleeding. However, the potential for a catastrophic event demands immediate hospitalization. If the fetus is more than 37 weeks gestation, then delivery is performed. Induction of labor can be attempted if a marginal or low-lying placenta is present. Continued heavy bleeding or a placenta covering the internal os demands an immediate cesarean delivery. Placenta previa with an immature fetus presents more difficult decisions. Strict bedrest and, if necessary, blood replacement can gain valuable time to allow the fetus to mature. The fetus should be monitored to detect signs of distress. Should intractable bleeding or fetal distress occur, the fetus must be delivered prematurely.

Abruptio placentae is managed according to the degree of severity and the gestational age. If the fetus is at term, delivery should be accomplished, usually induced by oxytocin. In the mild form of abruption, bedrest and monitoring of the fetus is the method of choice. Extension of a mild abruption to a more severe form is common, and the patient should be observed closely for increased pain or bleeding or both. A severe abruption demands immediate delivery by cesarean if the fetus is alive. A CVP catheter may be helpful in monitoring blood volume. Two large-bore intravenous catheters should be inserted, one for infusing crystalloids and medication and the other for infusing whole blood. Coagulopathy is common in severe abruption but is rapidly reversed after delivery of the fetus and placenta. A vaginal delivery of a dead fetus can be attempted if the patient's condition is stable.

PREGNANCY-INDUCED HYPERTENSION

Toxemia and preeclampsia-eclampsia are older terms for the current and more descriptive term pregnancy-induced hypertension. This disease is defined as hypertension with edema or proteinuria or both occurring after the 20th week of pregnancy. Hypertension is defined as a blood pressure above 140/90 mm Hg or a rise in systolic pressure of more than 30 mm Hg or in diastolic pressure of more than 15 mm Hg. Edema must be generalized and not dependent. Proteinuria is defined as more than 300 mg/24 hours). The diagnosis of severe pregnancy-induced hypertension requires one of the following: (1) a systolic blood pressure greater than 160 mm Hg, a diastolic blood pressure greater than 110 mm Hg, (2) proteinuria greater than 5 mg/24 hours, (3) oliguria (less than 400 ml/24 hours), (4) visual blurring or scotomas, (5) pulmonary edema or cyanosis, (6) severe thrombocytopenia or overt vascular hemolysis, (7) hepatocellular damage, and (8) epigastric or right upper quadrant pain or fetal growth retardation.

Pregnancy-induced hypertension is primarily a disease of the first pregnancy, occurring with higher frequency in the teenage and the older (older than 35 years) primigravida. Risk factors also include renal disease, pyelonephritis, diabetes mellitus, and a family history of hypertension.

CLINICAL SIGNS AND SYMPTOMS

One of the major objectives of prenatal care is to identify the impending pregnancy-induced hypertension patient. Often the first sign is a rapid weight gain (more than 6.6 kg per week), generalized edema being noted somewhat later. The blood pressure is then noted to be elevated above the baseline and is often labile in the

---

TABLE 106–2.
Clinical–Pathologic Correlations in Abortion and Placenta Previa

CLINICAL FINDINGS	PATHOLOGIC FINDINGS
In early stages may be asymptomatic	Hemorrhage into the decidua basalis from small maternal arterial vessels that show weakness in the medial layer. A thin layer of decidua is left on the myometrium and on the placenta.
Painless vaginal bleeding or in more severe cases lower abdominal pain (or back pain with a posteriorly implanted placenta)	Blood further splits the decidua and escapes to the vagina through the cervix or may remain trapped behind the placenta.
Fetal stress which may progress to fetal distress	Compromise in maternal-fetal exchange of gases and nutrients
Fetal distress	In some cases bleeding may be initiated from fetal placental vessels leading to elevated serum α-fetoprotein in the mother and, if more severe, an elevated fetal red cell count in maternal blood.

TABLE 106–3.
Clinical–Pathologic Correlations in Pregnancy-Induced Hypertension*

CLINICAL FINDINGS	PATHOLOGIC FINDINGS
Labile hypertension	Increased sensitivity of vasculature to pressor peptides and cathecholamines due to decreased production of E or I prostaglandins and eicosanoids
Rapid weight gain, edema	Decreased glomerular filtration rate secondary to swelling of intracapillary glomerular cells. Ability to excrete sodium is decreased.
Intrauterine growth retardation of fetus	Decreased uterine blood flow secondary to vascular spasm
Epigastric pain	Decreased hepatic blood flow with increased transaminase levels. "Swelling" of liver with tense Glisson's capsule in severe preeclampsia
Hemolysis and decreased platelet count	In severe disease and occasionally in patients with mild to moderate hypertension there is evidence of coagulopathy with intravascular platelet thrombi.
Convulsions (eclampsia), retinal hemorrhages. Exudates and papillary edema rare	Cerebral vasoconstriction, platelet thrombi in cerebral microcirculation

* From Lindheimer MD, Kat AT: Hypertension in pregnancy. *N Engl J Med* 1985; 313: 675.

early stages. Proteinuria is usually a late manifestation of the disease. Pregnancy-induced hypertension can be anticipated weeks in advance by the loss of resistance to angiotensin II infusion or by an elevated mean arterial pressure (more than 90 mm Hg) in mid-pregnancy.

Severe pregnancy-induced hypertension may result in epigastric pain, liver tenderness, visual disturbances, headache, obtunded sensorium, and dyspnea. Progressive hyperreflexia with clonus generally portends impending seizures (eclampsia).

PATHOPHYSIOLOGY

In normal pregnancy, the woman's arteries become more refractory to endogenous pressor peptides and catecholamines. Women with pregnancy-induced hypertension, for some unknown reason, have an intense sensitivity to these agents. This results in generalized peripheral vasospasm, increased peripheral resistance, hypertension, and decreased perfusion of organs such as the placenta and kidneys. The glomerular filtration rate is decreased because of swelling of the glomerular capillary endothelial cells (the pathognomonic lesion of pregnancy-induced hypertension). The ability to excrete sodium is also decreased, but the degree of impairment varies, and severe disease can occur in the absence of edema. One must remember that plasma volume is decreased and

hemoconcentration occurs even in the presence of interstitial edema. Eclampsia is attributed to the development of severe cerebral vasospasm and to platelet thrombi that obstruct the microcirculation.

DIAGNOSIS

The diagnosis of pregnancy-induced hypertension is usually straightforward: the blood pressure is elevated according to the above definition and is observed on two occasions more than 6 hours apart. Edema is more difficult to evaluate. Rings being tight on the finger and swelling of the hands and face upon arising in the morning are helpful signs. The urine should be checked for proteinuria throughout the course of hypertension because this phenomenon may be transient.

PRINCIPLES OF THERAPY

Hospitalization is often necessary once the diagnosis of pregnancy-induced hypertension is made. If the woman is at term, delivery of the fetus is the cure for the disease. Induction of labor, even with an unripe cervix, can result in the unexpected success of vaginal delivery. Mild pregnancy-induced hypertension can be expectantly managed in the preterm woman. Bedrest and careful monitoring of the fetus may result in a diuresis and ablation of the hypertension. Diuretics should not be given because these only compound the problem of hemoconcentration and poor peripheral circulation.

Severe pregnancy-induced hypertension is treated with strict bedrest, sedation, magnesium sulfate ($MgSO_4$) administration, and delivery. A 4-gm bolus of $MgSO_4$ is given intravenously over a 10-minute period. A maintenance dose of 2 to 3 gm/hour is required to achieve therapeutic levels of 4 to 7 mEq/L. Patellar reflexes should be checked every hour. These disappear at $MgSO_4$ levels of 8 to 10 mEq/L. A urine output of at least 25 ml/hour is required for adequate excretion of magnesium. If the diastolic blood pressure persists above 110 mm Hg, antihypertensive therapy in the form of hydralazine, 5 to 20 mg IV every hour, is given. This is one of the few antihypertensive medications studied that does not reduce uterine blood flow. Seizures are treated with intravenous diazepam (10 mg to 15 mg) or barbiturate (phenobarbital, 200 mg). Once the patient is stabilized, delivery is accomplished, usually by cesarean section. If, in the course of treatment, fetal distress is noted, immediate delivery is necessary.

REFERENCES

Chesley LL: *Hypertensive Disorders in Pregnancy.* New York, Appleton-Century-Crofts, 1978, p 628. *A scholarly and comprehensive dissertation on the subject with numerous references.*

Crenshaw C Jr, Jones DED, Parker RT: Placenta previa: A survey of twenty years' experience with improved survival by expectant therapy and cesarean delivery. *Obstet Gynecol Surv* 1973; 28:461. *One of the more extensive experiences with placenta previa.*

Lindheimer MD, Kat AT: Hypertension in pregnancy. *N Engl J Med* 1985; 313:675. *A concise current review of the subject.*

Lunan CB: The management of abruptio placentae. *J Obstet Gynaecol Br Commonw* 1973; 80:120. *A large case study recommending management to reduce perinatal mortality.*

Pritchard JA, MacDonald PC, Gant NF: *Williams Obstetrics,* ed 17. New York, Appleton-Century-Crofts, 1985, p 976. *An excellent, well-referenced, and up-to-date resource for general obstetric problems.*

Whittaker PG, Taylor A, Lind T: Unsuspected pregnancy loss in healthy women. *Lancet* 1983; 1:1126. *Pregnancy loss shortly after conception is identified on repeat BHCG assays in fertile women.*

107 MENOPAUSE AND CLIMACTERIC

John J. Halki, M.D., Ph.D.

Menopause is the time in a woman's life when menstruation ceases, whereas the climacteric is the period of life when the frequency of ovulation decreases and involution of the reproductive organs occurs. The climacteric period may span 30 to 40 years. The woman experiences diminished fertility, menopause, and symptoms of progressive aging and tissue atrophy. In the United States menopause occurs between the ages of 48 to 55 years with median age of 51.4 years. The climacteric period begins at approximately 40 years of age with gradually decreasing ovarian function. The primary factor in both the menopause and climacteric period is the decrease in estrogen production by the ovaries.

SIGNS AND SYMPTOMS

During the climacteric period, most women experience a variety of clinical manifestations. Early in the climacteric, at the time approaching menopause, a woman may complain of symptoms that are relatively acute (Table 107–1). Later in the climacteric period, following menopause, the symptoms or signs may be insidious and contribute to a diminished quality of life (Table 107–2).

As women approach menopause, the most common symptom is hot flashes, which occur in approximately 75% of women. This symptom is the hallmark of the climacteric. A hot flash, also called a hot flush, is a sudden sensation of heat that spreads over the upper body associated with a blushing of the skin and sudden sweating. Hot flashes usually occur during a 1- to 2-year period, but 25% to 50% of women may experience these symptoms for 5 or more years. The flashes frequently occur at night and may be of such severity as to impair sleep. Two other frequent symptoms related to the perimenopausal period are an irregularity or cessation of menses and insomnia.

The symptoms and signs of the middle to late stages of climacteric appear in the postmenopausal woman. As ovarian function is lost, the maturation process of estrogen-dependent tissue begins to wane. This results in atrophy of the vaginal epithelium which

TABLE 107–1.
Symptoms of the Early States of Climacteric

Hot flashes (vasomotor instability)
Menstrual dysfunction
Insomnia
Irritability
Lethargy/fatigue
Mood changes with crying spells
Worry
Anxiety
Depression
Decreased interpersonal relationships, especially with
  family members
Forgetfulness
Weight gain
Joint pain/backache
Palpitations
Constipation
Dysuria
Decreased or increased libido

often results in atrophic or senile vaginitis with symptoms of burning, pruritis, irritation, leukorrhea, and dyspareunia. Atrophic vaginitis accounts for approximately 15% of the cases of postmenopausal bleeding. The thinning of the vaginal epithelium parallels the lowering of estrogen levels and continues as the woman ages.

Atrophic changes in the urethra and bladder trigone may result in complaints of dysuria, urinary frequency, and stress incontinence.

The vulva undergoes atrophy characterized by dry, shriveled skin and often pruritis (kraurosis vulvae). A loss of the labia minora may occur by flattening into the surrounding skin or fusion to the labia majora. The introitus may become constricted, and the various vulva dystrophies may become evident.

The most disabling condition develops insidiously and is most prominent in the later postmenopausal period. This progressive condition is osteoporosis, a skeletal disorder due to a decrease in bone density. This disease state may result in shortening of stature due to compression fractures of the spine, particularly the thoracic vertebrae, and may be associated with severe back pain. This loss of height from approximately the waist upwards often leads to dorsal kyphosis or a dowager's hump. Twenty-five percent of Caucasian women over the age of 60 years have documented spinal fractures. Other osteoporotic fracture sites in these women are the distal forearm (Colles' fracture) and hip (fractures of the head of the femur). In the United States approximately 120,000 to 200,000 hip fractures occur annually in postmenopausal osteoporotic women. Hip fractures have a high risk of morbidity and mortality. Between 15% and 20% of women with hip fractures die due to complications from the fracture such as embolic, surgical, or cardiopulmonary sequelae. The survivor may be severely disabled and become an invalid.

Physical examination of the early climacteric woman in the premenopausal or immediate postmenopausal period will not reveal significant findings of lowered estrogen levels. Significant physical findings, however, are typically found later in the postmenopausal years. Frequently, the first sign is atrophic vaginitis. With loss of the normal vaginal rugae, the epithelium may appear dry, pale, cracked, and parchment-like with scattered hemorrhagic areas of varying degrees. The cervix may also have a similar pale and hemorrhagic appearance. The urethra may be inflamed, and a urethral caruncle is commonly present. Associated or later findings may be a drying or shrinking of the vulva with partial or complete disappearance of the labia minora. The labia majora may be smaller. There is constriction of the introitus especially in women who are not sexually active. Other findings are thinning of the pubic hair, the breasts are not as full, the nipples less erect, and the body figure is changed as fat is redistributed.

Physical changes due to postmenopausal osteoporosis are late findings in the climacteric process. Due to loss of trabecular bone density, there is a decrease in mobility, varying degrees of dorsal kyphosis, and a loss of height which may reach 4 to 5 inches. Height loss may be grossly estimated by measuring both the height and arm span. If the individual's span is substantially greater than the height, this usually indicates a loss of height. Back pain due to compression fractures of the vertebrae may be elicited on examination if there is acutely symptomatic osteoporosis.

TABLE 107–2.

Symptoms of the Middle to Late Stages of Climacteric

Atrophy of the vaginal epithelium resulting in atrophic or senile vaginitis
  Irritation
  Burning
  Pruritis
  Leukorrhea
  Dyspareunia
  Occasional vaginal bleeding
Atrophy of the urethra
  Dysuria
  Urinary frequency
  Cystitis with sterile urine cultures
  Urethral caruncles
  Noninflammatory urethritis
  Stress incontinence
Atrophy of the vulvar epithelium, which becomes thin and frequently irritated
  Vulvar dystrophies
  Introital constriction
  Loss of the labia minora or fusion with the labia majora
Postmenopausal osteoporosis
  Loss of height
  Dorsal kyphosis (dowager's hump)
  Compression fractures of the thoracic spine
  Forearm fractures (Colles' fractures)
  Hip fractures (head of femur)

CLINICAL–PATHOLOGIC CORRELATIONS (SEE TABLE 107–3.)

In the differential diagnosis of postmenopausal osteoporosis, one must rule out all other disease processes that can mimic this disease (Table 107–4). Women with osteoporosis should be examined for hypercortisolism, hyperthyroidism, hyperparathyroidism, neoplasms including metastatic carcinoma and multiple myeloma, diabetes mellitus, prolonged immobilization, and osteomalacia. The fasting urinary calcium-to-creatinine ratios may be significantly higher in postmenopausal women than in premenopausal women. Serum calcium and phosphate levels are usually normal. Carcinomatosis or osteomalacia are suspected if the alkaline phosphatase level is elevated. Parathyroid hormone levels are elevated in hyperparathyroidism but normal in postmenopausal osteoporosis. Thyroid function tests should be obtained if hyperthyroidism is suspected. In multiple myeloma, one should initially obtain serum and urine immunoglobulins.

DIAGNOSIS

Although the diagnosis of menopause is primarily made on the basis of clinical symptoms (i.e., hot flashes and a cessation of menses) the diagnosis can be confirmed by a pituitary gonadotropin assay of FSH and LH levels. In the first year following the last menses, evidence of ovarian failure is evidenced by an elevated FSH level of greater than 40 mIU/ml and an LH value within the normal adult range. Generally, 1 to 3 years after menopause, the levels of FSH and LH reach a maximum, with FSH levels of 100 mIU/ml or greater, and LH levels above 75 mIU/ml. Laboratory tests should only be used in conjunction with clinical findings. The diagnosis of premature menopause in a young woman may necessitate an ovarian biopsy. The ovarian biopsy, if postmenopausal, shows an absence of oocytes and follicles.

Suspicion of early osteoporosis may be confirmed by radiographic examination. The more precise radiographic techniques are com-

TABLE 107–3.
Clinical–Pathologic Correlations for Menopause and Climacteric

CLINICAL FINDINGS	PATHOLOGIC FINDINGS	
PREMENOPAUSE (EARLY CLIMACTERIC)		
Menstrual dysfunction	Ovaries become progressively refractory to FSH and LH stimulation	Ovarian follicles fail to mature
	Progressive degeneration of ovarian vasculature	Estrogen production insufficient to trigger ovulation but sufficient for endometrial proliferation
	Diminished numbers of FSH and LH receptors in ovaries	
Intervals of amenorrhea followed by heavy bleeding	Anovulation	No corpus luteum formed
Hot flashes		Unopposed estrogen may cause endometrial hyperplasia
MENOPAUSE		
Menstrual periods cease	Ovaries refractory to FSH and LH stimulation	Estrogen production insufficient for endometrial proliferation
Hot flashes		
Insomnia		
Irritability		
Lethargy/fatigue		
Mood changes		
Worry		
Anxiety		
Depression		
Decreased interpersonal relationships		
Forgetfulness		
Weight gain		
Joint pain/backache		
Palpitation		
Constipation		
Dysuria		
Decreased or increased libido		
POSTMENOPAUSE		
Vaginal burning	Ovaries totally refractive to FSH and LH	Increased levels of FSH and LH
Vaginal pruritis	Decreased serum levels of estrogen	Atrophy of urogenital structures
Vaginal irritation		Breast atrophy
Dyspareunia		Body fat redistribution
Leukorrhea		Thinning of pubic hair
Dysuria		
Frequency		
Stress incontinence		
Vulvar pruritis		
Back pain	Increased efflux of calcium from bone	Osteopenic
Loss of height		Decreased estrogen production
Dorsal kyphosis	Increased bone resorption	Osteoporosis
Distal forearm fracture (Colles' fracture)		
Hip fracture (head of femur)		

puter tomographic-quantitative osteoporosis analysis, single- or dual-photon absorptiometry, and densitometry. Standard x-ray films of the spine and bones of the appendages confirm only advanced bone loss and, therefore, are of extremely limited value.

PATHOPHYSIOLOGY

The decline in ovarian function is responsible for the clinical features of the menopause and climacteric period as well as the associated decreased steroidogenesis. The decreased steroidogenesis (primarily estrogen production) disturbs the pituitary-hypothalamic feedback mechanisms, which results in an increase in FSH and later LH levels and of the hypothalamic gonadotropin-releasing hormone (Gn-RH). Estrogen (estradiol) production by the ovaries does not continue beyond menopause. The estrogen level in the postmenopausal woman is primarily the result of extraglandular conversion of androstenedione to estrone. This estrogen milieu is less than that required for reproduction and with its progressive diminution throughout the climacteric woman's life eventually leads to a loss of vaginal and vulvar tissue turgor. Generalized atrophy of all estrogen-dependent tissues leads to the findings previously described.

The exact pathophysiology of postmenopausal osteoporosis is not well defined, except that the process is known to be associated with the decreased estrogen levels in the postmenopausal state. Certain contributory factors are associated with increased bone resorption in postmenopausal women (Table 107–5). The strength of bone results from a matrix principally of collagen combined with a crystalline hydroxyapatite containing calcium phosphate. In the postmenopausal woman, the decrease in calcium absorption and increase in calcium excretion are major factors contributing to a negative calcium balance. The primary abnormality is osteopenia due to proportionate losses of minerals to organic matrix, leading to mechanical fragility and the potential of subsequent compression and traumatic fractures (Table 107–3).

The relationships among estrogen, calcium, parathyroid hormone, and vitamin D in postmenopausal women have not been con-

TABLE 107–4.
Differential Diagnosis of Postmenopausal Osteoporosis

Diabetes mellitus
Hypercortisolism
   Cushing's syndrome
   Corticosteroid administration
Hyperthyroidism
Hyperparathyroidism
Neoplasm
   Metastatic carcinoma
   Multiple myeloma
Osteomalacia
Prolonged immobilization

TABLE 107–5.
Contributory Factors Associated with Increased Bone Resorption in Postmenopausal Women

Family history of osteoporosis
Status nulligravida
Aging
Lack of exercise
Cigarette smoking
Alcohol consumption
Genetic variables
   Small bones or low bone mass
   Caucasian or Oriental
Change in calcium metabolism
   Diet deficient in calcium and vitamin D
   Calcium malabsorption
Change in estrogen balance

clusively demonstrated nor do they explain the mechanism by which estrogen or its absence affects skeletal bone. Estrogen receptors have not been found in bone, and there is no evidence that physiologic amounts of estrogen can directly influence bone. For these reasons it is assumed that estrogen exerts an indirect action on the skeleton by possibly interacting in some manner involving the control of calcium metabolism. The most convenient hypothesis (Lindsay and Tohmé, 1987) for the action of estrogens on bone assumes that estrogen stimulates the production of endogenous calcitonin (Fig 107–1). The primary skeletal effect of calcitonin is to reduce bone resorption by osteoclast inhibition whereas the primary defect in osteoporosis is the increased bone resorption. It has been reported that estrogen increases plasma calcitonin in women.

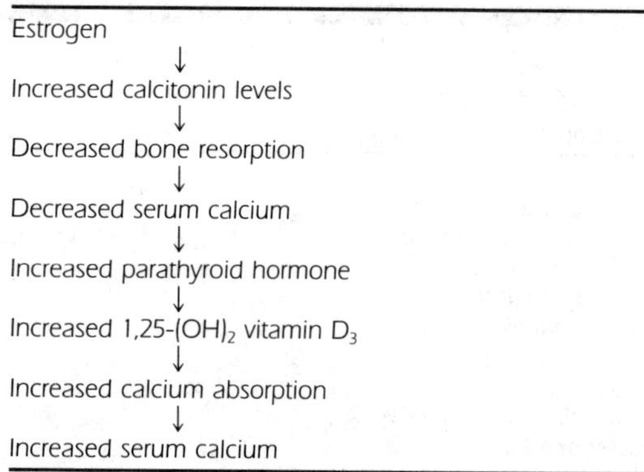

FIG 107–1.
Biochemical action of estrogen on bone: Current hypothesis of Lindsay and Tohmé (Adapted from Lindsay R, Tohmé JF: Alterations in skeletal homeostasis with age and menopause, in Mishell DR Jr (ed): *Menopause: Physiology and Pharmacology.* Chicago, Year Book Medical Publishers, 1987, p 87.)

PRINCIPLES OF THERAPY

Menopause per se does not require therapy. The major symptoms such as hot flashes and estrogen-dependent tissue atrophy can be alleviated or prevented by estrogen replacement therapy. Currently, the most common estrogen used for this purpose is the conjugated natural estrogen whose major components are sulfates or esters of estrone, equilin, and 17α-dihydroequilin. This estrogen is used either continuously or cyclically. With either mode of therapy, a progestin such as medroxyprogesterone acetate should be administered in conjunction with the estrogen to counter and reduce the adverse effect of tissue stimulation by estrogen only. The combined estrogen-progestin therapy also has substantial benefits in the prevention or slowing of the osteoporotic process. In addition, calcium intake must be maintained or increased if the daily calcium intake is insufficient. The daily recommended amount of calcium after menopause is 1500 mg daily. Because the diets of most women over 50 years of age are deficient in calcium, supplemental calcium may be necessary to ensure that the daily requirement is met.

REFERENCES

Edman CD. The climacteric, in Buchsbaum HJ (ed): *The Menopause.* New York, Springer-Verlag, 1983, pp 23–33. *Good overview.*

Estrogen replacement therapy. *ACOG Technical Bull,* Washington, DC, American College of Obstetrics and Gynecology, Inc, 1986; 93:1–5. *A concensus statement.*

Jones HW Jr, Jones GS: Management of the menopause, in *Novak's Textbook of Gynecology,* ed 10. Baltimore, Williams & Wilkins Co, 1981, pp 797–816. *A detailed discussion of therapy.*

Lindsay R, Tohmé JF: Alterations in skeletal homeostasis with age and menopause, in Mishell DR Jr (ed): *Menopause: Physiology and Pharmacology.* Chicago, Year Book Medical Publishers, 1987, pp 77–90. *A concise up-to-date discussion.*

Lobo RA, Brenner PF, Mishell DR Jr: Metabolic parameters and steroid levels in postmenopausal women receiving lower doses of natural estrogen replacement. *Obstet Gynecol* 1983; 62:94–98. *The effects of steroid replacement are studied.*

MacKay EV, Beischer NA, Cox LW, Wood C: Menopause and climacteric, in *Illustrated Textbook of Gynecology.* Artarmon, Australia, WB Saunders Co, 1983, pp 85–94. *A concise discussion.*

Osteoporosis. *ACOG Technical Bull,* Washington, DC, American College of Obstetrics and Gynecology, Inc, 1983; 72:1–5. *A concensus statement.*

Pak, CYC: Postmenopausal osteoporosis, in Buchsbaum HJ (ed): *The Menopause.* New York, Springer-Verlag, 1983, pp 35–54. *A detailed review of this major health problem.*

Shawky ZA, Badawy MD: Understanding the changes of menopause. *The Female Patient,* Secaucus, New Jersey. 1985; 10:66–74. *A discussion of pathophysiology.*

Speroff L, Glass RH, Kase NG: The ovary from conception to senescence, in *Clinical Gynecologic Endocrinology and Infertility,* ed 3. Baltimore, Williams & Wilkins Co, 1982, pp 101–140. *A detailed review of the ovary and its function.*

UTERINE CARCINOMA

Max A. Clark, D.O.

Cancer of the uterus is typically divided into two categories: cancer of the uterine corpus and cancer of the cervix.

CANCER OF THE UTERINE CORPUS

Today cancer of the endometrium is the most commonly encountered cancer of the female genital tract. About 2.4% of newborn white females and about 1.3% of newborn black females born in 1985 will be expected to develop endometrial cancer within their lifetimes. About 37,000 new cases will develop and approximately 3,000 will die annually. Approximately 75% to 80% of these uterine tumors occur in the postmenopausal years. Another 15% to 20% occur in the perimenopausal years, and about 5% of endometrial carcinoma occurs in patients under the age of 40 years.

CLINICAL SIGNS AND SYMPTOMS

Perimenopausal or postmenopausal bleeding is usually the first symptom of endometrial cancer. Any postmenopausal woman with vaginal bleeding is considered to have endometrial cancer until proven otherwise. Premenopausal bleeding that is abnormal in amount or timing needs to be investigated. This applies even to the patient who is bleeding from an obvious vaginal or cervical lesion, because more than one disease can be present simultaneously. A systematic and thorough investigation is required to delineate the source of the bleeding.

PATHOPHYSIOLOGY

Histologically 90% are adenocarcinomas; malignant tumors of the glandular epithelium. Other subtypes include adenoacanthomas, adenosquamous, clear cell, papillary, secretory adenocarcinoma, and mucinous adenocarcinoma. Adenoacanthomas with proliferation of benign squamous elements associated with an adenocarcinoma, and adenosquamous carcinomas with proliferation of malignant squamous elements associated with an adenocarcinoma are stage for stage not more aggressive than ordinary endometrial adenocarcinomas. Evidence suggests that papillary, secretory, and the rare mucinous adenocarcinomas may be more aggressive than adenocarcinoma of the endometrium and, thus, may need more aggressive therapy. Uterine sarcomas, tumors of mesenchymal origin in the myometrium or endometrium, comprise about 5% of all uterine tumors (Table 108–1).

The typical endometrial cancer spreads by direct extension into the uterine wall where it enters the lymphatic vessels. From there it may spread either along the infundibulopelvic ligament or by direct extension to the periaortic lymph nodes or the uterine cervix. Once the disease is no longer confined, it usually spreads rapidly and widely. Common sites for metastases are the lung, brain, skeleton, and abdominal viscera.

It is generally felt that the prolonged use of

TABLE 108–1.
Uterine Cancers: Histologic Classification

Adenocarcinoma
Adenocanthoma
Adenosquamous carcinoma
Clear cell carcinoma
Papillary carcinoma
Secretory carcinoma
Mucinous carcinoma
Undifferentiated carcinoma
Uterine sarcomas

an exogenous estrogen without a progestational agent increases a woman's risk of having endometrial cancer. When cyclical progesterone is added, the incidence of endometrial cancer drops to nonuser levels. Progestin use along with a regular gynecologic examination and periodic endometrial sampling should virtually eliminate mortality from endometrial cancer.

In patients who do not take exogenous estrogen, but develop endometrial cancer, unopposed estrogen secretion has been implicated as an etiologic agent. Because about 10% of the cases of estrogen-secreting ovarian tumors have been associated with cancer of the endometrium, there is some indirect support for this theory. In other cases, estrogen-secreting ovarian tumors are associated with uterine hyperplasia which is probably a precursor of endometrial cancer. A potent source of unopposed estrogen in some postmenopausal females is the conversion of adrenal androstenedione, to estrone in the liver and body fat. Estrone, a weak estrogen, can be converted to a potent estrogen, estradiol, by the endometrial cells. This conversion is increased in the postmenopausal woman. Other risk factors for endometrial carcinoma include menopause after age 52 years, obesity, hypertension, nulliparity, and diabetes, but these factors are most likely not causative. They frequently occur in conjunction with hypothalamic-pituitary axis abnormalities that lead to anovulation and unopposed estrogen secretion by the ovaries.

CLINICAL–PATHOLOGIC CORRELATIONS

Abnormal vaginal bleeding is the most common symptom of endometrial cancer. In advanced stages with diffused peritoneal spread massive ascites may cause pressure phenomena or pain (Table 108–2). Also, diffuse peritoneal metastases may lead to bowel obstruction, partial or complete, which can cause nutrition and electrolyte disturbances. Distant metastases to the skeleton may result in severe bone pain and lung metastases may produce pleural effusions.

DIAGNOSIS

Abnormal vaginal bleeding demands proper evaluation including endometrial sampling usually by fractional dilatation and curettage. Ultrasound, magnetic resonance imaging, and computerized tomography do not replace histologic sampling. Thus, negative noninvasive procedures do not rule out an endometrial cancer in patients with abnormal bleeding. Abnormal bleeding patterns in perimenopausal women should be viewed with a high index of suspicion. A careful history should be taken,

TABLE 108–2.
Clinical–Pathologic Correlations for Endometrial Carcinoma

CLINICAL FINDINGS	STAGE	PATHOLOGIC FINDINGS
Usually age > 40 yr; prolonged menses or intermenstrual spotting; perimenopausal menstrual; postmenopausal bleeding from the vagina	I	Tumor limited to uterus
	a	Length of uterine cavity—8 cm or less
	b	Length of uterine cavity—greater than 8 cm
	II	Tumor involves the cervix
	III	Tumor extends outside the uterus, but not outside the pelvis
Usually age > 40 yr; prolonged menses or intermenstrual spotting; perimenopausal menstrual incgs; postmenopausal bleeding from the vagina; ascites; pleural effusion; pain	IV	Tumor involves the bladder or rectum or extends outside the pelvis

and a pelvic examination should be performed with a Pap smear. Although the Pap smear can reveal endometrial cancer, a normal Pap smear and normal physical findings do not rule out endometrial cancer.

The best way to detect the disease is by fractional dilatation and curettage, which assesses what is in the endometrial cavity and whether cancer, if present, has involved the cervix. This procedure also helps differentiate adenocarcinoma of the endocervical canal from endometrial carcinoma. Cystoscopy, proctoscopy, and intervenous pyelography contribute little to the diagnostic evaluation and are not cost effective. Their use should be restricted unless pelvic examination indicates possible spread of the disease. Also of limited value are hysteroscopy and lymphangiography.

PRINCIPLES OF TREATMENT

The 5-year survival rate of patients with stage I endometrial carcinoma (tumor is confined to the uterine cavity) who receive prompt, accurate staging and contemporary treatment approaches 85% to 95%. Worldwide, however, the 5-year survival rate is only about 75% for stage I. The usual treatment for both stage Ia and Ib disease is total abdominal hysterectomy and bilateral salpingo-oophorectomy with peritoneal cytologic studies, palpation of the contents of the entire abdomen, and sampling of the periaortic and pelvic lymph nodes. After removal, the uterus is evaluated for tumor penetration of the myometrium and the histologic grade of the tumor. Grade I is the most differentiated and least aggressive, and grade III is the least differentiated and the most aggressive. If the tumor has not penetrated more than a third of the myometrial wall, if the tumor has not spread to the cervix, lymph nodes, or pelvic structures, if peritoneal cytologic washings during surgery are negative, and if the histologic grade is less than III, no further treatment is given to stage I, Ia, or Ib tumors. In stage Ia or Ib with grade III lesions, or with tumor penetration of the myometrial wall greater than the inner third, adjuvant pelvic radiation is recommended via external beam, following the surgery. Some also recommend treating histologic grade II endometrial cancers with postoperative external beam therapy. If the endometrial cancer involves the cervix (stage II),

preoperative or postoperative radiation accompanies hysterectomy and bilateral salpingo-oophorectomy as well as sampling the periaortic lymph nodes. Other centers treat stage II disease with radical surgery or full course radiation therapy. The value of preoperative versus postoperative radiation is controversial, but the general trend is away from preoperative radiation.

Stage III and IV lesions must be considered individually. Treatment may involve various combinations of surgery, radiation, chemotherapy, and progestins.

CANCER OF THE UTERINE CERVIX

Ninety-five percent of invasive cancers of the cervix are squamous cell carcinomas, with adenocarcinomas making up the remaining 5%. About 7,000 women die of cervical cancer and about 16,000 new cases are reported each year in the United States. Since 1945, mortality has declined from 15 to 6 per 100,000, and the incidence has dropped from 12 to about 6 per 100,000.

CLINICAL SIGNS AND SYMPTOMS

Cervical cancer produces no symptoms in its early stages. This underscores the key role played by the pelvic examination and Pap smear in detecting and diagnosing the disease. In the more advanced stages complaints of postcoital spotting, frank vaginal bleeding without any predictable frequency, serous vaginal discharge, cachexia, leg edema, and pain are not unusual.

Untreated, the cancer spreads and a pelvic mass may cause ureteral obstruction. Death usually results from the loss of kidney function, hemorrhage, or infection.

PATHOPHYSIOLOGY

Carcinoma of the cervix typically spreads by direct extension into the parametrial or vaginal fornices. Lymph node metastases are common and increase with the stage of the disease (Table 108–3). If the pelvic tumor continues to grow, bilateral ureteral obstruction may ensue, and death follows from uremia unless a ureterostomy or nephrostomy is performed.

TABLE 108–3.
Clinical–Pathologic Correlations for Cervical Carcinoma

CLINICAL FINDINGS	STAGE	PATHOLOGIC FINDINGS
	I	Tumor confined to cervix
Abnormal Pap smear	a	Microinvasion
Abnormal Pap smear	Ib occult	Invsasion not recognized clinically
Abnormal Pap smear	b	All other cancers of cervix
Abnormal Pap smear; vaginal bleeding	IIa	Involvement of upper 2/3 of vagina
Abnormal Pap smear	IIb	Involvement of parametria but not to side wall
Abnormal Pap smear; vaginal bleeding	IIIa	Involvement of the lower 1/3 of the vagina
Abnormal Pap smear; vaginal bleeding; ureteral obstruction; pelvic pressure	IIIb	Parametrial involvement to pelvic side wall
Abnormal Pap smear; vaginal bleeding; ureteral obstruction; pelvic pressure with pain	IVa	Involvement of bladder or rectum
Abnormal Pap smear; vaginal bleeding; ureteral obstruction; pelvic pressure with pain	IVb	Distant metastases outside pelvis

Distant metastases may involve the peritoneum, lung, and pelvic nerve plexi. It may also spread to the bony pelvis and to the vertebrae.

CLINICAL–PATHOLOGIC CORRELATIONS

The clinical–pathologic correlations are listed in Table 108–3. Other than an abnormal Pap smear, no early signs are seen. Recently, great interest has been generated in the human papilloma viruses, especially types 16 and 18. These viruses cause condolomata on the uterine cervix and external genitalia. When hysterectomy specimens with severe dysplasia (carcinoma in situ) are carefully reviewed condolomata are often seen adjacent to the dysplasia. In biopsy specimens from women with histologic dysplasia evidence of human papilloma virus infection is reported in about 25%. Other possible etiologic agents have been implicated such as the herpes type II virus, and the effect of a histone or protamine from sperm degradation on the cervical squamous epithelium of the cervix. However, there is no clear documentation that herpes virus, protamines, or histones cause cervical cancer. The same is true of the human papilloma virus, but accumulating evidence suggests more than a casual relationship with this virus.

Epidemiologically, the two most important risk factors for developing carcinoma of the cervix are multiple sexual partners and intercourse before the age of 20 years. These patients merit a careful annual evaluation and Pap smear.

DIAGNOSIS

A Pap smear for detecting cervical cancer should be a part of the routine gynecologic examination of women of childbearing potential. The recommended frequency of the examination, including a Pap smear, is yearly. Some have encouraged that Pap smears be taken in low risk populations about every 3 years. About 1 in 10,000 patients will not be detected by this procedure, but some studies have reported the false-negative rate for Pap smears to range from 15% to 40% in some laboratories. Consequently, most gynecologists still recommend a yearly Pap smear. Abnormal Pap smears should be investigated by colposcopy and biopsy of the abnormal areas. The colposcope can also identify epithelial abnormalities of the cervix in preinvasive or early invasive lesions that are not visible on pelvic examination.

If colposcopic-directed biopsies fail to explain an abnormal Pap smear, repeated biopsies or conizytion of the cervix is the next diagnostic step. In more advanced cases, eroded or ulcerated areas and indurated or exophytic areas may signify cervical cancer. A biopsy of any suspicious lesion is important.

PRINCIPLES OF TREATMENT

The goal of treatment of cervical dysplasia is to eradicate all abnormal cervical epithelial surfaces. Treatment may include biopsy, cryocautery, electrocautery, laser therapy, conization, or hysterectomy. Untreated cervical dysplasia may progress to cervical cancer.

Stages I and IIa invasive cervical carcinoma may be treated by radical surgery or by radiation therapy. The 5-year survival rates for both methods are similar in stage I disease, but the 5-year survival rate for stage IIa disease is higher with radiation therapy.

Large, bulky stage Ib cervical carcinomas or endophytic lesions that create the so-called barrel-shaped cervix are best treated with radiation and surgery. The hysterectomy is preceded with external and intracavitary radiation.

Stage IIb, IIIa, and IIIb cancers are treated by radiation therapy after the patient has undergone retroperitoneal lymph node dissection to ascertain the extent of the tumor. Stage IVa cervical cancer may be cured by a pelvic exenteration. Between 30% and 35% of patients with advanced cervical cancer respond to chemotherapy, but overall survival is poor and responders do not live longer than nonresponders. Thus, surgery and radiation are the mainstays of treatment for cervical carcinoma.

REFERENCES

Coppelson N (ed): *Gynecologic Oncology: Fundamental Principles and Clinical Practice*. New York, Churchill Livingstone, 1981. *A very comprehensive text, in two volumes, that discusses all aspects in depth of gyncecologic-oncology.*

DiSia J, Creasman WT: *Clinical Gynecologic Oncology*. St. Louis, The C.V. Mosby Co., 1984, pp 146–192. *Written for the student, resident, and practicing clinician alike, this readable text reviews all aspects of gynecologic cancer including treatment, immunology, and complications.*

Gambrell RD: Preventing endometrial cancer with progestin. *Contemp Obstet/Gynecol* 1981; 17: 133–143. *One of the early articles dealing with the addition of progestin to estrogen regimens in postmenopausal females.*

Rubin P, Bakemeier R, Krachov S: *Clinical Oncology: A Multidisciplinary Approach*. Rochester NY, American Cancer Society, 1983, pp 444–454. *A paperback review of cancer prepared for student and clinician alike.*

Silverberg E: Cancer statistics, 1985. *CA-A Journal for Clinicians* 1985; 35:19–36. *A review of the occurrence and death rates for cancer patients in the US prepared from American Cancer Society and US vital statistics.*

109 OVARIAN CARCINOMA

William A. Nahhas, M.D.

Carcinoma of the ovary occurs in approximately 8 of every 100,000 women worldwide and is the third most common female genital malignancy. Ten to 15 of every 1,000 women over the age of 40 years will develop ovarian carcinoma, and only 2 of every 10 will be cured. Only 8% of ovarian tumors occur in women under the age of 35 years. Ovarian cancer is the number one killer among genital tumors in women and is exceeded in mortality statistics only by breast, colon, and lung cancer. Each year in the United States, approximately 18,000 women will develop ovarian cancer, and 11,000 will die of this disease. Twenty percent of women with ovarian carcinoma have had prior pelvic surgery, including a hysterectomy without removal of the ovaries. The most common ovarian tumors are of the epithelial variety including serous, mucinous, endometroid, and clear cell carcinomas. Gonadal stromal tumors, germ cell tumors, and metastatic carcinomas are less common and will not be discussed in this chapter.

CLINICAL SIGNS AND SYMPTOMS

Epithelial ovarian carcinoma is an intra-abdominal disease with an insidious onset. Consequently there are no specific diagnostic early signs or symptoms. As the pelvic tumor enlarges and as metastatic deposits in the upper abdomen grow, the patient will complain of nonspecific gastrointestinal symptoms such as bloating, easy satiety, and postprandial discomfort, constipation, pelvic pressure, or increasing abdominal girth. Occasionally the patient may feel an abdominal or inguinal mass. Difficulty in breathing can occur due to abdominal distension or to pleural effusion. Some patients may develop swelling of the lower extremities.

A pelvic or abdominal mass with or without the presence of ascites should alert the physician to the diagnosis of ovarian carcinoma. Vaginal bleeding is not a common occurrence with hormonally inert ovarian tumors. Inguinal lymphadenopathy and lower extremity edema may be present.

If left untreated, ovarian carcinoma produces increasing ascites and enlarging pelvic and abdominal masses, causing intra-abdominal pressure, intestinal obstruction, inanition, cachexia, and eventually death.

PATHOPHYSIOLOGY

Epithelial tumors of the ovary may be of the serous, mucinous, endometroid, or clear cell variety. These tumors may involve one or both ovaries causing enlargement, irregularity, and surface excrescences. The ovaries can become densely adherent to the pelvic peritoneum and other pelvic structures. Ovarian carcinoma commonly metastasizes to the omentum causing a large upper-abdominal mass. The tumor can also implant on all intra-abdominal peritoneal surfaces including the undersurface of the diaphragm and the serosa and mesentery of the bowel. The gastrointestinal tract is the organ whose function is most commonly affected by ovarian carcinoma, resulting in obstruction of the small or large bowel. The disease can spread to pelvic and para-aortic lymph nodes and can occasionally obstruct the ureters or cause pressure on the urinary bladder. Patients with advanced ovarian carcinoma suffer from malnutrition and cachexia. Pleural effusion can cause breathing difficulties.

CLINICAL–PATHOLOGIC CORRELATIONS

The generally accepted stages of ovarian carcinoma with their clinical correlations are shown in Table 109–1.

DIFFERENTIAL DIAGNOSIS

Any pelvic mass can be ovarian carcinoma. The most common differential diagnosis is between ovarian carcinoma, benign adnexal masses, uterine fibroids, and diverticulosis. A

TABLE 109–1.
Clinical–Pathologic Correlations for Carcinoma of the Ovary

CLINICAL FINDINGS	STAGE	PATHOLOGIC FINDINGS
Pressure symptoms or palpable mass if tumor is large; pain if tumor twists or infarcts; hemoperitoneum if tumor ruptures	I	Growth limited to ovaries
	IA	Growth limited to one ovary, no ascites 1. No tumor on external surface, capsule intact 2. Tumor present on external surface and/or capsule ruptured
Pressure symptoms or palpable mass if tumor is large; pain if tumor twists or infarcts; hemoperitoneum if tumor ruptures	IB	Growth limited to both ovaries, no ascites 1. No tumor on external surface, capsule intact 2. Tumor present on external surface and/or capsule ruptured
If amount of tumor or ascites is large: abdominal distention, gastrointestinal dysfunction, difficult breathing, palpable mass	IC	Tumor either stage IA or IB, but with ascites or peritoneal washings positive for malignant cells
Similar to stage I; rarely uterine bleeding	II	Growth involving one or both ovaries with pelvic extension
	IIA	Extension and/or metastases to the uterus and/or fallopian tubes
	IIB	Extension to other pelvic tissues including the pelvic colon
	IIC	Tumor either stage IIA or IIB but with ascites or peritoneal washings positive for malignant cells
Abdominal distention, ascites, gastrointestinal or urinary dysfunction, palpable pelvic or abdominal mass, difficult breathing, leg edema; rarely uterine bleeding	III	Growth involving one or both ovaries with intraperitoneal metastases outside the pelvis and/or positive retroperitoneal nodes or with tumor limited to the true pelvis with histologically proven malignant extension to small bowel, omentum, or abdominal colon
Evidence of extra-abdominal metastases; vaginal bleeding; pleural effusion and breathing difficulty	IV	Growth involving one or both ovaries with distant metastases. If pleural effusion is present, there must be positive cytology of the pleural fluid. Parenchymal liver metastases equals stage IV.

pelvic kidney may be present rarely and may be felt as a pelvic mass.

DIAGNOSIS

Standard gynecologic screening techniques are not successful in the early diagnosis of ovarian cancer. Even though careful annual or semiannual examination is important, only one otherwise unsuspected ovarian cancer can be detected in 10,000 routine examinations. Liberal indications for prophylactic oophorectomy at the time of hysterectomy in women over 40 years are suggested.

The normal postmenopausal ovary should not be larger than $1.5 \times 1 \times 0.5$ cm and should not be palpable during routine pelvic examination. Therefore, a "normal-sized" or palpable ovary in a postmenopausal woman should be suspected of malignancy until surgically proven otherwise. Cervicovaginal cytologic smears may aid in the successful diagnosis of ovarian cancer in less than 5% of cases, and only when a uterus is present. In such cases, the disease is usually advanced at the time of diagnosis. Culdocentesis with aspiration of fluid from the pelvis is subject to the same drawback. Neither routine ultrasonography nor computed tomography (CT scanning) have provided conclusive diagnostic data. Recent monoclonal antibody studies are still experimental but may offer some hope for the future. An epithelial ovarian tumor antigen (CA 125) is currently under study. Detection of this antigen in serum may hold promise for early diagnosis and for follow-up after therapy. At present, periodic examination with prompt investigation of an abnormal ovary or of the presence of ascites continues to be the best diagnostic course.

Once a pelvic or abdominal mass is detected, further diagnostic tests are usually unnecessary even though intestinal x-ray films and an intravenous pyelogram are often performed. Preoperative evaluation consists of an electrocardiogram, chest x-ray films, and blood studies including measurement of serum electrolytes and liver and renal function tests. A liver scan may be indicated. Endoscopic examinations of the bladder and colon are rarely necessary. The definitive diagnosis and staging are usually made at the time of surgical exploration. Occasionally the diagnosis can be suspected if malignant cells are detected in pleural or abdominal fluid removed prior to surgery. Rarely, the diagnosis is made by biopsy of an enlarged inguinal lymph node.

PRINCIPLES OF PREVENTION AND THERAPY

The etiologic role of viruses, nutrition, environment, socioeconomic-cultural factors, genetics, familial tendencies, and psychic stress have been studied. No specific etiologic agents or circumstances have been uncovered for the development of ovarian cancer. Because the incidence of ovarian cancer is lower in women who have taken birth control tablets and in those of high parity, prolonged periods of anovulation appear to offer some protection against this disease.

Carcinoma of the ovary is most often detected when there is extensive intra-abdominal spread (stage III). Less often, the tumor can be found while confined to one or both ovaries (stage I) or with pelvic extension (stage II). Surgery is usually the initial approach and should be directed toward removing the maximum amount of tumor without compromising vital organs or creating life-threatening complications. The goal is to leave no visible or palpable tumor or to leave tumor masses less than 1 to 2 cm in diameter (optimal tumor-reductive surgery). Such surgery usually includes a total abdominal hysterectomy, bilateral salpingo-oophorectomy, omentectomy, and resection of large intra-abdominal tumor masses along with thorough surgical staging of the disease. Rarely, resection of portions of the bowel and bladder may be necessary for optimal surgical results. Ascitic fluid or peritoneal washings should be studied for the presence of malignant cells especially in the earlier stages. The presence of malignant cells in such situations can change the stage classification and, therefore, the therapy and prognosis.

Following maximal tumor-reductive surgery, courses of chemotherapy are administered for 6 to 12 months. Postoperative radiation therapy or intra-abdominal radioactive colloids may occasionally be used. The usual drug combinations for chemotherapy contain an alkylating agent (cyclophosphamide), an anthracycline (doxorubicin), and a platinum derivative (cisplatin). If the patient is clinically free of dis-

TABLE 109–2.
Principles of Therapy

1. Surgery alone usually does not cure the majority of patients with epithelial ovarian carcinoma.
2. Ovarian tumors are sensitive to various chemotherapeutic agents.
3. The effectiveness of chemotherapy is inversely related to the residual tumor burden.
4. Maximum tumor-reductive surgery is necessary to increase the response to chemotherapy.
5. Second-look laparotomy after completion of chemotherapy may be necessary to evaluate the response to treatment.

ease at the end of chemotherapy, a "second-look" laparotomy may be necessary to assess the intra-abdominal status of the tumor (Table 109–2).

The decision to manage stage IA ovarian carcinoma conservatively by unilateral oophorectomy must be based on careful evaluation and requires that stage IA be proven by thorough surgical staging. The tumor should be of borderline potential for malignancy or be a well-differentiated, pure cell type. The woman should be young, of low parity with informed desire for future reproduction. In addition, the carcinoma should be unruptured, less than 10 cm in diameter, and without surface excrescences, extensions, or adhesions. There should be no invasion of the tumor capsule or mesovarium, and ascites should be absent. Pelvic washings should contain no malignant cells. The contralateral ovary and the pelvic and para-aortic lymph nodes should be free of disease.

The cure rate of 20% to 30% has only mar-ginally increased through aggressive surgery and chemotherapy; however, this combination has increased the average symptom-free survival rate from about 1 year to 3 years. Most patients who undergo aggressive surgery followed by chemotherapy will be clinically free of disease at the end of treatment. Unfortunately, a large number are found to have persistent carcinoma at the time of second-look laparotomy. Even in this group, additional symptom-free survival time can be achieved by further chemotherapeutic treatment. The few patients who are found to be free of disease at the time of the second look may be cured. However, further follow-up will show that approximately 25% to 30% of the patients free of detectable disease at the time of a second look will develop further recurrent carcinoma. This recurrence rate may further increase with time; therefore, the management of patients following second-look laparotomy remains controversial and is currently the subject of clinical trials.

REFERENCES

Barber HRK, Graber EA: The PMPO syndrome. *Obstet Gynecol* 1971; 38(6):921–923. *A discussion of the importance of pelvic examination in postmenopausal women.*

Barber HRK, Graber EA, Kwon TH: Ovarian cancer. *CA* 1974; 24:339–350. *An overview of the disease.*

Creasman WT, Park R, Norris H, DiSaia PJ, Morrow CP, Hreshchyshyn MM: Stage I borderline ovarian tumors. *Obstet Gynecol* 1982; 59(1):93–96. *A description of the good prognosis of low-grade malignancies.*

DiSaia PJ, Creasman WT: The adnexal mass and early ovarian cancer. Advanced epithelial ovarian cancer, in DiSaia PJ, Creasman WT: *Clinical Gynecologic Oncology.* St Louis, CV Mosby Co, 1984, pp 254–285, 286–361. *A thorough review of diagnosis and treatment.*

Hacker NF, Berek JS, LaGasse LD, Nieberg RK, Elashoff RM: Primary cytoreductive surgery for epithelial ovarian cancer. *Obstet Gynecol* 1983; 61(4):413–420. *A review of the importance of aggressive tumor-reductive surgery.*

Lewis JL, Griffiths T, Morrow CP, Wharton T: Managing ovarian cancer: The second-look operation. *Contemp Obstet Gynecol* 1978; 12:137–155. *A discussion of the rationale for second-look laparotomy.*

Silverberg BS, Lubera JA: A review of American Cancer Society estimates of cancer cases and deaths. *CA* 1983; 33(1):2–26. *A review of incidence and death rates.*

part IX

Eye and Ear Disorders

COMMON SYMPTOMS OF OTOLOGIC DISEASE

Robert A. Goldenberg, M.D.

Otologic disease is an abnormal condition of the outer, middle, or inner ear. Six primary symptoms will be discussed: otalgia, otorrhea, hearing loss, vertigo, tinnitus, and facial paralysis. These symptoms will be correlated with the associated pathologic conditions.

CLINICAL SIGNS AND SYMPTOMS

OTALGIA

Otalgia may be sudden or long-standing. The sudden pain of acute otitis media is accompanied by fever, malaise, or an upper respiratory tract infection. The tympanic membrane is bright red, bulging, and demonstrates a loss of the normal landmarks. If the pain subsides abruptly and the ear begins to drain, the tympanic membrane has usually ruptured. Sudden otalgia may also be caused by an outer ear infection, in which the walls of the canal are swollen and edematous, and the tympanic membrane may not be visualized. A small furuncle or pimple in the outer ear may be missed by introducing the otoscope without first directly examining the outer canal. Long-standing pain may be associated with chewing in the presence of temporomandibular joint neuralgia. Crepitation over the joint may indicate this arthritic condition. Trauma, insect bites, or cotton-swab injuries must always be considered. The possibility of referred pain from the neck, larynx, or base of the tongue demands that these areas be carefully examined, especially for occult malignancy.

OTORRHEA

Otorrhea may be abrupt from a perforation of the tympanic membrane or otitis externa such as swimmer's ear. Drainage may also be long-standing with a chronic perforation of the tympanic membrane, osteomyelitis of the mastoid bone, or a cholesteatoma. Duration, increase or decrease in severity, odor, color, consistency, and amount of drainage are important considerations. A cholesteatoma may look like a simple perforation. It is actually an invaginated skin cyst growing into the middle ear and the mastoid cells that is filled with white cheese-like keratin. The tympanic membrane is usually quite scarred and shows a loss of the normal landmarks. The external auditory canal may be filled with debris or cerumen and must be cleaned to visualize the entire tympanic membrane in all cases in which these symptoms exist.

HEARING LOSS

Hearing loss may be sudden or gradual in onset, unilateral or bilateral, total or partial, fluctuating, progressive, or stable. Often the patient is not aware of the problem but is brought to the physician by a family member. With a conductive hearing loss, the patient often speaks softly because his own voice is heard more loudly; the opposite is true of nerve deafness. A physical examination may show normal tympanic membrane landmarks, but the results of a whisper test or the classic "watch tick" test will be abnormal. Tuning forks are helpful to distinguish between a conductive hearing and nerve deafness. In the Weber test, a tuning fork that vibrates at a frequency of 512 vibrations per second (512-tuning fork) is placed centrally on the forehead, glabella, or teeth; normally it is heard equally in both ears. If the sound lateralizes to one ear, a conductive hearing loss in that ear or a nerve hearing loss in the opposite ear is present. In the Rinne test, the 512-tuning fork is placed alternately on the mastoid area behind the ear and in front of the ear canal.

The sound should be heard louder in front of the ear; if it is louder when placed on the bone behind the ear, a conductive hearing loss should be suspected.

VERTIGO

Vertigo is the hallucination of rotatory movement. Either the patient is spinning and the environment is still or the environment is spinning and the patient is still. Dizziness, on the other hand, is the sensation of lightheadedness, falling, swimming in the head, imbalance, fainting, or occasional visual disturbance. This distinction is important because vertigo is almost always a symptom of labyrinthine dysfunction. There are few physical findings associated with this symptom. Nystagmus is often present during an acute vestibular crisis with the fast phase usually directed toward the diseased ear. Nystagmus from vestibular disease is usually horizontal; vertical or rotatory nystagmus may indicate central nervous system disease.

TINNITUS

Tinnitus may be unilateral or bilateral, low- or high-pitched, constant or intermittent, pulsatile or steady. Humming, cracking, ringing, buzzing, clicking, or roaring are terms often used by patients to describe this aggravating symptom. Unilateral tinnitus may be the only symptom of an acoustic neuroma, and this must be suspected when present. Many times there are no physical findings. Impacted cerumen can be easily diagnosed (and cured!). A glomus tumor of the middle ear causes pulsatile tinnitus. It appears as a pulsating red mass behind the tympanic membrane, which often blanches with direct pressure. A carotid bruit may indicate vascular disease.

FACIAL PARALYSIS

Facial paralysis may be partial or total, unilateral or bilateral, sudden or gradual in onset. Concomitant facial pain is often associated with a poor return of function; facial pain with a palpable parotid mass is often a sign of a malignant tumor. Facial paralysis associated with a bulging red tympanic membrane must be evaluated and treated immediately to prevent permanent facial paralysis. Facial paralysis must always be carefully evaluated to determine if it is peripheral or central in origin. A central paralysis due to an upper motor neuron lesion will affect only the lower branches of one side because the upper forehead branches have bilateral innervation. A peripheral or lower motor neuron lesion will cause a total paralysis of the involved side because the lesion is distal to the facial nerve nucleus. Peripheral facial paralysis almost always indicates temporal bone pathology. The parotid gland must always be carefully evaluated for a possible parotid tumor.

Otologic disease can lead to severe and life-threatening complications (Table 110–1). Otitis media, beginning in childhood, can progress to a total destruction of the hearing and balance mechanisms as well as some of the more severe complications described in Table 110–1. Meniere's disease can cause severe vertigo and hearing loss, but eventually subsides as the ear "burns itself out." Undiagnosed cerebellopontine angle tumors are catastrophic (fortunately not a common finding). Early diagnosis, because of a high index of suspicion, is a crucial factor in finding this ultimately fatal tumor early.

PATHOPHYSIOLOGY

The outer ear funnels sound waves to the tympanic membrane; vibrations are then transmitted through the middle ear where they are amplified by the hydraulic ratio of the tympanic membrane to the oval window, the lever action of the ossicles, and a phase differential between the oval and round windows. Mechanical energy is converted to electrical energy by several thousand inner hair cells of the organ of Corti located in the cochlea. Neural impulses are then transmitted through the auditory nerve, brain stem, and midbrain to the temporal lobe of the cortex. The specific neurotransmitter has not yet been identified.

A perforation, disruption of the ossicles, fixation of an ossicle, or fluid in the middle ear will decrease the vibratory energy of the amplifier mechanism and thus produce a conductive hearing loss. Ototoxic drugs, the normal aging process, acoustic trauma, and some systemic diseases may cause a loss of hair cells

TABLE 110–1.
Common or Life-Threatening Complications of Otologic Disease

Otitis media	Conductive hearing loss
	Sensorineural hearing loss
	Facial nerve paralysis
	Labyrinthine fistula
	Meningitis
	Brain abscess
	Epidural/subdural abscess
	Postauricular abscess
	Lateral sinus thrombosis
Meniere's disease	Severe sensorineural hearing loss
	Incapacitating vertigo
	Undiagnosed cerebellopontile angle tumor
Facial nerve paralysis	Permanent cosmetic disfigurement
	Exposure keratitis of eye
Cerebellopontile angle tumor	Death
	Total facial paralysis
	Neurologic defects
	Total hearing loss

in the organ of Corti and thus produce a nerve deafness.

The vestibular system is more complex. Its neural pathways are fully integrated with those of the visual and central nervous systems. The end organs of the vestibular system are the ampulla of the three semicircular canals plus the otoliths of the utricle and saccule. The neuroepithelia of these structures are sensitive to rotation and linear movements, respectively. Neural impulses then pass through specific pathways to the higher centers of the brain.

Inflammation of the labyrinth by a virus or bacteria can cause irritation of the ampula and thus produce vertigo. Increased pressure of the endolymph (inner ear fluid) or a biochemical change of this fluid may cause vertigo such as in Meniere's disease. Direct trauma by concussion or basilar skull fracture can damage the inner ear itself and cause symptoms.

CLINICAL–PATHOLOGIC CORRELATIONS

The clinical–pathologic correlations for otologic disease are shown in Table 110–2.

DIFFERENTIAL DIAGNOSIS

The differential diagnosis for the various otologic symptoms is shown in Table 110–3.

DIAGNOSIS

The basic tool for evaluation of hearing loss is the audiogram. This test consists of several parts. Pure tones (frequency specific) are presented to each ear individually or both ears together. The lowest level at which the patient can hear is recorded as the threshold of hearing; the stimulus is measured as a decibel, an arbitrary measurement of sound intensity. These stimuli are presented through earphones (air conduction), a bone oscillator (nerve conduction), or by free field speakers. Speech may also be used as a stimulus to document a speech reception threshold measured in decibels. Zero-decibel loss is a perfect score. A forty-decibel loss indicates a moderate hearing loss and usually some difficulty in hearing normal conversation. A ninety-decibel loss is severe and is often a significant handicap.

Speech discrimination can be measured by presenting phonetically balanced words (e.g., baseball, hot dog, cowboy) to each ear at levels well above threshold. Scores below 30% suggest severe inner-ear disease.

Tympanometry objectively measures the compliance of the tympanic membrane; lack of movement usually indicates middle-ear fluid such as in serous otitis media. The results of the stapedial reflex test, which measures the action of the stapedius muscle branch of the facial nerve, are abnormal if the stapes is fixed by otosclerosis.

TABLE 110–2.
Clinical–Pathologic Correlations for Otologic Disease

CLINICAL FINDINGS	PATHOLOGIC FINDINGS
Otalgia	Inflammation or infection of external ear
	Inflammation or infection of middle ear
	Soft tissue trauma of ear
	Referred pain from facial, trigeminal, glossopharyngeal, vagus nerves
	Neuritis of temporomandibular joint
Otorrhea (pus)	Infection of external auditory canal
	Infection of middle ear with perforation
	Osteomyelitis of mastoid cells
	Cholesteatoma of middle ear/mastoid
Otorrhea (clear)	Basilar skull fracture (cerebrospinal fluid)
Otorrhea (blood)	Traumatic perforation of tympanic membrane
	Basilar skull fracture
Hearing loss	Discontinuity or fixation of conductive mechanism (tympanic membrane, ossicles, fluid in middle ear, or mass of outer or middle ear)
	Loss of sensory epithelium of organ of Corti (cochlea)
Vertigo	Biochemical shift of Na^+ and K^+ in perilymph
	Increased pressure gradient of perilymph
	Inflammation of vestibular nerve
Tinnitus	Sensorineural hearing loss
	Irritation of primary neurons of auditory pathway
	Dysfunction of cochlea (organ of Corti)
	Changes in hemodynamics of carotid artery or jugular bulb
Facial nerve paralysis	Interrupted continuity of primary neurons of facial nerve
	Lesion of central nervous system at or above level of facial nerve nucleus
	Biochemical–electrical dysfunction of primary facial nerve neurons

Brain-stem evoked-response audiometry objectively measures the integrity of the entire hearing pathway. It is helpful in determining thresholds of hearing in infants or other patients who are difficult to test. It is also helpful in the diagnosis of an acoustic neuroma.

Electronystagmography precisely measures nystagmus by recording the electrical potentials of the extraocular muscles. Visual, positional, or caloric stimuli provoke a response that can be recorded and measured. Computerized electronystagmography uses harmonic acceleration to test the vestibular system.

Conventional radiography as well as polytomography can be used to evaluate the mastoid cell system and inner ear structures. Computerized tomography with a high-resolution technique and magnetic resonance imaging are more sensitive methods of demonstrating temporal bone abnormalities.

The facial nerve can be tested both functionally and topographically. Direct electrical stimulation of the facial nerve with a visually observed muscle response or graphically recorded action potential (electroneurography) gives the most information for predicting the return of facial function. Electromyography is accurate but late in predicting the return of function.

The site of a facial nerve lesion can be tested. Decreased tearing as measured by Schirmer's tear test places the lesion at the level of the geniculate ganglion or greater superficial petrosal nerve branches to the lacrimal gland. Positive results of the stapedial reflex test place the lesion at the facial nerve branch to the stapedius muscle. Positive results of the salivary flow test and taste test place the lesion at the chorda tympani nerve as it branches from the facial nerve.

PRINCIPLES OF PREVENTION AND THERAPY

The treatment of hearing loss depends entirely on whether it is conductive or sensorineural. Almost all cases of conductive deafness can and should be surgically corrected. Current mi-

TABLE 110–3.
Differential Diagnosis

SYMPTOM	POSSIBLE CAUSE
Otalgia	Perichondritis of auricle
	Hematoma of auricle
	Impacted cerumen
	Furuncle
	Acute otitis externa (bacterial or fungal)
	Chronic otitis externa (dermatologic)
	Malignant otitis externa
	Neoplasm
	Myringitis
	Acute otitis media
	Temporomandibular joint disease
	Temporal arteritis
	Headache
	Eagle's syndrome
	Carotodynia
	Sinus disease
	Trauma
Otorrhea	Chronic suppurative otitis media with perforation
	Chronic suppurative otitis media with cholesteatoma
	Cholesterol granuloma
	Basilar skull fracture
	Perforation of tympanic membrane
Hearing loss	Otitis externa—acute or chronic
	Otitis media—acute or chronic
	Impacted cerumen
	Congenital abnormality
	Traumatic perforation of tympanic membrane
	Glomus tumor of middle ear
	Malignancy
	Otosclerosis
	Foreign body in ear canal
	Temporal bone fracture
	Acoustic trauma
	Acoustic neuroma
	Presbycusis
	Ototoxic hearing loss
	Meniere's disease
	Tertiary syphilis
	Autoimmune inner ear disease
Vertigo	Meniere's disease
	Paroxysmal positional vertigo
	Traumatic (concussive) vertigo
	Cerebellopontine angle tumor
	Central nervous system disorders
	Perilymph fistula
	Vestibular neuronitis
	Basilar artery insufficiency
	Medication
Tinnitus	Sensorineural hearing loss
	Acoustic trauma
	Glomus tumor of middle ear
	Meniere's disease
	Altered hemodynamic flow of carotid or jugular vessels
Facial nerve paralysis	Bell's palsy
	Cerebellopontine angle tumor
	Temporal bone tumor/trauma
	Facial nerve neuroma
	Surgical lesion
	Salivary gland tumor
	Melkersson-Rosenthal syndrome
	Ramsay Hunt syndrome
	Congenital paralysis
	Central nervous system lesions

crosurgical techniques have high success rates with homograft tissue grafts to replace the tympanic membrane, synthetic or tissue prostheses for ossicular reconstuction, and elimination of mastoid disease with or without cholesteatoma. If the conductive hearing loss caused by middle ear effusion in children cannot be treated medically, myringotomy with or without insertion of pressure equalizing tubes should be advised.

Sensorineural hearing loss can be treated with use of a properly fitted hearing aid or other assistive listening device. Certain types of nerve deafness may be surgically stabilized or improved, such as with an endolymphatic shunt for cochlear hydrops, or medically, such as for syphilis or autoimmune inner ear disease. Patients with total bilateral nerve deafness who cannot wear even the strongest hearing aid may be candidates for cochlear implantation.

Vertigo can generally be treated with medication. Depending on the specific diagnosis, medical management may include diuretics, low-salt diet, vasodilators, tranquilizers, and other symptomatic treatment. Surgical procedures are available if medical management fails. Such procedures include the surgical treatment of the endolymphatic sac or inner ear itself, selective sectioning of the vestibular nerve, or, rarely, a destructive labyrinthectomy.

Tinnitus unfortunately eludes successful therapy at the present time unless a specific treatable cause can be found. Medication, surgical treatment, hypnosis, and biofeedback have all been recommended and may be beneficial in selected cases. A tinnitus masker or hearing aid for the other patients seems to be the only present treatment.

Surgical decompression of the facial nerve in idiopathic facial paralysis (Bell's palsy) is controversial treatment, but may be beneficial to patients who do not spontaneously recover. Primary surgery on the facial nerve for tumors or intrinsic disease has yielded increasingly satisfactory results. Microsurgical anastomosis of the nerve or nerve grafting techniques can currently be accomplished.

Neuro-otologic surgery of the cerebellopontine angle, middle fossa, skull base, and infratemporal fossa has developed into a specialized field where otologic and neurologic surgeons must work together.

REFERENCES

Goodhill V: *Ear Diseases, Deafness, and Dizziness.* Hagerstown, Maryland, Harper & Row, 1979, p 781. *A general textbook of ear disease.*

Hughes GB: *Textbook of Clinical Otology.* New York, Thieme Stratton, 1985, p 435. *A detailed textbook addressing the spectrum of otologic disease.*

Katz AE: *Manual of Otolaryngology: Head and Neck Surgery Therapeutics.* Philadelphia, Lea & Febiger, 1986, p 530. *A concise manual emphasizing the therapy for otologic conditions.*

Shambaugh GE, Glasscock ME: *Surgery of the Ear.* Philadelphia, WB Saunders Co, 1980, p 749. *A surgical treatise addressing all aspects of otologic surgery.*

111 OTITIS MEDIA

Sherman J. Alter, M.D.

The rapid and short onset of signs and symptoms of inflammation in the middle ear is termed acute otitis media. While symptomatic acute otitis media may quickly resolve, the inflammation of the middle ear mucoperiosteal membrane accompanied by the collection of liquid in the middle ear space may persist. Depending on how long this fluid persists, such otitis media with effusion may be classified as acute if the fluid persists less than 3 weeks, as subacute if it persists 3 weeks to 3 months, or as chronic if it persists longer.

CLINICAL SIGNS AND SYMPTOMS

Otitis media is primarily a disease of children. Several epidemiologic studies reveal a high incidence of this disease in infants and young children. Studies in the United States have shown that from 76% to 95% of all children will experience at least one episode of acute otitis media. Approximately 70% of children will have had one episode of acute otitis media by 3 years of age, and one-third of these will have experienced three or more episodes. The incidence of acute otitis media appears to peak during the periods of respiratory viral activity. Additionally, high-risk groups for the development of acute otitis media exist and include infants with cleft palates, children with Down's syndrome, and native American Indian or Eskimo children.

Acute otitis media is usually a self-limited illness that follows a characteristic clinical course. Symptoms generally consist of otalgia (ear pain) affecting one or both ears, with or without fever. Local symptoms occur primarily in older children and adults and usually will direct attention to the ear. Acute otitis media in the neonate and younger child, however, may not manifest itself through specific local symptoms. Otitis media in these groups may be seen initially as increased fretfulness and feeding problems or as systemic manifestations, such as vomiting and loose stools. One-fourth of children younger than 2 years of age may not have otalgia when they have ear infections. Symptoms of concomitant viral upper respiratory infections may exist in the child with acute otitis media. An element of hearing impairment is frequently present.

Left untreated, pain in the ear will increase, and generalized systemic symptoms become accentuated. Mild tinnitus and further impairment of hearing may occur. With progression of the infection, the tympanic membrane will eventually rupture with the release of purulent material, blood, or serosanguinous fluid from the ear. General symptoms of an increased toxic condition, ear pain, and ear discharge will usually subside within 48 hours of perforation. A recurrence of pain (frequently nocturnal), a large amount of purulent discharge that persists for more than 2 weeks, and continued fever may indicate mastoiditis.

Otitis media is a potentially serious disease because of its complications. In the preantibiotic era, serious intracranial complications, such as meningitis, epidural or subdural abscess, and extrameningeal brain abscesses developed in about 3% of cases. Extracranial complications include purulent labyrinthitis, mastoiditis, and cholesteatoma. A reversible mild to moderate conductive hearing loss is usually evident. Some children may have hearing loss for up to 6 months after an episode of acute otitis media. Significant hearing loss can be documented in many children with prolonged middle ear effusion. Some studies report that children 3 years of age who had recurrent or persistent acute otitis media scored less well on standard tests of speech and language than children who had had little or no middle ear disease.

On physical examination the appearance of the tympanic membrane is most important. The otoscope must provide magnification and a bright source of illumination. Pneumatic otoscopy should always be performed. The opening of the external ear should be completely occluded with the ear speculum. The tympanic membrane in otitis media will usually be injected or have a yellow or gray coloration. The normal light reflex will be absent. The tympanic membrane will be bulging, and the short process cannot be visualized. Movement of the eardrum elicits pain. A mild conductive hearing loss may be detected/measured. Ear drainage will occur after tympanic membrane perforation. Tenderness over the mastoid area suggests mastoiditis.

With persistance of middle ear effusion, the tympanic membrane will appear opaque and dull gray or yellow. It may appear retracted and display decreased mobility to pneumatic otoscopy. Occasionally an air fluid level or bubbles may be visualized behind the ear drum.

Associated physical findings of rhinitis or pharyngitis may frequently be present. A complete physical examination should be performed to rule out concomitant infectious processes or complications.

PATHOPHYSIOLOGY

Abnormal eustachian tube function appears to be the most important factor in the pathogenesis of otitis media. The eustachian tube has three important physiologic functions: ventilation of the middle ear, protection from nasopharyngeal secretions, and clearance (drainage) of middle ear secretions. While functionally collapsed at rest, the tube intermittently opens during swallowing because of the contraction of the tensor veli palatini muscle. This intermittent opening maintains ambient air pressure in the middle ear. A cartilaginous portion of the eustachian tube extends from the nasopharynx; the upper third of the tube is bony and extends into the middle ear opening of the upper anterior wall of the tympanic (middle ear) cavity. Ciliated columnar epithelium lines the eustachian tube and the middle ear.

Functional obstruction secondary to increased tubal compliance occurs primarily in infants and children. High pressures in the nasopharynx may insufflate the eustachian tube and result in reflux. Nasopharyngeal secretions and organisms may then traverse the eustachian tube and reflux into the middle ear. Intrinsic mechanical obstruction occurs when the mucosa of the eustachian tube swells as happens with upper respiratory infections in children. The eustachian tube may be extrinsically obstructed secondary to compression by nasopharyngeal tumors or adenoids.

Acute otitis media typically develops in association with an upper respiratory infection. Extension of the infection from the upper airway to the middle ear takes place through the eustachian tube, through the peritubal lymphatics or blood vessels, or by mucosal extension. In response to the infecting agents, an influx of polymorphonuclear leukocytes occurs in the middle ear, and purulent exudate fills the middle ear space. With continued tubal obstruction, the middle ear space and mastoid air cells become a closed cavity. The tympanic membrane becomes inflamed secondary to the local edema and increased number of leukocytes. The blood vessels become congested and Shrapnell's membrane bulges. Septic necrosis and thrombophlebitis of the tympanic veins result in a perforation of the tympanic membrane.

In response to the infection, the nonciliated cuboidal epithelium of the mastoid air cell system proliferates, desquamates, and obstructs drainage into the middle ear. Necrosis of tissues, osteitis, and further spread of infection may follow.

A persistent otitis media with effusion may occur with continued middle ear inflammation, infection, or tubal obstruction. The middle ear mucosa is transformed and characterized by round cell infiltration and develops into a secretory epithelium with formation of glands. The effusion may contain immunoglobulins and enzymes. Bacteria may or may not be present in these effusions.

Numerous studies have assessed the microbiology of middle ear infection, primarily in children aged 1 month to 6 years. Table 111–1 summarizes the bacterial isolates obtained by tympanocentesis in children. *Steptococcus pneumoniae* is the most common isolate, followed by *Hemophilus influenzae*, both typable, but, primarily nontypable. From 10% to 20% of *H. influenzae* in the ear is type b. The prevalence of *Branhamella catarrhalis* is important in that a majority of these organisms are beta-lactamase-producing. An effusion may contain up to 10^4 colony-forming units per milliliter in quantitative cultures. In studies utilizing viral isolation, a virus may be isolated from up to 25% of children with otitis media. *Chlamydia trachomatis* has not been isolated with any frequency in children with otitis media.

In older children and adults, the three most common agents causing otitis media and their order of prevalence are *S. pneumoniae, H. influenzae,* and *Streptococcus pyogenes.* Even in the neonate, *S. pneumoniae* and *H. influenzae* are the most important bacterial causes of otitis media. However, in very ill neonates and infants less than 6 weeks of age in intensive care units, especially in those with prolonged nasotracheal intubation, otitis media may be caused by staphylococci or gram-negative enteric bacilli in approximately 20% of cases. Similarly, such uncommon bacteria may be the cause of otitis media in immunocompromised patients. Occasionally, *Mycobacterium tuberculosis* can cause acute otitis media with perforation of the tympanic membrane.

CLINICAL–PATHOLOGIC CORRELATIONS

The clinical manifestations that occur with acute otitis media are primarily a direct result of the inflammatory process in the middle ear. The pain-sensitive structures of the middle ear and mastoid include the tympanic membrane, periosteum of the mastoid cortex, the visceral middle ear mucosa, and the mucoperiosteum of the middle ear and mastoid. The osseous structures of the middle ear and the other parts of the temporal bone do not appear to be supplied with pain receptors. The factors that stimulate these pain receptors are (1) stretching, (2) the volume and pressure of the middle ear effusion, and (3) the toxic products of infection. Disease involving the middle ear may potentially cause a large constellation of symptoms in addition to otalgia. In the infant, otalgia can be expressed clinically by crying, irritability, and sometimes scratching or pulling on the ear. Associated systemic symptoms of fever, vomiting, and a generalized toxic condition may be evident. Impairment of hearing occurs secondary to decreased mobility of the tympanic membrane because of associated middle ear fluid. This middle ear effusion may also elicit the description of additional symptoms such as blockage or fullness in the ears, "popping," or tinnitus. Perforation of the tympanic membrane results in otorrhea (Table 111–2).

TABLE 111–1.

Bacterial Isolates in Acute Otitis Media in Patients 1 Month to 6 Years of Age*

BACTERIAL ISOLATES	PERCENT OF CASES
Streptococcus pneumoniae	30–40
Hemophilus influenzae	20–30
Branhamella catarrhalis	8–18
Streptococcus pyogenes	4–8
Staphyloccus aureus	1–2
Staphyloccus epidermidis	1–2
Sterile	25–35

* From Wald, E, Changing Trends in the Microbiology of Otitis Media with Effusion, in *Pediatric Infectious Disease,* 1984; 3:381.

TABLE 111–2.

Clinical–Pathologic Correlations of Otitis Media

CLINICAL FINDINGS	PATHOLOGIC FINDINGS
Otalgia	Toxic products resulting from inflammatory response and infection
	Stretching of pain-sensitive middle ear structures by fluid
Systemic signs (fever, irritability, feeding problems)	Toxic products resulting from inflammatory response and infection
Otorrhea	Release of middle ear fluid through tympanic membrane perforation
Hearing impairment	Decreased mobility of tympanic membrane secondary to middle ear fluid

DIFFERENTIAL DIAGNOSIS

The diagnosis of acute otitis media is usually readily made by history and physical examination. External otitis media and furunculosis of the external ear, however, may be first seen as ear pain and may impair full evaluation of the tympanic membrane. Trauma or a foreign body in the ear canal may cause otalgia. Referred otalgia may be associated with infections or tumors in the pharynx or larynx. Dental infections may also cause a referred otalgia. Neoplasms involving the palate, nasopharynx, or base of the skull will occlude the eustachian tube and may cause ear pain. It should also be remembered that a tympanic membrane may appear red during an episode of crying or in association with a mild upper respiratory infection. Therefore, in the absense of associated signs or symptoms, an injected tympanic membrane is not diagnostic of otitis media.

DIAGNOSIS

The diagnosis should be easily made with pneumatic otoscopy. Tympanometry may be used to further measure the mobility of the tympanic membrane. Middle ear compliance varies as a function of the pressure differential across the tympanic membrane. With fluid in the middle ear, the compliance of the middle ear will be reduced or will be maximal toward a negative pressure (as with eustachian tube obstruction). Audiologic evaluation may show either low-frequency or high-frequency hearing loss or both. Tympanocentesis with a culture of middle ear fluid should be considered in cases of otitis media that occur in the following patients:

Neonates

Immunocompromised children

Children with suppurative complications

Children who fail to respond to usual drug regimens

Children with severe otalgia

Certain radiographs and computed tomography may be needed in cases involving suppurative complications, such as mastoiditis or brain abcesses.

PRINCIPLES OF PREVENTION AND THERAPY

Therapy of acute otitis media involves the use of antimicrobial agents. The selection of appropriate antibiotics mandates a familiarity with the most frequently encountered pathogens (Table 111–1). With the in vitro susceptibility data of these pathogens and information on middle ear penetration of antibiotics, a rational therapeutic choice can be made. Oral beta-lactam antibiotics or erythromycin–sulfonamide combinations are safe, effective, and tolerable to infants and young children. Antibiotics effective against beta-lactamase-producing bacteria are needed when these organisms are expected to be frequently encountered. In critically ill and selected neonatal patients, definitive antimicrobial therapy should be guided by culture results obtained from tympanocentesis. These patients may require further evaluation for concomitant systemic infections and may require parenteral antibiotics.

Ancillary treatment of acute otitis media may include myringotomy for severe persistent pain or for certain complications of otitis media, such as meningitis, abcess, or mastoiditis. Beyond providing relief of nasal symptoms, antihistamines or decongestants offer no additional benefit. Analgesia and antipyresis are important therapeutic modalities.

Patients with acute otitis media should be reevaluated 72 hours after the initiation of therapy. Symptomatic otitis media that persists after 72 hours of therapy warrants either diagnostic tympanocentesis or a change in antimicrobial therapy. At the end of a 10-day course of antibiotics, all patients should again be reevaluated. Persistent otitis media with effusion may be detected by otoscopy in approximately one-half of young children after a 10-day course of antibiotic therapy. Persistent otitis media with effusion appears in most cases to be a self-limited condition. The child with asymptomatic persistent effusion should be examined at 4- to 6-week intervals. Because bacteria similar to those in acute otitis media have been isolated from middle ear aspirates of some children with persistent otitis media with effusion, a trial of antibiotics appears to be appropriate in those children with an effusion persisting longer than 3 months. If such a trial fails, myringotomy and insertion of tympanostomy tubes may be indicated.

For infants and children with recurrent otitis media, that is, three or more episodes of middle ear infection within the preceding 6 months, a prolonged trial (at least 1 month) of prophylactic antibiotics may be warranted. If the condition is unresponsive to this, myringotomy with insertion of tympanostomy tubes may be indicated.

Audiologic evaluation should be performed in any child with recurrent otitis media or with otitis media that persists 3 months. Such evaluation is important in children with bilateral involvement and in the very young child.

REFERENCES

Bluestone CD: Surgical management of otitis media. *Pediatr Infect Dis* 1984; 3(4):392–396. *Discusses the indications for surgical intervention related to the type of disease encountered by the clinician.*

Bluestone CD, Klein JO: Otitis media with effusion, atelectasis, and eustachian tube dysfunction, in Bluestone CD, Stool SE (eds): *Prediatric Otolaryngology.* Philadelphia, WB Saunders Co, 1983, pp 356–512. *A thorough discussion of all aspects of acute otitis media.*

Casselbrant ML, Brostoff LM, Flaherty MR et al: Otitis media with effusion in preschool children. *Laryngoscope* 1985; 95:428–436. *A study of the incidence, prevalence, and natural history of otitis media with effusion in children followed for 2 years.*

Feigin RD, Kline MW, Spector G: Otitis media, in Feigin RD, Cherry JD (eds): *Textbook of Pediatric Infectious Diseases.* ed 2, Philadelphia, WB Saunders Co, 1987, pp 197–215. *An excellent review of the pathogenesis, diagnosis, and management of middle ear infection.*

Henderson FW, Collier AM, Sanyal MA: A longitudinal study of respiratory viruses and bacteria in the etiology of acute otitis media with effusion. *N Engl J Med* 1982; 306(23):1377–1383. *A 14-year study in a day-care center investigating the role of viral infection in the etiology of otitis media.*

McCracken GH, Jr: Antimicrobial therapy for acute otitis media. *Pediatr Infect Dis* 1984; 3(4): 383–386. *A discussion of antimicrobial therapy based on review of clinical efficacy studies.*

112   HOARSENESS

Blaine Block, M.D.
Joseph Stemple, Ph.D.

Hoarseness is the most important and common symptom of laryngeal disease. It is sometimes the only early symptom and occasionally the only manifestation of late diseases of the larynx. Other symptoms such as dysphagia, pain, and stridor are common in relatively few laryngeal diseases, while hoarseness seems to be the least common denominator of laryngeal function.

Hoarseness is caused by any condition that interferes with normal phonatory function. As the vocal cords close for phonation, they vibrate. The air passing through the larynx is variously affected by the size of the glottis, the thickness of the cords, the wave of motion along the cords, the tenseness of the cords, and several other factors. In most diseases of the larynx, the vocal cords fail to perform properly, resulting in hoarseness. There are about 50 separate causes of hoarseness. A determination of the cause of hoarseness can only be made by an examination of the larynx. Too often, hoarseness is attributed to a cold or "laryngitis" without direct visualization of the vocal cords and their function. Often this delays treatment, which can present problems with serious diseases such as cancer. As a general rule any patient who is hoarse for longer than 12 to 14 days and has not already had the larynx examined by direct vision should have this done.

The disorders that cause hoarseness can be divided into two categories. The first is organic pathology. The second is disorders of vocal function of which some are from abuse, whereas others are purely functional, many related to the patient's emotions.

The anatomy of the larynx succinctly described includes the vocal folds, the arytenoid cartilages, the muscle of the larynx, and the thyroid cartilage housing. The supraglottic portion of the larynx includes the epiglottis, the hyoid bone, and the supraglottic musculature, while the area below the cords primarily involves the cricoid cartilage and the mucosa leading to the upper trachea.

ORGANIC PATHOLOGIC DISORDERS

The organic pathology of the larynx can be classified into five categories: congenital, infections, hormonal, neoplastic, and paralytic.

CONGENITAL

The congenital disorder of the larynx that most commonly accounts for hoarseness is a laryngeal web, or laryngomalacia. A congenital laryngeal web occurs when the vocal fold fails to separate during the tenth week of embryonic development. Webbing may occur anywhere from the anterior to the posterior glottis. It is most often incomplete and may cause airway obstruction as a more important symptom than hoarseness. The voice qualities of infants and children with congenital webs may range from normal to severely dysphonic, depending on the extent of the web. Laryngomalacia causes stridor more than hoarseness, but in infants whose crying is their primary means of vocal communication, it often distorts the cry because of the airway obstruction. Laryngomalacia usually produces loud inspiratory stridor that becomes much worse as the child cries or breathes deeply. Usually it involves the epiglottis or the arytenoepiglottic folds which fold in on themselves with expiration to narrow the airway creating the stridorous sound. When the epiglottis is lifted with a laryngoscope, the stridor usually disappears. The condition is not fatal and usually clears spontaneously between the ages of 18 and 24 months when the larynx attains a firmer structure from continued growth. Parents of children with laryngomalacia need some reassurance, once the child has been watched long enough, to be sure that the airway is not obstructed.

INFECTIONS

Infectious diseases of the larynx are multiple, but the most common are usually related to short-term upper respiratory illnesses caused by a virus or bacteria. Such infections produce the condition known as acute laryngitis. It is a self-limited disease of no longer than 8-days to 10-days duration. The patient often totally loses his or her voice. The patient feels that the throat is tickly. Often a rough cough is an accompanying symptom, and pain may occur. Talking always makes the discomfort worse. If the infection becomes severe enough, stridor or dyspnea may also be present. Because this disease can theoretically be due to a whole spectrum of bacteria and viruses, there may be no associated fever. When viewed with the laryngeal mirror or laryngoscope, the vocal cords are usually quite erythematous with somewhat thickened and rounded rather than sharp edges. There is often some swelling of the arytenoid mucosa. Most patients with acute laryngitis require no specific treatment, but those who have a bacterial infection, such as a *Streptococcus* or *Hemophilus* infection, need to be treated with an appropriate antibiotic. Completely stopping smoking should be encouraged. Some long-term infectious diseases can cause hoarseness. Tuberculosis is probably the most common of these, but is rare today. Hoarseness can occur in virtually any stage of the tuberculous process and is usually, but not always, secondary to pulmonary tuberculosis.

HORMONAL

Many hormone diseases indirectly affect the larynx as a manifestation of the generalized overabundance or lack of a circulating hormone. The most common is hypothyroidism. With an insufficient amount of circulating thyroxine, changes occur in the vocal cord, as they do in other portions of the body, from the edema associated with the disease. The fluid that accumlates is primarily an acid mucopolysaccharide, which distorts the laryngeal tissues. The resulting voice is moderately hoarse and very husky. Hypothyroidism tends to be slow and insidious in its onset, and on direct examination the larynx shows a striking loss of the shininess of the true vocal cords. The cords appear to be edematous or polypoid, with some flabbiness of the cords' free margin. Hoarseness is sometimes the first symptom of hypothyroidism noticed by patients who have had other symptoms of hypothyroidism for some time and have been overlooked by the patient. Measuring serum thyroxine or triiodothyronine levels or both is appropriate; measuring thyroid-stimulating hormone (TSH) levels is particularly important. The treatment of the laryngeal problem is the treatment of the systemic disease.

Another hormone-related problem that causes hoarseness is hyperpituitarism, which produces enlargement of the larynx as well as bone, soft tissues, and cartilage in the rest of the body. Acromegaly with its secondary gigantism often leads to poor voice quality. Their voices are often hoarse with an excessively low pitch due to an enlargement of the entire laryngeal mechanism.

The most common hormone disorder leading to laryngeal dysfunction is probably in women who have had a hysterectomy. Many of these women experience vocal difficulties with a temporary or permanent lowering of vocal pitch. The patient often attempts to maintain her normal higher pitch, thus placing increased strain on the entire laryngeal mechanism and setting the stage for the development of hoarseness and other voice disorders.

NEOPLASTIC DISEASES

The neoplastic conditions involving the larynx are common and run the entire spectrum from benign lesions such as hyperkeratosis and leukoplakia to the aggressive malignant diseases of the hypopharynx and the glottis. Leukoplakia and hyperkeratosis describe a variety of nonmalignant neoplastic diseases that may result in organic and functional voice disorders. The etiologic factors appear to be chronic irritation from chemicals, tobacco, or smoke. Incessant coughing, throat clearing, and general voice abuse, however, also play a role. Both of these disorders are manifest by rather severe dysphonia, usually characterized by a low pitch, raspiness which progresses. Figures 112–1 and 112–2 show that hyperkeratosis can be a large lesion involving a substantial portion of one or both vocal cords or a small lesion involving only one small area of one vocal cord. It often appears as a patchy, white membrane with a growth build-up, which sometimes mimics the appearance of carcinoma. It can present as a whole spectrum of diseases from a very mild thickening of the laryngeal mucosa to a lesion with parakeratosis, dyskeratosis, marked change in the basement membrane, and a marked change in the basilar cells with rather severe dysplasia. The treatment is surgical stripping of the vocal cords. The growth almost always comes off freely without difficulty.

Other benign conditions involving the larynx include hemangiomas (which can occur anywhere in the larynx including subglottically), neurilemomas, fibromas, and chondromas; all

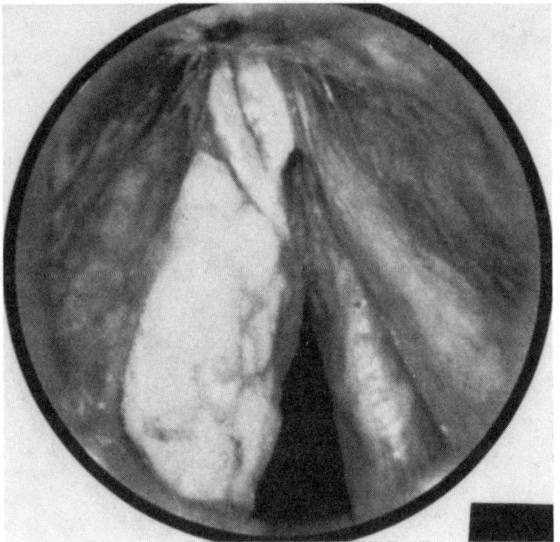

FIG 112–1.

Large hyperkeratotic lesion of left true vocal cord with carcinoma in situ.

are rare. The pathologic changes of these diseases are the same as the microscopic changes of these diseases in other parts of the body.

Carcinoma of the larynx appears to be occurring with increasing frequency. Hoarseness is often the first symptom. The disease is typi-

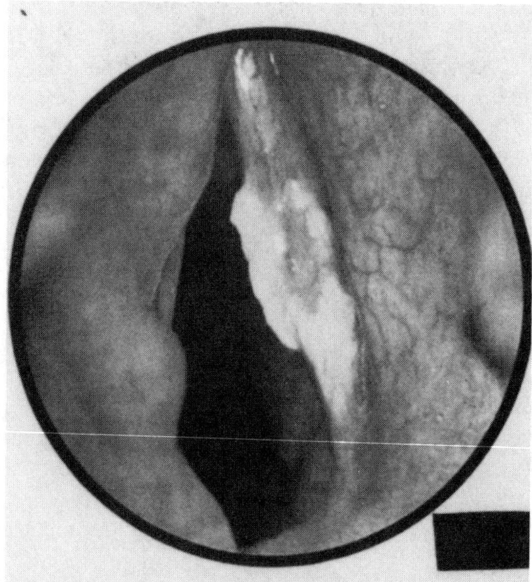

FIG 112–2.
Small hyperkeratotic lesion of right true vocal cord.

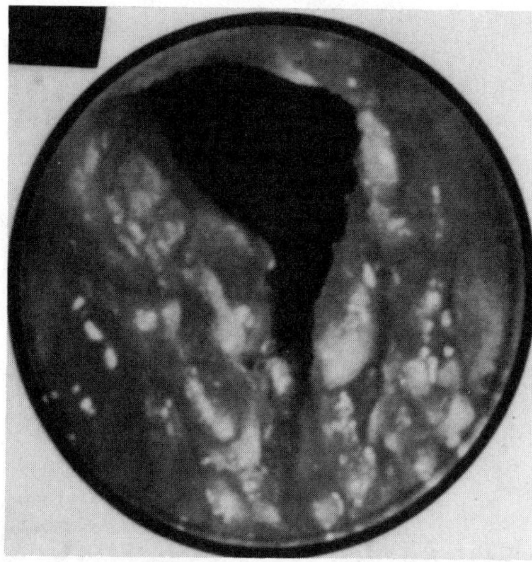

FIG 112–3.
Laryngeal carcinoma.

cally seen in men over age 50 who smoke. It is often associated with other carcinomas that affect smokers (i.e., bronchogenic carcinoma and esophageal carcinoma) as well as other head and neck cancers (i.e., mouth, tongue, tonsil, and pharnyx). The disease is usually clinically staged at the time of diagnosis, and the treatment is related to clinical stage. Figure 112–3 shows that carcinomas can be erosive or massively exophytic. A total loss of phonation has often been one of the major complications of the treatment of laryngeal carcinoma (laryngectomy). In recent years, however, the addition of new types of surgery as well as new phonatory restoration techniques has left only a small group of people aphonic after treatment.

PARALYTIC DISEASES

Basically, two nerves affect the function of the larynx—the superior and recurrent laryngeal nerves. The most common form of laryngeal paralysis is unilateral adductor paralysis (Fig 112–4). The paralyzed vocal fold rests in the paramedian position, and with phonation an air gap remains. The resultant voice is characterized as extremely breathy with air loss creating the sensation of shortness of breath as the patient must constantly inspire to get an expiratory flow past his cords to phonate. In bilateral adductor vocal cord paralysis, both cords rest in the paramedian position. The airway is good but voice quality is poor. Bilateral abductor paralysis (Fig 112–5) gives good voice with little hoarseness but extreme shortness of breath.

There are numerous causes of paralysis of the recurrent laryngeal nerve—bronchogenic carcinoma and carcinoma of the thyroid gland are two of the more common devastating causes. Surgical trauma, such as in thyroidectomy, carotid endarterectomy, or anterior spine surgery, is occasionally associated with injury to the recurrent laryngeal nerve resulting in paralysis. Diseases of the upper chest that involve the aorta can cause laryngeal paralysis on the left side because the recurrent nerve dips under and around the aorta on its course back into the neck to supply the vocal cord on the left. Neurologic disorders occasionally appear as recurrent nerve paralysis (i.e., MS, ALS).

Other forms of hoarseness include spastic dysphonia, a curious and serious voice disorder that is poorly understood. The several types of this disorder usually occur in middle-aged men and women. Many of these patients complain of physical fatigue, tightness of the chest, back, and shoulder muscles, and shortness of breath due to their efforts to phonate through a closed glottis. Some investigators have tried to relate this to psychologic disorders, other forms of spastic disorders, or multiple infections, but no definite cause has been found. Laryngeal papilloma probably can be placed in the infectious category because it appears to be caused by a virus. It occurs in both children and adults but is more devastating to children. It usually occurs between the ages of 2 years and 4 years and is seen about equally in boys and girls. It often causes extreme hoarseness. The wart is typical papilloma. They may spread from the larynx into the trachea and bronchi and become extremely difficult to treat. Usually this disease regresses with age and typically disappears by puberty. However, by that time many of these children have had multiple surgical procedures to remove the papillomas with resultant scarring that produces poor phonation and hoarseness.

DISORDERS OF VOCAL FUNCTION

Disorders of vocal function include abusive disorders, characterized by vocal cord nodules, polyps, and chronic laryngitis, as well as functional disorders including false cord phonation, conversion aphonia, dysphonia, and functional falsetto.

ABUSIVE

The most common vocally abusive behaviors include shouting, loud talking, screaming, vocal noises, coughing, and throat clearing. All of these actions force the vocal folds to adduct too vigorously, creating trauma between the cords. Sheer force, one of the main elements in the development of these vocal disorders, can take the form of sudden and violent straining or repetitive mild abuse.

Vocal nodules are in particular diseases of childhood. They typically occur in children who shout on a playground and yell at their siblings. They may also occur in adults, such as workers in a factory who must shout over the

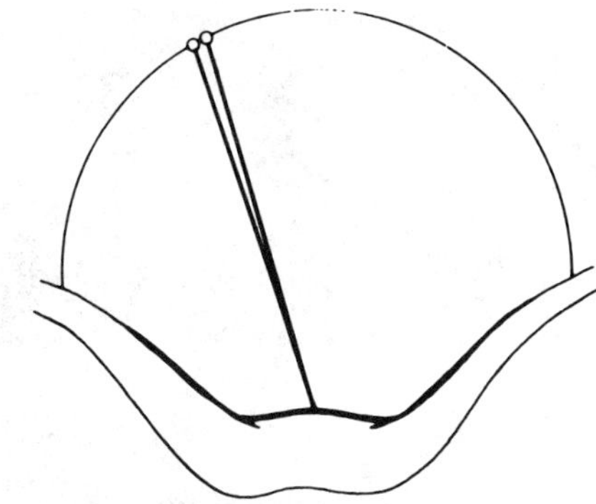

FIG 112–4.
Compensated unilateral vocal cord paralysis. Right cord paralyzed with left compensating for stronger phonation.

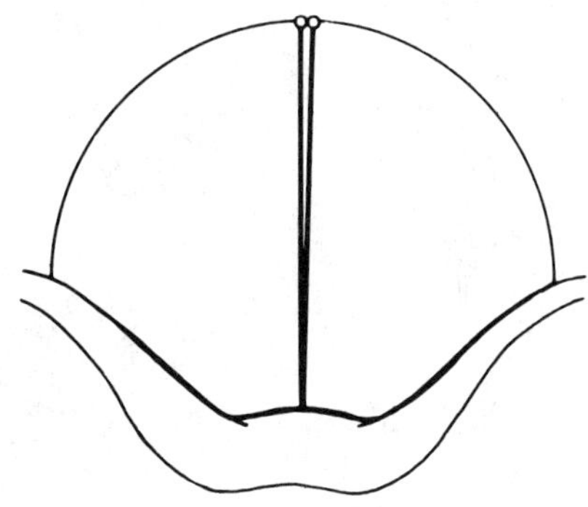

FIG 112–5.
Bilateral abductor paralysis. Voice is strong but patient has minimal laryngeal airway.

noise of machinery to communicate. Vocal nodules are small thickenings that occur at the junction of the anterior and middle one-third of both true vocal cords (Fig 112–6). They also tend to be associated with voice overuse. Professional singers, through long hours of rehearsal followed by performance after performance, frequently develop vocal nodules. When they occur in childhood, they tend to disappear during adolescence with the overall growth that occurs. Frequently the treatment of choice in childhood is voice therapy to reduce the abusive behavior until the adolescent laryngeal growth spurt. When the nodules occur in adults, reducing the abusive behavior is frequently inadequate, and surgical intervention, often with the laser, is required.

Vocal polyps tend to be fluid-filled sacs of tissue, similar to blisters. They can occur anywhere along the length of the vocal folds (Fig

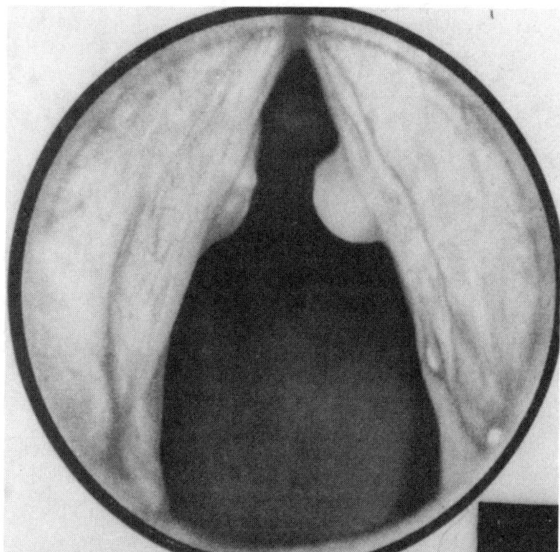

FIG 112–6.
Bilateral vocal cord nodules.

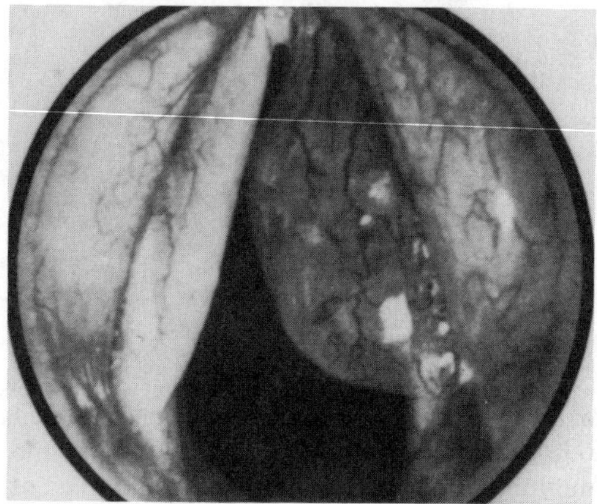

FIG 112–7.
Right true vocal cord polyp.

112–7). They can be pedunculated or sessile. They can be caused by a sudden violent incident of vocal abuse such as shouting at a sporting event, or they may be caused by many forms of long-term progressive abuse including improper respiration with phonation, talking at the wrong pitch, voice overuse, and smoking. Hoarseness is almost always a symptom. If, however, the polyps are pedunculated, the hoarseness may be intermittent. When the polyp falls below the level of the cords, the voice improves, and when stuck between the cords on phonation the hoarseness is at its worst. As this disease progresses, it often leads to polypoid degeneration caused by long-term misuse of the laryngeal mechanism, and both cords may undergo massive polypoid changes. The voice quality is typically severely dysphonic, usually with low pitch, breathiness, and extreme raspiness. One occupation in which polypoid degeneration often occurs is auctioneering. Chronic laryngitis can be a polypoid disorder but is often simple irritating thickening of the true vocal cords due to chronic irritative factors such as smoking and voice abuse. Some of the specific chronic laryngitides that can produce polypoid degneration are syphilis and tuberculosis. True chronic laryngitis is often associated with allergic and hypometabolic states as well as with other chronic respiratory disorders such as bronchiectasis and chronic bronchitis. Cough, as well as compulsive throat clearing, is often an important factor in chronic laryngitis.

FUNCTIONAL

One functional disorder is plica vestibularis, or people speaking with their false vocal cords, also called *ventricular phonation*. The false cords are really guardians of the laryngeal airway. They are not thin and fine like the true cords. Consequently, the voice produced by their use is very deep, harsh, and hoarse. The cause of ventricular phonation is unclear. It sometimes occurs as a compensatory voice when the true cords are affected by other serious disease. It is often a functional behavior related to physical and emotional tension and anxiety.

A subgroup of functional disorders is conversion aphonia and dysphonia. Patients with these disorders whisper or phonate inappropriately despite a neurologically and anatomically normal laryngeal mechanism. They are often almost totally aphonic. The onset is often sudden and sometimes accompanied by a short-lived sore throat. The majority of these patients are women. The disorder is almost always a physical manifestation of a psychologic disorder. Often the most appropriate treatment is voice therapy. Usually by the time these patients see the speech pathologist or the laryngologist, the need for the conversion reaction has disappeared, and they will quite easily convert back to using a normal voice. It is important to realize that these people are not malingerers. They truly do not realize they are capable of producing a normal voice.

The third functional voice disorder is a functional falsetto, sometimes called a *juvenile voice*. It is important to remember that the male voice lowers about one octave during maturation and the female voice by two to three semitones. When this acoustic change does not take place following physical maturation, a man is said to have a functional falsetto and a woman, a juvenile or childish voice. Many causes for this disorder have been suggested including attempts to resist the natural growth into adulthood, the desire to maintain a competent childhood soprano singing voice, and embarrassment when the voice lowers dramatically, perhaps earlier than that of their peers. The voice qualities associated with this disorder often include mild dysphonia and high-pitched low-intensity voice with some breathiness. Voice therapy is the treatment of choice.

The last functional disorder of voice has no apparent pathologic cause. Certain people who complain of intermittent hoarseness show no evidence of vocal cord neurologic or anatomic dysfunction when examined. The intermittent hoarseness was usually time- and place-dependent and associated with some form of laryngeal fatigue. Many of these patients become frustrated when their vocal symptoms persist and they are told that their laryngeal mechanism is normal. Often voice therapy by a speech pathologist will help them accept or remove the intermittent hoarseness.

In summary, many of the organic and functional disorders can affect the vocal mechanism and manifest as hoarseness. To associate the clinical findings with the symptom necessitates examination of the larynx through fiberoptic, indirect mirror, or videotape techniques. It must be stressed that, as a symptom of common illness, hoarseness should not last more than 14 days. If hoarseness is present for more than 2 weeks, it is incumbent on the clinician to attempt to define the etiologic mechanism.

REFERENCES

Aminoff MJ, Dedo HH, Izdebski K: Clinical aspects of spasmodic dysphonia. *Neurol Neurosurg Psychiatry* 1978; 41:361–365. *Current thinking on treatment of spasmodic dysphonia.*

Arnold GE: Advances in laryngeal physiology and our clinical application. *Eye, Ear, Nose, Throat Monthly* 1966; 45:78–84. *Understanding how the larynx works.*

Becker W (ed): *Atlas of Otorhinolaryngology and Bronchoesophagology.* Philadelphia, WB Saunders Co, 1969. *Concise pictorial and verbal descriptions of clinical otolaryngologic pathology.*

Ferguson CF: Congenital abnormalities of the infant larynx. *Otoloaryngol Clin North Am* 1970; 3: 185–200. *A discussion of pathology of the infant larynx.*

Green M: *The Voice and Its Disorders,* ed 3. Philadelphia, JB Lippincott Co, 1972. *A discussion of how our voice works and what affects its function.*

Stemple JC: *Clinical Voice Pathology, Theory and Management.* New York, CE Merrill, 1984. *A concise discussion of voice disorders for students.*

113

COMMON OCULAR DISORDERS

John A. Fleishman, M.D.
John D. Bullock, M.D., M.S.

The methods of proper bedside ocular examination are rarely taught adequately in medical school. This is unfortunate because examination of the visual system is remarkably straightforward and the data obtained are more objective than those for any other organ system. The importance of a cursory yet accurate ophthalmologic examination is even more important if one considers that 40% of all afferent information processed by the brain is visual.

The symptoms of ocular disease are few. Loss of vision, pain, proptosis, injection, photophobia, flashes and floaters, diplopia, and discharge are the primary possible complaints. (For a discussion of diplopia see Chap 115, Strabismus and Amblyopia.)

Obtaining the best corrected visual acuity is the first step in evaluating vision. This requires that any refractive error be overcome either by the use of spectacles or a pinhole, and if the visual acuity is obtained at near fixation in a patient over the age of 40 years proper near-correction must be provided (Chap 114, Refractive Errors). The patient should be queried regarding whether the loss of vision is monocular or binocular. Because the nasal retinal fibers decussate in the optic chiasm, lesions of or posterior to the chiasm involve loss of vision in both visual fields, although the patient is often aware of visual loss in only one eye. True monocular visual loss indicates disease involving either the eye or optic nerve. Evaluation of the peripheral visual fields may be obtained by having the patient cover one eye while fixating on the examiner's nose with the other eye. Fingers presented in each quadrant are counted to provide a rapid assessment of the visual field. If the patient is unable to count the fingers, the response to hand motion may be mapped. In general, loss of central vision oc-curs with ocular or optic nerve disease, bitemporal visual loss indicates chiasmal interference, and homonymous field loss indicates disease posterior to the chiasm.

ACUTE PAINLESS MONOCULAR VISUAL LOSS

Except when secondary to retinal disease, acute painless monocular visual loss is usually secondary to demyelinating disease in the young (optic neuritis) and vascular disease in the older patient (retinal vascular disease and ischemic optic neuropathy). See Table 113–1 for the symptoms and signs of acute painless monocular visual loss.

OPTIC NEURITIS

Optic neuritis causes a rapid loss of central vision. The disease usually occurs between the ages of 20 and 50 years. There may be retrobulbar pain on movement of the eye. The patient should be questioned regarding other symptoms of demyelinating disease (such as transient weakness, numbness, and loss of bowel or bladder control).

A central scotoma is usually present. The visual acuity may vary from mildly decreased (20/30) to no light perception. The color vision is decreased. An afferent pupillary defect is present. If the demyelinating lesion is retrobulbar, the optic disc will appear normal. If the lesion involves the optic disc, disc swelling will be noted. The former is more common. Weeks to months later optic disc pallor may develop.

Almost 90% of patients regain visual acuity to near premorbid levels within weeks to several months. Approximately 25% to 50% of

TABLE 113–1.
Acute Painless Monocular Visual Loss (Nonretinal)

AGE AT ONSET	SIGNS AND SYMPTOMS	COMMENTS
OPTIC NEURITIS		
Childhood–50 yr	Rapid central visual loss; ± pain; central scotoma, afferent pupillary defect; ± disc edema	90% of patients recover their sight; 25%–50% develop multiple sclerosis
AMAUROSIS FUGAX		
Any age—usually > 50 yr	Transient (< 5 min) visual loss with or without accompanying neurologic deficit, retinal arteriolar plaques, or carotid bruit/carotid murmur	Harbinger of cerebral stroke
TEMPORAL ARTERITIS		
70 yr–80 yr (may occur in younger patients as well)	Fever, weight loss; polymyalgia rheumatica, headaches, swollen painful temporal artery; sudden visual loss; second eye affected shortly thereafter; ± swollen disc; increased ESR; confirmed by temporal artery biopsy	Prognosis is good with treatment (high doses of corticosteroids). No treatment often results in bilateral blindness.
ANTERIOR IDIOPATHIC ISCHEMIC OPTIC NEUROPATHY		
50 yr–70 yr	Sudden visual loss—remains stable; swollen hemorrhagic disc; no systemic symptoms; normal ESR	No treatment necessary; must differentiate from temporal arteritis. Fellow eye affected in 25%–40% of patients

patients experiencing their first episode of optic neuritis will develop other signs of demyelinating disease in the future, indicating a diagnosis of multiple sclerosis. The other cases are usually idiopathic or postviral. In children optic neuritis is usually bilateral, involves both optic discs (bilateral disc edema mimicking papilledema), and is postviral in etiology.

There is no established therapy for optic neuritis. Systemic cortiocosteroids may shorten the course, yet the final outcome is probably unchanged.

AMAUROSIS FUGAX

Amaurosis fugax is a symptom complex rather than a disease; yet its recognition as a harbinger of cerebral stroke is so important, it deserves discussion. It is characterized by brief (less than 5-minute) episodes of monocular visual loss. The patient may often describe a dimming of the vision similar to a "curtain being drawn over the eye." Other transient neurologic deficits may accompany such episodes.

Amaurosis fugax is caused by the transient obstruction of the ocular circulation by microemboli. The most common source of such emboli is a carotid artery plaque or cardiac valve. The retinal arterioles should be examined for microemboli (Fig 113–1). Auscultation of the heart and carotid arteries should be performed.

Amaurosis fugax may herald impending cerebral stroke. Immediate neurologic consultation with appropriate studies, which may include carotid Doppler studies, digital subtraction angiography, cerebral angiography, or echocardiography, is recommended where appropriate.

ISCHEMIC OPTIC NEUROPATHY

Ischemic optic neuropathy can be divided into two categories, arteritic and anterior idiopathic. The former is much less common than the

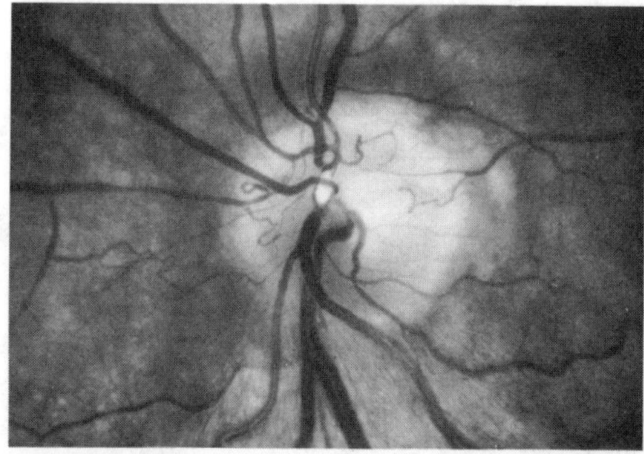

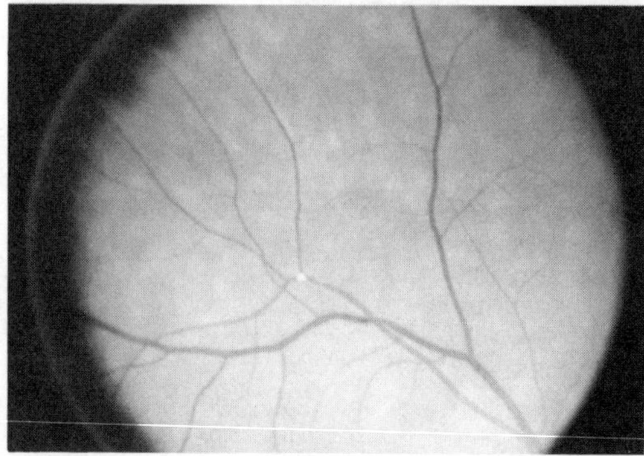

FIG 113–1.
Cholesterol plaques (Hollenhorst) of carotid origin lodged in central retinal artery *(top)* and in distal retinal arteriole *(bottom).*

latter and is an ocular manifestation of the systemic disease temporal arteritis.

Temporal Arteritis

Temporal arteritis generally occurs in elderly patients (70 to 80 years of age) and is characterized by fever, headache, malaise, weight loss, and myalgias (polymyalgia rheumatica). The headache is severe and may be temporal or suboccipital in location. Jaw claudication may occur. The visual loss is sudden and cataclysmic and may be preceded by fleeting visual symptoms similar to amaurosis fugax.

The temporal artery may be cordlike and tender. If the retrobulbar optic nerve is infarcted, the optic disc will appear normal; if the nerve is not infarcted, a clinical picture similar to central retinal artery occlusion may be found. The erythrocyte sedimentation rate (ESR) is often elevated (>40 mm/hour).

Giant cell arteritis resulting in vascular occlusion is noted histopathologically. Involvement of the posterior ciliary arteries is commonly responsible for the visual loss.

Rapid involvement of the fellow eye is the rule if therapy is delayed. If the diagnosis is suspected clinically and the ESR is elevated, high doses of systemic corticosteroids should be started immediately. The diagnosis is confirmed with a temporal artery biopsy; a negative biopsy, however, does not preclude the diagnosis. The response to steroid therapy is swift and dramatic, yet chronic use of steroids may be required. The vision loss is permanent.

Anterior Idiopathic Ischemic Optic Neuropathy (AION)

Anterior idiopathic ischemic optic neuropathy (AION) occurs in a younger age group (50 to 70 years of age) than the arteritic type and is much more common. This disease afflicts the eye only and must be differentiated from the devastating arteritic variety. A rapid loss of vision in the absence of systemic complaint is the rule. Premonitory visual symptoms are absent.

The visual loss is almost always stable and nonprogressive. More than one episode per eye is very rare, and involvement of the fellow eye occurs in about one-third of patients within a period of months to years. There is no treatment.

On physical examination the optic disc is seen to be swollen and hemorrhagic coincident to infarction of the optic nerve head (Fig 113–2). Altitudinal field defects are the rule; the loss of vision is mild to severe. An afferent pupillary defect is present. The ESR is normal.

THE RED EYE

Injection of the globe is a nonspecific sign that must be evaluated in light of the clinical setting. It is often a manifestation of ocular surface disease such as conjunctivitis, ocular trauma, or uveitis. The symptoms of ocular surface disease include decreased vision, foreign body sensation, photophobia, tearing, and discharge. The examination may be hindered by photophobia and foreign body sensation. Instillation of a topical anesthetic drop facilitates examination. Fluorescein dye will stain the epithelial

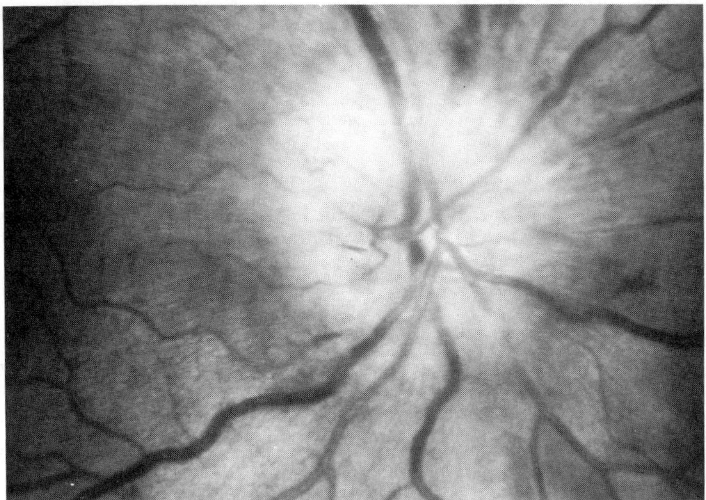

FIG 113–2.
Swollen, infarcted optic disc with perpapillary flame-shaped retinal hemorrhages characteristic of anterior idiopathic ischemic optic neuropathy.

basement membrane and, upon exposure to a Woods lamp, the dye fluoresces. Thus staining of the cornea indicates a corneal epithelial defect that exposes the underlying basement membrane.

CORNEAL SURFACE DISEASE

Corneal Abrasion

Corneal epithelial abrasion commonly occurs subsequent to minor ocular trauma. The eye is injected, and the patient complains of decreased vision, foreign-body sensation, photophobia, and tearing.

A corneal epithelial defect is noted on physical examination after applying fluorescein dye. A mild iritis with ciliary spasm and miosis may be noted on slit-lamp examination. The presence of a corneal foreign body should be ruled out. A small foreign body on the corneal surface may be safely removed at the slit lamp with topical anesthesia and a cotton swab.

With proper treatment, most corneal abrasions heal within 24 hours. Treatment consists of instillation of an antibiotic ointment with activity against *pseudomonas aeruginosa* (such as gentamicin or tobramycin) and the application of a tight pressure patch. A patched eye should be examined every 24 hours because bacterial infiltration of the defect may occur.

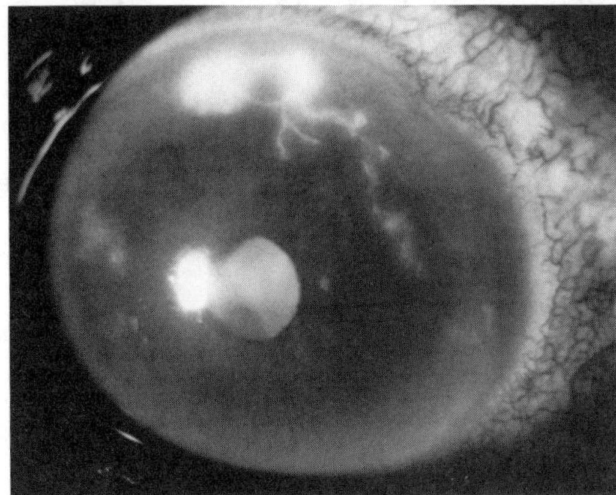

FIG 113–3.
Classic dendritic appearance of herpes simplex keratitis after instillation of fluorescein dye.

(NOTE: *Topical anesthetics are extremely toxic to the cornea when used repetitively and should never be prescribed to a patient.*)

Corneal Ulcer

Corneal ulceration may be viral (e.g., herpes simplex type 1), bacterial, or fungal. Herpes simplex keratitis is due to activation of the latent virus within the sensory nerves of the cornea. The corneal epithelial ulcer of herpes simplex has a classic dendritic appearance (Fig

113–3). A whitish infiltrate at the base of or surrounding a corneal epithelial defect may indicate bacterial ulceration. Patients with a compromised ocular surface, such as dry eyes from keratitis sicca, are particularly prone to corneal ulceration. Likewise, a chronic traumatic epithelial defect may be secondarily colonized by bacteria or fungi. The latter may occur particularly if vegetable matter is introduced into the defect at the time of the trauma.

Corneal ulceration, especially bacterial or fungal, is an ophthalmologic emergency, because ocular perforation may ensue. Immediate ophthalmologic consultation is required. (NOTE: *Because topical corticosteroid therapy may activate herpetic eye disease, the use of topical steroids should be reserved to the ophthalmologist.*)

CONJUNCTIVITIS

A red eye with marked conjunctival inflammation and discharge indicates conjunctivitis. Photophobia, foreign-body sensation, and decreased vision may be present, particularly if the cornea is involved (keratoconjunctivitis). A history of concurrent viral upper respiratory infection and a watery discharge are characteristic of viral conjunctivitis.

Fluorescein staining of the cornea should be performed to rule out significant corneal involvement (i.e., corneal ulceration). Mild punctate staining of the cornea is common. Cultures in cases of conjunctivitis of the newborn (ophthalmia neonatorum) should be done to rule out gonococcal disease. A mild chemical conjunctivitis may occur 24 hours to 48 hours after silver nitrate instillation.

Most cases of acute adult conjunctivitis are viral (adenovirus) and require no specific therapy. However, marked purulent discharge may indicate a bacterial cause and should be cultured. In such cases, ophthalmologic consultation should be sought.

Chronic conjunctivitis (exceeding 3 weeks) is often secondary to chlamydial disease and may require systemic antibiotic therapy. In the young sexually active patient, chlamydial conjunctivitis may be spread venereally; the patient's partner must be treated as well. *Chlamydia trachomatis* (trachoma) is one of the leading causes of blindness worldwide and is still endemic in some areas of the United States.

MAJOR OCULAR TRAUMA

Penetrating Ocular Injury

Every patient with a possible penetrating ocular injury should have an immediate ophthalmologic consultation. The vision should be checked; however, if the lids are swollen shut, an examination should be deferred because pressure transmitted to a ruptured globe through the lids may lead to extrusion of the intraocular contents (Fig 113–4). A rigid metal shield (or the bottom of a paper cup) should be

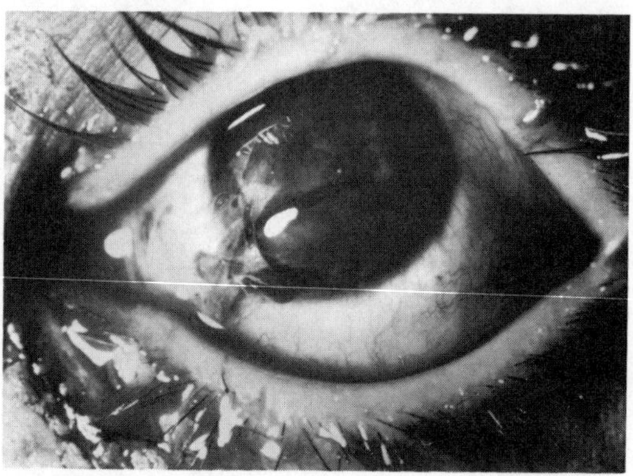

FIG 113–4.
Corneal laceration with extruded iris, flat anterior hemorrhage, hyphema, and traumatic cataract.

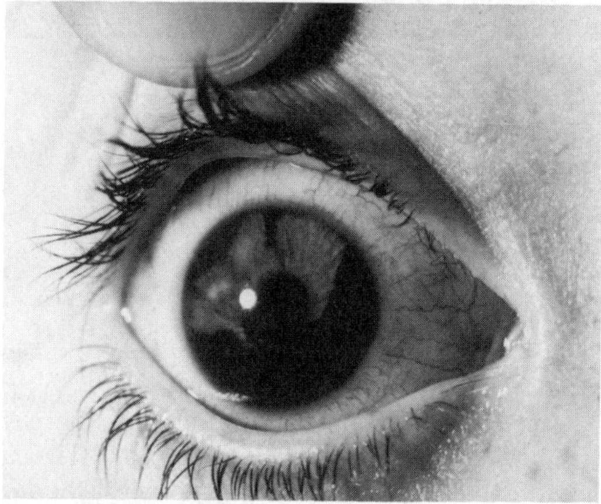

FIG 113–5.
Hyphema filling 40% of anterior chamber that occurred subsequent to blunt ocular trauma.

taped securely to the bony orbit until an ophthalmologist is available.

Hyphema

Hyphema, or anterior chamber hemorrhage, commonly occurs following blunt injury to the globe (Fig 113–5). The hemorrhage occurs subsequent to a tear in the anterior chamber angle. Retraction of the clot leads to rebleeding 3 days to 5 days later in about 30% of patients. Ophthalmologic monitoring is necessary to rule out glaucoma. The major complications include increased intraocular pressure and glaucomatous optic atrophy, rebleeding, and staining of the cornea with blood. The treatment is bedrest with the head of the bed elevated for 5 days (no reading, eye shielded) and oral aminocaproic acid, an antifibrinolytic agent that significantly reduces the incidence of rebleeding. Patients with sickle cell trait or disease may have a complicated course.

UVEITIS

The symptoms and signs of uveitis include decreased vision, ciliary flush and injection, photophobia, and ciliary spasm. Anterior chamber flare and cells are present. The term *uveitis* includes anterior uveitis (iritis) as well as posterior uveitis. Uveitis may occur as an ocular manifestation of many systemic diseases (see Table 113–2). Laboratory investigation in a child with uveitis may include an FTA-ABS, ESR, chest x-ray, PPD, and ANA. In the adult uveitis patient a chest x-ray, PPD, ESR, and FTA-ABS may be ordered. In male adults x-rays of the sacroiliac joints and HLA B-27 determination are useful in ruling out ankylosing spondylitis. The treatment of uveitis consists of cycloplegia and the use of topical, periocular, or systemic corticosteroids.

ORBITAL DISEASE

The principal symptoms of orbital disease include pain, proptosis, diplopia, visual loss, and periorbital changes. The common causes of orbital disease for children and adults are listed in Table 113–3.

PERIORBITAL AND ORBITAL CELLULITIS

Periorbital, or preseptal, cellulitis is an infection confined to the structures anterior to the orbital septum, a fibrous tissue extension of the

TABLE 113–2.
Uveitis Associated with Systemic Disease

SYSTEMIC DISEASE	CHARACTERISTICS
Ankylosing spondylitis	80% of patients are male
Juvenile rheumatoid arthritis	More female than male patients; Pauciarticular; + ANA
Reiter's syndrome	Males predominately
	Nonbacterial urethritis; polyarthritis; conjunctivitis; iritis
Inflammatory bowel disease	Ulcerative colitis: 5%–12%
	Crohn's disease: 2%
Syphilis	Many ocular findings
Sarcoidosis	Lacrimal gland involvement (dry eye) in 80% of patients
	Uveitis: 40%
	Anterior: 35%
	Posterior: 10%
	Combined: 55%
	Conjunctivitis: 35%
Tuberculosis	Many ocular findings
Behçet's syndrome	More common in Japan
	Hypopyon iritis; retinal vasculitis; aphthous stomatitis; genital ulceration

TABLE 113-3.
Common Causes of Orbital Diseases

CHILDREN
Orbital cellulitis
Capillary hemangioma
Lymphangioma
Dermoid/epidermoid cysts
Optic nerve glioma
Rhabdomyosarcoma
Pseudotumor
Metastatic neuroblastoma (often bilateral)
Leukemia
ADULTS
Grave's ophthalmopathy
Pseudotumor
Cavernous hemangioma
Lymphangioma
Meningioma
Dermoid/epidermoid cyst
Lacrimal gland tumors

orbital periosteum that extends into the lids. Despite marked edema of the lids, the intraorbital tissues are uninvolved. Periorbital cellulitis most often occurs subsequent to trauma. Extension of infection into the orbit results in orbital cellulitis. The symptoms of orbital cellulitis include proptosis, chemosis, restricted ocular motility, pain, and decreased vision. The patient is febrile, and the white blood count is elevated. In children, trauma and ethmoid sinusitis are the most common causes of orbital cellulitis. *Streptococcus, Staphylococcus,* and *Hemophilus influenzae* are common infectious agents. The differentiation of periorbital from orbital cellulitis may be difficult.

Admission of the patient to the hospital and administration of high doses of intravenous antibiotics are required. Adequate coverage against penicillinase-producing *Staphylococcus* and *H. influenzae* (in young children) is important. Close monitoring of the physical findings is mandatory. A failure to respond to therapy may indicate abscess formation requiring surgical drainage. Orbital cellulitis can be life-threatening; cavernous sinus thrombosis, meningitis, and brain abscess may ensue if adequate therapy is withheld.

REFERENCES

Beck RW, Smith CH: The neuro-ophthalmic examination. Symposium on Neuro-Ophthalmology in Neurologic Clinics 1(4): Nov. 1983. *An outstanding introduction to examination techniques.*

Duane TD, Jaeger EA (eds): *Clinical Ophthalmology.* Philadelphia, Harper & Row, 1985. *An excellent and detailed text.*

Fraunfelder FT, Roy FH (eds): *Current Ocular Therapy,* ed 2. Philadelphia, WB Saunders Co, 1985. *A book that provides easy access to indepth information.*

Scheie HG, Albert DM (eds): *Textbook of Ophthalmology,* ed 9. Philadelphia, WB Saunders Co, 1977. *An excellent overview of ophthalmology.*

114

REFRACTIVE ERRORS

John A. Fleishman, M.D.
John D. Bullock, M.D., M.S.

The eye is an optical instrument whose structure is designed to form a sharp image on the fovea of the retina. The net refractive power of the eye is about 60 diopters, 40 diopters of which are provided by the refractive power of the cornea and 20 diopters by the lens of the eye. In addition, the normal eye has the ability to increase its total dioptic power by increasing the convexity of its lens, a process referred to as accommodation. This is used to focus on objects as they shift in position relative to the eye. A detailed discussion of optics is beyond the scope of this section, and the reader is referred to Rubin's *Optics for Clinicians* (Rubin, 1977), an excellent review.

EMMETROPIA

Emmetropia refers to the condition in which objects at infinity are imaged at a point focus on the retina in the unaccommodated state. Emmetropia is the most common refractive state of the eye. Emmetropic patients require no correction with glasses until they reach the age of presbyopia.

AMETROPIA

Ametropia refers to the condition in which objects located at infinity are not imaged at a point focus on the retina. Ametropia includes myopia, hyperopia, and presbyopia.

MYOPIA

The myopic eye has too much refractive power; thus, objects viewed at infinity are imaged in front of the retina (i.e., in the vitreous). Myopia is also referred to as nearsightedness. As an ob-

ject approaches the myopic eye from infinity, the far point of the eye will be reached, and rays from this point will form a point focus on the retina. The refractive error of the myopic eye, in diopters, equals the reciprocal of the far point in meters (e.g., a patient with a 3-diopter

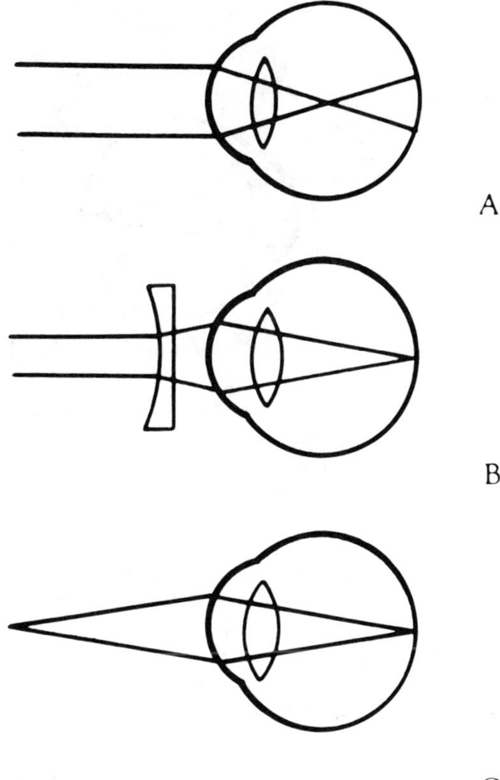

FIG 114–1.
Myopia. **A,** In axial myopia the eyeball is too long—parallel rays of light come to a point focus in front of the retina; **B,** A minus lens diverges the rays sufficiently so that parallel rays of light form a point focus on the retina; **C,** Divergent rays from the far point (FP) come to a point focus on the retina.

TABLE 114–1.
Conditions Associated with High Myopia

CONDITION	PATHOPHYSIOLOGY
Scleral crescent	Thinning of ocular coats: exposure of sclera
Posterior staphyloma	Thinning of ocular coats: scleral ectasia
Retinal detachment	Retinal hole formation
Lacquer cracks	Thinning of ocular coats: breaks in Bruch's membrane
Macular degeneration	Subretinal neovascularization
Increased cup/disc ratio	Enlarged scleral canal (may be confused with glaucomatous optic atrophy)

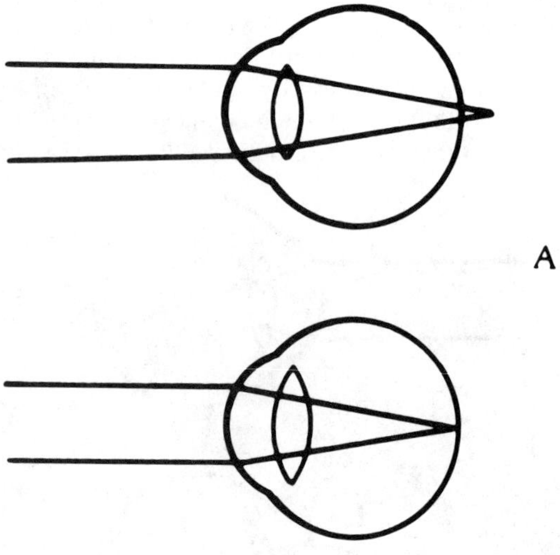

FIG 114–2.

Hyperopia. **A,** With relaxation of accommodation, parallel rays of light come to a point focus behind the retina; **B,** Accommodation increases plus power of eye bringing rays of light to a point focus on the retina.

myopia has a far point of 33 cm and thus sees an object in focus at this location; objects farther from the eye appear blurred).

Most myopia is axial, that is, the length of the eye is too great (Fig 114–1,A). The normal eye approaches 75% of its growth by age 4 years. However, the eye continues its growth at an abnormal rate in myopia. The average axial length of the eye is about 24.5 mm. The myopic eye may have an axial length between 26 and 36 mm. Another type of myopia is refractive myopia, in which the refractive power of the eye is too great (i.e., the corneal curvature is too steep or the refractive index (light-bending ability) of the lens is increased). The latter

often occurs with senile cataract. Myopia is treated with lenses that diverge light (minus lenses) (Figs 114–1,*B* and 114–1,*C*).

Clinical Signs and Symptoms

Defective distance vision is present. Myopic patients require correction with glasses to see past their far-points. Low myopia is not associated with significant pathologic changes and may be a benefit as the individual approaches presbyopic age because less accommodation is required for near work. High myopia can be associated with retinal degeneration, retinal detachment, and primary open-angle glaucoma (Table 114–1).

HYPEROPIA

Hyperopic eyes have too little refractive power (i.e., the hyperopic eye is too short) (Fig 114–2). In the unaccommodated state, all objects appear out of focus. Young hyperopic patients can accommodate and thus overcome their refractive error. However, this accommodation becomes a problem with prolonged close work which requires an increased accommodative effort. Patients with low hyperopia (1 or 2 diopters) are usually able to overcome their hyperopia by accommodating for distance vision. Most hyperopia is due to the eye being too short (axial hyperopia). Aphakia is an extreme form of hyperopia which occurs after the lens of the eye has been removed (i.e., after cataract extraction). Aphakia results in very high hyperopia. An eye that was previously emmetropic will usually require a spectacle lens of about 10 diopters to compensate for the loss of the crystalline lens. Hyperopia is corrected by converging or plus lenses.

Clinical Signs and Symptoms

Young hyperopic patients usually have normal visual acuity. They may complain of eye strain with prolonged near effort for the above reasons. As the patient ages and accommodative ability wanes, more and more of the hyperopia will require correction with glasses. In the pediatric age group, moderate to high degrees of hyperopia frequently causes accommodative esotropia or "crossed eyes." (See Chap 115, Strabismus and Amblyopia.)

ASTIGMATISM

In astigmatism the spherical refractive power of the cornea is not the same in all meridians. In regular astigmatism the principal meridians (the meridian with the most refractive power and the meridian with the least refractive power) are at right angles to each other. Astigmatism is corrected by a cylindric lense that refracts rays of light in only one meridian. Astigmatism is often associated with myopia or hyperopia, and the combination can be corrected by spherocylindric lenses, the sphere to correct the myopia or hyperopia and the cylinder to correct the astigmatism. Irregular astigmatism is not correctable with glasses because the principal meridians are not at right angles. Irregular astigmatism can be corrected with hard contact lenses if the corneal irregularity is not so severe as to preclude contact lens fitting.

ACCOMMODATION AND PRESBYOPIA

Objects closer than 6 m to the eye emit rays of light that are divergent to the eye. Such rays come to focus behind the retina and are thus seen as a blur. The crystalline lens has the ability to increase its curvature, which increases the refractive power of the eye and brings the divergent rays from objects closer than 6 m to the eye into sharp focus on the retina. This process of accommodation is mediated by contraction of the ciliary muscle, which is innervated by the parasympathetic fibers of the oculomotor nerve. Accommodation is an integral part of the synkinetic reflex, or near-reflex, which consists of miosis, convergence, and accommodation.

In all individuals, the ability to accommodate decreases with age due to a hardening of the crystalline lens. The resulting condition is presbyopia and typically becomes clinically significant at about age 45 years. Accommodative power decreases steadily until about the age of 70 years (Fig 114–3). The near point of accommodation (in meters) is the nearest point that a patient can see clearly. It is the reciprocal of the patient's accommodative power in diopters. Presbyopic individuals hold reading material farther away from their eyes as their accommodative ability decreases. Plus, or convex, glasses can be prescribed to replace the lost accommodative ability. Disorders associated with a loss of accommodation are listed in Table 114–2.

DIAGNOSIS

Testing visual acuity implies that the best-corrected acuity is recorded. Recording a distance visual acuity of 20/400 in a patient with an uncorrected myopia is meaningless because correction with proper glasses will result in a best-corrected acuity of 20/20. A fast and fairly accurate approximation of the best-corrected visual acuity in the patient with uncorrected ametropia can be obtained by having the patient look through a small pinhole. The pinhole allows only parallel rays that are not refracted to enter the eye, thus no corrective lens is required to overcome the refractive error of the

Age in years	1 5 10 15 20 25 30 35 40 45 50 55 60 65 70 75
Total accommodation	18 16 41 12 10 8 5 7.0 5.5 4.5 3.5 2.5 1.75 1.00 .75 .25 .00

FIG 114–3.
Donder's table demonstrating total accommodative amplitude and its relationship to age.

TABLE 114–2.
Disorders of Accommodation

DISORDER/AGENT	PATHOPHYSIOLOGY
Ciliary ganglion lesion (Adie's pupil)	Defective innervation
Third nerve palsy	Defective innervation
Midbrain lesions	Defective innervation
Botulism	Interruption of cholinergic transmission
Diphtheria	Toxin-induced demyelination
Diabetes mellitus	Sorbitol-induced osmotic lens changes and defective parasympathetic innervation
Myotonic dystrophy	Atrophy of ciliary body
Riley-Day syndrome	Generalized disorder of autonomic function
Shy-Drager syndrome	Generalized disorder of autonomic function
Anticholinergic agents	Interruption of cholinergic transmission

eye. This explains why ametropic patients squeeze their lids together in order to see clearly without their glasses; they are essentially using the eyelids as a pinhole. Pinhole visual acuity is rarely as good as the best-corrected visual acuity due to diffraction at the margins of the pinhole.

REFERENCES

Reinecke RD, Herm RJ: *Refraction*, ed 2. New York, Appleton-Century-Crofts, 1976. *A programmed text for the neophyte refractionist.*

Rubin M: *Optics for Clinicians*, ed 2. Gainesville, FA: Triad Scientific Publishers, 1977. *An excellent and easily understood text.*

115 STRABISMUS AND AMBLYOPIA

John A. Fleishman, M.D.
John D. Bullock, M.D., M.S.

The mechanisms required to maintain ocular alignment and bifoveal fixation involve a complex array of cerebral, brain stem, and orbital subsystems. Pathologic changes in any of these systems can result in ocular misalignment (i.e., strabismus).

A tropia is a constantly manifest ocular deviation. A phoria is a latent ocular deviation (i.e., it occurs only when bifoveal fixation is interrupted as in rapid alternate covering of the eyes). Phorias are overcome by fusion mechanisms. If fusion mechanisms decompensate (e.g., from fatigue or stress), a phoria may become a tropia. An exodeviation (exotropia or exophoria) refers to temporal deviation of the eye. An esodeviation (esotropia or esophoria) refers to a nasal deviation. A hyperdeviation refers to a superior deviation of the eye, a hypodeviation to an inferior deviation.

STRABISMUS IN THE CHILD

In childhood the retinal image of a deviating eye is ignored by the brain. This active cerebral process is called *suppression*. Suppression of the image of the nonfixating eye results in (1) the absence of diplopia or double vision because only the foveal image from the nondeviating eye is interpreted by the brain, and (2) the development of amblyopia. Amblyopia is a reduction in the best-corrected visual acuity in an eye that is being suppressed. Amblyopia develops only in childhood.

Clinical Signs and Symptoms

The incidence of amblyopia in the general population is about 2%. An adult with an amblyopic eye complains that the eye is "weak" or "lazy" and that the vision in the eye has been diminished since childhood. The child with an amblyopic eye has no complaints. Strabismus is usually, but not invariably, present.

The best-corrected visual acuity in the amblyopic eye can be mildly to profoundly decreased. A child will prefer to fixate with the sound eye and any attempt to force him or her to fixate with the amblyopic eye will greatly perturb the child.

A complete ophthalmologic examination is mandatory to determine the cause of amblyopia. In strabismic amblyopia, the amblyopia is due to a tropic deviation, which will be found on examination. In anisometropic amblyopia, the amblyopia is due to a large difference in the refractive errors of the two eyes with the eye with the greater refractive error usually becoming amblyopic. In anisometropic amblyopia, an ocular deviation may or may not be present; most often there is an associated ocular deviation. In this type of amblyopia, the tropia is a result of the amblyopia rather than its cause. Deprivation amblyopia (amblyopia ex anopsia) occurs from disuse of the eye as a consequence of upper lid ptosis or a congenital opacity of the cornea or crystalline lens.

Principles of Therapy

Treatment of amblyopia is only effective prior to age 6 years. Constant total occlusion of the sound eye (occlusion therapy) forces the cerebral mechanisms subserving the visual function of the amblyopic eye to develop. Almost miraculously the vision will improve in the affected eye. The younger the child, the shorter the period of required patching; a 6-month-old infant may require only 3 or 4 days of constant patching. In anisometropic amblyopia, proper correction with glasses must occur prior to occlusion therapy. Excessive patching may result in occlusion amblyopia (i.e., amblyopia in the previously sound eye). This, when it occurs, is easily treated by reversing the occlusion.

The visual prognosis is excellent in cases of strabismus and anisometropic amblyopia when therapy is commenced prior to the age of 6 years. After the age of 8 years, almost no improvement in visual acuity will occur with occlusion therapy. The prognosis in cases of deprivation amblyopia depends on the success with which the underlying problem is treated; again, early therapy is imperative.

ESODEVIATIONS IN CHILDREN

CONGENITAL ESOTROPIA

Large-angle esotropia in patients up to 6 months of age is classified as congenital esotropia. A family history of strabismus is commonly present. The child is usually otherwise normal, although congenital esotropia can be seen with hydrocephalus and cerebral palsy.

Usually the esotropia alternates between the two eyes with the child alternating fixation with the adducting eye. In this case, amblyopia does not develop. The esodeviation usually exceeds 30 prism diopters. The refractive error is usually minimal.

Principles of Therapy

Correction of refractive errors and, if needed, amblyopia therapy is imperative. Early surgical alignment of the eyes is the cornerstone of therapy.

Amblyopia is usually not present due to cross-fixation. Surgical therapy is, therefore, primarily cosmetic and seems to establish a small angle deviation (microstrabismus).

ACCOMMODATIVE ESOTROPIA

Accommodative esotropia is the most common form of childhood strabismus. The onset of variable-angle esotropia is characteristically between the ages of 6 months and 6 years. The deviation may initially be intermittent, but it becomes constant with time. Stress or illness may precipitate the onset of esotropia. A family history is often present.

Amblyopia is present in the deviating eye. Measurement of the angle of strabismus at near and at distance, as well as a cycloplegic refraction, is required.

In refractive accommodative esotropia, a large hyperopic refractive error is present. To overcome this hyperopia, the child accommodates. Because accommodation is closely linked to convergence (the synkinetic or near reflex), the child converges while accommodating, which results in the esodeviation. Usually the more hyperopic eye develops the esotropia.

In nonrefractive accommodative esotropia, there is no significant hyperopia; however, an abnormally large amount of convergence is stimulated for each unit of accommodation. This is referred to as a high accommodative convergence-to-accommodation ratio. The esodeviation is marked in near fixation and is minimal to absent in distance fixation.

Principles of Therapy

Correcting the hyperopic refractive error with glasses and patching is the proper treatment of refractive esotropia. Bifocal glasses correction (so the child does not have to accommodate at near fixation) and patching are proper treatment of nonrefractive esotropia. With both types, decompensated, or residual, esodeviations may occur after glasses correction. Surgical therapy

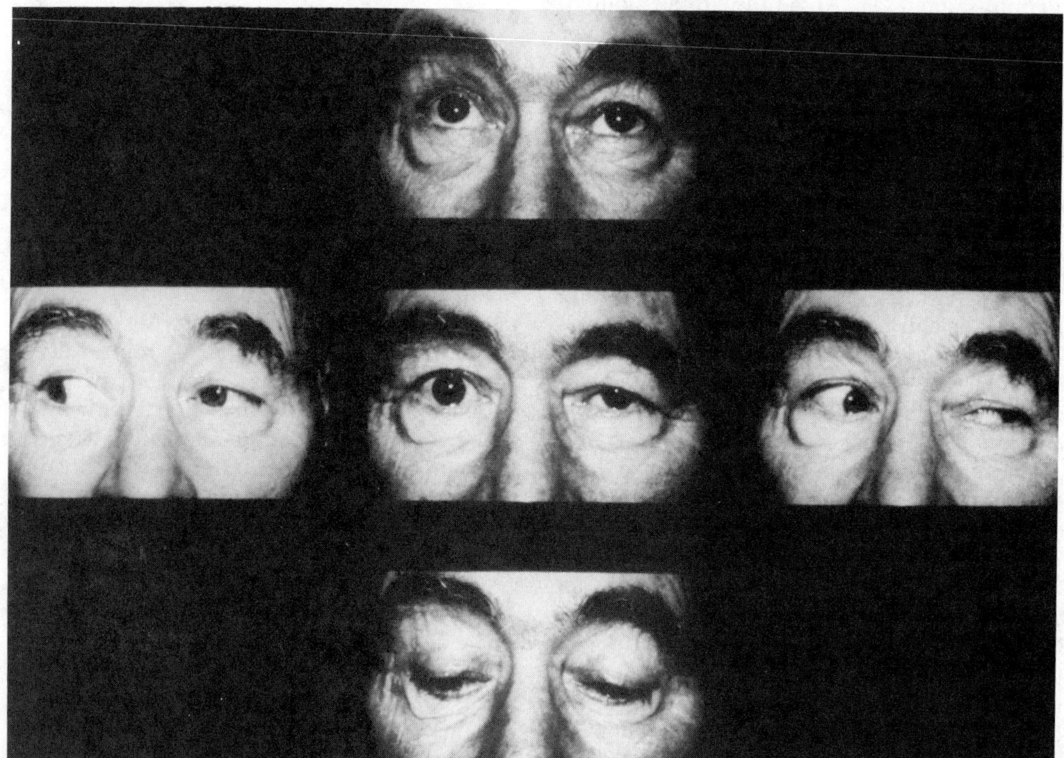

FIG 115–1.
A patient with a partial left third nerve palsy demonstrating left-sided ptosis and decreased adduction of the left eye. The pupil was not involved.

of the residual deviation is performed only after the amblyopia has been treated.

OCULAR DEVIATIONS IN ADULTS

Adult onset strabismus is associated with diplopia or double vision. Trauma or illness may cause a breakdown in normal fusion mechanisms resulting in a phoria becoming a tropia. Most adult strabismus is noncommitant (i.e., the angle of deviation varies in the cardinal positions of gaze). The deviation is often due to a palsy of one of the cranial nerves subserving the extraocular muscles (i.e., the oculomotor, trochlear, or abducent nerves) and is greatest when gaze is directed into the field of the paretic muscle. The palsy may involve only one cranial nerve or, as in the case of cavernous sinus lesions, may involve several cranial nerves in a variety of combinations.

OCULOMOTOR (THIRD NERVE) PALSIES

The oculomotor nerve innervates the pupillary sphincter, as well as the levator of the upper eyelid, superior rectus, medial rectus, inferior rectus, and inferior oblique muscles. Once inside the orbit, the third nerve divides into a superior division, innervating the superior rectus and levator muscles, and an inferior division, innervating the pupil and the medial rectus, inferior rectus, and inferior oblique muscles. External ophthalmoplegia refers to involvement of the extraocular muscles while internal ophthalmoplegia implies involvement of the pupil (Fig 115–1). In a total third nerve palsy, the upper lid is ptotic, the pupil dilated, and the eye deviated into a down (hypotropic) and out (exotropic) position. Table 115–1 lists the various types of third nerve palsies and their characteristics.

TROCHLEAR (FOURTH NERVE) PALSIES

Fourth nerve palsies result in weakness of the superior oblique muscles, the only muscle innervated by the trochlear nerve. The superior oblique is a depressor and intorter of the globe; thus a palsy of this muscle results in elevation (hypertropia) and extorsion of the eye. The fourth nerve has a long and circuitous path from the brain stem to the orbit and during trauma is often stretched or torn as it crosses

---

TABLE 115–1.
Oculomotor (Third Nerve) Palsies

SITE OF LESION	CHARACTERISTICS	
Nuclear lesion (very rare)	Obligatory nuclear lesion:	
	1. Unilateral third nerve with contralateral superior rectus palsy and bilateral partial ptosis	
	2. Bilateral third nerve with normal levator function	
Fascicular lesions	Associated brain stem signs:	
	Corticospinal tract	Weber's syndrome: third nerve with contralateral hemiplegia
	Red nucleus	Syndrome of Benedikt: third nerve with contralateral ataxia and intention tremor (usually cerebrovascular in origin)
Interpeduncular lesion	Caused by an aneurysm of the posterior communicating artery*; painful, often with signs of subarachnoid hemorrhage; pupil is involved	
Cavernous sinus lesions	Multiple cranial nerve involvement (III, IV, V, VI); pupil may be spared (? superimposed Horner's syndrome)	
Orbital lesions	Often caused by a secondary tumor or pseudotumor (inflammation); proptosis often present; superior and inferior divisions may be affected singly or together; ± pupillary involvement	
Diabetic (ischemic) Third nerve palsy	Often diabetes mellitus is an occult cause; painful third nerve palsy; pupil is spared*; resolves in weeks to 3 months; ischemic (demyelinating) lesion of peripheral third nerve fibers	

* An isolated third nerve palsy with pupil involvement is almost always secondary to an aneurysm of the posterior communicating artery. Immediate evaluation (angiography) is required. Isolated third nerve palsy with pupillary sparing is usually ischemic.

the tentorium prior to its entry into the cavernous sinus. The causes, symptoms, and signs of fourth nerve palsies are listed in Table 115–2.

TABLE 115–2.
Trochlear (Fourth Nerve) Palsies

CAUSES

Trauma, diabetes mellitus, congenital defect, myasthenia gravis

SYMPTOMS

Vertical diplopia; objects appear tilted

SIGNS

Head tilt to opposite side; ipsilateral hyperdeviation: worse on contralateral gaze and ipsilateral head tilt (three-step test)

Excyclotorision (on double Maddox Rod testing)

ABDUCENS (SIXTH NERVE) PALSIES

Isolated sixth nerve palsies are fairly common. The abducens nerve innervates only the lateral rectus muscle. Thus, an isolated abduction deficit occurs in a sixth nerve palsy. An esodeviation is always present and is characteristically greater at distance than at near fixation. The differential diagnosis of abduction deficits is listed in Table 115–3 and the causes and characteristics are listed in Table 115–4. Diagnostic tests useful in differentiating the various causes of abduction deficits are shown in Table 115–5.

TABLE 115–3.
The Differential Diagnosis of Abduction Deficits

CAUSE	CHARACTERISTICS
Sixth nerve palsy	See Table 115–4.
Grave's ophthalmopathy	Proptosis; lid retraction; defective upgaze and forced duction
Myasthenia gravis	Positive Tensilon test
Convergence spasm	Miosis during spasm/young patients
Orbital fracture (medial rectus entrapment)	Positive forced duction
Duane's syndrome (anomalous innervation)	Retraction of globe on adduction

---

TABLE 115–4.
Sixth Nerve Palsies

CAUSE	CHARACTERISTICS
Increased intracranial pressure	Nonspecific finding
Trauma	Recovery: variable
Ischemic (hypertension, diabetes mellitus)	Recovery in weeks to months
Pontine lesions	Ipsilateral seventh nerve palsy
Cerebellopontine angle lesions	Meningioma, acoustic neuroma
Clivus tumors	Clivus chordoma, nasopharyngeal carcinoma
Cavernous sinus lesions	Cranial nerves III, IV, and V also involved
Postviral conditions	Childhood occurrence—spontaneous recovery
Middle ear infection	Childhood occurrence

TABLE 115–5.
Diagnostic Tests for Abduction Deficits

TEST	CONDITIONS POSSIBLY RULED OUT BY TEST
Forced duction test	Grave's ophthalmopathy; orbital fracture (rectus muscle entrapment)
Tensilon test	Myasthenia gravis
Blood pressure measurement/glucose tolerance test	Ischemic causes (hypertension, diabetes mellitus)
Computed tomographic (CT) scan	Orbital or intracranial mass lesion
Erythrocyte sedimentation rate	Temporal arteritis
In Children:	
Middle ear examination	Petrositis from otitis media
Complete blood count	Viral infection (lymphocytosis)

REFERENCES

Duane TD and Jaeger EA (eds): *Clinical Opthalmology*, vol 1, chaps 1–20. Philadelphia, Harper & Row, 1986. *Comprehensive review of strabismus and amblyopia.*

Miller NR (ed): *Walsh and Hoyt's Clinical Neuro-Opthalmology*, ed 4, vol 2. Baltimore, Williams and Wilkins, 1985. *Excellent and in-depth discussion of strabismus and cranial nerve palsies.*

Opthalmology Basic and Clinical Science Course, Section 6: Binocular vision and ocular motility. San Francisco, American Academy of Ophthalmology, 1985. *Outline form of an excellent review.*

Parks MM (ed): *Atlas of Strabismus Surgery.* Philadelphia, Harper & Row, 1983. *Excellent overview of surgical techniques.*

Reinecke R: *Strabismus: A Programmed Text.* New York, Appleton-Century-Crofts, 1977. *An excellent introduction to strabismus.*

Von Noorden GK (ed): *Atlas of Strabismus*, ed 4. St Louis, CV Mosby Co, 1983. *Easy-to-follow pictorial guide.*

116 GLAUCOMA

John A. Fleishman, M.D.
John D. Bullock, M.D., M.S.

Glaucoma is an ocular disorder in which vision is lost in a characteristic pattern of nerve-fiber bundle defects of the visual field. The intraocular pressure is increased, resulting in cupping and atrophy of the optic disc as the retinal ganglion-cell axons that compose the disc are destroyed. The exact mechanism by which increased intraocular pressure causes optic disc damage is unknown, but probably involves mechanical as well as vascular changes at the lamina cribrosa where the axons exit the globe to form the optic nerve. Glaucoma is actually a group of diseases including primary open-angle glaucoma, angle-closure glaucoma, congenital glaucoma, and the secondary glaucomas.

PRIMARY OPEN-ANGLE GLAUCOMA

CLINICAL SIGNS AND SYMPTOMS

Primary open-angle glaucoma is typically a disease of older persons and is a major cause of blindness. The disease prevalence is about 5%. It often occurs in families, but the exact mode of inheritance is uncertain and probably involves the expression of several genetic factors. Visual loss is painless and insidious, occurring over a period of years or decades. It is characterized by the slow progression of nerve-fiber bundle defects. Patients are generally unaware of the visual loss until late in the disease process because the papillomacular bundle that subserves central vision is refractory to damage in the early stages. On a rare occasion, a patient with extremely high intraocular pressure may develop corneal edema and complain of halos around lights and blurred vision.

The intraocular pressure may be normal (see below) to severely increased. The eye is usually white and quiet. If the pressure is markedly elevated, the cornea may be edematous. Progressive, asymmetric cupping of the optic discs is an important sign. Glaucomatous cupping is often more pronounced in the vertical meridian (Fig 116–1). Notching of the rim of the disc represents a localized, severe loss of ganglion cell axons and usually corresponds to nerve-fiber bundle defects in the visual field.

Because intraocular pressure is characterized by diurnal variations that may be accentuated in glaucoma, one must not interpret a single normal reading as excluding a diagnosis of glaucoma. In the same eye at different times of the day, the pressure may be significantly elevated.

Untreated patients progressively lose vision over a period of years, usually remaining asymptomatic until a severe degree of peripheral field or central vision has been lost. Primary open-angle glaucoma appears to occur more frequently and may have a more aggressive course in black patients.

PRINCIPLES OF THERAPY

Although therapy is not curative, it is extremely effective in halting disease progression. Available evidence indicates that the increased intraocular pressure in primary open-angle glaucoma is caused by an increased resistance to aqueous outflow through the trabecular meshwork structures. Medical therapy is aimed at increasing aqueous egress from the eye or decreasing the rate of aqueous formation by the ciliary body.

Topical therapeutic agents include beta-adrenergic blocking agents, miotic agents, and epinephrine. Beta-blocking agents such as timolol or betaxolol act by decreasing the rate of aqueous formation. The former agent should be used with caution in patients with asthma or heart block because it is not beta-receptor selective. Miotic agents, such as carbachol and pilocarpine induce miosis and facilitate aqueous outflow. Systemic side-effects are rare, but some patients are unable to tolerate the miosis or ciliary spasm that may occur. The strong mi-

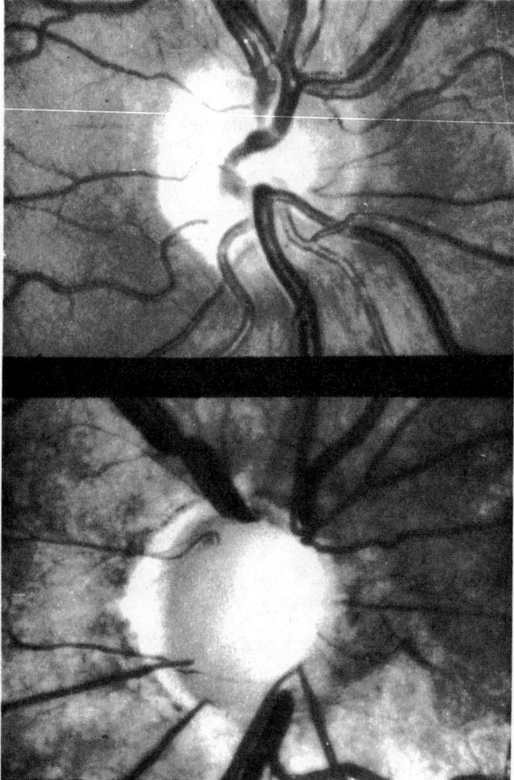

FIG 116–1.
Normal optic disc with healthy nerve fiber tissue is present in top photo. Severe loss of nerve fiber tissue resulting in glaucomatous cupping is shown in lower photo.

otic agents, acetylcholine esterase inhibitors (eserine, phospholine iodide, and demecarium bromide), may cause retinal detachment, cataracts, or iris cysts. Prolonged neuromuscular blockade from the use of depolarizing agents during anesthesia may occur in patients who have used topical acetylcholine esterase inhibitors prior to surgery.

If topical medical therapy is unsuccessful, systemic carbonic anhydrase inhibitors may be used. These agents (acetazolamide and methazolamide) are effective in lowering aqueous fluid formation. Systemic side-effects include metabolic acidosis, renal calculi, paresthesias, gastrointestinal disturbances, and mood swings, particularly in elderly patients.

Glaucoma surgery may be instituted if medical therapy is ineffective or poorly tolerated. Argon-laser trabeculoplasty involves the placement of small laser burns in the trabecular meshwork and is fairly effective in increasing fluid outflow. Modern filtering surgery (such as trabeculectomy) provides an artificial passage for the fluid to drain out of the globe into a subconjunctival bleb and is a moderately successful procedure.

DIFFERENTIAL DIAGNOSIS

The diagnosis of glaucoma requires that visual field loss be present. However, because this may only occur after years of elevated intraocular pressure, a subgroup of glaucoma "suspect" patients exists. The term "ocular hypertension" refers to the condition in which the intraocular pressure is elevated above statistical norms with no evidence of optic disc cupping or visual field loss. A percentage of such patients will ultimately develop frank glaucoma; many, however, will not. Because the intraocular pressure at which glaucomatous damage occurs may vary from individual to individual, there is no established "safe" level of intraocular pressure. In general, an intraocular pressure exceeding 21 mm Hg should be suspected, and these patients should be monitored for the development of glaucoma.

Patients with myopia have enlarged scleral canals and thus often have large optic cups that may mimic glaucomatous cupping. Visual field examination will, however, establish the presence of glaucoma.

PRIMARY ANGLE-CLOSURE GLAUCOMA

PATHOGENESIS

In angle-closure glaucoma, obstruction of fluid outflow is caused by apposition of the peripheral iris to the trabecular meshwork. Anatomically predisposed eyes have a shallow anterior chamber with a convex iris and an anteriorly placed lens-iris diaphragm. Conditions that may precipitate an attack of angle closure include pupillary dilation and relative pupillary block. Relative pupillary block of fluid flowing from the posterior to the anterior chamber may cause a forward bowing of the peripheral iris sufficient to close the angle. Dilation of the pupil (in darkness or after dilating drops) may cause the peripheral iris to block the trabecular meshwork, resulting in angle closure. Angle-closure glaucoma is rare compared to open-angle glaucoma.

CLINICAL SIGNS AND SYMPTOMS

The symptoms and signs of acute angle-closure glaucoma are listed in Table 116–1. In some patients, subclinical episodes of angle closure may result in the symptoms of halos around lights and mild ocular ache corresponding to short periods of angle closure that spontaneously abate. Such a history should be sought. The clinical picture may be dominated by nausea and vomiting; in such cases misdiagnosis is common.

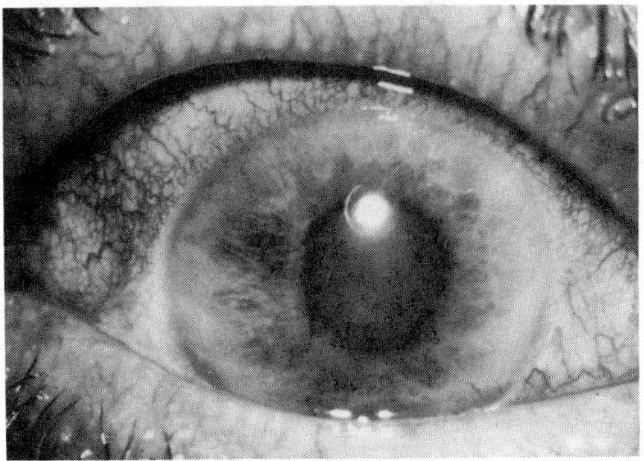

FIG 116–2.
Acute angle closure glaucoma with injected globe, cloudy edematous cornea, flat anterior chamber, and mid-position unreactive pupil.

An injected eye with corneal clouding from edema and mid-position, unreactive pupil is characteristic (Fig 116–2). The anterior chamber is shallow. The intraocular pressure is usually high (50 mm Hg–80 mm Hg); however, a low pressure is not unusual later in the attack as periods of aqueous hyposecretion supervene. The results of a gonioscopic evaluation of the anterior chamber angle by an ophthalmologist are diagnostic. The differential diagnosis is listed in Table 116–1.

PRINCIPLES OF THERAPY

Unlike for open-angle glaucoma, surgical therapy is curative for angle-closure disease. Prior to surgery, an attempt to break the angle-closure attack and lower the intraocular pressure is made. Intensive miotic therapy (pilocarpine, 2%) pulls the peripheral iris away from the angle. Topical beta-adrenergic blocking agents, carbonic anhydrase inhibitors, and intravenous hypertonic solutions are used to lower the pressure.

Surgical treatment is aimed at creating an alternate path for fluid to pass from the posterior to the anterior chamber. This is accomplished by making a hole in the peripheral iris with a laser (laser iridotomy) or surgically (peripheral iridectomy).

CONGENITAL GLAUCOMA

CLINICAL SIGNS AND SYMPTOMS

Congenital glaucoma occurs in about 1 in 10,000 infants. Inheritance is autosomal recessive with incomplete penetrance. It is bilateral in 75% of cases. The symptoms and signs of congenital glaucoma are listed in Table 116–2. The immature globe of the infant enlarges when subjected to increased intraocular pressure, a condition known as buphthalmos (Fig 116–3). Diagnosis is confirmed upon examination under anesthesia. A horizontal corneal dimension greater than 12.0 mm is highly suggestive. Gonioscopy reveals an abnormal anterior chamber angle with flat iris insertion and a translucent gelatinous membrane at the angle base (Barkan's membrane). Optic disc cupping occurs rapidly in congenital glaucoma and is the most important clinical sign. The cupping of congenital glaucoma may be reversible if therapy is instituted early.

PRINCIPLES OF THERAPY

Congenital glaucoma is an opthalmologic emergency, and suspected infants should be examined by an experienced ophthalmologist. Surgical therapy, including goniotomy or trabeculotomy, is highly effective only if treat-

TABLE 116–1.
Angle Closure Glaucoma

CLINICAL FINDINGS	PATHOLOGIC FINDINGS
SYMPTOMS AND SIGNS	
Blurred vision, halos	Corneal edema
Pain, redness	Increased intraocular pressure (rapid)
Nausea, vomiting	Increased intraocular pressure (vagally-induced)
Iris atrophy	Ischemic necrosis
Decreased vision	Increased intraocular pressure
	Corneal edema
	Optic atrophy
Midposition, fixed pupil	Angle closure and iridocorneal apposition
Shallow anterior chamber	Important sign in other eye
DIFFERENTIAL DIAGNOSIS	
Iritis	
Acute abdominal process	
Acute third nerve palsy	

TABLE 116–2.
Congenital Glaucoma

CLINICAL FINDINGS	PATHOLOGIC FINDINGS
SYMPTOMS AND SIGNS	
Tearing, photophobia, blepharospasm	Increased intraocular pressure
Corneal haziness, Descemet's tears	Corneal edema, buphthalmos (increased intraocular pressure)
Buphthalmos	Enlarged globe
Abnormal chamber angle	Anomalous development
Optic disc cupping	Increased intraocular pressure
DIFFERENTIAL DIAGNOSIS	
Corneal clouding: Forceps injury Mucopolysaccharidoses Viral or bacterial keratitis	
Corneal enlargement: Megalocornea	

TABLE 116–3.
Secondary Glaucomas

CAUSE	PATHOLOGIC MECHANISM
Corticosteroid-induced	Unknown (open-angle)
Iritis/uveitis	Inflammatory (open- and/or closed-angle)
Traumatic	Hyphema: obstructive (RBCs) occurring late: angle-recession
Lens-induced (phacomorphic)	Angle-closure (hypermature cataract)
Lens-induced (subluxation)	Angle-closure (homocystinuria, Marfan's syndrome, Weill-Marchesani syndrome)
Lens-induced (phacolytic)	Ruptured lens induces inflammation/obstruction
Intraocular tumor (retinoblastoma, malignant melanoma)	Angle-closure (mass effect or inflammatory)
Neovascular (proliferative diabetic retinopathy, central retinal vein occlusion)	Angle-closure (synechial)
Ghost-cell glaucoma (following vitreous hemorrhage)	Obstructive (RBCs)

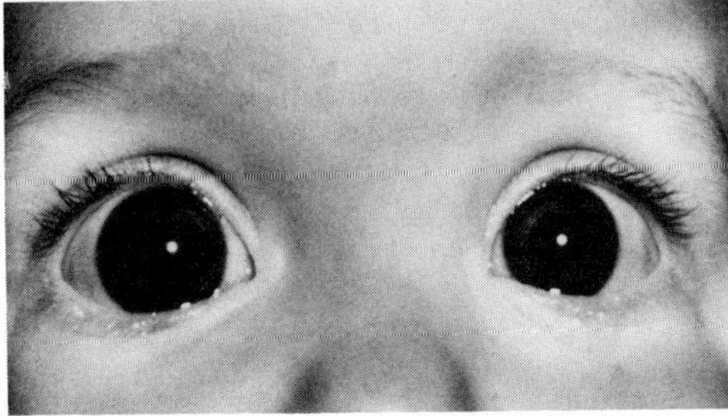

FIG 116–3.
External photograph of infant with congenital glaucoma demonstrating enlarged right globe, a condition known as buphthalmos.

ment is instituted prior to irreversible visual loss.

DIFFERENTIAL DIAGNOSIS

The differential diagnosis of congenital glaucoma is listed in Table 116–2. Ocular and systemic disorders associated with congenital glaucoma include aniridia, iridocorneal mesodermal dysgenesis syndromes, neurofibromatosis, and the Sturge-Weber syndrome.

THE SECONDARY GLAUCOMAS

Secondary glaucomas occur as a consequence of many ocular disorders including inflammation (iritis), trauma (angle recession), proliferative diabetic retinopathy (neovascular glaucoma), and lens subluxation. Elements of open-angle or closed-angle glaucoma or both may be present; thus, therapy must be individualized. A list of common causes of secondary glaucoma is presented in Table 116–3.

REFERENCES

Chandler PA, Grant WM: Glaucoma, ed 2. Philadelphia, Lea & Febiger, 1979. *An excellent in-depth discussion of the glaucomas.*

Fraunfelder FT, Roy FH (eds): *Current Ocular Therapy,* ed 2. Philadelphia, WB Saunders Co, 1985. *A brief and complete presentation of therapeutic information.*

Glaucoma, in Duane TD, Jaeger EA (eds): *Clinical Ophthalmology,* vol 3, chaps 41–57. Philadelphia, Harper & Row, 1985. *An in-depth overview.*

Kolker AE, Heatherington J (eds): *Becker and Shaffer's Diagnosis and Therapy of the Glaucomas.* St. Louis, CV Mosby Co, 1983. *An excellent in-depth review of the glaucomas.*

Kwitko ML: *Glaucoma in Infants and Children.* New York, Appleton-Century-Crofts, 1973. *In-depth overview of congenital and adolescent glaucoma.*

Shields MB: *A Study Guide for Glaucoma.* Baltimore, Williams & Wilkins, 1982. *Advanced clinical analysis.*

117 EYELID AND CONJUNCTIVAL DISEASES

Edward B. Feinberg, M.D.

The transparency of the cornea depends on the interrelated functions of the lids, lacrimal apparatus, and conjunctiva. The normal cornea has no vasculature, making oxygen delivery to the epithelium totally dependent on lacrimal transport.

Alterations of form and position of the eyelids are common. The typical complaint of the patient with abnormal lids and intact trigeminal nerve function is a foreign body-like sensation, which in its mildest form is often described as dryness. The foreign body-like sensation is typically described as pain, but appropriate questioning will reveal the foreign body sensation component.

In entropion, the lids turn inward and allow the eylashes to abrade the corneal epithelium. This is most common in elderly persons due to spasms of the lid musculature. There is a major association with chronic inflammation of the lash follicles (marginal blepharitis).

Treatment is directed first at an immediate

protection of the corneal epithelium with ocular lubricants and topical antibiotics to prevent opportunistic invasion of corneal stroma at the site of the damage. Antibiotics without epithelial toxicity are preferred. Corticosteroids are contraindicated.

Etiologic treatment involves control of the meibomian follicle inflammatory disease by a careful removal of sebaceous material and administration of appropriate local antibiotics. Surgical procedures to eliminate lid spasm and to protect the cornea may be required.

In ectropion, the lids turn outward and fail to redistribute the oxygen-carrying tear film with each blink. The symptoms are similar to those of entropion but are milder because there is no direct abrasion of the cornea by the lashes. The causes are categorized into cicatricial, spastic, paralytic, and senile. The principles of treatment are similar to those for entropion for corneal protection, but ultimate correction of the lack of lid protection is usually surgical.

Lagophthalmos occurs when closure of the lid fissure is incomplete. Common causes are facial nerve palsy, thyroid ophthalmopathy, and coma. Here, too, the symptom is that of a foreign body-like sensation when intact sensation and mentation are present. Primary treatment consists of ocular lubricants, and if the corneal epithelium is disrupted, prophylactic antibiotics. The use of corticosteroids, including the unfortunately ubiquitous steroid-antibiotic combinations, must be scrupulously avoided.

It is important to understand that lid closure fulfills only a part of the needs of the cornea. The cornea not only requires protection against drying but also a continuous circulation of tears to keep constant the oxygen supply to corneal epithelium. This is particularly applicable in the care of the comatose patient. In addition to meticulous lid closure with tape (or suture and tape), hourly manual blinking by nursing staff is essential to proper care.

Hordeolum and chalazion are common ophthalmic diseases. Both are manifestations of occluded meibomian gland drainage by sebaceous material. Hordeolum, stye, is acute, with a sudden appearance of a tender localized red swelling of the lid. Pointing of the abscess can often be seen on the internal surface of the lid. The untreated lesion will often spontaneously drain and resolve, but may convert to a chala-zion. A chalazion is a sterile chronic granulomatous sebaceous cyst in the tarsus of the lid.

The differential diagnosis in the adult must include meibomian squamous carcinoma, particularly in recurrent cases.

Treatment consists of warm compresses to encourage pointing and drainage and to soften the inspissated sebaceous obstruction. Lid hygiene is helpful as prophylaxis against further episodes. Topical antibiotics are often used but are of little value. Surgical drainage is effective.

THE CONJUNCTIVA

Conjunctivitis may be primary or secondary to an inflammation of deeper structures. Allergic conjunctivitis is the most common type.

Patients often have a strong personal and family history of atopic disease. The symptoms are burning and itching; photophobia is frequent. The allergen is usually airborne, such as dust, pollen, or animal dander.

Examination shows edema, injection, and a watery discharge. The discharge may have a mucopurulent component. Papillary hypertrophy of the palpebral conjunctiva may be seen. The Wright-stained smear shows mixed lymphocytic and granulocytic components with a predominance of eosinophils.

Treatment consists of cold compresses, vasoconstrictors, and antihistamines. Rarely corticosteroids may be needed. Complete cleansing of the body, including shampooing the hair with attention to the lashes and brows after each episode of outdoor exposure is helpful if the allergen is a pollen. Identification and subsequent avoidance of a specific allergen is desirable, if possible.

Infectious conjunctivitis, or keratoconjunctivitis, can be due to a wide spectrum of viral and bacterial agents. Pain, photophobia, and a draining red eye are presenting complaints.

Examination reveals decreased acuity when keratitis is a significant component. The conjunctiva is red and injected. The discharge ranges from watery to purulent with fibrin membranes adhering to the conjunctiva. A Wright-stained smear will contain mostly lymphocytes if the infection is viral and mostly granulocytes if it is bacterial. Gram's stain may reveal the offending organism. A sample of the drainage should be cultured. Many viral agents are highly contagious, and strict precautions will help prevent infection of the examiner or transmission by the examiner to patients subsequently examined.

Herpes simplex keratoconjunctivitis is an important entity. Eye involvement is rare in primary herpes simplex infections but may occur as an acute follicular conjunctivitis. The initial symptoms of recurrent herpetic keratitis are photophobia, lacrimation, and pain.

Recurrent herpes simplex may occur following a variety of triggering stimuli and can first be seen as a variable spectrum of corneal, conjunctival, and lid involvement. Corneal involvement has several characteristic clinical features (e.g., a branching, superficial corneal epithelial ulcer, with a unique dendritic shape). The cells adjacent to the ulcer can be seen with biomicroscopy to be swollen with vesicles. The ulcer takes up fluorescein dye, and Wood's light or cobalt illumination will dramatically reveal the characteristic dendritic shape of the ulcers. A loss of corneal sensation can easily be demonstrated by checking each cornea with a wisp of cotton.

Frequently there are fine keratic precipitates under the lesion. Recurrent attacks may cause corneal scarring and a loss of vision. Herpetic endophthalmitis essentially never occurs in the natural course of the disease. However, it is frequently seen as a complication of corticosteroid treatment.

Herpes simplex keratitis is an infection of fixed tissues with the herpes simplex virus, and

---

TABLE 117–1.

Clinical–Pathologic Correlations in Common Diseases of the Eyelids and Conjunctivae

CLINICAL FINDINGS	PATHOLOGIC FINDINGS
LIDS	
Hordeolum (stye): Discrete, elevated erythematous, tender papule or pustule Usually near lid margin.	Acute purulent inflammation of skin adenexae of lids—sebaceous glands and hair follicle
Internal hordeolum: Diffuse, deep tender erythematous area Usually involves most of lid	Acute purulent inflammation of meibomian gland within tarsal plate of lid
Chalazion: Hard, painless module in eyelid	Chronic inflammation of meibomian gland with granulomatous reaction around lipid material
CONJUNCTIVA	
Papillary hypertrophy of chronic allergy conjunctivitis	Vascular hypertrophy and dilation with edema and lymphocyte and plasma cell infiltration Conjunctival epithelium thrown into folds
Follicular reaction due to allergic reaction and chronic infection, especially trachoma. Follicles are smaller and paler than papillae.	Lymphoid hyperplasia of subepithelial conjunctiva with minimal vascular response
Bacterial conjunctivitis	Acute conjunctivitis with edema and neutrophils
Acute allergic conjunctivitis	Acute conjunctivitis with edema and eosinophils
Acute viral conjunctivitis, especially adenovirus (epidemic kerato-conjunctivitis.	Acute conjunctivitis with edema and mononuclear cells Fibrin and cell debris membrane on epithelium possible
Acute viral conjunctivitis, especially herpes.	Acute conjunctivitis with edema and mononuclear cells with many multinucleated forms
Trachoma	Chronic lymphocyte infiltration with prominent fibroblastie response Basophilic inclusion bodies in epithelial cells
CORNEA	
Herpes simplex keratitis	Lymphocytes and plasma cells in corneal stroma. Intranuclear inclusion bodies in epithelial cells. Epithelial ulceration, including involvement of stroma, possible.

thus recurrence and neurotropism are anticipated manifestations. Pharmacologic treatment of the virus is possible with the nucleic acid analogues iododeoxyuridine and adenosine arabinoside.

Although there are indications for giving corticosteroids to suppress the intracorneal immune reactions that lead to scarring, this must be supervised by an ophthalmologist and is beyond the scope of this book. Steroids should never be used in uncomplicated herpes simplex keratitis because the potential for catastrophic complications is high.

CLINICAL–PATHOLOGIC CORRELATIONS

Table 117–1 shows the clinical–pathologic correlations in the common diseases of the eyelids and conjunctivae.

REFERENCES

Duane D (ed): *Clinical Ophthalmology.* Philadelphia, Harper & Row, 1985. *A good general text.*

Fraunfelder FT, Roy FH: *Current Ocular Therapy,* ed 2. Philadelphia, WB Saunders Co, 1985. *A brief overview of therapy.*

Hedges III, TR, Schwartz B (eds): *Consultation in Ophthalmology.* Chicago, Year Book Medical Publishers, 1986. *The indications for evaluation.*

Newell FW (ed): *Ophthalmology: Principles and Concepts,* ed 6. Chicago, Year Book Medical Publishers, 1986. *An in-depth discussion of the diseases of the eyelid and conjunctivae.*

Vaughan D, Asbury T (eds): *General Ophthalmology,* ed 11. Norwalk, Conn, Appleton-Century-Crofts, 1986. *A good general overview.*

118 RETINAL DISEASES

John A. Fleishman, M.D.
John D. Bullock, M.D., M.S.

DIABETIC RETINOPATHY

Diabetic retinopathy is the leading cause of new onset blindness in the 20- to 64-year-old group. It can be classified into nonproliferative and proliferative phases (Table 118–1). Of all patients with diabetes mellitus, about 30% have some form of retinopathy. About 5% have severe proliferative retinopathy. The prevalence of retinopathy increases with the duration of the diabetes. By 7 years, about 50% of patients will have some form of retinopathy; by 25 years almost 90% of patients will be affected. The importance of yearly retinal examination cannot be overemphasized because treatable disease may progress to irreversible damage in an asymptomatic patient.

CLINICAL SIGNS AND SYMPTOMS

Nonproliferative diabetic retinopathy is characterized by closure of the retinal capillaries and retinal vascular leaking. The funduscopic changes are listed in Table 118–1. Macular edema is the most important cause of decreased vision in diabetic retinopathy. Prolif-

TABLE 118–1.
Diabetic Retinopathy

CLINICAL SIGN	PATHOPHYSIOLOGY
NONPROLIFERATIVE RETINOPATHY	
Microaneurysms, dilated capillaries, and focal capillary closure	Increased platelet adhesiveness, increased erythrocyte aggregation, defective fibrinolysis, thickening of vascular endothelial basement membrane
Retinal edema and exudates, intraretinal hemorrhages	Retinal vascular leakage (defect in tight junctions between capillary endothelial cells)
Cotton-wool spots	Widespread capillary closure (nerve fiber layer infarcts)
Intraretinal microvascular abnormalities (IRMA)	Retinal ischemia
Venous beading	Vascular stasis
Large blot hemorrhages	Vascular incompetence
PROLIFERATIVE RETINOPATHY	
Retinal neovascularization	Retinal ischemia (diffusible vasoproliferative factor)
Rubeosis iridis/neovascular glaucoma	Retinal ischemia (diffusible vasoproliferative factor)
Vitreous hemorrhage	Contraction of fibrous tissue or vitreous detachment (tearing of delicate new vessels)
Tractional retinal detachment	Retinal traction by contracting preretinal fibrous membranes

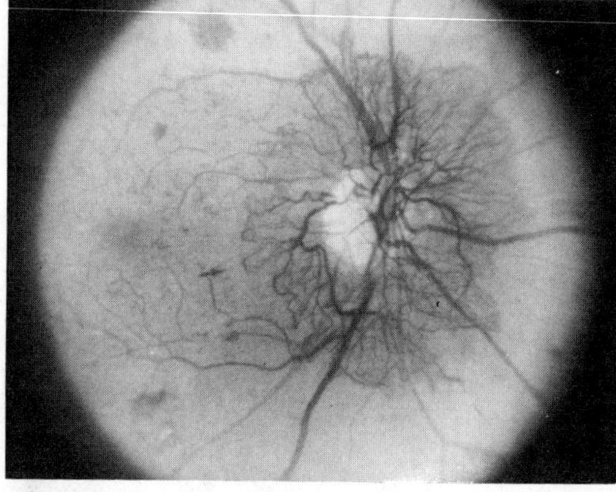

FIG 118–1.
Fundus photograph of posterior pole demonstrating severe diabetic neovascularization. Neovascular fronds are elevated and extend into vitreous body.

erative retinopathy is often preceded by preproliferative changes (Table 118–1). Presumably, the retina produces a diffusable factor in response to ischemia. This factor is postulated to stimulate the new vessel growth (i.e., neovascularization). These vessels are delicate and leaky and grow from the retina or optic disc forward into the vitreous (Fig 118–1). Fibrous tissue deposition follows neovascularization. Subsequent contraction of the fibrous component can result in bleeding and retinal traction, which can manifest clinically as vitreous hemorrhage and tractional retinal detachment. In addition, neovascularization can involve the iris (rubeosis iridis) with anterior chamber angle neovascularization occurring shortly thereafter. The latter results in neovascular glaucoma, a type of angle-closure glaucoma.

PRINCIPLES OF THERAPY

It is not well established that tight control of blood glucose in the diabetic patient will prevent diabetic retinopathy. Pan-retinal laser photocoagulation destroys the ischemic retina resulting in a decrease in new vessel growth. Regression of the neovascularization following laser therapy can be dramatic. Photocoagulation of discrete areas of vascular leakage may reduce retinal edema. Vitreous hemorrhage and tractional retinal detachment may require surgical vitrectomy.

HYPERTENSIVE RETINOPATHY

Hypertensive retinopathy represents an ocular manifestation of the systemic vascular response to sustained, severe elevation in blood pressure. The retinal pathologic changes visible ophthalmoscopically mirror the vascular changes occurring in other organs.

CLINICAL SIGNS AND SYMPTOMS

The ocular history of patients with hypertensive retinopathy varies considerably depending on the severity of the retinal changes. Patients with early hypertensive retinopathy and no macular edema have no visual complaints.

The initial retinal arteriolar response to high blood pressure is vasoconstriction. Attenuation of retinal arterioles with focal narrowing and concealment, or "nicking," of retinal venules at arteriovenous crossing sites can be observed by routine ophthalmoscopic examination. The pathologic and clinical changes of retinal arteriolar sclerosis are listed in Table 118–2.

Severe prolonged hypertension may result in vascular leakage and a characteristic picture of hypertensive retinopathy (Table 118–2). Optic disc edema, when it occurs, usually does so in later stages. Decreased vision due to hypertension is primarily the result of retinal hemorrhage(s) and macular edema.

PRINCIPLES OF THERAPY

Treatment of the systemic hypertension is imperative. Local photocoagulation of discrete areas of vascular leakage may effectively reduce macular edema.

BRANCH RETINAL VEIN OCCLUSION

Branch retinal vein occlusion refers to an occlusion of a retinal venule. Such an occlusion may occur in a major tributary or very small retinal vein.

CLINICAL SIGNS AND SYMPTOMS

Acute branch retinal vein occlusion is usually accompanied by a painless loss of vision that may range from mild to severe. The systemic diseases associated with branch vein occlusion are listed in Table 118–3.

The superior-temporal branch vein is most often involved, while nasal vein obstruction is rare. Occlusion occurs at arteriovenous crossing sites, where the arteriole and venule share a common adventitia. Arteriosclerotic changes in the arteriole obstruct blood flow in the venule resulting in a thrombotic venular occlusion. The funduscopic picture is characterized in Table 118–3. Macular edema is the most important cause of vision loss. Ultimately, collateral vessels develop to drain the affected sector of retina, and edema regression may occur. Significant retinal ischemia may result in retinal neovascularization and subsequent vitreous hemorrhage.

PRINCIPLES OF THERAPY

Fluorescein angiography is invaluable in evaluating retinal ischemia and macular edema. Laser photocoagulation is effective in treating neovascularization as well as macular edema.

TABLE 118–2.
Hypertensive Retinopathy*

DISORDER	PATHOPHYSIOLOGY
Retinal arteriolar sclerosis	Intimal hyalinization, media hypertrophy, and endothelial hyperplasia
Classification Grade 1—Broadening of arteriolar light reflex and mild AV crossing changes Grade 2—Marked broadening of arteriolar light reflex and AV crossing changes Grade 3—Copper-wire arterioles and more severe AV crossing changes Grade 4—Silver-wire arterioles (vascular occlusion)	
Hypertensive retinopathy	Retinal arteriolar sclerosis and retinal vascular incompetence
Classification Grade 1—Mild attenuation of retinal arterioles Grade 2—Moderate to severe arteriolar attenuation with focal areas of narrowing Grade 3—Grade 2 plus retinal exudates, hemorrhages, and cotton-wool spots Grade 4—Grade 3 plus optic disc edema	

* Scheie HG: Evaluation of ophthalmoscopic changes of hypertension and arteriolar sclerosis. *Arch Ophthalmol* 1953; 49:117–138.

TABLE 118–3.
Retinal Venous Occlusion

BRANCH VEIN OCCLUSION	
Systemic associations:	Systemic hypertension
	Diabetes mellitus
	Arteriosclerosis
Funduscopic Signs	*Pathophysiology*
Hemorrhages, retinal edema, cotton-wool spots	Vascular incompetence/leakage; retinal ischemia
Retinal neovascularization	Retinal ischemia (diffusible factor)
Venous collateral formation	
CENTRAL VEIN OCCLUSION	
Systemic associations:	Systemic hypertension, diabetes mellitus, cardiovascular disease, blood dyscrasias, dysproteinemias, vasculitis
Ocular association	Primary open-angle glaucoma (20%)
Funduscopic Signs	*Pathophysiology*
Hemorrhages, retinal edema, cotton-wool spots, disc edema	Vascular incompetence/leakage; retinal ischemia
Rubeosis iridis/neovascular glaucoma	Retinal ischemia (diffusible factor)

About 50% of patients will have at least 20/40 vision 1 year post-therapy. Permanent vision loss can result from chronic macular edema, subretinal fibrosis, and epiretinal membrane formation.

CENTRAL RETINAL VEIN OCCLUSION

There are two types of central retina vein occlusion. One is associated with mild or no retinal ischemia and mild vision loss; the other is associated with severe retinal ischemia and severe vision loss.

CLINICAL SIGNS AND SYMPTOMS

A painless loss of vision occurs in central vein occlusion. The systemic associations that may accompany central retinal vein occlusion are listed in Table 118–3. In most cases arteriosclerotic changes in the central retinal artery result in compression and thrombotic occlusion of the central retinal vein at the lamina cribrosa. Primary open-angle glaucoma often precedes central retinal vein occlusion and may be undiagnosed prior to the vascular event.

The funduscopic findings of central retinal vein occlusion are listed in Table 118–3. Fluorescein angiography is important in assessing the degree of retinal ischemia. If severe, retinal ischemia can be associated with rubeosis iridis and neovascular glaucoma. Macular edema is the most important cause of vision loss (Fig 118–2).

PRINCIPLES OF THERAPY

There is no therapy for the milder nonischemic type of central vein occlusion. Pan-retinal laser photocoagulation is effective in cases of ischemia with rubeosis iridis.

The prognosis is fairly good in the nonischemic variety, where partial or complete resolution of macular edema may occur. The visual prognosis in cases with severe ischemia is poor.

BRANCH RETINAL ARTERY OCCLUSION

Branch retinal artery occlusion refers to an occlusion of a retinal arteriole with subsequent infarction of the retinal tissue supplied by the involved vessel.

CLINICAL SIGNS AND SYMPTOMS

Acute, painless loss of vision resulting in altitudinal visual field loss is characteristic. Disorders associated with branch retinal artery occlusion are listed in Table 118–4.

Superior-temporal branch artery occlusion is

most common; nasal artery occlusions occur less frequently. The involved retina is opaque and edematous. Emboli within the retinal arterioles may be seen on funduscopic examination. Visual loss corresponding to the infarcted areas of the retina is permanent.

CENTRAL RETINAL ARTERY OCCLUSION

CLINICAL SIGNS AND SYMPTOMS

Acute, severe, painless loss of vision is characteristic. A history of transient ischemic attacks or amaurosis fugax may accompany branch and central artery occlusions. Disorders associated with central retinal artery occlusion are listed in Table 118–4.

The retina appears opaque and edematous due to the infarction of the nerve fiber layer. A cherry red spot at the fovea results from the intact choroidal vasculature being visible beneath the surrounding opaque retina (Fig 118–3). An intact cilioretinal artery may spare the macula. There is blood flow stasis within the retina vessels. Intraretinal plaques may be present suggesting an embolic cause. In many cases, atherosclerotic changes within the central retinal artery at the lamina cribrosa will result in thrombotic occlusion of the artery.

PRINCIPLES OF THERAPY

Central retinal artery occlusion is an emergency. Animal studies show that irreversible retinal damage occurs after 100 minutes of anoxia. Therapy is aimed at reducing intraocular pressure by anterior chamber paracentesis or by ocular massage. Inhalation of a 95% oxygen/5% carbon dioxide mixture may successfully dilate the central retinal artery. Therapy is usually unsuccessful in cases with an atherosclerotic cause.

Eyes with an intact cilioretinal artery may retain central vision. Vision in infarcted areas of the retina is permanently lost.

SENILE MACULAR DEGENERATION

Senile macular degeneration is the leading cause of new onset blindness in the United States. A spectrum of pathologic processes may

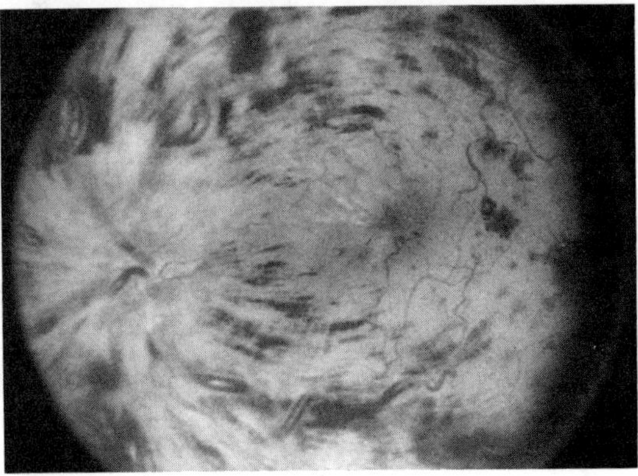

FIG 118–2.
Central retinal vein occlusion demonstrates extreme tortuosity of retinal veins, hemorrhages, and retinal edema.

TABLE 118–4.
Retinal Arterial Occlusion: Branch Artery Occlusion and Central Artery Occlusion

SYSTEMIC ASSOCIATION
Atherosclerosis
Systemic hypertension
Carotid occlusive disease (cholesterol emboli)
Arteriosclerosis (platelet-fibrin emboli)
Cardiac valvular disease (endocarditis, mitral valve prolapse)
Atrial myxoma
Hemoglobinopathies
Vasculitis
Oral contraceptives
Hypercoagulable states
Migraine
Orbital emphysema (rare)

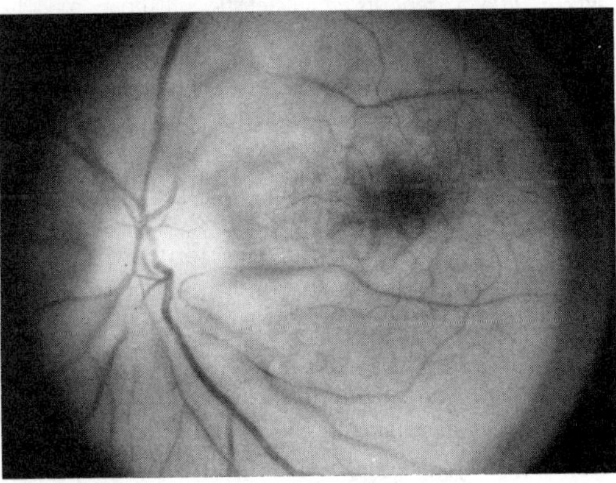

FIG 118–3.
Central retinal artery occlusion demonstrates milky-white coloration of infarcted retina and cherry red spot at fovea.

TABLE 118–5.
Senile Macular Degeneration (SMD)

FUNDUSCOPIC SIGN	PATHOLOGY
DRY (ATROPHIC, NONEXUDATIVE) SMD	
Drusen deposition	Hyaline deposits within Bruch's membrane degeneration/decompensation of retinal pigment epithelium (RPE)
RPE atrophy (geographic or areolar atrophy)	Drusen deposition, photoreceptor degeneration, RPE clumping
WET (EXUDATIVE) SMD	
Serous and/or hemorrhagic detachment of sensory retina and RPE	Subretinal neovascularization (vessel ingrowth from choroid through breaks in Bruch's membrane)
Disciform degeneration	Cicatricial changes within areas of old subretinal hemorrhage

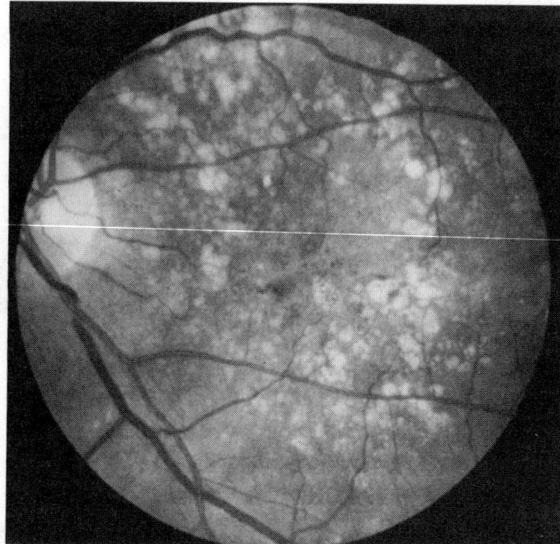

FIG 118–4.
Diffuse drusen deposits characteristic of senile macular degeneration.

occur in the aging macula, and a variety of funduscopic changes may be found. The basic pathogenesis is uncertain; however, a metabolic defect in the retinal pigment epithelium and its interaction with the photoreceptors is postulated. Drusen are hyaline depositions that are deposited on Bruch's membrane and are the hallmark of senile macular degeneration. They may appear as discrete yellowish lesions (hyaline drusen), as calcific crystalline deposits (calcific drusen), or as diffuse deposits (Fig 118–4).

CLINICAL SIGNS AND SYMPTOMS

Clinically, senile macular degeneration can be divided into a nonexudative (dry or atrophic) type and an exudative type characterized by subretinal neovascular membrane formation. The characteristics of each type are listed in Table 118–5. Disruption of Bruch's membrane by drusen deposition can result in choroidal vascular in-growth into the subretinal or subretinal pigment epithelial spaces causing serous or hemorrhagic retinal detachment or both as leakage and hemorrhage from the abnormal vessels occur. Disciform degeneration (macular scar formation) can result.

PRINCIPLES OF THERAPY

There is no treatment for the atrophic or nonexudative type of macular degeneration. Laser photocoagulation for subretinal neovascular membranes that have not extended into the foveal avascular zone can be effective. A delay in therapy may result in irreversible damage. Thus elderly patients who complain of central visual disturbance should be promptly examined. Fluorescein angiography is indispensable in diagnosis and determining the treatment of subretinal neovascular membranes.

Loss of central vision results in visual acuity in the 20/200 to "count fingers" range. Fortunately, peripheral vision is almost always spared, and patients are able to maintain most of the activities of daily living.

RETINOPATHY OF PREMATURITY

Retinopathy of prematurity is a proliferative retinopathy that occurs in premature and low-birth-weight infants. Infants with birth weights less than 1,000 gm are at particular risk. The disease occurs because the peripheral temporal retinal vasculature in the premature infant is susceptible to oxygen-induced capillary endothelial cell cytotoxicity. High partial pressures of oxygen lead to obliteration of vascularization in the temporal retinal periphery.

CLINICAL SIGNS AND SYMPTOMS

The optimal time for examination is at 7 weeks to 9 weeks of age. A mesenchymal arteriovenous shunt develops at the junction between the peripheral avascular retina and the posterior vascularized retina. Temporal dragging of the optic disc and posterior retina may occur as a result of tractional retinal detachment. In severe cases neovascularization supervenes, and vitreous hemorrhage and/or retinal detachment may result.

PRINCIPLES OF THERAPY

The role of vitamin E therapy is uncertain; it may reduce the severity, but not the incidence of the retinopathy of prematurity. In severe cases, surgical vitrectomy and cryopexy are occasionally successful

Over 80% of cases are mild and undergo spontaneous regression. Severe cases have a poor prognosis. The long-term ocular complications in eyes with regressed retinopathy of prematurity include myopia, cataract, retinal detachment, glaucoma, and strabismus.

RETINAL DETACHMENT

Retinal detachment refers to a separation of the neurosensory portion of the retina from the retinal pigment epithelium. A retina detachment may be associated with a retinal hole (rhegmatogenous detachment) or may be associated with subretinal exudate or retinal traction with no accompanying retinal hole (nonrhegmatogenous detachment).

The symptoms of retinal detachment are flashes of light, "floaters," or loss of peripheral visual field and/or loss of central vision. The patient may give history of high myopia or ocular trauma.

Indirect ophthalmoscopy is mandatory because the significant pathologic changes (retinal holes and tears) in the peripheral retina cannot be seen by direct ophthalmoscopy. The detached retina is opaque and often floating in the middle of the vitreous space.

PRINCIPLES OF THERAPY

Laser photocoagulation, cryopexy, and most often, scleral buckling surgery are the primary treatment modalities.

Retinal detachment is an emergency. Once the macula has detached, central vision never returns to premorbid levels even in the presence of an anatomically successful operation. Thus, early treatment is associated with an excellent visual prognosis while delayed treatment yields significantly less satisfactory results.

REFERENCES

Duane TD, Jaeger EA (eds): The retina, in *Clinical Opthalmology*, vol 3. Philadelphia, Harper & Row, 1985. *An in-depth analysis of retinal diseases.*

Fraunfelder FT, Roy FH: *Current Ocular Therapy*, ed 2. Philadelphia, WB Saunders Co, 1985. *An excellent general text.*

Gass JDM: *Stereoscopic Atlas of Macular Disease*, ed 2. St. Louis, CV Mosby Co, 1977. *The standard text for macular diseases written by the world's leading expert on the subject.*

Macular Photocoagulation Study Group: Argon laser photocoagulation for senile macular degeneration: Results of a randomized clinical trial. *Arch Ophthalmol* 1982; 100:912. *A controlled study examining the efficacy of photocoagulation in the treatment of senile macular degeneration.*

Scheie HG: Evaluation of ophthalmoscopic changes of hypertension and arteriolar sclerosis. *Arch Ophthalmol* 1953; 49:117–138. *The standard classification of retinal hypertensive retinopathy.*

Scheie HG, Albert DM (eds): *Textbook of Ophthalmology*, ed 9. Philadelphia, WB Saunders Co, 1977. *An excellent general text for the beginner.*

119

OCULAR MALIGNANCY

John A. Fleishman, M.D.
John D. Bullock, M.D., M.S.

Retinoblastoma is a primary tumor of the retina. Retinoblastoma is the most common intraocular malignancy of childhood with an incidence of about 1 in 25,000 live births. About 250 new cases occur each year in the United States. Approximately 6% of those will have a family history, the remainder resulting from sporadic mutations. In familial cases, the tumor is inherited as an autosomal dominant with high penetrance. Of the sporadic cases, 25% are due to a germinal mutation and 75% to a somatic mutation. Almost all bilateral cases are due to a germinal mutation. Thirty percent are bilateral. Normal parents with one affected child have a 6% chance of producing another affected child. If more than one child is affected, then there is a slightly less than 50% chance that subsequent children will be affected.

CLINICAL SIGNS AND SYMPTOMS

Ninety percent of cases are seen before the age of 2 years with an average age at diagnosis of 17 months. The common initial signs are listed in Table 119–1. Patients with small tumors often present with strabismus, while those with moderate size tumors usually present with leukocoria (white pupil) (Fig 119–1). Patients with extraocular extension may present with orbital signs or distant metastases. Two types of tumor growth may determine the clinical appearance. Endophytic growth implies that the tumor grows from the retina into the vitreous. These tumors are often visible as whitish-pink masses. Exophytic tumors grow in the subretinal space and may appear as a total retinal detachment with subretinal exudates. The tumor is often multicentric, and more than one tumor per affected eye is quite common. Calcification of the tumor often occurs and can be identified radiographically in 70% of cases. Vitreous seeding with tumor cells is common.

The common histopathologic appearance of retinoblastoma is uniform round or polygonal cells with scant cytoplasm and a large nucleus with abundant chromatin. Pseudorosette formation is common. Large columnar cells radially arranged around a central lumen (Flexner-Wintersteiner rosettes) probably represents differentiation into primitive rod and cone elements and is a favorable prognostic sign. The clinical–pathologic correlations are shown in Table 119–2.

DIAGNOSIS

The funduscopic appearance of an endophytic retinoblastoma with "cottage cheese" calcification is diagnostic. Exophytic tumors in eyes with retinal detachment, vitreous hemorrhage, or inflammation may be difficult to diagnose. A complete fundus examination under anesthesia is required. X-ray films to detect calcium and B-scan ultrasonography are often helpful. Aqueous humor may be obtained by paracen-

TABLE 119–1.
Retinoblastoma (*N* = 235)

INITIAL SIGNS	PERCENTAGE OF CASES*
Leukocoria	61
Strabismus	22
Decreased vision	5
Routine exam	4
Orbital signs (proptosis)	2
Red, painful eye with glaucoma	2
Unilateral dilated pupil	1
Spontaneous hyphema	0.5
Heterochromia iridis	0.5

* Howard GM, Ellsworth RM: Differential diagnosis of retinoblastoma. Relative frequency of lesions which simulate retinoblastoma. *Am J Ophthalmol* 1965; 60:610–618.

TABLE 119–2.
Clinical–Pathologic Correlations

CLINICAL FINDINGS	PATHOLOGIC FINDINGS
RETINOBLASTOMA	
Leukocoria	Endophytic or exophytic growth with retrolenticular mass
Strabismus, decreased vision	Tumor growth involving visual axis
Whitish-pink mass in vitreous	Endophytic growth pattern
Nonrhegmatogenous retinal detachment	Exophytic growth pattern
Proptosis, lid edema	Extraocular extension
CHOROIDAL MELANOMA	
Visual loss	Tumor obstructing visual axis, intraocular hemorrhage, retinal detachment, secondary glaucoma
Hyphema, heterochromia, glaucoma	Extension of tumor into anterior segment
Retinal detachment (nonrhegmatogenous)	Subretinal growth of tumor
Dark epibulbar mass	Scleral invasion by tumor
Proptosis, lid edema	Extraocular extension by tumor

tesis for a lactic dehydrogenase (LDH) assay. An aqueous-to-plasma ratio of LDH concentration that is greater than 1.0 is common in patients with retinoblastoma. Retinoblastomas accumulate ^{32}P in a characteristic fashion and in difficult cases, a ^{32}P-uptake test may be used. Family members should be examined for evidence of regressed retinoblastoma. Every patient with retinoblastoma should have skull and chest x-rays, bone and liver scans, bone marrow aspiration, and cerebrospinal fluid cytologic studies to identify possible metastatic disease. The tumor is highly metastatic.

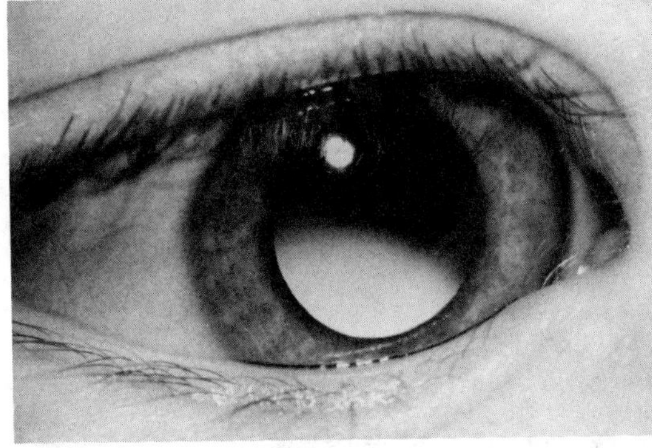

FIG 119–1.
Leukocoria (white pupil) in a patient with retinoblastoma.

PRINCIPLES OF THERAPY

In cases of unilateral tumor, prompt enucleation following studies showing no evidence of metastases is advisable. In bilateral cases the more severely affected eye is enucleated and the other eye is irradiated. Supervoltage radiation through temporal ports (3.0 × 4.0 cm) with a total dosage of 3500 rads to 4500 rads is recommended. Radiation-induced cataracts and retinopathy are minimal at such dosages. Within 2 weeks to 3 weeks most tumors begin to shrink and display calcification. Systemic chemotherapy with Cytoxan and vincristine is indicated in advanced unilateral or bilateral disease with or without metastases. Because involved eyes have a high rate of new tumor development during the first 6 months of life, frequent examinations under anesthesia are advisable to assess for new tumor involvement. Other modes of therapy include photocoagulation, cryotherapy, and cobalt 60 plaques and are usually reserved for solitary retinoblastomas smaller than 10 mm.

The prognosis for survival in the United States today appears to be almost 90% with the prognosis for unilateral and bilateral almost equal. The degree of cellular differentiation of the tumor and the presence of optic nerve and choroidal involvement are important factors in estimating survival. Cases with metastasis have a very poor prognosis. The potential of saving vision in treated eyes depends primarily on tumor size and location. In about 1% of cases, the tumor undergoes spontaneous regression.

Sarcomatous tumors of the orbit following irradiation may occur. Osteogenic sarcoma is the most common. Children with bilateral retinoblastoma may have an increased susceptibility to radiation-induced tumors. In addition, unrelated neoplasia may develop years later in these patients. Osteogenic sarcoma of the femur has been seen most frequently.

MALIGNANT MELANOMA

Malignant melanoma is a highly aggressive neoplasm originating from melanocytes. Malignant melanoma involving the eye represents a spectrum of disease with the location, size, and tumor cell-type determining the general clinical presentation, type of therapy, and prognosis. Melanoma may involve the conjunctiva, iris, ciliary body, or choroid.

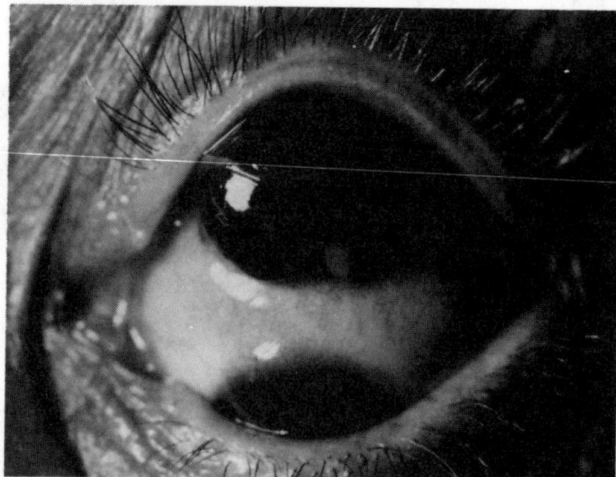

FIG 119–2.
A large elevated conjunctival malignant melanoma protruding from the superior conjunctival fornix.

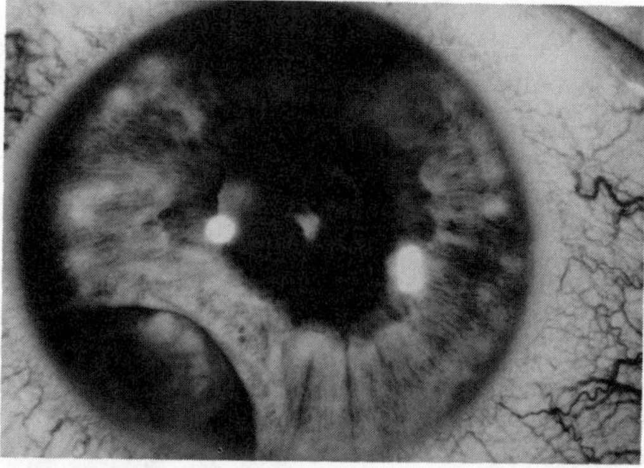

FIG 119–3.
A pigment iris melanoma growing from the iris base. Note the distortion of the pupil.

MELANOMA OF THE CONJUNCTIVA

Melanoma involving the conjunctiva has a better prognosis than cutaneous melanoma, but it is still a potentially lethal neoplasm.

CLINICAL SIGNS AND SYMPTOMS

About 40% of conjunctival melanomas develop from preexisting nevi, 25% from acquired melanosis, and 25% de novo. The lesion may be asymptomatic and first noted on routine ophthalmologic examination, or the patient may complain of an enlarging pigmented mass on the interpalpebral bulbar conjunctiva.

On physical examination, a variably pigmented, highly vascular mass involving the bulbar conjunctiva in the interpalpebral zone is typically seen. Although less common, the tumor may occur in the conjunctival fornices or the palpebral conjunctiva (Fig 119–2). Fixation to the surrounding tissues may occur when invasion has occurred. Lesions in an early stage may be difficult to differentiate from conjunctival nevi. The rapid growth rate and vascularity of melanomas are distinguishing characteristics.

PRINCIPLES OF THERAPY

Therapy of conjunctival melanomas involves total excision of the lesion(s). Cryotherapy of the bed of the excised lesion may be used to lessen the chance of recurrence. With intraocular or intraorbital spread, enucleation or exenteration may be required.

The prognosis for long-term survival is quite good. In one series, long-term survival was 78%. Tumors in the conjunctival fornices are usually larger when discovered and usually have a worse prognosis.

MELANOMA OF THE IRIS

CLINICAL SIGNS AND SYMPTOMS

Iris melanomas are often an incidental finding on slit-lamp examination. Alternatively, the patient may complain of an enlarging pigmented mass on the iris associated with decreased vision (sector cataract).

On physical examination the tumor may be highly pigmented or amelanotic. Differentiation from an iris nevus may be difficult. Observation in such cases may be prudent because melanomas will invariably grow. Melanomas of the iris may be highly vascular. Other signs of malignancy include ectropion iridis, cataract, glaucoma, and pupillary distortion (Fig 119–3). Rarely, a diffuse growth pattern may produce a syndrome of unilateral acquired hyperchromic heterochromia and secondary glaucoma.

PRINCIPLES OF THERAPY

Management is usually simple excisional iridectomy. With extension of the tumor into angle structures, an iridocyclectomy may be required. Tumors with diffuse growth patterns, although rare, often require enucleation.

The prognosis for survival in cases of iris melanomas is excellent. The tumors usually consist of spindle A or spindle B tumor cells, with epithelioid cells being rare.

MELANOMA OF THE CILIARY BODY

Melanomas involving the ciliary body vary widely, depending on the size and growth rate of the tumor. Cryptically placed behind the iris, these tumors often achieve large size prior to discovery.

CLINICAL SIGNS AND SYMPTOMS

The patient may be asymptomatic, and the diagnosis may be made incidentally. Alternatively, refractive changes due to displacement and pressure on the lens, focal cataract, or a dark epibulbar mass (when the tumor invades the sclera) may be the initial symptoms. Dilated episcleral vessels in the quadrant of the tumor may be present. Rarely, diffuse tumor growth may involve the entire ciliary body, a "ring" melanoma.

DIAGNOSIS

Transillumination and indirect ophthalmoscopy are useful in delineating the extent of the tumor. A ^{32}P-uptake test may be helpful.

PRINCIPLES OF THERAPY

Therapy is highly variable and should be tailored to the individual situation. Small tumors may be observed over time if the patient's vision remains good. Large tumors can be treated by iridocyclectomy. Large tumors with scleral extension and "ring" melanomas usually require enucleation. The prognosis is variable depending on the size and extension of the tumor.

MELANOMA OF THE CHOROID

CLINICAL SIGNS AND SYMPTOMS

The symptoms produced by a choroidal melanoma depend on the location. Anterior tumors may reach considerable size before affecting vision; posterior lesions situated near the macula tend to produce visual loss earlier. The patient, however, is often asymptomatic, and the diagnosis is made on routine examination.

Indirect ophthalmoscopy is needed to visualize the entire retina. Classically an elevated, variably pigmented, oval-shaped choroidal mass is observed. Orange pigment (lipofuscin) or drusen may be present in the overlying retinal pigment epithelium, but these are not diagnostic. A surrounding serous or hemorrhagic retinal detachment may be present (Fig 119–4). As the tumor expands, it will often rupture through Bruch's membrane, resulting in a characteristic mushroom-shaped growth pattern. See Table 119–2 for clinical–pathologic correlations.

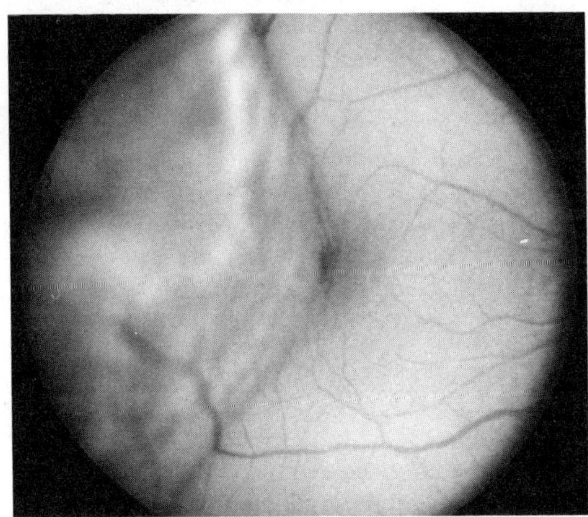

FIG 119–4.
A large malignant melanoma with overlying retinal detachment. The tumor extends toward the fovea at center of the photograph.

DIAGNOSIS

The diagnosis is often clinically obvious on indirect ophthalmoscopic examination. Numerous lesions may mimic a choroidal melanoma such as choroidal nevus, retinal detachment, disciform macular degeneration, choroidal hemangioma, metastatic tumor to the choroid and retinoschisis. Fundus photographs are useful in following the course of small lesions that resemble nevi because melanomas invariably grow. Fluorescein angiography may be useful in selected cases. Ocular ultrasonography is helpful because the pattern on ultrasound is characteristic. The ^{32}P-uptake test is occasionally helpful but cannot differentiate choroidal metastasis from melanoma.

All patients should be evaluated for metastatic disease including a general physical examination, measurement of serum LDH and alkaline phosphatase levels, chest x-ray, and liver, spleen, and bone scans.

PRINCIPLES OF THERAPY

The therapy of choroidal melanomas is controversial. Enucleation has been the primary mode of therapy. However, recent data suggest that the death rate from metastatic disease peaks about 2 years to 3 years after enucleation. Whether this means that enucleation disseminates the tumor or changes host-defense mechanisms or that metastasis would have occurred in the absence of enucleation is uncertain. Prudent observation of small melanomas over time in older patients is acceptable. Small tumors may respond to laser photocoagulation. Irradiation therapy with proton beam or cobalt 60 or iodine 125 plaques has become increasingly popular. Chemotherapy is indicated in cases with metastasis.

The prognosis is highly variable and depends on tumor size and extension and cell type.

RHABDOMYOSARCOMA

Orbital rhabdomyosarcoma is the most common primary orbital malignant tumor of childhood. These are tumors of striated muscle cells which typically occur in the peripheral skeletal muscles of adults and of the head, neck, and orbit in children. The tumor develops from pluripotential mesenchymal tissue possessing the ability to develop into striated muscle.

CLINICAL SIGNS AND SYMPTOMS

The average age at diagnosis is 7 years to 8 years. Typically the sudden onset of unilateral proptosis with periorbital edema and discoloration of the lids is found. The tumor is often located superonasally in the orbit, but it can occur anywhere in the orbit. The regional lymph nodes should be palpated for possible metastasis.

DIAGNOSIS

Orbital computed tomographic (CT) scanning, tomograms, and ultrasonography are all useful. Destruction of the bony walls of the orbit is characteristic. Suspected lesions should be biopsied. Electron microscopy may be important in establishing a histopathologic diagnosis.

PRINCIPLES OF THERAPY

Radiation therapy alone or combined with systemic chemotherapy is the most effective therapy and has replaced exenteration. The prognosis depends on the extent of the tumor, the presence or absence of metastases, and the cell type. Metastases generally occur in the lungs, cervical lymph nodes, and occasionally bone.

METASTATIC OCULAR TUMORS

Metastatic carcinoma involving the eye may be the most common intraocular tumor. Most cases involve the posterior uvea. Decreased vision, pain, photopsia, red eye, photophobia, and floaters are common symptoms and signs. The lesions are usually mottled, yellow-white, elevated masses which are often associated with a nonrhegmatogenous retinal detachment. Table 119–3 lists the common primary tumors that may metastasize to the eye. The treatment is usually external beam irradiation, 3000 rads to 4500 rads, in divided doses.

TABLE 119–3.
Metastatic Carcinoma of the Eye and Adnexae
($N = 227$)

SITE OF METASTATIC TUMOR	PERCENT OF TOTAL CASES*
Intraocular	196
Orbital	28
Optic nerve	3

PRIMARY TUMOR

SITE OF PRIMARY TUMOR	PERCENT OF TOTAL CASES*
Breast†	40
Lung†	29
Kidney	4
Testicle	3
Prostate	1
Pancreas, stomach, ileum, and colon	<1
Unknown	18

* Ferry AP, Font RL: Carcinoma metastatic to the eye and orbit. *Arch Ophthalmol* 1974; 92:276–286.

† In women, breast carcinoma accounts for 77% of cases, and in men lung carcinoma accounts for 49%.

REFERENCES

Ferry AP, Font RL: Carcinoma metastatic to the eye and orbit. *Arch Ophthalmol* 1974; 92:276–286. *A review of 227 cases of metastatic carcinoma involving the eye and adnexae.*

Howard GM, Ellsworth RM: Differential diagnosis of retinoblastoma. Relative frequency of lesions which simulate retinoblastoma. *AM J Ophthalmol* 1965; 60:610–618. *A comprehensive review of 235 cases of retinoblastoma.*

Reese AB: *Tumors of the Eye*, ed 3. New York, Harper & Row, 1976. *A detailed text about all ocular tumors.*

Shield JA: Diagnosis and management of intraocular tumors. St Louis, CV Mosby Co, 1982. *A standard, detailed text of all intraocular tumors.*

Zimmerman LE, McLean IW, Foster WD: Does enucleation of the eye containing a malignant melanoma prevent or accelerate the dissemination of tumor cells? *Br J Ophthalmol* 1973; 62:420–425. *An excellent discussion of the controversy regarding enucleation in choroidal melanoma.*

part X

Nervous System and Psychiatric Disorders

120

STROKE: OCCLUSIVE CEREBRAL VASCULAR DISEASE

Samuel E. Pitner, M.D.

Stroke is an extremely common problem in our aging population. Vascular disease of the brain is the third leading cause of death in the United States. Considered as a group, all types of stroke have a fatality rate of 20%. Over 1% of living Americans are believed to have had a stroke at some time in their lives.

Strokes are brain lesions caused by diseased blood vessels. Whatever the exact pathologic condition of a cerebral artery, it produces symptoms only by interrupting blood flow or by rupturing to produce hemorrhage into the parenchyma of the brain (intracerebral hemorrhage) or over its surface (subarachnoid hemorrhage). These types of hemorrhage are considered in Chap 121, Intracranial Hemorrhage. We will be concerned here only with cerebral thrombosis or embolism.

CLINICAL SIGNS AND SYMPTOMS

The acute onset of localized (as opposed to diffuse) brain dysfunction is the hallmark of stroke. The abrupt onset of any condition is sometimes spoken of as apoplectic, from the old term for stroke, apoplexy. If the vascular obstruction is temporary and circulation to an area is restored before actual infarction occurs, the symptoms are completely reversible. Transient cerebral ischemic attacks, most often referred to as transient ischemic attacks or TIAs, by definition can last only 24 hours; however, a typical attack usually lasts for only several minutes. Unfortunately, the most common initial manifestation of cerebral vascular disease is that of a completed stroke, where actual infarction occurs. In this instance, symptoms remain at the same level or even increase for a few days, after which there is usually gradual but often incomplete improvement in the patient's neurologic deficit. Occasionally, there

seems to be a stepwise progression of the deficit while the patient is under observation, a situation known as stroke-in-evolution. The course of these and other cerebral vascular syndromes is shown in Table 120–1.

Due to the distribution of the blood supply of the brain, occlusion of a vessel nearly always produces asymmetric and localized (focal) neurologic dysfunction. Symptoms of diffuse (global) cerebral ischemia such as syncope or giddiness are not localizing and cannot be considered due to cerebral vascular disease unless they are associated with focal dysfunction.

In considering the anatomy of the cerebral circulation from a clinical standpoint, we must begin with the great vessels in the neck, the two carotid arteries and the two vertebral arteries, because extracranial occlusive cerebral vascular disease produces symptoms that in most cases are indistinguishable by history and examination from those of intracranial arterial occlusion. To a great extent, the part of the cerebral circulation from the vertebral arteries remains separate from that from the carotid arteries, so the first step in localizing an ischemic cerebral lesion is deciding which of these two systems is involved.

Eighty percent of the cerebral blood flow comes through the carotid arteries, which supply the bulk of the cerebral hemispheres and approximately 80% of the brain by weight. This sometimes is referred to as the carotid system and also is called the anterior circulation. The velocity of blood flow in this system generally is greater than in the vertebral artery circulation; in the latter, the vertebral arteries join to form the basilar artery and, in most people, also provide blood to the occipital cortex through the posterior cerebral arteries. Thus, this second arterial system (also called the vertebrobasilar or posterior circulation) supplies the brain stem and, through the posterior cere-

TABLE 120–1.
Temporal Profile of Occlusive Cerebral Vascular Syndromes

SYNDROME	DURATION AND COMMENT
Transient cerebral ischemia (transient ischemic attack, TIA)	Typically 20 minutes Never over 24 hours Often multiple Usually stereotyped
Completed stroke (cerebral vascular accident, CVA)	Neurologic deficit of variable severity lasting over 24 hours Nearly half preceded by TIAs Unfortunately, most stroke patients seeking medical attention have this type.
Reversible ischemic neurologic deficit (RIND)	Minimal neurologic deficit for more than 24 hours but with complete recovery (a type of completed stroke)
Stroke-in-evolution	Progressively worsening deficit over hours or days
Cerebral embolism	Can mimic any of above

bral arteries, the posterior part of the mesial surface of the cerebral hemispheres.

Table 120–2 lists the most frequent symptoms and signs in circulatory disturbances in these two systems and the anatomical structures whose involvement produces them. Remember that the temporal profile of the illness varies with the pathologic changes induced; ischemia usually reverses and the patient recovers, whereas actual infarction produces a longer lasting impairment.

The patient with transient cerebral ischemia only rarely is seen by a physician during an episode so that this diagnosis of necessity is based primarily on the history. Continuing neurologic abnormalities (unless less than 24 hours old) observed on examination would exclude a diagnosis of TIAs. As can be seen from Table 120–2, a wide variety of findings can be seen on neurologic examination, and those observed depend on the exact location of the lesion. The patient's state of consciousness may be impaired. Occasionally, this is a direct result of the stroke in individuals with lesions in the territory of the basilar artery and who have primary involvement of the reticular activating formation. More often, this is the result of a shift of supratentorial brain structures due to edema produced during the course of a large infarction of the cerebral hemispheres themselves; this makes impaired consciousness an ominous prognostic sign (see Chap 7, Coma and States of Diminished Consciousness).

The neurologic examination alone does not allow differentiation of an intracranial from an extracranial arterial occlusion; nearly one-third of all cerebral infarctions are believed to be due to a lesion of one of the large arteries in the neck. In just under half of patients with an extracranial arterial lesion, there will be some finding on the examination of the head and neck that will give a clue to the site of the arterial lesion. Probably the most common of these are bruits over the carotid bifurcation or elsewhere about the head or neck. Some patients with complete occlusion of their internal carotid artery will show a Horner syndrome ipsilateral to the arterial lesion. Apparent decreased carotid pulses to palpation are not reliable findings.

A general physical examination, particularly the cardiac examination, is very important, especially in the differential diagnosis of thrombosis and embolism. The presence of an arrhythmia or valvular heart disease can be particularly important in suggesting embolism as opposed to thrombosis as the source of a cerebral infarction.

PATHOPHYSIOLOGY

Following occlusion of an intracranial artery, complete ischemia produces neuronal and glial cell death within several minutes. Tissue acidosis occurs, producing maximal dilation of the blood vessels in and around the ischemic area. Breakdown of the blood–brain barrier follows, which allows an uptake of radiopaque material by the brain that is seen in CT scans in

TABLE 120–2.
Clinical–Pathologic Correlation: Localization of the Common Sites of Ischemia or Infarction

CAROTID ("ANTERIOR") CIRCULATION		VERTEBROBASILAR ("POSTERIOR") CIRCULATION	
SYMPTOM	ANATOMICAL STRUCTURE	SYMPTOM	ANATOMICAL STRUCTURE
Hemiparesis or hemiplegia	Corticospinal tract—cortical or in internal capsule	Hemianopsia Cortical blindness Blurred vision	Occipital cortex (posterior cerebral arteries)
Hemihypesthesia	Sensory pathways—thalamic or cortical	Diplopia	Cranial nerve nuclei III, IV, or VI or their connections
Aphasia	Cortex and/or subcortical connections of dominant hemisphere		
Nondominant parietal lobe syndromes	Parietal lobe structures, right hemisphere	Ataxia	Cerebellum or cerebellar connections
Amaurosis fugax (transient monocular blindness)	Retinal ischemia via ophthalmic artery	Vertigo	Vestibular nuclei or connections
		Facial numbness (often tongue or perioral)	Spinal tract of cranial nerve V or its nucleus

Note: Symptoms are listed in order of decreasing frequency.

over half of the cases. Cytotoxic cerebral edema then develops, usually reaching a peak in 72 hours. This produces localized decreases in brain density and a shift of intracranial structures that may be seen on a CT scan. If the cerebral hemisphere is involved, edema may progress to cause progressive distortion of the brain stem. Increasing involvement of the ascending reticular formation decreases consciousness and finally ends with secondary brain stem hemorrhage, coma, and death. Lesions involving the brain stem directly can have the same course.

The same general sequence of events occurs in the infarcted areas in embolic strokes. However, emboli generally are much more friable than thrombi and tend to break up and be swept distally after lodging at bifurcations. Be-

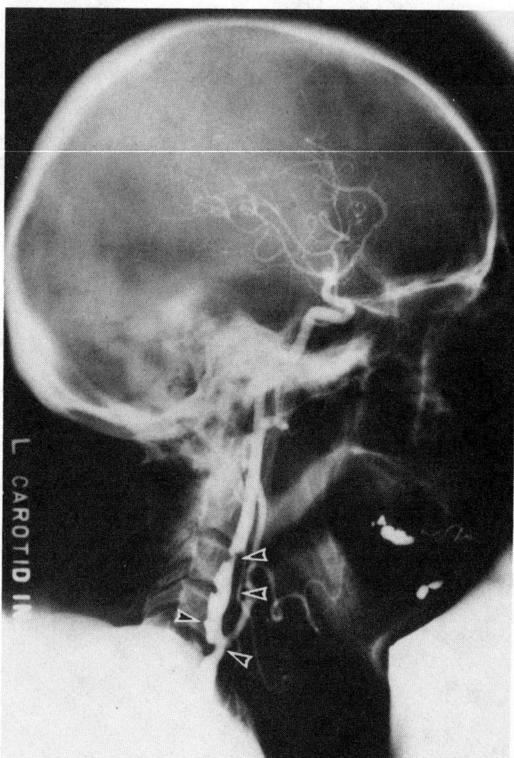

FIG 120–1.
Cerebral angiogram showing bifurcation of common carotid into external and internal carotid arteries. Negative filling defects at right arrows are stenotic lesions. Contrast media at the left arrow is filling an ulcerated lesion (Courtesy of Dr. Rich Carroll, Miami Valley Hospital Radiology Department, Dayton, OH).

cause this means a return of cerebral blood flow with full arterial pressure into an area with damaged endothelium, infarcts due to embolism are much more likely to be hemorrhagic than pale. (A hemorrhagic infarct on a CT scan always strongly suggests a diagnosis of embolism.)

Transient cerebral ischemic attacks differ from completed strokes in that cerebral ischemia stops short of actual infarction and recovery of function occurs. TIAs are more likely to occur when the vascular disturbance is in one of the great vessels in the neck rather than an intracranial artery. Because of the circle of Willis and some potential for development of collateral circulation, occlusion of a single internal carotid or vertebral artery usually does not cause symptoms itself. If enough vessels are involved, a rapid drop in cardiac output can produce a focal ischemic stroke, but this is relatively rare. Most TIAs are believed to result from artery-to-artery embolism arising from an ulcerated plaque in a stenotic neck vessel (see Fig 120–1). Erosion of an atherosclerotic plaque exposes collagen to the circulating blood and attracts platelets. Because these platelet emboli are very friable, they tend to break up and pass through to the venous circulation in the course of a few minutes, thus explaining the transient nature of TIAs. Although this never has been observed directly in the cerebral circulation, of course, this sequence of events has been observed by ophthalmoscopy in the retinal circulation in cases of amaurosis fugax. This is the basis for the use of drugs to decrease blood platelet reactivity in transient cerebral ischemic attacks.

CLINICAL–PATHOLOGIC CORRELATIONS

The clinical–pathologic correlations are listed in Table 120–2.

DIFFERENTIAL DIAGNOSIS

The differential diagnosis varies widely, depending on the patient's symptoms. Transient ischemic attacks (TIAs) must be differentiated from other episodic or paroxysmal disorders.

TABLE 120–3.
Differentiating Cerebral Vascular Disease from Other Disorders

TYPE OF VASCULAR DISEASE	NONVASCULAR DISORDERS TO BE CONSIDERED
Transient ischemic attacks	Focal seizures
	Migraine auras
	Cardiac arrhythmias
	Syncope
	Generalized seizures
Completed stroke	Intracranial hemorrhage
	Brain tumor (primary or metastatic)
	Brain abscess
	Traumatic lesions
	Degenerative disorders
	Demyelinating disease

The other major conditions that must be ruled out are shown in Table 120–3. Special considerations apply to vertebrobasilar TIAs. First, even true vertigo as opposed to giddiness itself does not warrant a diagnosis of vertebrobasilar TIA; inner ear disease can produce this symptom also. Consciousness is practically never affected in carotid system TIAs and only rarely in vertebrobasilar disease. Nevertheless, at times it may be difficult to differentiate vertebrobasilar insufficiency from a generalized or global decrease in cerebral circulation, such as from an abrupt fall in cardiac output due to an arrhythmia. Generally speaking, an overall (global) decrease in cerebral blood flow produces syncope or near syncope but only rarely produces focal neurologic signs.

The differential diagnosis of completed stroke also is presented in Table 120–3. The conditions to be considered are the major neurologic disorders that produce persistent (as opposed to transient) focal neurologic deficits. Usually these conditions have a different history, including progression over days or even months rather than an abrupt onset. Occasionally, such events as hemorrhage into a brain tumor can mimic a stroke.

The differential diagnosis of thrombosis and embolism as causes of cerebral infarction can be difficult. The diagnosis of cerebral embolism generally is based on the presence of a likely source for emboli. This diagnosis is more definite if there is evidence of embolization elsewhere in the body. Hemorrhagic infarction on a CT scan suggests embolism. Multiple episodes in a short period of time favors embolism, as half of all cases of cerebral embolism show multiple areas of infarction.

LABORATORY DIAGNOSIS

The laboratory, including radiologic, studies required for a given stroke patient will vary in each case depending on the exact clinical situation. When the patient has findings compatible with completed stroke, studies directed to ruling out other conditions considered in the differential diagnosis (Table 120–3) may be necessary. Intracranial hemorrhage is best ruled out by computed tomography (CT scan), but some cases will require spinal fluid examination.

Once the occurrence of an infarction has been established, it may be necessary to exclude nonatherosclerotic causes of arterial thrombosis in some patients. In addition to embolism, these include (but are not limited to) arteritis (including syphilitic), blood dyscrasias, and numerous other possibilities. Finally, coexistent disease must be investigated. For example, in some studies 10% of patients presenting with an acute stroke have a coexisting acute myocardial infarction.

Particularly in the case of TIAs, but also in minor completed strokes, studies to evaluate the extracranial part of the cerebral arterial circulation for possible vascular surgery may be indicated. Studies used to evaluate the carotid arteries also are shown in Table 120–4. The most accurate of these is cerebral angiography. However, this has a serious complication rate of just under 1% and is not indicated in all stroke patients by any means.

TABLE 120–4.
Diagnostic Studies in Stroke

I. Studies to exclude nonvascular lesions:
   CT scan*
   Chest x-ray films*
   Skull x-ray films*
   CSF examination
   Radioisotope scan
   EEG
   Angiography
II. Studies to define type of vascular disease:
   CT scan*
   ECG*
   Echocardiogram*
   Angiography*
   Serologic tests for syphilis
   CSF examination
   Erythrocyte sedimentation rate, antinuclear antibody level, etc.
   Coagulation studies
III. Studies to diagnose, locate, or define extracranial arterial lesions: (These apply primarily to patients with TIAs)
   Cerebral angiography
   Ultrasound imaging of neck vessels
   Ophthalmodynamometry
   Digital venous imaging
   (Also called digital subtraction angiography)
   Phonoangiography
   Ocular plethesmography

* Asterisks denote the most useful studies in each group.

PRINCIPLES OF THERAPY

The treatment of completed stroke consists primarily of physical therapy and other measures to hasten the restoration of such neurologic function as will return. Positioning in bed and the early initiation of passive range-of-motion exercises for paralyzed or paretic limbs are important. Depressed consciousness requires special nursing care to prevent pulmonary and other infectious complications. Attempts to control brain swelling in the deteriorating patient usually are futile. Corticosteroids have never been clearly demonstrated to be effective in this type of cerebral edema. Neither are osmotic diuretics usually practical because of the frequent "rebound" of pressure when their effect wears off. Anticoagulants (or endarterectomy in the case of extracranial arterial disease) are not effective once cerebral infarction has occurred. Most studies have shown that anticoagulants and operation are not helpful in completed stroke and may be harmful with one exception; in cerebral embolism, recent studies indicate that (in spite of the prevalence of hemorrhagic infarction) the risk of further systemic or cerebral embolization is greater than the risk of expanding a hemorrhagic infarction by anticoagulant treatment.

Unfortunately, stroke-in-evolution usually is recognized after deterioration has occurred. In

TABLE 120–5.
Suggested Guidelines for Management of Transient Ischemic Attacks

TYPE OF TIAS	ISCHEMIC ATTACKS GUIDELINES*

Carotid system TIAs	Potential surgical candidates with definite TIA:
	   Angiography
	   Other patients: medical treatment (see below)
	Patients with favorable arterial lesion as shown by
	   angiography
	   Thromboendarterectomy
	   Other patients: medical treatment (see below)

Vertebrobasilar TIAs	Medical treatment (see below)
	   (Angiography has a high risk-to-benefit ratio in these
	   patients.)

Both types of TIAs	Medical Treatment:
	   Symptoms for less than 3 months:
	      Anticoagulants for 3 months, then aspirin for 1 year
	   Symptoms for over 3 months:
	      Aspirin therapy for 1 year
	   No TIAs for 1 year:
	      No therapy indicated

* Modified from Sandok BA, Furlan AJ, Whisnant JP, Sundt TM Jr: Guidelines for the management of transient ischemic attacks. *Mayo Clin Proc* 1978; 53:665–674.

the patient who is deteriorating under observation, aggressive treatment is warranted. Patients who make a good recovery from a completed stroke may be candidates for investigation for vascular surgery later in the course of their illness.

No controlled study has ever shown a significant difference in outcome in patients with TIAs treated with carotid arterial surgery, anticoagulants, or agents to reduce platelet aggregation. A recent international collaborative study of surgical anastomosis of branches of the external carotid artery with intracranial arteries for cerebral ischemia showed that the procedure failed to alter the course of the disease. The treatment of TIAs is controversial. One approach to the management of these patients is shown in Table 120–5. Of the patients with TIAs, relatively few (30%–40%) suffer a completed stroke within 5 years of the first TIA. A disproportionate percentage (25%) of these patients who do have completed strokes do so in the first 3 months after the onset of TIAs. Therefore, the recommended medical therapy varies with the time since the onset of transient cerebral ischemic attacks.

REFERENCES

American Heart Association: *Current Concepts of Cerebrovascular Disease: Stroke.* Published bimonthly by the American Heart Association, Inc, Dallas. *Each issue of this newsletter contains a review of an important topic in the area of stroke by an authority in the field. The companion to Current Concepts of Cardiovascular Disease, it is published every other month. Single copies usually are available without charge from local AHA affiliates.*

American Heart Association: *Stroke: A Journal of Cerebral Circulation.* Published bimonthly under the auspices of the AHA. *This subscription journal publishes the bulk of the latest clinical and laboratory research on stroke in North America.*

The EC/IC Bypass Study Group: Failure of extracranial-intracranial arterial bypass to reduce the risk of ischemic stroke: Results of an international randomized trial. *N Engl J Med* 1985; 313: 1191–1200. *This international cooperative study demonstrated no significant difference in outcome in patients with TIAs or minor strokes treated medically and treated by microsurgical anastomosis of branches of the superficial temporal artery via a hole in the skull to branches of the middle cerebral artery.*

Kistler JP, Ropper AH, Heros RC: Therapy of ischemic cerebral vascular disease due to atherothrombosis. *N Engl J Med* 1984; 311:27–33 (Part I) and 100–105 (Part II). *This article is a good, recent review of the topic in a widely circulated general medical journal.*

Sandok BA, Furlan AJ, Whisnant JP, Sundt TM Jr: Guidelines for the management of transient ischemic attacks. *Mayo Clin Proc* 1978; 53: 665–674. *This approach to the patient with TIAs as described by one of the best known cerebral vascular neurologic-neurosurgical groups active in the field is still valid.*

Toole JF: *Cerebrovascular Disorders,* ed 3. New York, Raven Press, 1984. *This is the long-awaited third edition of this authoritative monograph. It is highly readable but provides enough depth to serve as a reference. Each chapter is followed by references conveniently grouped by specific topic.*

Samuel E. Pitner, M.D.

Intracranial hemorrhage occurs either spontaneously, and thus must be differentiated from occlusive strokes, or following trauma, although in some cases there may be no history of this. The term "intracranial hemorrhage" encompasses hemorrhage occurring at all sites within the skull, ranging from bleeding within the substance of the brain itself (intracerebral hemorrhage) to bleeding between the various layers of the meninges (subarachnoid, subdural, and epidural hemorrhage).

INTRACEREBRAL HEMORRHAGE

Patients with intracerebral hemorrhage make up about 10% of all cases of cerebrovascular disease and present with the acute onset of focal neurologic signs; thus, these patients must be differentiated from patients with cerebral infarctions. In one-third of these patients, the neurologic deficit is truly apoplectic because it is maximal from its onset, but in most patients the deficit rapidly progresses within minutes to a few hours. Sudden death is rare, but 25% to 40% of patients are in coma on arrival at the hospital. Generally, vomiting and headache at the onset and a fairly rapid decrease in the state of consciousness are more likely to be associated with intracerebral hemorrhage than with a cerebral infarction, whereas the occurrence of transient ischemic attacks (TIAs) before the main episode suggests infarction (see Chap 120, Stroke).

Cerebral hemorrhage is particularly likely to occur in certain areas of the brain. These are, in order of decreasing frequency, the basal ganglia-thalamus area, pons, and cerebellum. The usual picture of hemorrhage into the basal ganglia-thalamic area is quite similar to that of an occlusive stroke in the carotid arterial system (anterior circulation) with rapid develop-ment of hemiparesis or hemihypesthesia or both. Because of the rather abrupt development of mass effect, decreased consciousness usually occurs quickly; in fact, in the average emergency room, intracerebral hemorrhage is the most common supratentorial mass lesion that produces coma (see Chap 7, Coma and States of Diminished Consciousness). Pontine hemorrhage produces the onset of coma with quadriparesis. Patients with cerebellar hemorrhage usually have a history of severe headache and ataxia followed in minutes or a few hours by coma as acute hydrocephalus develops from compression of the fourth ventricle by the hematoma. The cerebellum is an infrequent but particularly important site of hemorrhage because this is the one location from which surgical evacuation of the clot clearly improves survival.

Findings on physical examination vary with the site of the hemorrhage. In thalamic hemorrhage, a minimal lesion produces hemihypesthesia, but extension of the lesion into the internal capsule produces hemiplegia. In putaminal hemorrhage, hemiplegia is present from the onset. If the hemorrhage extends down into the upper brain stem, the eyes often are deviated down and in, and the pupils are small but reactive. Very early in pontine hemorrhage there may be facial paresis on one side of the body and hemiplegia on the other. By the time most of these patients are seen medically, however, they usually are profoundly comatose with quadriplegia, decerebrate rigidity, and pinpoint pupils. If patients with cerebellar hemorrhage are seen very early in the course of the illness, they present with headache and truncal ataxia. However, most of these patients will be unconscious when seen. One important finding in many cases of cerebellar hemorrhage is forced conjugate deviation of the eyes to one side *in the absence* of hemiplegia. (In most large infarctions involving the frontal lobes, there is forced conjugate deviation of the eyes to the side of the lesion, but almost invariably accompanied by contralateral hemiplegia.)

The most important factor in the pathogenesis of most cases of spontaneous intracerebral hemorrhage is hypertension. This produces hyaline necrosis of the walls of the cerebral arterioles which causes the weakened vessel to rupture. These arteriolar lesions in hypertensive patients are most frequent in the areas of predilection for intracerebral hemorrhage (basal ganglia-thalamus area, pons, and cerebellum). (Occlusion as opposed to rupture of these arterioles produces small infarcts called lacunes.) Intracerebral hemorrhages from causes other than hypertension tend to occur at various sites. These include hemorrhages due to trauma, blood dyscrasia, and various types of necrotizing arterial or arteriolar lesions. Cerebral amyloid angiopathy is increasingly recognized as a cause of intracerebral hemorrhage in elderly, nonhypertensive patients.

By far the best laboratory technique for diagnosis of intracerebral hemorrhages is computed tomography (CT scan). Cerebral hemorrhage is nearly always visible from its outset on a CT scan (Fig 121–1); in contrast, infarctions may be invisible for a few days until enough edema develops to make them show up as a low-density area on the CT scan. In 50% to 80% of patients with intracerebral hemorrhage, blood ruptures through the ependymal lining into the ventricles and thus into the cerebrospinal fluid (CSF). Examination of the CSF is the second choice as a diagnostic study, but only if CT scanning is not available.

The treatment of most forms of intracerebral hemorrhage is conservative. The incidence of the condition, 10% of all strokes, is unchanged,

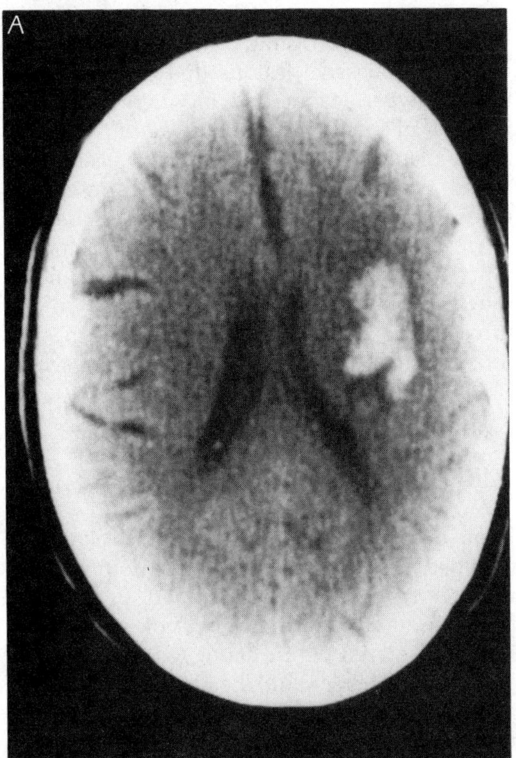

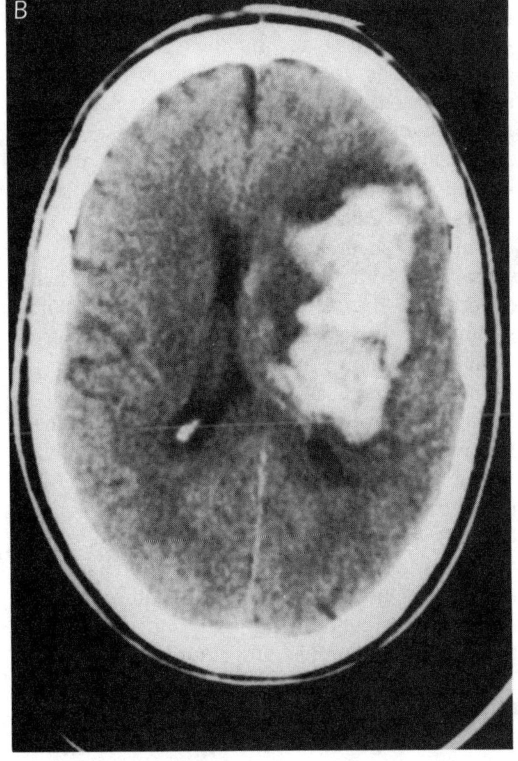

FIG 121–1.
A, CT scan showing intracerebral hemorrhage (white, high-contrast areas) visible against the darker outline of the brain. **B,** CT scan in the same patient whose condition worsened a few hours later. Note how the hemorrhage has enlarged and now is causing the brain to herniate across the midline with distortion of the opposite ventricular system. (Courtesy of Dr. Rich Carroll, Miami Valley Hospital Radiology Department.)

yet the death rate is down. This probably reflects both an overall decrease in the incidence of massive lesions due to better therapy of hypertension and an increase in the number of smaller lesions seen only on CT scans that previously would have been diagnosed as infarctions. Surgical therapy clearly can save some patients with cerebellar hemorrhage; some clinicians report reducing the mortality from over 80% to around 50%. Some of the few intracerebral hemorrhages not in the three major locations listed also may be appropriate for surgical removal if they are accessible.

SUBARACHNOID HEMORRHAGE

If one defines stroke as brain disease secondary to blood vessel disease, subarachnoid hemorrhage certainly has to be included. In contrast, however, to all other types of stroke, it usually is not first seen as an acute focal neurologic deficit. In subarachnoid hemorrhage, bleeding is over the surface of the brain in the subarachnoid space and does not cause localized disruption of cerebral pathways. Instead, the effects of subarachnoid hemorrhage are diffuse and range from severe headache and little else in mild cases, to the abrupt onset of coma in severe cases. Unlike other strokes, subarachnoid hemorrhage is a significant cause of sudden death, and up to 20% of patients may be dead on arrival at an emergency room.

The usual history is of an abrupt onset of an extremely severe headache, usually during physical activity of some sort. With increasing severity of the hemorrhage, there is a corresponding increase in obtundation, and the patient may become comatose. Occasionally patients will have a history of recent onset of headaches, indicating minor ("sentinel") bleeding a few days or weeks previously. Even when the cause of the subarachnoid hemorrhage is an aneurysm, only 10% of patients will have a history of pain coming from an unruptured aneurysm before the onset of the hemorrhage. Patients in whom subarachnoid hemorrhage is from an arteriovenous anomaly may have a history of unexplained seizures. Only occasionally does one encounter focal neurologic signs or symptoms, such as hemiparesis; these findings

usually indicate that there is an associated intracerebral hematoma as well as subarachnoid hemorrhage.

On physical examination, mildly affected patients often will have only a severe headache with a stiff neck and other signs of meningeal irritation. Severely affected patients may be so profoundly comatose that signs of meningeal irritation cannot be demonstrated. In most patients, however, the state of consciousness and the degree of meningeal irritation are intermediate between these two extremes. A small percentage of patients may show localized cranial nerve dysfunction; the most common of these is the presence of a third nerve palsy of varying degrees of completeness associated with an aneurysm of the junction of the internal carotid artery and posterior communicating artery. As noted, lateralized neurologic dysfunction, such as hemiparesis, is infrequent. On ophthalmoscopy, evidence of preretinal (subhyaloid) hemorrhage should be sought; only about 20% of patients have this finding, but in adults it is practically pathognomonic of subarachnoid hemorrhage.

The most common pathogenesis of subarachnoid hemorrhage, as determined at autopsy, is trauma. Hence, the term "spontaneous" or "primary" subarachnoid hemorrhage sometimes is used to indicate nontraumatic subarachnoid hemorrhage. The most common cause of spontaneous subarachnoid hemorrhage is rupture of an aneurysm, which is found clinically in 60% of cases and at autopsy in 80% of cases. Congenital, or berry, aneurysms, located at major cerebral arterial bifurcations near the circle of Willis, are most often responsible. (By contrast, mycotic aneurysms, which are due to indolent infection in the blood vessel wall and are associated largely with subacute bacterial endocarditis, tend to occur in the more distal branches of the middle cerebral artery.) Atherosclerosis and hypertension probably are factors in the development and rupture of berry aneurysms, even though the defect in the media of the vessel is believed to be congenital. The peak age for rupture of a cerebral aneurysm is approximately 55 years. The next most frequent cause of spontaneous hemorrhage, a congenital arteriovenous anomaly, can rupture at any age and, indeed, is the most common cause of spontaneous subarachnoid hemorrhage below the age of 30 years. Various blood dyscrasias, including sickle cell anemia, also can cause subarchnoid hemorrhage.

The differential diagnosis of subarachnoid hemorrhage depends on the initial clinical findings. A minority of patients will have a bad headache and no neurologic impairment, but usually will have a stiff neck. The most severely involved patients arrive in coma (see Chap 7, Coma and States of Diminished Consciousness). Most patients are between these two extremes. Because of the frequency of meningeal irritation, meningitis and encephalitis enter into the differential diagnosis of subarachnoid hemorrhage in most patients. In this regard, it must be emphasized that the majority of, but by no means all, patients with subarachnoid hemorrhage show evidence of bleeding on a CT scan. If one is suspicious of subarachnoid hemorrhage, a lumbar puncture should be performed, even if the CT scan is negative. With rare exceptions, all patients with subarachnoid hemorrhage should have complete cerebral angiography in an effort to demonstrate an aneurysm or arteriovenous anomaly as the source of bleeding.

Treatment of subarachnoid hemorrhage must be acknowledged as not completely satisfactory; the patient's state of consciousness on admission is much more important as a prognostic factor than is the method of treatment. In aneurysmal subarachnoid hemorrhage, mortality from recurrent bleeding is extremely high; 35% of patients die in the first 2 weeks after the initial hemorrhage, with chances of recurrence diminishing after that. Patients with aneurysmal subarachnoid hemorrhage are a particular challenge to the neurosurgeon because early operation obviously is necessary if any of the patients who would otherwise die in the first 2 weeks are to be saved. However, severe postoperative arterial spasm producing a secondary cerebral infarction is a problem after early operation. Late operation has fewer complications, but many patients die awaiting surgery if this approach is taken. Once an arteriovenous anomaly has bled, excision is the treatment of choice. If for any reason it cannot be removed, treatment by intra-arterial injection of glass microspheres and other forms of artificial emboli to induce thrombosis of the lesion may be helpful. In cases of inoperable lesions or of hemorrhage without obvious cause, medical treatment with antithrombolytic agents, such as ϵ-aminocaprolic acid, or with agents that control systemic hypotension may be used.

SUBDURAL HEMORRHAGE

Clinically, subdural hemorrhage is best approached as acute subdural hemorrhage or chronic subdural hematoma. Acute subdural hemorrhage is seen mainly in individuals with known and obvious head trauma who also have brain lacerations and intracranial hemorrhages and who have a poor prognosis even with surgical drainage because of these associated injuries. On the other hand, most patients with chronic subdural hematomas either do not have a history of trauma or at most give a history of apparently trivial trauma, even though trauma is the most common cause. This discussion of subdural hemorrhage will be concerned only with this group of patients who give no history of major trauma and who therefore are more likely to be admitted to medical or psychiatric services than to trauma services.

Most cases of chronic subdural hematomas occur in patients under 18 months of age or over 60 years of age. Chronic subdural hematomas between these ages are most frequently in patients with coexistent alcoholism, dementia, or chronic epilepsy. Most conscious patients complain of headache. Most patients have a history of some alteration of consciousness and also may have a history of confusion. Focal and generalized seizures are not uncommon.

On physical examination, patients with chronic subdural hematomas often have altered consciousness or are demented. Although signs of diffuse neurologic dysfunction predominate, patients usually show some evidence of a focal lesion, such as a mild hemiparesis. Because the lesion covers the surface of the brain (and involves both hemispheres in half the cases) and produces primarily diffuse pressure effects, findings indicating marked disruption of parenchymal pathways are infrequent. For example, both hemiplegia and homonymous hemianopsias are rare. In contrast to patients with acute subdural hemorrhage, patients with chronic subdural hematomas only rarely show any evidence of trauma about the head or neck on examination. Because some cases are associated with some subarachnoid leakage as well as the mass effect, a few patients will show a stiff neck or other signs of meningeal irritation.

The pathogenesis of chronic subdural hematoma usually is rupture of a bridging vein passing from the brain through the potential subdural space to one of the venous sinuses. Presumably the risk is greater in infants and the elderly, as well as in patients with pathologic cerebral atrophy, because of a relatively greater space between the brain and skull. Blood dissects the arachnoid from the dura, possibly causing further venous rupture and bleeding. After a period of time, fibroblasts enter the clot and a so-called neomembrane is formed over the surface of the clot. Some believe that at this point the hematoma grows by taking in spinal fluid by osmosis through the neomembrane and arachnoid. Subdural hematomas usually cover the convexity of one or both cerebral hemispheres, but occasionally may be in the posterior fossa or in the interhemispheric sulcus. Bleeding disorders may give rise to subdural hematomas as may infiltration of the meninges by tumor cells or leukemic cells.

At present CT scanning is the best method for the diagnosis of chronic subdural hematomas. At a certain stage of development of these hematomas, they may have the same amount of penetrance to x-rays as the adjacent brain ("isodense") and may be missed on CT scanning. Likewise, the hematoma may cover the brain surface adjacent to the skull and confound the CT-scan diagnosis of these lesions. As nuclear magnetic resonance becomes more widely available, it probably will be a better diagnostic technique for chronic subdural hematoma. A high percentage of these lesions also can be seen on radioisotope brain scans. The spinal fluid pressure in these cases often is not elevated, but the spinal fluid has a high protein concentration, at times even being xanthochromic. Some small subdural hematomas clearly will resolve themselves. Others will resolve if the fluid between the dura and arachnoid is removed; this is most practical, of

course, in infants where the subdural space can be tapped directly through the corner of the fontanel. Many neurosurgeons believe that more established hematomas require a complete craniotomy with removal of the neomembrane in order to prevent reaccumulation. Occasionally a shunt must be placed to keep the fluid from reaccumulating.

EPIDURAL HEMORRHAGE

Patients with epidural hemorrhage nearly always have a history of trauma. In about half of the cases, trauma is limited to the temporal area, such as a blow to the side of the head by a pitched ball, usually of sufficient force to produce a loss of consciousness. Many patients remain unconscious from the moment of impact, but about half have only a concussion and arouse, only to lose consciousness again later as the blood clot expands. This time of transient improvement often is referred to as the "lucid interval."

On examination these patients usually do show evidence of trauma, as well as alteration of consciousness. As epidural hematomas usually are located laterally in the temporal area, these patients typically show the syndrome of uncal herniation (see Chap 7, Coma and States of Diminished Consciousness). The pupil ipsilateral to the lesion is dilated. Usually the patient also has contralateral hemiparesis.

Epidural hematomas nearly always are due to arterial bleeding, and brain compression thus develops faster than is usual in subdural bleeding, which is of venous origin. Fracture of the squamous portion of the temporal bone with depression causing laceration of the middle meningeal artery is the most common cause of this lesion. Usually skull fractures can be seen on standard skull x-ray films as well as on CT scans. As with subdural hematomas, nontraumatic cases of epidural hematomas are rarely seen. Epidural hematomas are a true neurosurgical emergency. Evacuation of the hematoma through a burr hole usually is life-saving, whereas undiagnosed and untreated lesions almost invariably are fatal.

REFERENCES

Pevehouse BC, Bloom WH, McKissock W: Ophthalmologic aspects of diagnosis and localization of subdural hematoma: An analysis of 389 cases and review of the literature. *Neurology* 1960; 10: 1037–1041. *The definitive clinical study of eye signs in subdural hematomas.*

Pitner SE, Johnson WW: Chronic subdural hematoma in childhood acute leukemia. *Cancer* 1973; 32:185–190.

Plum F, Posner JB: *The Diagnosis of Stupor and Coma*, ed 3. Philadelphia, FA Davis, 1980. *The definitive work on the differential diagnosis of disorders of consciousness.*

Sahs AL, Nibbelink DW, Tomer JC: *Aneurysmal Subarachnoid Hemorrhage.* Baltimore, Urban and Schwarzenberg, 1981. *The report of a large national cooperative study that is a gold mine of clinical information on this topic.*

Toole JF: *Cerebrovascular Disorders*, ed 3. New York, Raven Press, 1984. *The long-awaited third edition of this authoritative monograph. Highly readable, but provides depth to serve as a reference. Each chapter is followed by references conveniently grouped by specific topic.*

122 SEIZURE DISORDERS

Thomas Mathews, M.D.

Seizures are the result of transient excessive cerebral neuronal discharges. The clinical expression of the abnormal discharge depends on its location and spread and may consist of loss of consciousness, motor, sensory, or behavioral phenomena. Epilepsy, one of the most common neurologic disorders in clinical medicine, is the condition of chronic recurrent seizures in which the primary defect is in the brain (i.e., it is a cerebral disorder). Metabolic seizures such as seizures associated with hypoglycemia, alcohol withdrawal, or Stokes-Adams attack may be recurrent, but do not have a primary cerebral defect. The prevalence of chronic recurrent seizures is 0.5% to 1%. However, 7% to 8% of the population will experience at least one seizure.

PATHOPHYSIOLOGY AND CLASSIFICATION

The physiologic basis of the epileptic neuronal discharges is not clearly understood. The repetitive volleys of impulses from the involved neurons may be due to episodic depolarization from the movement of ions across abnormal cell membranes. This disorderly paroxysmal discharge may be limited to a small area or may be propagated to involve the entire brain.

The traditional classification into grand mal, petit mal, focal, and psychomotor seizures based primarily on semiology has been replaced by an international classification that correlates clinical features with EEG patterns and pathophysiologic changes (Table 122–1). The epilepsies are divided into two categories: generalized seizures and partial seizures.

GENERALIZED SEIZURES

There is clinical and EEG involvement of both cerebral hemispheres simultaneously. Consciousness is lost from the onset. In generalized seizures the discharge involves the reticular nuclei in the diencephalon and is projected to the cerebral hemispheres. It is uncertain if the discharge originates in the reticular nuclei (centrencephalic theory, Fig 122–1,A) or if there is diffuse or multifocal cortical hyperexcitability, with the diencephalic nuclei only playing a subordinate role in projecting the discharge to the hemispheres (modified corticoreticular theory, Fig 122–1,B). If excitatory motor systems are involved, generalized tonic-clonic seizures result. If inhibitory systems are activated, there is loss of consciousness without motor activity (absence seizures).

TABLE 122–1.
Classification of Epileptic Seizures*

GENERALIZED SEIZURES

(loss of consciousness at onset; clinical and EEG
  involvement of both hemispheres simultaneously)
  Tonic-clonic (grand mal)
  Absence (petit mal)
  Myoclonic
  Tonic
  Clonic
  Atonic

PARTIAL SEIZURES

(localized cortical focus)
  Simple (consciousness preserved)
  Complex (consciousness impaired)
  Simple or complex partial seizures evolving to
    generalized tonic-clonic seizures

* Modified from Commission on Classification and Terminology of the International League against Epilepsy: Proposal for revised clinical and electroencephalographic classification of epileptic seizures. Epilepsia 1981; 22:489–501.

PARTIAL SEIZURES

Clinical and EEG findings indicate origin of the discharge from a discrete area of the brain (Fig 122–1,C). Partial seizures indicate focal pathologic changes in the brain (tumors, anoxic tissue, or traumatic scars). Partial simple seizures are characterized by intact consciousness. Partial complex seizures are characterized by impaired consciousness. In partial seizures evolving into generalized tonic-clonic seizures, the focal epileptic discharge spreads to the diencephalon and is projected to both hemispheres (Fig 122–1,C).

CLINICAL SIGNS AND SYMPTOMS

GENERALIZED SEIZURES

In tonic-clonic seizures, the ictus, or attack, lasts 1 minute to 3 minutes and is stereotypical. In the tonic phase, the patient abruptly loses consciousness, falls to the ground, and is rigid. The clonic phase is heralded by rhythmic contractions. There may be tongue biting, cyanosis, incontinence, tachycardia, and mydriasis. Postictal flaccidity and coma are followed by confusion, drowsiness or sleep, myalgia, and headaches. Many generalized tonic-clonic seizures are secondary to spread of partial seizures. Primary tonic-clonic seizures

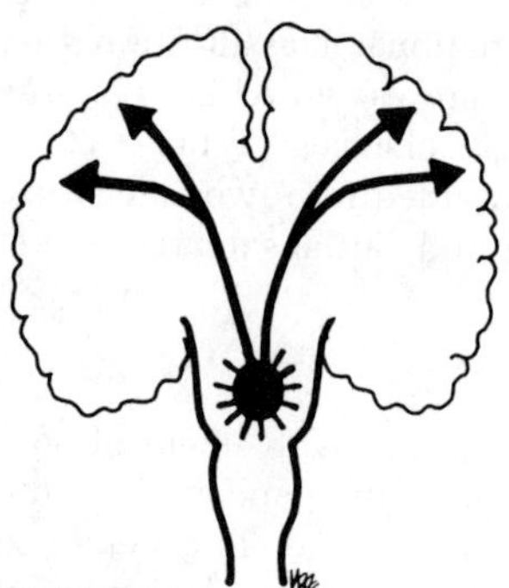

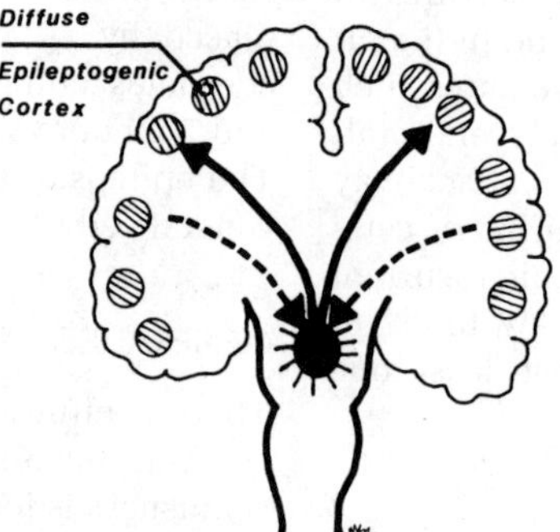

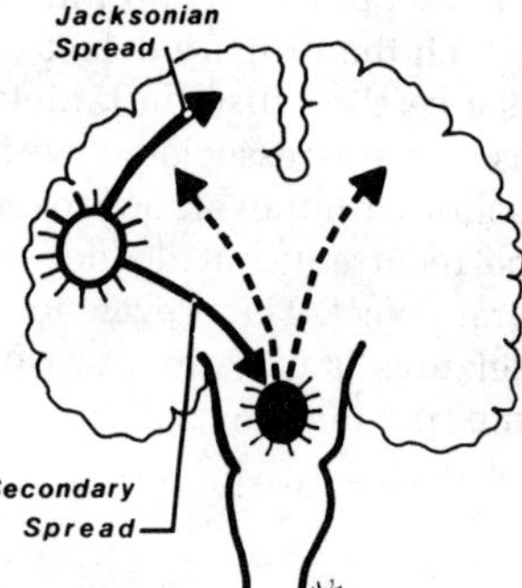

FIG 122–1.
A, generalized seizures (centrencephalic theory). The epileptic discharge originates in the diencephalic reticular system and is projected to the hemispheres. **B,** generalized seizures (modified cortico-reticular theory). Diffuse or multifocal epileptogenic cortex interacts with the reticular projection system. **C,** partial seizures. The epileptic focus is localized to a discrete area of the cortex. It may spread cortically (jacksonian) or to the diencephalon and subsequent projection to the hemispheres (secondary generalized epilepsy). (Modified from Luders S, Lesser R P, et al: Cleveland Clinic Quarterly, 1984; 51:205–226.)

are less common, are often familial starting in childhood or adolescence, are not associated with structural defects in the brain. With rare exception, metabolic seizures are generalized tonic-clonic seizures.

Absence seizures (petit mal) consist of abrupt arrest of consciousness, a blank stare, unresponsiveness, and arrest of ongoing activity without falling to the ground. There may be a few clonic jerks and lip-smacking automatisms. The attack lasts 5 seconds to 20 seconds and terminates abruptly without postictal confusion. Absence seizures (absences) occur frequently, as many as 50 to 100 attacks daily. Absences begin between 3 years and 10 years and are often familial; onset in adulthood is rare. In typical absences, intellectual development is normal, and there are no structural abnormalities in the brain.

Myoclonic, tonic, and atonic seizures are usually seizures of childhood. Myoclonic seizures are characterized by sudden generalized or focal shocklike muscle contractions. Tonic seizures are characterized by rigidity and extensor posturing. Atonic seizures ("drop" attacks) are characterized by a brief loss of postural tone and falling to the ground. In clonic seizures there are rhythmic contractions of extremities without any tonic rigidity. These childhood seizures are often associated with severe brain disorders and mental retardation (except for the myoclonic seizures of adolescence).

PARTIAL SEIZURES

In partial simple seizures consciousness is preserved. The precise clinical features depend on the location of the epileptic focus. A partial seizure originating in the motor cortex causes contralateral tonic-clonic jerking. Spread of the discharge to adjacent areas results in a jacksonian seizure (epileptic march). Motor seizures may consist of head turning or speech arrest. Partial simple seizures originating in the sensory cortex may manifest with contralateral numbness and tingling, flashing lights and colors.

Partial complex seizures (temporal lobe or psychomotor seizures) are one of the most common types of epilepsy. The patient's awareness and responsiveness are impaired. The aura (initial or remembered part of the seizure) consists of psychic phenomena. Cognitive symptoms such as deja vu, dreamy states, forced thinking, and depersonalization or affective states such as fear, anger, or pleasure may be experienced. Olfactory, gustatory, visual, and auditory hallucinations, sensory illusions, and abnormal visceral sensations are characteristic psychosensory aurae of partial complex seizures. The hallmark of the partial complex seizure ictus is the psychomotor automatism, a trancelike state of clouded consciousness and responsiveness for which the subject is amnesic. During an automatism the patient may exhibit stereotypical motor activity (e.g., lip-smacking, chewing, and swallowing), or other nonpurposeful movements. Automatisms may be reactive to the environment, including verbalization, gestures, or continuation of ongoing activity. Complicated, integrated, purposeful activity may sometimes be carried out. The attacks last 1 minute to 5 minutes and are followed by postictal confusion. Partial complex seizure is distinguished from absence seizure by the psychic aura, the postictal confusion, and a longer duration.

Partial simple and partial complex seizures can evolve into generalized tonic-clonic seizures (Fig 122–1,C). The partial origin of these seizures may be clinically unapparent, but may be identified by focal EEG abnormalities. Postictal hemiparesis (Todd's paralysis), a unilateral Babinski's sign, or aphasia, signifies that the seizure had a focal origin.

DIFFERENTIAL DIAGNOSIS

Many episodic cerebral events can mimic epilepsy. Common misdiagnoses are syncope and psychiatric disorders (hysteria, anxiety, panic and rage attacks, fugue states, and malingering). Transient cerebral ischemia, breath holding, migraine, narcolepsy-cataplexy, and hyperventilation can be mistaken for epilepsy. Psychogenic seizures (pseudoseizures) should be considered in epilepsies refractory to treatment and may need prolonged video-EEG monitoring for accurate diagnosis.

DIAGNOSIS

The diagnostic studies in a case of seizure are designed to determine the type and the cause of the seizures. The seizure type (classification) can be determined from the patient's history, and the EEG.

The cause of the seizure should be determined before initiating long-term treatment (Table 122–2). Seizures due to metabolic (extracerebral) causes do not need long-term anticonvulsant drugs. Seizures due to a structural cerebral lesion such as a tumor may need specific treatment directed to the cause, in addition to anticonvulsant therapy. In a substantial number of patients the cause will remain unknown despite extensive investigation.

Laboratory tests such as a complete blood cell count (CBC), urine analysis, blood chemistry, serologic studies, and drug screening will help detect metabolic and toxic causes. Cerebrospinal fluid samples taken by lumbar puncture may be analyzed for suspected infections (e.g., syphilis or encephalitis).

Computed tomography (CT scan) is the radiographic procedure of choice to detect structural brain lesions (e.g., tumors, malformations, calcification, and contusions). Rarely, angiography is needed for vascular lesions. Special tests include magnetic resonance imaging, which may be more sensitive than CT scanning in detecting structural lesions, position emission tomography, which can help to localize epileptic foci for surgical resection, and special biochemical assays and biopsies in suspected cases of inborn errors of metabolism such as lipid storage diseases.

The EEG helps to document and classify the type and cause of the seizures. In generalized seizures, there are bilateral synchronous spike and wave or polyspike discharges. Typical absence seizures show characteristic bilateral spike-and-wave bursts that occur three per second. In partial seizures, focal spikes and sharp or slow waves may be seen. In metabolic seizures, the interictal EEG may be normal or show diffuse slowing. The EEGs may be normal in 10% to 20% of epileptic patients. Prolonged recordings, activation procedures such as photic stimulation, hyperventilation, sleep deprivation, and nasopharyngeal electrode placements will increase the number of abnormal EEGs. Special EEG procedures such as prolonged closed-circuit video-EEG and telemetry and ambulatory EEG are useful in difficult cases where diagnosis is uncertain or the seizures are refractory to therapy.

PRINCIPLES OF THERAPY

With developments in diagnosis, new anticonvulsant drugs, and therapeutic drug-level monitoring, seizures can be well controlled in 70% to 80% of patients. Selection of the anticonvulsant drug depends on the seizure type as determined by the clinical features and the EEG (Table 122–3). Phenobarbital and primidone are effective antiepileptic drugs but should not be the initial drug of choice because of their sedative properties. Therapy with one drug is preferred to polypharmacy. The doses of the single drug should be increased slowly until control is achieved or toxicity develops. If seizures are frequent despite therapeutic plasma levels of the drug, a second drug may be added or substituted. Poor control and low plasma levels are usually due to noncompliance and cannot be corrected by multiple drugs. Therapeutic drug level monitoring is essential to determine the optimal dosage, to detect toxicity and abnormal drug metabolism, and to monitor noncompliance. Blood drug levels must be combined with clinical judgment in adjusting antiepileptic medications.

Knowledge of anticonvulsant drug pharmacology is essential. Drug absorption, binding, and metabolism may be altered by drug–drug interaction, disease states, or genetic differences. Such effects may cause altered blood levels of the anticonvulsant, leading to drug toxicity or poor control of the seizures. The half-life and the steady state plasma concentrations of a drug determine the frequency and amount of drug intake. Drugs with short half-lives such as valproate, primidone, and carbamazepine are administered three to four times daily, and the drug dosage can be increased every 2 days to 3 days (five elimination half-lives). Drugs with long half-lives such as phenytoin, phenobarbital, and ethosuximide can be administered once or twice daily for better compliance, and changes in dosage should be done every 2 weeks to 3 weeks.

Refractory seizures should be periodically reevaluated. Common causes of refractoriness are noncompliance, erroneous diagnosis (especially of syncope and psychogenic seizures), and progressive CNS diseases (e.g., a low-grade glioma). Refractory partial seizures may benefit from surgical excision of the epileptic focus.

TABLE 122–2.
Clinical–Pathologic Correlations

SEIZURE TYPE	AGE	INTERICTAL EEG	ETIOLOGY/PATHOLOGY
GENERALIZED SEIZURES			
Tonic-clonic	All ages	Polyspikes or spike and wave discharges over *both* *hemispheres* *Note:* EEG is normal in metabolic seizures.	Major etiologies: (1) idiopathic (i.e., No structural brain lesions; has genetic predisposition); (2) *Diffuse brain* diseases (e.g., lipid storage disease, tuberous sclerosis); (3) *Toxic-metabolic* (e.g., alcohol withdrawal, drug intoxications, electrolyte derangements [Ca^+, Na^+, Mg^+, PO_4], hypoglycemia, hyperosmolar states, liver and kidney failure, cerebral hypoxia or ischemia)
Absence	Childhood	Three Hz spike and wave discharges over *both* *hemispheres*	Idiopathic. Usually no structural brain pathology; has genetic predisposition.
Atonic, tonic, myoclonic, clonic, and mixed generalized seizures	Childhood	Polyspikes and spike and wave discharges over *both* *hemispheres*	Diffuse and severe brain pathology is frequent.
PARTIAL SEIZURES			
Simple, complex and secondary generalized epilepsy	All ages, but more common in adults	Focal spike discharges in localized area of *one hemisphere;* may spread to involve whole brain (secondary generalized epilepsy)	*Childhood:* Birth trauma, anoxia, congenital malformations, infection, tumors *Adulthood:* Post-traumatic, tumors, stroke, infection, anoxia *Note:* In many partial seizures the etiology remains unknown.

TABLE 122–3.
Antiepileptic Drugs for Seizure Disorders

SEIZURE TYPE	ANTIEPILEPTIC DRUG	
	FIRST CHOICE	SECOND CHOICE
Tonic-clonic, primary (genetic)	Valproic acid	Phenytoin
Absence*	Ethosuximide	Valproic acid
Myoclonic, clonic atonic, tonic	Valproic acid	Phenytoin
		Clonazepam
Partial simple, complex and	Carbamazepine†	Phenytoin
secondary generalized	Phenytoin†	Primidone
		Phenobarbital

* Valproic acid is drug of choice for mixed generalized seizures (absence with tonic-clonic or myoclonic seizures).

† Phenytoin is as effective as carbamazepine but has more chronic toxicity.

Attention must be paid to the social, vocational, and psychologic complications that are common in many epileptic patients.

Cessation of drug therapy may be considered in selected patients who are seizure-free for 5 years.

STATUS EPILEPTICUS

Status epilepticus refers to a series of seizures without recovery of consciousness or to continuous seizures lasting more than 30 minutes. This medical emergency has a direct mortality of 10% to 15%. Convulsive status epilepticus may be a generalized tonic-clonic or partial motor status epilepticus. Nonconvulsive status epilepticus is much less common and may be absence status or partial complex status epilepticus. Generalized tonic-clonic status epilepticus causes cardiorespiratory complications and metabolic derangements such as hypoxia, lactic acidosis, hyperpyrexia, hypotension, pulmonary edema, cardiac arrhythmias, and rhabdomyolysis. Even partial convulsive status epilepticus and nonconvulsive status epilepticus must be terminated quickly because prolonged epileptic discharges can result in neuronal death and permanent neurologic sequelae.

The management of status epilepticus includes general measures to maintain the airway and to stabilize cardiorespiratory function. Generalized tonic-clonic status epilepticus must be terminated immediately and is best achieved by intravenous diazepam followed by a loading dose of phenytoin. Intravenous phenobarbital is used if the status epilepticus persists. General anesthesia is indicated if status epilepticus persists beyond 60 minutes. Diagnostic tests are used to determine the cause of the status epilepticus. It is often caused by an acute cerebral insult or by a metabolic derangement that requires specific investigation and therapy.

REFERENCES

Commission on Classification and Terminology of the International League against Epilepsy: Proposal for revised clinical and electroencephalographic classification of epileptic seizures. *Epilepsia* 1981; 22:489–501.

Delgado-Escueta AV: The epilepsies: New developments of the 1980s. *Current Neurology* 1986; 6:235–288. *This article reviews recent developments on basic mechanisms and current concepts of treatment, and explores future research challenges in the epilepsies.*

Delgado-Escueta AV, Trieman DM, Walsh GO: The treatable epilepsies. *N Engl J Med* 1983; 308: 1508–1514, 1576–1584. *A simple and succinct review of drug treatment of epilepsy.*

Lothman EW, Collins RC: Seizures, in Pearlman AL, Collins RC, (eds): *Neurological Pathophysiology.* New York, Oxford University Press 1984, pp 229–249. *Good description of basic pathophysiologic mechanisms.*

Luders H, Lesser RP, Dinner DS, Morris HH: Generalized epilepsies. A review. *Cleve Clin Q* 1984;

51:205–226. *Describes the pathophysiology and classification of epileptic seizures.*
Porter RJ: Epilepsy: 100 elementary principles, in Major *Problems in Neurology,* no 12. Philadelphia, WB Saunders Co, 1984. *One hundred indispensable clinical "pearls" about the diagnosis and*

treatment of epilepsy.
Solomon GE, Kutt H, Plum F: *Clinical Management of Seizures.* Philadelphia, WB Saunders Co, 1983. *This book is recommended as a concise and inexpensive reference text on epilepsy.*

123 INTRACRANIAL TUMORS

Thomas Mathews, M.D.

Space-occupying lesions in the CNS include neoplasms, abscesses, granulomas, and hematomas. The consequences of these diverse lesions are often quite similar, despite differences in their onset and rate of growth. Both neoplastic and non-neoplastic masses can result in increased intracranial pressure, cerebral edema, and hydrocephalus, and can cause irritation, compression, and destruction of brain tissue.

CLASSIFICATION EPIDEMIOLOGY AND BIOLOGY

Tumors of the CNS may be primary or secondary to a systemic malignancy. Metastatic brain tumors are more common than primary tumors. Brain tumors arise from the glial or neuronal elements of the brain and spinal cord or from the meninges, nerves, and blood vessels. Classifications have been based on cell type, embryologic origin, degree of anaplasia, or anatomical location (Table 123–1). There is no uniformly accepted nomenclature or classification because of uncertainty about the ancestry of undifferentiated cells in many tumors such as medulloblastoma and glioblastoma, as well as the heterogeneity of cell types in many tumors.

The incidence of primary brain tumors is about five cases per 100,000. Brain tumors account for only 2% of all deaths from cancer. Brain tumors are more common in childhood. In

this age group it is the second most common malignancy after leukemia. Brain tumors have a predilection for certain age groups and anatomical locations (Table 123–2). In children most neoplasms are infratentorial, whereas in adults only 10% to 20% are in this location. Medulloblastomas and cerebellar astrocytomas are the most common childhood tumors, whereas meningiomas, schwannomas, and pituitary tumors usually occur in adults.

Malignancy of brain tumor is based on the extent of dedifferentiation, pleomorphism, and mitoses. Gliomas have been graded on a 1 to 4 scale of increasing malignancy depending on the degree of anaplasia. The biologic behavior and prognosis of brain tumors depend not only on the degree of anaplasia, but also on the location and invasiveness of the tumor. Many benign gliomas are diffusely infiltrative and are not circumscribed or encapsulated as are benign tumors outside the CNS. Histologically benign tumors in the brain stem and diencephalon may behave like malignant tumors because of involvement of vital areas and inaccessibility to surgical resection.

The causes of brain tumors are unknown. Hereditary factors may play a role in the dysgenetic syndromes or phakomatoses. There is a high incidence of brain tumors in Von Recklinghausen's disease, tuberous sclerosis, and von Hippel-Lindau syndrome. Retinoblastomas may also be familial, but the vast majority of

TABLE 123–1.
Classification of Primary Brain Tumors*

I. Neuroectodermal
  A. Glial origin (gliomas)
    • Glioblastoma multiforme
    • Astrocytoma
    • Oligodendroglioma
    • Ependymoma
    • Choroid plexus papilloma
  B. Neuronal origin
    • Medulloblastoma
    • Neuroblastoma
    • Ganglioneuroma
II. Mesodermal
  • Meningioma
  • Sarcoma
III. Nerve sheath tumors
  • Schwannoma (neurilemmoma)
  • Neurofibroma

IV. Congenital/maldevelopmental
  • Craniopharyngoma
  • Dermoid and teratoma
  • Germ cell tumors
  • Chordoma
  • Hamartoma

V. Vascular
  • Hemangioblastoma
  • Vascular malformation

VI. Pituitary tumors

VII. Miscellaneous and unclassified

* Modified from WHO International Histologic Classification of Tumors, No 21, Geneva, Switzerland, 1979; and Russell DS, Rubenstein LJ: *Pathology of Tumors of the Nervous System*, ed 4. Baltimore, Williams & Wilkins, 1977.

TABLE 123–2.
Frequency and Kinds of Primary Brain Tumors in Different Locations and Age Groups

AGE GROUP	INFRATENTORIAL	SUPRATENTORIAL
Childhood-Adolescence	60% to 70% of cases Medulloblastoma Cerebellar astrocytoma Brain stem glioma Ependymoma	30% to 40% of cases Astrocytoma Craniopharyngioma Ependymoma
Adulthood	10% to 20% of cases Schwannoma Meningioma	80% to 90% of cases Glioblastoma Astrocytoma Meningioma Pituitary adenoma Oligodendroglioma

brain tumors are not hereditary. Radiation to the head can lead to the development of brain tumors many years later. The role of chemical carcinogens and viruses has not been established, although hydrocarbons, nitrosourea, and several viruses can cause brain tumors in animals.

PATHOPHYSIOLOGY

INCREASED INTRACRANIAL PRESSURE (ICP)

The cranium is a rigid container that has no capacity to expand. It is filled with brain, blood, and CSF, which are relatively non-compressible. Any increase in brain volume can initially be accommodated by displacement of CSF or blood or by compression of the brain. When its capacity to compensate is exceeded, the intracranial pressure begins to rise (Fig 123–1). Even modest increases in cerebral volume (e.g., caused by hypoxia or hypercarbia) may cause dramatic elevation of intracranial pressure if the patient's pressure is on the steep portion of the pressure–volume curve.

Note: A spinal tap is contraindicated in suspected mass lesions because it may alter intracranial dynamics and precipitate a catastrophic herniation.

The intracranial contents can be increased by

a mass itself, cerebral edema, obstructive hydrocephalus, and vascular engorgement. The contribution of the mass to the intracranial pressure depends on size, histologic character, and rate of growth of the mass. Benign neoplasms such as meningioma can grow to a very large size with little effect on the pressure, whereas acute or malignant lesions such as hematoma or metastasis rapidly increase the intracranial pressure.

Cerebral edema often contributes more to the intracranial pressure than does a mass itself. In edema the water content and the bulk of the brain are increased. Cerebral edema may be seen with tumor, stroke, trauma, infection, and toxic-metabolic insults. There are two types of cerebral edema. In cytotoxic edema (e.g., hyponatremia), water accumulates intracellularly, and the blood–brain barrier is intact. In vasogenic edema the blood–brain barrier is breached, and water and plasma proteins extravasate through the tight junctions of the capillary endothelium into the extracellular space. The edema of tumors, strokes, and trauma is vasogenic. Different lesions produce different degrees of edema. Malignant tumors, abscesses, and hematomas often provoke massive edema, whereas low-grade gliomas and meningiomas show little brain swelling. Vasogenic edema occurs in white matter and is maximal around the lesion (Fig 123–2).

Obstruction of CSF circulation may also contribute to increased intracranial pressure. Even small intraventricular or posterior fossa tumors can obstruct the aqueduct or fourth ventricle and produce hydrocephalus (Fig 123–3).

A potential consequence of increased intracranial pressure is herniation of brain tissue. The cranial cavity is divided into supratentorial and infratentorial compartments. There is an opening in the tentorium to accommodate the brain stem. The falx cerebri further divides the supratentorial compartment for the two cerebral hemispheres. Both the cranium and its dural reflections are rigid and unyielding. When a mass in one compartment cannot be accommodated the brain will be forced under the falx or into the tentorial opening or the foramen magnum. Such brain shifts are referred to as herniation.

There are several herniation syndromes (Fig 123–4). In subfalcial herniation hemispheric masses produce side to side shifts pushing the cingulate gyrus under the free edge of the falx.

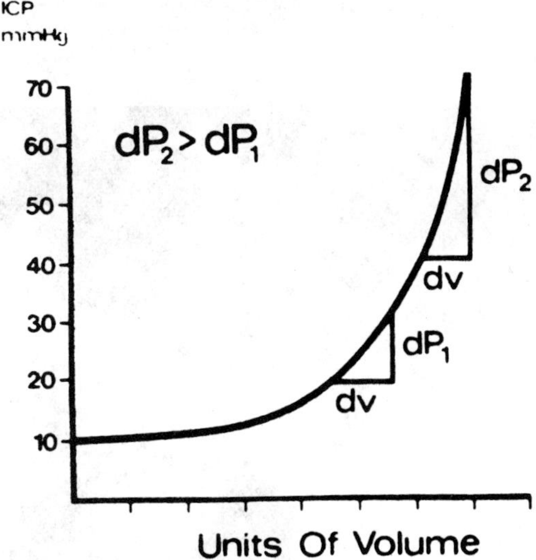

FIG 123–1.
Relationship between intracranial pressure and volume of mass. After initial compensation, a small increase in the volume of mass may cause a large increase in intracranial pressure. (From Jennett B: An Introduction to Neurosurgery, ed 3. Chicago, Year Book Medical Publishers, 1977. Reproduced by permission.)

In uncal herniation, the uncus of the temporal lobe is displaced downward through the tentorial notch with compression of the third cranial nerve and ipsilateral pupillary dilatation. Medially placed or bilateral masses cause central or diencephalic herniation. Uncal and central herniations often occur together. The caudal displacement and compression of the diencephalon and brain stem result in deteriorating consciousness, pupillary, ocular, cardiac, and respiratory dysfunction; death can occur if herniation is not reversed promptly (Table 123–3). In tonsillar herniation the cerebellar tonsils are displaced through the foramen magnum with compression of the medulla. This is common with infratentorial masses.

CLINICAL–PATHOLOGIC CORRELATIONS

Mass lesions produce progressive symptoms. Benign tumors such as meningiomas and low-grade gliomas may progress over years or decades, whereas malignant neoplasms can develop rapidly in days or weeks. Glioblasto-

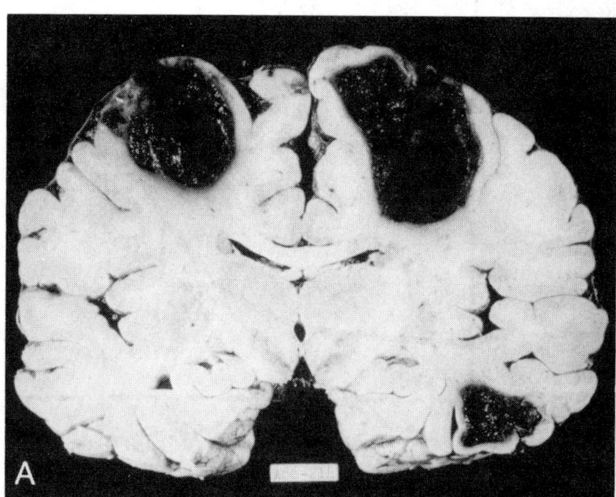
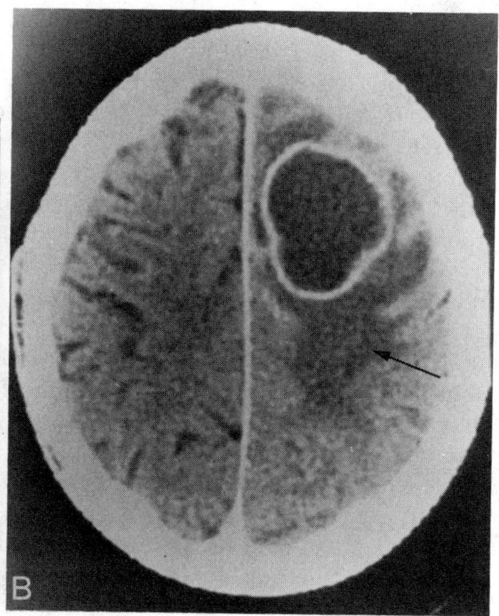

FIG 123–2.
Cerebral metastases. **A,** metastasis are round, circumscribed and often multiple. Necrosis or hemorrhage is common. **B,** CT scan shows a single circumscribed metastasis with central necrosis (low density) and peripheral ring enhancement. Low density in the white matter around the mass indicates cerebral edema.

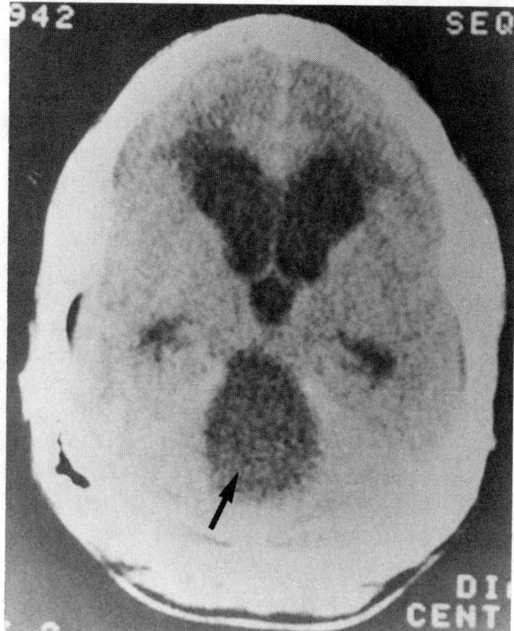

FIG 123–3.
Cerebellar astrocytoma. A cranial CT scan of an 18-year-old man who had severe headaches and gait ataxia. The cerebellar mass is circumscribed and cystic and can be completely extirpated. Note the hydrocephalus, which developed early due to obstruction of the fourth ventricle.

mas and metastases may have an abrupt onset, mimicking a stroke due to hemorrhage or necrosis in the tumor. Clinical manifestations of mass lesions may be attributed to increased intracranial pressure (Table 123–3), herniation (Table 123–3), or focal symptoms due to irritation, compression, and destruction of brain tissue (Table 123–4).

DIAGNOSIS

Computerized tomography (CT scanning) is a sensitive diagnostic tool for brain masses. Tumors may appear either as low- or high-density lesions. Contrast enhancement indicates vascularity or breakdown of the blood–brain barrier and is striking in cases of malignant tumors (e.g., glioblastoma, Fig 123–5) and vascular tumors (e.g., meningioma and hemangioblastoma).

Calcification seen as high-density foci in unenhanced scans is common in oligodendroglioma, meningioma, maldevelopmental tumors, and granulomas. Cerebral edema appears as hypodense areas in the white matter around the mass (Fig 123–2). Shift of the brain and hydrocephalus is readily evident on CT scans (Fig

123–3 and 123–5). Erosion of the skull by meningiomas and metastases and expansion of the sella turcica by pituitary adenomas and of the internal auditory meatus by acoustic schwannomas can be detected by x-ray films, polytomography, or CT scanning. Magnetic resonance imaging (MRI) may be superior to CT scanning for low-grade gliomas and tumors in the posterior fossa and craniocervical junction.

PRINCIPLES OF THERAPY

Radical resection reduces tumor bulk, relieves the high intracranial pressure, and often prolongs survival. Benign tumors that are circumscribed and favorably located can be completely extirpated. These include meningiomas, schwannomas, pituitary adenomas, and cerebellar astrocytomas. Brain tumors in vital or inaccessible locations cannot be totally resected without serious neurologic impairment. Radiation is useful for glioblastoma, pituitary adenoma, and medulloblastoma. For low-grade gliomas, radiation may prolong survival and delay recurrence. It is usually the treatment of choice for brain metastasis. Drugs for treating brain tumors must cross the blood–brain barrier and are only of limited value for most brain tumors. Cerebral edema can be reduced by mannitol, corticosteroids, or furosemide. Intubation and hyperventilation with lowering of P_{CO_2} reduces cerebral blood volume and can dramatically reduce cerebral edema. Obstructive hydrocephalus can be relieved by shunting the CSF.

COMMON BRAIN TUMORS

GLIOBLASTOMA MULTIFORME

Glioblastoma multiforme is the most common primary brain tumor in adults. It is usually supratentorial and rarely originates in the cerebellum or spinal cord. Most glioblastoma multiforme arise from anaplastic dedifferentiation of gliomas. Glioblastoma multiforme has a characteristic appearance with multicolored areas of hemorrhage, necrosis, and vascularity

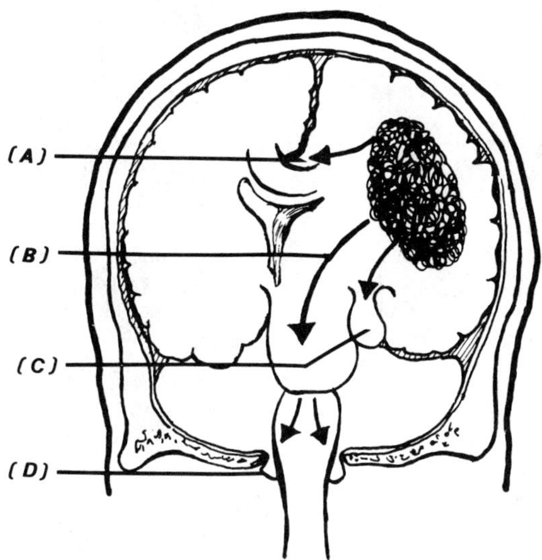

FIG 123–4.
Brain herniations secondary to mass lesions. **A,** subfalcial herniation where the cingulate gyrus shifts under the falx; **B,** central herniation with downward displacement of the diencephalon; **C,** uncal herniation in which the medial temporal lobe is displaced through the tentorial opening; **D,** herniation of the cerebellar tonsils through the foramen magnum. (Modified from Plum F, Posner JB: *Diagnosis of Stupor and Coma,* ed 3, Philadelphia, FA Davis, 1980; and Adams, RD, Victor, M: *Principles of Neurology,* New York, McGraw Hill, 1985.)

TABLE 123–3.
Symptoms and Signs of Mass Lesions

DUE TO INCREASED INTRACRANIAL PRESSURE	DUE TO HERNIATION
Mental changes	Deteriorating consciousness
Headache, vomiting	Changes in pupillary size and reaction
Dizziness	Abnormal "doll's eye" reflexes and caloric tests
Papilledema	Abnormal respiration
Bradycardia, increased blood pressure	Decerebrate and decorticate postures
Enlarging skull (children)	
Bulging fontanelle (infants)	

TABLE 123–4.
Clinical–Pathologic Correlations for Intracranial Tumors

LOCATION	COMMON TUMOR TYPES	CLINICAL FINDINGS
Cerebral hemispheres; basal ganglia; thalamus	Glioblastoma multiforme Metastatic carcinoma Meningioma Astrocytoma Oligodendroglioma	Headaches; dementia; personality and behavior changes; seizures; hemiplegia; aphasia/apraxia; homonymous hemianopsia
Brain stem	Astrocytoma	Cranial nerve palsies; pyramidal dysfunction; sensory impairment; ataxia; bulbar and pseudobulbar palsies
Cerebellum	Medulloblastoma Astrocytoma Hemangioblastoma Metastasis	Nuchal and occipital headache; gait ataxia; incoordination of extremities; nystagmus; early obstructive hydrocephalus
Cerebellopontine angle	Acoustic schwannoma Meningioma	Unilateral tinnitus, deafness; dizziness, vertigo; ipsilateral fifth and seventh cranial nerve signs; ipsilateral ataxia
Sellar and parasellar	Pituitary adenoma Craniopharyngioma Meningioma Teratoma	*Neurologic:* Optic atrophy; bitemporal hemianopsia; oculomotor palsies *Endocrine:* panhypopituitarism; dwarfism, gigantism, acromegaly; amenorrhoea/galactorrhea, impotence; Cushing's disease, diabetes insipidus
Spinal canal	Metastasis Schwannoma Meningioma Ependymoma Astrocytoma	Vertebral or radicular pain; paraplegia/quadriplegia; sensory loss; ataxia; sphincter dysfunction

(Fig 123–5). It infiltrates widely, through the corpus callosum to the opposite hemisphere or into subcortical regions. Glioblastoma multiforme is pleomorphic and is highly cellular with abundant mitoses and admixtures of undifferentiated and more mature glial cells. Computed tomography shows a contrast-enhancing mass, edema, and mass effect (Fig 123–5). Despite aggressive subtotal resection, radiation, and chemotherapy, most patients die in 1 year to 2 years.

ASTROCYTOMA

Astrocytomas may be benign or malignant. Biologically the anaplastic astrocytoma is similar to glioblastoma. Astrocytomas in children are located in the cerebellum, brain stem, hy-pothalamus, and optic nerves, whereas in adults most are in the cerebral hemispheres. Benign astrocytomas are slow growing and diffusely infiltrative without clear-cut boundaries. Microscopically the astrocytoma consists of well-differentiated mature astrocytes. However, the cerebellar astrocytoma is well circumscribed and often cystic and can be extirpated completely (Fig 123–3). Brain stem and diencephalic astrocytomas have a 5-year survival rate of 20% to 30%, and hemispheric astrocytomas have a 5-year survival rate of 50%.

OLIGODENDROGLIOMA

Oligodenrogliomas are benign, slow growing, infiltrative supratentorial neoplasms. They occur in adults, usually with seizures as the first

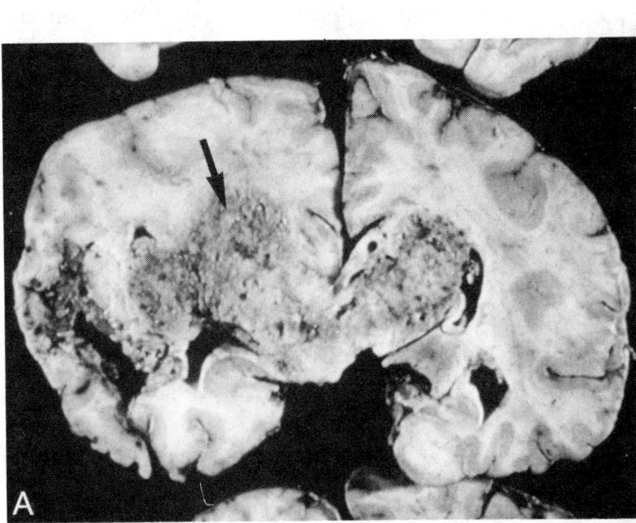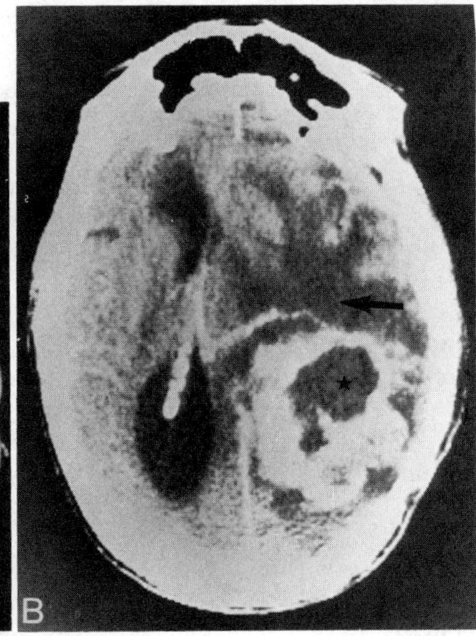

FIG 123–5.
Glioblastoma multiforme. **A,** diffusely infiltrative tumor with areas of necrosis and hemorrhage; **B,** CT scan showing striking contrast enhancement due to tumor vascularity. Central low density indicates necrosis. Note the edema in the white matter (low density) and shift of ventricles.

manifestation. Calcification occurs in 75% of these tumors. Aggressive surgical resection and radiation result in a 5-year survival rate of 85%.

MEDULLOBLASTOMA

Medulloblastoma is the most common brain tumor in childhood. It usually arises in the cerebellar vermis and extends into the fourth ventricle causing early obstructive hydrocephalus. Medulloblastoma is highly malignant and consists of poorly differentiated anaplastic cells. Treatment consists of surgical removal, chemotherapy, and radiation of the entire neuraxis because this neoplasm seeds through the CSF into the ventricles and spinal canal. A 5-year survival rate of 50% can be achieved with aggressive treatment.

MENINGIOMA

Meningiomas constitute 20% of all primary brain tumors. They arise from arachnoid cells particularly in the arachnoid villi protruding into the dural sinuses. Meningiomas tend to be located parasagittally, over the convexity, in the sphenoid wing, olfactory groove, and para-

sellar regions. Meningiomas are benign, well-circumscribed, ovoid, and they compress but do not invade the brain. Meningiomas frequently calcify and are highly vascular with intense enhancement on a CT scan. Most meningiomas can be cured; basal meningiomas may be difficult to remove completely and may recur years later.

NERVE SHEATH TUMORS (schwannoma, neurofibroma)

Nerve sheath tumors (schwannoma, neurofibroma) form 8% of primary brain tumors. They are thought to arise from Schwann's cells or perineural fibroblasts. Most schwannomas arise from the vestibular branch of the eighth cranial nerve. Trigeminal schwannomas are much less common. Schwannoma is the most common primary tumor in the spinal canal. Multiple schwannomas or occurrence at an early age is highly suggestive of Von Recklinghausen's disease. Acoustic schwannomas result in unilateral tinnitus, hearing loss, and dizziness. As the tumor grows out of the internal auditory canal, it compresses structures in the cerebellopontine angle (Table 123–4). A surgical cure is possible in most cases.

PITUITARY ADENOMAS

Pituitary adenomas account for 10% of brain tumors. Microadenomas may be confined to the sella turcica. As they enlarge, they distend and distort the sella turcica and emerge in the suprasellar region compressing the optic chiasm or the ocular nerves in the cavernous sinus. The endocrine effects may consist of panhypopituitarism with decreased secretion of growth hormone, the gonadotropins, thyroid-stimulating hormone, and ACTH. Secretion of prolactin by the tumor results in amenorrhea and galactorrhea, and impotence. Excessive growth hormone levels cause acromegaly and gigantism, and excessive ACTH level results in Cushing's disease. In pituitary apoplexy, hemorrhage or necrosis in the tumor causes abrupt onset of headache, blindness, and impaired consciousness. Treatment consists of surgical removal, radiation, and life-long hormone replacement.

PRIMARY SPINAL NEOPLASMS

The primary spinal tumors in decreasing order of frequency are schwannoma, meningioma, ependymoma, and astrocytoma. The clinical manifestations are listed in Table 123–4. Meningiomas and schwannomas are surgically curable. Ependymoma and astrocytoma are intramedullary and cannot be resected completely.

CNS METASTASIS

Metastasis to the CNS by hematogenous spread occurs in 15% of cases of systemic cancer. Cancers from the lung, breast, and kidney and melanoma frequently metastasize to the CNS, whereas cancers of skin, ovaries, uterus, bladder, pancreas, thyroid, and larynx and the sarcomas seldom involve the brain. Prostate cancer frequently involves the spine but rarely spreads to the brain. The hematologic malignancies involve the meninges but seldom form solid metastases. Metastases may involve any part of the neuraxis, and multiple lesions are seen in 50% to 60% of cases. Metastases are circumscribed, "punched-out," necrotic masses surrounded by edema (Fig 123–2). Treatment consists of corticosteroids and radiation. Accessible solitary lesions may be surgically excised. In leptomeningeal carcinomatosis, there is diffuse spread of cancer in the subarachnoid space causing multiple cranial nerve palsies, radioculopathy, hydrocephalus, and focal cerebral or spinal dysfunction. Diagnosis is confirmed by finding malignant cells in CSF cytologic studies.

The most common cause of spinal cord compression is epidural metastatic cancer. The vertebra is first involved with subsequent extension into the extradural space. Pain and vertebral tenderness are the earliest clinical findings (Table 123–4). X-ray films and radionuclide scans show bony destruction, and myelography confirms the diagnosis. Treatment consists of corticosteroids and radiation or decompressive laminectomy. Early diagnosis and immediate treatment are necessary to avoid permanent paraplegia.

REFERENCES

Jennett B: *An Introduction to Neurosurgery*, ed 3. Chicago, Year Book Medical Publishers, 1977. *This text provides an introduction to surgical aspects of brain tumors.*

Plum F, Posner JB: *The Diagnosis of Stupor and Coma*, ed 3. Philadelphia, FA Davis, 1980. *The most comprehensive and well-known text on coma; refer to this for a detailed description of the pathophysiology and clinical recognition for the herniation syndromes.*

Posner JB: Neurologic complications of sytemic cancer. *Disease-a-Month* 1978; 25(2):1–60. *Should be read by all physicians who deal with cancer. More than 15% of cancer victims will have secondary CNS involvement.*

Russell DS, Rubenstein LJ: *Pathology of Tumors of*

the *Nervous System*, ed 4. Baltimore, Williams & Wilkins, 1977. *The standard reference text on the neuropathology of brain tumors.*

Shapiro WR: Intracranial neoplasms, in Rosenberg RN, Grossman RG (eds): *The Clinical Neurosciences*. New York, Churchill Livingstone, 1983; 1:233–283. *This chapter is recommended as the best current reference. It provides an overview of*

the biology, clinical manifestations, and treatment of brain tumors.

Walker RW, Posner JB. Central nervous system neoplasms. *Current Neurology* 1986; 6:285–322. *A current review that emphasizes recent research in biology and treatment especially radiation and chemotherapy of malignant gliomas.*

124 MENINGITIS

John S. Czachor, M.D.
H. Bradford Hawley, M.D.

Meningitis can be defined as inflammation of the tissues, the leptomeninges, that surround the brain. It is a true medical emergency with significant mortality and long-term morbidity. The causative organism may be varied and includes bacteria, viruses, fungi, amoebas, and parasites. Meningitis may be broadly grouped into *pyogenic meningitis* and *aseptic meningitis*, based on culture reports. This chapter will focus on pyogenic meningitis, specifically bacterial pyogenic meningitis.

CLINICAL SIGNS AND SYMPTOMS

The patient's history can provide several clues for determining the cause of the meningitis. Certain factors increase the potential for the host to acquire this infection. Extremes of age, crowded living conditions, the black race, nasopharyngeal carriage of virulent factors by newborns, and chronic diseases such as alcoholism, cirrhosis, and diabetes are all predisposing factors.

Headache, nausea, vomiting, nuchal pain, fever, and various degrees of neurologic involvement are usually present. Photophobia and other ophthalmologic symptoms secondary to ocular nerve palsies can be seen. Other cranial nerves may be similarly affected. Papilledema may be present, but it is unusual in meningitis. Confusion and lethargy may be hallmarks of meningitis for both young and elderly persons. Any histories of head trauma, leading of cerebrospinal fluid, cranial surgery, central nervous system shunts, or suppurative parameningeal infection are important historic points to obtain. It is important to realize that the very young and the very old may not present with the classic history associated with meningitis because their immune systems are either immature or incompetent, respectively (Table 124–1).

The typical patient may appear to be in a toxic condition, diaphoretic, and prostrate, and may complain of generalized weakness, myalgias, and occasionally arthralgias. A global headache is usually present, and the pain of the headache may be out of proportion to the physical findings. Papilledema is seldom present but must always be sought. Neck rigidity is noted after Kernig's maneuver (straight-leg raise causing painful neck) and Brudzinski's maneuver (dorsiflexion of neck resulting in

TABLE 124–1.
Presumptive Diagnosis and Treatment Classified by Age*

AGE RANGE	PREDOMINANT ORGANISMS	ANTIBIOTIC	ANTIBIOTIC FOR PATIENTS WITH PENICILLIN ALLERGY
0–2 months	Gram-negative bacilli Streptococci *Listeria monocytogenes*	Ampicillin and aminoglycoside or ampicillin and a third-generation cephalosporin	Third generation cephalosporin
>2 months–<5 years	*Hemophilus influenza*	Ampicillin and chloramphenicol or third-generation cephalosporin	Third generation cephalosporin
>5 years–<30 years	*Neisseria meningitidis*	Penicillin G	Chloramphenicol
Adult	*Streptococcus pneumoniae*	Penicillin G	Chloramphenicol

* Adjustments made after culture results were final.

pain); most patients will avoid movements that cause pain. The results of the neurologic examination generally do not provide a focus, but mental confusion, either secondary to fever or to meningeal irritation, is sometimes noted. Extracranial sites of infection such as pneumonia, cellulitis, and abscesses are important indicators of potential sources of bacteremia that lead to meningitis. Otitis media and mastoiditis are important cranial infections to document. Rashes, purpura, or petechiae may be seen in various types of meningitis.

Fatality is the usual outcome of untreated bacterial meningitis. Despite adequate antibiotic therapy and the development of newer antibiotics, mortality is still significant, in the range of 10% to 30%. Complications of meningitis are listed in Table 124–2. Because 90% of all meningitis occur between ages 7 months and 5 years, the long-term morbidity becomes significant.

PATHOPHYSIOLOGY

Bacteria gain access to the CNS by three pathways: (1) hematogenous spread, (2) contiguous contamination, and (3) direct implantation. Usually, the most common route of infection is by the bloodstream. The latter two types are the result of intimate contact between the infecting organism and the CNS.

The hematogenous spread involves several steps before the bacteria can set up an infection. Colonization of a new serotype in the nasopharyngeal or oropharyngeal mucosa begins the process. Occasionally, distant foci are involved. Next, the organisms transgress the mucosal barrier and gain access to the bloodstream. Dissemination after access to the bloodstream is probably a rare event dependent on a number of host and organism factors including immunologic factors, such as IgA secretion, and microbial virulence characteristics, particularly capsular surface serotype. Once within the blood, the organisms invade the cerebrospinal fluid (CSF). The mechanism is unclear, but the organism probably gains passage at the junction of the bloodstream and choroid plexus. The organism is then spread through the usual CSF flow.

Logarithmic growth increases bacterial numbers; early in the infection, host-defense mechanisms are absent in the CSF. As the bacteria multiply, they damage surrounding tissue and eventually disrupt the blood–brain barrier allowing diapedesis of phagocytic cells and leakage of proteins such as complement and immunoglobulin into the CSF. The usual mechanism of humoral immunity can then occur. It is important to administer *bactericidal* antibiotics early in the infection to decrease the absolute number of bacteria present. As the infection progresses, the blood–brain barrier

TABLE 124–2.
Complications Associated with Meningitis

EARLY COMPLICATIONS

Death
Sepsis
Dehydration
Hyponatremia
  • Syndrome of inappropriate secretion of antidiuretic hormone (SIADH)
  • Overhydration
Seizures
Disseminated intravascular coagulation (DIC)
Cerebral edema
Cerebral infarction

LATE COMPLICATIONS

Persistent fevers
  • Concurrent extracranial infections
  • Febrile reaction to drug
  • Serum-sickness type reaction secondary to antibody formation to capsular polysaccharide of infecting
    organism
Subdural effusions
Cortical vein thrombosis
Septic arthritis
Selective nerve deficits
Mental retardation and learning disabilities
Hydrocephalus
Seizures

TABLE 124–3.
Clinical–Pathologic Correlations for Meningitis

CLINICAL FINDINGS	PATHOLOGIC FINDINGS
Hypoglycorrhachia	Blocked facilitated diffusion of glucose
CSF pleocytosis	Disruption of blood–brain barrier
Elevated protein level in CSF	Disruption of blood–brain barrier
Headache	Inflamed meninges with increased intracranial pressure
Nuchal rigidity	Inflamed meninges

becomes more disrupted, resulting in greater passage of both humoral factors and antibiotic agents. Eventually the infection is suppressed with the restoration of the integrity of the blood–brain barrier and the resolution of leakage into the CSF.

CLINICAL–PATHOLOGIC CORRELATIONS

The clinical features of meningitis result from the entry of microbial agents into the CSF, an area of impaired host resistance. These agents then exert their action in a relatively local area with notable effects (Table 124–3).

DIFFERENTIAL DIAGNOSIS

Meningitis must first be distinguished from conditions that may mimic it including parameningeal suppurative foci, carcinomatous meningitis, meningoencephalitis, sarcoidosis, cerebral vasculitides, and chemical meningitis.

Because papilledema is unusual in meningitis, its presence should alert the physician to other causes of infection. In conjunction with focal neurologic defects, the differential diagnosis includes brain abscess, epidural abscess, subdural empyema, and meningoencephalitis. With findings of papilledema or focal defects, intracranial imaging for mass effect is indicated prior to any CNS invasive procedure. A special situation exists when an initial diagnosis of meningitis is made but the patient fails to improve with treatment. If fever persists and repeated spinal taps reveal continued infection, a diagnosis of parameningeal infection rather than meningitis must be considered. Repeated CSF invasion by microbes occurs from the abscess that abuts on the subarachnoid space, thus simulating meningitis. In patients known to have cancer, fever plus an abrupt change in mental status leads the physician to consider meningitis as the cause. Carcinomatous meningitis may be the actual problem and can be confirmed by CNS cytologic studies. Chemical meningitis is usually diagnosed by the typical meningeal findings plus a history of antecedent spinal anesthesia or diagnostic studies involving the subarachnoid space. Sarcoidosis, cerebral vasculitides, and Behçet's syndrome are usually diagnoses of exclusion.

Neonatal meningitis has a specific spectrum of bacterial pathogens that are different from those associated with other ages. Neonatal meningitis is associated with prematurity, birth trauma, and premature rupture of membranes and is related to maternal perineal and vaginal flora. Common signs and symptoms may be absent because of the immature immune system. Gram-negative bacilli, Group B *Streptococcus,* enterococci, and *Listeria monocytogenes* are the usual pathogens.

Meningitis tends to be a disease of children when its incidence is considered. Approximately 60% to 70% of all bacterial meningitis cases are found in children less than 5 years of age. Several pathogens are common in children and adolescents after the neonatal period. Most prevalent up to age 6 years is meningitis caused by *Hemophilus influenzae.* Also present, but less common in childhood, is *Neisseria meningitidis* meningitis, which tends to occur seasonally primarily in the winter and spring. *N. meningitidis* has at least six disease-causing serogroups, the most common serogroups are labeled A, B, C, and Y. Pneumococcal meningitis may occasionally occur, but generally is found in older children.

H. influenzae is the leading cause of meningitis in any age group. The overall mortality rate for this meningitis is 3% to 8%. Pharyngitis and otitis are associated with this meningitis. A major problem is the emergence of plasmid-mediated β-lactamase-producing strains of *H.*

influenzae. These have been isolated with increasing frequency over the past few years, and now some 10% to 30% of all isolates are β-lactamase positive. A major problem with meningococcal meningitis is the absence of a significant prodrome. However, an initial sign may be petechiae. This is not limited to meningococcal meningitis and can also occur with echovirus type 9 meningitis and pneumococcal meningitis (usually in asplenic patients). Disseminated intravascular coagulation may accompany meningococcal meningitis if meningococcemia is present.

Adulthood generally is the key time period for *Streptococcus pneumoniae* meningitis. However, in young adults meningococcal meningitis is known and is common among military recruits. Another common cause of meningitis at the young-adult age is aseptic or viral meningitis which occurs seasonally, commonly during the summer and in the early autumn months. It can be confused with bacterial meningitis because the CSF findings are variable.

Cases of viral meningitis usually resolve in 2 days to 5 days without significant sequelae. There are many causative organisms for viral meningitis, including enterovirus (causing more than 50% of all cases of viral meningitis), mumps virus, echovirus, cytomegalovirus, Epstein-Barr virus, and the herpes family of viruses. Most notable of all viral meningitides are Herpes simplex 1 and 2 infections. They are the only treatable types of viral meningitis (using acyclovir). Other antiviral agents are either in development or unnecessary because some viral infections have minimal virulence and do not require treatment.

Pneumococcal meningitis is the most frequent type of meningitis in adults after the age of 30 years. The mortality rate for pneumococcal meningitis is 30% to 60%. Pneumonia may precede this type of meningitis, and sinusitis, otitis, leaking CSF, trauma, and neurosurgical procedures all are associated with S. *pneumococcus* meningitis. There seems to be greater alteration in consciousness in this type of meningitis than in other types. Two percent of all pneumococcal strains are penicillin resistant.

The immunocompromised patient is especially vulnerable to other types of meningitis. Fungal and tuberculous meningitis are most prevalent in these patients. Steroid dependency increases the risk for both of these infections, as does the presence of neoplasm. Common fungal meningitis agents include *Cryptococcus neoformans* and *Candida* species. Amphotericin in combination with 5-fluorocytosine is the usual treatment. Tuberculous meningitis usually occurs in the setting of miliary tuberculosis or subependymal tubercle rupture. The clinical signs of *tuberculosis* may be absent in tuberculous meningitis. Typical CSF findings include a lymphocytic pleocytosis. Some physicians use corticosteroid treatment when the CSF protein level is over 500 mg/dl which may help reduce post-treatment adhesive arachnoiditis. Both fungal and tuberculous meningitis can be chronic. In one subgroup of immunocompromised patients, renal transplant patients, *Listeria monocytogenes* is the predominant organism. Ampicillin is the drug of choice for treating this infection.

DIAGNOSIS

The diagnosis of meningitis remains contingent on the retrieval of a CSF sample by lumbar puncture. Studies of the fluid with Gram's stain and appropriate cultures help to secure the diagnosis and are a guide to treatment (Table 124–4). Extra fluid should be held for further testing if the preliminary tests fail to yield a diagnosis. Viral or cytologic studies or repeat evaluation for confirmation of abnormal laboratory findings may be needed. A spinal tap (lumbar puncture) should not be performed if there is evidence of increased intracranial pressure such as papilledema or focal neurologic findings unless intracranial imaging has been obtained to exclude any anatomic abnormality because brain stem herniation may result.

The laboratory findings in the CSF have been a source of frustration to physicians for years. The findings indicative of bacterial and aseptic infection overlap considerably. Generally, a white cell count greater than $1000/\text{mm}^3$, with the majority being polymorphonuclear neutrophil leukocytes (PMNs), hypoglycorrhachia, and an elevated protein level suggest a bacterial cause. However, early viral meningitis may have a predominant PMN pleocytosis. This eventually will shift to a monocytic predominance. Decreased glucose levels and elevated protein levels may exist in aseptic meningitis, but not in most cases. If there is some confusion as to the diagnosis, then collection of another CSF sample by lumbar puncture is indicated 6 hours to 12 hours later.

Another problem rests with patients who are suspected of having meningitis but who have received prior treatment with various amounts of antibiotics for various durations. Approximately 50% of all patients with suspected meningitis have had prior antibiotic therapy at the

TABLE 124–4.
Spinal Fluid Examination

LABORATORY TEST	RESULT
Gram's stain	Positive in bacterial infection; negative in other kinds
India ink	Positive in *Cryptococcus neoformans* infection
Acid-fast stain	Positive in 80% of cases of tuberculous meningitis with multiple lumbar punctures
Wet-mount	Positive in amoebic meningitis *(Nacglcria)*
Cell differential count	≥ 5 leukocytes/mm^3 is abnormal
	≥ 1 PMN/mm^3 is abnormal
	$\leq 50\%$ PMNs suggests nonbacterial infection origin, but is not diagnostic
Glucose level	$\leq 60\%$ of concurrent blood sugar or < 30 mg/dl suggests bacterial infection
Protein level	≥ 150 mg/dl suggests bacterial infection
Lactic acid level	> 35 mEq/L suggests bacterial infection
Counterimmunoelectrophoresis (CIE)	Specific for antigens of pneumococci, meningococci, or *H. influenza*
Latex agglutination	More sensitive than CIE; specific for antigens of pneumococci, meningococci, *H. influenzae*, group B streptococci, cryptococci

time of lumbar puncture. This has been shown to decrease the chance of recovering a causative bacterial agent by almost 30%. However, based on the spinal fluid chemistry studies, the diagnosis of meningitis still can be made. Collection of another CSF sample by lumbar puncture is indicated if the original sample fails to confirm the diagnosis. Several tests have been advocated in order to help eliminate this confusion and include measurement of CSF lactate levels and counterimmunoelectrophoresis (CIE) and latex agglutination to identify specific bacterial antigens. However, these tests can be insensitive with false-negative results. Again, collection of another CSF sample is indicated if the first examination is unable to separate bacterial, partially treated bacterial, and viral meningitis.

PRINCIPLES OF TREATMENT

Early administration of antibiotics is essential in bacterial meningitis. The diagnosis of the specific bacterial type is frequently not known immediately after lumbar puncture. Therefore, the presumptive choice of antibiotics is made on the basis of the history and the results of the physical examination and the laboratory examinations, including the information obtained about the CSF. Uncertainty secondary to prior antibiotic treatment as an outpatient or secondary to nondiagnostic results of the CSF studies may play a part in the decision-making process. This uncertainty may be reduced with careful clinical correlation and observation. Repeated lumbar puncture to collect CSF samples may be necessary. Various aspects of treatment are presented in Table 124–1 and Figure 124–1.

When considering the treatment of meningitis, the use of blood cultures can help with the etiologic diagnosis. Positive blood cultures are found in a majority of meningitis cases and can provide additional information for choosing an antibiotic.

The duration of treatment varies with the causative organism, and the individual situation must be considered as a whole. Generally, treatment of meningitis is continued for 4 days to 5 days after the patient is afebrile. For the three major bacterial meningitis agents (*H. influenzae*, *N. meningitidis*, and *S. pneumoniae*), antibiotic therapy consists of a 10-day course. The duration of treatment of other *Steptococcus* and *Staphylococcus* species ranges from 7 days to 14 days, 10 days being the average. Enterococci and *Listeria* have slightly longer courses of therapy, ranging from 14 days to 20 days. Gram-negative enteric organisms have the longest course of treatment, lasting 21 days to 28 days.

When gram-negative organisms are the cause of meningitis, several points must be remembered. First, these organisms can be multiresistant. Second, the antibiotic chosen must cross the blood–brain barrier. If the use of an aminoglycoside is deemed necessary, the route of administration remains a difficult decision because aminoglycosides do not pass easily through the blood–brain barrier. In order to achieve good concentrations of this drug in the CSF, daily intrathecal or even intraventricular administration may be needed. Also, when choosing a cephalosporin, remember that all of these agents do not penetrate well into the spinal fluid. No first-generation agent will be an acceptable choice for treatment. Of the second-generation cephalosporins, only cefuroxime crosses the blood–brain barrier in therapeutic concentrations. Moxolactam, ceftazidime, ceftriaxone, and cefotaxime are third-generation cephalosporins that are acceptable choices. Cefoperazone does not cross the blood–brain barrier in concentrations sufficient to treat meningitis.

Prolonged fevers during the treatment of meningitis can also cause concern for the physician. This fever is often not a continuation of the original meningitis. To determine whether or not the problem is related to meningitis, repeat lumbar punctures to collect CSF samples are indicated. At 48 hours, CSF samples from patients responsive to treatment will have no organisms with Gram's staining, it will be sterile on culture and will have chemistry values that approach normal. Thus, the fever is not from meningitis if the CSF meets these criteria. If the CSF is not sterile, parameningeal foci of infection must be sought. Causes of persistent fever are listed in Table 124–2 under late complications. Such fevers can modify treatment and should be considered during the course of treatment.

Meningitis in conjunction with a CSF shunt presents a special problem. Treatment usually consists of systemic antibiotics along with re-

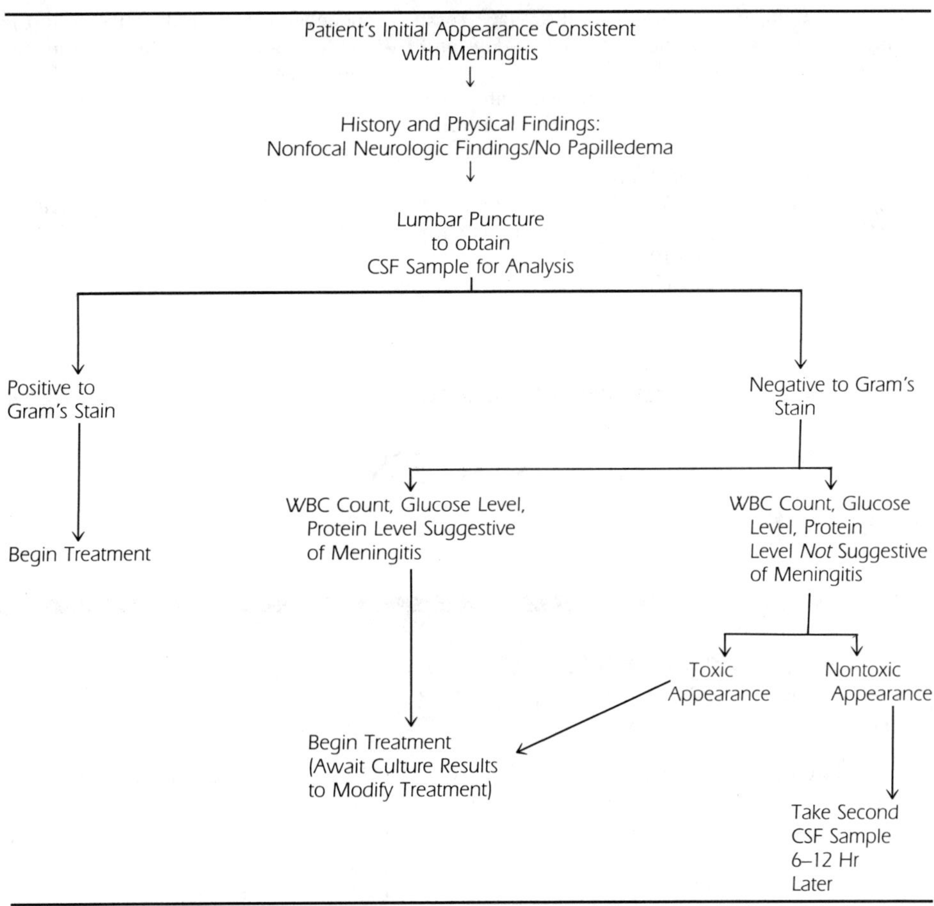

FIG 124–1.
Treatment plan for uncomplicated meningitis.

moval of the infected shunt. The use of systemic antibiotics alone has been shown to have a lower cure rate and even increase mortality. The shunt probably harbors the infecting organism, and its removal will increase the chance for cure.

Finally, a post-treatment lumbar puncture is not indicated. The CSF findings in a cured patient at the end of antibiotic therapy cover a range, and, if the clinical appearance of the patient is good, further CSF studies may only serve to confuse the situation.

REFERENCES

Balagtas RC, Levin S, Nelson KE, Gotoff SP: Secondary and prolonged fevers in bacterial meningitis. *J Pediatr* 1970; 77:957–964. *Gives an excellent differential diagnosis for prolonged fever in meningitis.*

Dalton HP, Allison MJ: Modification of laboratory results by partial treatment of bacterial meningitis. *Am J Clin Pathol* 1968; 49:410–413. *This is an excellent review on partially treated meningitis.*

Kass EH, Platt R: Current therapy in infectious disease 1983–1984. St Louis, CV Mosby Co, 1983. *More than just therapy included here, including epidemiology and pathophysiology.*

Mandel GL, Douglas RG, Bennett JE: *Principles and*

Practice of Infectious Diseases, ed 2. New York, John Wiley and Sons Inc, 1985. *Up-to-date and in-depth review of the subject.*

Molavi A, LeFrock JD (eds): Symposium on infections of the central nervous system. *Med Clin North Am* 1985; 69(2). *Current references for a range of topics covering CNS infections.*

Scheld WM: Bacterial meningitis in the patient at risk: Intrinsic risk factors and host defense mechanisms. *Am J Med* 1984; 76(5A):193–207. *Excellent pathophysiologic discussion about meningitis.*

Schoenbaum SC, Gardner P, Shillito J: Infections of cerebrospinal fluid shunts: Epidemiology, clinical manifestations and therapy. *J Infect Dis* 1975; 131:543–552. *Discusses the problem of meningitis and shunts.*

Swartz MN, Dodge PR: Bacterial Meningitis—A review of selected aspects. *N Engl J Med* 1965; 272:725–731, 779–787, 842–848, 898–902, 954–960. *Another excellent series that reviews the subject.*

125 BRAIN ABSCESS

Michael P. Coyle, M.D.
Timothy B. Sorg, M.D.

Encapsulated or free pus within the parenchyma of the brain is termed brain abscess. Although technologic advances have aided in reducing the morbidity and mortality of this entity, much remains to be done to improve the outlook of those afflicted. Predisposing factors for the development of brain abscess include acute and chronic otitis media, pulmonary and cardiac infections, trauma, congenital heart disease, sinusitis, and the acquired immunodeficiency syndrome (AIDS). Predilection for different sites of the brain have been noted and are related to the primary source of infection. The frequencies of abscesses in various locations are listed in Table 125–1. Often the classic signs and symptoms are not present or are subtle, and a high index of suspicion is needed to make the diagnosis. Brain abscess remains a serious diagnostic problem that often is difficult to manage.

CLINICAL SIGNS AND SYMPTOMS

Brain abscess should be considered in any patient with headache and focal neurologic signs, or an impaired level of consciousness. The classic triad of brain abscess manifestations is fever, headache, and focal neurologic deficits, but all three are present in fewer than 50% of patients. In general, signs of increased intracranial pressure and focal neurologic deficit predominate over signs of infection. The specific neurologic manifestations depend on the size of the abscess and which part of the brain is affected. The most common signs and symptoms are listed in Table 125–2. Almost half of the patients with brain abscesses present with no signs or symptoms of an infectious process and are diagnosed as having a space-occupying lesion. Most patients give a history of a previous infection, usually a chronic ear or sinus infection that is either recurrent or partially treated.

The clinical course of brain abscess is variable. In most patients, the onset of symptoms is gradual over 2 days to 14 days. Fever may be absent, and neurologic findings may be subtle. Changes in mental status are frequent and range from lethargy to coma. Although many patients present with a gradual onset of symptoms and signs, a subset of patients can present with manifestations of meningitis and a rapidly fulminating course.

The patient with a brain abscess may have only a low-grade fever or papilledema. A variety of localizing neurologic signs such as aphasia, visual field defect, contralateral motor or sensory deficits, nystagmus, or ipsilateral cerebellar ataxia may be found. Sometimes, only mild changes in intellectual function are noted. Other findings include cranial nerve palsies or signs of meningeal irritation such as nuchal rigidity. Evidence of a primary source of infection often is apparent, such as an ear or sinus infection or perhaps a pulmonary infection including bronchiectasis or lung abscess. Frequently, a change in a patient's level of consciousness is seen, and occasionally signs of brain herniation occur.

Brain abscess left untreated leads to a mortality rate of nearly 100%. Death is caused either by herniation of the brain or rupture of the abscess into the cerebrospinal fluid. Occasionally, if an abscess is well encapsulated, mild symptoms may be present and persist for years.

PATHOPHYSIOLOGY

The early stages of brain infection with its associated inflammatory changes produce a typical response, with edema and infiltration of polymorphonuclear leukocytes, plasma cells, and mononuclear cells. A necrotic center forms early in the course of cerebritis, gradually enlarges, and then decreases in size with capsule formation. The capsule is composed mainly of collagen and usually is completed by the second or third week of abscess formation. As the capsule forms around the necrotic center of the brain abscess, there is less cerebritis and cerebral edema surrounding the capsule.

With computed tomography (CT), the characteristic appearance of a brain abscess in its mature stages is demonstrated by three discernable regions. A hypodense area representing the necrotic center is located centrally. Surrounding this is an area of ring enhancement, which has been equated with abscess encapsulation but which is thought actually to represent brain inflammation or cerebritis. Injection of a contrast agent makes this ring more visible on CT and is felt to be due to an altered blood-brain barrier. A hypodense region of variable width is peripheral to the ring and signifies cerebral edema.

TABLE 125–1.
Frequencies of Brain Abscesses in Various Locations*

LOCATION	FREQUENCY (% OF CASES)
Temporal	32
Frontal	25
Parietal	18
Occipital	10
Cerebellar	10
Basal ganglia	3
Brain stem	2

* Based on data from Beller AJ, Sahar A, Praiss I: Brain abscess: Review of 89 cases over a period of 30 years. *J Neurol Neurosurg Psychiatry* 1973; 36:757–768; Nielsen H, Glydensted C, Harmsen A: Cerebral abscess: Aetiology and pathogenesis, symptoms, diagnosis and treatment. *Acta Neurol Scand* 1982; 65:609–622; and Yang S-Y: Brain abscess: A review of 400 cases. *J Neurosurg* 1981; 55:794–799.

TABLE 125–2.
Incidences of Common Signs and Symptoms of Brain Abscess*

SIGN OR SYMPTOM	INCIDENCE (% OF CASES)
Headache	70
Nausea and vomiting	57
Fever	52
Focal neurologic deficit	52
Hemiparesis	50
Impaired consciousness	48
Papilledema	48
Visual impairment	34
Seizures	28
Nuchal rigidity	25
Nystagmus	19
Ataxia	19
Aphasia	8

* Based on data from Nielsen H, Glydensted C, Harmsen A: Cerebral abscess: Aetiology and pathogenesis, symptoms, diagnosis and treatment, *Acta Neurol Scand* 1982; 65:609–622; Scheld WM, Winn HR: Brain abscess, in Mandell GL, Douglas RG Jr, Bennett JE (eds): *Principles and Practice of Infectious Diseases.* New York, John Wiley & Sons, 1985, pp 585–592; and Yang S-Y: Brain abscess: A review of 400 cases. *J Neurosurg* 1981; 55:794–799.

Brain abscess of the frontal lobe, commonly preceded by sinusitis or influenza, usually is associated with a streptococci infection. Otogenic infections may lead to temporal lobe abscesses; mixed flora, including anaerobes, are involved. *Bacteroides, Streptococcus,* and *Enterobacter* are the usual isolates. Trauma, either surgical or accidental, is associated with staphylococcal and clostridial infections. Metastatic brain abscesses harbor the organisms found in the primary source of infection and often are located in the frontal or parietal lobes. An important cause of metastatic brain abscess is pulmonary infection, and *Streptococcus, Bacteroides, Actinomyces,* and *Nocardia asteroides* have been implicated as the causative organisms. Staphylococcal endocarditis is another important cause. Various protozoa, fungi, and yeasts are assuming a more important role as the pathogens found in brain abscesses, especially in immunocompromised patients such as those with the acquired immunodeficiency syndrome.

CLINICAL–PATHOLOGIC CORRELATIONS

The clinical features of brain abscess are associated primarily with the region of the brain affected and the subsequent increase in intracranial pressure. The main clinical–pathologic correlations are shown in Table 125–3.

DIFFERENTIAL DIAGNOSIS

A tumor of the brain, either primary or metastatic, should be a primary consideration in the differential diagnosis, especially in the patient without evidence of an antecedent or concurrent infection. Other possibilities include cerebral infarction, intracerebral hemorrhage, meningitis or encephalitis, and subdural hematoma. The presence of focal neurologic deficits should prompt cerebral CT scanning, if available. If the classic clinical picture of brain abscess is seen, together with a CT scan which is characteristic, the diagnosis is usually brain abscess. Abnormalities that may mimic brain abscess on CT scan include cystic glioma, metastasis, an infarct related to bacterial endocarditis, granuloma, infarction, and changes from recent brain surgery. If there is a mass lesion in the brain that is thought to be related to an infectious process, secondary brain destruction from viral encephalitis, subdural em-

pyema, or intracranial vasculitis should be considered.

DIAGNOSIS

An important consideration in the diagnostic evaluation of a brain abscess is that lumbar puncture may not be helpful and may be fatal if herniation occurs. When focal neurologic deficits or papilledema are present, lumbar puncture should be deferred until a CT scan is performed if pyogenic meningitis is suspected. The most common findings in the CSF are elevated pressure and white blood cell count (usually less than 200/mm^3) and elevated protein levels (usually less than 200 mg/dl). A white blood cell count greater than 50,000/ml suggests an abscess which has ruptured into the ventricular system. Bacterial cultures of the CSF are positive most often when the abscess is contiguous with the ventricular system.

Computed tomography scanning is the most valuable diagnostic method to evaluate a brain abscess, and with its introduction the mortality from this CNS infection has decreased. CT scanning should always include a contrast study. The ring enhancement with injection of contrast material is seen partially on the first day of early cerebritis and becomes well developed by the third day. For the next 5 days or 6 days, ring enhancement and diffusion of contrast material into the central lucent zone are seen. During the second week less diffusion of contrast material into the lucent center is seen, with even less diffusion after 14 days. By 2 weeks, a well-encapsulated brain abscess has formed, and after that, ring enhancement persists with less diffusion, which signifies less surrounding cerebral edema.

If CT scanning is not available, brain scan is the diagnostic modality of choice and offers a high degree of sensitivity. Skull x-ray films may be abnormal with a shift of a calcified pineal body or evidence of osteomyelitis of the skull. Other x-ray films that may be helpful are those of the sinuses, mastoids, and chest. An EEG may show focal abnormalities. Cerebral angiography can be useful and may help differentiate an abscess from a tumor but may not be reliable if encapsulation has not occurred. A test that is nonspecific but often elevated is the

TABLE 125–3.
Clinical–Pathologic Correlations for Brain Abscess*

CLINICAL FINDINGS	PATHOLOGIC FINDINGS
1. Fever (may decrease with abscess encapsulation), leukocytosis with shift, elevated ESR	1. Bacterial invasion

2. Signs and symptoms of increased intracranial pressure:
  a. Headache—usually on same side if temporal lobe abscess, and in occipital lobe if cerebellar abscess
  b. Nausea and vomiting
  c. Papilledema
  d. Impaired consciousness
	2. Cerebritis

3. Number 2 and/or neurologic deficit according to specific region of the brain affected
  a. Seizures, aphasia, visual field deficit, contralateral motor or sensory deficit, limb and/or facial weakness
  b. General intellectual impairment, focal or generalized seizures
  c. Ataxia, nystagmus
  d. Aphasia, visual field deficit, contralateral weakness, seizures
  e. Difficulty swallowing, cranial nerve palsies, pyramidal tract signs
	3. Abscess formation in specific region of the brain
	  a. Temporal
	
	  b. Frontal
	
	  c. Cerebellar
	  d. Parietal
	
	  e. Brain stem

4. Headache, nuchal rigidity	4. Rupture of abscess into cerebrospinal fluid
5. Coma, third nerve palsy, extensor plantar response	5. Brain herniation

* Based on data from Harter DH: Parameningeal infections, in Wyngaarden JB, Smith LH (eds): *Cecil Textbook of Medicine,* ed 17. Philadelphia, WB Saunders Co, 1985, pp 2111–2114; and Scheld WM, Winn HR: Brain abscess, in Mandell GL, Douglas RG Jr, Bennett JE (eds): *Principles and Practice of Infectious Diseases.* New York, John Wiley & Sons, 1985, pp 585–592.

erythrocyte sedimentation rate. Evaluation of the peripheral blood and urine is not useful in the diagnosis. Nuclear magnetic resonance (NMR) may be a valuable diagnostic tool in the future for the detection and assessment of brain abscess.

PRINCIPLES OF PREVENTION AND THERAPY

As indicated previously, certain infections predispose to brain abscess, and it would seem prudent to provide adequate treatment and follow-up for patients with these infections. Strict aseptic technique and prophylactic measures should be used when surgery is performed in the head and neck region, especially when done in association with trauma. Young patients found to have congenital heart disease are at risk for developing a brain abscess, and appropriate antimicrobial therapy should be used when indicated.

Fortunately, since the advent of antibiotics, the incidence of brain abscess has decreased. Especially in the early stages of cerebritis, before encapsulation occurs, appropriate antibiotics can be used alone. Most of the responsible microorganisms are penicillin-sensitive, and this drug remains the antibiotic of choice for empiric therapy. Metronidazole or chloramphenicol are often added to the regimen because of their excellent anaerobic activity and penetration into abscess cavities. Staphylococcal infections may occur, especially in endocarditis and in cases associated with trauma. In this setting, a penicillinase-resistant penicillin should be used. When brain abscess is treated by medical means alone, parenteral therapy should continue for approximately 6 weeks, followed by an additional 2 months of oral antibiotics.

Many patients with brain abscess require some form of surgical intervention. In the patient with clinical deterioration, surgery is indicated. Aspiration may be performed in this situation and when a specific bacteriologic diagnosis is required. Later, after the abscess is encapsulated, the area may be evacuated. Some studies indicate no significant difference in mortality between those managed by aspiration alone, repeated aspiration, aspiration followed by excision, or excision alone. A deep-seated abscess, multiple abscesses, or a debilitated condition of the patient may preclude surgery.

The use of corticosteroids in the treatment of brain abscess is controversial, but generally they are employed to diminish cerebral edema when increased intracranial pressure is life-threatening. It should be recalled that ring enhancement on CT scan is associated with cerebritis, and termination of or inadequate steroid treatment also may result in increased ring enhancement. It follows that ring enhancement may not indicate treatment failure and may persist for several weeks after adequate therapy. Computed tomography must be used with either medical or surgical therapy to evaluate the progress of the abscess.

When antibiotics were introduced, the mortality from brain abscess decreased, but not to the level that was expected. More scrupulous microbiologic evaluation and earlier diagnosis with CT scanning have had a significant impact on morbidity and mortality. With treatment, the mortality rate ranges from 10% to 20% and depends on various factors such as the type of organism involved, location of the abscess, timing of surgery if performed, and general condition of the patient. Other important factors include the level of consciousness at the time of presentation and whether there is a single abscess or multiple abscesses. The space-occupying aspect of a brain abscess is related directly to mortality. As alluded to above, diminished level of consciousness at the time of presentation, multiple abscesses, and brain abscesses that have ruptured are all situations in which the prognosis is regarded as poor. Fortunately, more people are recovering from brain abscess with continued technologic advancements and conscientious medical care. However, among those who do recover, some are faced with residual neurologic impairment, and many require chronic anticonvulsant therapy.

REFERENCES

Beller AJ, Sahar A, Praiss I: Brain abscess: Review of 89 cases over a period of 30 years. *J Neurol Neurosurg Psychiatry* 1973; 36:757–768. *A detailed and comprehensive review of brain abscess.*

Britt RH, Enzmann DR, Yeager AS: Neuropathological and computerized tomographic findings in experimental brain abscess. *J Neurosurg* 1981; 55:590–603. *Excellent comparison of CT scan changes and corresponding pathologic changes in experimentally induced brain abscess.*

de Louvois J: The bacteriology and chemotherapy of brain abscess. *J Antimicrob Chemother* 1978; 4:395–413. *An important discussion of the microbiology of brain abscess including antimicrobial therapy.*

Harter DH: Parameningeal infections, in Wyngaarden JB, Smith LH (eds): *Cecil Textbook of Medicine,* ed 17. Philadelphia, WB Saunders Co, 1985, pp 2111–2114.

Nielsen H, Glydensted C, Harmsen A: Cerebral abscess: Aetiology and pathogenesis, symptoms, diagnosis and treatment. *Acta Neurol Scand 1982;* 65:609–622. *An extensive review of 200 cases of patients with brain abscess over a period of 40 years.*

Scheld WM, Winn HR: Brain abscess, in Mandell GL, Douglas RG Jr, Bennett JE (eds): *Principles and Practice of Infectious Diseases.* New York, John Wiley & Sons, 1985, pp 585–592. *A contemporary approach to the diagnosis and management of the patient with brain abscess.*

Yang S-Y: Brain abscess: A review of 400 cases. *J Neurosurg* 1981; 55:794–799. *A discussion with emphasis on diagnosis and treatment including comparative data for various surgical methods used to treat brain abscess.*

PARKINSON'S DISEASE

Patrick A. Kelley, M.D.

Parkinson's disease is an extrapyramidal syndrome caused by an alteration of neurotransmitters in the brain. The major alteration is a deficiency of dopamine, an inhibitory neurotransmitter, found predominantly in the striatum (caudate nucleus and putamen) and substantia nigra of the midbrain. A relative excess of acetylcholine, an excitatory neurotransmitter, is also present. In idiopathic Parkinson's disease this neurotransmitter imbalance is caused by a progressive neuronal degeneration primarily involving the pigmented cells of the substantia nigra. This neurotransmitter imbalance can also be caused iatrogenically. The use of neuroleptic agents (e.g., phenothiazines, butyrophenones) may cause a clinical parkinsonian syndrome by blocking dopamine receptors. Reserpine may cause parkinsonian symptoms by depleting dopamine in the striatum. Metoclopramide also may cause parkinsonian symptoms. Recently it has been discovered that Parkinson's disease can be induced by the neurotoxin 1-methyl-4-phenyl-1,2,3,6-tetrahydropyridine (MPTP) which causes dopamine deficiency and severe destruction of the zona compacta of the substantia nigra.

After an interval of months to years following the pandemic of encephalitis lethargica in 1914, a high proportion of survivors developed Parkinson's disease. Postencephalitic parkinsonism has essentially disappeared.

CLINICAL SIGNS AND SYMPTOMS

The classic triad of symptoms in Parkinson's disease is tremor, rigidity, and bradykinesia. Other frequent symptoms are listed in Table 126–1. All patients should be asked about their use of neuroleptics. The typical patient with Parkinson's is elderly (onset is most frequent between 50 and 70 years of age) and complains of progressive tremor and slowness of movement. The tremor of Parkinson's disease is a rhythmic oscillation, or pill-roll, of the hands at rest. The tremor is less prominent with action, is increased with anxiety, and absent during sleep. Tremor of the feet may occur, but tremor of the head is rare.

Rigidity and bradykinesia may inhibit any type of movement. The stooped-over gait becomes slow and shuffling with poor arm-swing. Initiation of gait may become difficult. A tendency to fall backward (retropulsion) or forward (festination) may be seen. The patient has difficulty arising from a chair or getting out of bed. As the disease progresses, simple daily tasks such as eating and brushing the teeth may become impossible.

At physical examination, the typical patient exhibits a resting tremor of the hands, a blunted facial expression, and generalized bradykinesia. Symptoms are usually bilateral, but commonly one side predominates. Cogwheel rigidity is detected by passively flexing and ex-

TABLE 126–1.
Frequent Symptoms of Parkinson's Disease*

Tremor
Rigidity
Bradykinesia
Masking of facies
Stooped posture
Shuffling gait
Difficulty standing from a seated position
Retropulsion
Festination
Constipation
Dementia
Micrographia
Slow eyelid flutter with eyes closed
Diminished speech volume
Saccadic eye movements
Infrequent eye blinking

* Data from personal experience.

tending the wrists, elbows, or other joints. This phenomenon may also be observed by testing rapidly alternating movements such as hand rotation. Cogwheeling is considered to represent tremor superimposed on rigidity. Other features such as mild dementia, retropulsion, and a shuffling gait may be observed. If there is associated dementia, frontal-lobe release phenomenon such as grasping may be elicited. A glabellar reflex may also be present (persistence of eyelid blinking to rhythmic midforehead tapping). The findings of the remainder of the neurologic examination are unremarkable.

Symptoms in the untreated patient with idiopathic Parkinson's disease slowly progress over years. Tremor often predominates initially, followed later by rigidity and bradykinesia. Initial unilateral predominance often becomes bilateral. The stooped-over shuffling gait progressively deteriorates. The patient is prone to falling as retropulsion and festination become more severe; the use of a cane or walker may become necessary. If the disease progresses to an advanced stage, rigidity predominates and the patient may become bedridden and immobile with the arms, legs, and trunk flexed into a fetal position. This degree of severity, however, is relatively rare.

With appropriate treatment, patients with idiopathic Parkinson's disease can be expected to improve significantly. Patients with relatively mild disease show the greatest degree of improvement. Patients with more severe disease may receive only partial relief. A degree of adverse effects from medication might have to be tolerated for continued symptomatic relief. Eventually, symptoms may become refractory to antiparkinsonian medications. Progression of the disease is highly variable.

Not all patients receiving neuroleptic agents develop iatrogenic Parkinson's disease. Parkinsonian symptoms may be seen shortly after the onset of neuroleptic use or may take time to develop. Parkinsonian symptoms are usually reversible by withdrawal of the neuroleptic drug. Tardive dyskinesia, resulting from chronic denervation of dopaminergic receptor sites, begins only after prolonged use of neuroleptic drugs and is often irreversible.

PATHOPHYSIOLOGY

A proper neurotransmitter balance is essential for the maintenance of normal body tone and movement. If the normal dopamine-acteylcholine balance is disrupted, abnormal involuntary movements occur. Dopamine deficiency results in a clinical parkinsonian syndrome, whereas a relative dopamine excess results in choreiform movements as seen in Huntington's disease.

The striatum (caudate nucleus and putamen) receive afferent fibers from the cerebral cortex, thalamus, and the substantia nigra. Nigrostriatal fibers send dopamine to the striatum where it is contained in synaptic nerve endings. The striatum in turn projects upon the globus pallidus which projects onto the thalamus. The main projection of the ventrolateral nucleus of

---

TABLE 126–2.
Clinical–Pathologic Correlations*

| | PATHOLOGIC FINDINGS | |
CLINICAL FINDINGS	MACROSCOPIC	MICROSCOPIC
IDIOPATHIC PARKINSONISM		
Tremor	Depigmentation of the substantia nigra	Neuronal loss of substantia nigra
Rigidity	Depigmentation of the locus ceruleus	Lewy body formation in substantia nigra
Bradykinesia	Cerebral atrophy (in some cases)	
Stooped posture		
Shuffling gait		
IATROGENIC PARKINSONISM		
Same as above	None detected	None detected

* Data from personal experience.

the thalamus is to the motor cortex of the brain. Rubral and cerebellar connections also influence basal ganglionic function. In Parkinson's disease, levels of dopamine are markedly depressed in the striatum and substantia nigra.

Parkinsonian symptoms evolve because of a deficiency of the inhibitory neurotransmitter, dopamine, in the striatum. Hence, parkinsonian features arise because of the relative disinhibition of neurotransmitters on the striatal receptor cells.

CLINICAL–PATHOLOGIC CORRELATIONS

On sectioning the brain of a parkinsonian patient, one observes an absence of normal pigmentation of the substantia nigra and locus ceruleus (see Table 126–2). Generalized cerebral atrophy may be apparent in some patients. Microscopically, there is a marked depletion of the normal cell population of the substantia nigra. The remaining cells may contain eosinophilic cytoplasmic inclusions called Lewy bodies. Secondary transneuronal degeneration of cells in the striatum is inconsistently found.

The amount of cell degeneration, Lewy body formation, and pigment loss of the substantia nigra correlates well with the severity of the parkinsonian symptoms. In patients with unilateral symptoms, pathologic changes are detected in the substantia nigra contralateral to the affected side of the body. Similar pathologic changes are not detected in iatrogenic Parkinson's disease where dopamine production is normal or even excessive. In neuroleptic-induced Parkinson's disease, the chemical blockade of striatal dopamine receptors is not detected morphologically.

DIFFERENTIAL DIAGNOSIS

The tremor of Parkinson's disease is a rhythmic oscillation of the hands at rest. Any organic tremor is augmented by anxiety. Tremor should be distinguished from tremulousness where the movement is much faster and of lower amplitude. Tremulousness is seen in anxiety, hyperthyroidism, hypoglycemia, and other metabolic states. Tremulousness may be caused by caffeine, amphetamine, lithium, and other

medications. Patients who are tremulous may also demonstrate hyperhydrosis and tachycardia and complain of dizziness and anxiety. They do not exhibit rigidity, bradykinesia, or other parkinsonian symptoms.

Patients with an organic tremor usually have Parkinson's disease or a benign (familial) essential tremor. The latter is similar to that of Parkinson's disease, but is more prominent with action than at rest, is often familial, may involve a side-to-side tremor of the head, and often begins at a younger age than the tremor of Parkinson's disease. Such patients do not exhibit other parkinsonian features. The benign essential tremor may be improved by the ingestion of ethanol, minor tranquilizers, or propranolol.

Bradykinesia, rigidity, and masking of facies can be confused with a number of conditions. Emotional depression often causes apathy, slowness of movement, and blunted expression. With associated anxiety, tremulousness might also be observed, making the distinction more difficult. Structural disturbances of the frontal lobes such as subdural hematoma, meningioma, Alzheimer's disease, and normal-pressure hydrocephalus may cause progressive dementia, blunted facial expression, and gait apraxia (slow shuffling gait).

Manganese intoxication may produce parkinsonian features. Progressive supranuclear palsy results in dementia, masking of facies, retropulsion, and rigidity, but may be distinguished from Parkinson's disease by the presence of supranuclear ophthalmoplegia and pseudobulbar palsy. Parkinsonian features may also be seen in Jakob-Creutzfeldt disease, which is caused by a "slow" virus, but here there is associated subacute dementia, myoclonus, motor degeneration, ataxia, and possibly seizures. Hypothyroidism, which may cause progressive dementia and bradykinesia, might also be confused with parkinsonism.

DIAGNOSIS

Parkinson's disease is a clinical diagnosis. There is no laboratory test to confirm or exclude parkinsonism. At times, depending on the initial findings, other conditions must be excluded. If the patient primarily demonstrates dementia, rigidity, and gait apraxia and there is no tremor, computerized tomography (CT scan) of the brain should be obtained to exclude tumor, communicating hydrocephalus, cerebral atrophy, or subdural hematoma. If the distinction between tremor and tremulousness is difficult, testing might be obtained to exclude anemia, hypoglycemia, hyperthyroidism, or other metabolic abnormalities.

PRINCIPLES OF PREVENTION AND THERAPY

There is no known treatment that will alter the progressive neuronal degeneration in idiopathic Parkinson's disease. Treatment is symptomatic and is based on an attempt to normalize the neurotransmitter imbalance in the brain. Dopamine, the primary neurotransmitter deficient in Parkinson's disease, does not cross the blood–brain barrier. Its precursor, levodopa, crosses the blood–brain barrier and is then converted to dopamine, which stimulates the dopamine receptors in the striatum. The dosage of levodopa is titrated for the individual patient to produce the maximum benefit and minimum adverse effect. The dopa decarboxylase inhibitor, carbidopa, may be administered concurrently to counteract the peripheral side-effects of levodopa. Adverse effects of levodopa, which are dose related, include nausea, orthostatic hypotension, depression, confusion, and choreoathetoid movements. After prolonged levodopa therapy, some adverse effects which may not become apparent for years include dyskinetic movements and the on–off phenomenon (sudden deterioration of function due to Parkinson's disease despite stable drug dosage). The dopaminergic agonist, bromocriptine, is also effective in Parkinson's disease. Its side-effects are similar to those of levodopa.

Because of the relative excess of acetylcholine in Parkinson's disease, anticholinergic drugs are also effective antiparkinsonian agents. They are generally more effective for tremor than for rigidity or bradykinesia. The dosage must be individualized. The adverse effects include dry mouth, blurred vision, confusion, memory impairment, and urinary retention.

Amantadine, an antiviral agent effective against influenza A_2 virus, also exhibits antiparkinsonian activity. The adverse effects are infrequent but include nausea, memory loss, depression, confusion, and livedo reticularis mottling of the lower extremities.

Amantadine, the anticholinergic drugs, levodopa (with or without carbidopa), or bromocriptine each may be used alone or in combination with other antiparkinsonian agents.

The stereotaxic placement of a surgical lesion in the ventrolateral nucleus of the thalamus is rarely used today. Surgical treatment is considered only for patients unresponsive to medical therapy.

Iatrogenic Parkinson's disease may often be prevented by the simultaneous administration of an anticholinergic drug in conjunction with the neuroleptic drug. Once established, iatrogenic Parkinson's disease is best treated with withdrawal of the neuroleptic agent, if possible, along with administration of an anticholinergic drug or amantadine. Levodopa should not be used in neuroleptic-induced Parkinson's disease.

REFERENCES

Adams RD, Victor M: *Principles of Neurology*, ed 2. New York, McGraw-Hill Book Co, 1981. *An excellent text of clinical neurology.*

Baker AB, Joynt R: *Clinical Neurology*. Philadelphia, Harper & Row, 1985. *An excellent text of clinical neurology.*

Ballard PA, Tetrud JW, Langston JW: Permanent human parkinsonism due to 1-methyl-4-phenyl-1,2,3,6-tetrahydrophyridine (MPTP): Seven cases. *Neurology* 1985; 35:949–956.

Blackwood W, Corsellis JAN (eds): *Greenfield's Neuropathology*. Chicago, Year Book Medical Publishers, 1976. *An excellent text of neuropathology.*

Iankovic J (ed): *Movement Disorders. Neurologic Clinics*. Philadelphia, WB Saunders Co, 1984. *An excellent review of the movement disorders.*

Indo T, Ando K: Metoclopramide-induced parkinsonism. *Arch Neurol* 1982; 39:494–486.

Truex RC, Carpenter MD: *Human Neuroanatomy*. Baltimore, Williams & Wilkins, 1969. *An excellent text of neuroanatomy.*

Hytham A. Kadrie, M.D.

Myasthenia gravis is a neuromuscular disorder manifested by fatigability and weakness of one or more voluntary muscles. Myasthenia gravis has a predilection for the cranial muscles, especially the ocular muscles, varies in severity, and is partially and temporarily relieved by cholinergic drugs or rest. About 25% of cases show spontaneous remissions sometime during their course. The severity of systemic involvement is variable. A classification recognizing the variability of myasthenia gravis has been developed by Osserman (Osserman and Whipple, 1966) to allow a comparison of the prognosis and results of the various treatment modalities (Table 127–1).

Myasthenia gravis is a disease of the neuromuscular junction. The basic defect in the disease is a reduction of available acetylcholine receptors at the neuromuscular junctions, probably as a result of a destructive autoimmune process.

CLINICAL SIGNS AND SYMPTOMS

Myasthenia may affect individuals of any age, but most frequently affects young adults. It is three times more common in women than men up to age 40 years; after that, both sexes are affected about equally.

The typical patient usually presents with complaints of diplopia and ptosis or weakness that fluctuates in severity, especially the proximal muscles. Other initial symptoms can include dysarthria, dysphagia, or difficulty chewing food. The symptoms are usually least severe in the morning (i.e., after the muscles rest during sleep) and most severe in the evening (i.e., after the muscles are fatigued). Symptoms will commonly vary from day to day and may sometimes disappear completely (spontaneous remissions). Serious exacerbations or crises can occur suddenly and usually unpredictably but may occur in association with infections, stress, pregnancy, or anesthesia.

Typically the presenting patient is a young woman or an elderly man. When examined, the patient will have: double vision in various directions of conjugate gaze; drooping of one or both eyelids which increases with effort; or proximal muscle weakness that increases with repetitive testing. These physical findings are temporarily reversible with intravenous cholinesterase inhibitors. Therefore, a commonly used diagnostic test for myasthenia is an intravenous injection of 10 mg of edrophonium, which quickly but temporarily relieves the muscle weakness. Nerve conductions are sometimes used to confirm the diagnosis (i.e., myasthenia gravis causes a decremental response with repetitive nerve stimulation at three stimuli per second).

The incidence of myasthenia is about 1 in 20,000 population. Remissions, if they occur, tend to do so during the early stages (about 25% remit during the first 2 years). Unfortunately remissions are usually only partial and not prolonged. Patients with the purely ocular form of myasthenia often do not develop generalized myasthenia, especially when the symptoms remain confined to the extraocular

TABLE 127–1.
Osserman Classification of Myasthenia Gravis*

1. Ocular involvement only
2. Mild generalized myasthenia with ocular involvement
3. Moderate generalized myasthenia, usually with some bulbar involvement
4. Early stages of severe myasthenia developing over weeks to months with severe bulbar involvement
5. Late severe myasthenia, with severe bulbar involvement

* From Osserman KE, Whipple HE: Myasthenia gravis. *Ann NY Acad Sci* 1966; 135:679–680.

muscles for more than a year. The highest mortality rate for myasthenia gravis appears to be during the first year of the disease and is usually due to bulbar and/or respiratory muscle involvement.

The long-term prognosis for myasthenia has greatly improved over the past two decades with the advent of several available treatment modalities such as anticholinesterase drugs, corticosteroids and other immunosuppressive agents, and thymectomy. The mortality rate was estimated to be approximately 20% before these treatment modalities, compared to about 3% or less now.

PATHOPHYSIOLOGY

Myasthenia gravis appears to be an autoimmune disease in which specific IgG antibodies attack and destroy acetylcholine receptors at the neuromuscular junction. What actually triggers this autoimmune response is unknown.

Pathologically, one sees very little with ordinary light microscopy of an affected muscle. Electron microscopy, on the other hand, shows the postsynaptic membrane to have sparse, shallow folds with markedly simplified abnormal geometric patterns.

Approximately 10% of patients with myasthenia have a thymoma, of which a few are malignant. Another two-thirds of patients will have hyperplasia of the thymus gland's germinal centers. This pathologic relationship between myasthenia and the thymus gland first led investigators to suspect an autoimmune process as the cause of the disease.

CLINICAL–PATHOLOGIC CORRELATIONS

The clinical features of myasthenia gravis are a result of the destruction of the motor end-plate acetylcholine receptors by a specific IgG antibody. Why the extraocular muscles and proximal muscles are so sensitive or selected over distal muscles is not understood.

DIFFERENTIAL DIAGNOSIS

A number of conditions can clinically simulate the presentation of myasthenia gravis. Probably the most common pseudomyasthenic syndrome

is functional fatigue and weakness due to depression and/or chronic anxiety. These patients will have no organic weakness on physical examination, a negative edrophonium test, and no decremental response on the EMG with repetitive nerve stimulation.

Patients with the "myasthenic syndrome," Eaton-Lambert syndrome, typically present with proximal limb weakness and respond to intravenous edrophonium. However, they usually have reduced or absent deep-tendon reflexes plus an *incremental* rather than decremental response to rapid repetitive nerve stimulation. This condition is often associated with oat cell cancer of the lung. The underlying pathology is a reduction in the quanta of acetylcholine released at the axon terminal. It can be treated with guanidine, a drug that increases the release of acetylcholine at axonal terminal endings.

Botulism can imitate myasthenia. The bacterium, *Clostridium botulinum*, produces a toxin which apparently blocks the release of acetylcholine at the axon's terminal ending. This anaerobic bacteria may be found in improperly canned or bottled foods. Symptoms of poisoning by this toxin usually develop within 48 hours of ingestion and may initially consist of diplopia and dysarthria. Treatment consists of antitoxin administration, guanidine, and artificial ventilation if necessary.

Thyrotoxicosis can produce a myopathy causing proximal muscle weakness. About 5% of patients with myasthenia gravis develop hyperthyroidism at some time during their course. Thyrotoxic myopathy does not respond to edrophonium and does not show a decremental response to repetitive stimulation.

DIAGNOSIS

The diagnosis of myasthenia gravis can be made by pharmacologic, electrophysiologic, and immunologic tests. The best test to confirm the diagnosis is pharmacologic, by injecting intravenously 10 mg of edrophonium chloride and observing for dramatic improvement in the strength of involved muscles within 1 minute.

Electrophysiologically, the diagnosis may be confirmed by a specific abnormality in the effect of repetitive stimulation of the evoked compound muscle action potential. For a patient with generalized myasthenia, it is convenient to stimulate the median nerve at the wrist and record the responses of the thenar muscles. If the weakness is restricted to facial muscles it is better to record from these muscles while stimulating the facial nerve at the angle of the jaw. Typically the first response will have a normal amplitude with a sequential decrease in subsequent responses. A low-frequency stimulus, usually 3 Hz, is used, with a decrease in amplitude of greater than 7% being normal. Decremental responses are found in 95% of patients with generalized myasthenia when three or more different muscles are tested. Unfortunately fewer than 50% of patients with pure ocular myasthenia show a decremental response.

The decremental response results from progressive failure of more and more neuromuscular junctions in which transmission is impaired. During repeated stimulation of normal human motor nerves, the amount of acetylcholine released per impulse declines after the first few impulses because the nerve terminal is not able to sustain its original release rate. Because the neuromuscular junctions in patients with myasthenia have reduced numbers of acetylcholine receptors as compared to normal individuals, there is less of a safety margin for reaching threshold and thus the activation of fewer and fewer muscle fibers occurs with each successive nerve impulse.

Immunologic tests are now being used in several laboratories as aids in the diagnosis of myasthenia gravis. In the past 6 years myasthenia patients have been shown to have a reduced number of acetylcholine receptors which appears to be the result of an autoimmune attack on the receptors by an IgG antibody. A sensitive radioimmunoassay based on the binding of an antibody to radioactively labeled acetylcholine receptors has been developed. By this method, receptor-binding antibodies have

---

TABLE 127–2.
Treatment Plan for Myasthenia Gravis

I.   Definitive diagnosis
II. Initial treatment
    A. Anticholinesterase medication (pyridostigmine bromide)
    B. If results are not satisfactory, consider thymectomy or corticosteroid.
III. Thymectomy
    A. Indications
       1. Thymoma
       2. Generalized myasthenia gravis
          a. Patient < 50 years of age
          b. Wait long enough to exclude early spontaneous remission (usually 6–12 months after onset of myasthenia).
    B. Preoperative preparation: If operation is a major risk because of patient's state of weakness, give corticosteroids until condition is satisfactory.
    C. Surgery should be done in an institution with the facilities and experience for postoperative management of the thymectomy patient.
IV. Corticosteroid therapy
    A. Indications
       1. After thymectomy for invasive thymoma
       2. Any of the following in an uncontrolled patient:
          a. Older age group (> 50 years of age)
          b. Declines thymectomy
          c. Status post-thymectomy
          d. Pure ocular involvement
    B. Method
       1. Adjust anticholinesterase drug dosage to maximum.
       2. Begin daily administration of small doses and increase gradually until optimal response or as tolerated.
       3. Gradually switch to alternate-day schedule.
       4. Maintain dosage until improvement reaches plateau (usually 6–12 months).
       5. Taper gradually until minimal maintenance dose is established.
       6. Observe for side-effects.
       7. Anticholinesterase dosage may be cautiously decreased, as tolerated.
V. Immunosuppressive drugs: Reserved for unusual patients resistant to thymectomy and corticosteroids

been found in about 87% of patients with myasthenia gravis. The antibody titers corresponded, but not exactly, to the clinical status of the patient.

PRINCIPLES OF THERAPY

Long-term treatment is successful and can essentially abolish most if not all of the physical findings.

The primary goal of therapy is to reduce the amount of weakness to a tolerable level whereby the myasthenic patient can lead a relatively normal life. The treatment involves the careful use of two groups of drugs, the anticholinesterases and corticosteroids, and occasionally thymectomy.

Pyridostigmine bromide is probably the most widely used oral anticholinesterase drug. The effect begins within 30 minutes and lasts approximately 4 hours.

Corticosteroids produce a good response in over 60% of patients, but long-term corticosteroid use has problem side-effects. Recently, other immunosuppressive drugs (e.g., azothioprine, 6-mercaptopurine) have been used in myasthenia with some success. They have been used along with plasmapheresis as a last resort in a small group of patients with severe myasthenia who have not previously responded to corticosteroids or thymectomy.

Thymectomy has been used as a treatment since the early 1940s. It is thought to induce a greater rate of remission or at the least reduce the severity of the disease.

A rational approach to the treatment of a myasthenic patient is summarized in Table 127–2.

REFERENCES

Adams RD, Victor M: *Principles of Neurology.* New York, McGraw-Hill Book Co, 1977. *A general clinical neurology review textbook.*

Baker LH: *Clinical Neurology.* Hagerstown, Md, Harper & Row, 1978. *An extensive neurology textbook for neurology residents.*

Drachman DB: Myasthenia gravis. *N Eng J Med* 1978; 298:136–143, 186–192. *Excellent review article on etiology of myasthenia gravis.*

Lindstrom JM, Seybold ME, Hennon VA, et al: Antibody to acetylcholine receptor in myasthenia gravis; prevalence, clinical correlates, and diagnostic value. *Neurology* 1976; 26:1054–1059. *Paper on the discovery of antibodies to muscle acetylcholine receptors.*

McComas AJ: *Neuromuscular Function and Disorders.* London–Boston, Butterworths, 1977. *An excellent textbook reviewing disorders of nerve fibers, neuromuscular junction and muscle fibers.*

Osserman KE, Whipple HE: Myasthenia gravis. *Ann NY Acad Sci* 1966; 135:679–680. *A review of the clinical findings in myasthenia gravis including the classification.*

Patrick J, Lindstrom J: Autoimmune response to acetylcholine receptor. *Science* 1973; 180:871–872. *Original paper regarding the discovery of antibodies to muscle acetylcholine receptors in myasthenia gravis.*

Simpson JA: An evaluation of thymectomy in myasthenia gravis. *Brain* 1958; 81:112–144. *A review article on the indications and value of thymectomy in patients with myasthenia gravis.*

Thomas Mathews, M.D.

Multiple sclerosis (MS) is a chronic incurable and often disabling neurologic disorder of young adults. The disease affects multiple sites in the white matter of the brain, spinal cord, and optic nerves and is characterized by motor, sensory, visual, and sphincter dysfunction. The cause of MS is unknown, and there is no specific treatment.

CLINICAL SIGNS AND SYMPTOMS

The onset of MS is between age 20 and 40 years; it is uncommon in the first decade and after age 60 years. Multiple sclerosis is more common in females, and there is a family history of an afflicted relative in 10% to 15% of patients. The symptoms and signs of MS are extremely variable. In the early stages, MS symptoms are often evanescent or bizarre without objective signs, and the condition is commonly misdiagnosed as hysteria. Neurologic symptoms and signs are often worsened by elevation of body temperature or in hot weather. Common initial or early signs and symptoms of MS include motor weakness, sensory and visual symptoms, cerebellar and sphincter dysfunction.

Monoplegia, hemiplegia, or paraplegia may be slowly progressive, subacute, or abrupt. Pyramidal tract signs are ubiquitous and include hyperreflexia, spasticity, clonus, absent abdominal reflexes, and Babinski's sign. Corticobulbar involvment may eventually result in pseudobulbar palsy. Atrophy and areflexia are associated with dorsal root entry zone or anterior horn cell involvement and are uncommon. Generalized fatigue out of proportion to motor weakness is frequent and disabling.

Numbness, paresthesias, dysesthesias, and girdle sensations without objective sensory findings may be mistaken for hysteria. In Lhermitte's phenomenon, neck flexion causes shocklike electric sensations down the spine or extremities due to plaques in the posterior columns.

Visual symptoms are common in MS. There is optic nerve involvement at the onset in 15% to 30% of MS cases. Optic or retrobulbar neuritis is characterized by orbital pain, blurred vision, central scotomas, and abnormal pupillary light reflexes (Marcus Gunn pupils). The discs may be normal, edematous, or atrophic. Diplopia is common, reflecting brain stem involvement. Common ocular motility disturbances include internuclear ophthalomoplegia due to involvement of the medial longitudinal fasciculus; there is ipsilateral paresis of the medial rectus and nystagmus in the contralateral abducting eye. Bilateral internuclear ophthalmoplegia in a young adult is highly characteristic of MS.

Cerebellar involvement is common. Gait ataxia is often due to a combination of cerebellar, pyramidal, and proprioceptive defects. Incoordination and intention tremor of the extremities can be very disabling. Cerebellar and pyramidal involvement contribute to dysarthric speech. Vestibulocerebellar involvement causes vertigo and dizziness and may be the initial symptom in 5% of MS patients.

Sphincter problems such as impotence, constipation, urinary urgency, and incontinence are common and disabling. Incomplete bladder emptying predisposes to recurrent urinary tract infection.

Mental changes are frequent in established MS. Depression and euphoria are common affective changes. Cerebral plaques cause mild cognitive impairment early in the illness. Dementia is seen rarely in the advanced stages.

The clinical course of MS is quite variable. Of the several patterns seen, relapsing and remitting MS in the most common, particularly in young patients. The frequency and duration of the relapses and remissions are quite unpredictable. Remissions may be complete or incomplete leading to increasing disability. Between 10% and 20% of multiple sclerosis patients have a steady chronic progressive course. This is commonly seen in older patients with the spinal form of MS. Patients may begin with a relapsing form and later develop a progressive course. Between 10% and 20% of patients have a benign course and a normal life span. Attacks resolve with little or no disability, and clinical manifestations are mild. About 5% of patients have a fulminant course with many relapses, severe disability, or death within months to a few years. Death from MS itself is uncommon. Decubitus ulcers and intercurrent urinary and respiratory infections are common contributory causes. With modern medical care, the survival in MS is reduced by only 10 years.

PATHOPHYSIOLOGY

Multiple sclerosis is a primary demyelinating disorder. Normally formed myelin is selectively destroyed, but neurons and axons are

TABLE 128–1.
Clinical–Pathologic Correlations

CLINICAL MANIFESTATIONS	COMMON PLAQUE SITES
Optic/retrobulbar neuritis Central scotomata Marcus Gunn pupils	Optic nerve
Pyramidal tract dysfunction Sensory symptoms and signs Sphincter dysfunction Lhermitte's phenomenon	Spinal cord
Pyramidal tract dysfunction Sensory symptoms and signs Internuclear ophthalmoplegia Diplopia Vertigo Nystagmus	Brain stem
Incoordination Tremor Gait ataxia	Cerebellum
Cognitive impairment Depression Euphoria	Cerebral white matter

preserved. Myelin forms the sheath that envelops the axon. Myelin in the CNS is derived from and maintained by the oligodendrocyte, and myelin in the peripheral nervous system by the Schwann cell. In demyelination the primary site of injury may be in the myelin membrane or the oligodendrocyte. Myelin facilitates impulse transmission by saltatory conduction. In unmyelinated and demyelinated fibers, transmission is by the slower process of continuous conduction.

Demyelination may have several different effects on impulse transmission. It may block conduction completely, resulting in loss of function (e.g., paralysis or blindness). Slow conduction of impulses may still be possible in demyelinated areas. Lesions that only partially block conduction may be clinically "silent" but may become symptomatic during altered physiologic states such as an elevated body temperature. Asymptomatic lesions may be demonstrated by brain imaging or evoked potential testing (Fig 128–1). Demyelination may cause abnormal or ectopic impulse generation or transmission ("short circuit" of naked axons) resulting in irritative and paroxysmal symptoms such as dysesthesias, Lhermitte's phenomenon, and trigeminal neuralgia.

In multiple sclerosis, multiple focal areas of demyelination (plaques) are scattered throughout the white matter of the brain, spinal cord, and optic nerves (hence the term *disseminated* or *multiple.*) The peripheral nervous system is not clinically involved, although biopsies and nerve conduction velocities may show subtle abnormalities. Plaque vary from a few millimeters to several centimeters in diameter and are characteristically located in the white matter around the ventricles (Fig 128–2). Chronic plaques are gray, retracted, and firm because of extensive reactive astrocytosis (hence the term *sclerosis*). In acute plaques, there is an intense perivascular infiltration of lymphocytes, plasma cells, and lipid-laden macrophages. The increased amount of the immunoglobulin IgG found in the CSF is synthesized by lymphocytes in the plaques.

The cause of multiple sclerosis is unknown. It may be an autoimmune disorder. A leading hypothesis is that T-lymphocytes sensitized to a CNS antigen initiate the myelin destruction. Experimental allergic encephalomyelitis is an animal model of multiple sclerosis. Injection of the brain antigen myelin basic protein results in a cell-mediated demyelination that is very similar to acute MS. T-lymphocytes are abundant in MS plaques and synthesize immunoglobulins. The finding of abnormal subsets of T-lymphocytes in the blood and in the CNS of MS patients during relapses also points to cell-mediated immune mechanisms in the pathogenesis of MS. Many other abnormalities in both cellular and humoral immune responses have been described in MS, but their significance remains uncertain.

Viruses have also been implicated in multiple sclerosis. Direct viral infections of the CNS are known to produce chronic demyelination in humans (progressive multifocal leukoencephalopathy, subacute sclerosing panencephalitis) and in animals (visna, scrapie). However, in MS no viruses have been consistently demonstrated by electron microscopy or culture, and studies of brain, CSF, and blood have been inconclusive for a specific virus. Viruses may also cause demyelination indirectly, by altering or triggering an immune response (e.g., a demyelinating encephalomyelitis may follow a viral exanthem or vaccination).

Genetic factors also play a role in multiple sclerosis. Relatives of MS patients have a 15-fold increased risk of the disease. There is also a racial predisposition for MS. Whites of northern European stock have a higher prevalence whereas Asians and Africans have a relative resistance to this disease. The major histocompatibility leukocyte antigens HLA-A3, HLA-B7, and HLA-Dr2 are more prevalent in MS. These antigens also influence immunologic function. These findings support an immunogenetic predisposition to MS.

There is a striking geographic variability in the prevalence of MS with high prevalence (40 to 100 per 100,000) in the northern United States, Canada, and northern Europe and low prevalence (5 per 100,000) in Asia and Africa. Immigrants from high prevalence areas of Europe to low prevalence regions such as Israel and South Africa have a lowered risk of MS if the migration occurred before adulthood. There are foci of unusually high prevalance (Orkney and Shetland Islands off northern Scotland) and clusters of cases resembling epidemics. For example, in the Faroe Islands during the three decades following the arrival of British troops, unusual numbers of MS cases were recorded.

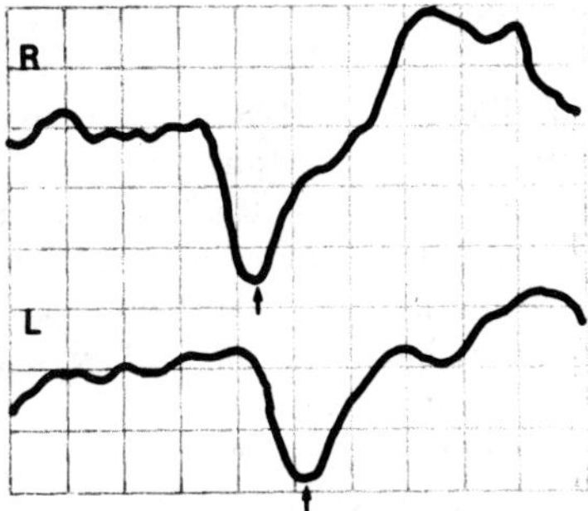

FIG 128–1.
Visual evoked potentials in a patient with spastic paraplegia without ocular symptoms or signs. Visual stimulation produced evoked responses (arrows) in the occipital cortex. The latency in the left eye is prolonged, indicating "silent" left retrobulbar neuritis.

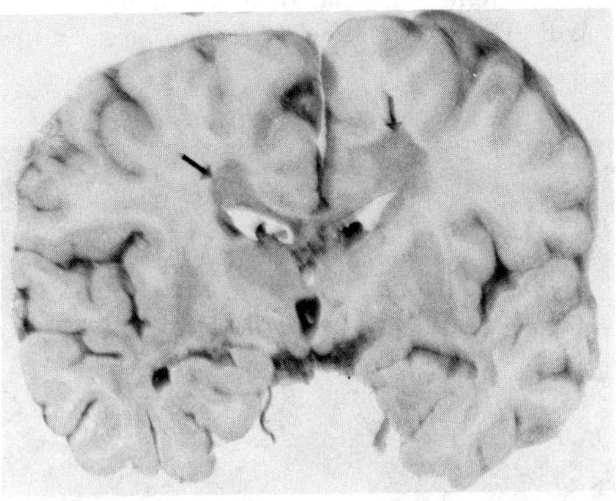

FIG 128–2.
Multiple plaques (arrows) in a patient with multiple sclerosis. Note the characteristic periventricular location.

These epidemiologic data suggest an infectious eitology, perhaps a childhood virus infection with a long incubation.

CLINICAL–PATHOLOGIC CORRELATIONS

Any part of the brain, spinal cord, or optic nerves can be affected, resulting in a rich diversity of clinical presentations. Many plaques are clinically silent. Brain imaging, evoked potential testing, and autopsy frequently reveal many more plaques than would have been expected from the clinical picture. Common sites of plaques and their clinical correlates are listed in Table 128–1.

DIAGNOSIS

A definite diagnosis of MS requires lesions to be disseminated in space and time (i.e., involving multiple areas of the CNS [space] and distinct and separate episodes of neurologic dysfunction [time]). There are no specific or pathognomonic laboratory tests for MS, and the results of all investigations may be negative even in definite MS. However, laboratory tests are important adjuncts to support the clinical diagnosis, identify clinically silent or multiple plaques, and rule out other neurologic disorders that can mimic MS.

Cerebrospinal fluid may show a number of changes in MS. Lymphocytes may be increased (10 to 100 cells/ml^3) during acute relapses. The total protein is normal or elevated up to 100 mg/dl. The IgG fraction of total protein is increased, and the IgG index (CSF IgG/albumin expressed as a ratio of serum IgG/albumin) is abnormal in 80% to 90% of MS. Qualitatively, CSF IgG by agarose electrophoresis will show oligoclonal banding in 80% to 90% of MS. In normal CSF, IgG migrates as a diffuse band. Oligoclonal banding is the most sensitive IgG test for MS. Myelin basic protein levels are increased during relapses, reflecting myelin breakdown and activity of the disease.

Note: IgG abnormalities are not specific for MS because they occur in other inflammatory and degenerative disorders of the CNS.

Evoked potentials testing permits measurement of impulse conduction in CNS pathways. Stimulation of visual, auditory, or somatosensory pathways will elicit responses in appropriate areas of the brain. Lesions involving these pathways will alter the wave form or delay the latency of the evoked responses (Fig 128–1).

CT scans show multiple hypodense or contrast enhancing white matter lesions in 25% of patients. Contrast enhancement indicates breakdown of the blood–brain barrier due to active demyelination. Magnetic resonance imaging (MRI) is much more sensitive than CT scan in detecting plaques and has become the imaging procedure of choice for MS (Fig 128–3).

PRINCIPLES OF THERAPY

There is no specific treatment that will arrest or reverse the course of MS. The most widely used drugs are aimed at modifying the immune responses. Corticosteroids or ACTH may shorten the duration of the acute attack but do not alter the long-term course of MS. The value of immunosuppressive drugs (e.g., azathioprine or cyclophosphamide) has not been clearly established in long-term controlled studies.

While a cure is not possible, many associated conditions and complications can be treated. Special attention must be paid to the psychologic, social, and rehabilitation needs of the patient. Depression should be treated vigorously with drugs and psychotherapy. Spasticity and painful flexor spasms may be relieved by baclofen, diazepam, and physical therapy or by surgical procedures. Bladder care involves urodynamic evaluations, treatment of incontinence

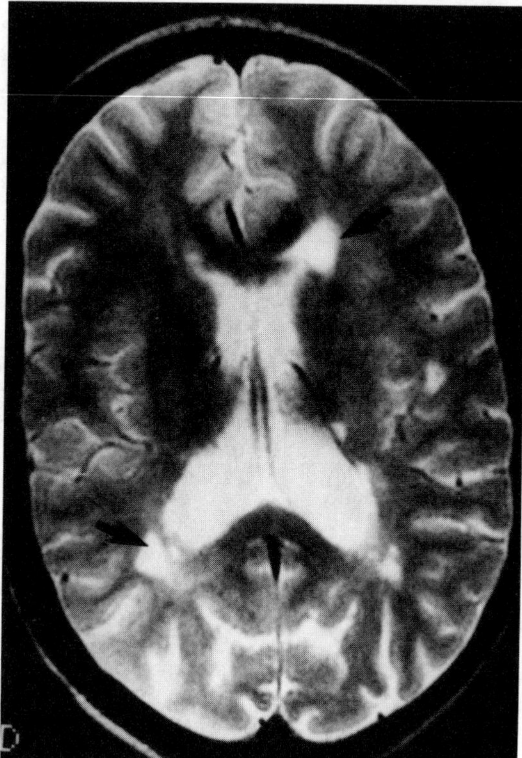

FIG 128–3.
Magnetic resonance image showing multiple lesions in the cerebral white matter. Magnetic resonance is the imaging procedure of choice in multiple sclerosis. (Courtesy of Technicare Corporation.)

and urgency with drugs, self-catheterization, and vigorous treatment of urinary infection. Erectile impotence is common and requires marital counseling. General measures (e.g., good nutrition, rest, and avoidance of heat) are important.

REFERENCES

Hart RG, Sherman DG: The diagnosis of multiple sclerosis. JAMA 1982; 247:498–502. *A good review of diagnostic procedures in MS.*

Hashimoto SA, Paty DW: Multiple sclerosis. *Disease-a-Month* 1986; 32(9):519–589. *This is the most current and readable monograph on multiple sclerosis.*

Matthews WB (ed): McAlpine's Multiple Sclerosis. New York, Churchill Livingstone, 1985. *Encyclopedic monograph; excellent description of clinical and epidemiologic aspects of MS.*

McFarlin DE, McFarland HF: Multiple sclerosis (parts 1 & 2). N Engl J Med 1982; 307:1183–1188, 1246–1251. *Reviews current viral and immunologic theories of pathogenesis of MS.*

Poser C (ed): *Diagnosis of Multiple Sclerosis.* New York, Thieme Stratton, 1984. *Readable chapters on latest advances in brain imaging, CSF and evoked potential testing for MS.*

Weiner HL, Hafler DA: Multiple sclerosis, in Appel S (ed): *Current Neurology,* vol 6. Chicago, Year Book Medical Publishers, 1986. *An excellent overview of basic immunologic concepts and immunotherapy of multiple sclerosis.*

Whittaker JN: Demyelinating diseases, in Pearlman AL, Collins RC (eds): *Neurological Pathophysiology.* New York, Oxford University Press, 1984.

129 NEUROMUSCULAR DISORDERS

Samuel E. Pitner, M.D.
Margaret A. Turk, M.D.

Neuromuscular disorders are diseases affecting the motor unit, which consists of the anterior horn cell and its axon (in the nerve root, plexus, and peripheral nerve), the neuromuscular junction, and the skeletal muscle itself. The terms *amyotrophies* and *atrophies* usually denote disorders of the anterior horn cells or motor nerves. The term *radiculopathy* refers to disorders of the nerve root (radicle); radiculopathies most frequently are due to compression and are considered in Chapter 149, Intervertebral Disc Disease. If multiple nerve roots are involved, the condition is referred to as a *polyradiculopathy.* The term *neuropathy* (or the older and usually less correct term *neuritis*) refers to disorders of peripheral nerves. A lesion of a single nerve, as in the case of the median nerve in the carpal tunnel syndrome, is referred to as a *mononeuropathy.* In polyneuropathy or peripheral neuropathy, there is not isolated involvement of a single large peripheral nerve. Instead, the more distal portions of several peripheral nerves are affected. This chapter does not address mononeuropathy.

There is no generic name for disorders of the neuromuscular (myoneural) junction; many pharmacologic and toxic agents affect the function of the neuromuscular junction, but only one condition, myasthenia gravis, generally is considered to be a neuromuscular disorder. Finally, there are the primary diseases of skeletal muscle, which as a group are called myopathies.

The clinical course of all neuromuscular disorders varies from a slowly progressive condition taking many years to become symptomatic to a fulminant paralysis complete in 24 hours. Of necessity, only a very limited number of these disorders can be considered in this chapter. Emphasis is placed on determining the portion of the motor unit affected rather than on the specific disease entities.

CLINICAL SIGNS AND SYMPTOMS

Diseases affecting primarily the anterior horn cells generally tend to be slowly progressive and painless, at least since the virtual elimination of poliomyelitis (polio), and are without any sensory changes. The most common condition affecting the anterior horn cells in adults, amyotrophic lateral sclerosis (ALS), also affects the upper motor neurons. Hence the British term for this disorder, motor neuron disease, is quite apt. Usually the disease shows symptoms classically associated with diseases of the lower motor neuron, that is, wasting of muscle and flaccidity, as well as weakness. Fasciculations, which consist of barely visible twitching movements in relaxed muscles are usually not large enough to cause any movement and are characteristic of anterior horn cell disease, particularly this disorder. The patient may complain of twitching or cramping. Occasionally, the disease starts with symptoms due to weakness of the muscles innervated by the motor cranial nerves. Slowly progressive weakness is the primary complaint of ALS patients. A similar disorder, infantile progressive spinal muscular atrophy or Werdnig-Hoffmann disease, occurs in infants and may even begin in utero; multiparous women may recognize diminished fetal movements.

In most patients with polyneuropathy, the more distal portions of the legs are affected first and then the arms. These patients often complain of dragging their feet or stumbling when walking, and later may lose strength in the intrinsic muscles of the hands and have difficulty with such tasks as opening wide-mouthed jars. Most, but not all, of these patients also have sensory symptoms. In addition to numbness

(paresthesia), there may be actual pain or even the perception of a light touch as a disagreeable burning feeling (dysesthesia). Some slowly progressive, often genetically determined, polyneuropathies take many years to develop. On the other hand, some acute polyneuropathies such as seen in some poisonings and the Guillain-Barré syndrome (technically a polyradiculopathy, but a condition that in most ways behaves like a polyneuropathy) can develop in a matter of hours or days. An important historic point to differentiate very rapidly developing neuropathies from spinal cord disease is that sphincter disturbances and impotence are only rarely seen in polyneuropathy.

Myasthenia gravis is a disease characterized by fatigability as opposed to continuing weakness. At its onset, these patients have normal strength, but they fatigue rapidly. Typically, the disease fluctuates from hour to hour during the day; generally the patients say they are stronger in the morning and weaker at the end of the day. The vast majority of these patients present with a complaint related to dysfunction of muscles innervated by the motor cranial nerves, particularly the extraocular or the pharyngeal muscles. Thus ptosis, diplopia, and dysphagia are the most common initial complaints. When there is general involvement beyond the cranial nerves, the patients' complaints (except for the fluctuating degree of weakness) are similar to those of patients with myopathies.

The term myopathy refers to primary disorders of muscle, most of which have a slowly progressive course. Myopathies tend to involve the large proximal muscle groups such as the shoulder and pelvic girdles. A typical history of a patient with a myopathy is of difficulty climbing stairs or arising from a chair and, if the upper extremities are primarily affected, difficulty in putting parcels on a shelf or in elevating the arms to comb the hair. Although some anterior horn cell disorders and polyneuropathies are hereditary, the family history is of particular importance in diagnosing myopathy. The muscular dystrophies, nearly all of which have a biochemical–genetic basis, make up a large proportion of the myopathies.

The primary findings on physical examination in neuromuscular disorders are shown on Table 129–1. The first site of weakness and the

TABLE 129–1.
Clinical–Pathologic Correlations of Disorders of the Motor Unit

SITE OF LESION	DISTRIBUTION OF WEAKNESS	SENSORY CHANGE	DEEP TENDON REFLEXES	OTHER CLINICAL FEATURES
Anterior horn cell (Lower motor neuron)	Variable	None	Decreased (may be increased early in ALS)	Fasciculation frequent
Multiple peripheral nerves (Polyneuropathy; peripheral neuropathy)	Distal and symmetric	Usually distal and symmetric distribution	Distal and symmetric loss or decrease	Often have dyesthesia
Neuromuscular junction (Myoneural junction, e.g., myasthenia gravis)	Cranial nerve involvement prominent	None	Normal	Weakness fluctuates
Skeletal muscle (Myopathy)	Proximal and symmetric	None	Preserved until late	Frequently familial

progression are much too variable in diseases involving the anterior horn cell to have a typical distribution. Weakness in polyneuropathy tends to be distal and symmetric, while that in myopathy is proximal and symmetric. In arising from a chair, patients with myopathies involving the pelvic muscles often must use their arms to extend the thighs on the legs and pelvis ("climb up their legs"). This is known as Gower's sign.

The deep tendon reflexes in cases of anterior horn cell diseases tend to diminish with the progression of the disorder. In amyotrophic lateral sclerosis, where there is upper motor neuron involvement, spasticity may be seen early in the course of the disease. Because most peripheral neuropathies also have a sensory component, deep tendon reflexes tend to be lost very early in the course of polyneuropathy. Of all the neuromuscular disorders, polyneuropathy alone causes sensory changes. Early and prominent motor cranial nerve involvement is present in myasthenia gravis. One expects to see fasciculation only in anterior horn cell disease.

TABLE 129–2.
Common Causes of Peripheral Neuropathy

METABOLIC
Diabetes mellitus*
Uremia
Acute intermittent porphyria
Ischemia of multiple peripheral nerves

TOXIC
Heavy metals (lead, arsenic, etc.)
Certain organic compounds—Tri-orthocresyl
    phosphate poisoning—jake leg paralysis
Drugs (particularly vinca alkaloids, furantoins)

NUTRITIONAL
Chronic alcoholism*
Thiamine, B_{12}, folate, or pyridoxine deficiency

INFECTIOUS/POSTINFECTIOUS
Guillain-Barré syndrome
Chronic relapsing polyneuropathy
Neuropathies of leprosy and diphtheria

GENETIC (USUALLY CHRONIC)
Charcot-Marie-Tooth disease*
Familial sensory neuropathy
Various hypertrophic neuropathies

* Asterisks denote the most common causes of peripheral neuropathy. In spite of intensive investigation, no definite cause can be identified in about 30% of clinical cases.

Special pharmacologic testing, more closely related to the physical examination than to laboratory studies, is necessary to establish the diagnosis of myasthenia gravis. Repetitive movements (including repeated closure of the eyes) often can be used to bring out fatigability. In the patient with persisting weakness, intravenous injection of edrophonium (Tensilon test) may markedly but transiently improve the weakness.

PATHOPHYSIOLOGY

The pathogenesis of amyotrophic lateral sclerosis and other anterior horn cell diseases remains unknown. Many of these diseases that occur in infancy and childhood have an autosomal recessive inheritance.

The common causes of peripheral neuropathies are listed in Table 129–2. Specific biochemical defects have been discovered in a few of the chronic familial peripheral neuropathies. In some peripheral neuropathies, there is loss of the peripheral myelin sheath, a so-called demyelinating polyneuropathy; in others, the axon itself slowly "dies back" from the periphery. It seems quite remarkable that polyneuropathy is not more common than it is, when we consider that the axon of a microscopic structure, the anterior horn cell, may extend for nearly a full meter. (One analogy that has been given is that if the neuron were a size of a pea, the axon would stretch the length of a football field!) Most nutritional or toxic polyneuropathies tend to be axonal rather than demyelinating.

Over the past decade, the pathogenesis of myasthenia gravis has been worked out in detail. Although the condition shows up clinically as disordered neuromuscular junction physiology, the basic defect is immunologic. Patients with myasthenia gravis have antibodies to the postsynaptic acetylcholine receptor (AChR) site. These antibodies can be transmitted transplacentally, hence the syndrome of transient myasthenia gravis seen in infants of myasthenic mothers. These antigen–antibody reactions eventually produce anatomical changes in the postsynaptic receptor site, dramatically reducing the area of the receptor membrane available to molecules of acetylcholine. This produces what is, in effect, too little

TABLE 129–3.
The Major Types of Muscular Dystrophy

TYPE	INHERITANCE	AGE OF ONSET	COMMENT
Duchenne type muscular dystrophy	X-linked recessive (carrier tests available)	Boys only Onset by age 7 yr	Survive to early twenties 1:10,000 births affected
Myotonic muscular dystrophy	Autosomal dominant	Adults usually, but any age, including congenital	Commonly have multiple associated endocrinopathies
Limb-girdle muscular dystrophy	Autosomal recessive (usual) (highest spontaneous mutation rate)	Onset any age	Type most difficult to distinguish from other, nondystrophic myopathies
Facioscapulohumoral muscular dystrophy	Autosomal dominant (usual) (lowest mutation rate)	Onset any age	Congenitally absent muscles common Very specific weakness distribution

Note: Types listed in order of estimated declining frequency. Most authorities recognize four or five rare types in addition to the above.

postsynaptic acetylcholine. Agents that inhibit acetylcholinesterase have been used for 50 years in the treatment of myasthenia because these tend to improve the situation by prolonging the action of acetylcholine at the remaining receptor sites.

The pathogenesis is known for only a few diseases of muscle. For example, muscle phosphorylase, phosphofructokinase, and carnitine or enzymes involved in its metabolism may be deficient and produce myopathies. An autoimmune basis is strongly suspected in polymyositis and dermatomyositis. Because of the frequent family history and the known genetic basis, most of the muscular dystrophies (see Table 129–3) are presumed to be due to a biochemical–genetic defect. One of the most exciting recent research breakthroughs has been identification of the exact gene locus on the X chromosome for Duchenne type muscular dystrophy.

DIAGNOSIS

The history and physical examination alone should allow one to decide which type of disorder of the motor unit one is dealing with. However, other studies may be necessary at times, and some of these are shown in Table 129–4. Electromyography (EMG) and nerve conduction velocity studies are particularly useful in confirming the anatomical site of involvement. In general, the EMG findings are essentially the same in anterior horn cell disease and peripheral nerve disease, showing a so-called neurogenic pattern. This differs from a typical myopathic pattern, so the EMG further helps to distinguish these conditions from myopathies. Generally speaking, nerve conduction velocities are normal until late in anterior horn cell disease and normal in myopathies, but tend to be abnormal early in the course of peripheral neuropathies. Repetitive nerve stimulation studies in combination with EMG are particularly helpful in the diagnosis of myasthenia gravis, as is "single-fiber" EMG.

A number of laboratory studies may be necessary to establish the diagnosis in any one case (Table 129–4). In patients with a myopathy there may be elevation of various serum enzymes, particularly creatine phosphokinase (CPK), lactic dehydrogenase (LDH), SGOT, and aldolase. Hundred-fold elevations of the serum CPK level are typical of early Duchenne type muscular dystrophy. Measurement of serum CPK levels also can be useful in attempting to define carrier states in this disorder.

PRINCIPLES OF PREVENTION AND THERAPY

The treatment of most neuromuscular disorders necessarily is only symptomatic because the exact pathogenesis and means to reverse the defect are known only for a few disorders. Bracing and occupational and physical therapy are very important in most of these conditions. Corticosteroid therapy seems to be helpful in a few cases of peripheral neuropathy; its use in the Guillian-Barré syndrome, however, is highly controversial. Meticulous control of diabetes mellitus seems to help diabetic neuropathy, as does abstinence from alcohol in alcoholic neuropathies. Obviously, the removal of responsible toxins is important in the treatment of toxic polyneuropathies.

The treatment of myasthenia gravis can be considered as both pharmacologic and immunologic. Because of its very short action, edrophonium is useful only in the diagnosis of myasthenia gravis. Longer-acting compounds such as pyridostigmine and physostigmine may be helpful as acetylcholin-esterase antagonists. (Unfortunately, an overdose of this type of medication also produces weakness, a situation known as "cholinergic crisis.") Therapy directed to the immunologic aspects of this disease, including treatment with ACTH, prednisone, or plasmapheresis, may be effective. The association of myasthenia gravis with pathologic changes in the thymus was recognized long before all of the immunologic functions of the thymus were understood. Surgical removal of the thymus (thymectomy) continues to be a treatment of severe myasthenia.

Only a few of the primary diseases of muscle, excluding those associated with systemic metabolic defects, are susceptible to specific therapy. Corticosteroids and occasionally immunosuppressive medication is useful in the therapy of polymyositis. Generally, one relies on bracing and physical therapy for treating most of these conditions.

TABLE 129–4.
Laboratory Studies to Localize Disorders of the Motor Unit

SITE OF LESION	EMG FINDINGS	NERVE CONDUCTION VELOCITY (NCV)	MUSCLE BIOPSY FINDINGS	OTHER STUDIES
Anterior horn cell (lower motor neuron)	Neurogenic pattern	Normal early; decreased late	Neurogenic	Myelogram may be needed to exclude spinal mass lesion
Multiple peripheral nerves (polyneuropathy; peripheral neuropathy)	Neurogenic pattern	Decreased early Sensory NCV usually slow also	Neurogenic	Total protein content of cerebrospinal fluid may be increased
Neuromuscular junction (myoneural junction, e.g., myasthenia gravis)	Single-fiber EMG can be diagnostic	Normal; repetitive stimulation study characteristic	Usually normal May show lymphorrhages	Edrophonium (Tensilon) test usually positive; AChR antibodies usually present
Skeletal muscle (myopathy)	Myopathic pattern	Normal	Myopathic May be diagnostic	Certain serum enzymes (CPK, SGOT, LDH) may be elevated

REFERENCES

American Association of Electromyography and Electrodiagnosis: *Muscle and Nerve* (9 issues yearly). New York, John Wiley & Sons. *This journal publishes exclusively clinical research and basic science articles on the neuromuscular disorders and related conditions.*

Brooke MH: *A Clinician's View of Neuromuscular Diseases.* Baltimore, Williams & Wilkins, 1977. *A readable, reasonably short overview of the field from a clinical perspective.*

Dyck PJ, Thomas PK, Lamberg EH (eds): *Peripheral Neuropathy.* Philadelphia, WB Saunders Co, 1984. *Bulky and not easy to read, but still the ultimate reference work on this topic.*

Kakulas BA, Adams RD: *Diseases of Muscle*, ed 4. Philadelphia, Harper & Harper, 1985. *The most current reference work in this area. Stresses the pathology of the conditions, but not to the detriment of their clinical aspects.*

Walton JN (ed): *Disorders of Voluntary Muscle.* Edinburgh, Churchill Livingstone, 1974. *Long the standard reference work on all aspects of the myopathies.*

130 CEREBRAL PALSY

Margaret A. Turk, M.D.
Samuel E. Pitner, M.D.

Cerebral palsy is defined as a disorder of movement and posture resulting from a nonprogressive injury affecting the immature brain. The underlying neuropathologic lesion is static and nonprogressive; it may involve single or multiple locations of the brain. Because the injury is to an immature system, there can be changes in signs and symptoms from infancy through childhood as development proceeds. Injury to the central nervous system that results in cerebral palsy can occur prenatally, perinatally, or postnatally in early childhood. The disorder is defined by the motor involvement, but there often are associated disabilities of cerebral function that can prove to be the major limiting factor in development and later independent function.

The incidence is reported as one to two per 1,000 live births; cerebral palsy is the most frequent childhood disability. There are approximately 500,000 individuals with cerebral palsy in the United States today.

The most common causes of cerebral palsy are noted in Table 130–1. Prenatal and perinatal factors account for up to two-thirds of cases. Acquired cerebral palsy (i.e., caused by postnatal factors) accounts for about 5% of cerebral palsy cases. Any illness or trauma complicated by cerebral anoxia, ischemia, or hemorrhage can account for a residual neuromotor deficit. In approximately 30% of patients diagnosed as having cerebral palsy, there is no identifiable cause.

Cerebral palsy is classified by the type of motor dysfunction, specifically by the abnormality of muscle tone (Table 130–2) and also by the location of involvement (Table 130–3). Spastic cerebral palsy is the most common type; within that category, hemiparetic and spastic diplegia (Little's disease) are the majority. Hemiparesis used to be the most common presentation, but with improved obstetric care, it is decreasing. Diplegia most commonly is seen as a result of prematurity, particularly in infants with birth weights under 1500 gm. Athetosis is due to damage to the basal ganglia. This was due in the past mainly to kernicterus, caused by the very high bilirubin levels associated with neonatal hemolytic syndromes. With modern management of disorders such as Rh incompatibility, the incidence of athetoid cerebral palsy has declined markedly. Hypotonia is often seen as an early sign of cerebral palsy, but usually evolves into the other motor dysfunctions by the age of 12 months.

CLINICAL SIGNS AND SYMPTOMS

Generally, the physician is alerted to the possibility of a central nervous system insult by the mother's history of complicated pregnancy and labor and by the neonatal course. The developmental history of the child is important to elicit, even for an infant. Infants who have very short periods of alertness, a weak cry, difficulty feeding, and show little interest in their environment should be suspected of having cerebral palsy. High-risk infants as well as infants who have difficulties initially should be observed closely. Cerebral palsy may be indicated by feeding disorders, which may arise from difficulties with oral motor functions and in how to position the infant for feeding.

As development progresses, further developmental history can show a delay or abnormality of movement and posture. An early preference for one hand is often the first sign of motor dysfunction. An inability to maintain sitting at 6 months when placed in the sitting position is also an indication of delay. The classic "W" sitting position (hips and knees in flexion with internal rotation at hips) is often used by children with lower extremity spasticity to maintain a wider base of support. Abnormal crawling patterns can point to motor dysfunction. The age at which the child begins standing and walking and also the quality of these movements can show poor motor control. Delay in motor milestones is the prevailing symptom of children with cerebral palsy. Actual loss of previously acquired abilities suggests the pressure of degenerative disorders or brain tumors as opposed to the static lesions of cerebral palsy. Usually the late acquisition of sitting first alerts parents and physicians. More specific questions can show difficulties in other areas of development, but these are not often noted by parents. For premature infants, development must be modified and matched for gestational age rather than chronologic age. The physician must be knowledgeable in normal develop-

TABLE 130–1.
High-Risk Factors for Cerebral Palsy

PRENATAL

Maternal/fetal infections
Maternal ingestion of toxic substances
Chromosomal abnormalities
Maternal hypertension
Abruptio placentae
Placenta previa
Maternal malnutrition
Poor prenatal care

PERINATAL

Prematurity (especially birth weight < 1500 gm)
Prolonged/precipitous labor
Intrauterine asphyxia
Cephalopelvic disproportion
Umbilical cord prolapse/compression
Abnormal presentations
Cardiopulmonary diseases of infancy/prematurity
Hyperbilirubinemia

POSTNATAL

Head trauma (accident or abuse)
Cerebral vascular accidents
Intracranial infections
Toxic exposure

TABLE 130–2.
Cerebral Palsy: Classification by Abnormality of Muscle Tone

TYPE	PERCENT OF PATIENTS
Spastic	70–80
Athetoid	10–12
Rigid	4–5
Hypotonic	rare
Mixed	10–20

TABLE 130–3.
Cerebral Palsy: Classification by Site of Involvement

TYPE	EXTREMITIES INVOLVED
Hemiparesis	One side, upper > lower
Diplegia	Lower >> upper
Quadriparesis	All four extremities involved, lower > upper
Double hemiplegia	All four extremities involved, upper > lower

ment, the parameters of late normal development, and the quality of movement in order to evaluate the history appropriately.

Infants at risk for having cerebral palsy must

be observed closely to detect early signs of the disorder. The early physical examination includes evaluation of muscle tone, reflexes, and postural responses. The muscle tone may be increased or decreased, as well as asymmetric. Volitional movement may be difficult to recognize until after 4 months of age, but response to examination may indicate an asymmetric or decreased response. Persistent primitive reflexes can be diagnostic, but are not prognostic. The early signs noted within the first 6 months of life can later confirm a diagnosis of cerebral palsy at age 12 months to 18 months as motor development continues to lag and neuromotor deficits become more obvious. The subtle signs in mild cases may not become manifest until more advanced milestones, particularly walking, are to be achieved.

Evaluation of muscle tone is difficult below the age of 6 months, and oftentimes alterations of tone are the earliest signs. Tone is evaluated by the resistance to movement and the range of motion of the joints. The infant or child who is irritable and crying will superimpose tonal changes, and this must be taken into account. An increased range of motion seen most easily at the shoulders and hips, indicates hypotonia. When the infant is held in vertical suspension, there will be poor head control and no shoulder stabilization. Head control is also noted to be a problem in prone position and when being pulled to sit. In contrast, increased resistance to range denotes hypertonia. Extensor posturing is the activity used to test function. When the child is held in vertical suspension, there may be scissoring of the lower extremities, which is abnormal after 2 months of age. Head control in an infant with cerebral palsy may be managed through an extensor posture, which often is interpreted as early head and trunk control. When being pulled to sit, an infant will show extreme extension of the lower extremities, which may bring the child to a full standing position. Throughout development, there can be fluctuating tone with changes from hypotonicity to hypertonicity, depending on use of reflexes and tone for movement. Often there can be a mixture of abnormal tones such as hypotonic trunk and neck and hypertonic extremities.

Deep tendon reflexes are often difficult to elicit in normal infants. Ease in obtaining more than the quadriceps and Achilles reflexes may

indicate upper motor neuron involvement. Hyperreflexia with clonus and overflow may also be present. Sustained clonus should be considered pathologic.

Primitive reflexes are present in all infants, and their delayed presentation or prolonged existence can assist in the diagnosis of cerebral palsy. As of yet, these reflexes have not been shown to give prognostic information. Persistence of the Moro reflex and asymmetric tonic neck reflexes may indicate cerebral palsy, particularly of the spastic or athetoid type. Positive supporting and grasp reflexes generally persist with spasticity. Abnormal reflexes can be obligatory and inhibit voluntary motor control, or can have subtle influences on muscle tone and the quality of motor activities. Often, these reflexes come into play more strongly in one position than another.

Abnormalities in tone, reflexes, or posture responses indicate a possible upper motor neuron disorder. The presence of all three abnormalities is significant.

The clinical course in cerebral palsy is quite diverse and depends on the motor function, associated complications, and cognitive level. The course is also influenced by growth and development resulting in fluctuation of function and dysfunction. Development remains delayed, although continued maturation improves functional activities. The more extensive the brain injury, the more likely motor function will remain limited. Table 130–4 outlines the typical courses of the four major classifications of cerebral palsy.

The incidences of the associated handicaps and complications vary. Infants and children with cerebral palsy should be screened regularly for these associated findings. Generally, the more severe the motor dysfunction, the more likely are multiple handicaps. The most commonly associated handicaps are listed in Table 130–5.

CLINICAL–PATHOLOGIC CORRELATIONS

Injury to the immature brain can result from hypoxia, ischemia, hemorrhage, or kernicterus. The lesions may be single or multiple, and good clinical correlation with the site of the lesion is often difficult. Laboratory and diagnos-

TABLE 130–4.
Cerebral Palsy—Natural Course

CLASSIFICATION	EARLY DEVELOPMENTAL FINDINGS	HAND FUNCTION	GROSS MOTOR FUNCTION	COMMUNICATION	ASSOCIATED HANDICAPS
Spastic hemiparesis	Asymmetry of motor function	Fisted hand shows early preference Eventual self-care and independence Involved hand is helper only	Asymmetric crawl Toe-walking one side with short stance Independent Walking by age 3 yr usually	Usually normal Aphasia if onset > age 2 yr in right hemisphere	Contractures—upper > lower Surgical release at ankle common Shortened limbs on involved side Low incidence MR*
Spastic diplegia	Hypotonia Use extensor thrust Spasticity by 6 mo of age	May have fisting of hands Eventually adequate hand function Usually independent with self-care	"W-sitting" "Commando crawl" Toe-walking, bilateral 85% walk independently or with aid	Often normal	Contractures—hip pathology Tendon releases Scoliosis Low incidence MR Low incidence seizures
Spastic quadriparesis	Hypotonia or hypertonia Asymmetry can be present Spasticity > 6 mo old in hypotonics	Fisted hand initially 33% can be independent, with self-care 25% dependent for all care	Diverse outcomes 33% walk with assisting devices 25% never walk	Dysarthria Oral motor dysfunction	More problems with contractures Severe hip contractures Scoliosis most progressive High incidence MR High incidence seizures High incidence dependency
Athetosis	Hypotonia	Movement disorders noted > 12 mo Upper more involved Fanning of fingers with immature grasp	Favorable prognosis for walking	Dysarthria common	Rare deformities Low incidence seizures Low incidence MR Hearing loss Spondylosis (especially cervical) in early adulthood

* MR = mental retardation

TABLE 130–5.
Deficits Commonly Associated with Cerebral Palsy

Mental retardation
Seizures
Visual defects
Hearing loss
Learning disability
Oral motor dysfunction
   Feeding
   Communication
   Language
Behavior disorders
Skeletal deformities
   Limb growth discrepancy
   Contractures
   Hip subluxation/dislocation
   Scoliosis

tic procedures may delineate areas of involvement, but frequently studies are negative and no specific causative factor is found. Hypoxic-ischemic encephalopathy is the most common cause of cerebral palsy, particularly in term infants. Hypoxia can develop prenatally in cases of intrauterine anoxia due to poor transplacental gas exchange, and perinatally with respiratory complications during or after birth. Ischemia arises either intrauterine or postnatally as a consequence of the abnormal cardiovascular function that accompanies asphyxia, congenital heart disease, apneic spells, or sepsis.

Intracranial hemorrhage can also cause cerebral palsy. However, because of improved obstetric care, subdural hemorrhage because of birth trauma has become less significant. Periventricular and intraventricular hemorrhage is the most common cause of neurologic morbidity among premature infants of less than 32 weeks gestation. Other causes are septic embolization, venous thrombosis with polycythemia, or hemorrhage secondary to an atrioventricular malformation, aneurysm, or coagulation difficulties.

The area of cerebral involvement can determine motor involvement. The premature brain has a low resistance to hypoxia or ischemia in the germinal matrix juxtaposed to the ependymal lining of the lateral ventricles. Hypoxia and often secondary hemorrhage into this area, seen very frequently in premature infants, can cause spastic diplegia. The pyramidal tracts controlling the lower extremities are closer to the lateral ventricles than are the tracts to the upper extremities, so the classic diplegic picture is seen. If a single hemisphere is affected, contralateral hemiparesis results. Involvement of the cortex of both hemispheres or severe and diffuse damage results in quadriparesis.

Bilirubin neurotoxicity is seen less often because of prenatal testing for Rh incompatibility and exchange transfusions of the newborn. Kernicterus occurs with a total serum bilirubin over 16 mg to 18 mg/dl. Bilirubin cannot cross the blood–brain barrier when it is bound to serum albumin. With a rise in the free bilirubin fraction, there may be increased permeability or increased susceptibility to the free bilirubin. Bilirubin has a propensity for deposition in the basal ganglia and other subcortical nuclei. Therefore, the clinical presentation of kernicterus is disorders in movements associated with these areas.

DIFFERENTIAL DIAGNOSIS

The vast majority of infants with cerebral palsy have hypotonia in the early months of life. At this stage of the illness, it usually is not possible to localize the lesion to the brain, and other causes of hypotonia such as anterior horn cell, nerve, or muscle lesions must be excluded. With the evolution of upper motor neuron signs such as increased reflexes and persistence of primitive reflexes, one can be pointed to the diagnosis of cerebral palsy. The eventual evolution of tone changes help to solidify this diagnosis. However, progressive cerebral and spinal lesions such as tumors and degenerative disorders must be considered.

In progressive CNS disorders, the developmental dysfunction or actual loss of functions including involuntary activities such as feeding may be limited initially. Increased seizure activity can also indicate a progressive lesion. Enlarged head circumference should be evaluated further to rule out congenital hydrocephalus or a tumor. Organomegaly suggests a storage disease. Dysmorphic features may indicate specific syndromes or cerebral malformations. Endocrine and metabolic disorders also should be considered; other clinical features may also alert the physician to these disorders.

The evolution of tone and reflexes can assist in the diagnosis. Spastic evolution in cerebral palsy usually becomes evident after about 6 months. Movement disorders become obvious at 12 months or later. Injury to the spinal cord secondary to birth trauma can initially appear as hypotonia during the phase of spinal shock. There may be associated brisk flexor withdrawal responses, lack of supraspinal primitive reflexes, and urinary retention. Spasticity may develop in the face of a cognitively alert infant sooner than by 6 months of age. Chromosomal abnormalities can cause hypotonia, particularly persistent hypotonia; the Prader-Willi syndrome is an example of such a condition that can now be more consistently diagnosed with chromosomal analysis.

Mental retardation alone can cause delay in motor milestones in early development and is often confused with cerebral palsy. A full developmental history can eventually lead to the diagnosis of a primary cognitive deficit. The reflexes remain normal or mildly decreased, and muscle tone increases as would be expected through maturation, not evolution of spasticity or movement disorder.

DIAGNOSIS

The diagnosis of cerebral palsy is made based on the initial history and physical examination and on serial examinations. Laboratory studies can be helpful in ruling out other suspected causes that would be treatable or would significantly alter the prognosis. There is no definitive laboratory test to make a diagnosis of cerebral palsy. A definite diagnosis of cerebral palsy is difficult to make within the first year of life, and it can only be made with the objective evidence of compatible findings in the history, the upper motor neuron signs, and the typical developmental progress. Laboratory data are often negative.

Metabolic and endocrine disorders can be diagnosed through laboratory data, and chromosomal abnormalities can also be noted. Cerebral palsy can be associated with some of these.

With the recent advancement in brain imaging, central pathologic changes can sometimes be documented. Computed tomography scans and radioisotope brainscans may localize lesions when cerebral palsy is suspected. Ultrasonography is widely used in infants to visualize hemorrhage, encephalomalacia, hydro-cephalus, and porencephalic cysts. Some fetal CNS abnormalities may even be detected in utero. Although the EEG is of little value unless seizures are present, other studies such as evoked potentials can also give supporting evidence of CNS dysfunction. Somatosensory evoked potentials and brain stem auditory evoked potentials can outline competency of the central pathways. Visual evoked potentials can also indicate early dysfunction of visual pathways.

These studies support the diagnosis of cerebral palsy and can indicate localization of an injury. The CT scans are most often positive in hemiparesis. Most signs of cerebral palsy, however, can localize the area of injury by examination alone.

PRINCIPLES OF THERAPY

The management of a child with cerebral palsy necessitates an interdisciplinary team approach. Motor deficits may not be the only abnormality, and all systems should be developed to their highest level of function. A developmental approach should anticipate possible complications and should educate the family for preventive or anticipatory treatment. The psycho-social aspects of the family and the child should be addressed whenever possible. Fostering reasonable expectations of function can assist families in accommodating to their child's disability. The habilitation plan is a joint involvement of the family, physicians, and other professionals working with the child.

Therapeutic intervention strategies vary, and opinions differ regarding appropriate types of therapies. Objective evidence regarding timing and type of therapy as well as the benefit of therapy is as yet unavailable. Working through these issues with the family is very important. Selecting the therapy appropriate for the goal and realizing the need for a home program are also important.

The amount of therapy necessary is often a controversial point for parents. To gain benefit from therapy, infants and children must participate at some level. More therapy is not necessarily better, and care must be taken to individualize a program to meet specific goals. The need for therapy will change with growth and development, depending on the needs of the child and areas to be stressed. A maintenance program, particularly of range of motion, should be managed at home with appropriate follow-up. A home program is of utmost importance to maintain the activities learned in therapy sessions and to make them a part of daily activities. The function at home, school, and in other situations in life must be consistent. Functional tasks need to be geared toward age-appropriate skills, guided more by cognitive function than chronologic age. The range of therapy includes physical, occupational, and speech therapy. Orthopedic surgery might be required. At times medication is employed to reduce spasticity.

Cognitive function generally limits the final outcome. Psychosocial adaptations to the disability including the patient's self-esteem and body image also contribute to this. There is normal or near-normal intelligence in 30% to 40% of cases and long-term studies show that about 10% of adults with cerebral palsy are employed or achieving their highest level of independence. The adolescent and young adult with cerebral palsy often find assimilation into society extremely difficult, and therefore manage a more sheltered existence. Physical ability, cognitive status, and psychosocial function ultimately influence the cerebral palsy patient's achievements in life.

REFERENCES

Batshaw ML, Perret, Y: *Children with Handicaps: A Medical Primer.* Baltimore, Paul H. Brooks Publishing Co, 1981. *This book gives limited clinicopathophysiology of cerebral palsy, with emphasis on therapy and reflex development, although in a superficial manner.*

Developmental Medicine and Child Neurology. Spastics International Medical Publications. Philadelphia, JB Lippincott Co. *This journal is published bimonthly with original articles on specific topics in developmental disabilities.*

Finnie NR: *Handling the Young Cerebral Palsied at Home.* New York, EP Dutton & Co, 1968. *This book is often given as a reference text for parents. It deals strictly with appropriate handling of the infant/child with cerebral palsy. Practical information is presented in a manner that is easily understood.*

Martin EW: Pediatrician's role in the care of disabled children. *Pediatrics in Review* 1985; 6:275. *This article specifically deals with identifying appropriate roles for pediatricians as a central resource for families with a disabled child.*

Molnar GE (ed): Cerebral palsy. *Pediatric Rehabilitation* 1985; 17:420. *This is the best recent reference on cerebral palsy, particularly long-term management of this disease process.*

Scherzer AL, Tscharnuter I: *Early Diagnosis and Therapy in Cerebral Palsy: A Primer on Infant Developmental Problems.* New York, Marcel Dekker, Inc, 1982. *This book discusses the clinico-pathophysiology of cerebral palsy.*

Taft LT, (editorial advisory board): Cerebral palsy. *Pediatr Ann* 1986; 15:3. *The journal devotes issues to specific topics for CME credit. The topic of this issue is cerebral palsy with in-depth articles on multiple areas, including diagnosis, reflex development, rehabilitation, and counseling.*

131 ANXIETY DISORDERS

Abraham Heller, M.D.
Arnold Allen, M.D.

Anxiety is an emotion, a state of feeling, common to everyday experience. It is related to fear, the emotion that arises when danger threatens the individual. The autonomic nervous system response to anxiety is adrenergic—with dry mouth, increased pulse rate and blood pressure, muscular tension, and sweating—preparing the individual for the "fight or flight" reaction. Anxiety becomes clinical when it is maladaptive, as when it arises without an identified threat or when the emotional intensity is disproportionate to the reality of the threat. Clinically, anxiety may be an incidental symptom in many disorders, physical and psychiatric, or it may be a primary or the dominant symptom of a group of psychiatric disorders. In all of these situations, the individual suffers intense discomfort, in the extreme, sheer panic, without ever losing grasp of reality. The primary types of anxiety disorders are shown in Table 131–1.

SIMPLE PHOBIA

Persistently excessive and irrational fear of a specific object or situation is the basis of simple phobia. The condition is common. The impairment is limited by avoidance behavior, exemplified by the common children's street rhyme—"step on a crack, break your mother's back!"—as a dire caution against behavior to be avoided at all cost. Commonly feared objects are snakes, animals, insects; commonly feared situations are being in closed places (claustrophobia) or being in high places (acrophobia).

SOCIAL PHOBIA

A persistent, excessive, and irrational fear of public humiliation or embarrassment is the basis of social phobia. Most common of these phobias are fear of speaking or performing in public. The necessity for performance in public gives rise to very distressing anticipatory anxiety. Avoidance limits the impairment; the need to avoid and the difficulty in meeting one's professional responsibility may complicate one's career. Psychotherapy, particularly employing behavioral methods, and anxiolytic medication, or a combination of these, can be helpful in this condition.

AGORAPHOBIA (FEAR OF WIDE-OPEN PLACES)

An excessive, irrational fear of being alone in public places, of being caught in public and subjected to intolerable distress or incapacitation without avenue of escape or without access to help is the basis of agoraphobia. Typi-

TABLE 131–1.
Types of Anxiety Disorders

PHOBIC DISORDERS
Simple phobia
Social phobia
Agoraphobia
ANXIETY STATES
Generalized anxiety disorder
Panic disorder
Obsessive-compulsive disorder
Post-traumatic stress disorder

cally, avoidance and anticipatory anxiety promote a step-by-step constriction of the individual's sphere of activity to the point that some individuals become unable to venture out of the home. In less severe cases, individuals may be able to tolerate the phobic situation if accompanied by a familiar person. Cases of agoraphobia may occur with or without panic attacks.

Treatment modalities for agoraphobia include psychotherapy, especially with the use of behavioral methods. Anxiolytic medication may be helpful. In line with the revelation of recent research that many agoraphobics have significant episodes of depression or a persistent underlying depression, antidepressive medication may be helpful in some cases.

GENERALIZED ANXIETY DISORDER

In generalized anxiety, the mood of the individual is suffused with anxiety without identifiable external source and beyond conscious explanation on the part of the sufferer. Morbidity and impairment are in proportion to the anxiety and may range from mild to very severe. The disorder is manifested by signs of motor tension, autonomic hyperactivity, apprehensiveness, and vigilance (Table 131–2). Treatment approaches include psychotherapy or behavioral therapy, anxiolytic medication, and at times combinations of these.

PANIC DISORDER

Attacks of panic are characterized by a sudden onset of intense apprehension, intense fear to the point of terror, loss of control, and helplessness, all accompanied by a feeling of doom. The attacks occur both predictably and unpredictably. A typical panic-producing situation is driving a car, particularly in traffic. This condition is accompanied by a great deal of anticipatory anxiety. The common symptoms are shown in Table 131–3.

A clinically objective and helpful understanding of panic disorder (PD) has begun to unfold only in the last 10 to 15 years through a growing volume of research. A number of salient characteristics have been identified:

Sex Distribution: Female:Male   4:1

Prevalence: 2%–5% in the general population
10%–40% in patients seen in cardiology practice
Increased prevalence among first-degree relatives
Increased concordance in monozygotic twins

Onset: Typically in early adulthood

Clinical Course: Fluctuates throughout rest of life
Over 1/4 are symptomatic 20 years after onset
50% have some level of disability

Biologic Differentiation: Sodium lactate infusion precipitates panic in patients and not in normal subjects.

TABLE 131–2.
Diagnostic Criteria for Generalized Anxiety Disorder*†

MOTOR TENSION
Shakiness, jumpiness
Muscle tension, trembling
Fidgeting, restlessness
Strained face
Inability to relax
AUTONOMIC HYPERACTIVITY
Sweating
Palpitations
Dry mouth
Increased pulse rate
Increased respiratory rate
Dizziness
Lightheadedness
Upset stomach
Discomfort in pit of stomach
Hot and cold spells
Lump in throat
Pallor
Cold clammy hands
Tingling in hands or feet
APPREHENSIVENESS
Anxiety
Fear
Worry with anticipations of misfortune
VIGILANCE AND SCANNING
Hyperattentiveness resulting in distractability
Difficulty in concentration
Feeling "on edge"
Irritability
Impatience

* These criteria are highlights from the *Diagnostic and Statistical Manual*, ed 3. Washington, DC, American Psychiatric Association, 1980, pp 225–239.
† These manifestations are for a pervasive anxiety lasting a period of at least 1 month.

Associated Depression: One-half or more patients have a history of overt or underlying depression.

Associated Mitral Valve Prolapse: A significantly high association (as high as 50%) in patients with panic disorder, compared to 4%–7% in the general population

Several factors support the conclusion that there is a significant biologic component in panic disorder. The disorder is chronic and potentially quite disabling. Patients with undiagnosed panic disorder are seen for physical complaints in primary care and cardiology practice. Panic disorder is not uncommon among cardiology patients.

Research indicated and clinical experience has confirmed that antidepressant medication can be effective in panic disorder by blocking the panic attacks. The anticipatory anxiety, which becomes entrenched over the years, requires separate treatment—anxiolytic medication (alprazolam [Xanax] is frequently specifically recommended), psychotherapy, behavioral therapy, or some combination of these. Beta-blocking medication is sometimes used adjunctively to control the target symptoms of tachycardia and palpitations. Support groups may be helpful to supplement other therapy and to promote rehabilitation of patients with chronically entrenched panic disorder.

OBSESSIVE-COMPULSIVE DISORDERS

Obsessions are intrusive and preoccupying thoughts that are ego-alien. The thoughts are senseless or repugnant to the individual. They are so pervasive as to defy any attempt by the individual to ignore them. Common themes are violence (thoughts of killing one's child, as an example), prurience, contamination (thought of becoming infected by shaking hands), and an endless need to reassure. Doubt as an ever-present component of obsessive thinking is a tip-off of an ambivalent, underlying conflict.

Compulsions are intrusive acts that are highly ritualistic and stereotyped. These acts appear to be designed to make magical intercession to forfend some dire event which exists at a subconscious level in the mind of the sufferer and is evidenced by unexplainable but unshakable feelings of worry and anxiety. Examples of compulsive behaviors include repetitive hand washing, counting, and touching.

Validations of effective treatment of obsessive-compulsive disorders are sparse. In some cases target symptoms have diminished or remitted during the course of analytic therapy or of behavioral therapy using desensitization. Antidepressant medication may be helpful in occasional cases in which obsessions or compulsions are symptoms of what is primarily a case of depression. In most cases the results with antidepressive medication have not been impressive.

POST-TRAUMATIC STRESS DISORDER

A post-traumatic stress may develop after a psychologically traumatic event of such extraordinary degree that it could be expected to produce marked symptoms of distress in virtually anyone. Enduring or surviving personal assaults, rape, war experiences, or other disasters or catastrophes may set the stage for the development of the disorder. These strains may overwhelm psychologic integrity or stability on an immediate or delayed basis. Survivors may live with the festering, unresolved psychologic remnants of the event and, therefore, be vulnerable to recurrent, painful reexperiences. Common symptoms are shown in Table 131–4.

Treatment approaches include individual or group psychotherapy, antianxiety or antidepressant medication, and at times a combination of psychotherapy and medication.

TABLE 131–3.
Common Symptoms and Characteristics of Panic Disorder

Dyspnea
Choking, smothering sensations
Hyperventilation
Palpitations
Chest pains
Unsteadiness, dizziness, vertigo
Feelings of unreality
Tingling in hands or feet
Hot or cold flashes
Trembling, shaking
Feeling of helplessness
Fear of collapse, dying, "going crazy"
Fear of loss of control

TABLE 131–4.
Symptoms of Post-traumatic Stress Disorder

TRAUMATIC REEXPERIENCE
Obsessional recollection of the original event
Recurrent nightmares involving the event
Dissociative states—environmental stimuli associated with the event trigger reactions and behaviors as if the event were recurring
Numbing or reduced involvement in or responsiveness to one's external world

IMPAIRING INDIVIDUAL SYMPTOMS
Impaired concentration and memory
Distracted by hypervigilance
Vulnerable to overreaction, jumpiness
Hypersensitive to and avoidance of experiences that symbolize or resemble the traumatic event
Survival guilt

REFERENCES

Breier A, Charney DS, Heninger GR: Major depression in patients with agoraphobia and panic disorder. *Arch Gen Psychiatry* 1984; 41: 1129–1135. *This article explores significant depression coincident with some cases of phobic and panic disorders.*

Hartman N, Kramer R, Brown WT: Panic disorder in patients with mitral valve prolapse. *Am J Psychiatry* 1982; 139:669–670. *The empirical coincidental relationship in many cases of panic disorder and mitral valve prolapse is presented.*

Spitz R, et al: Anxiety disorders, in *Diagnostic and Statistical Manual of Mental Disorders*, ed 3. Washington DC, American Psychiatric Association, 1980, pp 225–239. *The definitive coverage of classification of mental disorders.*

Symposium. Panic disorders: Clinical update 1984. *Psychosomatics* 1984; 25(Suppl):10. *Clinical and biologic aspects of panic disorders are comprehensively covered in this symposium.*

132   DEPRESSION

Arnold Allen, M.D.
Abraham Heller, M.D.

Depression as used in the psychosocial sphere describes a lowering of mood, affect, or feeling state. This can occur normally as a part of the normal stresses of everyday life (affect), as a manifestation of a variety of psychiatric or physical illnesses (symptom, or secondary depression), or as the major component of a group of distinct psychiatric disorders subsumed under the term *affective disorders* (syndrome). In the last of these, the depressed state may or may not alternate with periods of pathologic elevations of mood (mania). The classification of the more severe depressive disorders (syndromes) is outlined in Figure 132–1 (Webb, DiClemente, et al., 1980) in which Zone 1 represents the normal ups and downs of mood, Zone 2 a more severe condition, and Zone 3 a full-blown major disorder. Other components to consider in making the diagnosis are the presence of highs and lows

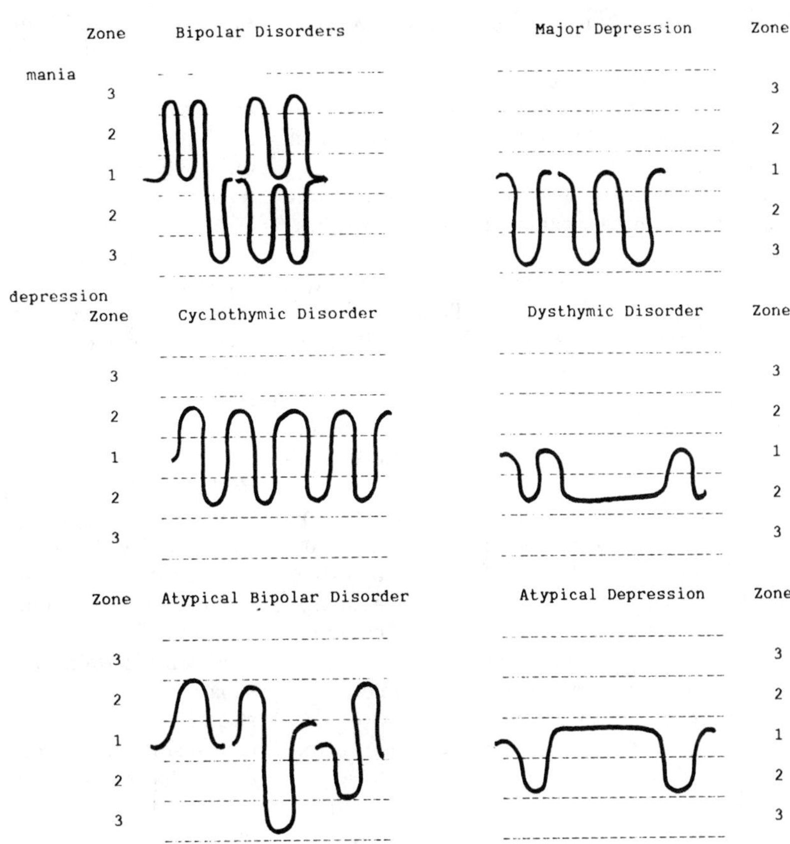

FIG 132–1.

Classification of syndromes. [From Webb LJ, DiClemente CC et al: *Training Guide to Diagnostic and Statistical Manual of Mental Disorders,* ed 3. Washington DC, Brunner/Mazel, Inc, American Psychiatric Association, 1980, p 987. Used by permission.]

and the duration of the syndrome. The normal condition is considered to blend into the pathologic when the intensity, duration, or appropriateness of the mood change exceeds normal expectations, interferes with an individual's everyday social and occupational functioning, or creates a hazard either to himself or herself (suicide) or to others (homicide).

As a result of different systems of diagnosis and classification, comparable incidence rates are difficult to obtain. Estimates suggest that the lifetime expectancy of developing an affective disorder ranges from 10% to 30% affecting 1% to 2% of the population and, further, that a considerable proportion of persons with de-pression never see a physician and that only 20% to 25% of depressed people receive treatment. The typical age of onset is reported by some to be early in adult life and by others to be at any time in adult life. Increasingly more attention is being focussed on depression in childhood and early adolescence. No convincing correlation has been found between social class and depressive illness, and women outnumber men by two to one as estimated for major depressive disorders and by five to one as estimated for dysthymic disorders. Opinions vary as to differentials about whether the incidences are different in married and in single people (Kaplan and Sadock, 1981).

CLINICAL SIGNS AND SYMPTOMS

The onset of depression varies considerably. In some it follows closely upon and is clearly related to an external precipitant (such as loss of a loved one or a financial or occupational loss), while in others its onset appears to be insidious with no demonstrable external connection. In some older classification systems the former was labeled as *reactive depression* and the latter *endogenous depression*. This differentiation has currently been discarded based on the concept that the depressive condition is multifactorially determined and is the final common pathway for a variety of biologic, psychologic, and sociologic influences (Kolb and Brodie, 1982).

Symptoms of depression seldom occur alone but in clusters of varying combinations in any of five categories including affective, cognitive, vegetative, activity-related, and physical symptoms. Table 132–1 lists some of the common initial symptoms of depression.

The symptoms of a major depressive episode usually develop over a period of days or weeks, but may have a quite sudden onset as, for example, following a severe stress such as a loss or a reversal. The onset may be preceded by several months of milder symptoms such as anxiety or panic attacks. Most acute depressive episodes are self-limiting, have a good prognosis, and subside within 6 months to 8 months even without specific therapy. With the advent of somatic therapies such as antidepressants and electroconvulsive therapy (ECT), not only can the recovery be hastened, but the intensity of the symptoms can be ameliorated. Depression can also occur in patients who do not meet all of the criteria for an affective disorder. Some examples are affective disorders of childhood, uncomplicated bereavement reactions, personality disorders (especially in histrionic and borderline disorders), and organic affective disorders.

PATHOPHYSIOLOGY

The cause of depression is unknown, probably because there is no one cause. The most likely scenario is that a genetic predisposition resulting in biochemical imbalances in the body coupled with certain early life experiences (loss, separation, parenting deficit) and later life stresses (loss, reverses, injury to self-esteem) can result in depression. There seems little doubt that the incidence of both unipolar and bipolar affective disorders is considerably increased in families of patients. Studies comparing monozygotic to dizygotic twins lend further

TABLE 132–1.
The Symptoms of Depression*

AFFECTIVE	COGNITIVE
Depressed mood	Difficulty in concentrating
Feelings of failure	Indecisiveness
Feelings of worthlessness	Reduced interest
Feelings of wrongdoing	Impaired judgment
Excessive guilt or shame	**PHYSICAL**
Wish to be dead	Fatigue
Inability to experience pleasure	Impotence
VEGETATIVE	Physical complaints
Insomnia (or excessive sleep)	**ACTIVITY-RELATED**
Anorexia (or excessive eating)	Slowed
Constipation	Trouble starting
Decreased libido	May be agitated
Weight loss	

* Adapted from Waldinger RJ: *Psychiatry for Medical Students.* Washington, DC, American Psychiatric Press, Inc, 1984, p 104.

evidence to this. Just what it is that is inherited is not clear.

Opinions vary as to whether the defect is in the neurohormonal control mechanisms (inherited) or in the ego (the executive portion of the personality) resulting from early childhood experiences. Recent research in the area has focused on neurotransmitters, the chemicals that transmit nerve impulses from one neuron to another. The primary ones being studied are norepinephrine and serotonin (the catecholamine-indoleamine hypothesis of depression). In some forms of depression there appears to be a CNS deficiency of norepinephrine, a substance normally found in the central and peripheral nervous systems. In these depressions 3-methoxy, 4-hydroxy-phenylglycol (MHPG), the metabolite of norepinephrine is found in abnormally low levels in the urine. This deficiency can be remedied by the administration of tricyclic antidepressants such as imipramine and desipramine, which block the reuptake of norepinephrine in presynaptic neurons thus increasing the amount that remains active as a neurotransmitter. A deficiency in serotonin has also been found in some depressed patients indicated by low levels of its metabolite, 5-hydroxyindoleacetic acid (5HIAA), in the CSF. At the same time these patients show normal or elevated urinary MHPG. This group has been found to respond clinically to amitriptyline, another tricyclic antidepressant that blocks serotonin reuptake by presynaptic neurons, thus increasing the amount of serotonin available for transmission. Unfortunately, not all clinically depressed patients demonstrate norepinephrine or serotonin deficiencies, nor do they respond to antidepressant medication. Much further study of the biology of depression is needed (Fawcett, 1985).

The psychosocial factors are also a vast field for study, and as yet no single sociologic factor or personality trait has been identified as predisposing to depression. Factors that have been implicated at different times in various studies have included such things as a defect in the early mother–child relationship with a failure to promote in the child a feeling that he or she is good and loved; early failure to develop a sense of self-esteem; and separation from a loved object, expecially as a result of loss of a parent by death or divorce of a parent.

DIAGNOSIS

A diagnosis of an affective disorder as the diagnosis of any disorder should be based on a compilation of history, direct examination (including physical examination and mental status examination), laboratory tests, and where indicated, psychologic tests. The initial interview should demonstrate the initial signs and symptoms of depression and should make particular inquiry about predisposing and precipitating factors, familial illness, current medications, and physical illnesses. A thorough physical examination should rule out any underlying physical cause. The patient's history should be confirmed by someone close to the patient. Various other conditions that can resemble depressive disorders should be differentiated because of the treatment and prognostic implications. The differential diagnosis should rule out other psychiatric conditions or underlying organic causes of which depression is a secondary manifestation. Some of the more common organic causes are shown in Table 132–2.

Clinically useful laboratory tests currently used for screening for depression include the dexamethasone-suppression test (DMST), the thyrotropin-response test, measurement of urinary levels of MHPG, and sleep studies. Measurement of CSF concentrations and of 5HIAA and of imipramine-binding sites, are still considered investigational. The DMST is currently the most popular laboratory screening device for depression, although its value is considered controversial because it is insensitive in close to 50% of major depressions, is flawed in depressions connected with senile dementias, and can yield false-positive results. Its use is based on the fact that many depressed patients are hypersecretors of cortisol and that dexamethasone fails to suppress this.

Many patients with tricyclic responsive depression also demonstrate sleep abnormalities such as early REM latency (before 60 minutes to 70 minutes) and increased REM density. One theory is that the increased REM activity may be the result of an imbalance between cholinergic (increased) and monoamine (decreased) activity. Sleep laboratory recordings can aid in distinguishing primary from secondary depression and in determining the likelihood of an

TABLE 132–2.
Organic Disorders That Produce Depression*

DRUG-ASSOCIATED DISORDERS	INFECTIOUS DISEASES
Reserpine use	Hepatitis
Propranolol use	Pneumonia
Corticosteroid use	Mononucleosis
Oral contraceptive use	**NEOPLASTIC DISORDERS**
Alcohol use	Cancer of head of pancreas
Marijuana use	Brain tumor
Hallucinogen use	**SYSTEMIC DISEASES**
Alcohol withdrawal	Anemia
Amphetamine withdrawal	Nutritional deficiency
Barbiturate withdrawal	**GENERAL**
Nicotine withdrawal	Dementias
Benzodiazepine withdrawal	Psychologic reaction to physical illness
ENDOCRINE DISORDERS	
Thyroid	
Adrenal	
Pituitary	
CENTRAL NERVOUS SYSTEM DISORDERS	
Cerebral vascular accidents	
Multiple sclerosis	

* Data from a variety of sources including personal experience.

early response to tricyclic drugs. An increase in REM latency and a decrease in total REM sleep time within 2 days of the initiation of medication predicts a good response.

PRINCIPLES OF THERAPY

The initiation of treatment of the depressed patient should be based on a correct diagnosis, an assessment of the severity of the condition, the degree of suicidal risk, available social support systems, the need for further studies, the advisability of hospitalization, and a decision as to whether the patient should be treated by his or her physician or by referral to a psychiatrist. Suicidal potential should always be a primary concern, because suicide is in fact the eighth most common cause of death in the United States, and apparently half of these are by depressed patients. Consideration should also be given to the fact that tricyclics are the most prescribed medication used in suicide (National Poison Control statistics). General measures to be initiated include attention to the patient's nutritional state (avoid starvation, dehydration) and providing active leadership in decision making, because these patients' condi-

tions often render them indecisive, without further damaging their self-esteem. Not infrequently, prescribing a mild sedative to be taken in the evening may be helpful in treating sleep disturbances. It is important also to convey to the patient the fact that his or her pain is being understood and to give the patient a feeling of hope. Current available therapies especially in acute depressions afford patients the prospect of a good prognosis.

Two major classes of antidepressants are currently in use. The most widely used are the tricyclic antidepressants (TCAs), whose action seems to be related to their capacity to potentiate the CNS actions of norepinephrine and serotonin. The most commonly used of these are imipramine and amitriptyline. The other class includes the monoamine oxidase inhibitors (MAOIs) such as tranylcypromine and phenelzine. The antidepressant action of the MAOIs is thought to be related to their ability to block the metabolism (degradation) of norepinephrine and serotonin. Adverse reactions are more common with the MAOIs than the TCAs. The choice of a particular antidepressant will depend on the patient's initial clinical picture, what has worked well for the patient or similarly affected family members in the past, the

TABLE 132–3.
Commonly Used Tricyclic and Related Antidepressants and Their Characteristics*

GENERIC NAME	TRADE NAME	EFFECT	DAILY DOSAGE RANGE (MG)	COMMENTS
Amitriptyline	Elavil and others	Mostly serotonergic	75–300	Sedatives
Imipramine	Tofranil and others	Mostly noradrenergic	75–300	
Desipramine	Norpramin	Noradrenergic	75–300	Metabolite of imipramine; least anticholinergic
Nortriptyline	Aventyl	Both	40–100	Metabolite of amitriptyline
Protriptyline	Vivactil	Both	15–60	Least sedating
Doxepin	Sinequan, Adapin	Both	75–300	Very sedating; least cardiotoxic
Amoxapine	Asendin	Both	200–300	Rapid onset of action of neuroleptics also extra-pyramidal symptoms and other side-effects
Trazodone	Desyrel	Serotonergic	200–300	Little cardiotoxicity

* Adapted from Waldinger RJ: *Psychiatry for Medical Students.* Washington, DC, American Psychiatric Press, Inc, 1984, p 373.

anticholinergic and cardiovascular effects of the antidepressant, and the degree of sedation desired. The commonly used tricyclics and related antidepressants, their characteristics, ranges of daily dosage, and other effects are shown in Table 132–3.

Side-effects are generally related to autonomic, anticholinergic, CNS, and cardiovascular effects. Postural hypotension, urinary retention, narrow-angle glaucoma, and paralytic ileus are some of the more troublesome side-effects. Such complications as drowsiness, sweating, and imbalance can often be managed by drug reduction or change to another drug in the same class. The MAOIs are generally second choices particularly because of their potentially dangerous side-effects (hypertensive crisis) precipitated by the ingestion of foods containing tyramine (certain chceses, wines, and herring).

All medications should begin with a low dose gradually raised to the recommended effective dosage range or until undesirable side-effects signal a need to change or stop. Typical lag time is 3 weeks to 4 weeks. These precautions are especially important in the geriatric population in whom such drug use should be carefully titrated. Doses may be divided into two or three daily doses or later a single daily dose given at bedtime. Measurements of serum drug levels can be helpful in adjusting to a proper therapeutic range.

Electroconvulsive therapy (ECT) is an effective and rapid treatment for patients who are severely depressed, agitated, and suicidal. This therapy induces a seizure by passing a controlled electric current through the brain. Fracture and other undesirable side-effects are avoided by the use of a muscle relaxant (succinylcholine) and general anesthesia. The course of treatment varies, with the usual number of treatments between six and twelve at a rate of three to four per week. A series of treatments (of as many as three treatments at one time) to hasten recovery has been reported, but this procedure is not generally recommended.

Psychologic therapies can include individual, group, or cognitive psychotherapy and can be either supporting or uncovering. Supportive psychotherapy is aimed more at the treatment of the current disability consequent to the illness (symptomatic treatment). Uncovering psychotherapy is aimed at helping the individual gain a deeper understanding of his or her mental functioning and coping mechanisms, with the intent of avoiding depressions in the future. Group psychotherapy is designed to help depressed persons improve their social skills and self-esteem in a mutually supportive environment. Cognitive therapy has the intent of correcting a tendency to think in negative and pessimistic terms about one's self and the world and is based on the premise that the depressive mood is consequent to depressive thinking rather than concomitant to it. This premise is open to question.

Recent studies have shown the superiority of combined psychotherapy and pharmacotherapy over the use of either by itself. No one treatment is universally effective, and none has been shown to be the treatment of choice for all depressions. Pharmacotherapy can be useful in preventing relapses, and psychotherapy in adding to interpersonal and social functioning. Decisions about treatment should be based on the availability of resources, on the patient's willingness to comply, and on the patient's motivation.

REFERENCES

Fawcett J: DSM III and the treatment of depressive disorders. In, *Psychiatry: Clinical Update Monograph for 1985.* Kalamazoo Mich, Upjohn Co, 1985. *A concise presentation of the treatment of depressive states.*

Garfinkel P, Emmanuel P: Affective disorders, in Greben SE, Rakoff VM, Voineskos G (eds): *A Method of Psychiatry.* Philadelphia, Lea & Febiger, 1985, pp 158–172. *A good review of the entire subject of affective disorders.*

Kaplan HI, Sadock BJ: *Modern Synopsis of Comprehensive Textbook of Psychiatry, III.* Baltimore, Williams & Wilkins, 1981. *A good, very brief overview of affective disorders.*

Kolb LC, Brodie KH: *Modern Clinical Psychiatry,* ed 10. Philadelphia, WB Saunders Co, 1982, pp 404–443. *A very good concise review of the subject of depression.*

Waldinger RJ: *Psychiatry for Medical Students.* Washington DC, American Psychiatric Press, Inc, 1984. *A good diagrammatic presentation of the symptoms and pharmacotherapy of depressive disorders.*

Webb L.J., DiClemente CC et al: *Training Guide to Diagnostic and Statistical Manual of Mental Disorders,* ed 3. Washington DC, Brunner/Mazel, Inc, American Psychiatric Association, 1980. *An excellent graphic presentation of the range of the classification of affective disorders.*

133 SCHIZOPHRENIA

Abraham Heller, M.D.
Arnold Allen, M.D.

Modern concepts of schizophrenia, a psychosis and the most serious of all psychiatric disorders, originated with Emil Kraepelin in 1896. This German psychiatrist, after studying and minutely describing thousands of cases of severely ill patients, drew together in one disease entity those distinguished by early onset of gross disorganization of thought, expression, and behavior, and who followed a course ending in apparent dementia. Kraepelin drew upon earlier contributions that delineated types of the common disease entity he proposed. Kahlbaum in 1863 had delineated *dementia paranoides,* characterized by delusions with disorganized thought and behavior; and in 1868, described *catatonia,* in which patients remained mute, unreactive, and in fixed and sometimes bizarre postures. Morel, in 1856, had described *demence precoce*, an illness with teenage onset and a course leading to intellectual and behavioral deterioration. Hecker, in 1870, described an illness with early onset and profound disorganization of thought and behavior, which he termed *hebephrenia*, after Hebe, the Greek goddess of youth, reflecting the childlike and often silly character of these patients. Kraepelin saw the diseases delineated by his predecessors as forms of a common disorder, starting in the teenage years or young adulthood, with gross disorganization of thought and behavior, and a downhill course to dementia. Kraepelin, borrowing from Morel, named this common disorder *dementia praecox*.

Eugen Bleuler, a Swiss psychiatrist, saw the clinical picture more broadly. In many cases there was a later age of onset, extending into the fifth decade. The spontaneous course did not always end in deterioration. Many cases, especially those of later and more acute onset, went on to remit spontaneously, partially or wholly. Bleuler's concepts were propounded in 1911 in his classic text, *Dementia Praecox or the Group of Schizophrenias*, in which he theorized that the basic entity was a syndrome in which all cases manifested four primary symptoms, and that secondary or accessory symptoms distinguished the different forms of these disorders (Table 133–1). Bleuler theorized further that these accessory symptoms were restitutive and represented efforts at coping, though manifestly maladaptive. His term, *schizophrenia*, conveys a sense of splitting of mental processes, a lack of congruence, and

consequent fragmentation of the various mental functions.

The current conventional criteria for the diagnosis of schizophrenia are carefully and extensively outlined in the *Diagnostic and Statistical Manual*, DSM-III, of the American Psychiatric Association (Table 133–2). The clinical manifestations involve various mental functions, several simultaneously:

Thinking: is predominantly affected, manifested in persecutory or grandiose delusions, looseness of logical associations of one thought with another, concrete or literal interpretations, with resulting incoherence and irrationality.

Perception: may be disturbed, manifested in hallucinations, most commonly of the auditory type.

Feeling: (affect) is either inappropriate in relation to thought and behavior, or is blunted or flat.

Behavior: may be strange, irrational, and sometimes stereotyped in fixed, odd patterns.

These clinical manifestations make up the surface evidence of the impairment—ranging from mild to profound according to the severity of the illness—that affects the sufferer's sense of self and interpersonal, social and economic competence, and fosters the tendency for the patient to lead a life of isolation and withdrawal.

The cause of schizophrenia is yet unknown. Current theories center on biologic—hereditary and neurochemical—and psychosocial factors.

TABLE 133–1.
Bleuler's Symptoms of Schizophrenia

PRIMARY SYMPTOMS

Association of thoughts which are loosely connected and become illogical or fragmented
Affect (feeling or emotion) which is blunted, flat, or inappropriate
Autism in which thinking is grossly idiosyncratic and out of touch with common, consensual reality
Ambivalence of thinking, feeling, or behaving, in which opposite extremes are manifested simultaneously or in rapid alternation without apparent subjective contradiction

SECONDARY SYMPTOMS (ACCESSORY, RESTITUTIVE, AND PATHOLOGIC ATTEMPTS AT ADAPTATION)

Paranoid type, characterized by grandiose or persecutory delusions with or without hallucinations
Hebephrenic type, characterized by grossly disorganized, regressed thinking and behavior
Catatonic type, characterized by stupor, rigidity, motionless posturing, and muteness
Simple type, without distinguishing secondary characteristics

TABLE 133–2.
Criteria for the Diagnosis of Schizophrenia*

Thought disorder: In form, by loosening of logical associations so that meaning becomes strained, idiosyncratic, or more or less incomprehensible and incoherent. Manifestations may be in the form of *neologisms* (made-up words), *perseveration* (repeated words or thoughts), *clanging* (association of thoughts by similar sounds), or *blocking* (up a blind alley, hanging in air)
Thought disorder: In content, with delusions (fixed, irrational beliefs) of gradiose or persecutory character and/or ideas of reference (belief that unrelated events are specially focused on the patient)
Perceptual disorder: With hallucinations, usually auditory, associated with the delusional thinking
Disorder of affect: Feelings or emotions are blunted, flattened, or inappropriate.
Psychomotor disorder: Poverty of spontaneous movements and reactivity, or purposeless, manneristic, stereotyped behavior
Disordered sense of self: Impaired personal identity, impaired ego boundaries, and differentiation of self from environment
Disordered volition: Impairment of self-initiated, goal-directed behavior; with deterioration from previous level of functioning; with onset before age 45 years, and of at least 6 months duration

SUBTYPES OF SCHIZOPHRENIA

Paranoid type: Characterized by grandiose or persecutory delusions with or without hallucinations
Catatonic type: Characterized either by stuporous unreactivity, rigid immobility and posturing, and muteness, or by purposeless, excited hyperactivity
Disorganized type: Characterized by marked disorganization and incoherence, and flat, incongruous, or silly affect
Undifferentiated type: With disorganization of thought and behavior, without differentiating characteristics of the foregoing subtypes

* Adapted from *Diagnostic and Statistical Manual of Mental Disorders,* ed 3. Washington, DC, American Psychiatric Association, 1980.

TABLE 133–3.
Frequency of Schizophrenia*

POPULATION	PERCENT AT RISK
Lifetime risk of schizophrenia in the general population	1
Frequency of schizophrenia in parents of an affected child	5–10
Frequency of schizophrenia in other full siblings of an affected child	10–15
Frequency of schizophrenia in offspring of two affected parents	40–65
Concordance rates for schizophrenia in dyzygotic twins	10–15
Concordance rates for schizophrenia in monozygotic twins	40–70

* Summarized from studies of risk in families and twins compared to risk in general population.

Family studies consistently show elevated risk of schizophrenia among biologic relatives (Table 133–3). Compared to the established lifetime risk in the general population of 1%, family and twin studies have shown greatly increased risk among biologic relatives.

The evidence for a genetic factor is strong, but one should note that even among monozygotic twins, in perhaps half of the cases, one twin remains free of the disease although the other is affected. Therefore, the prevailing opinion is that there is a genetic, predisposing, loading factor requiring something additional for the eventuation of the disease.

Among psychosocial factors, restrictive over-controlling, overprotective parenting, or conversely, cold, indifferent, or detached parenting, has been implicated in various studies. Distortion in roles of family members or in the manner of communication between family members has been implicated in other studies. In a famous study of the relation of schizophrenia to social class, prevalence rates were shown to increase progressively in successively lower social classes.

Psychopharmacologic investigations of possible mechanisms for the effectiveness of antipsychotic medications have produced the widely discussed dopamine hypothesis. Among many neurotransmitters involved in normal brain chemistry, excessive activity of the dopamine neurotransmitter has been implicated in schizophrenia. The effective medications, it has been found, block dopamine transmission.

Newer brain-imaging techniques are producing significant findings. Computed tomography (CT scan) has found evidence of brain atrophy in a significant minority of schizophrenic patients. Other, newer techniques—positron-emission tomography (PET) scans and nuclear magnetic imaging—demonstrate metabolic as well as anatomical aberrations.

All of the evidence put together is changing the impression about schizophrenia so that it may eventually be recognized as an organic, neurologic disorder.

PRINCIPLES OF THERAPY

Treatments of schizophrenia are empirically based. Studies of the results of treatment influence the currently accepted theories of etiology of the disorder or group of disorders; and treatment methods are in turn influenced by updated etiologic theories. Biologic intervention is predominantly psychopharmacologic. Psychologic treatments are directed toward the individual, group, or family, and at times, some combination of these. Social and vocational interventions are adjunctive to the primary therapies and are the major aspects of rehabilitation.

Earlier studies of schizophrenia and methods for its treatment were based mainly on institutionalized populations of patients. In the present day, with a broader clinical view of schizophrenia, impairment ranges from mild to very serious. The earlier and the more insidious the onset, the more likely a chronic course. The later and more dramatic the onset, the better the prognosis for remission and possible sustained functional recovery. As many as 20% of patients recover and do not go on to a chronic course. The need for the prolonged, institutional hospitalization of former years, even for the chronically impaired, has been greatly reduced by effective antipsychotic medications and sociotherapies. The question of hospital treatment arises in the initial crisis or acute exacerbations in the course of many patients. In many other patients with a less dramatic course of illness but with steady progression of impairment, especially those without constructive family or community supports, the need for hospitalization emerges sooner or later. These patients are likely to be hospitalized for longer periods of time and more often.

The acute cases are apt to develop in the context of crises in the lives of affected patients. For them, crisis intervention therapy is often effective in averting hospitalization. In this method, a combination of medication, individual and family therapy and counseling, and mobilization of interpersonal and community supports is brought to bear intensively over a brief period of time. Still today, when family or community supports are unavailable or not adequate for the requirements, or when the patient is too severely disordered, psychiatric hospitalization becomes an overriding necessity.

Among the elements of the treatment armamentarium on the hospital ward, antipsychotic medication is of prime importance (Table 133–4). Sociotherapies make meaningful additional contributions to hospital treatment. For a long time, occupational therapy and psychiatric social work with families of affected patients have been included in hospital programs. After World War II, milieu therapy became widely instituted in hospital practice with the recognition that the total patient experience in the hospital could contribute positively to the therapeutic process. In the therapeutic community hospital treatment, staff and patients interact in the shared social experience of the ward. Patients as a group are helped by staff to understand the aberrant behavior of individual patients. The patients as a group, with staff encouragement and guidance, provide potent peer pressure on individual patients to relate and behave more appropriately.

TABLE 133–4.
Antipsychotic Medications

Phenothiazines:	chlorpromazine (Thorazine)
	thioridazine (Mellaril)
	mesoridazine (Serentil)
	perphenazine (Trilafon)
	prochlorperazine (Compazine)
	trifluoperazine (Stelazine)
	fluphenazine* (Prolixin)
	acetophenazine (Tindal)
Thioxanthines:	chlorprothixene (Taractan)
	thiothixene (Navane)
Loxapine:	dibenzoxazepine (Loxitane)
Butyrophenone:	haloperidol (Haldol)

* As ester salts, fluphenazines are long-acting, injectable, intramuscular (IM) preparations, useful in managing noncompliant patients.

With the various combinations of methods, the need for institutional care of schizophrenic patients has been vastly reduced. Schizophrenic patients contributed about half of the 560,000 total patients in state and county hospitals in the United States in 1956; today they represent about half of the number, which has been reduced to 130,000. The frequency and length of hospitalization in the treatment careers of schizophrenic patients have also been drastically reduced. Between crisis intervention therapy and hospital treatment, most schizophrenic patients can be stabilized, frequently within days or a few weeks, and seldom longer than a month or two. But despite these treatments which enable these patients to return to families and life in the community, the disorder is in no sense cured.

Clinical responsibility shifts to posthospital care, that is to follow-up ambulatory care for treatment over time, to maintain or improve the gains of the acute treatment, to prevent acute exacerbations, and for social or economic rehabilitation. Medication is still a major element of treatment, although its manifest benefits must be carefully weighed against the potential side-effects (the most serious of which is tardive dyskinesia, a very morbid and often irreversible neuromuscular disorder). Clinical caution is required; doses of medication are to be kept in the lower ranges of effectiveness, with periodic tests of the possibility of lowering dosage or eliminating medication. Psychotherapy—individual, group, or family— is potentially useful in the extended time of outpatient treatment. Social and vocational rehabilitation, aimed at improving functional skills of patients, are of exquisite importance.

Compliance with the regimen of prescribed medication and a living situation with adequate social support in the community are the critical factors in maximizing the patient's capacity for independent living in the community, or for preventing exacerbation and need to return to hospital care.

With proper treatment, the chances of individuals suffering from schizophrenia fulfilling instrumental and self-supporting roles in families and in their respective communities are greatly improved. As befits treatment of any chronic condition, the principle of continuity of care is vital. Acute care, hospital treatment, and posthospital, outpatient treatment and rehabilitation must be coordinated and integrated if the requisite continuity of care system is to work the way that it can.

In summary, the efficacy of antipsychotic medications, well demonstrated in many research studies, makes them the mainstay of treatment. The efficacy of psychosocial therapies by themselves is not so impressively demonstrated in research studies, but they appear to add therapeutic benefits when combined with medication. Although the available therapies are effective in containing their target symptoms and greatly improving the lot of patients, the rate of development of some level of chronicity is little changed. Clinicians and researchers discern that the current, antipsychotic agents selectively affect the acute, target symptoms but do little for the patient's negative symptoms—apathy, isolation, and withdrawal. This is the frontier along which the clinician-investigator must next focus attention.

REFERENCES

Arieti S: *Interpretation of Schizophrenia*. New York, Brunner, 1975. *A most comprehensive clinical coverage of schizophrenia.*

Gregory I, Smeltzer DJ: Schizophrenia, paranoid and similar psychotic disorders, in *Psychiatry, essentials of clinical practice.* ed. 2, Boston, Little Brown, & Co, 1983, pp 245–261. *A concise textbook coverage of schizophrenia.*

Schizophrenic disorders, in *Diagnostic and Statistical Manual of Mental Disorders*, ed 3. Washington, DC, American Psychiatric Association, 1980, pp 181–203. *The definitive classification of mental disorders.*

Special Report: *Schizophrenia 1980*. Washington, DC, US Dept of HHS, PHS, ADAMHA, GPO, 1980. *An authoritative update of significant research and clinical aspects of schizophrenia.*

Abraham Heller, M.D.
Arnold Allen, M.D.

Substances of abuse are, in a chemical sense, drugs taken in the begining for their mind-altering effects. In current clinical usage, substance abuse is diagnosed on the basis of its impairment of health or social or economic functioning. With progression of substance abuse, in some users and with some drugs, tolerance supervenes (metabolic accommodation so that greater amounts of the drug are necessary to maintain the same level of effects), and eventually in some users and with some drugs substance dependence may develop. "Addict" and "addiction" are terms now considered pejorative and outdated; they are too judgmental and associated with the historic neglect by medical services and practitioners of those who suffer the conditions of substance abuse or dependence.

As a model for understanding the sufferers of their conditions, it is completely inadequate to focus on the "offending" substances as if "addiction" is to be understood solely in terms of substance "x." Rather, a more objective and comprehensive model is one of triangular interaction among the drug of abuse, the host-user, and the psychosocial setting. Just as in the case of any stressor—for example, any infectious agent or any stressful life event—the effect on the host is highly variable, and both the stressor and host are very much affected in turn by the context, the ecology (Fig 134–1).

Use of drugs varies widely among individuals in American culture. Among the majority, some drug use, particularly alcohol in various forms, is considered appropriate, normal, and a boon to living. Drugs are taken to heighten individual mood and sense of well-being and for social and recreational purposes. Some drugs are safer than others, but all have potential for abuse by some users and under some social pressures. Alcohol is far and away the predominant drug in American society, partly because it is legally approved and for the important reason that the great majority can use alcohol with more or less moderation and relative safety. Yet 10% to 15% of users become "problem drinkers," alcohol abusers, and alcohol-dependent individuals. These users all together number over 10,000,000 Americans, 5% to 10% of the entire adult population, individuals from every sector and stratum, not excluding professionals and other elite elements of society. Contrary to popular belief, most of these 10,000,000 people are living with their families and working, although they are accruing difficulties and miseries of many varieties for themselves, their families, and for society. Healthwise—since alcohol is a very toxic substance adversely affecting virtually all tissues of the body—the population of abusers are exorbitant overutilizers of health services. It is estimated that 20% to 40% of all hospital admissions (higher rates apply to

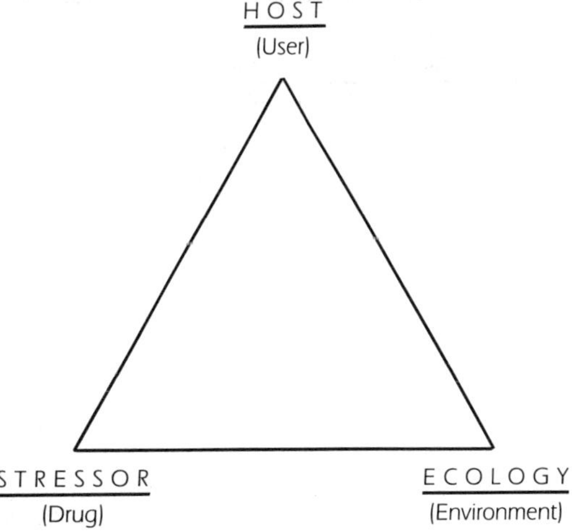

FIG 134–1.
Drug–user–environment interactional model.

emergency room admissions) are for conditions involving drug abuse, mainly of the alcoholic type, and this datum implies a fourfold concentration of abusers in the hospital patient population.

TABLE 134–1.

Characteristics of the Full Syndrome of Alcohol Withdrawal

Coarse tremors
  Hands
  Tongue
  Eyelids
Delirium
  Impaired consciousness
  Impaired memory
  Impaired thinking
  Disorientation
Agitation
Delusions
  Frightening paranoid-type
Hallucinations
  Auditory
  ± visual
  ± tactile
Autonomic hyperactivity
  Tachycardia
  Sweating
  Blood pressure elevation
Insomnia
Nausea and vomiting
Hyperpyrexia
  The ominous, ultimate manifestation of a
  hypermetabolic state

TABLE 134–2.

Physical Health Problems of Alcohol Abusers

Malnutrition and vitamin deficiency
Gastric disorders
Hepatic disorders
Cardiac disorders
Pancreatic disorders
Dermatologic disorders
Encephalopathy
Peripheral neuropathy
Skeletal muscle inflammation, weakness, atrophy
Anemia
Bleeding tendency
Esophageal varices
Testicular atrophy
Proneness to infections
Increased risk of malignancies
Increased risk of suicide
Increased risk of accidental injury
Foreshortened life span (6–10 yr)

Toxic effects of substances of abuse are of two kinds: intoxication (inebriation) and, in the case of some substances but not all, withdrawal syndromes. The common types of toxic effects are the basis of the major groupings of abuse, which are (1) depressants, (2) opioids, (3) stimulants, (4) cannabinoids, and (5) hallucinogens.

DEPRESSANTS

Alcohol and hypnotic-sedative drugs are all neuropharmacologically cross-tolerant. They achieve their effects by depression of the higher centers of the central nervous system. All of the depressants are likely to produce tolerance and psychologic and physiologic dependence if the use is consistent, prolonged, and of sufficient dosage. For individuals, the pattern, amount, and duration all vary widely. Central nervous system effects include dulling of consciousness; impairment of perception, cognition, and judgment; alteration of mood; increased action and reaction times; disinhibition and regression of behavior. Behavior regression is facilitated and may, for example, result in increased conviviality and recreative enjoyment, or may be maladaptive with poor social judgment, inappropriate aggressiveness, risk taking, accidents, destructiveness, and so forth.

As for alcohol, for legal purposes, a blood alcohol level of 100 mg/dl is considered prima facie evidence of intoxication. This legal cut-off point is calculated to eliminate virtually all false positives. In clinical fact, the blood alcohol level correlated with inebriation is broadly variable, and many individuals are impaired by alcohol intoxication at blood concentrations far below the conventional legal designation.

With the development of tolerance, with sustained and heavier drinking, the risk of alcohol withdrawal supervenes. The individual has to maintain a level of drinking to keep ahead of withdrawal manifestations, which threaten to erupt. The early signs and symptoms of alcohol withdrawal include insomnia, shakiness, nausea, anorexia, irritability, and difficulty in concentration. As the severity of withdrawal progresses, typically within 48 hours of cessation of alcoholic intake, or with falling blood level regardless of intake, generalized seizures may occur. Within a week after cessation of intake the full syndrome may emerge (Table 134–1).

Outlined above is the full-blown syndrome of delirium tremens, an extraordinarily morbid condition with a 10% mortality risk. The common "DTs" of alcohol dependence is also the withdrawal syndrome seen with all members of the depressant group of drugs. Other health problems are greatest from alcohol abuse. Its physical problems are outlined in Table 134–2, and its mental problems are listed in Table 134–3.

Diagnosis of substance abuse depends greatly on physician awareness and attention to the possibility of substance abuse in the differential diagnosis of a broad list of physical and mental conditions with which it is correlated. Knowledge of the personal background and life-style of the patient significantly increases the ability of the physician to discern problem use of drugs. Treatment starts with attention to the general physical and mental health of the patient and to any specific drug-related disorders. Withdrawal from the drug of abuse should follow at the earliest possible time. Detoxification—the treatment to withdraw or the treatment of those already undergoing withdrawal—is usually carried out in the hospital setting. Benzodiazepine medication is very effective in achieving physical stability and reducing morbidity while also providing some protection against potential seizures. After the patient's withdrawal, many physicians engage and follow the patient in a therapeutic regimen. Others refer the patient to specialists or to special rehabilitation programs. The personal physician can do much, often more than others, to encourage and mobilize the patient, the family, or important others to face the problem of drug abuse and undertake treatment and rehabilitation.

OPIOIDS (NARCOTICS)

Naturally occurring opium alkaloids and their derivatives, in addition to purely synthetic compounds with similar pharmacologic effects and cross-tolerance, form the opioid group of drugs (Table 134–4).

These drugs are used medically for their potent analgesic-sedative effects. In illicit use,

TABLE 134–3.
Mental Health Problems of Alcohol Abusers: Organic (Brain Syndrome) Disorders

Intoxication
  Memory blackouts
Amnestic
  Korsakoff's disease
  Wernicke's encephalopathy
Delusional
  Paranoid delusions without clouding of consciousness
Hallucinosis
  Auditory ± visual without clouding of consciousness
Affective
  Mood disturbance
  Depression
  Mania
Personality
  Out-of-character behaviors
  Poor judgment
  Loss of impulse control
Dementia
  Loss of intellectual ability
  Impaired memory
  No clouding of consciousness

TABLE 134–4.
Opioid Drugs

Natural opium alkaloids
  Morphine
  Codeine
Derivatives of natural alkaloids
  Oxycodone (Percodan)
  Dihydromorphinone (Dilaudid)
  Oxymorphone (Numorphan)
  Diacetylmorphine (heroin)
Synthetic opioids
  Meperidine (Demerol)
  Methadone (Dolophine)
  Pentazocine (Talwin)
  Dextropropoxyphene (Darvon)

they are taken to achieve a comfortable passive state in which the individual is "on the nod" enjoying peaceful imaginations or dreams. Intravenous heroin, the traditional choice of opiate users for recreational purposes, is taken to enjoy the thrill, however evanescent, of the abdominal "rush," an experience described as of orgastic intensity. Historically, in medicine, long before more appropriate medications became available, opiate drugs were used to relieve depression or to pacify psychotic patients.

Intoxication from the opioids is marked by many of the signs and symptoms listed in Table 134–5.

Opioids have a high addictive potential. With extended and consistent use, increased tolerance and in turn psychologic and physiologic dependence are achieved. The opioid withdrawal syndrome is intensely morbid. Several of the symptoms together mimic a severe flu-like disorder. The manifestations of the syndrome are lacrimation, coryza, rhinorrhea, yawning, pupillary dilatation, piloerection and vermification, sweating, nausea, vomiting, diarrhea, abdominal colic, muscle and bone pain, tachycardia, hypertension, fever, and insomnia. For the patient in relatively good general health, however, withdrawal carries virtually no mortality risk. Health risks derive partly from suppression of appetite and resulting malnourishment. The abuser, with lowered resistance and heedless of asepsis, injects himself or herself with various infectious agents. Infectious hepatitis is common among this drug-abusing group; local and systemically disseminated abscesses are frequent; in occasional cases, subacute bacterial endocarditis is seen. These individuals are prone to accident and injury. Depression is common with a substantial risk of suicide.

Opiate antagonists—naltrexone (Trexan), naloxone (Narcan), nalorphine (Nalline)—by precipitating withdrawal manifestations, provide a diagnostic test for the toxic presence of a narcotic and are also an aid in maintaining a drug-free state (rendering drug intake useless by blocking its effects). Many rehabilitation programs have been based on methadone maintenance; methadone as a substitute for street drugs is dispensed under controlled conditions, provides stabilization, and in appropriate dosage blocks the effects of heroin. Residential treatment programs use behavioral methods reinforced by group and community pressures to achieve a drug-free state and alteration of the individual's outlook and life pattern.

STIMULANTS

The stimulant drugs are taken to achieve euphoria, enhanced sensations, a sense of heightened ability and power, and other, more ineffable aspects of a thrilling "high." The components of the group are phenylethylamines (amphetamine, dextroamphetamine, methamphetamine or "speed"), methylphenidate (Ritalin), coca leaf alkaloid (cocaine), and anorectics (nonamphetamines).

The symptoms of toxicity and the organic and withdrawal syndromes are outlined in Table 134–6.

Adverse health effects result first from the anorexic effects (malnourishment) and sleep deprivation. With lowered resistance, infections are common; when the subject "shoots speed" (injects it intravenously), the grave risks of abscesses and subacute bacterial endocarditis are faced. With elevated blood pressure and cerebrovasospasm, the central nervous system risks are cerebrovascular accident in the short term and dementia in the long term. Psychiatric complications are equally dire and include psychoses, depression, and suicide.

CANNABINOIDS

Marijuana and hashish are preparations of the hemp plant, *Cannabis sativa*. The principal mind-altering constituent is tetrahydrocannabinol (THC). The routes of intake are smoking, ingestion, and occasionally in purified form, intravenously. As usually used, intoxication from marijuana produces mild euphoria, relaxation, an altered sense of time, and increased introspection. Conjunctival inflammation and tachycardia may be observed. With higher doses, depersonalization may be experienced along with hallucinations, confusion, and disorganization of mental functions. Occasionally, users experience panic attacks and may

---

TABLE 134–5.
Characteristics of Opioid Intoxication

Euphoria, dysphoria, or apathy
Drowsiness
Slurred speech
Pin-point pupils
Impaired attention
Impaired memory
Psychomotor retardation
Insensitivity to pain or injury
Impaired judgment

behave in grossly irrational ways. Tolerance to cannabinoids without physiologic withdrawal syndrome is seen. Psychologic dependence on cannabinoids is recognized with everyday drug use and characterized by social and vocational impairment, the "amotivational syndrome."

HALLUCINOGENS

Hallucinogenic drugs are referred to as "psychedelics" for their supposed mind-expanding properties and "psychotomimetics" for their assumed ability to mimic functional psychoses. Some common hallucinogens are synthetic (lysergic acid diethylamide [LSD], dimethyltryptamine [DMT], phenylisopropylamine [DOM or STP], phencyclidine [PCP]), and some are from natural sources (peyote cactus [mescaline], mushrooms [psylocybin], morning glory seeds, nutmeg).

These drugs are taken for their subjective effects, for the increase in sense of awareness and vivid perception, and for the feeling of "tripping," expanding into the universe, and experiencing it more wonderfully. The clinical manifestations are listed in Table 134–7. In the aftermath of hallucinogen use, some individuals experience "flashbacks," a repetition of the intoxication hallucinations with their attendant thoughts and feelings, most often intense fear or panic. PCP ("angel dust"), a veterinary anesthetic, is an anomalous member of the hallucinogen group. Its toxic psychosis is often more intense and enduring with gross distortion of bodily image and disorganization of thought. Violent behavior may be unleashed. The patient in a severe state of PCP toxicity is at risk of coma and death.

Treatment of hallucinogen intoxications involves first reassurance, limitation of environmental stimuli, and helping the patient to feel safe while drug effects wear off. With PCP intoxication particularly, some major antipsychotic medications should be avoided because they might dangerously complicate the anticholinergic propensity of PCP. When psychotic agitation from hallucinogen intoxication forces the use of medication to control it, diazepam can be given safely, or haloperidol can be considered because it is a low-dose, high-potency antipsychotic.

TABLE 134–6.
Clinical Manifestations of Stimulant Drug Abuse

Intoxication symptoms
  Euphoria
  Elation, grandiosity
  Pupillary dilation
  Tachycardia, palpitations
  Increased blood pressure
  Perspiration
  Nausea, vomiting
  Headache
Organic brain syndromes
  With persistent, heavy use
Organic delusional disorder
  With paranoia and hostile aggressiveness
Organic delirium
  With confusion and incoherence
Organic dementia
  With intellectual and other deterioration
Withdrawal syndrome
  Fatigue, apathy, depression, somnolence, disturbed sleep, increased dreaming

TABLE 134–7.
Clinical Manifestations of Hallucinogenic Drug Abuse

Intoxication, various combinations of:
  Vivid perception
  Synesthesia ("seeing" sound in color)
  Depersonalization/derealization
  Distorted body image
  Loss of boundary between self and universe
  Illusions
  Hallucinations
  Delusions
  Depression, anxiety, or elation
  Pupillary dilation
  Tachycardia
  Palpitations
  Sweating
  Tremors
  Increased blood pressure
  Increased body temperature
  Increased blood glucose level
Tolerance
  Develops rapidly
Dependence
  None
Adverse reactions
  Panic
  Risk of suicide

POLYDRUG ABUSERS

Another group of users in a sense are the polydrug abusers. These individuals use combinations of drugs, which may vary from time to time according to availability. "Street" drugs may be in a combination unknown to the consumer. Patients who are given prescriptions of analgesics and antianxiety agents may iatrogenically become dependent on both.

SCREENING

The physician is in a unique position to screen and identify those with drug use problems. Awareness of drug-related disorders together with a knowledge of the patient's life-style and experiences will bring forth attention to substance abuse in the differential diagnosis. The physician may supplement his or her clinical skill by increasingly sensitive, practical, affordable, and available laboratory screening tests for substance abuse.

REFERENCES

Cohen S: *The Substance Abuse Problems.* New York, Haworth Press, 1981. *An authoritative text on substance abuse.*

Diagnostic and Statistical Manual of Mental Disorders, ed 3. Washington, DC, American Psychiatric Association, 1980. Organic brain syndromes (pp 103–128). Substance-induced organic mental disorders (pp 128–139). *The definitive coverage with clinical criteria for the diagnosis of mental disorders associated with substance abuse.*

National Council on Alcoholism: Criteria for the Diagnosis of alcoholism. *Ann Intern Med* 1972; 77:249–258. and *Am J Psychiatry* 1972; 129: 127–135. *This presentation of a strategy of assessment and of the criteria for diagnosis of alcohol dependence was published simultaneously in these two prestigious journals. The article provides authoritative diagnostic criteria.*

Schuckit MA: *Drug and Alcohol Abuse, a Clinical Guide to Diagnosis and Treatment.* New York, Plenum, 1979. *A concise coverage of substance abuse.*

part XI

Joint, Connective Tissue and Skeletal Disorders

Alice Faryna, M.D.

Rheumatoid arthritis (RA) is a systemic disease of unknown etiology, which is characterized by the way it affects the joints clinically and radiographically. Typical adult rheumatoid arthritis may be defined as a seropositive (for rheumatoid factor), symmetric, large and small joint polyarthritis plus one of the following: subcutaneous nodules or radiographic erosions of the joints. The prevalence of rheumatoid arthritis is about 1% with a peak incidence in the age group 25 to 55 years and a female:male ration of 2.5:1.

CLINICAL SIGNS AND SYMPTOMS

In approximately two-thirds of patients, rheumatoid arthritis begins insidiously. Fatigue, malaise, and generalized myalgia or stiffness may precede overt joint symptoms by weeks or months. Up to 15% of patients may have an explosive acute onset of polyarticular synovitis. Rarely, adult patients may present with Still's disease (high remittent fever in association with an evanescent macular rash, followed by joint pain and swelling). Another rare representation is that of palindromic rheumatism. This syndrome resembles gout in that the patient experiences pain and swelling in one to three joints, which spontaneously resolve in a few days only to recur weeks or months later. The remainder (15% to 20% of patients) have a subacute onset with progression of symptoms over a period of several weeks.

The pattern of joint involvement also varies. Monoarticular onset, usually in the knee, occurs in 20% of patients; oligoarticular onset occurs in over 40%, while polyarticular (defined as greater than four joints) onset occurs in only 35%. Typically, the wrist and small joints of the hands are affected first, with involvement of large joints and lower extremities proceeding in an additive rather than migratory fashion. Morning stiffness lasting from 30 minutes to several hours is an almost universal feature. Anorexia and weight loss are common. As the disease progresses, patients experience greater difficulty in performing tasks such as personal grooming, dressing, writing, or vocational duties. A small percentage develop overt systemic manifestations such as numbness, chest pain, dyspnea, ocular discomfort, or leg ulcers.

A low-grade fever may be present at physical examination. Affected joints show tenderness on palpation and movement. Soft tissue swelling is present over the affected joints, and may extend over tendon sheaths. Effusion may be detectable, except in deeply situated joints such as the shoulder and hip. The overlying skin may be warm, but redness is less commonly detected. Muscle atrophy near affected joints is common. Range of motion is often restricted. Subcutaneous nodules over pressure points and joints are present at onset in less than 20% of patients, but appear at some time during the course of the disease in up to 35%. Lymphadenopathy and splenomegaly may be present in early stages of the disease.

Initially, the distribution of involved joints may be asymmetric, but eventually most patients develop widespread symmetric synovitis (Table 135–1). Although any synovial joint may be affected, it is unusual to find inflammatory changes in the distal interphalangeal joints or the thoracolumbar spine.

If the inflammatory process is not checked, deformities are likely to occur. Subluxation of the metacarpophalangeal and metatarsophalangeal joints leads to ulnar deviation of the fingers and "cock-up" toes, respectively. Stretching, rupture, or displacement of finger extensors leads to swan-neck and boutonnière deformities of the fingers. Flexion contractures of the elbows and fingers are common. Popliteal cysts may be palpable behind the knees and may rupture into the calf, simulating thrombophlebitis.

Extra-articular manifestations are generally associated with severe destructive joint disease and high titers of rheumatoid factor (RF). Because these manifestations may be clinically asymptomatic, their exact incidences in rheu-

matoid arthritis are not known, and they may not be detected during ordinary clinical examinations (Table 135–2). The most common sites are the skin, eyes, lung, pericardium, and peripheral nerves. Skin lesions include subcutaneous nodules, leg ulcers, and small digital infarcts, usually of little clinical consequence. The neuropathy may be a direct consequence of the rheumatoid process (vasculitis or a rheumatoid nodule occurring in a nerve trunk) or an indirect effect such as entrapment neuropathy or secondary amyloidosis. The most common site of entrapment occurs in the carpal tunnel, but other sites such as the elbow, popliteal space, and tarsal tunnel are not rare. Central nervous system involvement is rare. Catastrophic events are rare, but may be prevented if the physician is alert to early symptoms (Table 135–3). Renal disease occurring in a patient with rheumatoid arthritis suggests a drug reaction, an alternate diagnosis such as systemic lupus erythematosis, or a complication (amyloidosis or necrotizing vasculitis).

Spontaneous remissions are reported to occur in approximately 10% of cases. Reliability of such statistics depends on the method of the original diagnosis. Only 30% of patients origi-

TABLE 135–1.

Joints Commonly Involved in Rheumatoid Arthritis*

JOINTS	PERCENT OF PATIENTS (%)
Metacarpophalangeal	87
Wrist	82
Proximal interphalangeal	63
Knee	56
Cervical spine	54
Ankle	53
Cricoarytenoid	50
Metatarsophalangeal	48
Shoulder	47
Elbow	21

* Data from Kelly et al., 1985; McCarty, 1985; and Winfield G, Young A, Williams P, Corbett M: Prospective study of the radiological changes in hands, feet and cervical spine in adult rheumatoid disease, *Ann Rheum Dis* 1983; 42:613–618.

TABLE 135–2.

Extra-articular Manifestations of Rheumatoid Arthritis

FEATURES	FREQUENCY OF CLINICAL DETECTION (% OF ALL PATIENTS)	FREQUENCY OF DETECTION SELECTED SERIES OF PATIENTS
Subcutaneous nodules	25–35	
Sicca complex	9–34	
Neuropathy		
Diffuse sensory	Not available	35% to 40% by electromyogram
Entrapment	>30	
Myelopathy	1–10	
Lymphadenopathy	12–29	
Splenomegaly	15	
Pericarditis	10	30% to 50% at autopsy or echocardiography
Digital or leg ulcers	8–10	
Pleuritis/effusions	5	40% to 50% at autopsy
Felty's syndrome	<5	
Interstitial fibrosis	1.6–4.5	20% in hospital RA cases
Necrotizing vasculitis	<1	
Lung nodules	<1	35% in miners with RA
Episcleritis/scleritis	Rare	
Necrotizing bronchiolitis	Rare	
Myocarditis/valvulitis	Rare	5% to 10% at autopsy
Myositis	Rare	33% on biopsy
Amyloidosis	Rare	5.2% of hospital RA; 14% to 26% at autopsy

TABLE 135–3.
Clinical–Pathologic Correlations of Rheumatoid Arthritis

CLINICAL FINDINGS		PATHOLOGIC FINDINGS
FEATURE	COMPLICATION	
Episcleritis	Perforation of globe	Nodulosis and vasculitis
Pericardial effusion	Cardiac tamponade	Pericarditis
Dyspnea	Cor pulmonale	Interstitial fibrosis
Weakness, hyperreflexia, sensory loss; occipital pain	Quadriplegia	Cervical subluxation
Felty's syndrome	Sepsis; 5-year mortality rate of 36%	Sequestration of neutrophils; possible immune destruction;
Hoarseness/stridor	Respiratory failure	Fixation of cricoarytenoid joints in adduction
Rash, abdominal pain, mononeuritis multiplex	2-year mortality rate of 24%	Necrotizing vasculitis
Amyloidosis	Renal failure, neuropathy, congestive failure	Infiltration of kidneys, peripheral nerves, heart, skin, gastrointestinal tract

nally classified as definite rheumatoid arthritis by the criteria of the American Rheumatism Association (Table 135–4) appear to have rheumatoid arthritis on follow-up 3 years to 5 years later. When the more stringent New York criteria were applied to the original cohort, only 43% were designated as having rheumatoid arthritis. Of this group 65% could still be classified as having rheumatoid arthritis on follow-up. Possible explanations are that mild and early disease has a better prognosis, or that the criteria are not sufficiently specific. Between 20% to 30% of patients have an intermittent course characterized by partial or complete but temporary remissions. The majority (60% to 70%) have a chronic progressive course leading to decreased functional ability. From 3% to 5% are unresponsive to any form of therapy and are severely disabled. Patients with high titers of RF tend to have a more severe and complicated course. A slight decrease in longevity has been reported for patients with rheumatoid arthritis and is attributed to the small subset of patients with unresponsive disease. Deaths directly related to rheumatoid arthritis are primarily from infection, necrotizing vasculitis, and amyloidosis. Additional morbidity and mortality result from adverse drug reactions (gastrointestinal bleeding, bone marrow suppression, renal failure), extra-articular infections, and surgical complications. Recently, a slight excess of mortality from lymphoid malignancy has been reported.

PATHOPHYSIOLOGY

Immunopathogenesis is suggested by the strong association of rheumatoid arthritis with the HLA type Dr4 (a gene product of the immune response region of chromosome 6) and by evidence of the activation of macrophages, T cells, and B cells in the synovium. The earliest synovial lesions are hyperemia, synovial cell proliferation, neutrophil infiltration, and obliteration of small vessels by thrombi. Lymphocytes form perivascular aggregates, at times resembling lymphoid follicles. T cells predominate, but there is controversy about the relative proportions of helper and suppressor-cytotoxic cells. A variety of immunoglobulins are produced by the plasma cells. It is postulated that IgG or low molecular weight IgM rheumatoid factors form immune complexes with other IgG molecules, activating the complement cascade. Chemotactic molecules (C5a, C3a) cause an influx of neutrophils. During phagocytosis of immune complexes, destructive lysosomal enzymes and oxygen radicals are released. Other inflammatory mediators include prostaglandins and leukotrienes produced by injured cells, histamine from mast cells, complement fragments, and monocyte products, notably interleukin 1. Components of the coagulation system are also activated, contributing to the microvascular thrombosis that is part of the rheumatoid lesion. Collagenases participate in the degradation of cartilage. In addition, the hypertrophied synovium may form a chronic granulomatous mass (pannus), which invades and destroys cartilage and bone providing the typical erosive lesion. The inciting antigen for this process is unknown. Type II collagen, viruses, *Mycoplasma* organisms, IgG, and bacterial cell wall products are among potential etiologic agents under investigation.

CLINICAL–PATHOLOGIC CORRELATIONS

The earliest joint symptoms, pain, stiffness, and swelling, are the result of local inflammation, synovial hypertrophy, and effusion. Mediators involved in these events are vasoactive amines, arachadonic acid products, lymphokines, and complement products. Destruction of articular cartilage, tendons, and bone results from the effects of collagenases, elastases, and oxygen radicals produced by phagocytes. Monocyte products induce fever (interleukin 1) and synovial proliferation (angiogenesis factor, interleukin 1). An indolent non-necrotizing small vessel vasculitis is an integral part of the rheumatoid process in both the synovium and extra-articular sites. Complement components and immunoglobulin have been identified in vessel walls of the synovium and other involved organs, supporting the theory that immune complex disease plays a central role in rheumatoid arthritis. A wide array of clinical complications may occur as a consequence of the articular and extra-articular lesions (Table 135–3).

DIFFERENTIAL DIAGNOSIS

The conditions most easily confused with rheumatoid arthritis are primarily osteoarthritis, systemic lupus erythematosus, polymyalgia rheumatica, fibrositis, and the spondylarthropathies. A summary of the distinctive features of these and other polyarticular disorders is given in Table 135–5.

DIAGNOSIS

The classification criteria for RA of the American Rheumatism Association were revised in 1987 (Table 135–4), greatly simplifying the

TABLE 135–4.
Classification Criteria for Rheumatoid Arthritis

1. Morning stiffness of at least 1 hour for at least 6 weeks
2. Swelling of 3 or more joints for at least 6 weeks
3. Swelling of wrist, proximal interphalanageal or metacarpophalangeal joints for at least 6 weeks
4. Symmetry of swelling
5. Typical hand x-ray changes
6. Subcutaneous nodules
7. Presence of rheumatoid factor in the serum

Source: Arnett EC, Edworthy S, Bloch DA, et al: The revised ARA criteria for rheumatoid arthritis. *Arthritis Rheum* 1987; 30(suppl)S17:45.

1958 criteria without any loss of sensitivity or specificity. The presence of any 4 of the 7 criteria have a sensitivity of 93% and a specificity of 90% (compared to 92% and 85%, respectively, of the old criteria). The qualifying terms "classical," "definite," and "probable" are no longer used.

There are no laboratory tests specific for rheumatoid arthritis. It is common to find mild leukocytosis, increased erythrocyte sedimentation rate, and elevation of a variety of acute phase reactants such as the C-reactive protein. The urinalysis is normal. In cases of relatively aggressive disease, a mild normochromic, normocytic anemia and thrombocytosis are common. Rheumatoid factor is found in only one-third of patients at onset, but ultimately appears in 70% to 80%, usually by the end of the first year. Rheumatoid factor is not specific for rheumatoid arthritis, so that if the initial features are atypical, other causes of RF formation such as viral infections, chronic bacterial infections (e.g., subacute bacterial endocarditis), tuberculosis, syphilis, parasitic disease, sarcoidosis, and connective tissue diseases should be considered. A mild polyclonal increase in gamma globulin may be found. Serum complement levels are normal or slightly elevated. Cryoglobulins are found in up to 26% of patients overall, but in virtually all RA patients with necrotizing vasculitis. The antinuclear antibody test is positive in 15% to 25%.

The earliest radiographic changes are periarticular soft tissue swelling and osteopenia. When cartilage loss occurs, the joint space will show uniform narrowing. Erosions ultimately occur in over 70% of patients, but may not be apparent for the first 1 to 2 years. The erosions usually begin in the "bare" areas where the ar-

TABLE 135–5.
Differential Diagnosis of Rheumatoid Arthritis

DISORDER	RHEUMATOID ARTHRITIS-LIKE FEATURES	DIFFERENCES WITH RHEUMATOID ARTHRITIS
Osteoarthritis	Symmetric deformities of digits	Bony rather than soft tissue prominences; morning stiffness lasts less than 15 min; x-ray film shows osteophytes and subchondral sclerosis; no erosions; normal ESR
Polymyalgia rheumatica	Symmetric pain; prolonged morning stiffness	Rarely detectable synovitis; small joints spared; very high ESR
Fibrositis	Symmetric pain; complaints of stiffness	Normal results of joint examination, laboratory tests and x-ray films; tender points in characteristic sites
Systemic lupus erythematosus	Symmetric arthritis; RF-positive in 20%; similar hand deformities	Rarely erosive; anti-DNA and low complement levels in 60% of patients; skin, renal, and CNS features
Spondylarthropathy	Inflammatory joint effusions and ocular inflammation may occur.	Usually RF-negative; sacroiliitis and enthesopathy; oligoarticular and asymmetric; skin lesions
Psoriatic arthritis	Inflammatory joint effusions and ocular inflammation may occur.	RF-negative; may have erosions of distal interphalangeal joints Nail lesions common
Gout	May become polyarticular; tophaceous nodules; bony erosions	Asymmetric; erosions often beyond bare area; urate crystals in fluid Negative RF despite nodules
Pseudogout	Polyarticular in 5% of patients	Chondrocalcinosis; calcium pyrophosphate crystals in fluid
Rheumatic fever	Polyarticular; subcutaneous nodules	High fever; migratory rather than additive arthritis; resolves in 4 weeks; rash and carditis
Sjögren's syndrome (primary)	RF-positive; polyarthritis; sicca complex	History of parotitis; may affect gastrointestinal tract, kidney

ticular cartilage joins the bone and the synovial membrane attaches. Rheumatoid arthritis patients are not good bone-formers, so it is unusual to see ankylosis or osteophytes. Synovial fluid examination reveals type 2 inflammatory fluid (a WBC count of 2,000 to 50,000 with 75% neutrophils or greater). Complement levels are usually depressed. The glucose level varies from 40% to 90% of serum levels.

Synovial biopsy shows villous hypertrophy with proliferation of synovial cells and infiltration by mononuclear cells. The vessels show focal infiltration by neutrophils. Microthrombi may be found, and immunoglobulins plus complement may be found within the vessel walls. The villi often have areas of necrosis and fibrin deposition. Older lesions are relatively acellular and fibrotic.

Histologic study of the rheumatoid nodules shows central necrosis surrounded by a pallisade of elongated cells, which are surrounded by chronic inflammatory cells. The synovial and nodular histopathologic changes are not specific for rheumatoid arthritis.

PRINCIPLES OF PREVENTION AND THERAPY

There are no known preventive measures. Early treatment consists of full anti-inflammatory doses of salicylate or other nonsteroidal anti-inflammatory drugs. Acutely inflamed joints should be rested or splinted, but periodic range-of-motion exercises should be done to prevent atrophy and contractures. Progressive disease despite these measures may require slow-acting drugs such as gold, penicillamine, shows central necrosis surrounded by a palisade of elongated cells, which are surrounded by chronic inflammatory cells. The synovial and nodular histopathologic changes are not specific for rheumatoid arthritis.

PRINCIPLES OF PREVENTION AND THERAPY

There are no known preventive measures. Early treatment consists of full anti-inflammatory doses of salicylate or other nonsteroidal anti-inflammatory drugs. Acutely inflamed joints should be rested or splinted, but periodic range-of-motion exercises should be done to prevent atrophy and contractures. Progressive disease despite these measures may require slow-acting drugs such as gold, penicillamine, or azathioprine. Because these drugs are more toxic, their use must be monitored for side-effects according to established protocols and should be given only to patients with potentially reversible joint disease. Corticosteroids are used only as adjunctive therapy in doses not exceeding 10 mg of prednisone per day. Occasional intra-articular injections of corticosteroids can be beneficial. Cytotoxic drugs and total lymphoid irradiation are experimental therapies reserved for aggressive and unresponsive disease. Splinting, physical therapy, and education in joint protection are valuable adjunctive measures. Rehabilitative surgery plays a major role in improving the functional capacity of patients with deformities, disabling pain, or unrelenting synovitis. Involved joints are more susceptible to infection than normal joints. Synovial fluid culture and Gram's stain should be done when there is disproportionate pain and swelling in a particular joint.

REFERENCES

Blechman WJ, Gottlieb NL (eds): Oral gold therapy in rheumatoid arthritis. *Am J Med* 1983; 75(suppl) (6A):1–164. *Contains sections on oral gold and methotrexate as well as on conventional second-line drugs for the treatment of rheumatoid arthritis.*

Gordon DA, Stein JL, Broden I: The extra-articular features of rheumatoid arthritis. *Am J Med* 1973; 54:445–452. *This valuable report details 127 rheumatoid patients who were examined for extra-articular features according to a standardized protocol and followed for 5 years. Because the original cohort was a hospital population, the prevalence figures cannot be generalized to all rheumatoid patients.*

Kelley WN, Harris ED, Ruddy S, Sledge CB: *Textbook of rheumatology*, ed 2. Philadelphia, WB Saunders Co, 1985, pp 725–857, 879–955. *Most comprehensive text on pathogenesis and treatment.*

Masi AT, Feigenbaum SL: Seronegative rheumatoid arthritis: Fact or fiction? *Arch Intern Med* 1983; 143:2167–2172. *A helpful essay on the problem of the atypical rheumatoid arthritis patient.*

McCarty DJ: *Arthritis and Allied Conditions*, ed 10. Philadelphia, Lea & Febiger, 1985, pp 453–667. *Good overall textbook. The section on salicylates and nonsteroidal anti-inflammatory drugs is current and eminently readable.*

136 SYSTEMIC LUPUS ERYTHEMATOSUS

Robert A. Hawkins, M.D.

Systemic lupus erythematosus is a chronic inflammatory disease of unknown cause characterized by multiorgan involvement. Although many immunologic abnormalities are present, a hallmark of the disease is the presence in the serum of antinuclear antibodies (ANA) and other autoantibodies participating in immunologically mediated tissue injury. A limited form of the disease, discoid lupus erythematosus is usually confined to the skin. In contrast, systemic lupus erythematosus commonly involves the skin, joints, kidneys, nervous and cardiopulmonary systems, and other organs. It is also characterized by periods of exacerbation and remission.

CLINICAL SIGNS AND SYMPTOMS

The typical patient is female (the incidence ratio is 9:1, women to men), between the ages of 15 and 45 years, complaining of fatigue, low-grade fever, and joint pain, although any of the features listed in Table 136–1 may be present at onset of disease. Skin rashes are common and may take many forms. The typical acute lesion (butterfly rash) is a mildly edematous erythematous rash over the cheeks and bridge of the nose resembling the malar mask of the wolf (*lupus* in Latin means wolf). Frequently precipitated by sun exposure, it may be present only intermittently, and heals without scarring. Similar photosensitive rashes may occur on other parts of the body commonly exposed to the sun. Other cutaneous manifestations include bullae, purpura, hives, and discoid lesions.

Discoid lupus erythematosus represents the chronic, scarring form of skin disease, initially seen as scaling red papules on the face, scalp, shoulders, and arms. These resolve as atrophic depigmented plaques. The discoid form of the disease usually occurs entirely without other abnormalities; however, in about 5% of the patients, the systemic form of disease develops. A subacute cutaneous lesion occurs that is intermediate in severity between the acute maculopapular eruption and the chronic discoid lesion. Mucous membrane lesions in systemic lupus erythematosus consist of oral and nasal ulcers, which may or may not be painful. Alopecia occurs and is usually diffuse, but may be patchy. Raynaud's phenomenon of the fingers and toes occurs in a minority of patients.

Arthralgias and, less commonly, arthritis are the most common initial complaints. The joints may appear normal or may be warm, tender, and swollen. Articular pain is usually transient and migratory and involves the joints of the hands, wrists, and knees more often than other joints. In contrast to the findings in rheumatoid arthritis, the synovial fluid white blood cell counts are usually low, and destruction and deformities of the joints are rare. Because of the transient nature and paucity of physical findings characteristic of joint involvement, patients with systemic lupus erythematosus who have fatigue, fever, and arthralgias when they are first seen are frequently diagnosed as having psychogenic disease.

Renal involvement is common and usually of mild severity. Diffuse proliferative glomerulonephritis, however, can cause irreversible renal failure and represents one of the most serious complications of systemic lupus erythematosus. Most patients have lesser degrees of renal parenchymal inflammation, which may be clinically silent or cause mild to moderate proteinuria, hematuria, or a reduced creatinine clearance. Hypertension and urinary tract infections may complicate this process and, if untreated, accelerate the underlying renal disease.

Cardiopulmonary manifestations include pul-

TABLE 136–1.
Clinical Abnormalities in Systemic Lupus Erythematosus*

ABNORMALITY	FREQUENCY IN SYSTEMIC LUPUS ERYTHEMATOSUS (% OF PATIENTS)
Constitutional	
Fever	70–80
Fatigue	80–90
Weight loss	60–80
Arthritis, arthralgia	80–90
Skin	
Butterfly rash	40–60
Photosensitivity	30–40
Alopecia	25–35
Raynaud's phenomenon	5–10
Purpura	10–20
Oral or nasal ulcers	20–30
Renal	40–60
Gastrointestinal	30–35
Pulmonary	10–30
Serositis	
Pleuritis	40–60
Pericarditis	25–35
Peritonitis	25–35
Cardiac	30–40
Lymphoreticular	
Lymphadenopathy	40–50
Splenomegaly	15–25
Hepatomegaly	20–25
Central nervous system	
Seizures	15–30
Psychosis	10–20
Personality changes	20–50
Migraine headaches	5–15
Peripheral neuropathy	10–15
Hematologic	
Hemolytic anemia	10–20
Thrombocytopenia	10–15
Circulating anticoagulant	5–15
Leukopenia	40–50

* Data primarily from Rodnan, 1983.

monary infiltrates, pleuritis, and pericarditis. Pulmonary parenchymal infiltrates may mimic pulmonary infection. They occur frequently and may be transient. Pleuritis, manifest as pleurisy and exudative pleural effusions, occurs in over half of patients. Pericarditis may be asymptomatic or be present as pericardial pain. Cardiac tamponade is a rare complication. Myocarditis and verrucous endocarditis (Libman-Sacks endocarditis) are rare but should be suspected when there is evidence of congestive heart failure or a new heart murmur develops.

Serious neurologic abnormalities include seizures, psychosis, coma, and organic brain syndrome. Neuropathies of the cranial and peripheral nerves occur infrequently. Lesser degrees of neuropsychiatric involvement are common, including depression, anxiety, and psychoneurosis. Headaches, movement disorder, and paralysis are also features of the disease.

Hematologic abnormalities are common and may be the initial manifestation of systemic lupus erythematosus. The hypoproliferative anemia of chronic disease is the most frequent abnormality and usually reflects the general disease activity. A positive Coombs' test may occur but is often not accompanied by a hemolytic anemia. Leukopenia, with a white blood cell count below 4,000 cells/mm^3, is common. Thrombocytopenia is also frequent but is usually not severe.

Despite the broad spectrum of potential complications in systemic lupus erythematosus, an individual patient will usually have only four to six of the features listed in Table 136–1, and the severity is characteristically mild, but can be severe. Some patients may have progressive and fatal disease with renal failure, seizures, and coma, while others have mild arthralgias, skin rashes, and fatigue as their only manifestations of systemic lupus erythematosus. The disease tends to be more severe with onset in childhood (under 16 years of age) and less severe with onset in older adults (over 40 years of age). The course of the disease in an individual patient is also highly variable. A patient with pleuropericarditis, thrombocytopenia, and hemolytic anemia and requiring intensive care when first seen may subsequently be free of symptoms for months or even years.

PATHOPHYSIOLOGY

Although the etiology of systemic lupus erythematosus remains obscure, there is evidence of abnormal immune regulation characterized by hyperactive B-lymphocytes producing multiple autoantibodies. These autoantibodies are directed against nuclear, cytoplasmic, and cell membrane antigens. ANA are present in the serum of greater than 95% of patients with systemic lupus erythematosus. Circulating immune complexes are also a feature of disease.

A defective ability of the immune system to control self-tolerance mechanisms appears to be central to autoantibody production in systemic lupus erythematosus. Apparently, normal individuals have B-lymphocytes capable of producing antibodies to self constituents including nuclear, cytoplasmic, and cell membrane components, but production of significant quantities of these antibodies is prevented in the normal state. This state of immune tolerance to self antigens requires suppression of B-lymphocytes from differentiation and proliferation into antibody-secreting cells. The control of B-lymphocyte antibody production resides primarily in immunoregulatory T-lymphocytes. Thus, either a primary defect in T-cell immunoregulation or spontaneous activation of B-cells could bring about a loss of tolerance to self antigens and a production of previously suppressed autoantibodies. A multitude of defects in T-cell and B-cell function have been described in systemic lupus erythematosus. It appears that, rather than there being a single defect responsible, any of a number of defects in immune regulation may lead to polyclonal B-cell activation, autoantibody production, and the clinical syndrome of systemic lupus erythematosus.

Several predisposing and environmental factors appear to be important in the development of systemic lupus erythematosus. A genetic predisposition has been observed; if one identical twin has systemic lupus erythematosus, the other has a 70% chance of developing the disease. Individuals with congenital deficiencies of complement components are at greater risk for development of systemic lupus erythematosus. Sex hormones are also important; the incidence in women is greater than that in men, 9:1. Ultraviolet light exposure and certain drugs (see Table 136–2) are also capable of inducing the disease. The possibility of viral infection inducing and maintaining systemic lupus erythematosus has been explored for years, yet remains unproven.

Regardless of the underlying cause, autoantibodies to cell membrane, cytoplasmic, and nuclear constituents remain the immunologic hallmarks of systemic lupus erythematosus. Examples of ANA include antibodies directed against native (double-stranded) DNA, single-stranded DNA, deoxynucleoprotein, and ribonucleoprotein.

A number of other ANA have now been

TABLE 136–2.
Drugs Implicated in Inducing Systemic Lupus Erythematosus

Hydralazine
Procainamide
Isoniazid
Phenytoin
Penicillamine
Methyldopa
Quinidine
Sulfonamides
Chlorpromazine
Practolol
Acebutolol
Propylthiouracil
Lithium carbonate
Carbamazepine
Nitrofurantoin
Penicillin

described (Table 136–3). They are not intrinsically harmful, presumably because they cannot penetrate the membrane of living cells to interact with nuclear antigens. In the form of immune complexes, however, they appear to be directly responsible for the immune-mediated tissue damage which resembles serum sickness.

When cells die, their membranes rupture, and the intracellular constituents are exposed to the circulation. If ANA are present, these antibodies combine with their respective nuclear antigens, and these circulating immune complexes are removed by the mononuclear phagocytic system in the liver, spleen, and other lymphoid tissues. The rate of removal of these circulating immune complexes depends on their size, concentration, the ratio of antibody to antigen, and the intrinsic ability of the mononuclear phagocytic system to remove them by phagocytosis.

If not removed from the circulation, circulating immune complexes are trapped by vascular and basement membranes. There they activate the complement system, with subsequent production of a variety of vasoactive and chemotactic factors. These agents promote local vascular dilatation and the influx of inflammatory cells including neutrophils and macrophages, resulting in local tissue damage. The major sites of immune complex deposition in systemic lupus erythematosus are the joints, kidneys, choroid plexus of the brain, lungs, and skin. There is not always a good correlation between the level of circulating immune complexes and the degree of disease activity in systemic lupus erythematosus, nor is it under-

TABLE 136–3.
Autoantibodies Present in Systemic Lupus Erythematosus

ANTIGEN SPECIFICITY	SIGNIFICANCE (OR DISEASE SPECIFICITY)
Antinuclear antibodies to	
Double-stranded (native) DNA	Systemic lupus erythematosus
Single-stranded DNA	
Deoxynucleoprotein	Responsible for LE prep
Nucleolar	Scleroderma
Histone	Systemic lupus erythematosus, drug-induced systemic lupus erythematosus
Sm antigen	Systemic lupus erythematosus
Ribonucleoprotein	Mixed connective tissue disease
SS-A (also known as Ro) antigen	Sjögren's syndrome, systemic lupus erythematosus, neonatal lupus syndrome
SS-B (also known as La) antigen	Sjögren's syndrome, systemic lupus erythematosus, neonatal lupus syndrome
SS-C	Rheumatoid arthritis
Centromere	CREST* (syndrome)
Scl-70 antigen	Scleroderma
PM-1 antigen	Polymyositis
Anticytoplasmic antibodies to	
Mitochondria	Autoimmune hepatitis
SS-A (antigen)	Sjögren's syndrome, systemic lupus erythematosus
SS-B (antigen)	Sjögren's syndrome, systemic lupus erythematosus
Anti-cell-membrane antibodies to	
Erythrocytes	Autoimmune hemolysis
Leukocytes	Autoimmune leukopenia
Platelets	Autoimmune thrombocytopenia
Miscellaneous autoantibodies to	
Cardiolipin	False-positive serologic test for syphilis
Phospholipid	Elevated partial thromboplastin time Spontaneous thrombosis, abortion
Clotting factors (multiple)	Hemorrhage

* CREST = Calcinosis, Raynaud's, esophageal dysmotility, sclerodactyly, telangiectasia.

stood why some organs are severely affected while others are spared in the same patient.

Although present at some time during the disease course in only 75% of patients, antibodies to native (double-stranded) DNA appear to be particularly important in causing tissue damage in systemic lupus erythematosus, especially in the kidneys. Circulating immune complexes composed of native DNA and its antibody preferentially localize next to the glomerular basement membrane, initiating inflammatory damage. Titers of circulating antibody to native DNA have been shown to generally correlate with disease activity in systemic lupus erythematosus, especially renal disease. Additionally, antinative DNA antibodies are rarely found in other diseases; thus, their presence in an individual patient strongly suggests the diagnosis of systemic lupus erythematosus.

Autoantibodies directed against cell membrane constituents provide another and more direct mechanism for tissue damage. Anti-red cell antibodies can cause positive Coombs' tests and hemolytic anemia, and antiplatelet antibodies are responsible for platelet dysfunction and thrombocytopenia in some patients. Autoantibodies to lymphocyte membrane antigens have recently been shown to cross-react with antigens on neuronal tissues, suggesting that these autoantibodies may be responsible for some of the neuropathic changes in systemic lupus erythematosus. By selectively depleting certain subpopulations of lymphocytes, these lymphocytotoxic antibodies may also cause a more fundamental defect in immune homeostasis in systemic lupus erythematosus by disturbing T-cell helper/suppressor ratios. Autoantibodies to clotting factors alter coagulation homeostasis as well.

The pathologic changes in systemic lupus erythematosus are variable both in terms of severity and organ involvement. In organs affected by vasculitis, neutrophilic and lymphocytic accumulations and edema are observed around the blood vessels, which may be occluded. With cell death, eosinophilic debris (composed of fibrin, immunoglobulins, and complement components) accumulates. Hematoxylin bodies are basophil-staining bodies scattered throughout affected tissues and represent nuclear debris combined with ANA. These are said to be pathognomonic of systemic lupus erythematosus.

The degrees of renal lesions range from mild to severe. In mesangial glomerulonephritis there is proliferation of mesangial cells, increased mesangial matrix, and local deposition of immune complexes. Proliferative glomerulonephritis is distinguished by endocapillary cell proliferation, infiltration of inflammatory cells, irregular thickening of capillary loops, and deposits of immune complexes in the mesangium and along the peripheral capillary loops. In membranous glomerulonephritis, the capillary loops are uniformly thickened; however, there is little cellular proliferation, and immune complex deposits are usually confined to the mesangium. Variable inflammatory and degenerative changes are also seen in the renal interstitium.

Onion skin lesions, consisting of periarterial fibrosis, occur in the spleen and may represent scars from previous vasculitis. Sterile vegetations, the verrucous Libman-Sacks lesions, develop on the heart valves and chordae tendineae.

Pathologic changes in the skin are variable, ranging from a leukocytoclastic vasculitis of small venules in purpuric skin lesions to epidermal thinning, dermal–epidermal junction disruption, and lymphocytic infiltrations seen in the acute lupus rash. Lymphocytic infiltrations and villus hypertrophy are present in synovial tissue, and muscle biopsy usually shows perivascular lymphocytic infiltration. Lesions of the CNS vary. The most common lesion is the microinfarct. Large intracerebral hemorrhage and true vasculitis are rare.

CLINICAL–PATHOLOGIC CORRELATIONS

Immune complex deposits and autoantibodies to tissues and circulating cells are responsible for the majority of clinical manifestations of systemic lupus erythematosus (Table 136–4). Virtually any organ system of the body can be affected.

DIFFERENTIAL DIAGNOSIS

Systemic lupus erythematosus is known as the great mimic of diseases because the full differential diagnosis encompasses most diseases

TABLE 136–4.
Clinical–Pathologic Correlations for Systemic Lupus Erythematosus

CLINICAL FINDINGS	PATHOLOGIC FINDINGS
IMMUNE COMPLEX DEPOSITION	
Proteinuria	Glomerulonephritis
Hematuria	
Elevated serum creatinine levels	
Arthralgias, arthritis	Synovitis
Chest pain	Serositis
Pleural effusion	
Pericardial effusion	
Abdominal pain	
Varied skin rashes	Skin inflammation
Infarcts of involved organ	Vasculitis
AUTOANTIBODIES TO CELLULAR CONSTITUENTS	
Leukopenia	Antileukocyte antibody
Hemolytic anemia	Antierythrocyte antibody
Thrombocytopenia	Antiplatelet antibody
CNS dysfunction	Antineuronal antibody
AUTOANTIBODIES TO OTHER CONSTITUENTS	
Abnormal partial thromboplastin time	Antiphospholipid antibody
Hemorrhagic phenomenon	
Clotting factors	
False-positive serologic test for syphilis	Anticardiolipin antibody
Rheumatoid factor	Anti-immunoglobulin Fc receptor antibody

in internal medicine. The diagnosis of systemic lupus erythematosus is always a consideration in patients with multisystem disease, especially diseases associated with joint or muscle aches and pains. Systemic lupus erythematosus must be distinguished from infections such as syphilis, bacterial endocarditis, bacterial pneumonias, tuberculosis, Rocky Mountain spotted fever, disseminated gonococcemia, meningococcemia, and leptospirosis. Other diseases of the immune system with overlapping clinical features include acquired immunodeficiency syndrome, idiopathic thrombocytopenic purpura, sarcoidosis, thrombotic thrombocytopenic purpura, and other forms of vasculitis such as polyarteritis nodosa and Wegener's granulomatosis. Neuropsychiatric manifestations of systemic lupus erythematosus may mimic or be seizures, organic brain syndrome, or acute psychosis caused by tumors, drugs, or metabolic or electrolyte disturbances. Systemic lupus erythematosus must also be distinguished from other connective tissue diseases that frequently have a positive ANA such as rheumatoid arthritis, progressive systemic sclerosis, polymyositis, dermatomyositis, and Sjögren's syndrome. The key differentiating features of these diseases are listed in Table 136–5.

DIAGNOSIS

The diagnosis of systemic lupus erythematosus requires the presence of several clinical or laboratory features of the disease in the absence of other known causes. The American Rheumatism Association has devised a set of diagnostic criteria that allows 95% confidence in the diagnosis of systemic lupus erythematosus if four or more features are present out of 11 possible categories (Table 136–6). Although the original intent of this system was to allow uniformity of diagnosis in clinical investigation of systemic lupus erythematosus, it has also proven a useful tool for clinicians considering systemic lupus erythematosus in patients with multisystem disease. Thus a patient with a positive ANA test, pleurisy, malar rash, and arthritis can be diagnosed as having systemic lupus erythematosus with 95% confidence. It is important to emphasize, however, that all the criteria in Table 136–6 do not carry identical weight when being used to diagnose systemic lupus erythematosus and that it is not always necessary to have a minimum of four criteria in order to establish the diagnosis. For example, a young woman with pleuopericarditis, a positive ANA test, and high titers of antibody to na-

TABLE 136–5.
Differential Diagnosis of Diseases With a Positive ANA Test

DISEASE	CLINICAL FEATURES	LABORATORY FEATURES
Systemic lupus erythematosus	Incidence: women:men, 9:1 Onset: age 15–40 yr Skin rashes, fever Arthralgias Vasculitis Nephritis Seizures, psychosis Pleuropericarditis	Antibodies to native DNA 　or Sm antigen Thrombocytopenia Leukopenia Hemolytic anemia Positive Coombs' test Low serum complement level High serum creatinine level Abnormal urinalysis results
Rheumatoid arthritis	Incidence: women:men, 2:1 Onset: age 30–50 yr Polyarthritis, symmetric, 　joint swelling Morning stiffness Deformities of joints Subcutaneous nodules	Rheumatoid factor Thrombocytosis Neutropenia
Progressive systemic sclerosis	Incidence: women:men, 2:1 Onset: age 20–50 yr Scleroderma Raynaud's phenomenon in 　90% Esophageal dysmotility Intestinal dysmotility Malignant hypertension Pulmonary fibrosis	Skin biopsy, shows fibrosis
Polymyositis, 　dermatomyositis	Incidence: women:men, 2:1 Onset: age 10–50 yr Proximal muscle weakness Heliotrope rash Gottren's papules	Elevated serum levels of CK, 　LDH, SGOT, aldolase Abnormal electromyogram Muscle biopsy with inflammation 　and muscle necrosis
Sjögren's syndrome	Incidence: women:men, 2:1 Onset: age 30–60 yr Dry, irritated eyes Dry mouth Arthralgias	Rheumatoid factor Salivary gland biopsy shows 　lymphocytic infiltrate Positive Schirmer's test Abnormal scintiscan of salivary 　glands

tive DNA, undoubtedly has systemic lupus erythematosus, the diagnosis being based on the high specificity of antinative DNA for systemic lupus erythematosus. Other findings strongly suggestive of systemic lupus erythematosus include low levels of serum complement and the presence in the serum of antibody to Sm nuclear antigen.

PRINCIPLES OF THERAPY

There is no cure for systemic lupus erythematosus; therefore, therapy is directed at control of inflammation caused by the underlying immune defect. Treatment must be individualized because of the variability of manifestations in the individual patient as well as the natural history of the disease characterized by spontaneous exacerbations and remissions.

In many instances no treatment is required. If no serious organ involvement is present, management may consist of reassurance and instruction to obtain adequate rest, avoid overexertion, and avoid excessive exposure to the sun. There is debate regarding potential harmful effects of estrogen and progesterone compounds in women with systemic lupus erythematosus. If birth control pills or postmenopausal estrogen replacement therapy appear to worsen the activity of lupus in a patient, they should be withdrawn.

Milder symptoms such as arthralgias and myalgias may be treated with nonsteroidal

TABLE 136–6.
Preliminary Diagnostic Criteria for Classification of Systemic Lupus Erythematosus*

CRITERION	DEFINITION
Malar rash	Fixed erythema, flat or raised, over the malar eminences, tending to spare the nasolabial folds
Discoid rash	Erythematous raised patches with adherent keratotic scaling and follicular plugging; atrophic scarring may occur in older lesions
Photosensitivity	Skin rash as a result of unusual reaction to sunlight, by patient history or physician observation
Oral ulcers	Oral or nasopharyngeal ulceration, usually painless, observed by a physician
Arthritis	Nonerosive arthritis involving two or more peripheral joints, characterized by tenderness, swelling, or effusion
Serositis	Pleuritis—rub heard by a physician or evidence of pleural effusion or convincing history of pleuritic pain or Pericarditis—documented by ECG or rub or evidence of pericardial effusion
Renal disorder	Persistent proteinuria greater than 0.5 gm or greater than 3+ if quantitation not performed or Cellular casts—may be red cell, hemoglobin, granular, tubular, or mixed
Neurologic disorder	Seizures—in the absence of offending drugs or known metabolic derangements (e.g., uremia, ketoacidosis, or electrolyte imbalance) or Psychosis—in the absence of offending drugs or known metabolic derangements
Hematologic disorder	Hemolytic anemia—with reticulocytosis or Leukopenia—less than 4000/mm^3 total on two or more occasions or Lymphopenia—less than 1500/mm^3 on two or more occasions or Thrombocytopenia—less than 100,000/mm^3 in the absence of offending drugs
Immunologic disorder	Positive LE cell preparation or Anti-DNA: antibody to native DNA in abnormal titer or Anti-Sm antigen: presence of antibody to Sm nuclear antigen or False-positive serologic test for syphilis and known to be positive for at least 6 months and confirmed by *Treponema pallidum* immobilization or fluorescent treponemal antibody-absorption test
Antinuclear	An abnormal titer of antinuclear antibody by immunofluorescence or an equivalent assay at any point in time and in the absence of drugs known to be associated with "drug-induced lupus erythematosus" syndrome

*Data from Rodnan, 1983.

anti-inflammatory drugs. The antimalarial drugs, chloroquine and hydroxychloroquine, have proven especially useful in the treatment of discoid lupus erythematosus and may also be of benefit for more severe musculoskeletal complaints. Major organ involvement such as diffuse proliferative glomerulonephritis, hemo- lytic anemia, severe thrombocytopenia, sei- zures, coma, and pleuropericarditis require corticosteroid treatment. In instances where life-threatening complications fail to respond to corticosteroids, immunosuppressive drugs such as cyclophosphamide and azathioprine may be indicated.

REFERENCES

Beary JF III, Christian DL, Sculco TP (eds): *Manual of Rheumatology and Outpatient Orthopedic Disorders*. Boston, Little, Brown & Co 1981, pp 183–196.

Hughes GRV (ed): Systemic lupus erythematosus. *Clin Rheum Dis* 1982: 8:1–323. *A collection of articles addressing current aspects of systemic lupus erythematosus, with extensive references.*

Kelley WN, Harris ED, Ruddy S, Sledge CB (eds): *Textbook of Rheumatology*, ed 2. Philadelphia, WB Saunders Co, 1985, pp 1042–1114. *A comprehensive textbook discussion of the pathophysiology, clinical course, and treatment of systemic lupus erythematosus with extensive references.*

Rodnan GP, Schumacher HR (eds): *Primer on the Rheumatic Diseases*, ed 8. Atlanta, Arthritis Foundation, 1983, pp 49–58. *A useful synopsis of rheumatic disease, with basic information regarding diagnosis and treatment of systemic lupus erythematosus.*

Smolen JS, Chused TM, Leiserson WM, Reeves JP, Alling D, Steinberg AD: Heterogeneity of immunoregulatory T-cell subsets in systemic lupus erythematosus. *Am J Med* 1982; 72:783–790. *Discusses various abnormalities of T-lymphocyte subsets responsible for B-cell hyperactivity in systemic lupus erythematosus.*

Tan EM: Antinuclear antibodies in diagnosis and management. *Hosp Pract* 1983; 18:79–83. *A clear explanation of the "family" of antinuclear antibodies that have the greatest clinical relevance for the diagnosis of rheumatic conditions.*

Woolfe D (ed): Rehabilitation in the rheumatic diseases. *Clin Rheum Dis* 1981; 7:289–553. *A complete review of the various modalities of treatment of rheumatic disorders with emphasis on a multidisciplinary approach.*

137 SYSTEMIC VASCULITIS

Alice Faryna, M.D.

Systemic vasculitis refers to a diverse group of syndromes characterized by inflammation and necrosis of blood vessels involving more than one organ system. Prognosis depends largely on the size and extent of vessels affected. The syndromes are named according to the principal clinicopathologic manifestations, but there is no entirely satisfactory classification system. Specific labels are less important than recognition of the potential for irreparable organ damage.

CLINICAL SIGNS AND SYMPTOMS

Clinical manifestations reflect target organ ischemia. Assessment of the pattern of organ involvement is a useful diagnostic aid (Table 137–1).

HYPERSENSITIVITY VASCULITIS

This small-vessel vasculitis receives its name from the strong association it has with infections or the administration of drugs. The clinical picture is dominated by cutaneous lesions with various degrees of visceral involvement.

Patients usually present with small, palpable, purpuric lesions chiefly on the dependent portions of the body, often accompanied by edema and a burning or stinging discomfort. The lesions appear rapidly and usually clear within 3 weeks to 4 weeks. Less commonly, urticarial, macular, or papular erythematous lesions may be found. Several syndromes are recognized:

Henoch-Schönlein purpura (HSP) occurs most commonly in children or adolescents fol-

TABLE 137–1.
Comparison of Organ Involvement in the Vasculitides*

CLINICAL FEATURE	HYPERSENSITIVITY VASCULITIS	POLYARTERITIS NODOSA	ALLERGIC GRANULOMATOSIS	WEGENER'S GRANULOMATOSIS	KAWASAKI DISEASE	TEMPORAL ARTERITIS	TAKAYASU'S ARTERITIS
			FREQUENCY OF ORGAN INVOLVEMENT (%) PATIENTS WITHIN DISEASE CATEGORIES				
Fever/malaise	20—adult 70—children	50–70	>50	>30	95	40–50	20–50 (early phase)
Skin lesions	100	>40	>60	45–50	>90	NR†	Erythema nodosum
Mucosal lesions	>10	NR	(allergic rhinitis = 70%)	>60 (nasopharynx)	>90	NR	NR
Musculo-skeletal symptoms	40	>60	20–50	>60	25	45–50	50
Renal	30–45	70–85	30–50	80–85	30	NR	60
Gastrointestinal	15	45–60	60	NR	40	NR	10–20
Catastrophic	rare	5–15	rare	NR	NR	NR	rare
Peripheral neuropathy	>10	50–80	>60	25–50	NR	NR	NR
Central nervous system symptoms	?5	20–40 perhaps secondary to increased BP	30	rare	5	10–15	50 (primarily syncope)
Ocular lesions	NR	10–20	NR	>50	90	25–50	15–60
Cardiac Disease	rare	30–80	30–50	12–30	> 20	NR	35–45
Hypertension	13 (HSP)	> 50	30–50	NR	NR	NR	60–70
Pulmonary lesions	>15	rare	>70 (Asthma = 100)	>90	40 (autopsy)	NR	15
Other			Eosinophilia: 100 Prostatitis: 10	Sinusitis: >90 Otitis: 40–60	Lymphade-nopathy: 75	Headache or facial pain: >60	Absent pulses: >90 Claudication: 30–45 Bruits: 80–90

* Data from Cupps TR, Fauci AS: The vasculitides, in Smith LH (ed): *Major Problems in Internal Medicine*, vol 21. Philadelphia, WB Saunders Co, 1981, pp 1–211; Fan PT, Davis JA, Somer T, Kaplan L, Bluestone R: A clinical approach to systemic vasculitis. *Semin Arthritis Rheum* 1980; 9:248–304; and Landing BH, Larson EJ: Are infantile periarteritis nodosa with coronary artery involvement and fatal mucocutaneous lymph node syndrome the same? Comparison of 20 patients from North America with patients from Hawaii and Japan. *Pediatrics* 1977; 59(5):651–662.
† NR - not reported.

lowing an upper respiratory infection. The purpuric rash is accompanied by colicky abdominal pain, microscopic hematuria, and arthralgia or arthritis. Gastrointestinal bleeding may occur, but serious hemorrhage or renal failure is unusual. Hypertension occurs in up to 13% of patients.

In cases of *serum sickness*, 1 week to 2 weeks following the administration of heterologous serum, affected patients commonly develop fever, myalgia, lymphadenopathy, abdominal pain, and a rash that is usually urticarial, but may be purpuric. Polyarticular synovitis is common. Recovery over a period of 2 weeks to 3 weeks is usual, but life-threatening nephritis, carditis, or CNS disease may rarely occur. Although serum is rarely used now, a similar syndrome may result from a variety of drugs, especially penicillins.

The initial features of the *mixed essential cryoglobulinemia syndrome* are palpable purpura, arthralgia, and nephritis in association with cold-precipitable globulins in the serum for which no primary cause can be found. Raynaud's phenomenon or cutaneous ulcers are less common (in 25% to 30% of patients), but gangrene is rare. The condition may be persistent or recurrent. Progressive renal deterioration may occur.

The initial feature of *erythema nodosum* is painful erythematous tumors, up to 5 cm in diameter, over the extremities, especially the lower. Synovitis and mild systemic symptoms are common. The lesions resolve over a period of 4 weeks to 6 weeks and usually do not recur. There is a strong association with streptococcal or granulomatous infections, inflammatory disorders such as ulcerative colitis or sarcoidosis, and drugs such as sulfa and oral contraceptives.

In most cases, hypersensitivity vasculitis is a self limited disorder, and although there are occasional recurrences, the course is generally benign. Rarely, major gastrointestinal hemorrhage, bowel perforation, or renal failure ensues. Hypersensitivity vasculitis may complicate the course of a connective tissue disease or malignancy. In those situations, the prognosis depends on the underlying condition. A benign course cannot be expected when hypersensitivity vasculitis occurs along with a medium vessel vasculitis (see below).

POLYARTERITIS GROUP

Classic polyarteritis nodosa (PAN) is usually heralded by fever, malaise, and weight loss followed by evidence of ischemia or infarction in major organs. Frequent manifestations are polyneuropathy, hematuria, proteinuria, acute abdomen, gastrointestinal bleeding, and chest pain. Hypertension is a common feature and contributes to the late sequelae of congestive heart failure, myocardial infarction, uremia, and stroke. Primary involvement of the heart or CNS by vasculitis may occasionally occur as well, leading to pericarditis, angina, arrhythmia, or focal neurologic deficits. Mononeuritis multiplex is the most common form of peripheral neuropathy. The painful subcutaneous nodules, which give the disorder its name, actually occur in only 10% to 15% of cases and are often associated with livedo reticularis.

The Churg-Strauss variant of PAN, allergic granulomatosis, is characterized by involvement of the respiratory tract, a feature not seen in classic PAN. Patients present with a recent onset of asthma, pulmonary infiltrates, eosinophilia, and, occasionally, allergic rhinitis. Any features of classic PAN may also occur, but serious renal or gastrointestinal disease is unusual.

Unfortunately, many patients do not fit neatly into these categories, but exhibit overlapping features of hypersensitivity vasculitis, PAN, and allergic granulomatosis.

Mucocutaneous lymph node syndrome (Kawasaki disease) is a vasculitic syndrome of young children characterized by fever, acute enlargement of one or more cervical nodes, bilateral conjunctivitis, erythema of the lips, and oral mucosa, and edematous erythema of the hands and feet. Desquamation of the digits occurs in the second week. A macular rash, diarrhea, and synovitis are also common features. Arrhythmias, gallop rhythm, and cardiomegaly may occur.

For untreated patients, the 5-year survival rate in PAN is only 10%, with most deaths due to renal failure or cardiac events. The 5-year survival in allergic granulomatosis is 25%, with most deaths due to cardiac events, pneumonia, or status asthmaticus. The risk for acute catastrophic events is high in these two forms of vasculitis: mononeuritis multiplex occurs in up to 23% of patients; bowel hemorrhage, perforation, or infarction in up to 20%; cholecystitis in 17%; and myocardial infarction in 6%. Recovery is usual in Kawasaki disease, but a 1% mortality occurs between the third and fifth weeks from thrombosis or rupture of coronary artery aneurysms.

WEGENER'S GRANULOMATOSIS

The initial symptom of Wegener's granulomatosis usually is a nasal or sinus discharge, which may be purulent or bloody. Although pulmonary nodules or infiltrates are very common, they are symptomatic in only one-third of the cases. The pulmonary nodules may cavitate. Nodular, purpuric, or ulcerative skin lesions occur in half of the cases. Destruction of nasal cartilage and adjacent sinuses leads to facial deformities. Extension into and infection of the ears and CNS may complicate the course. Glomerulonephritis, which may be fulminant, occurs in 85%.

Prior to effective therapy, the course was uniformly fatal, usually from renal failure, with only 10% surviving at the end of 2 years.

GIANT CELL ARTERITIS

Temporal arteritis is predominantly a disorder of women over the age of 50 years. Although any large or medium vessels may be involved, typically branches of the carotid artery are affected. Headache, fever, malaise, tender temporal arteries, and jaw claudication are common initial features. Polymyalgia rheumatica (stiffness and aching of shoulder and hip girdle areas) occurs in about 40% of patients, though not necessarily concurrently. An almost equal number have nonspecific joint complaints. Visual blurring or diplopia occurs in up to half of patients. Ischemic retinopathy may be found if the patient is examined shortly after an episode of amblyopia. Swollen temporal arteries or diminished pulsations occur in up to half of patients, but may not be present early in the disease. Upper extremity bruits suggest involvement of the subclavian or brachial arteries (occurs in 15% of patients).

Takayasu's arteritis has a predeliction for young women of Oriental or Latin extraction, with the majority of cases having an onset between the ages of 10 years and 30 years. Initially, nonspecific symptoms of fever, malaise, night sweats, nodular skin lesions, proximal myalgias, or polyarthritis may recur for 5 years or 10 years before occlusive vascular disease is appreciated, at which time patients complain of dizziness, syncope, claudication, dypsnea, chest pain, and visual blurring. Physical findings include bruits, absent peripheral pulses, hypertension, tender central arteries, retinopathy, and a peculiar head-down posture to alleviate CNS symptoms. Although both systemic and pulmonary circuits may be involved, the most common sites are the aortic arch branches and the renal arteries.

Although there have been reports of fatalities in temporal arteritis, the overall mortality rate does not appear to be increased. The disease appears to be self-limited (2 years to 4 years). Currently, permanent blindness occurs in 10% to 15% of untreated cases. In series reported before 1960, partial or permanent visual loss occurred in 27% to 60%.

The 5-year survival rate for Takayasu's arteritis has been estimated to be 85%. Acute catastrophic events are rare because the size of the vessels involved permits the development of collateral circulation. Late complications from hypertension (congestive failure, stroke, and angina) occur in over 30% of patients.

PATHOPHYSIOLOGY

The pathologic findings result from injury to the vessel wall followed by inflammation, ischemia, and infarction of the involved organs. Saccular aneurysms commonly occur at bifurcations of medium-sized vessels. Segmental or focal areas of vascular inflammation are characteristic of medium- and large-vessel syndromes. Pathologic features are summarized in Table 137–2.

A major role for immune complex deposition in the pathogenesis of hypersensitivity vasculitis and the PAN group of systemic necrotizing vasculitis is supported by the similarity of the lesions to experimental models (serum sickness and the Arthus phenomenon) and by the reports of hypersensitivity vasculitis or PAN occurring during the course of a connective tissue disease. Multiple factors are involved in the pathogenesis: (1) formation of antigen–anti-

TABLE 137–2.
Pathologic Features of Vasculitis

TYPE	MACROSCOPIC FEATURES	MICROSCOPIC FEATURES
Hypersensitivity vasculitis	Edema; superficial hemorrhages; superficial ulcerations	Infiltration of venules and small arterioles by polymorphonuclear cells (PMN); nuclear debris; immune complexes in vessel walls; focal or diffuse glomerulonephritis; all lesions of same age
PAN	Scars and/or hemorrhagic infarcts; saccular aneurysms of small to medium vessels at bifurcations	Segmental infiltration of vessel wall by PMNs; fibrinoid necrosis; thrombosis; mural fibrosis and scarring; immune complex deposits rare; renal arteritis more common than glomerulonephritis; lesions vary in age
Allergic granulomatosis	Granulomas of lung, pericardium, omentum; infarcted tissue; few aneurysms; small arteries and veins affected	As in PAN, but eosinophils predominate; perivascular and extravascular granulomas; occasional giant cells and immune complex deposits
Kawasaki disease	Coronary aneurysms; widespread medium-vessel arteritis	Inflammation and destruction of the media; fibrinoid necrosis and intimal thickening rare; thrombosis, sclerosis
Wegener's granulomatosis	Pulmonary nodules and cavities; destruction of nasal cartilage	Necrotizing vasculitis and granulomas of upper and lower respiratory tracts involving small arteries and veins; glomerulonephritis
Temporal arteritis	Segmental thickening and occlusion of carotid or aortic arch branches	Mononuclear cell infiltration with destruction of elastic lamina; giant cells; intimal thickening and fibrosis
Takayasu's arteritis	Segmental stenosis of aorta and arch branches; occasionally pulmonary arteries; plaques and wrinkling of intima	Granulomas, giant cells and fibrosis of entire wall; necrosis of media and elastic laminae

body complexes with sedimentation coefficients > 19S during periods of slight antigen excess; (2) increased vascular permeability from activated platelets and products of IgE-sensitized basophils and mast cells; (3) deposition of immune complexes at sites of increased vascular permeability; (4) complement activation with release of chemotactic complement fragments; (5) influx of polymorphonuclear cells and phagocytosis of immune complexes; (6) release of lysosomes and oxygen radicals from phagocytes; (7) activation of coagulation factors by damaged endothelium; (8) release of leukotrienes and prostaglandins by damaged cells; and (9) defective clearance of immune complexes.

Bacterial, fungal, and viral antigens have been identified within immune complexes or cryoglobulins in some cases of PAN and hypersensitivity vasculitis. Hepatitis B antigen is a particularly likely offender. Other implicated antigens include penicillin, sulfa, intravenously administered street drugs, serum proteins, immunizations, insect venoms, and a variety of other drugs. *Propionibacterium acnei* is being investigated as a possible trigger for Kawasaki disease. The pathogenesis in the other forms of vasculitis is not clear. Macrophages and cell-mediated immunity are thought to play an important role in granulomatous forms. The role of genetic disorders of immunoregulation via the HLA system is being studied.

TABLE 137–3.
Clinical–Pathologic Correlations of the Vasculitides

CLINICAL FINDINGS	PATHOLOGIC FINDINGS
Fever, leukocytosis	Macrophage activation; release of interleukin 1; cell injury with release of prostaglandins
Edema, urticaria	Increased vascular permeability from (1) amines released from platelets, IgE-sensitized mast cells and basophils, (2) complement fragments, and (3) leukotrienes
Headache	Cranial arteritis; hypertension
Purpura	Diapedesis of red cells in areas of increased permeability
Ulceration	Occlusion of arterioles in subdermal/submucosal regions
Claudication	Muscle ischemia from small to medium artery occlusion
Arthralgia	Synovitis, probably from immune complex deposition
Hypertension	Reduced renal blood flow from occlusion of arcuate or renal arteries
Proteinuria/hematuria	Immune complex nephritis; renal infarcts
Abdominal pain	Mucosal ulcers, infarction, perforation of viscus; pancreatitis; cholecystitis
GI bleeding	Mucosal ulceration; bowel infarction; ruptured vessel
Chest pain	Pericarditis; coronary arteritis; pleuritis
Dypsnea	Congestive failure; pleural effusion; interstitial pulmonary fibrosis; bronchospasm
Hemoptysis	Pulmonary infarct; rupture of vessel into bronchus
Numbness/motor loss	Vasculitis of vasa vasorum of peripheral nerves
Amblyopia	Occlusion of ophthalmic or central retinal artery; hypertensive retinopathy
Stroke/transient ischemic attack	Hypertension; CNS vasculitis

CLINICAL–PATHOLOGIC CORRELATIONS

Intimal thickening or thrombosis or both in the inflamed vessel segments are responsible for the ischemic effects in the target organs. Necrosis of the media and disruption of the elastic layers contribute to the formation of aneurysms, although turbulence is also thought to be important in localization of aneurysms at bifurcation points. The major clinical–pathologic correlations are presented in Table 137–3.

DIFFERENTIAL DIAGNOSIS

The disorders most likely to mimic vasculitis are infections, malignancy, and a connective tissue disease (Table 137–4). Appropriate cultures should be done to exclude sepsis or focal infection. Serologic tests are helpful in identifying viral infections. Pulmonary lesions require a search for granulomatous infections and malignancy. The key points in distinguishing other multisystem diseases from a primary vasculitis are summarized in Table 137–5.

DIAGNOSIS

There are no specific tests for the vasculitides; diagnosis rests on histologic or arteriographic findings interpreted in the light of clinical manifestations. Other laboratory tests serve mainly to search for underlying causes, associated illness, or to identify other disorders that resemble vasculitis. The erythrocyte sedimentation rate (ESR) is elevated, often above 100 mm/hour, and is useful in monitoring activity of the more serious vasculitides. Other nonspecific abnormalities include normochromic, normocytic anemia, leukocytosis, thrombocytosis, and elevation of acute phase reactants. Rheumatoid factor may be present and should prompt a search for cryoglobulins. Complement levels may be normal or elevated, but when depressed, suggest the presence of cryoglobulinemia. The antinuclear antibody test (ANA) is occasionally positive, but titers are generally low. Appropriate screening tests for the evaluation of hypersensitivity vasculitis or a PAN-like syndrome include a complete blood count, measurement of the ESR, BUN/creatinine levels, creatinine phosphokinase levels,

TABLE 137–4.
Differential Diagnosis of Vasculitis

TYPE OF VASCULITIS	DIFFERENTIAL DIAGNOSIS
Hypersensitivity vasculitis	Bacterial sepsis, CTD*, malignancy, multiple myeloma, Waldenström's macroglobulinemia, platelet disorders, viral infections, inflammatory bowel disease
Polyarteritis nodosa	CTD, subacute bacterial endocarditis, atrial myxoma
Allergic granulomatosis	Bronchopulmonary aspergillosis, sarcoidosis, hypereosinophilic syndrome, lymphomatoid granulomatosis, Wegener's granulomatosis
Kawasaki disease	Juvenile arthritis, rheumatic fever, scarlet fever, toxic shock, viral infection
Wegener's granulomatosis	Goodpasture's syndrome, allergic granulomatosis, tuberculosis, bronchogenic cancer, relapsing polychondritis, (lethal) midline granuloma, sarcoidosis
Temporal arteritis	Migraine, occult infection, rheumatoid arthritis, transient ischemic attacks, trigeminal neuralgia
Takayasu's arteritis	Coarctation of aorta, granulomatous infections, syphilis, CTD

* CTD = Connective tissue disease.

tests for cryoglobulins, ANA, rheumatoid factor, and hepatitis BsAg, a urinalysis, chest x-ray films, and blood cultures. Platelet counts, prothrombin time, and partial thromboplastin time (PTT) should be obtained when purpura is noted. Thrombotic events in association with a prolonged PTT suggest a diagnosis of systemic lupus erythematosus.

The most useful diagnostic procedures are biopsy and angiography. Skin biopsy shows leukocytoclastic vasculitis (Table 137–2) in almost 100% of cases of hypersensitivity vasculitis. This diagnosis warrants a search for a concurrent medium-vessel vasculitis and connective tissue disease. Because the cost of investigating a case of systemic vasculitis can range from $6,000 to $36,000, the diagnostic tests should be selected carefully to increase the likelihood of a definitive result. In patients with localizing findings, a biopsy of the symptomatic site should be done if possible (i.e., of the sural nerve or a muscle). If this is unrewarding, abdominal arteriography is indicated. In patients without localizing findings, the arteriography is recommended first. If small aneurysms are not demonstrated, biopsies of organs in the following order may be useful: testicle, muscle, kidney. The sensitivity and specificity of this strategy have both been calculated to be 90%.

In Wegener's granulomatosis, biopsies of sinus or skin lesions have a lower yield of definitive information than biopsy of a lung lesion. The renal lesion is glomerulonephritis; granulomas are rarely found in the kidney. Temporal artery biopsy is the preferred procedure for suspected temporal arteritis. Specificity is high (>90%), but sensitivity (50% to 80%) depends on whether the biopsy is done unilaterally or bilaterally, and on the size of the excised segment (4 cm to 5 cm in length is recommended). Patients with only polymyalgia rheumatica should not have routine temporal artery biopsies. Aortography is the preferred diagnostic procedure for Takayasu's arteritis, showing stenosis, occlusion, saccular aneurysms, or tapered narrowing of involved arteries. Biopsies are not helpful in Kawasaki disease. Echocardiography is a noninvasive procedure that can sometimes demonstrate the coronary artery aneurysms.

PRINCIPLES OF PREVENTION AND THERAPY

Reducing the opportunities for hepatitis B infection through immunization of high-risk groups, along with precautions against inadvertent transmission, may reduce the incidence of vasculitis triggered by this agent. Conservative prescribing of drugs may reduce the incidence of some forms of hypersensitivity vasculitis. A conservative approach should also be employed in treatment of those vasculitides with low potential for serious complications. Many

TABLE 137–5.
Features of Multisystem Diseases Resembling Vasculitis

DISEASES	CLINICAL MANIFESTATIONS	LABORATORY/X-RAY FILM FINDINGS
Rheumatoid arthritis	Symmetric, additive large and small joint polyarthritis; prolonged morning stiffness; subcutaneous nodules; systemic vasculitis occurs in those with severe destructive disease and high titers of RF.	Rheumatoid factor (RF) in 70%–80%; ANA in 30%; no renal abnormalities; periarticular osteopenia and soft tissue swelling; erosions and deformities later
Systemic lupus erythematosis	Malar or discoid rashes; photosensitivity; arthralgia/arthritis; pleuritis/pericarditis in 50%; neuropsychiatric effects in 20%–25%; vasculitis may occur at any time.	ANA in 95%; anti-DNA in 60%; anti-Sm in 30%–40%; RF in 15%; renal abnormalities in 50%–60%; leukopenia, hemolytic anemia or thrombocytopenia; false-positive VDRL; focal or diffuse glomerulonephritis with "lumpy" immunofluorescence
Goodpasture's disease	Hemoptysis; hematuria; renal failure	Iron-deficiency anemia; hematuria; elevated creatinine; antibody to glomerular basement membrane; homogenous immunofluorescence of basement membrane
Juvenile arthritis	Onset may be systemic (fever and rash), polyarticular, or pauciarticular; latter two groups at risk for iridocyclitis; myocarditis, pleuritis in systemic form	RF in 10%–20% of polyarticular; ANA in 30%–50% of pauciarticular group
Rheumatic fever	Migratory polyarthritis; erythema marginatum; carditis; murmurs; subcutaneous nodules; chorea	Elevated ASO titer; ECG abnormalities; cardiomegaly; pulmonary edema
Sarcoidosis	Erythema nodosum; skin plaques and nodules; uveitis; arthralgia; dyspnea; muscle weakness; parotid swelling; anergic skin tests	Bilateral hilar adenopathy; interstitial lung disease; elevated globulin and calcium levels; noncaseating granulomas on biopsy; elevated CPK level
Infective endocarditis	History of valvular disease or drug abuse; mild fever; murmur in > 50%; petechiae upper half of the body; arthralgia; clubbing; congestive failure; metastatic infections in any area of body	Leukocytosis; anemia; nephritis; low complement; RF test often positive; blood cultures positive
Toxic shock	Fever, headache, vomiting, diarrhea, myalgia with refractory hypotension; erythroderma with later desquamation	Increased WBC count; decreased number of platelets; elevated CPK level; focus of staphylococcal infection
Syphilis (secondary)	Mucocutaneous lesions; lymphadenopathy; arthralgias; headache; focal neurologic deficits; seizures	Positive VDRL test and FTA-ABS; CSF pleocytosis; occasionally positive RF and ANA tests
Atrial myxoma	Dyspnea; syncope; peripheral edema; congestive failure; acute limb ischemia; focal neurologic deficits; third heart sounds; rarely, fever and malaise	Echocardiogram reveals atrial mass.
Hypereosinophilic syndrome	Muscle tenderness and weakness; peripheral neuropathy; congestive failure; neuropsychiatric symptoms; hepatosplenomegaly; urticarial or maculopapular rashes	Peripheral eosinophils > 1500/ml; increased CPK and SGOT levels; pulmonary infiltrates and effusions; eosinophilic infiltrate on biopsy

patients with mild forms of hypersensitivity vasculitis require only symptomatic treatment, if any. In the presence of gastrointestinal bleeding or nephritis, a short course of corticosteroids may be indicated. Necrotizing vasculitis of medium-sized arteries requires the use of high doses of corticosteroids, and cytotoxic drugs should be added to the regimen when vital organs are affected. Current survival rates are about 50% with corticosteroid treatment, and up to 80% with corticosteroids plus cytotoxic drugs. Cyclophosphamide is the drug of choice for Wegener's granulomatosis, which, with this treatment, has resulted in a 5-year survival rate of 93%. A diagnosis of definite or probable temporal arteritis mandates high doses of corticosteroids to prevent blindness. Corticosteroids have not been helpful in treating advanced Takayasu's arteritis, but there is hope that if given in the early systemic phase, the late complications may be prevented. At present, high doses of salicylates are considered the drug of choice for Kawasaki disease, because this appears to reduce the incidence of coronary artery aneurysms. Intravenous gamma globulin shows promise.

REFERENCES

Alarcon-Segovia DJ (ed): *Clinics in Rheumatic Diseases.* Philadelphia, WB Saunders Co, 1980, vol 6(2). *The chapters are not of uniform quality, but the one on temporal arteritis is excellent.*

Cupps TR, Fauci AS: The vasculitides, in Smith LH (ed): *Major Problems in Internal Medicine,* vol 21. Philadelphia, WB Saunders Co, 1981, pp 1–211. *Excellent in-depth review of pathophysiology with concise clinical descriptions.*

Fan PT, Davis JA, Somer T, Kaplan L, Bluestone R: A clinical approach to systemic vasculitis. *Semin Arthritis Rheum* 1980; 9:248–304. *Most comprehensive review of a wide spectrum of vasculitides. Good illustrations.*

Fauci AS, Haynes BF, Katz P, Wolff SM: Wegener's granulomatosis: Prospective clinical and therapeutic experience with 85 patients for 21 years. *Ann Intern Med* 1983; 98:76–85. *The best long-term study of the natural history and treatment of a rare but potentially devastating disease. Remissions induced in 85% with cyclophosphamide.*

Hall S, Lie JT, Kurland LT, Persellin S, O'Brien PC, Hunder GG: The therapeutic impact of temporal artery biopsy. *Lancet* 1983; 2:1217–1220. *A good summary of the natural history of temporal arteritis and the utility of biopsy.*

Landing BH, Larson EJ: Are infantile periarteritis nodosa with coronary artery involvement and fatal mucocutaneous lymph node syndrome the same? Comparison of 20 patients from North America with patients from Hawaii and Japan. *Pediatrics* 1977; 59(5):651–662. *A useful study of fatal cases that demonstrates the widespread nature of this usually benign vasculitis.*

Lupi-Herrera E, Sanchez-Torres G, Marcushamer J, Mispireta J, Horwitz S, Vela JE: Takayasu's arteritis. Clinical study of 107 cases. *Am Heart J* 1977; 93(1):94–103. *Informative clinical analysis of an unusually large series, with illustrative angiograms.*

138 RAYNAUD'S PHENOMENON

Alice Faryna, M.D.
Kim Goldenberg, M.D.

Raynaud's phenomenon is an episodic and reversible ischemic event due to vasospasm occurring in acral areas of the body, manifested by sudden onset of pallor or cyanosis or both.

CLINICAL SIGNS AND SYMPTOMS

Classically, patients with Raynaud's phenomenon describe triphasic color changes in the hands or feet precipitated by emotional stress or exposure to the cold. Initially, the skin blanches, then becomes cyanotic. During rewarming or recovery, which may take minutes to hours, the cyanosis is replaced by rubor. Few patients regularly exhibit all three phases; episodic pallor with or without cyanosis of the digits is the more common initial symptom. Other acral sites such as the ears and tip of the nose may be affected. There may be pain or numbness during the episode, but claudication is not a feature. Rarely, patients present with distal extremity pain without color changes.

The attacks may recur for many years without complications. Some patients, however, may develop trophic skin changes, progressive joint stiffness, and small skin ulcerations. A history of associated rash, joint swelling, muscle weakness, malaise, fever, or weight loss is often obtained in those with Raynaud's phenomenon secondary to a systemic disease. A history of repetitive trauma to the hands should be sought, particularly in men.

In cases of primary Raynaud's phenomenon (no underlying disease or identifiable cause), the physical examination is usually completely normal when performed between attacks. During an attack, the color changes described above can be observed. Typically, the affected areas show uniform pallor or cyanosis sharply demarcated from the adjacent normal skin. Bilateral, symmetric involvement of the distal two-thirds of the digits is the most common finding, although occasionally the color change can extend to the entire digit or include the palm. Initially, the attacks may be unilateral. Severe cases may later develop atrophy of the tufts of the digits and cutaneous infarcts or ulcers. Thickening of the skin resembling that in scleroderma occurs in 10% of patients. Gangrene is rare.

In cases of secondary Raynaud's phenomenon, the abnormal physical findings that suggest the presence of an underlying connective tissue disease include scleroderma proximal to the metacarpophalangeal joints, telangiectasia, calcinosis, abnormal nail-fold capillaries, erythematous patches over the knuckles, malar rash, joint swelling or deformity, and proximal muscle weakness. Underlying occlusive vascular disease is suggested by unilateral symptoms, the presence of bruits, or diminished pulses. Special maneuvers (Table 138–1) may be required to elicit these.

An estimated 5% to 10% of the general population and about 20% of women will give a history of Raynaud's phenomenon when carefully questioned. The median age of onset is 39 years, with women predominating (3:1). Early studies suggested that 70% of cases had a benign course. The term *Raynaud's disease* was applied to patients with Raynaud's phenomenon in whom no systemic disease appeared within 2 years of onset, but it is now apparent that many years can elapse between the onset of Raynaud's phenomenon and a connective tissue disease.

In studies of patients referred for evaluation of Raynaud's phenomenon, 32% to 77% are reported to have the primary type initially. About

"

TABLE 138–1.
Tests for Occlusive Vascular Disease

1. Elevate the extremity above the level of the heart—definite pallor within 60 seconds or less suggests occlusive disease.
2. Thoracic outlet syndrome:
   Adson maneuver: With the patient seated, the radial pulse is palpated as the arm is abducted; the head is extended and turned first away from and then toward the examined arm. Pulse quality should be observed and the supraclavicular space auscultated for bruits.
   Costoclavicular maneuver: The patient is instructed to stand in exaggerated military posture with the shoulders pulled backward and down. Check for radial pulse diminution.
   Hyperabduction maneuver: Check pulses after the arms are laterally circumducted and clasped above the head.
3. Palmar arch occlusive disease:
   Allen's test: After the fist is firmly clenched, the radial artery is manually compressed. The fist is then opened; if the ulnar artery is patent, the color should rapidly return to the palm. The test is then repeated with compression of the ulnar artery to test for patency of the radial artery.
4. Carpal tunnel syndrome:
   Phalen's maneuver: The wrists are acutely flexed by pressing the dorsum of the hands together for 30 seconds to 60 seconds. Reproduction of pain and paresthesia in the fingers suggests carpal tunnel syndrome.

8% of those followed for several years will develop a connective tissue disease. In up to 25%, trophic changes will develop in the digits, but gangrene occurs in less than 1%. In about 16%, the attacks eventually cease. Up to 22% of patients with primary Raynaud's phenomenon can be shown to have associated abnormalities in the skin, lungs, kidneys, or joints, but do not initially meet criteria for diagnosis of a systemic disease. Such patients are often classified as having "undifferentiated connective tissue disease." About 35% of these patients will later develop a recognizable connective tissue disease, usually systemic sclerosis. Onset of Raynaud's phenomenon in childhood is considered to be secondary to connective tissue disease in most cases, although prospective studies are lacking.

PATHOPHYSIOLOGY

Vasospasm occurs either when increased arterial tone exceeds intraluminal pressure or when normal arterial tone acts on a reduced blood volume. Raynaud originally proposed that excessive sympathetic activity was the cause of the syndrome. Central thermoregulatory mechanisms appear to be intact, however, and vasomotor tone is probably not increased because nerve blocks do not abort an attack. Local vascular defects are thought to be the central pathologic change, but the mechanism remains unknown.

Most of the blood flow through the fingertips passes through arteriovenous shunts rather than through capillaries. Normal subjects maintain capillary flow when cooled but have reduced shunt blood flow. Primary Raynaud's phenomenon patients reduce flow in both systems upon cooling but maintain the reduction in capillary flow even after rewarming.

Studies of blood viscosity show conflicting results. Increased production of prostaglandins and thromboxane has been documented, raising the possibility that local abnormalities in vasomotor regulation and platelet function may play a role. Repeated episodes of intravascular coagulation with release of vasoactive amines from platelets, and impaired release of histamine from perivascular mast cells have also been postulated as potential mechanisms of local defects.

There are few histopathologic studies of dermal vessels in primary Raynaud's phenomenon. Endothelial swelling and narrowing of the vessel lumen have been reported, but these changes may be age related. Intimal proliferation and fibrosis without inflammatory reaction or fibrinoid necrosis are the most common findings in systemic sclerosis patients with Raynaud's phenomenon. Nail-fold biopsies in primary Raynaud's phenomenon show a capillary density that is diminished and intermediate

TABLE 138–2.
Clinical–Pathologic Correlations for Raynaud's Phenomenon

DISORDER	CLINICAL FINDINGS	PATHOLOGIC FINDINGS	
		MECHANISM OF RP*	PATHOLOGIC CHANGES
Primary RP	Bilateral symmetric and triphasic color changes of digits; reversible; induced by cold or emotion; primarily in young women	Vasospasm due to local vascular defect	Exaggerated response to normal sympathetic tone postulated
Connective tissue disorders	History of rash, joint, or muscle pain; multisystem signs and symptoms; auto-antibodies	Structural changes in small vessels with reduced local flow	Intimal thickening, fibrosis, thrombosis in systemic sclerosis; vasculitis in other disorders
Occlusive arterial disorders	Large and small vessel involvement; claudication; faint or absent pulses; positional pallor and rubor; bruits; risk factors for atherosclerosis	Vessel-narrowing with reduced flow distally	Atheromata with local thrombi or distal emboli
Thromboangiitis obliterans	Upper and lower extremity ischemia; primarily in young men; smoking history; migratory thrombophlebitis	Vessel-narrowing with reduced local flow	Segmental inflammation of small/medium arteries and veins; hypersensitivity to tobacco postulated
Trauma	Ischemia may be unilateral or involve single digits; occupational history of repetitive trauma	1. Endothelial injury 2. Vasospasm at vibratory frequencies near 125 Hz	1. Thrombosis or aneurysm 2. Endothelial damage
Entrapment	Symptoms related to position or activities; paresthesia or weakness may be persistent.	Compression of neurovascular bundle; vasospasm	Sympathetic nerve irritation, extraluminal compression
Hematologic disease	Systemic signs and symptoms, purpura, renal failure	Particulate occlusion of small vessels	Hyperviscosity from cryoglobulins, monoclonal gammopathy, polycythemia, cold agglutinin disease
Drugs	Ischemia, gangrene, or claudication; history of drug exposure	Vasoconstriction or fibrosis	Direct action on vessel walls or mediated by alpha-adrenergic receptors
Reflex sympathetic dystrophy	Chronic pain and edema of hands; often unilateral; history of infarct, myocardial infarct, stroke, trauma	Vasospasm	Sympathetic nerve irritation

* RP = Raynaud's phenomenon

between that found in normals and that in patients with the CREST variant of systemic sclerosis (calcinosis, Raynaud's, esophageal dysmotility, sclerodactyly, telangiectasia). Clinical–pathologic correlations are presented in Table 138–2. The most common cause of secondary Raynaud's phenomenon is a connective tissue disease, accounting for about 50% of this type of the disease.

DIFFERENTIAL DIAGNOSIS

In young, otherwise asymptomatic women with a normal physical examination, Raynaud's phenomenon is most likely the primary type. In children, adults over the age of 40 years, and men of all ages, Raynaud's phenomenon is more likely to be secondary. Most cases of Raynaud's phenomenon in the general population are primary, but this form is likely to be under-represented in referral centers where the more complicated cases are sent. Features that favor a diagnosis of secondary Raynaud's phenomenon are persistent unilateral or single digit involvement; history of repetitive trauma to the hands or use of vibratory tools; exposure to certain toxins or drugs; progression to chronic ischemia or gangrene; and symptoms or signs of a systemic disease. The sensitivity of Raynaud's phenomenon is high in systemic sclerosis and mixed connective tissue disease, but because of the high prevalence of primary Raynaud's phenomenon (up to 20% in females), the specificity is low (see Table 137–3). The presence of immune system abnormalities on laboratory testing is suggestive of an underlying systemic disease, even if the patient is asymptomatic, because the latent period may be several years. Regular follow-up of such patients is recommended.

DIAGNOSIS

The diagnosis of Raynaud's phenomenon is made from the history and physical findings. In doubtful cases, a cold challenge may be done by immersing the hands in ice water for 20 seconds to 30 seconds and observing for typical color changes. (This should not be done when trophic changes of the digits have occurred.)

Normal subjects will return to pre-immersion skin temperature and color in less than 10 minutes, while patients with Raynaud's phenomenon require 20 minutes or more. As noted above, distinguishing primary from secondary Raynaud's phenomenon is more difficult.

There are no laboratory markers of Raynaud's phenomenon. A complete blood count, sedimentation rate, urinalysis, tests for rheumatoid factor, ANA, and cryoglobulins, and serum electrophoresis are a reasonable screen for an underlying systemic disease. Other laboratory tests should be selected on the basis of clues derived from the history and physical findings.

X-ray films of the cervical spine may reveal a cervical rib causing a thoracic outlet obstruction. The ability to rapidly restore skin temperature after cold exposure and rewarming may help exclude occlusive disease. Doppler blood-flow study is a noninvasive method for evaluating possible occlusive disease. Arteriography is the most definitive way to identify vascular occlusion, but should not be done routinely.

PRINCIPLES OF PREVENTION AND TREATMENT

For some patients, wearing warm apparel and avoiding cold exposure may be sufficient to prevent attacks. Mild attacks can sometimes be aborted by whirling the arms around or through biofeedback techniques. Tobacco use should be discouraged, and vasoconstricting drugs should be discontinued. In more severe cases, more aggressive therapy is required. A variety of drugs have been used with variable results. Alpha-adrenergic blockers (phenoxybenzamine, tolazoline) and catecholamine depletors (reserpine and methyldopa) have all been reported to be of benefit to some patients. Intra-arterial reserpine has occasionally successfully reversed severe ischemia. Recently, the calcium-channel blockers have shown promising results. Stanozolol, a fibrinolytic enhancer, has been reported to be beneficial in some patients. Sympathetic nerve block has had variable results, with better response in lower extremities than in upper extremities. Cervical sympathectomy has not been effective.

TABLE 138–3.
Differential Diagnosis of Secondary Raynaud's Phenomenon

	INCIDENCE OF RP (% OF CASES)	COMPLICATIONS
Connective tissue disorder		
Systemic sclerosis	98	Gangrene of digits,
Mixed connective tissue disease	85	pulmonary hypertension,
Dermatomyositis	12–45	"scleroderma kidney"
Systemic lupus erythematosus	15–20	Rarely gangrene of digits
Rheumatoid arthritis	10	Cutaneous ulcers
		Occasional evolution into systemic sclerosis
		Rarely necrotizing vasculitis
Arterial occlusion		
Arteriosclerosis obliterans	NA*	Gangrene; amputation
Thromboangiitis obliterans	NA	Gangrene; amputation
Entrapment syndromes		
Thoracic outlet obstruction	NA	Chronic pain, paresthesia
Carpal tunnel syndrome	0.1	Weakness, atrophy of hand
Trauma		
Vibratory tools	50	Rarely gangrene
Cold exposure	Up to 90% in some occupations	Rarely gangrene
Hematologic disorder		
Cryoglobulins	Rare	Low potential for gangrene
Monoclonal gammopathy	Rare	with all types
Polycythemia	Rare	
Drugs		
Ergot	NA	Occasionally gangrene or
Methysergide	NA	trophic changes
Beta-blockers	Up to 50% in some series	
Bleomycin	NA	
Polyvinylchloride	Infrequent	
Miscellaneous	NA	
Reflex sympathetic distrophy		
Pheochromocytoma		
Primary pulmonary hypertension		
Variant angina		
Myxedema		

* NA = Not available.

In secondary Raynaud's phenomenon, the underlying disorder should be treated when possible. Neurovascular compression syndromes can be treated with postural exercises or occasionally surgery (resection of a cervical rib, carpal tunnel release, thrombectomy). Raynaud's phenomenon associated with vasculitis may be responsive to corticosteroids. Plasmapheresis may be beneficial in the rare cases due to hyperviscosity. Studies are currently being conducted on the efficacy of vasodilatory prostaglandins and inhibitors of thromboxane.

REFERENCES

Blunt RJ, Porter JM: Raynaud syndrome. *Semin Arthritis Rheum* 1981; 10:282–308. *Most comprehensive review of all aspects of Raynaud's phenomenon, with over 250 references.*

Spencer-Green G: Raynaud phenomenon. *Bull Rheum Dis* 1983; 33(5). *Very concise summary of the entire subject, and more up-to-date than Blunt and Porter, 1981, on treatment.*

Spittel JA: Clinical vascular disease, in Brest AN (ed): *Cardiovascular Clinics.* Philadelphia, FA Davis, 1983, pp 62–80. *An indispensable guide to the recognition of occlusive vascular diseases that may mimic vasospastic disease.*

Wyngaarden JG, Smith LH (eds): *Cecil Textbook of Medicine,* ed 17. Philadelphia, WB Saunders Co, 1985, pp 353–356. *Best textbook presentation of Raynaud's phenomenon; brief but thorough.*

139 PROGRESSIVE SYSTEMIC SCLEROSIS

John G. Paty, Jr., M.D.

Progressive systemic sclerosis (PSS or scleroderma) is a rare systemic disorder characterized by tightening and induration of the skin of the hands (sclerodactyly), arms, legs, trunk, and face. It is four times as common in women as men. Esophageal motility disturbance and pulmonary involvement occur in over 90% of patients. Other internal organs may be involved such as the small bowel, colon, kidneys, and heart. Cardiac involvement with cardiomyopathy and associated arrhythmias and kidney involvement with accelerated hypertension are often life threatening.

CLINICAL SIGNS AND SYMPTOMS

The patient with PSS usually presents with Raynaud's phenomenon, skin involvement, dysphagia, dyspepsia, or arthritis. The arthritis is similar to that in rheumatoid arthritis but with less joint swelling. During the early phase, diffuse edema of the hands and forearms may occur and may be confused with other types of arthritis. Later, as the skin becomes indurated, tightness and stiffness of the hands are common complaints. Patients often complain of food "hanging up" in the middle of their chest. Dysphagia occurs with solid foods and, as the motility disturbance progresses, patients report having to "wash their food down" with liquids. Bowel involvement may cause chronic diarrhea due to bacterial overgrowth, malabsorption, or obstruction. Less often patients present with the new onset hypertension or dyspnea on exertion. Some patients have a limited form of progressive systemic sclerosis, the CREST syndrome, which includes calcinosis, Raynaud's phenomenon, esophageal motility disturbance, sclerodactyly, and telangiectasia.

In PSS, the sclerodactyly and limited motion of the digits often result in a decreased hand grip. An indurated "hide-bound" texture to the skin may be present, and the face may appear pinched with a limited ability to open the mouth ("tobacco-pouch" mouth). Telangiectasis may be present on the lower lip, face, palms, buccal mucosa, or periungual areas. Ulcerated or even gangrenous fingertips with auto-amputation secondary to Raynaud's phenomenon may be present. Chest auscultation may reveal coarse basilar crackles. With renal involvement, hypertension is usually present and the eyegrounds may demonstrate findings of malignant hypertension.

The natural history of scleroderma depends on the organs involved. Pulmonary, renal, and cardiac involvement indicate a poor prognosis, and failure of these systems or associated complications are the major causes of death. With renal involvement, a clinical picture of malignant hypertension usually ensues, with most patients surviving less than 6 months. However, recent experience with aggressive management of the hypertension, including the use of the angiotensin-converting enzyme inhibitor (captopril) and hemodialysis, appears to improve this grim outlook. Cardiac involvement (including cardiomyopathy with congestive heart failure, conduction defects with associated arrhythmias including complete heart block secondary to fibrosis of the conduction system) is also a major cause of mortality. Ninety percent of the patients with scleroderma will at some time during their course have pulmonary involvement characterized by restrictive lung disease due to an interstitial fibrosis. Impairment of gas exchange is common, particularly of the CO diffusing capacity. When the involvement is extensive, respiratory failure ensues. Intimal hyperplasia of the pulmonary arteries may accompany the pulmonary disorder, setting the stage for chronic respiratory failure and cor pulmonale. Although patients with the CREST syndrome have little internal organ involvement, eventual death from pulmonary hypertension is not uncommon.

DIFFERENTIAL DIAGNOSIS

When "hide-bound" skin on the back of the hand is absent, other diagnoses must be considered. Patients with Raynaud's disease may have sclerodactyly distal to the proximal interphalangeal joints secondary to ischemic atrophy of the distal phalanges. However, proximal to the metacarpal-phalangeal joints skin abnormalities are not present, and internal organ involvement, except for the distal esophagus, is absent. Mixed connective tissue disease may appear quite similar to the early edematous phase of scleroderma. These mixed patients may have features of several connective tissue disorders including polymyositis, systemic lupus, scleroderma, and rheumatoid arthritis. Diffuse swelling of hands and digits and Raynaud's phenomena are also common in these patients, but the more proximal skin changes are absent. Serologically they have high titer (> 1:640), speckle-patterned antinuclear antibodies with positive ribonuclear protein (RNP) antibodies. Moreover, some ultimately develop typical scleroderma during the several-year course of their disease. Patients with polymyositis or dermatomyositis lack the typical skin changes of scleroderma, but some

patients with scleroderma may have a myocytic component (scleromyositis). Patients with systemic lupus will not have scleroderma skin involvement, but, as previously noted, a positive ANA will be present in about 50% of PSS patients.

DIAGNOSIS

The diagnosis of progressive systemic sclerosis is based on the history and typical skin changes. Occasionally, patients with bowel involvement will have minimal skin changes (progressive systemic sclerosis *sine* scleroderma). Fifty percent or more of patients will have a positive antinuclear antibody test, and about 30% a positive rheumatoid factor test. The antinuclear antibody is generally of a speckled pattern and moderate ($\leq$ 1:640) titer. An elevated erythrocyte sedimentation rate and hypergammaglobulinemia are seen in about half of these patients. Cryoglobulins and cryofibrinogens may also be found. At least 90% of patients will have an abnormality of their pulmonary function studies including a decrease in vital capacity and carbon monoxide diffusion capacity. The echocardiogram may show a pericardial effusion or dilated ventricles with poor contractility or both. In patients with dyspnea, a Muga scan may be helpful in evaluating left ventricle function. The ECG may show supraventricular or ventricular arrhythmias, heart block, or low voltage. Chest x-rays may show an enlarged heart and interstitial fibrosis. The upper GI series may show poor motility of the distal third of the esophagus. Esophageal motility disturbances may not be seen with x-ray studies. Manometric esophageal motility evaluation, when available, is the most sensitive method of evaluating esophageal function. Duodenal involvement can usually be demonstrated by the "loop sign" (dilated duodenum) on the upper GI series. Wide-mouthed diverticulae of the small bowel and the colon may be seen on the small bowel series and barium enema.

PATHOPHYSIOLOGY

Microcirculatory studies in patients with scleroderma, including muscle biopsy and nail-fold capillary measurements, demonstrate a decreased number of small arterioles and a loss of capillaries with secondary hypertrophy of other capillaries. Scleroderma, therefore, may be promulgated by an abnormality in the microcirculation. The organ fibrosis and the deposition of increased collagen in the dermis, characteristic of scleroderma, may occur as a result of these abnormal microcirculatory changes. Histologically, the collagen appears to be immature but otherwise normal. In the early edematous phase, excessive mucopolysaccharide production (glycosaminoglycans) by skin fibroblasts has been postulated. Recent data have implicated the production of lymphokines chemotactic for fibroblasts, the perpetrators of the fibrosing process, by T-cells.

The critical clinical–pathologic correlations for scleroderma are shown in Table 139–1.

PRINCIPLES OF THERAPY

Treatment depends on the specific organ involved. Antibiotics may be helpful in cases of chronic diarrhea due to bacterial overgrowth resulting from hypomotility. Cimetidine may be of benefit in preventing esophageal stricture. The treatment of renal disease must be vigorous. Encouraging results have recently been reported using the angiotensin-converting enzyme inhibitor, captopril. In spite of vigorous antihypertensive management, however, some patients develop progressive renal failure and require dialysis. A permanent pacemaker may be required if complete heart block or a sick sinus node is present. There is little or no place for corticosteroids in the management of scleroderma. Reports of the benefits of penicillamine therapy are anecdotal and unproven at this time.

TABLE 139–1.
Clinical–Pathologic Correlation of Scleroderma

ORGAN SYSTEM INVOLVED	CLINICAL FEATURES	PATHOLOGIC CORRELATION
Heart	Cardiomegaly, congestive heart failure, arrhythmia	Intimal proliferation of intramyocardial coronary vessels and perivascular and contraction band fibrosis
	Asymptomatic or symptomatic pericardial effusion	Pericardial inflammation or fibrosis
Kidney	Hypertension, azotemia, decreased glomerular filtration rate, proteinuria, renal failure	Arteriolar intimal hyperplasia with medial thinning and adventitial fibrosis or necrotizing fibrinoid necrosis of renal arterioles (malignant hypertensive changes)
Lung	Dyspnea, chest pain, cough, rales, cor pulmonale, interstitial lung markings or pleural effusion on chest x-ray	Intimal hyperplasia of small pulmonary arteries or arterioles, alveolar inflammation and/or fibrosis or inflammation of the pleura
GI	Dysphagia, abnormal esophageal motility	Smooth muscle atrophy and fibrosis of the lower esophagus
	Diarrhea, malabsorption, obstruction, large mouth diverticulae on small bowel series or barium enema	Small bowel or colon smooth muscle atrophy and fibrosis
Skin	Edema (early phase)	Subcutaneous lymphoid and mononuclear cell infiltration
	Hide-bound (late) and depigmentation or hypopigmentation	Increased dermal collagen and loss of dermal appendages

REFERENCES

Follansbee WP, Curtiss EI, Medsger TA et al: Physiologic abnormalities of cardiac function in progressive systemic sclerosis with diffuse scleroderma. *N Engl J Med 1984; 310:142–148, Scintigraphic evaluation of coronary circulation of myocardial function in scleroderma.*

Huffstutter JE, LeRoy EC: Scleroderma as a fibrotic disorder, in Gupta S, Talal N (eds). *Immunology of Rheumatic Diseases.* New York, Plenum Publishing Corp, 1985, pp 397–423. *Review of investigations into the pathogenesis of scleroderma.*

LeRoy EC: Scleroderma (systemic sclerosis), in Kelly WN, Harris ED, Ruddy S, Sledge CB (eds). *Textbook of Rheumatology,* vol II. Philadelphia, WB Saunders Co, 1981, pp 1211–1230. *Excellent review of clinical and pathologic features and medical treatment of patients with scleroderma.*

Lopez-Overjero JA, Saal SD, D'Angelo WA, Cheigh JS, Stenzel KH, Laragh JH: Reversal of vascular and renal crises of scleroderma by oral angiotensin-converting enzyme blockade. *N Engl J Med 1979; 300:1417–1419. Successful reversal of scleroderma renal crises using angiotensin-converting-enzyme inhibitor.*

Maricq HR, LeRoy EC, D'Angelo WA et al: Diagnostic potential of in vivo capillary microscopy in scleroderma and related disorders. *Arthritis Rheum 1980; 23:183–189. Nail-fold capillary loop microscopy in connective tissue disease.*

Masi AT, Rodnan GP: Preliminary criteria for the classification of systemic sclerosis (scleroderma). *Bull Rheum Dis 1981; 21:1–6. American Rheumatism Association's criteria for scleroderma demonstrating sensitivity and specificity greater than 90% in diagnosing scleroderma.*

Medsger TA, Masi AT, Rodnan GP, Benedek TG, Robinson H: Survival with systemic sclerosis (scleroderma). A life-table analysis of clinical and demographic factors in 309 patients. *Ann Intern Med 1971; 75:369–376. Scleroderma survival in Pittsburgh, Pa and Memphis, Tenn showing decreased survival with renal, cardiac, and pulmonary involvement with worse prognosis correlated with older age, males, and blacks.*

Roberts NK, Cabeen WR, Moss J, Clements PJ, Furst DE: The prevalence of conduction defects and cardiac arrhythmias in progressive systemic sclerosis. *Ann Intern Med 1981; 94:38–40. Analysis of conduction defects and arrhythmias in 50 patients with progressive systemic sclerosis.*

Rodnan GP, Fennell RH: Progressive systemic sclerosis with scleroderma. *JAMA 1962; 180:665–670. Four patients who died with progressive systemic sclerosis with minimal skin involvement.*

140 POLYMYALGIA RHEUMATICA AND GIANT CELL ARTERITIS

John G. Paty, Jr., M.D.

Polymyalgia rheumatica (PMR) and giant cell arteritis (GCA) (temporal arteritis) are disorders of unknown cause that occur almost exclusively in the elderly. They are rare before the seventh decade. Polymyalgia rheumatica is a pain disorder primarily affecting the proximal limbs with an accompanying high erythrocyte sedimentation rate (ESR). It may occur as an isolated entity or as a presenting manifestation of giant cell arteritis or other collagen vascular disease. Giant cell arteritis is a granulomatous vasculitis affecting medium and large vessels. It may initially appear as polymyalgia rheumatica, headache, fever of unknown origin, or disturbance of vision.

CLINICAL SIGNS AND SYMPTOMS

Polymyalgia rheumatica is characterized by pain in the shoulder and hip girdles *(pseudopolyarthrite rhizomelique)*. Its onset may be sudden or insidious. The patient may experience a viral-like illness followed by persistent pain in the shoulders, upper arms, hips, or thighs. The pain may last throughout the day with only minimal improvement with activity. Alternately patients may awaken with a sudden onset of severe pain having had no prodromal illness. They often have to be helped out of bed. In either instance, patients will usually have been ill for several weeks before seeing a physician (Table 140–1).

Giant cell arteritis, granulomatous angiitis, particularly involves the vessels branching from the aortic arch. In addition to polymyalgia rheumatica, patients may present complaining of an onset (often sudden) of a headache. The headache is usually unilateral and/or temporal with an accompanying tenderness of the involved temporal artery. The headache may also be bilateral or less often generalized or occipital. Visual symptoms, when present, tend to follow the headache and usually indicate ophthalmic artery involvement. Blurred vision, diplopia, or transient blindness are the most common of these complaints. Intermittent claudication involving the muscles of mastication or very rarely the calf muscles is a less common early manifestation of giant cell arteritis. Fever of unknown origin with weight loss and anemia may be another clinical appearance of giant cell arteritis. Occasionally malignancy is initially invoked as the underlying cause of the patient's debility (Table 140–2).

The physical findings in polymyalgia rheumatica are few. Joint motion is normal. Trigger points are usually absent, but some patients complain of pain when the involved area is palpated. Muscle strength is usually normal. A mild synovitis may be present in the wrists, knees, or metacarpophalangeal (MCP), and proximal interphalangeal (PIP) joints. When polymyalgia rheumatica is the initial manifestation of another collagen vascular disease such as rheumatoid arthritis or systemic lupus erythematosus, the physical examination may demonstrate findings suggestive of the other disorder. When accompanied by a history of headache, and a palpable tender temporal artery, there is presumptive evidence for temporal arteritis. If vision is impaired, papilledema associated with optic neuritis may be seen.

In giant cell arteritis, the positive physical findings, if present, are limited to a diminished or absent temporal pulse and/or tender temporal artery (or carotid rarely), an abdominal bruit, or bruit over the involved vessel. Patients may have signs of recent weight loss or pallor.

The natural history of polymyalgia rheumatica depends on its disease association. If giant cell arteritis is present, the ultimate outlook depends on the course of the arteritis. If it occurs in its purest form, without an associated collagen vascular disease, the prognosis is excellent, and most patients with treatment will become asymptomatic within 2 years. When polymyalgia rheumatica is the initial manifes-

TABLE 140–1.
Clinical–Pathologic Correlation for Polymyalgia Rheumatica

CLINICAL FINDINGS	PATHOLOGIC FINDINGS
Shoulder and hip girdle pain	Unknown Negative biopsy
High erythrocyte sedimentation rate	

TABLE 140–2.
Clinical–Pathologic Correlation for Giant Cell Arteritis

CLINICAL FINDINGS	PATHOLOGIC FINDINGS
Headache	Arteritis of medium and large sized vessels, particularly those off the aortic arch; inflammatory response involves intima, media, and adventitia
Visual symptoms	
Jaw claudication	Disruption of internal elastic laminae with infiltration of histiocytes, lymphocytes and giant cell
Polymyalgia rheumatica	
Fever, weight loss, anemia	Partial or complete occlusion of vessels by inflammatory process

tation of another collagen vascular disease, the ultimate prognosis depends on the outcome of the associated disease.

The natural history of giant cell arteritis depends on the presence or absence of visual symptoms. Visual impairment or blindness (amaurosis fugax) is its most frequent and serious complication. If treatment is begun before the onset of visual symptoms, the outlook is good. If not, a permanent loss of vision may occur. Central nervous system and other vascular complications are rare.

DIFFERENTIAL DIAGNOSIS

In polymyalgia rheumatica the differential diagnoses include fibrositis, giant cell arteritis, or other collagen vascular disease. Both systemic lupus erythematosus and rheumatoid arthritis may initially present as polymyalgia rheumatica. Antinuclear antibody (ANA) and rheumatoid factor (RF) tests are negative in cases of "pure" polymyalgia rheumatica. Fibrositis is rare after the age of 60 years, and the ESR is normal. Giant cell arteritis can be presumed to be absent if headache and the visual symptoms or other vascular symptoms (e.g., jaw claudication) as well as systemic symptoms such as fever and anemia are absent. In this clinical setting, a temporal artery biopsy can be deferred. However, patients should be instructed to notify the physician if a headache, visual problems, or other vascular symptoms occur.

The differential diagnoses of giant cell arteritis, particularly when it appears as polymyalgia or a fever of unknown origin includes systemic infection, carcinoma, drug fever, or other collagen vascular disease. When it appears as a headache, a central nervous system infection or tumor and migraine headache (rare in the elderly) should be considered. In the elderly patient it may be difficult to clinically distinguish functional headaches from giant cell arteritis, particularly if the ESR is moderately elevated (30 mm to 80 mm/hour Westergren method) and temporal artery tenderness is mimicked by functional cephalgia and tenderness.

DIAGNOSIS

The diagnosis of polymyalgia rheumatica is based on one or more of the characteristic findings in the history and physical examina-

tion plus an elevated ESR of 50 mm/hour or more (usually higher, often above 70 mm/hour). The laboratory findings are otherwise unremarkable. A dramatic improvement with low doses of prednisone (10 mg/day) may be used as a therapeutic trial to aid in diagnosis.

The diagnosis of giant cell arteritis is based on the history, the physical findings, the presence of an elevated ESR by the Westergren method of 50 mm/hour (frequently 100 mm/hour or more) and the characteristic histology of granulomatous angiitis on examination of a temporal artery biopsy. Often a low-grade fever and normocytic, normochromic anemia are present.

PATHOPHYSIOLOGY

The causes of both polymyalgia rheumatica and giant cell arteritis are unknown. Levels of circulating immune complexes may be elevated. Immunoglobulin particles of IgA, IgG, and complement have been found in the involved arteries of patients with giant cell arteritis and in the synovial phagocytic cells of patients with polymyalgia rheumatica. Circulating immune complexes usually decrease following treatment with corticosteroids and in general correlate with the erythrocyte sedimentation rate (ESR) (i.e., the higher the ESR, the higher the level of circulating immune complexes). The precise role of immune complexes in the disease, however, is not known. Circulating lymphoblasts suggesting turned-on lymphocytes, as reported in rheumatoid arthritis, have also been reported in polymyalgia rheumatica. This is not specific for the disorder but may be interpreted as evidence of an ongoing immune response. Tests of cellular immunity in patients with giant cell arteritis and polymyalgia rheumatica have shown no consistent abnormality. Serum from patients with polymyalgia rheumatica and giant cell arteritis have been reported to be cytotoxic for human endothelial cells which decreases with disease remission in most patients. Only one study has shown an association of HLA antigens with polymyalgia rheumatica and giant cell arteritis. In that study an increased incidence of HLA/B8 was reported, but in general no haplotype has been found significantly increased above controls in either disease. The higher incidence of these diseases in the rather homogeneous population of northern Europe and the relative infrequent occurrence in blacks, however, suggests a genetic factor. Finally there is one report of a husband and wife with GCA/PMR which invokes the potential of an infectious etiology.

PRINCIPLES OF THERAPY

Patients with polymyalgia rheumatica improve dramatically within a few hours or days following the institution of daily low dose of corticosteroids. The dosage can be slowly tapered while monitoring the patient's symptoms and the ESR for evidence of reactivation. Failure to respond to low doses of prednisone or worsening in a patient who initially improves, requires a careful investigation for other causes including giant cell arteritis.

Treatment of giant cell arteritis is directed at controlling the inflammatory vasculitis; therefore, initial high doses of corticosteroids are required. When the diagnosis is suspected, treatment should begin immediately, prior to obtaining the biopsy results. Monitoring the ESR is usually a reliable method for assessing the activity of the vasculitis and adjusting the corticosteroid dose. However, the observation of a patient's symptoms is the most important because occasionally the ESR will be normal (< 30 mm/hour) in the presence of active polymyalgia rheumatica or giant cell arteritis.

REFERENCES

Fernandez-Herlihy L: Polymyalgia rheumatica. *Semin Arthritis Rheum* 1971; I:236–245. *Review of clinical features of polymyalgia rheumatica.*

Hamilton DR, Shelley WM, Tumulty PA: Giant cell arteritis: Including temporal arteritis and polymyalgia rheumatica. *Medicine* 1971; 50:1–27. *Clinical and pathologic features of giant cell arteritis including prognosis and treatment.*

Hauser WA, Ferguson RH, Holley KE et al: Temporal arteritis in Rochester, Minnesota, 1951 to 1967. *Mayo Clin Proc* 1971; 46:597–602. *Demographic features and incidence of giant cell arteritis in Rochester, Minnesota.*

Healey LA: Polymyalgia rheumatica and giant cell arteritis, in McCarty DJ (ed): *Arthritis and Allied Conditions*, ed 10. Philadelphia, Lea & Febiger, 1985, pp 901–904. *Textbook of rheumatology chapter on polymyalgia rheumatica and giant cell arteritis.*

Healey LA, Parker F, Wilske KR: Polymyalgia rheumatica and giant cell arteritis. *Arthritis Rheum* 1971; 14:138–141. *Guidelines on diagnosis of polymyalgia rheumatica and giant cell arteritis.*

Healey LA, Wilske KR: Manifestations of giant cell arteritis. *Med Clin North Am* 1977; 61:261–270. *Excellent article on treatment of giant cell arteritis.*

OSTEOPOROSIS

Gilbert L. Wergowske, M.D.

Osteoporosis is a decrease in bone mass associated with an increased susceptibility to fractures. Although bone mass normally decreases with age, osteoporosis is not a normal aging phenomenon. Juvenile osteoporosis is a rare, self-limited disease of prepuberty associated with vertebral collapse and metaphyseal injury. The regional osteoporoses are local disorders related to disuse, inflammation, necrosis, or idiopathic causes. Pain in regional and juvenile osteoporosis may occur in the absence of fracture, whereas pain in postmenopausal osteoporosis is almost always associated with a fracture. The term osteopenia denotes decreased bone mass without reference to etiology.

CLINICAL SIGNS AND SYMPTOMS

Early in the disease process there may not be symptoms, and history may be limited to risk factors for osteoporosis. Pain usually is not present without a recent fracture. Loss of height or a previous fracture (usually of the wrist) with minimal trauma may be reported. Risk factors for osteoporosis are listed in Table 141–1, with their pathologic correlations.

When physical signs are present, the disease is far advanced. Examination may reveal thoracic kyphosis with compensatory increased lordosis of the cervical and lumbar spine or scoliosis from vertebral compression fractures. Tenderness and pain may be present along the spine due to muscle spasm, recent fracture, or irritation of the skin from bone prominences unprotected by adequate soft tissue.

Many osteoporotic patients suffer progressive compression fractures of the thoracic and upper lumbar vertebrae, and fractures of the distal radius and of the neck of the femur. Although radial fractures usually precede femoral fractures by about 25 years, it is impossible to predict the course of the disease in the individual patient. Some severely osteopenic patients never suffer any fracture. Fracture of the wrist limits activity only temporarily, but may produce a fear of falling that perpetuates inactivity. Vertebral fractures, which reduce activity and mobility through pain and deformity, most often occur in women aged 55 years to 75 years because of an accelerated loss of trabecular bone.

Fractures of the hip tend to occur in men and women over 65 years of age, from gradual, combined cortical and trabecular bone loss. These fractures often result in prolonged immobilization and progression of the osteoporosis. About 20% to 30% of patients with hip fractures suffer immediate morbidity from such complications as pulmonary emboli or infection, but even without these complications the 2- to 10-year survival after a hip fracture is significantly less than expected for usual age and sex of these patients. Over 8 million people in the United States have osteoporosis, and about 40,000 people each year require long-term care for a hip-fracture-related disability.

PATHOPHYSIOLOGY

Peak bone mass occurs at about age 35 years for cortical bone and somewhat earlier for trabecular bone. Bone mass is about 30% higher in men than women and about 10% higher in black people than white people. Bone mass decreases rapidly for 3 years to 7 years after menopause, and accelerated trabecular loss begins before menses actually cease.

Thinning of the trabeculae in the vertebral bodies is pronounced, and loss of strength is out of proportion to trabecular loss. The horizontal trabeculae are particularly affected. Vertebral compression fractures are common, but

TABLE 141–1.
Risk Factors for Osteoporosis

RISK FACTOR	CLINICAL CORRELATION	PATHOLOGIC CORRELATION
Age	Bone mass normally decreases with age for all population groups.	Decreased bone mass, increased susceptibility to accelerated bone resorption
Sex	Female peak bone mass is less.	Less bone mass from which to lose
	Menopause accelerates bone resorption.	Accelerated bone loss
Race	Less peak bone mass in white and Oriental patients than in black patients	Less bone mass from which to lose
Heredity	Fair-skinned patients of European descent more susceptible	Not well understood
		Possibly less peak bone mass
Body habitus	Thin, underweight	Less peak bone mass
		Possibly decreased stress stimulation of bone formation
Nulliparity	Less peak bone mass	Less bone mass from which to lose
Early menopause (natural or surgical)	Estrogen deficiency accelerates bone resorption.	Bone loss may begin with less peak bone mass; longer exposure to accelerated resorption
Decreased calcium intake	Decreases calcium available for absorption	Less peak bone mass
		Increased requirements from bone stores
Malabsorption (disease or surgical)	Decreases absorption of available calcium	Less peak bone mass
		Increased requirements from bone stores
Cigarette smoking	Accelerates menopause	Bone loss begins earlier
	Possibly accelerates estrogen metabolism	Decreased protective effect from estrogen therapy
Medications	Interferes with calcium or vitamin D metabolism; accelerates bone resorption	Less peak bone mass
Heparin		Increased requirements from bone stores; increased susceptibility to accelerated resorption
Corticosteroids		
Antacids		
Dilantin		
Alcoholism	Malabsorption; liver disease, increased calcium excretion	Less peak bone mass
		Increased requirements from bone stores; increased susceptibility to accelerated resorption
Coffee drinking	Decreases bone mass	Lower bone mass from which to lose
High protein intake	Increases calcium excretion	Increased requirements from bone stores
Sedentary life-style	Decreases stress-related bone formation	Less peak bone mass
		Accelerated resorption of bone
Lack of exposure to sunlight	Possibly interferes with vitamin D production	Decreased calcium absorption

usually are limited to the thoracic and upper lumbar vertebrae (T8 to L3) Intervertebral discs may herniate through a disrupted cartilaginous plate into the weakened vertebral body producing Schmorl's nodes. Thinning also occurs in the five groups of trabeculae of the proximal femur where the radiographic appearance (the Singh Trabecular Pattern Index) of the bone has been used to estimate the severity of the disease.

The mineral content of cortical bone is lost at a much slower rate than that of trabecular bone in the normal aging process. This difference may result from the high surface-to-volume ratio and more rapid turnover of trabecular bone or to independent modulation of the two bone compartments. The outer diameter of the marrow cavity usually increases. Cortical bone resorption occurs at endosteal (the primary site in adults), intracortical, and subperiosteal sites. Extensive subperiosteal resorption may suggest hyperparathyroidism; the other patterns are less specific.

Osteoporotic bone is histologically normal. There is simply less bone tissue per volume. Dynamic studies that label the bone with tetracycline and quantitative histologic measurements have revealed decreased bone formation, increased bone resorption, or both, suggesting that osteoporosis may be the common expression of a number of different diseases.

Serum calcium and phosphorus levels remain normal after menopause and in osteoporosis, although intestinal calcium absorption decreases. Parathyroid hormone (PTH) levels in the serum/plasma are normal to slightly lower.

Calcitonin levels in the serum/plasma in osteoporosis are controversial, possibly because of difficulties with the hormone assay. The bulk of evidence suggests that osteoporosis does not result from calcitonin deficiency. Accelerated skeletal calcium release may even stimulate calcitonin secretion in osteoporotic patients.

Serum/plasma levels of 1,25-dihydroxy vitamin D_3 (1,25-$(OH)_2D$) are lower in osteoporotic patients. Treatment with calcitrol has been shown to increase calcium absorption in the gut, but vitamin D supplements alone have not dramatically reduced vertebral fractures. Estrogen therapy increases 1,25-$(OH)_2D$ levels and has decreased vertebral fracture rates independent of associated changes in PTH secretion.

Estrogen secretion decreases dramatically with menopause. Women then derive endogenous estrogens through peripheral conversion of androgenic steroids. The increased peripheral conversion of androgens in adipose tissue may help explain the protective effect of obesity against osteoporosis. Smoking cigarettes may hasten menopause and accelerate hepatic metabolism of the exogenous estrogens.

CLINICAL–PATHOLOGIC CORRELATIONS

The common clinical features of osteoporosis are fractures of the distal radius, vertebral bodies (T8 to L3), and the femoral necks. Fractures of the vertebral bodies are the most common and produce pain and deformity of the spine. Deformity of the chest wall predisposes to some pulmonary and cardiovascular diseases and decreases mobility. Although fractures of the distal radius and femoral neck are common, healing of long bone fractures is not impaired. These fractures produce a fear of falling and, by decreasing mobility, may accelerate bone loss.

The pathologic correlation is the thinning of trabecular and cortical bone. Normal age-related loss of bone mass results from decreased osteoblast activity or life span. Osteoporosis results when accelerated bone resorption adds to demineralization. Accelerated skeletal calcium release decreases PTH secretion and possibly 1,25-$(OH)_2D$ formation. The deficit of 1,25-$(OH)_2D$ results in decreased calcium absorption from the gut. Decreased effective calcium intake, low peak bone mass, and heredity also predispose to osteoporosis. Estrogen has not been shown to directly affect bone, but probably works through its stimulation of 1,25-$(OH)_2D$.

DIFFERENTIAL DIAGNOSIS

Osteoporosis is only one of a number of diseases that cause osteopenia. Because some of the other processes are more easily treated (osteomalacia) or more immediately life threatening (multiple myeloma), it is important to establish the diagnosis. When the distinction cannot be made on the basis of the history and physical examination, and cannot be confirmed by commonly available laboratory procedures (e.g., hemogram, serum calcium and phosphorus levels, serum and urine protein electrophoresis, hormone levels), bone biopsy may be necessary. Bone biopsy is generally safe and has few complications, but requires some surgical and pathologic expertise that may not be available in some areas. Features of differentiation are listed in Table 141–2.

DIAGNOSIS

There are no specific laboratory indicators for osteoporosis in its early stages. The diagnosis rests on the history (risk factors) and physical examination. Radiologic procedures may help demonstrate osteopenia, but they are often quite expensive and correlation with fractures is not yet optimal. Vertebral compression fractures and osteopenia may be obvious on the standard chest or other x-ray films in advanced disease. The Singh Trabecular Pattern Index for the proximal femur described earlier is cumbersome for use in routine quantitative assessment of bone mass and has limited predictive value.

Radiography is the measure of cortical thickness on standard x-ray and films, usually of metacarpal bones or the radius. Photodensitometry compares bone density on the x-ray film with that of a standard. Lack of precision limits the usefulness of these procedures.

Photon absorptiometry measures the attenuation of a single or dual photon beam (sources, iodine 125 or gadolinium 153) as it passes through bone. The reproducibility of measurements with this technique is good (2% to 5%). Single beam densitometers are portable and may be used for screening large populations; however, they are limited to analysis of appendicular bone density because they cannot correct for soft tissue distribution. Dual beam studies may be made of the axial skeleton, but are expensive and not widely available.

Computerized tomography allows assessment of cortical and trabecular bone and permits verification of position of the bone independent of the x-ray beam, a source of error in attenuation measurements. This method

TABLE 141–2.
Differential Diagnosis of Osteoporosis

DISEASE	DIFFERENTIATING FEATURES

Malignant diseases
  Multiple myeloma
  Lymphoma
  Leukemia
  Carcinomatosis
	Fever, weight loss, and other signs and symptoms of the malignancy
	Abnormal hemogram or peripheral blood smear, abnormal serum or urine proteins, abnormal findings from bone biopsy

Osteomalacia and rickets	Features of underlying disorders predominate, pseudofractures on x-ray films, abnormal findings from bone biopsy
Paget's disease	High alkaline phosphatase level in plasma, increased urinary hydroxyproline level, sclerotic areas on x-ray films

Endocrine disorders
  Hyperparathyroidism
  Cushing's disease
  Thyrotoxicosis
  Estrogen deficiency
  Panhypopituitarism
	Features of underlying disorder usually predominate, individual hormone levels are elevated or decreased, and their metabolic consequences are apparent on levels of serum glucose, calcium, etc.

Connective tissue diseases
  Osteogenesis imperfecta
  Homocystinuria
  Ehlers-Danlos syndrome
  Marfan's syndrome
  Rheumatoid arthritis
	Features of underlying disorder usually predominate (e.g., ectopia lentis, scleral coloring, bone deformity, cutaneous abnormality, mental retardation, homocystine in urine)

Calcium deficiency and malabsorption	Features of underlying disorder usually predominate (e.g., sprue or other malabsorption syndrome, gastrointestinal bypass surgery)
Miscellaneous disorders Hemochromatosis	Features of underlying disorder usually predominate (e.g., skin coloration, diabetes, iron stores increased)

can measure small changes in bone mass over time.

Neutron activation analysis, a research tool, uses irradiation with fast neutrons to provide a measure of total body calcium. There is good correlation of total body calcium values with cortical bone mass, but not with trabcular bone mass.

PRINCIPLES OF PREVENTION AND THERAPY

Osteoporosis is largely preventable. Estrogen replacement is the mainstay in the prevention and treatment of postmenopausal osteoporosis. Estrogen will retard bone loss but will not restore bone mass. The benefit is greatest with early treatment but has been seen when therapy is delayed for up to 6 years. The required estrogen dose is reduced by calcium supplementation. This may be important when the risks of estrogen/progestin therapy are considered.

The average daily intake of calcium in the United States is 450 mg to 550 mg. Men, premenopausal, and estrogen-treated postmenopausal women require about 1,000 mg of elemental calcium per day. Estrogen deficiency raises the requirement to 1,500 mg per day. Milk and dairy products are the major dietary source of calcium. Each 8-ounce (240 ml) glass of milk contains 275 mg to 300 mg of calcium. Commercial additives for milk now allow adequate consumption even for those with lactase deficiency.

Calcium tablets can be given to those who cannot ingest the recommended level through dietary means. Adequate intake must begin up to 10 years before the menopause to have any protective effect. Higher levels of intake produce no added benefit and may cause urinary stones in predisposed individuals.

Adequate vitamin D is required for absorption of calcium. The requirement increases with age and inadequate sunlight exposure. Vitamin D toxicity may develop with an intake as low as 2,000 IU daily, so recommended doses are about 1,200 IU daily. Calcitrol, a synthetic vitamin D analogue, has also been employed with some success.

Inactivity accelerates bone loss. Modest weight-bearing exercise is useful in therapy, and exercise may still help if weight bearing is not possible. Eliminating home hazards such as throw rugs and exposed electric cords and being alert for the effects of prescribed medications are important. When fractures do occur, rapid return to function must be encouraged.

Sodium fluoride, with high calcium intake and estrogen therapy, is effective in reducing vertebral fractures in osteoporotic women, but severe gastrointestinal side-effects often limit its usefulness.

Calcitonin has recently been approved for use in osteoporosis. It has shown some promise in slowing or even reversing osteoporosis, but requires injections. Experience with this regimen is too limited to recommend widespread use. Other agents are under investigation.

REFERENCES

Albright F, Smith PH, Richardson AM: Postmenopausal Osteoporosis. *JAMA* 1941; 116:2465–2474. *The first description of postmenopausal osteoporosis in humans.*

Avioli LV (ed): *The Osteoporotic Syndrome. Detection, Prevention, and Treatment.* New York, Grune & Stratton, 1983. *A short, but complete text covering all aspects of postmenopausal osteoporosis.*

Grubb SA, Jacobson PC, Awbrey BJ, McCartney WH, Vincent LM, Talmage RV: Bone density in osteopenic women: A modified distal radius density measurement procedure to develop an "at risk" value for use in screening women. *J Orthopaedic Res* 1984; 2:322–327. *A discussion of bone densitometry and presentation of a screening technique using widely available equipment.*

Johnson CC Jr, Hui SL, Witt RM, Appledorn R, Baker RS, Longcope C: Early menopausal changes in bone mass and sex steroids. *J Clin Endocrinol Metab* 1985; 61:905–911. *Evidence that accelerated bone loss in menopausal osteoporosis actually begins before menses cease.*

Meier DE, Orwoll ES, Jones JM: Marked disparity between trabecular and cortical bone loss with age in healthy men. *Ann Intern Med* 1984; 101:605–612. *A comparison of bone compartment losses by readily available methods.*

National Institutes of Health: Osteoporosis. Consensus Development Conference Statement, vol 5,

1984. US Government Printing Office: # 1984-421-132:4652. *A succinct review of risk factors and current recommendations for detection, prevention, and treatment from recognized experts in osteoporosis.*

Resnick D, Niwayama G: *Diagnosis of Bone and Joint Disorders. Philadelphia, WB Saunders Co, 1981, pp 1638–1681. A well-referenced, excellent histologic, radiographic, and pathophysiologic correlation of osteoporosis.*

Riggs BL, Seeman E, Hodgson SF, Taves DR, O'Fallon WM: Effect of the fluoride/calcium regimen on vertebral fracture occurrence in postmenopausal osteoporosis. N Engl J Med 1982; 306:446–450. *A comparison of most of the accepted therapeutic options.*

Sandler RB, Herbert DL: Quantitative bone assessments: Applications and expectations. J Am Geriatr Soc 1981; 29:97–103. *Limited description of readily available bone assessment studies and their predictive values for fractures.*

Wilson PF, Garrisons RJ, Castelli WP: Postmenopausal estrogen use, cigarette smoking, and cardiovascular morbidity in women over 50: The Framingham study. N Engl J Med 1985; 313:1038 –1043. *A recent assessment of the risks of estrogen therapy in menopausal women.*

142 OSTEOARTHRITIS

Ronald D. Foster, M.D.
Robert A. Hawkins, M.D.

Osteoarthritis is a chronic, degenerative disease of joints characterized by loss of articular cartilage and formation of osteophytes. In contrast to the marked inflammation of the synovium present in rheumatoid arthritis, osteoarthritis is primarily noninflammatory. Osteoarthritis can be classified into a primary form, in which no predisposing abnormality can be found, and a secondary form, in which several factors appear responsible for initiating cartilage deterioration (Table 142–1). Synonyms for osteoarthritis are degenerative joint disease and osteoarthrosis.

CLINICAL SIGNS AND SYMPTOMS

The typical patient is between the ages of 40 and 60 years and complains of pain of insidious onset in one or a few joints. Although both sexes are equally affected, under age 45 years, men are more likely to be affected, and over age 45, women are more likely.

Initially deep aching in the joint occurs after normal use, however, with progressive joint deterioration, pain is also present at rest. Other cardinal features of osteoarthritis include joint stiffness following inactivity (gel phenomenon) and morning stiffness lasting no more than a few minutes, in contrast to the morning stiffness of rheumatoid arthritis, which may last for an hour or longer. Limitation of motion occurs due to joint space narrowing, surrounding osteophyte formation, and loose bodies within the joint, which may cause it to lock in flexion.

Weight-bearing joints commonly affected by osteoarthritis include the hips, knees, and cervical and lumbar spine. Hip-joint pain is usually felt in the inguinal region or inner thigh, although it may radiate to the anterior or lateral thigh or to the knee. Osteoarthritis of the knee is frequently the result of damage to ligaments

TABLE 142–1.

Classification of Osteoarthritis

I. Primary
  A. Idiopathic
  B. Primary generalized osteoarthritis
  C. Erosive osteoarthritis
II. Secondary
  A. Traumatic
    1. Acute
    2. Chronic
    3. Neuropathic arthropathy
  B. Pre-existing inflammatory joint disease
  C. Endocrine and metabolic
    1. Diabetes mellitus
    2. Acromegaly
    3. Intra-articular corticosteroid injections
    4. Wilson's disease
    5. Hemochromatosis
    6. Ochronosis
    7. Gout
  D. Congenital and developmental defects
    1. Hip dysplasias
    2. Legg-Calvé-Perthes disease
    3. Slipped capital femoral epiphysis
    4. Multiple epiphyseal dysplasia
    5. Osteochondritides
  E. Miscellaneous disorders
    1. Avascular necrosis
    2. Bleeding dyscrasias
    3. Paget's disease

or menisci from previous occupational or sports injuries. Neck pain radiating to the shoulders and neck stiffness with limitation of motion are the most common symptoms of cervical osteoarthritis. With lumbar spine involvement, the patient complains of low back pain, which may radiate into the buttocks or posterior aspect of the legs. More severe disease may result in motor and sensory abnormalities in the legs.

The distal interphalangeal (DIP) joints, proximal interphalangeal (PIP), and the first carpometacarpal joints of the hands are also commonly involved. Although significant bony enlargement and limitation of motion are common in these joints, pain is usually less severe and debilitating when compared to that in the weight-bearing joints. Enlarged DIP joints are called Heberden's nodes, and enlarged PIP joints are called Bouchard's nodes.

Osteoarthritis of the shoulder is usually limited to the acromioclavicular joint. In osteoarthritis of the foot, the first metatarsophalangeal joint is affected, while the remaining joints are not typically involved. Other joints including the metacarpophalangeal joints, wrists, elbows, shoulders, and ankles are generally spared in osteoarthritis, and their involvement should suggest a process causing secondary osteoarthritis, such as trauma to the joint (Table 142–1).

Joint examination in the early stages of osteoarthritis may reveal only pain with motion. Physical findings in later stages include crepitus, limitation of motion, and gross bony deformities. Valgus and varus deformities of the knees develop due to asymmetric loss of cartilage. Joint contractures and, rarely, bony ankylosis indicate severe and long-standing disease. Synovial effusions, especially of the knees, are common. Significant joint inflammation is unusual in osteoarthritis unless another rheumatologic disorder, such as gout or pseudogout, coexists. An exception to this rule is the variant known as erosive (inflammatory) osteoarthritis, in which the DIP and PIP joints are warm, erythematous, and tender.

PATHOPHYSIOLOGY

Knowledge of the structure and function of articular cartilage is useful in understanding the processes responsible for its destruction. The chondrocyte is responsible for synthesis of the two major extracellular macromolecules, collagen and proteoglycan. The unique properties of these tightly aggregated molecules account for the tensile strength and compressibility of cartilage. Type II collagen is the only form of collagen found in normal cartilage and provides the framework for the tissue.

Superficially, the collagen fibrils are oriented parallel to the joint surface, providing protection from shear forces during joint motion. Deeper, the collagen fibrils are oriented perpendicular to the bone-cartilage interface, anchoring the cartilage to the subchondral bone.

Proteoglycans are interspersed within the collagen framework. They are composed of a linear protein backbone and the glycosaminoglycan side chains, keratan sulfate, and chondroitin sulfate. These negatively charged glycosaminoglycans are strongly hydrophilic accounting for the 75% water content of cartilage. When cartilage is compressed during normal joint loading, water is displaced forming a lubricating "squeeze film" between the opposing articular surfaces. With release of compression, the hydrophilic nature of the proteoglycans promotes rapid water reabsorption resulting in cartilage reexpansion. Interspersed within this avascular matrix, the chrondrocytes are nourished by diffusion from the synovial fluid, which is assisted by the displacement and reabsorption of the water.

The intrinsic capability of the cartilage to withstand sudden compressive forces (impulse loading) and shear forces is limited. Subchondral bone and surrounding soft tissue have important protective roles in dissipating forces on the joint. Thus processes that alter their ability to absorb loads place the cartilage at risk for damage. The chondrocyte, unfortunately, has a limited capability to effect repair. Osteoarthritis, then, results when an imbalance exists between cartilage degradation and synthesis.

The earliest microscopic change of osteoarthritis is fibrillation of the articular surface with loss of integrity of the protective layer of superficial collagen. At this stage, there is disaggregation of proteoglycans from collagen in the deeper layers with their subsequent loss from the cartilage. The factors responsible for these events are not well understood but may include chondrocyte dysfunction, entry of proteolytic enzymes into the cartilage matrix through the damaged superficial collagen layer, and abnormal joint stress with insufficient ability to effect repair. With progression, the cartilage thins and fissures appear at the surface and may extend to the subchondral bone. Synovial fluid entering through these fissures under pressure may cause pressure necrosis of the subchondral bone resulting in subchondral cyst formation. Excessive impulse loading also causes microfractures in the subchondral bone, which heal with sclerosis. Sclerotic bone is less able to absorb compressive forces; thus the cartilage is forced to bear greater loads, accelerating the degenerative process. Bony and cartilaginous osteophytic overgrowths appear at the joint margin. These may represent compensatory phenomena to increase the joint's load-bearing area or to stabilize the joint in response to ligamentous laxity. Mild synovitis and synovial effusions develop.

Genetic factors are important in influencing the development of osteoarthritis and in the pattern of joint involvement. For example, in generalized osteoarthritis with Heberden's nodes, the disease has autosomal dominant inheritance in women but autosomal recessive inheritance in men. There are also racial and ethnic differences in disease susceptibility. For example, there is a higher prevalence of osteoarthritis in American Indians compared with the general population.

Although the initiating event in primary osteoarthritis is not known, there are several processes that induce secondary osteoarthritis by virtue of their ability to alter normal joint biomechanics or the biochemical make-up of cartilage or subchondral bone (Table 142–1). Thus osteoarthritis is frequently the final common pathway for virtually any other form of arthritis.

CLINICAL–PATHOLOGIC CORRELATIONS

Because articular cartilage lacks innervation, damage to it is not directly preceived as pain; thus only one-third of joints with radiographic evidence of osteoarthritis produce symptoms. However, there are several other pathologic features that produce pain, including subchondral microfractures, osteophyte impingement on soft tissues, synovitis, joint capsule distension, muscle spasm, intra-articular ligamentous disease, and periarticular soft tissue inflammation. These features are summarized in Table 142–2.

The physical findings reflect the underlying pathology. Progressive roughening and thinning of the articular cartilage result in crepitus, loss of mobility, and ligamentous laxity causing joint instability. Intra-articular loose bodies formed from fragments sheared off of the articular surface can cause the joint to lock in flexion. Periarticular osteophytes cause bony enlargement and mechanically interfere with joint mobility. Mild synovitis is manifested by joint swelling due to synovial effusions and villous hypertrophy.

DIFFERENTIAL DIAGNOSIS

Osteoarthritis may be first seen in either a monoarticular or polyarticular pattern and must be distinguished from a variety of other

TABLE 142–2.
Clinical–Pathologic Correlations for Osteoarthritis

CLINICAL FINDINGS	PATHOLOGIC FINDINGS
Crepitus	Cartilage roughening and loss
Joint instability	
Joint deformity	
Joint enlargement	Osteophyte formation
Heberden's nodes	
Bouchard's nodes	
Loss of range of motion	
Pain	
Pain	Subchondral microfractures
Swelling	Synovitis
Synovial effusions	
Joint warmth	
Pain	
Loss of range of motion	Loose bodies
Joint locking	
Loss of range of motion	Muscle spasm
Pain	
Loss of range of motion	Flexion contractures
Pain	

forms of chronic arthritis (Table 142–3). With the exception of osteoarthritis and systemic lupus erythematosus, these disorders result in an inflammatory synovial effusion characterized by elevation of white cell counts and a poor mucin clot. Additionally, pigmented villonodular synovitis, neoplastic synovitis, juxta-articular bone tumors, avascular necrosis, and osteochondritis dessicans resemble monoarticular osteoarthritis. However, the radiographic and synovial fluid abnormalities of these other disorders allow for their differentiation from osteoarthritis.

DIAGNOSIS

The diagnosis of osteoarthritis is based on the history and physical examination and is aided by radiographs. The results of laboratory tests, including erythrocyte sedimentation rate, rheumatoid factor, and antinuclear antibody assays, are normal or negative. Radiographs are useful for diagnosis, as changes mirror the pathologic findings. Cardinal radiographic features include joint space narrowing, subchondral bone sclerosis, marginal osteophytes, and subchondral bone cysts. Synovial fluid white cell counts are low, and synovial fluid glucose levels approximate serum values.

PRINCIPLES OF THERAPY

Unfortunately, no therapy exists that can reverse the changes of osteoarthritis. Therapy is directed at alleviating pain, controlling the minor degree of inflammation that may accompany the process, and maintaining stability and range of motion of joints. Nonsteroidal anti-inflammatory drugs provide pain relief and reduce inflammation. Other mild analgesics may be used concomitantly. Judicious use of intra-articular corticosteroids is beneficial. Physical therapy aids in maintaining joint mobility and muscle strength. Activities that may damage the joint are discouraged. Selective surgical procedures including prosthetic joint replacement, especially of the hips and knees, are useful in relieving pain in advanced stages.

REFERENCES

Beary JF III, Christian CL, Sculco TP (eds): *Manual of Rheumatology and Outpatient Orthopedic Disorders*. Boston, Little, Brown & Co, 1981, pp 183–196. *A concise pocket manual of key pathologic findings, clinical features, and therapy.*

Howell DS, Talbott JH (eds): Osteoarthritis symposium. *Semin Arthritis Rheum* 1981; 11(1):1–149. *A collection of recent contributions toward understanding the pathogenesis of osteoarthritis.*

Kelley WN, Harris ED, Ruddy S, Sledge CB: *Textbook of Rheumatology*, ed 2. Philadelphia, WB Saunders Co, 1985, pp 1417–1458. *A comprehensive textbook discussion of the pathophysiology, clinical course, and treatment of osteoarthritis, with extensive references.*

Rodnan GP, Schumacher HR (eds): *Primer on the Rheumatic Diseases*, ed 8. Atlanta, Arthritis Foundation, 1983, pp 104–108. *A useful synopsis of rheumatic disease, with basic information regarding diagnosis and treatment of osteoarthritis.*

Sokoloff L (ed): Osteoarthritis. *Clin Rheum Dis* 1985; 11:175–445. *A collection of articles addressing current aspects of osteoarthritis.*

Woolfe D (ed): Rehabilitation in the rheumatic diseases. *Clin Rheum Dis* 1981; 7:289–553. *A complete review of the various modalities of treatment of rheumatic disorders with emphasis on a multidisciplinary approach.*

Differential Diagnosis

DISEASE	FINDINGS		
	CLINICAL	LABORATORY	RADIOGRAPHIC
Osteoarthritis	Polyarticular or oligoarticular Incidence equal in women and men Onset: age 30–70 yr Bony enlargement	Normal	Joint space narrowing Osteophytes Osteosclerosis
Systemic lupus erythematosus	Polyarticular or oligoarticular Incidence: women:men, 9:1 Onset: age 15–40 yr Skin rashes Seizures, psychosis Nephritis Pleuropericarditis	Positive ANA Thrombocytopenia Leukopenia Anemia Abnormal urinalysis Low serum complement level	Normal
Rheumatoid arthritis	Symmetric, polyarticular Incidence: women:men, 2:1 Onset: age 30–50 yr Morning stiffness Rheumatoid nodules	Positive rheumatoid factor Thrombocytosis Elevated ESR Neutropenia Anemia	Erosions Periarticular osteopenia
Gout	Monoarticular or polyarticular Incidence: women:men, 1:8 Onset: age 30–60 yr Tophi	Elevated serum uric acid Synovial fluid Crystals of monosodium urate	Erosions Tophi Periarticular osteopenia
Pseudogout	Monoarticular or polyarticular Incidence: women:men, 1:2 Onset: age 50–70 yr	Synovial fluid Crystals of calcium pyrophosphate dihydrate	Chondrocalcinosis
Ankylosing spondylitis	Axial, occasional monoarticular Incidence: women:men, 1:2 Onset: age 20–50 yr	Elevated ESR Anemia	Vertebral fusion Sacroileitis Erosions
Reiter's syndrome	Oligoarticular, axial involvement Incidence: women:men, 1:9 Onset: age 20–50 yr Urethritis Conjunctivitis Oral mucosal erosions Skin rash	Elevated ESR Anemia	Sacroileitis Erosions Bony spurs
Psoriatic arthritis	Oligoarticular, axial involvement Incidence equal in women and men Onset: age 20–50 yr Psoriasis Onycholysis, nail pits	Elevated ESR Anemia	Erosions "pencil in cup" Sacroileitis Bony spurs
Tuberculosis or fungal infection	Monoarticular Pulmonary infiltrates	Microbial cultures Fungal serology	Bony destruction

GOUT AND PSEUDOGOUT

Toni I. Evans, M.D.

GOUT

Gout is a multisystem disease resulting from prolonged hyperuricemia. Its most frequent manifestation is acute arthritis, often recurrent, at which time monosodium urate monohydrate crystals are demonstrable in the joint fluid. These crystals can be deposited periarticularly (tophi), in the kidneys (gouty nephropathy), or as kidney stones.

CLINICAL SIGNS AND SYMPTOMS

There are four stages to the full spectrum of joint disease in gout: asymptomatic hyperuricemia, acute gouty arthritis, intercritical gout, and chronic tophaceous gout. Hyperuricemia, detected on routine laboratory work, may remain asymptomatic for the life of the patient; however, the higher the serum urate level, the more likely the patient is to develop symptoms. The patient with acute gouty arthritis presents with the acute onset of severe joint pain, redness, and swelling; the condition is typically monoarticular and is more common in the lower extremities. Classically it involves the first metatarsal-phalangeal joint (podagra), but it can involve any and multiple joints. The acute attack may last days to weeks and then completely resolve. The next stage, intercritical gout, is asymptomatic. Some patients never have another acute attack, but the usual course is recurrent acute attacks at progressively more frequent intervals, alternating with asymptomatic periods (intercritical gout), occasionally with fever and constitutional symptoms.

The untreated patient may progress to chronic tophaceous gout, marked by aching, stiff, deformed joints accompanied by tophi. The degree and duration of hyperuricemia determine when this stage occurs. The use of drugs to lower plasma urate has decreased the percentage of patients who progress to this stage.

Other possible complications of prolonged hyperuricemia are renal complications that may lead to renal insufficiency, acute renal failure, and renal stones (see Pathophysiology).

In acute gouty arthritis, the affected joint is red, hot, swollen, and very tender. Later during the chronic tophaceous stage, the patient's joints are deformed, stiff, and aching and are accompanied by tophi, which appear as painless soft masses that can be found in various locations, usually periarticularly.

PATHOPHYSIOLOGY

Hyperuricemia and gout may be classified as primary, secondary, or idiopathic. In primary gout, the disorder is innate, while in secondary gout it is secondary to another disease process or to drugs. In addition, the hyperuricemia may be due to uric acid overproduction, renal underexcretion, or both. The majority of patients are underexcretors (90%). (See Table 143–1 for the different types.) Gout tends to run in families and serum uric acid is probably controlled by multiple genes.

Uric acid is the end product of purine metabolism. One of the principle regulators of uric acid synthesis is the intracellular concentration of 5-phosphoribosyl-1-pyrophosphate (PRPP). Therefore, any condition leading to increased levels or increased availability or PRPP will lead to increased production of uric acid. The mechanism of increased uric acid production in the following inborn errors of metabolism is believed to result from the increased PRPP levels: increased PRPP synthetase, hypoxanthine-guanine-phosphoribosyl-transferase (HGPRTase) deficiency (complete or partial), and glucose-6-phosphatase deficiency (complete or partial). These enzyme defects only account for a small percentage of gout cases. See Table 143–1 for the classification of these disorders and Figure 143–1 for a schematic of purine metabolism.

Acute Gouty Arthritis

When plasma becomes supersaturated with uric acid, crystals are deposited in the synovium, on the surface and within the articular cartilage, in bursa, in tendons, and in tendon sheaths. When the crystals are released into the synovial fluid, they are coated with immunoglobulins and phagocytized by neutrophils, causing chemotactic factors to be produced, which attract more neutrophils. The engulfed crystals cause the neutrophil to degranulate, releasing lysosomal enzymes that cause inflammation and joint damage. The role of other mediators, such as Hageman factor and prostaglandins, is unclear at the present time, but may be important.

Kidney Disease in Gout

There are three types of kidney disease associated with gout: gouty nephropathy, acute uric acid nephropathy, and renal stones. In gouty nephropathy, monosodium urate monohydrate crystals are deposited in the medulla. The consequences of these deposits are unknown. Decreased concentrating ability, proteinuria, and chronic renal insufficiency are all common in gouty patients, but the exact correlation (after taking into account other medical problems in these patients) is unclear. Acute uric acid nephropathy, which is the intratubular deposition of uric acid crystals, can occur in patients with increased cell turnover (i.e., leukemia, lymphoma) and leads to acute renal failure. Renal stones from gout are of three types: uric acid, mixed uric acid–calcium oxalate, and calcium oxalate stones. The microscopic and macroscopic changes in the kidneys and joints are described in Table 143–2.

CLINICAL–PATHOLOGIC CORRELATIONS

The signs and symptoms of acute and chronic gouty arthritis as well as gouty renal disease are primarily the result of the deposition of monosodium urate crystals and the resultant inflammatory reaction. See Table 143–2 for the clinical–pathological correlation.

DIFFERENTIAL DIAGNOSIS

The intense joint inflammation and possible fever of acute gouty arthritis make differentiation from septic arthritis difficult at times. The periarticular as well as articular inflammation

---

TABLE 143–1.
Classification of Hyperuricemia and Gout

TYPE	METABOLIC DERANGEMENT
PRIMARY	
Enzyme defect	
Increased activity of PRPP synthetase	Overproduction of uric acid
Partial HGRPT deficiency	Overproduction of uric acid
Unknown defect	Overproduction of uric acid
	Underexcretion of uric acid
SECONDARY	
Enzyme defect	
Complete HGPRT deficiency	Overproduction of uric acid (Lesch-Nyhan syndrome)
Glucose-6-phosphatase deficiency	Both overproduction and underexcretion of uric acid
Drugs (i.e., diuretics, salicylates)	Underexcretion of uric acid
Increased turnover of nucleic acid	Overproduction of uric acid
(myeloproliferative and	
lymphoproliferative disorders)	
Renal defect	Underexcretion of uric acid
IDIOPATHIC	

TABLE 143–2.
Clinical–Pathologic Correlations of Gout

CLINICAL FINDINGS		PATHOLOGIC FINDINGS	
		MACROSCOPIC	MICROSCOPIC
Nontender masses, asymptomatic	Tophus	Soft tissue masses	Deposits of radially arranged urate crystals surrounded by mononuclear cells as well as multinucleated giant cells
Erythematous, hot swollen, painful joints	Acute arthritis	Congested, swollen synovium	Synovium infiltrated with crystals, neutrophils, and mononuclear cells
Aching, stiff, deformed joints	Chronic arthritis	Congested, hypertrophied synovium, whitish deposits with uneven surface of articular cartilage, cysts in subchondral bone	Pannus formation of synovium Urate deposits in the intercellular matrix of the articular cartilage
Symptoms of renal colic or asymptomatic	Kidney	Radiolucent stones in pelvis	Urate deposits, possibly with calcium oxalate also
Symptoms of renal insufficiency		Kidney may be small with a granular surface and decreased cortex	Urate deposits in medullary interstitium, pyramids, papillae
Symptoms of acute renal failure			Intratubular urate deposits

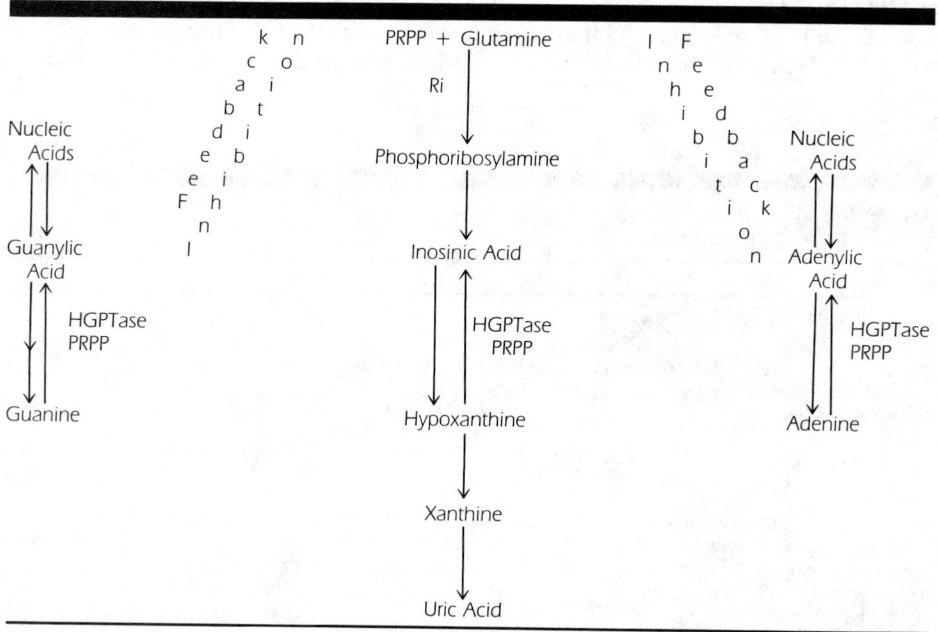

FIG 143–1.
Scheme of purine metabolism—PRPP = 5-phosphoribosyl-1-pyrophosphate, HGPRTase = hypoxanthine-guanine-phosphoribosyl-transferase.

as well as the possible fever that can occur with gout may be confused with cellulitis or thrombophlebitis. The serum uric acid level, a prior history of attacks of gout, the joints involved, and ultimately the chemical analysis of the synovial fluid make differentiation possible.

DIAGNOSIS

The definitive diagnosis of gout is made by demonstrating with polarizing light microscopy negatively birefringent needle-shaped crystals in synovial fluid or in an aspirate of a gouty tophus. Hyperuricemia, a history of uric acid stones, a family history of gout, or great toe involvement in a patient with acute arthritis make gout a likely possibility, but these findings are not definitive. A dramatic clinical response of the joint inflammation to colchicine is also strongly suggestive.

Radiographic abnormalities in gout usually occur only after many years of the disease. Some of the characteristic findings in x-ray films are: asymmetric polyarticular disease (particularly of the appendicular skeleton), bony erosions (intra-articularly or periarticularly and often outlined by a bony lip), preservation of the joint space until late in the disease, lack of appreciable osteoporosis, and soft tissue swelling including nodular masses (tophi).

PRINCIPLES OF PREVENTION AND THERAPY

Whether asymptomatic hyperuricemia of any degree should be treated is controversial, recognizing that the higher the uric acid level the more likely gout is to develop. Acute gouty arthritis is treated with colchicine or nonsteroidal anti-inflammatory drugs, most notably indomethacin. Correction of predisposing factors to gout should be initiated (i.e., obesity, alcohol ingestion, intake of drugs that cause hyperuricemia). Moderate purine restriction may be helpful.

The point in the course of the disease at which uricosuric drugs or xanthine oxidase inhibitors should be initiated is also controversial. Some clinicians start them after the first acute arthritis attack has resolved, whereas others wait to see if acute gouty attacks will recur and implement nonpharmacologic measures in the meantime. In the patient with symptomatic hyperuricemia (recurrent gout, kidney disease, tophi, or joint disease) the uric acid excreted in a 24-hour urine collection should be measured. If the patient is an underexcretor (less than 700 mg uric acid in 24 hours) and does not have severe renal insufficiency or a history of uric acid stones, uricosuric agents can be started after the acute attack has resolved. Allopurinol, a xanthine oxidase inhibitor, should be used if the patient has any of the above contraindications to uricosuric agents. With treatment of symptomatic hyperuricemia, the incidence of kidney stones, renal insufficiency, and permanent joint damage (including tophi) can be substantially decreased.

PSEUDOGOUT

Pseudogout (or calcium pyrophosphate deposition disease [CPPD] disease) refers to any one of several clinical syndromes characterized by the deposition of calcium pyrophosphate dehydrate crystals in cartilage, joints, and other periarticular tissues.

CLINICAL SIGNS AND SYMPTOMS

There are five clinical patterns of CPPD disease. Type A (also called pseudogout because it clinically mimics gout) refers to acute or subacute attacks of arthritis lasting days to weeks. The knee joint is most commonly affected, followed in frequency by other large joints, but any joint and occasionally several joints may be involved. Like in gout, there may be low-grade fever or leukocytosis, but the attacks are usually not as sudden or painful as in gout, and generally affect different joints preferentially. Type B or pseudorheumatoid arthritis involves several joints and consists of subacute attacks of arthritis lasting weeks or months, accompanied by morning stiffness, synovial thickening, flexion contractures, and an elevated erythrocyte sedimentation rate. Differentiating points from rheumatoid arthritis include: a decreased likelihood of the pseudorheumatoid patient to have rheumatoid factor (only 10% of patients have rheumatoid factor) and asymmetric joint involvement. Types C and D, or pseudo-osteoarthritis, consist of degeneration of several, usually symmetrical joints. Type C patients also have superimposed acute arthritic attacks, whereas type D patients do not. The joints preferentially affected are usually different from those affected in osteoarthritis when there are multiple joints affected, however. Type E refers to asymptomatic CPPD disease discovered by x-ray studies. Type F, or pseudoneurotrophic joints, is uncommon but consists of a neurotrophic-like arthropathy with CPPD disease. Normal results of a neurologic exam differentiate it from a true neurotrophic joint.

CPPD disease may be hereditary, sporadic, or it may be associated with a metabolic abnormality. (See Table 143–3).

The natural course of CPPD disease is variable. A patient may start out with one clinical pattern and convert to another pattern later. Treatment improves symptoms, but does not appear to affect the course of the disease. In the case of CPPD associated with metabolic disorders, treatment of the associated disorder does not appear to improve the course of the CPPD disease.

PATHOPHYSIOLOGY

Calcium pyrophosphate crystals are deposited in articular cartilage, synovium, tendons, and bursa. An acute attack of CPPD disease appears to occur similarly to that of gout. CPPD crystals are shed into synovial fluid, where they are coated with immunoglobulins, after which they are phagocytized by neutrophils. This leads to release of lysosomal enzymes and attraction of more neutrophils, both contributing to the inflammation.

TABLE 143–3.
Classification of CPPD Disease (Pseudogout)

1. Hereditary
2. Sporadic
3. Associated with metabolic disorders
   a. Hyperparathyroidism
   b. Hypothyroidism
   c. Hemochromatosis
4. Possibly associated with metabolic disorders
   a. Gout
   b. Diabetes mellitus
   c. Wilson's disease
   d. Hypophosphatasia

Inorganic pyrophosphate levels are increased in the synovial fluid of patients with CPPD disease, but they are also increased in patients with osteoarthritis as well as in patients with other joint diseases, so the significance is unclear.

CLINICAL–PATHOLOGIC CORRELATIONS

In general, radiologic and pathologic changes do not appear to correlate with symptoms in CPPD disease. See Table 143–4 for the clinical and pathologic changes that occur in CPPD disease.

DIFFERENTIAL DIAGNOSIS

As previously mentioned, depending on the clinical pattern, CPPD disease may mimic gout, rheumatoid arthritis, degenerative joint disease, or neurotrophic joint disease. (See Clinical Signs and Symptoms for the differentiating points.)

DIAGNOSIS

The definite diagnosis of CPPD disease is made by finding weakly positive birefringent crystals by synovial biopsy or in synovial fluid using polarized light microscopy. (See Table 143–5 for diagnostic criteria of CPPD disease.)

Radiographically, there are two types of changes: characteristic articular or periarticular calcification and structural joint damage. The structural joint damage (i.e., bony sclerosis and joint space narrowing) can mimic degenerative joint disease, but may involve different joints than degenerative joint disease, and may also show more severe joint destruction than is seen in degenerative joint disease.

PRINCIPLES OF THERAPY

Aspiration of synovial fluid followed by injection of steroids provides symptomatic relief of acute attacks. Anti-inflammatory drugs are also effective and can be used chronically, if necessary. Colchicine has also been used for CPPD disease, and although it is not as predictably effective as in gout, it may be effective, especially if given intravenously. As mentioned previously, no treatment to date has been found to affect the course of the disease.

TABLE 143-4.
Clinical-Pathologic Correlations of CPPD Disease (Pseudogout)

CLINICAL FINDINGS	SITE	PATHOLOGIC FINDINGS	
		MACROSCOPIC	MICROSCOPIC
Range from asymptomatic to acute arthritis (swollen, painful, hot, erythematous joints) to chronic arthritis (painful, stiff joints) to concomitant acute and chronic arthritis	Synovium	May have calcific deposits May have embedded fragments of cartilage and bony spicules	Calcium pyrophosphate crystals
	Articular cartilage	May be thinned, have calcific deposits	Stromal reaction and multinucleated giant cells Calcium pyrophosphate crystals
	Tendons, ligaments, soft tissues, bone	May have calcific deposits	Calcium pyrophosphate crystals
	Bone	May have thickened trabeculae, cystic degeneration	

TABLE 143-5.
Revised Diagnostic Criteria for CPPD Disease (Pseudogout)*

1. Demonstration of calcium pyrophosphate crystals (obtained by biopsy, necropsy, or aspiration of synovial fluid) by definitive means (e.g., characteristic "fingerprint" in x-ray diffraction powder pattern or by chemical analysis).
2. a. Identification of monoclinic and/or triclinic crystals showing no or a weakly positive birefringence by compensated polarized light microscopy
   b. Presence of typical calcifications in roentgenograms
3. a. Acute arthritis, especially of knees or other large joints, with or without concomitant hyperuricemia.
   b. Chronic arthritis, especially of knees, hips, wrists, carpus, elbow, shoulder, and metacarpophalangeal joints, especially if accompanied by acute exacerbations. The chronic arthritis shows the following features helpful in differentiating it from osteoarthritis.
      1. Uncommon site (e.g., wrist, MCP, elbow, shoulder)
      2. Appearance of lesion radiologically (e.g., radiocarpal or patellofemoral joint space narrowing, especially if isolated [patella "wrapped around" the femur])
      3. Subchondral cyst formation
      4. Severity of degeneration—progressive, with subchondral bony collapse (microfractures)
      5. Osteophyte formation—variable and inconstant
      6. Tendon calcifications, especially achilles, triceps, obturators
      7. Involvement of the axial skeleton with subchondral cysts of apophyseal and sacroiliac joints, multiple levels of disc calcification and vacuum phenomenon, and sacroiliac vacuum phenomenon.

CATEGORIES OF CPPD DISEASE

    A. Definite—Criteria 1 or (2a + 2b)
    B. Probable—Criteria 2a or 2b
    C. Possible—Criteria 3a or 3b

* From McCarty DJ: *Arthritis and Allied Conditions.* Philadelphia, Lea & Febiger, 1985, p 1522.

REFERENCES

Boss GR, Seegmiller JE: Hyperuricemia and gout: Classification, complications, and management. N Engl J Med 1979; 300:1459–1468. *Complete, comprehensible review article on gout.*

Kelley WN, Howell DS: Section thirteen: Crystal-induced synovitis, in Kelley WN, Harris ED, Ruddy S, Sledge C (eds): *Textbook of Rheumatology.* Philadelphia, WB Saunders Co, 1981, pp

1397–1454. *Detailed and complete chapters on gout and pseudogout.*

Krane SM: Crystal-induced joint diseases, in Rubenstein E, Federman DD (eds): Scientific American Medicine. New York, Scientific American, 1984. *Well-referenced brief summary of gout and pseudogout.*

McCarty DJ: Calcium pyrophosphate dehydrate crystal deposition disease—1975. Arthritis Rheum 1976; 19:185–275. *Comprehensible review article on the clinical manifestations of pseudogout.*

McCarty DJ: Arthritis and Allied Conditions. Philadelphia, Lea & Febiger, 1985, p 1522. *Diagnostic criteria of CPPD disease.*

Resnick D: Crystal-induced arthropathy: Gout and Pseudogout. JAMA 1979; 242:2440–2443. *Good summary of the radiographic changes in gout and psuedogout.*

Resnick D, Niwayama G, Goergen TG et al: Clinical, radiographic, and pathologic abnormalities in calcium pyrophosphate dehydrate deposition disease (CPPD): Pseudogout. Radiology 1977; 122:1–15. *Good discussion of the range of pathologic and radiographic changes in pseudogout.*

Robbins SL, Angell M (eds): Basic Pathology. Philadelphia, WB Saunders Co, 1976, pp 142–144. *Good description of the pathology of gout.*

Rodnan GP, Schumacher HR (eds): Primer on the Rheumatic Diseases, ed 8. Atlanta: Arthritis Foundation, 1983, pp 120–130. *Good brief overview of gout and pseudogout.*

Seegmiller JE: Gout: A biochemical perspective, in Gutman AB (ed): Gout: A Cinical Comprehensive. Research Triangle Park, NC, Medcom, 1971, pp 27–35. *Good chapter on purine metabolism and the enzyme deficiencies in gout.*

Wyngaarden JB, Kelley WN: Gout and Hyperuricemia. New York, Grune & Stratton, 1976, pp 179–210. *A good discussion of the pathogenesis and pathologic changes of gout.*

144 SEPTIC ARTHRITIS

Alice Faryna, M.D.
Kim Goldenberg, M.D.

Septic arthritis is an acute or chronic synovitis resulting from invasion of the joint space by microbial organisms.

CLINICAL SIGNS AND SYMPTOMS

Pain and swelling of one or more joints are the most commonly reported symptoms. Fever, when present, is usually less than 39°C, and chills are uncommon. Infants in particular are unlikely to be febrile, presenting with irritability, lethargy, and pseudoparalysis of a limb. The mean duration of symptoms prior to diagnosis is 12 days to 14 days for an intact joint, and 1 month for a prosthetic joint, with a range of 1 day to several months. Tuberculous infections typically produce indolent effusions with minimal pain and no fever and may go undiagnosed for 6 months or more. Migratory polyarthralgia is characteristic of disseminated gonococcal infection and viral infections.

The large extremity joints are the most frequent sites of monoarthritis, with a predeliction for the hips in children and the knees in adults (Table 144–1). Patients who use illicit drugs intravenously are more likely to acquire infections of the sternoclavicular or sacroiliac joints than of the extremity joints.

Nongonococcal arthritis is usually monoarticular. Risk factors (Table 144–2) are often present. Migratory polyarthralgia is present in 70% of cases of disseminated gonococcal infection, and about 40% of all cases will have ef-

TABLE 144–1.
Initial Signs and Symptoms in Septic Arthritis

| | FREQUENCY (% OF CASES) | |
FEATURE	ADULTS	CHILDREN
Joint pain	70–95	>50
Joint swelling	40–45	Not available
Fever	45–75	33 (neonate)
Joint involved:		
Knee	50	35–40
Hip	20	60
Shoulder	15	4
Ankle	10	5
Wrist	5	Rare
Metatarsals/Metacarpals	5–10	10
Elbow	5	4

TABLE 144–2.
Risk Factors in Nongonococcal Arthritis

RISK FACTOR	EXAMPLES
Joint trauma	Joint surgery; intra-articular steroids; puncture wounds; femoral venipuncture
Preexisting arthropathy	Rheumatoid arthritis; gout; pseudogout
Impaired host defenses	Cancer; diabetes; use of corticosteroids; use of immunosuppressive drugs; leukopenia
Hereditary host defects	Complement deficiencies; phagocyte defects; agammaglobulinemias
Foreign bodies	Joint prosthesis; penetrating joint wounds
Bacteremia	Intravenous drug abuse; indwelling catheters; instrumentation of body cavities; skin ulcers
Antecedent infections	Urinary tract infections; pneumonia; meningitis; infective endocarditis; sepsis

fusions, of which 10% are polyarticular. The typical patient with disseminated gonococcal infection is a young healthy woman who is pregnant or menstruating and rarely has symptoms of a genital infection. The average duration of symptoms of gonococcal arthritis, prior to diagnosis, is 5 days.

In virtually all cases of acute septic arthritis, the affected joints will be very painful to palpation and movement. Fever has been documented in about half the cases, generally in those with septic arthritis of hematogenous origin. Swelling is apparent in less than half the cases because effusions in deeply situated joints such as the hip and shoulder are often not clinically detectable. Superficial joints such as the knee, elbow, ankle, and hand joints commonly reveal swelling and warmth, less commonly redness. Purulent drainage is rarely found except at surgical sites. Evidence of a

portal of entry, such as dermatitis or a decubitus ulcer, or a primary focus of infection elsewhere, such as the lung, urinary tract, or meninges, may be apparent on physical examination in up to half of the patients. Tenosynovitis with a sparse eruption of red papules with necrotic centers is strongly suggestive of disseminated gonococcal infection. Macular, urticarial, or purpuric rashes suggest a viral origin, while erythema nodosum suggests tuberculosis or a mycosis.

Untreated infections of the joints have a poor prognosis. The death rate in the preantibiotic era was 6% to 12%. Current series show variable outcomes depending on the subject population. Mortality rates vary from less than 1% to 20%, with most deaths occurring in severely immuno-compromised patients. Overall, a good outcome can be anticipated in 70% of cases, with full recovery in almost all cases of disseminated gonococcal infection. Poor outcomes (joint destruction, ankylosis, chronic pain, limited motion, recurrent infection) are associated with advanced age, infected prosthetic or rheumatoid joints, hospital-acquired infections (infants), mixed aerobic–anaerobic infections, and underlying chronic diseases or immunosuppression. The relationship of duration of symptoms prior to diagnosis to outcome varies according to the virulence of the organism. Poor outcomes have, however, been shown to be more likely when the time required to achieve a sterile joint after starting treatment exceeds 2 days.

PATHOPHYSIOLOGY

In experimental models of septic arthritis in which virulent microbes are injected directly into the joint, the bacteria can be found in the synovium within 1 to 2 hours. Over the next 2 days, the synovium becomes hyperemic and is infiltrated by neutrophils, and the lining cells begin to proliferate. After 48 hours, the infiltrate becomes mononuclear, abcesses form, and the effusion becomes purulent. After 7 days, irreversible changes begin to take place; proteolytic enzymes released from neutrophils and synovial cells destroy the cartilage and then the bone. A thick layer of granulation tissue (pannus) derived from the hypertrophied synovium adds to the destruction by invading adjacent bone. In tight compartments such as the hip, pressure necrosis can result from tense effusions, which contain metabolic products that also contribute to cartilage degradation. Bacterial antigens have been shown to induce a chronic synovitis in the absence of living organisms, suggesting that immune mechanisms may perpetuate the inflammatory response after living organisms are no longer present.

CLINICAL–PATHOLOGIC CORRELATIONS

Microorganisms invading the joint are usually disseminated by hematogenous spread from a remote focus and less often from direct innoculation. Compared to the incidence of bacteremia, joint infections are relatively rare, owing to the protection afforded by the reticuloendothelial system and periarticular structures. Table 144–3 shows selected microorganisms, their potential pathologic effects, and the clinical manifestations of those effects. The pathogenesis of septic arthritis is often related to an immune system compromised either by chronic disease, drugs, trauma, age, or endocrine factors in the host. In infants, for example, metaphyseal capillaries, which lack phagocytic cells, extend into the epiphyseal growth plate, increasing the likelihood of seeding the adjacent joint. Staphylococci, group B streptococci, and gram-negative bacilli are the most likely organisms in this age group. Children between the ages of 1 and 5 years lack antibodies for *Hemophilus influenzae*, which is a common pathogen in this age group. *Neisseria gonorrhoeae* predominates in the septic arthritis of sexually active adolescents and young adults, whereas the staphylococci and group A beta-hemolytic streptococci predominate in the joint infection of children ages 5 to 15 years and adults more than 30 years old. *Pseudomonas* and *Serratia* species are the most common pathogens in drug abusers. Although the relationship of host age and the pathogenicity of various organisms is not known, their ubiquitous and invasive nature may be important, given a susceptible host.

DIFFERENTIAL DIAGNOSIS

MONARTICULAR FORM

The most common causes of acute monoarthritis are trauma, infection, and crystal synovitis. The initial signs and symptoms of crystal synovitis are identical to those of septic arthritis, including fever, malaise, and leukocytosis in many patients. Gout has a predilection for the first metatarsophalangeal joint and the ankle. Pseudogout favors the knees and wrists and may follow a subacute or chronic course. The presence of intracellular crystals of urate or calcium pyrophosphate in the synovial fluid establishes the diagnosis, but does not exclude the possibility of a superimposed infection.

The peripheral arthritis that may occur in patients with one of the spondyloarthropathies (Reiter's syndrome, ankylosing spondylitis, psoriasis, inflammatory bowel disease) has

TABLE 144–3.
Clinical–Pathologic Correlations for Septic Arthritis

| CLINICAL | PATHOLOGIC FINDINGS | |
	MICROBIAL ORGANISMS	PATHOGENESIS
	BACTERIA	
Joint pain and swelling (monoarticular in 90% of cases)	*Staphylococcus aureus*/streptococci	Hematogenous; local inoculation
Fever, chills; presence of risk factors (see Table 144–2)		Complement activation by cell-wall peptidoglycans suggesting antibody-independent inflammation
Tenosynovitis and vasculitic rash; monoarticular or polyarticular arthritis	*Neisseria* sp	Dissemination more likely with deficiency of late complement proteins (C5–C8); deposition of immune complexes
Sepsis more common; affinity for sacroiliac, sternoclavicular and symphysis pubis; history of intravenous drug abuse	*Pseudomonas/Serratia* sp	Multiple host defense-mechanism deficiencies; phagocytic, cellular, complement
	MYCOBACTERIA	
Monarticular (85% of the cases) common in the knee (24%); hip (20%); wrist (20%)	*Mycobacterium tuberculosis*	Hematogenous, lymphatic; reactivation of primary site
Rarely pulmonary; in tendon sheaths of hand or wrist (50% of cases)	*M. kansasii*	Prior trauma or surgery (45% of cases); corticosteroid injection (36%)
Rarely pulmonary; in tendon sheaths of hand or wrist (50% of cases)	*M. marinum*	Exposure to marine life; local inoculation
Rarely pulmonary; in tendon sheaths of hand or wrist (50% of cases)	*M. fortuitum*	Inoculation from soil
	FUNGI	
Extremities affected, sparing hips and shoulder; chronic, progressive; usually afebrile	*Sporothrix schenckii*	Local inoculation; hematogenous from pulmonary site
Knee (75% of cases); less often in hips and shoulders; rarely in small joints; lesions on scalp and pubis in drug abuse	*Candida albicans*	Hematogenous; corticosteroid injection; almost always in a immunocompromised host
	VIRUSES	
Migratory or additive symmetric or asymmetric joint signs; favors small joints of hand, then large joints; urticarial or purpuric rash; signs of hepatitis	Hepatitis B	Immune complex deposition of IgM, C3, and hepatitis B surface antigen; complement activation
Symmetric effects on fingers, wrists, knees, carpal tunnel; rubella rash	Rubella	Replication in synovium; immune complexes

some features in common with septic arthritis: it usually involves fewer than four joints and has a predeliction for large joints of the lower extremity. Extra-articular features involving the eyes, skin, genital tract, and gastrointestinal tract help distinguish this group from nongonococcal arthritis.

POLYARTICULAR FORM

For those disseminated gonococcal infection patients who present with a polyarticular pattern, the differential diagnosis includes acute rheumatic fever, acute onset of rheumatoid arthritis, Reiter's syndrome, systemic lupus erythematosis, and polyarticular gout or pseudogout. The dermatitis-arthritis syndrome is not unique to disseminated gonococcal infection and has been reported in a variety of bowel disorders such as inflammatory bowel disease and postoperative blind-loop conditions.

The key features differentiating these other diseases from either monoarticular or polyarticular infection are the absence of organisms on Gram's stain or culture and the failure to respond to appropriate antibiotics.

DIAGNOSIS

The peripheral WBC count is elevated in only half of the cases. Acute-phase reactants and the erythrocyte sedimentation rate are usually elevated, but are nonspecific findings. Blood cultures may be positive in about 50% of nongonococcal arthritis cases, but in only 20% to 30% of those with disseminated gonococcal infection, almost exclusively in those with the polyarticular-dermatitis presentation. Antibody titers to viral antigens, measured at an early stage and during convalescence, may give presumptive evidence of a viral origin.

A definitive diagnosis can only be made by examination of the synovial fluid. This should be done without delay in any patient with a recent onset of pain and swelling in one or two joints. The first portion of the aspirate should be analyzed by staining with Gram's stain and culturing for aerobic and anaerobic organisms. A drop of fluid should be analyzed under polarized light for crystals. Any remaining fluid should be sent for a WBC count, a differential count, and a glucose determination. Septic arthritis generally yields type III fluid (Table 144–4), but there can be considerable overlap with type II. The classification of joint fluid depends mainly on the synovial fluid WBC count, which is usually more than 50,000 cells/ml in septic arthritis. Ranges of 3,600 to 905,000 cells/ml have been reported. A low cell count may be due to prior administration of antibiotics or the use of immunosuppressive drugs.

In nongonococcal arthritis, the result of a Gram's stain will be positive in 50% of the cases, but the culture will be positive in over 80%. In disseminated gonococcal infection, the result of a Gram's stain will be positive in less than 25%, and the culture will be positive in less than 50%, but culture of samples from anogenital and oral sites will identify gonococcus in over 80%. In the remainder, typical signs and symptoms and a rapid response to appropriate antibiotics will support the diagnosis.

Gram's stain and culture of synovial fluid samples may have negative results when an adjacent bursa with a "sympathetic" inflammatory but sterile effusion is inadvertently sampled instead of the infected joint.

High levels of lactate in the synovial fluid have been found in nongonococcal infections, but are no more specific than a synovial WBC count of more than 50,000 cells/ml. Succinic acid may be a more specific indicator of bacterial infection. Counterimmunoelectrophoresis (CIE) can sometimes detect bacterial antigens derived from *Streptococcus pneumoniae*, *N. meningitidis* and *H. influenzae*, but not from gonococci. Synovial biopsy for specific culture and special stains is the procedure of choice when mycobacteria or fungi are suspected, and the laboratory should be alerted to the need for special techniques.

X-ray studies taken during the first week of

TABLE 144–4.
Classification of Synovial Fluid in Septic Arthritis

FEATURE	TYPE II FLUID (INFLAMMATORY)	TYPE III FLUID (SEPTIC)
Appearance	Turbid; yellow-white	Opaque; purulent
Viscosity	Poor	Poor
WBC/ml	2,000–50,000 or more	50,000–300,000
Cell type	Neutrophils > 50%	Neutrophils > 75%
Glucose level	< 40 mg/dl in 10% of cases	< 40% mg/100 ml in 60% of cases
Lactate level	Increased in 8% of cases	Increased in 50% of cases
Succinic acid	Rarely elevated	Increased in all

joint infection show only soft tissue swelling and effusion. Later, periarticular osteopenia develops, followed by joint-space narrowing as cartilage is lost. Bony destruction is a late finding. CT scans and radionuclide imaging may be helpful in localizing inflammation in axial or deep extremity joints, but are not specific.

PRINCIPLES OF PREVENTION AND TREATMENT

Aseptic technique during joint surgery or aspiration is the major preventive measure. Identifying and treating asymptomatic carriers of gonococcal infection should be carried out in high-risk populations, especially young, sexually active women because these individuals are at greater risk for disseminated gonococcal infection.

Patients with acute monoarthritis and type III synovial fluid should be given antibiotics pending culture results even if the Gram's stain result is negative because failure to rapidly sterilize a septic joint is associated with poor outcomes. The initial choice of antibiotic is dictated by either the Gram's stain result or the clinical signs and symptoms. Intravenous penicillin or a cephalosporin are indicated for a clinical picture of disseminated gonococcal infection. Tube-dilution susceptibility tests should be done for nongonococcal organisms. Monoarthritis is usually due to *Staphylococcus* and should be treated with a penicillinase-resistant drug. Vancomycin is recommended for infected prosthetic joints because *Staphylococcus epidermidis* is a common pathogen in this setting. Septic arthritis in the elderly or the immunocompromised patient requires broad coverage for resistant staphylococci and gram-negative bacilli. Drug addicts should be given antipseudomonas drugs. Isoniazide plus rifampin usually suffice for *Mycobacterium tuberculosis*, but some would add ethambutal. Atypical mycobacteria are difficult to treat, and there are no standard regimens. Amphotericin B, 5-fluorocytosine, or both are used for fungal infections.

The joint should be aspirated daily until the synovial fluid WBC count falls and fluid no longer reaccumulates. Intra-articular antibiotics are not recommended. Repeated cultures are necessary to ensure that the infection is responding. If the patient is not improving after 5 days of appropriate antibiotics, surgical drainage may be indicated. Infected joint prostheses usually require removal to effect a cure. Hip and shoulder infections, particularly in children, require surgical drainage. The affected joint should be splinted, and adequate analgesia prescribed. As soon as the synovitis improves, passive and then active range-of-motion exercises should be instituted. In disseminated gonococcal infection, oral antibiotics may be given to complete the treatment after an initial response to parenteral antibiotics has been established.

REFERENCES

Dan M: Septic arthritis in young infants: Clincal and microbiologic correlations and therapeutic implications. *Rev Infect Dis* 1984; 6:147 155. *An interesting analysis of hospital vs community-acquired infections.*

Goldenberg DL, Reed JI: Bacterial arthritis. *N Engl J Med* 1985; 312:764–771. *A concise and up-to-date summary of common bacterial infections.*

Holmes KK, Counts GW, Beaty HN: Disseminated gonococcal infection. *Ann Intern Med* 1971; 74: 979–993. *An analysis of gonococcal syndromes with excellent color photographs of the skin lesions.*

McCarty DJ (ed): *Arthritis and Allied Conditions*, ed 10. Philadelphia, Lea & Febiger, 1985, pp 1627–1712. *An excellent comprehensive presentation of the pathophysiology and clinical aspects.*

Newman JH: Review of septic arthritis throughout the antibiotic era. *Ann Rheum Dis* 1976; 35:198–205. *The epidemiology and outcomes of hematogenous septic arthritis are well presented.*

Roca RP, Yoshikawa TT: Primary skeletal infection in heroin users. *Clin Orth Related Research* 1979, 144:238–248. *Description of the clinical and microbial characteristics of skeletal infections of heroin users who do not have endocarditis.*

145

OSTEOMYELITIS

John S. Czachor, M.D.
H. Bradford Hawley, M.D.

Osteomyelitis can be defined as the infection of any bone. The etiology of this entity is varied because bacteria or fungi may cause the inflammation. The mortality associated with osteomyelitis has decreased dramatically since the advent of the antibiotic era, but significant morbidity exists in the chronic forms of this disease. Osteomyelitis is divided into the acute form and the chronic form. Acute osteomyelitis may be considered to be the first bone infection, while chronic osteomyelitis may be any relapse after the original infection.

CLINICAL SIGNS AND SYMPTOMS

The history often alerts the physician to the presence of osteomyelitis. Risk factors for the development of this disease include a history of underlying disease (e.g., sickle cell disease, diabetes), a history of penetrating or blunt trauma, or a history of a preceding infection. Intravenous drug abuse is also a risk factor. Patients with long-term indwelling catheters for vascular access such as Broviac and Hickman catheters may be prone to bacteremia with eventual seeding of the bony skeleton. Chronic hemodialysis may also provide a portal of entry for hematogenous spread of microorganisms with eventual osteomyelitis. See Table 145–1 for characteristics of acute osteomyelitis. When considering a diagnosis of chronic osteomyelitis, a history of previous osteomyelitis, a history of previous surgery, or the presence of foreign bodies or metallic hardware in direct contact with bony structures are important points to elicit.

The physical findings are varied, but the usual hallmarks of infection are generally present in acute osteomyelitis (Table 145–2). Patients with chronic osteomyelitis often have nonacute presentations marked by the absence of high-grade fever, erythema, and swelling, but have increased drainage from sinus tracts and more pain in the affected area.

The mortality rate used to be in the range of 15% to 25%. Now, with the availability of antibiotics, this percentage has declined to only 1% to 2% of all cases. The complications of osteomyelitis are listed in Table 145–3. Delayed or improper treatment of acute osteomyelitis will increase the number of recurrent episodes and will subsequently lead to or result in the formation of a chronic osteomyelitis.

PATHOPHYSIOLOGY

Acute osteomyelitis may be divided into three categories according to the source or means of infection: hematogenous spread, direct inoculation, and associated with peripheral vascular disease. The key element is the introduction of the organism into the blood supply of the bone. Once present in the local vascular environment, the infection can begin to run its course.

Bone is an active metabolic tissue that requires a good blood supply to accomplish its tasks of synthesis and growth. Hematogenous osteomyelitis usually attacks bones of children at the rapidly growing metaphysis. The nutrient arteries tend to have circuitous capillary loops near the epiphyseal growth plates in the metaphysis. These then empty into an area of low-flow sinusoids that eventually involve the medullary cavity. It is here that blood flow is greatly reduced, which can aid bacterial deposition. The afferent capillary loops lack phagocytic lining cells; the efferent capillaries contain phagocytic cells, but they are functionally inactive. Thus, once bacteria are deposited, re-

TABLE 145–1.
Characteristics of Acute Osteomyelitis Classified According to Source of Infection*

| | SOURCE OF INFECTION | | |
CHARACTERISTICS	HEMATOGENOUS	DIRECT INOCULATION	VASCULAR INSUFFICIENCY

Age distribution
Precipitating factors
	≤ 20 yr and ≥ 50 yr
	Bacteremia
	Blunt trauma (nonpenetrating)
	Underlying diseases
	  Sickle-cell disease
	  Other hemoglobinopathies
	  Chronic granulomatous disease
		Any age (surgical) (Peak > 50 yr)
		Surgery
		Penetrating trauma
		  Puncture wound of foot
		  Bites
		  Diagnostic procedures
			≥ 50 yr
			Diabetes mellitus
			Peripheral vascular disease
			Contiguous spread of soft-tissue infections

Bones involved	Long bones Vertebrae	Femur Tibia Skull Mandible	Feet

Organisms
  involved
	Usually one organism
	  Staphlococcus aureus (60%)
	  Gram-negative rods
	  Salmonella sp
		Often mixed infection
		  Staphylococcus aureus
		  Gram-negative rods
		  Anaerobic organisms
			Usually mixed infection
			  Staphylococcus aureus or
			  Staphylococcus epidermidis
			  Streptococci
			  Gram-negative rods
			  Anaerobic organisms

* Modified from Norden CW, in Mandel GL et al: Principles and Practice of Infectious Diseases, ed. 2, p 705.

TABLE 145–2.
Clinical Findings of Acute Osteomyelitis

CLINICAL FINDINGS	FREQUENCY (% OF CASES)
PHYSICAL FINDINGS	
Tenderness	70–90
Erythema	15–60
Fever	50–60
Decreased range of joint motion	40–50
Preceding infection	30–55
Warmth over area	30–40
Fluctuation	11
Drainage	5
LABORATORY FINDINGS	
Bone cultures positive	90
Blood cultures positive	50–60
Positive radiographic signs at 1 week	30
Positive radiographic signs at 4 weeks	90

TABLE 145–3.
Complications of Osteomyelitis

ACUTE OSTEOMYELITIS

Sepsis
Septic arthritis
Destruction of epiphyseal growth cartilage (prepubertal)
Chronic osteomyelitis
Coexistent infections secondary to dissemination
Local abscesses/local extension of infection

CHRONIC OSTEOMYELITIS

Pathologic fracture
Sinus tract formation
Transformation to cancer from a chronic draining sinus
Amyloidosis (rare)
Formation of sequestrum and involucrum
Brodie's abscesses

moval mechanisms are limited. These capillary loops are also end-artery branches, and any occlusion of this area will result in avascular necrosis. These factors make the metaphysis the favored site of blood-borne osteomyelitic infection.

In patients from age 1 year until puberty, the initial insult is thought to begin in the metaphyseal sinusoidal veins. The pus is restricted by the growth plate, causing lateral spread. Thus the bony cortex is breeched, and the loose periosteum is lifted. A subperiosteal collection of pus is the final result.

Postpubertal osteomyelitis occurs in much the same manner except that the periosteum is firmly attached to the bone. Because of this attachment, there is less subperiosteal abscess formation and less periosteal proliferation. Instead necrosis of bony tissues, breakdown of bone structures, and demineralization results from the acute suppurative inflammation. The bacteria, changes in pH, local edema, and leukocyte reaction all contribute to the aforementioned changes. The local process may then spread by way of Haversian and Volkmann's canals. This compromises vascular supply further and causes more bone cell death. Postpubertal osteomyelitis may also spread to the epiphysis because some capillaries perforate the growth plate. Septic arthritis and destruction of the epiphyseal growth cartilage are complications of this spread.

If untreated or inadequately treated, acute osteomyelitis can become chronic. The avascular bone becomes separated from viable bone and is known as sequestra. If the infection is contained and a line of demarcation exists, a subperiosteal collection of pus may remain and is known as a *Brodie's abscess*. Once subperiosteal abscess formation is complete, it may induce exuberant growth of the periosteum. This growth may surround either the sequestra or Brodie's abscess and is known as the *involucrum*.

In osteomyelitis caused by direct inoculation, the mechanism is rather simple. Organisms are in intimate contact with bone, and then the infectious process begins. This scenario accounts for a minority of cases in children, but a significant proportion in adults. Precipitating factors include open fracture, open reduction and internal fixation of fractures, wound infections, and direct penetrating trauma.

Osteomyelitis may also be seen in patients with peripheral vascular insufficiency. Osteomyelitis develops from extension of a local infection or trophic ulcers. Diabetic patients generally have this type of osteomyelitis. Marginal soft tissue viability and poor bone vascularity limit the local inflammatory response, predisposing the involved region to infection and eventually necrosis.

The mechanism of chronic osteomyelitis relies on the prolongation of acute osteomyelitis. A delay in diagnosis, inappropriate antibiotic choice, inappropriate antibiotic duration, inadequate surgical drainage, or any combination of the factors is responsible for continued infection and eventual chronicity. A major risk factor for chronic osteomyelitis is the presence of a large amount of necrotic bone. This will inhibit bone healing and may harbor organisms. Continued or new infection may occur with resultant vascular thrombosis and further bone necrosis. Thus, the self-perpetuating cycle is complete (Fig 145–1).

CLINICAL–PATHOLOGIC CORRELATIONS

The clinical features of osteomyelitis result from the entry of microorganisms into a highly vascular area. The local effects are secondary to the interruption of the blood flow and the inability of the body to transfer adequate host defenses to this region. The body then reacts in specific ways to cause the clinical features noted in Table 145–4.

DIFFERENTIAL DIAGNOSIS

The differential diagnosis of osteomyelitis includes conditions that may be independent or coexistent with osteomyelitis. Cellulitis, septic arthritis, fasciitis, and pyomyositis all may be coincident infectious processes. Also, any inflammatory joint disease such as rheumatoid arthritis could be confused with a local osteomyelitis. Ewing's sarcoma has often been confused with osteomyelitis both histologically and radiographically. Osteomyelitis itself has many different presentations and can be separated into clinical entities with different characteristics.

Neonatal osteomyelitis tends to be preceded by a complication of pregnancy, delivery, or the neonatal period. Any complicated birth

TABLE 145–4.
Clinical–Pathologic Correlations for Osteomyelitis

CLINICAL FINDINGS	PATHOLOGIC FINDINGS
Periosteal elevation	Infection contained by epiphyseal growth plate; lateral spread. The cortex becomes perforated resulting in a subperiosteal collection of pus.
Sequestrum	Bone necrosis secondary to infection encroaching on vascular channels. Blood supply is interrupted resulting in osteocyte death.
Involucrum	Exuberant growth of new bone under the periosteum secondary to the subperiosteal abscess, resulting in the encasement of sequestrum.
Brodie's abscess	Demarcation of the necrotic area of bone with containment of infection, resulting in a subperiosteal accumulation of pus.

Acute Osteomyelitis → Bone Necrosis → Poor Healing → Persistent Organisms → Infection

FIG 145–1.
Process by which acute osteomyelitis develops into chronic osteomyelitis.

process usually leads to intensive and invasive monitoring of the infant. Procedures such as fetal scalp monitoring during labor, umbilical catheterization, or heel sticks may be the source of a skeletal infection. However, there usually are no preceding complications when Group B *Streptococcus* is the offending bacterial species. *Staphylococcus aureus* and *Escherichia coli* along with Group B *Streptococcus* are common in this age group. With no growth plate to limit the spread of the infection, the joint may be destroyed or the usual bone growth may cease.

Hematogenous osteomyelitis is predominantly a disease of children younger than age 16 years. Another peak incidence is in adults age 50 years and older who most frequently have vertebral osteomyelitis. Blood-borne osteomyelitis generally attacks long tubular bones, specifically the femur, tibia, and humerus, which are the site of most hematogenously disseminated infections. Multiple bone involvement is not uncommon and can be seen in 15% of cases. *S. aureus* is still the most common etiologic agent and is found in about 50% of cases. As in other infectious processes, gram-negative bacilli are playing an increasing role as pathogens. Specifically, *E. coli*, *Klebsiella*, and *Pseudomonas* species are being isolated in increasing frequency.

Several specific types of hematogenously spread osteomyelitis can be differentiated. Intravenous drug abuse has been found to be associated with osteomyelitis in young adults. The clinical course generally is indolent. *Pseudomonas aeruginosa* is responsible for many of the infections. Yeast, other gram-negative bacilli, and staphylococci are also common. The vertebrae, pelvis, and clavicles are prime targets of infection. Indwelling catheters such as Hickman, Broviac, and other types of central venous catheters may have bacteremias associated with their use, and may eventually lead to skeletal seeding. Subclavian catheters may be associated with infections that spread directly to the adjacent clavicles, producing osteomyelitis. Osteomyelitis of the ribs and thoracic vertebrae in hemodialysis patients with indwelling cannulas must be differentiated from renal osteodystrophy.

Underlying diseases such as sickle cell disease can be associated with osteomyelitis. *Salmonella* osteomyelitis is common in patients with sickle cells and is responsible for 80% of all bone infections in these patients. Gram-negative bacilli account for nearly 100% of these osteomyelitis cases. Sickle-cell disease, hemoglobin SC cell disease, and sickle beta-thalessemia are also noted to have a predisposition to *Salmonella* bone infections.

Hematogenously spread osteomyelitis may occur in patients suffering minor nonpenetrating trauma. Local trauma has been noted to occur in up to one-third of acute hematogenous osteomyelitis cases. The pathogenesis is uncertain, but it is felt that the infection is set up secondary to local ischemia and necrosis, which leads to a focus of bacterial invasion.

Osteomyelitis may be spread by direct inoculation of the bone. This may occur from an exogenous source or spread from a contiguous source. The most common precipitating factor is the development of an open or compound fracture as the result of penetrating trauma. The bone may be seeded by direct entry of either skin organisms or flora present on the penetrating object. Also, if a contiguous soft-tissue injury is present, this may spread and set up an osteomyelitis after penetration. Direct inoculation into bone from contiguous infection not necessarily related to penetrating trauma may also result in osteomyelitis. Soft-tissue infections (especially in the fingers and toes), infected teeth, and sinus infections are all well-known infections that lead to osteomyelitis. Surgically induced inoculation also accounts for a substantial number of cases of osteomyelitis. Generally orthopedic procedures such as open reduction or internal fixation are risk factors for the development of an infection. External fixation or traction also is a predisposing factor. Animal or human bites and closed-fist injuries are other sources of penetrating injury that may lead to osteomyelitis from direct inoculation. This can occur in patients at any age. Any bone in the body may be involved, but the tibia and femur are most frequently infected because these bones are most often the site of fracture and orthopedic manipulation. Once again *S. aureus* is still the most common infecting organism, but the occurrence of infections from multiple organisms account for more than half of the infections. *S. aureus* usually is one of the organisms in mixed infections. Foot puncture wounds in children have a high incidence of *Pseudomonas aeruginosa* osteomyelitis.

Osteomyelitis associated with vascular

insufficiency is usually seen in diabetic patients who have complications such as retinopathy, nephropathy, and neuropathy or who have severe atherosclerosis. Children rarely have this type of osteomyelitis because this disease is associated with changes occurring over the years. The disease usually occurs in patients 50 to 70 years of age. The small bones of the feet, the phalanges and metatarsals, are involved. This type of osteomyelitis also is often caused by multiple organisms. Staphylococci, both S. epidermidis and S. aureus, are most commonly isolated. Streptococci, anaerobic bacteria, and gram-negative bacilli are also frequently isolated.

Vertebral osteomyelitis has been noted to be increasing in incidence. This infection is prevalent in drug addicts, in patients with hematogenous spread from other foci of infection, or after trauma, usually surgical trauma. When the infection spreads from the genitourinary tract, it probably does so by ascending through the posterior venous plexus to the vertebral venous system known as *Batson's plexus*. This is usually a disease of adults and generally affects the vertebrae in decreasing frequency from lumbar to thoracic to cervical vertebrae. However, drug addicts have an increased incidence of cervical osteomyelitis. The manifestations of vertebral osteomyelitis are quite diverse and can present as a myriad of symptoms. The differential diagnosis includes low-back pain syndrome, radiculopathy, epidural abscess, meningitis, or disc herniation. S. aureus remains the predominant infecting organism, but gram-negative bacilli such as P. aeruginosa are becoming more prevalent.

Anaerobic osteomyelitis has apparently been increasing in frequency because of greater physician awareness and proper culture techniques. Anaerobes are a large part of many fixed infections causing osteomyelitis and are especially prevalent in the type of osteomyelitis associated with diabetes and vascular insufficiency. Predisposing factors include trauma, fractures (usually open fractures), and human bites. Long bones such as the tibia and femur are the sites of approximately 40% of all anaerobic osteomyelitis, while facial bones are involved in approximately 27% of cases. Small bones of the feet are also very commonly infected in anaerobic osteomyelitis. When there is a foul-smelling purulent exudate or organisms seen with Gram's stain but not cultured or

both, the physician should be alert to the possibility of an anaerobic infection. Other settings in which a suspicion of anaerobic osteomyelitis should be high are infection of the pelvis after abdominal sepsis and infections from sacral decubiti. Generally, multiple organisms are isolated. Over 80% of anaerobic infections involve multiple organisms, whether they be several anaerobes or a mixture of both aerobes and anaerobes. *Bacteroides fragilis* and *B. melaninogenicus* are the most frequent isolates. *Peptococcus* species and *Peptostreptococcus* species are also recovered in significant amounts. Patients with mixed aerobic and anaerobic infections often have been noted to fail to respond to treatment.

Fungi may cause osteomyelitis; these infections generally appear as a cold abscess overlying an osteolytic lesion. Immunocompromised hosts are a prime target for the fungi. Indwelling catheters, hyperalimentation, and steroid dependency are risk factors for the development of fungal infections that may lead to skeletal deposition and osteomyelitis. Amphotericin B in combination with surgery is the usual mode of therapy.

Tuberculous osteomyelitis usually results from hematogenous dissemination from the initial infection, but can also be spread from contiguous structures. The onset of tuberculous osteomyelitis may be insidious because the symptoms are usually nondescript. Pain is often the most common complaint, and usually some arthritis is associated with the osseous lesion. Any bone may be involved, but the most common sites are weight-bearing areas. The spine is the greatest site of tuberculous osteomyelitis; the lower thoracic vertebrae are most often involved with the lumbar spine next most often. The hip, knee, ankle, and small bones of the hands and feet are usual sites of infection. The use of systemic chemotherapy with antituberculous drugs has eliminated the need for surgery and immobilization in uncomplicated cases of tuberculous osteomyelitis.

DIAGNOSIS

The diagnosis of osteomyelitis may be difficult because both acute and chronic osteomyelitis may appear in many ways. The history and physical examination, as usual, lend important information to the physician. Acute hematogenous osteomyelitis appears as a febrile, toxic episode with local suppuration around the involved bone. These manifestations are usually seen in children, but less often in adults. An indolent presentation of osteomyelitis may also be seen. Drainage is an infrequent occurrence in blood-borne osteomyelitis. In direct-inoculation osteomyelitis, about 50% of patients appears to be in a toxic condition. Most osteomyelitis associated with vascular insufficiency has local symptoms rather than toxic episodes. Fever and septicemia are unusual, while chronic drainage is common.

A leukocytosis with a left shift may be found, as may be an elevated ESR. These have no predictive value when considering the outcome of the disease. Because treatment is based on identification of a specific organism, it is necessary to isolate the causative pathogen. Blood cultures are usually positive in 50% to 60% of the cases of hematogenous osteomyelitis. Bone cultures are positive in up to 90% of all osteomyelitis infections. However, all cultures can be negative in 3% to 15% of cases. Culture of a sample from draining sinus can give a positive identification; however, it may not accurately represent the true infecting organism responsible for the osteomyelitis. These sinuses may be contaminated by colonizing bacteria, further confusing identification of the etiologic agent. Sinus tract cultures also have been shown to correlate poorly with bone biopsy cultures.

Radiographic information helps to confirm the diagnosis of osteomyelitis. After 7 days to 10 days, radiographic evidence is scant. It usually takes 3 weeks to 4 weeks for radiographic findings to appear. The delay is due in part to the time needed for half of the bone matrix to be resorbed in order to visualize a lytic process. Before new bone is formed, the destructive changes need to be completed. Radiologic signs of osteomyelitis include deep soft-tissue swelling, periosteal reaction, cortical irregularity, demineralization, and sequestrum formation. Radionuclide scanning, however, may reveal the changes of osteomyelitis in 3 days to 4 days and remain up to 1 week to 2 weeks after the acute process has resolved. Identification is earlier because the scanning isotope is laid down at the sites of increased osteoblastic activity and increased blood supply to the bone in osteomyelitis. Radionuclide scanning can give false-positive results in conditions that lead to bone injury and repair. Surgery in the recent past or trauma can mimic osteomyelitis and can lead to an incorrect diagnosis. The role of computed tomography remains to be defined in the diagnosis of osteomyelitis.

PRINCIPLES OF THERAPY

The treatment of osteomyelitis depends on the specific identification of the causative organism. Because of the great amount of staphylococcal osteomyelitis, empiric therapy usually will include antibiotics against this organism. Once the final determination of pathogen and its sensitivities is complete, appropriate antibiotics are ordered.

The treatment of acute osteomyelitis is purely medical unless there is no response to the treatment in 48 hours to 72 hours. If this occurs, then surgical treatment, most likely a bone biopsy or debridement for organism identification and abscess drainage is indicated. The length of therapy should be 4 weeks to 6 weeks with the appropriate specific antibiotic given parenterally. In acute osteomyelitis peak serum bactericidal titers have no predictive value, but trough titers of 1:2 or greater accurately predict a cure. Trough titers less than 1:2 predict therapeutic failure. Generally, no oral antibiotic is indicated after parenteral therapy.

The prognosis is good in acute osteomyelitis. Variables that influence outcome are the duration of the symptoms, the early start of antibiotics, and the duration of the antibiotic therapy. The sooner antibiotics are started, the better the outcome. Making the diagnosis of osteomyelitis with subsequent administration of antimicrobial agents should occur within 3 days to 5 days after the onset of symptoms to ensure a good outcome. Treatment failures are found to occur when patients have received a short course (less than 3 weeks total) of antibiotics. The usual duration of antibiotic therapy is 6 weeks.

Treatment of chronic osteomyelitis remains controversial. Bone necrosis may be the central issue. Sequestra may be the nidus for continued infection even after starting antibiotic treatment. Therefore, surgical treatment is an integral part of therapy in chronic situations.

First, intravenous antibiotic therapy is begun, and approximately 10 days to 14 days later, surgery can be performed. Removal of avascular tissue, necrotic bone, and lingering abscesses is mandatory. Antimicrobial agents then are continued parenterally for a total of 4 weeks to 6 weeks after the surgery. In chronic osteomyelitis peak serum bactericidal titers of 1:16 or greater and trough titers of 1:4 or greater predict cure; peak titers less than 1:16 and trough titers less than 1:2 accurately predict failure in therapy. Up to 2 months of oral antibiotics may then be prescribed.

One of the difficulties in treating chronic osteomyelitis is attaining adequate antibiotic concentrations in the infected area. Because it is an area of avascular necrotic bone, delivery of the antibiotic is decreased. Several techniques to increase the concentration of antibiotics have been tried with varying amounts of success. These include regional perfusion of the antimicrobial agent to the affected area either by mechanical means or by muscle flap, irrigation of the wound with antibiotic solutions at the time of surgery, and installation of antibiotic-impregnated polymer beads. Hyperbaric oxygen with its high oxygen environment under pressure has also been used in conjunction with antibiotics and surgery to help in the treatment of chronic osteomyelitis. Not only does it promote better wound healing, but it also inhibits the growth of the bacteria.

If any metallic foreign body such as orthopedic hardware remains in the site of chronic osteomyelitis, it must be removed. Only after all hardware has been removed and antibiotics have been given for a total of 4 weeks to 6 weeks after hardware removal can subsequent orthopedic procedures be successful. Joint stability may indeed be a problem before the orthopedic treatment, but nonunion of the bone secondary to a continued chronic osteomyelitis infection is common unless the above steps are followed.

REFERENCES

Fitzgerald RH: Antibiotic distribution in normal and osteomyelitic bone. *Orthop Clin North Am*, 1984; 15(3):537–546. *Where does that antibiotic go? This article tells you.*

Hall BB, Rosenblatt JE, Fitzgerald RH: Anaerobic septic arthritis and osteomyelitis. *Orthop Clin North Am* 1984; 15(3):505–516. *A good description of anaerobic pathology.*

Mandel GL, Douglas RG, Bennett JE: *Principles and Practice of Infectious Diseases*, ed 2. New York, John Wiley & Sons, 1985. *Up-to-date, extensive and well written. An excellent reference.*

Wald ER: Risk factors of osteomyelitis. *Am J Med* 1985; 78(suppl 6B):206–212. *This will allow the reader to know all the risks leading to osteomyelitis.*

Waldvogel FA, Medoff G, Swartz MN: Osteomyelitis: A review of clinical features, therapeutic considerations and unusual aspects. *N Engl J Med* 1970; 282:198–206, 260–286, 316–322. *The articles on the subjects. Complete and time honored.*

Waldvogel FA, Vasey H: Osteomyelitis: The past decade. *N Engl J Med* 1980; 303:360–370. *This article updates the above reference (Waldvogel, Medoff, and Swartz, 1970).*

Weinstein MP, Stratton CW, Hawley HB et al: Multicenter collaborative evaluation of a standardized serum bactericidal test as a predictor of therapeutic efficacy in acute and chronic osteomyelitis *Am J Med*, 1987; 83:218–222. *Recently published reference that helps to determine the adequacy of therapy.*

Wheat J: Diagnostic strategies in osteomyelitis. *Am J Med* 1985; 78 (suppl 6B):218–224. *A relevant discussion on "how to" diagnose osteomyelitis.*

146

COMMON FRACTURES

Hobart E. Klaaren, M.D.

A fracture is a break in the continuity of the cortex of a bone. Fractures are usually caused by an injuring force, applied directly or indirectly to a bone. A direct force crushes a bone by compression (e.g., a "compression fracture" of a vertebra sustained in a fall). An indirect force fractures by leverage, and the bone fails from torque, tensile, or shear strain, (e.g., a forearm fracture from a fall on an outstretched hand).

PATHOPHYSIOLOGY

Fractures vary in response to the severity and direction of the injuring force and to the strength and structure of the affected bone.

Many adjectives are used to describe specific fractures. Open fractures have external wounds communicating to the disrupted bone, and closed fractures do not (though in either case the fracture may be minor or severe). A fracture may be complete (e.g., an offset, overriding transverse fracture of a long bone) or incomplete (a greenstick fracture, or a torus fracture). A fracture may be undisplaced or displaced. It may be rotated, angulated, offset, or overriding. It may be comminuted (in multiple fragments) or segmental (a double fracture separated by a long segment). The direction of the fracture may be longitudinal, transverse, oblique, or spiral. A chip fracture is a small avulsion fracture, usually pulled off by a ligament or tendon attachment. A fracture-dislocation is a fracture accompanied by a dislocation of an adjacent joint. Thus the possible variations of fractures and involved bones are numerous.

Fractures that occur in diseased or weakened bone with minimal or no injuring force applied are called pathologic fractures. Bone may be weakened by congenital disease (e.g., osteo-genesis imperfecta) or acquired disease (e.g., metastatic cancer or osteoporosis). Fatigue or stress fractures are caused by repetitive applied forces. Fractures may occur from unrecognized or denied trauma (e.g., child abuse) or from falls due to intoxication or drug abuse.

Fractures in children usually heal faster than similar fractures in adults. Children's bone is more elastic, and the periosteum is tougher; therefore, incomplete fractures (e.g., greenstick fractures) are more common. Interruption of growth lines is very important in treatment and prognosis. Growth line fractures which extend into a joint require very accurate open reduction and internal fixation.

All tissues and organs near major fractures must be evaluated for possible simultaneous injury. Skin, vascular function, and nerve function (motor and sensory) must be assessed. Major organ or neural injuries or both may be associated with fractures of the central skeleton.

Bone healing is an orderly process initiated by a fracture. A hematoma forms. Fibrous connective tissue grows in from the marrow, periosteum, and surrounding tissues. Pluripotential cells grow in and convert to cartilage-producing and bone-producing cells, which form a callus. Callus is reshaped to cortical and cancellous bone as a structural response to applied mechanical stress, and this process appears to be mediated by electrical stimuli carried to the osteoblasts. Apposition and immobilization of the bone ends and a good blood supply to the bone fragments are the usual basic requirements for fracture healing. Extensive skin and soft tissue damage, bone fragmentation, tissue dead space, contamination, and infection can be major deterrents to healing. Cortical and tubular bone heals less rapidly than cancellous (trabecular) bone.

Fractures in certain locations have a propensity for slow union or nonunion. These include the diaphyses of long bones (especially the distal humerus and the tibia) and certain intra-articular fractures where the blood supply is cut off to the joint fragments (e.g., subcapital hip fractures and midcarpal-scaphoid fractures).

DIAGNOSIS

The diagnosis of a fracture is made by the history of an injury and examination of the injured part. Localized tenderness and deformity are usually apparent. X-ray films should be made in at least two planes (usually anterior-posterior and lateral) and should include the full length of the bone and the joint at each end of it. Occasionally, planograms, computed tomography (CT) scans, and radioactive technetium scanning may be helpful in diagnosis.

PRINCIPLES OF TREATMENT

The principles of treatment are to restore and maintain fracture alignment and apposition, to maintain blood supply, to avoid contamination and infection, and to immobilize the fractured bone sufficiently well until healing occurs. Treatment methods include splints, casts, braces, traction, and various external and internal fixation devices (e.g., pins, plates, screws, wires, intramedullary rods).

The complications include delayed union, malunion, nonunion, infection and osteomyelitis, traumatic arthritis, and associated vascular, neural and organ injuries. The blood supply may be compromised in a fascial compartment by edema and hemorrhage leading to necrosis of all tissues within that compartment ("compartment syndrome"). Patients must be monitored adequately to prevent, recognize, or correct these problems.

SPECIFIC FRACTURES

Finger fractures are common. If they involve the joints, the permanent disability may be severe. Specialized internal fixation techniques are often necessary. Boxer's fractures of a metacarpal occur from striking a person or object.

Colles' wrist fractures, which are common, especially in older osteoporotic women, are fractures of the distal radius with dorsal displacement of the distal fragment.

Forearm fractures usually occur by indirect force from a fall and may involve one or both bones (radius and ulna).

Elbow fractures and dislocations occur in many varieties and combinations. Careful x-ray evaluation is essential, and x-rays may be difficult to interpret, especially in children who have multiple ossific growth nuclei. Comparison x-ray views of the unaffected elbow may be helpful in detecting differences, showing a fracture or dislocation.

Humeral neck fractures are common in older people and alcoholics who fall and try to catch themselves. Some of these fractures are impacted (jammed together) and heal readily. Others are severely displaced and comminuted.

Clavicle fractures are common and usually heal adequately with simple splinting plus a sling. Commercially available clavicle straps are used.

Spinal injuries may be of many types and severity. Stability of the injured spine must be ensured. Spinal cord function must be assessed.

Displaced unstable pelvic fractures are being treated more aggressively in recent years with internal or external fixation. The pelvic organs and structures must be evaluated for function and integrity.

Hip fractures are usually best treated by internal fixation to allow the patient to be mobile.

Femoral shaft fractures are often treated by closed intramedullary nailing under image-intensifier control without opening a wound to the fracture site.

Tibial fractures are a common aspect of major trauma, and many types of treatment are used depending on the fracture and the orthopedist's preference.

Ankle fracture-dislocations often require open reduction and very accurate internal fixation.

Crush fractures of the os calcis are common and serious injuries, often with prolonged disability. Reduction by either closed or open techniques is difficult.

REFERENCES

Rockwood CA Jr, Green DP: *Fractures in Adults,* vols 1, 2, and 3. Philadelphia, JB Lippincott Co, 1984. Chapters:

1. Harkness JW, Ramsey WC, Ahmadi B: Principles of fractures and dislocations.
2. Green DP, Rowland SA: Fractures and dislocations in the hand.
3. Anderson LD: Fractures of the shafts of the radius and ulna.
4. DeLee JC, Green DP, Wilkins KE: Fractures and dislocations of the elbow.
5. Epps CH Jr: Fractures of the shaft of the humerus.
6. Stauffer ES, Kaufer H, Kling TF: Fractures and dislocations of the spine.
7. Kane WJ: Fractures of the pelvis.
8. DeLee JC: Fractures and dislocations of the hip.
9. Mooney V, Claudi BE: Fractures of the shaft of the femur.
10. Leach RE: Fractures of the tibia and fibula.
11. Wilson FC: Fractures and dislocations of the ankle. *A comprehensive reference on fractures and dislocations. Volume 3 is devoted to fractures in children.*

147 SCOLIOSIS AND SPINAL DEFORMITIES

James T. Lehner, M.D.

This chapter deals with scoliosis, kyphosis, lordosis, and some specific deformities of the spine that cause these angular deformities. Scoliosis can be defined as a lateral curvature of the spine. It is not normally found in any area of the spine. Kyphosis is an anterior flexion of the spine. It is normal in the sacral coccygeal elements and in the thoracic spine of developed human beings and can exist as either an increased flexion in these areas or an abnormal flexion in either the lumbar or cervical spine. Lordosis is the opposite of kyphosis, or posterior flexion of the spine. It is normal in the lumbar and cervical area but can exist to a pathologic degree in these areas or in the thoracic or sacral coccygeal areas.

SCOLIOSIS

The broad term *scoliosis* refers to a lateral curvature of the spine. It is not a specific disease, but has many causes. Scoliosis can be classified into two basic types. A nonstructural scoliosis is a reversible lateral curvature of the spine without any vertebral rotation. It can be due to poor posture, muscle spasm, underlying tumors, other pathologic changes, or most commonly, lower limb length discrepancies (such as shortening of one limb). Structural scoliosis is a true structural vertebral problem. It is usually associated with vertebral rotation in the area of the curve. Thus, shoulder heights can be uneven, scapular heights can be uneven, and rib humps and lumbar humps become evident. Patients can compensate and carry their shoulders, head, and neck directly above the pelvis or not compensate and lean when upright. The curves are identified by the convex side of the curve (such as "right thoracic curve" or "left lumbar curve").

Structural scoliosis can be classified into four groups: idiopathic, neuromuscular, congenital scoliosis, and a miscellaneous category. Idiopathic scoliosis makes up at least 75% of all cases of structural scoliosis and is always present before full growth is achieved. The infantile form appears before age 3 years; the juvenile form appears between ages 4 years and 9 years; and the adolescent form appears from age 10 years and on. Of these, the most common is the adolescent variety.

The pathogenesis of idiopathic scoliosis is not clearly defined. Anthropometric studies show that girls with idiopathic scoliosis have increased trunk and lower extremity height compared to age-matched controls. These would indicate that an abnormal, accelerated growth pattern could be a provoking factor in scoliosis. Since the intervertebral discs become wedged in scoliosis, biochemical abnormalities have been studied and found. There are abnormalities in skin collagen and disc collagen in patients with idiopathic scoliosis which are consistent with a generalized collagen defect. No abnormality of glycosaminoglycan metabolism is known. Genetic studies have been confusing but indicate that there is a hereditary predisposition to the disease. This may be either a dominantly inherited single gene abnormality with variable penetration or a multiple genetic factor disorder. Muscle biopsies reveal differences in fast twitch fiber content between concave and convex sides of curves. Postural equilibrium has been measured, and abnormal postural reactions are noted in the idiopathic scoliosis population, particularly of oculo-vestibular interactions. While all of these do not add up to a clear-cut picture of the true etiology of idiopathic scoliosis, they point out that children with idiopathic scoliosis do have differences from the general population in their basic makeup.

Neuromuscular scoliosis includes cases of neurologic or muscular origin, such as those due to primary neurologic problems including myelomeningocele, poliomyelitis, and cerebral palsy and those due to muscular disorders including Duchenne's muscular dystrophy as well as the other myopathies. In congenital scoliosis the formation of the vertebrae is defective so that vertebrae are formed asymmetrically (hemivertebrae) or abnormally fused together (congenital bars). These can cause a variety of skeletal and neurologic complications due to the resultant bizarre structural deformity. The miscellaneous group includes many syndromes associated with scoliosis including neurofibromatosis, chest wall deformities, and deformities resulting from metabolic, traumatic, infectious, and other conditions including many forms of dwarfing.

IDIOPATHIC SCOLIOSIS

Idiopathic scoliosis is by far the most common type of structural scoliosis. It occurs in up to 8% of the population, but is clinically significant in approximately 0.5%. It is a hereditary disorder, and the most common, adolescent scoliosis, progresses to significant problems in girls much more commonly than in boys (8:1).

Clinical Signs and Symptoms

Idiopathic scoliosis is painless when it first starts. Usually children do not notice any deformity at all. Families notice problems such as elevation of the shoulder, asymmetry of the rib or waistline, or problems fitting pants due to the waistline abnormality. Diagnosis is simply made on physical examination by looking for deformities, both from behind and the side with the child standing and bending over (i.e., for a neckline abnormality, shoulder height discrepancy, scapular imbalance, waist-line asymmetry, thoracic and lumbar humps, and asymmetry in the position of the arms relative to the chest cavity).

The radiographic examination should be done with the patient standing. The Cobb method of measuring the curvature in degrees has become accepted internationally. Any curve under 10 degrees is considered clinically insignificant. Curves over 10 degrees have variable prognoses due to their tendency to progress. In general, the younger the child is and the more severe the curve is when first seen, the more significant the chance is for that child's curve to get worse with continued growth. An immature child with a curve from 20 degrees to 29 degrees has a 68% chance of having a very significant progression of the curve, whereas a mature child with a curve of 10 degrees to 18 degrees has only a 2% chance of having that curve progress. In general, curves under 30 degrees at the end of growth do not progress.

SCOLIOSIS AND BACK PAIN

Often patients with scoliosis are seen for backache, but scoliosis is rarely a source of backache in childhood. Patients with severe scoliotic curvatures (over 60 degrees) often develop degenerative arthritis secondary to the deformity and thus develop arthritic pain later. Conversely, though, many people with backache from herniated discs, spine tumors, and other conditions will develop spastic scoliosis. It is important to differentiate these conditions from idiopathic scoliosis. The presence of a mild scoliosis or other spinal deformity does not necessarily help in making a diagnosis in the patient with backache.

PROGNOSIS

The complications of untreated scoliosis are directly related to the severity of the curve. If the curve is over 30 degrees, the chances of significant problems are increased. People with thoracic curves over 60 degrees die 15 years earlier than the average population and usually die from cardiac and pulmonary compromise. The severe deformity of the chest wall secondary to scoliosis leads to restrictive pulmonary disease and then secondary "cor pulmonale" and heart failure. Adults with severe curves develop arthritis and pain. Progression of these symptoms occurs in direct relationship to the severity of the curve. In general, all curves over 60 degrees worsen regardless of the patient's maturity. Curves between 30 degrees and 60 degrees have a variable chance of getting worse. Curves under 30 degrees usually are stable in adulthood. The amount of cosmetic deformity can vary, but, in general, curves over 30 degrees have a readily detectable cosmetic deformity, which worsens as the curve gets worse.

Women with severe curves have a compromised quality of life in adulthood. Statistics show that women with 60-degree curves have only a 24% chance of getting married, have up to a 90% incidence of back pain, and have a 47% chance of having the disease severe enough to qualify for disability compensation. Very few patients with significant curves are able to engage in heavy manual labor.

FORMS OF TREATMENT

To be treated, the disease must first be detected. Screening is done in the schools for adolescent idiopathic scoliosis which is by far the most common type of scoliosis. The screening is usually initiated in the sixth grade and is done by school nurses or gym teachers who are trained in looking for scoliosis. With early detection of scoliosis, it is possible to lower the need for surgical procedures for scoliosis and also to lessen the complexity of those procedures. Often up to 8% of the children screened in school will be judged "positive." Most of these children have a postural problem only, but a significant number, 1% to 3%, have structural scoliosis or other deformities. The vast majority of those with scoliosis can be treated with observation and for most patients by the primary care physician (Table 147–1).

X-ray Studies

Some of the children who are judged "positive" on screening require x-ray films, although very mild curves can be followed by visual examination only. The best x-ray film is a single anteroposterior or posteroanterior x-ray picture of the spine with the patient standing and the breast and gonadal areas shielded. In general, curves that are progressing and those that are over 20 degrees in growing children should be referred to an orthopaedist.

Management of Progressive Curves

Observation is the best management procedure for patients with curves that are under 20 degrees and those between 20 degrees and 30 degrees that are not showing any signs of progression. The variable clinical course of individual curves has shown that many of these curves will not progress and thus do not need any form of treatment. Since each curve acts individually, it is difficult to predict on one visit what these milder curves will do, and a period of observation of 3 months or 4 months with follow-up x- ray films may be indicated. If a curve shows 5 degrees of progression from the initial films to any follow-up films, it should be classified as a progressive curve. Once a curve reaches 30 degrees, its chance of progression becomes quite significant. If an exercise program is advised, children should engage in interscholastic or intramural athletic programs rather than assigned physical therapy programs or regimented exercises.

For those children who require active treatment, bracing is very effective in preventing

TABLE 147–1.

Evaluation and Treatment of Idiopathic Scoliosis and Kyphosis: Suggested Guidelines for the Primary Care Physician*

GROWTH STATUS	CURVE MEASUREMENT (COBB METHOD)	RECOMMENDATION
IDIOPATHIC SCOLIOSIS		
Prepubertal (No secondary sex characteristics)	5°–10°	Follow-up every 6 months; x-ray every 6–12 months
	> 10°	Refer to orthopedist
Pubertal	5°–10°	Follow-up every 6 months
	10°–20°	Follow-up every 4 months with x-ray
	> 20°	Refer to orthopedist
Postpubertal	10°	No follow-up
(Menses or secondary sexual development for ≥ 18 months)	10°–20°	Follow-up in 6–12 months with x-ray (Discontinue if no progression)
	> 20°	Refer to orthopedist
KYPHOSIS	< 40°	Postural exercises if indicated
	> 40°	Refer to orthopedist

Notes:
1. The above are general guidelines only; each case must be treated individually.
2. All growing siblings (including brothers) over the age of 8 years should be examined for scoliosis yearly, and an x-ray film should be taken if there is any question of asymmetry.
3. X-ray films for scoliosis should be PA or AP T1–S1 with patient standing; x-ray films for kyphosis should be lateral T1–S1 with patient standing.

* From Ohio Postural Screening Program.

progression of the curve. The philosophy of bracing is to keep the curves from getting worse, but a modest amount of correction may be obtainable with bracing. Currently two types of braces are used. Braces work on a three-point principle, pushing on the center (apex) of the curve and on points opposite the curve above and below this area. Thus, a right thoracic curve has to be pushed at three points: on the left side of the neck, the right side of the deformity, and on the left side of the lumbar area or pelvis. Underarm orthoses are efficacious for thoracolumbar and lumbar curves. These braces need to be used full-time initially and then on a part-time basis until the child is fully grown. The average duration is 3 years, but the duration in each case is based on the individual needs of the child.

Electrical stimulation of the paraspinal muscles is now used for the same indications as bracing, that is, for progressive curves between 20 degrees and 29 degrees and for most curves between 30 degrees and 40 degrees. Early results suggest that electrical stimulation is less efficacious than bracing. Children must be selected individually for bracing or electrical intervention. Those curves which are over 60 degrees when seen, or over 40 degrees and still progressing are best handled with surgical stabilization. This can be done with either anterior (lumbar curves) or posterior (most other curves) surgery. Instrumentation is used to correct the deformity, and a spinal fusion is performed in the area of the curve. This stabilizes the spine and is highly successful in preventing progression.

After successful orthotic or surgical management, scoliosis patients can interact normally in society. They carry on normal social, economic, and reproductive lives.

TREATMENT OF INFANTILE AND JUVENILE SCOLIOSIS

The curves in infantile and juvenile scoliosis are different from the much more common adolescent variety in that boys are more often affected than in the adolescent variety and the curves can be progressive, stable, or resolving. These patients need to be observed, and if their condition requires treatment, the treatment period will be much longer. While these cases are harder to treat than those of the adolescent variety, the same general guidelines should be used.

TREATMENT OF OTHER FORMS OF SCOLIOSIS

Neuromuscular scoliosis is caused by impaired neurologic function, muscular weakness, or imbalance of the spinal muscles. All children who develop a thoracic level paraplegia under the age of 10 years will develop a scoliosis. The more severely involved patients with myelomeningocele and the more severely involved cerebral palsy patients with spastic quadriplegia have very high incidences of scoliosis. Scoliosis is common in Duchenne's muscular dystrophy as children get weaker and rely more on sitting in wheelchairs than walking. The scoliosis quickly becomes structural and further impairs the children's ability to function, even in a chair, and may make them bedridden. Pelvic obliquity (one side of the pelvis higher than the other) develops and leads to pressure sores on the sitting areas, pelvis, and hips. A striking pulmonary compromise may occur. These children are best treated before a deformity becomes significant with adequate adaptations made to their wheelchairs or with bracing to prevent rapid progression of the curves. Often the scoliotic curves are amenable to surgical stabilization. In these situations it is much better for the child to have surgery, which allows him or her to sit up and enjoy even a limited view of the world than to have the child lie in bed because of the severe spinal problems. Many forms of rigid fixation of the spine are employed to assure stabilization in this group of patients.

Congenital scoliosis is often associated with other congenital anomalies. In one-third of the children, an abnormality of the urogenital system is present and an intravenous pyelogram is recommended. This will often reveal an absence of kidneys, duplication of excretory systems, or other abnormalities.

In general, congenital scoliotic problems worsen at a rate dependent on the child's ability to growth. If there is a hemivertebra present on the left side of the spine and no balancing segment on the right side, the deformity will grow in direct relationship to how that "keystone" vertebra grows. If a level is not segmented correctly, it cannot grow at all, so the curve will not grow. Congenital spine problems basically become worse at a linear rate with growth. Usually bracing is not helpful; milder curves can be observed only; curves with significant rate of progression need surgical treatment.

OTHER SPINAL DEFORMITIES

KYPHOSIS (Round Back Deformity)

Kyphosis is seen as a clinical problem one quarter as often as scoliosis. Kyphosis up to 40 degrees is normal in the thoracic spine, and kyphosis is also normal in the sacral coccygeal segment. Most kyphotic problems occur as hyperkyphosis of the thoracic spine (over 40 degrees). The main kyphotic diseases to be differentiated in children are postural roundback and Scheuermann's disease. These two entities can be differentiated by the tremendous flexibility of the postural roundback and the stiffness of a Scheuermann's patient. In Scheuermann's disease, the lateral x-ray film of the spine will show vertebral wedging. The postural roundback is usually treated with an exercise program to increase muscle tone and to encourage the child to stand more erect. Scheuermann's disease often requires the use of a Milwaukee brace for moderately severe curves and combined anterior and posterior surgical treatment for more severe deformities.

LORDOSIS (Swayback Deformity)

Lordosis is rarely seen as a clinical problem. Lordosis is normal in the cervical and lumbar spine. Lumbar lordosis can be accentuated in some of the neuromuscular disorders. True lordosis in the thoracic spine is a very significant problem that severely compromises pulmonary function. Most lordosis, however, is in the lumbar spine, which is quite flexible, and is usually not a clinical problem.

FRACTURES AND DISLOCATIONS OF THE VERTEBRAL COLUMN

Fractures and dislocations of the spine post two problems: first, compromise of musculoskeletal stability, and second, a compromise of neurologic function. Neurologic compromise may include complete or incomplete spinal cord damage with paraplegia or quadriplegia or nerve root lesions. If a neurologic lesion does not correspond to the anatomical radiographic findings, an answer for the discrepancy must be sought through myelography, computed tomographic (CT) evaluations, and other techniques. Reduction of a fracture has been shown to have the greatest benefit in maximizing the neurologic function by reestablishing the spinal canal.

For fractures in the cervical spine, reduction has been obtained with traction through skull tongs or halo devices. In many of these injuries halo casts or halo braces allow the patient to get out of bed and start a rehabilitation program. In the surgical treatment for cervical spine injuries, posterior ligamentous instability problems require posterior stabilization with wiring of the unstable area and local fusion. Anterior burst-type injuries with bone in the spinal canal require anterior debridement and fusion. Complex situations may require both anterior and posterior approaches.

Thoracolumbar injuries may be stable or unstable injuries. Stable compression fractures are more common. These injuries are equivalent to stepping on a cardboard box. The bony structure is actually as stable after the fracture as it was beforehand, only deformed. The spinal column is usually in a kyphotic position afterwards Unstable fractures and dislocations in the thoracolumbar area are more significant injuries. The use of CT scanning has shown many of these injuries to be more complicated than plain x-ray films and planar tomography have been able to show in the past. Any fracture becomes unstable when ligamentous structures are disrupted or vertebral segments are displaced more than 3 mm, as seen on the x-ray films or when a vertebra collapses to less than 50% of its normal height.

Stable injuries can be treated with bedrest until the patient is comfortable and then mobilized. The original injury may be associated with intestinal ileus, but this usually clears rapidly. Most of these patients should be admitted to the hospital for observation and pain control. Braces are controversial for "stable" injuries, but many patients feel more comfortable wearing some type of simple orthotic device.

Unstable spinal injuries can be treated in two ways. First, for those patients with no neurologic involvement or for completely paraplegic patients, nonoperative treatment with bedrest and gradual ambulation or a body cast or body polypropylene jacket may be appropriate when the injury seems to involve a bone with the ability to heal. Secondly, patients with partial paraplegia with bone impinging on the spinal canal, or ligamentous injuries or other injuries which do not have the potential to heal spontaneously, require surgical stabilization. This can be done with various anterior, posterior, or combined anterior/posterior approaches to the spine. Unstable injuries usually are treated with some form of internal fixation of the spine that allows the patient to be mobilized and rehabilitated quickly (Fig 147–2, A, B, C, D).

SPONDYLOLISTHESIS

Spondylolisthesis is a translational shift of one vertebra over the next vertebra below it. Most commonly it is an anterior shift of the fifth lumbar vertebra on the sacrum, although it can occur at other levels. It can be due to congenital, developmental, traumatic, or other causes. The most important categories of spondylolisthesis are the isthmic and the degenerative varieties.

The isthmic variety is most commonly a defect in the pars interarticularis area of the L5 vertebra. It allows the L5 vertebral body to slip forward on the sacrum and can start causing pain in childhood. These patients usually have tight hamstring muscles. Many of them (such as weight lifters, gymnasts, linemen) give a history of heavy physical exercise, which includes hyperextension of the lumbar spine. If a defect in the pars interarticularis is not associated with a forward slip, it is called a spondylolysis. If a slippage is present in childhood, it can worsen as the child grows.

Most patients with spondylolysis and mild spondylolisthesis can be treated with symptomatic care. Muscle irritability can be treated with rest, analgesics, exercise programs, and intermittent bracing. Failure to respond to these or progression of slippage of the vertebra forward necessitates surgical stabilization with a posterior fusion. This is quite successful in reducing these patients' symptoms and in stopping further slippage. Extremely severe slippage requires a radical surgical approach to obtain reduction.

The degenerative variety of spondylolisthesis is an aging process and occurs most commonly at the L4–5 interspace. Degeneration of the intervertebral disc and arthritis of the facet joints can be sources of localized pain and radicular pains. The wearing out of these joints can lead to a foraminal narrowing and segmental instability allowing degenerative spondylolisthesis with forward slippage of a vertebra on the one below it. This most commonly occurs at the L4–5 interspace, but can occur at numerous levels. This arthritic condition affecting the lumbar spine usually does not occur until age 40 years. The same condition in the cervical spine usually occurs a decade later than that. Whenever there are hypertrophic ligamentous or bony structures or where there is a foraminal narrowing or a relative narrowing of the spinal canal by degenerative spondylolisthesis, neurologic symptoms can occur. They can result from a single-root neurologic disorder in the cervical spine, various upper motor neuron disorders, or various types of lower motor-neuron claudication, which mimic vascular claudication in the lumbar spine. This latter entity has to be differentiated from a vascular claudication, and typically the patients have pain in the back and the legs after activity. They can be differentiated from the patients with vascular claudication by the more common association with back ache, presence of good peripheral pulses, a very stiff lumbar area on examination, and relief of symptoms obtained by bending forward (reducing lumbar lordosis). Vascular claudication patients get relief of their symptoms by stopping activity, but do not have to bend over.

BACK PAIN IN CHILDREN

Back pain in children should be treated as a serious complaint; it is very rare in comparison to adult backache, because children have a lot more important things to do than complain of pain. Back pain in children can be mechanical, developmental, inflammatory, traumatic, or neoplastic. Mechanical derangements include postural deformities, muscular strains, or (rarely) herniated nucleus purposes. Developmental abnormalities include spondylolysis and spondylolisthesis, Scheuermann's kyphosis, and severe scoliosis. Inflammatory processes includes disc space infections, calcification, vertebral osteomyelitis, rheumatoid disorders, and sacroiliac joint infections. Neoplastic diseases of the vertebral column or the spinal canal can cause back pain, spasm, and a painful scoliosis. An example of this is a 10-year-old boy with severe backache, mild scoliosis, and a history of severe pain at night relieved by aspirin. X-ray films showed an absence of a pedicle. The bone scan findings were positive in the area of the defect, and the CT scan showed a nidus of a benign osteoid osteoma. Resection of the tumor resulted in complete relief of symptoms immediately.

REFERENCES

Blount WP, Moe JH: *The Milwaukee Brace*, ed 2. Baltimore, Williams & Wilkins Co, 1980. *An in-depth discussion of the brace and its use.*

Bradford D, Hensinger RM: *The Pediatric Spine*. New York, Thieme, 1985. *In-depth focus on the child's spine growth and problems.*

Bradford D, Lonstein JE, Oglivie JW, Winter RR: *Mobe's Textbook of Scoliosis and Other Spinal Deformities.*, ed. 2, Philadelphia, WB Saunders Co, 1987. *Comprehensive text.*

Dickson RA, Bradford D (eds): *Management of Spinal Deformities*, Woburn, Mass, Butterworth, 1984. *Excellent discussion of therapy.*

Jacobs RR (ed): *Pathogenesis of Idiopathic Scoliosis.* Chicago, Scoliosis Research Society, 1984. *Detailed discussion of pathogenesis.*

Lonstein JE: The prediction of curve progression in untreated idiopathic scoliosis during growth. *Am J Bone Joint Surg* 1984; 66A:1061–1071. *Prognosis in idiopathic scoliosis.*

Luque ER: *Segmental Spinal Instrumentation.* Thorofare, NJ, Slack Publishers, 1984. *Extensive discussion, well referenced.*

MacNab IM: *Backache*. Baltimore, Williams & Wilkins Co, 1977. *A full breadth discussion of this common problem.*

148 BURSITIS AND TENDONITIS

John G. Paty, Jr., M.D.

Bursae and tendon synovial sheaths are found where structures move relative to each other and are in tight apposition. This relationship applies particularly to sites where tendons are deflected around bones or under retinacula around joints. The arrangement at its simplest is the olecranon and the patella where the skin must move freely over subcutaneous bony surfaces usually under conditions of pressure. The bursae at the latter sites are simply flattened sacs of synovial membrane supported by dense irregular connective tissue. They are interposed in the loose areolar tissue (superficial fascia) between skin and bone. Because of their position they are usually known as subcutaneous bursae. The degree of bursal flattening is obscured by the term *sac*. Its opposed walls are separated merely by a film of fluid, making the bursa more of an enclosed cleft. These walls are to some extent tethered to periosteum and dermis, moving with these structures and hence sliding over each other. This arrangement reduces friction, but its fundamental characteristic is creating absolute discontinuity between tissues, yielding complete freedom of movement over a limited range. Each bursa contains a capillary film of synovial fluid acting as a lubricant and providing the synovial membrane cells with a wet environment on their free surfaces and is a metabolic intermediary between tendons and their surroundings.

Most synovial bursae occur between tendons and bone, tendons and ligaments, or between a tendon and another bursae. They may, however, be located between muscle and bone, tendon or ligament (submuscular synovial bursae). Some also separate aponeurotic areas from bone (subfascial bursae) or interligamentous areas from bone. Not only are most bursae near joints, but they may communicate with them making the synovial membrane of the bursa and joint continuous. There are approximately 156 bursae.

Tendon synovial sheaths, primarily found in the wrist, hand, ankle, and foot, surround tendons where they pass under ligamentous bands or retinacula or through fascial slings or osseofibrous tunnels. They consist of two concentric layers separated by a capillary film of synovial fluid and are continuous at their extremities (i.e., a closed double-walled cylinder in which the internal, visceral layer is attached to the tendon by loose areolar tissue and the external, parietal layer is attached to the neighboring connective tissue or periosteum).

Where skin is subjected to repetitive lateral displacement under pressure, as in forearm or elbow in writing or in the buttock in certain sedentary occupations, "adventitious" bursae may appear, providing the skin with more freedom of movement. Adventitial bursae lack a true synovial, endothelial lining but are subject to the same pathologic changes as true bursae.

PATHOPHYSIOLOGY AND DIAGNOSIS

Anatomically and physiologically, bursae and tendon sheaths are similar, and both are similar to the synovial lining of joints. They are all subject to such disturbances as acute and chronic trauma, acute or chronic infection, and inflammatory conditions like gout, tuberculosis, or rheumatoid arthritis. The function of the digits may be affected by constriction of the tendon from fibrous thickening of the tendon sheath (stenosing tenovaginitis). A variety of conditions embraced by bursitis, tenosynovitis (tendon synovial sheath inflammation), and tendonitis (tendon inflammation or strain) are grouped together here by anatomical location for simplicity (Tables 148–1 and 148–2).

867

TABLE 148–1.

Clinical–Pathologic Correlations of Bursitis/Tendonitis

CLINICAL FINDINGS	PATHOLOGIC FINDINGS
Shoulder pain on abduction, external and internal rotation and tenderness over the proximal humeral head	Inflammatory reaction involving the rotator cuff, sometimes associated with subacromial bursitis
Shoulder pain through the painful arc, (60 degrees to 120 degrees abduction) and tenderness over the greater tuberosity of the humerus	Supraspinatous tendinitis or impingement of supraspinatous tendon under coracoacromial arch
Shoulder pain on resisted supination of the forearm (Yergason's sign) and tenderness over the bicipital groove	Inflammatory reaction involving the longhead of the biceps tendon sheath (tenosynovitis)
Swelling and tenderness over the olecranon	Inflammatory (aseptic or septic) reaction or bleeding into the olecranon bursa
Pain with wrist extension with the elbow straight and tenderness of the lateral epicondyle. Pain in the elbow associated with tennis, lifting a skillet or a cup of coffee and repetitive activities of the forearm	Inflammation of the subtendinous space of the common extensor tendon attachment to the lateral epicondyle of the elbow
Wrist pain and tenderness proximal to the anatomical snuff box and a positive Finkelstein's test, (de Quervain's disease)	Inflammatory reaction (tenosynovitis), involving the sheath of the long abductor and short extensor tendons of the thumb and fibrous thickening of the tendon sheath at the radial styloid often restricting tendon motion (stenosing tenovaginitis)
"Locked" digit with tender nodule involving flexor tendon and palpable "snapping" with extension of digit (trigger finger or thumb)	Stenosing tenovaginitis (fibrous thickening of tendon sheath with tendon constriction and secondary swelling) of the flexor tendon at or near the metacarpal head
Painful hip with normal motion and tenderness over the posterior greater trochanter. Pain often occurs when lying on the affected side	Inflammation of the bursa around the gluteal insertion on the greater trochanter of the femur
Painful swollen knee cap (housemaid's knee)	Nonseptic or septic prepatellar bursitis
Knee pain going up and down stairs and tenderness over the medial proximal tibia (anserine bursitis)	Inflammation of the anserine bursa
Knee pain with running, squatting, or jumping, with tenderness at the inferior pole of the patella	Inflammation of the patellar tendon sheath
Heel pain with swelling and tenderness, sometimes crepitus of the Achille's tendon or tenderness behind the calcaneous	Peritendonitis of the Achilles tendon or inflammation of the bursa between the Achilles tendon and calcaneous (retrocalcaneal bursitis). Inflammation of the subcutaneous bursa between the skin and Achilles attachment to the calcaneous may occur as a result of direct trauma (pump bumps)
Pain under heel on walking, particularly after inactivity with tenderness to palpation under the heel	Inflammation of the bursa or fascia at the attachment of the plantar fascia. Periostitis of the calcaneous may occur in Reiter's syndrome or ankylosing spondylitis

SHOULDER

Pain associated with restricted motion may result from any of the common intrinsic shoulder syndromes. The patient with bicipital tendonitis (tenosynovitis) will usually first complain of pain in the arm near the insertion of the pectoralis major on the humerus. Pain may radiate down the arm. Shoulder motions are usually somewhat limited, especially arm elevation with 90 degrees of abduction. This disorder results from a nonspecific inflammation of the tendon sheath of the long head of the biceps tendon sheath where it emerges anteriorly from the capsule of the shoulder joint. A diagnosis can usually be made by having the patient flex the elbow to 90 degrees and

TABLE 148–2.
Etiology of Bursitis/Tendonitis

BURSITIS/TENDONITIS	ETIOLOGY
Acute calcific and noncalcific tendonitis of the rotator cuff	Spontaneous or overuse of the shoulders as in lifting or overhead use of the arm
Chronic rotator cuff tendonitis	May follow acute tendonitis or occur in occupations requiring overhead use of the arm as in painting, powerline climbing, or secondary to impingement of the supraspinatous tendon under the coracoacromial arch
Subacromial bursitis	Secondary to calcific rotator cuff tendonitis
Biceps tenosynovitis	Spontaneous, overuse, occasionally secondary to arthritis in the shoulder
Tennis elbow (lateral epicondylitis)	Repetitive activity of the hands requiring extension at the wrists, for example, tennis, carpentry, gardening, clipping hedges, or carrying luggage
Olecranon bursitis	Trauma, infectious gout, or rheumatoid arthritis
de Quervain's disease (abductor tenosynovitis, tendonitis, and stenosing tenovaginitis of the thumb)	Repetitive adduction of the thumb with radial deviation of the wrists (washer woman sprain)
Trochanteric bursitis	Excessive walking or running, rarely spontaneous
Prepatellar bursitis	Trauma resulting from prolonged pressure over the knee (housemaid's knee). Occasionally infectious
Patellar tenosynovitis or tendonitis	Excessive running or basketball (jumper's knee)
Achilles tenosynovitis or tendonitis	Excessive running or secondary to the spondyloarthropathies, or rheumatoid arthritis
Plantar fasciitis	Occasionally spontaneous but usually associated with excessive walking or running or secondary to the spondyloarthropathies, or rheumatoid arthritis

pronate the forearm. The examiner then grasps the patient's hand and asks him or her to supinate against resistance. If this maneuver produces pain in the anteromedial aspect of the shoulder, a positive Yergason's sign, the diagnosis of bicipital tendonitis is confirmed.

Calcific tendonitis, subacromial bursitis, and rotator cuff tendonitis without calcification are so closely related that their signs and symptoms can be discussed together. In fact, calcific tendonitis of the supraspinatus is frequently associated with subacromial bursitis. The acute irritation of the bursa is usually a secondary reaction produced by the calcific tendonitis of the supraspinatus or one of the other rotator cuff tendons. After the offending calcific material escapes into the subdeltoid bursa, it is absorbed, and spontaneous clinical recovery usually ensues within a few days or weeks.

The amount of diffuse perihumeral tenderness or localized tenderness at the greater tuberosity just distal to the tip of the acromion will vary with the stage of the disorder. During the hyperacute or acute stage, the anguished patient will characteristically hold the affected arm against the chest wall. The pain may be incapacitating and the tenderness exquisite. All ranges of motion are restricted with internal rotation the first lost and the last to return. When calcium is visualized on the x-ray, the shadow will have a hazy appearance. Nighttime pain may be intolerable. Acute or hyperacute calcific tendonitis is most often a self-limited disease. Tendonitis involving the supraspinatus, teres minor, or infraspinatus may cause pain in the posterior region of the shoulder. Constitutional symptoms are rare, but in the hyperacute form swelling may occasionally be visible and there may be a low grade fever and some elevation of the ESR. If resolution does not occur within 2 weeks, progression to a subacute or chronic stage may develop.

In the subacute or chronic stages, the loss of motion is frequently associated with a "painful arc," demonstrated by passive abduction of the arm. Pain will be evoked as the arm passes the horizontal line but will be absent before and after this point is reached. When positive, this sign indicates a "pinching" (impingement sign) of the involved tissue between the greater tuberosity and the acromion process. Supraspinatous tendonitis may be inferred if pain is elicited by patient resistance to adduction with the arm at 90 degrees abduction and 30 degrees forward flexion.

ELBOW

Olecranon bursitis (miner's elbow, student's elbow, beer drinker's elbow) is apparent when the elbow is inspected and palpated during flexion and extension. Trauma, infection, other inflammation, rheumatoid arthritis, or gout may produce an accumulation of fluid in the olecranon bursa. In rheumatoid arthritis or gout, nodules or tophi may be palpable within the bursa. Idiopathic or traumatic olecranon bursitis is usually painless unless there has been bleeding into the bursa or due to extremely tense swelling of the bursa. Fluid may be aspirated for synovial analysis to help distinguish noninflammatory from inflammatory bursitis.

Bicipital bursitis is characterized by antecubital pain and tenderness. A bursa beneath the biceps brachii tendon may become inflammed from repeated trauma as in pitching a ball. There is no swelling. Localized tenderness is present at the insertion of the tendon. Pain is accentuated by flexion and supination.

Lateral humeral epicondylitis (tennis elbow), tendonitis of the wrist and finger common extensor insertion, is characterized by a throbbing pain in the lateral aspect of the elbow accentuated by extension of the wrist. Palpation reveals tenderness over the lateral epicondyle. A clinical sign supporting the diagnosis is the provocation of pain when the patient attempts dorsiflexion (elevation) of the middle finger against resistance with the wrist and elbow held in extension (Maudsley's test). Pain on forced ulnar deviation of the wrist with the elbow in extension is an additional confirmatory test (Mill's sign).

Radiohumeral bursitis occurs at the juncture of the radial head and lateral epicondyle of the elbow. It is most often found in combination with tennis elbow. The symptoms are similar to tennis elbow with pain in the elbow, but the tenderness is located over the radiohumeral groove.

WRIST

Chronic stenosing tenovaginitis, deQuervain's disease, affects the long abductor and short extensor tendons of the thumb. This disorder occurs more commonly in women, often following repetitive activities of the involved hand especially a wringing motion. In the past the syndrome was called washer-woman's sprain. The patient complains of pain on palpation just proximal to the anatomical "snuff box" of the wrist. Finkelsteins's test, in which the fist is clenched over the flexed thumb and forceful ulnar deviation of the hand by the examiner elicits pain at the radial styloid, can be useful in diagnosis.

DIGITS

Stenosing tenovaginitis can affect the digital flexor tendons to cause "trigger" or "snapping" finger. Flexion of the finger usually feels normal, but extension is accompanied by a painful snap. The tendon has a fusiform swelling. Motion usually catches at a point at the tendon sheath on the flexor surface of the finger over the base of the metacarpal head. Characteristically, tenderness is confined to this site.

HIP REGION

Trochanteric bursitis may simulate hip joint disease and sciatica. The involved bursa is between the gluteus maximus muscle and the posterolateral surface of the greater trochanter. Pain is usually near the greater trochanter and radiates down the lateral or posterolateral aspect of the thigh. A so-called gluteal limp may be present. Although abduction and internal rotation may be uncomfortable, complete passive range of motion is usually present in contrast to a condition in which there is true hip involvement.

Ischiogluteal bursitis (weaver's bottom) is characterized by pain over the center of the buttocks. Adjacent to the ischial tuberosity is a bursa that overlies the sciatic nerve and the posterior femoral cutaneous nerve. Sitting on hard surfaces produces pain. Nighttime pain may disturb sleep. Palpation of the ischial tuberosity when the patient is prone elicits tenderness.

Iliopectineal bursitis (psoas) is a rarely described condition with relatively vague, poorly localized symptoms. The iliopectineal bursa is the largest synovial bursa in the body and is situated between the deep surface of the iliopsoas muscle and the anterior surface of the hip joint. The clinical picture includes hip or groin pain with difficulty in walking due to a painful lower extremity. The extremity is held in flexion and moderate external rotation. Point tenderness may be present just inferior to Poupart's ligament lateral to the femoral pulse, and pain may result with hyperextension of the hip.

KNEE

There are numerous bursae in the region of the knee but only specific ones require consideration in the differential diagnosis of knee pain.

Prepatellar bursitis (housemaid's knee) is manifested by swelling and effusion of the superficial bursa overlying the patella. It is usually an obvious abnormality that is the result of chronic bursae reaction to repetitive activity or pressure, such as kneeling on a firm surface. The pain is minimal except when direct pressure is applied. Passive flexion and extension are usually unaffected. Patellar tendonitis (jumper's knee) often occurs in runners and basketball players. Tenderness at the origin of the tendon from the inferior pole of the patella is characteristic. Suprapatellar bursitis is usually associated with synovitis of the knee.

Semimembranosus bursitis is called a Baker's or popliteal cyst when distended with fluid. In the adult, popliteal cysts are frequently associated with rheumatoid arthritis or an internal derangement of the knee. Fullness in the popliteal fossa may cause an inability to fully extend the knee and hence interfere with walking.

Infrapatella bursitis (clergyman's knee) is characterized by a swelling on both sides of the patella ligament near the tibial tuberosity. This condition is usually caused by repeated trauma to the area of the tibial tuberosity and occurs in a variety of occupations, such as roofers, floor-layers, and painters.

Anserine bursitis (cavalryman's disease) now occurs mainly in obese women with disproportionately heavy legs. The anserine bursa lies deep to the tendons of the sartorius, gracilis, and semitendinosus that form the pes anserinus which is superficial to the tibial collateral ligament on the medial aspect of the knee. Clinical features include knee pain, particularly going up or down stairs, palpable swelling, and tenderness over the site of the bursa. The lesion may simulate or coexist with osteoarthritis of the knee.

ANKLE, FOOT, AND HEEL

Tenosynovitis or tendonitis about the ankle is a relatively uncommon condition, but when present, the tendons most commonly involved are the peroneus longus, peroneus brevis, and posterior tibial tendons. Inversion of the foot while palpating the ankle just posterior to the lateral malleolus is painful when tendonitis of the peroneus tendons is present. Eversion of the foot causes pain when posterior tibial tendonitis is present. Not uncommonly in rheumatoid arthritis, the tendons about the ankle have enlarged tendon sheaths and are crepitant on motion.

Painful heels may be caused by a number of conditions that include Achilles peritendonitis (the Achilles has no tenden synovial sheath) or tendonitis, calcaneal bursitis, or plantar fasciitis. The bursae around the heel that are of potential clinical significance include the bursa between the skin and the Achilles tendon, the retrocalcaneal bursa (between the Achilles tendon and the calcaneus), and the calcaneal bursa (between the skin and the calcaneus). A precise differential diagnosis is sometimes impossible because of the intimate relationship of the structures in the heel region. Achilles tendonitis or retrocalcaneal bursitis is associated with tenderness and swelling over the back of the heel. Subcutaneous involvement is frequently traumatic in origin (pump bumps), whereas inflammation of the deeper bursa between the calcaneus and Achilles tendon is more likely caused by excessive running or a systemic disease such as rheumatoid arthritis. Calcaneal bursitis (policeman's or soldier's heel) is frequently associated with a calcaneal spur. Symptoms may not be related to the presence of a spur. Asymptomatic spurs are frequently seen on x- ray. Fluffy exuberant spurs associated with erosions may be found in Reiter's syndrome or ankylosing spondylitis. Plantar fasciitis is usually manifested by pain and tenderness beneath the posteromedial border of the heel. An x-ray may show a bony spur at the site of attachment of the plantar fascia to the calcaneous. Occasionally an adventitious bursa may form around the bony spur.

SEPTIC BURSITIS

Superficial bursae such as the olecranon and prepatellar are the most commonly affected by septic bursitis. The predisposing factors include trauma or occupation-related pressure, corticosteroid therapy, uremia, or diabetes mellitus. Infected bursa are characterized by being red, hot, and exquisitely tender. These can be aspirated to obtain material for Gram's stain and culture to establish an etiologic diagnosis.

PRINCIPLES OF THERAPY

There are many proposed treatments for noninfected bursitis, tendonitis, and tenosynovitis. These include rest, massage, ultrasound, antiinflammatory drugs, splints, and several surgical procedures. The most common approach, however, is local corticosteroid injection which is usually successful. Extreme caution should be used when injecting steroids around tendons. Steroids should not be injected directly into a tendon or near a tendon when a complete or partial rupture is suspected because rupture may occur with intra-tendinous injection of corticosteroids.

REFERENCES

Conn HF, Conn RB (eds): Diagnosis of extremity pain, in *Current Diagnosis*, ed 6. Philadelphia, WB Saunders Co, 1980, pp 61–66. Diagnosis of extremity pain.

DeGowin EL, DeGowin RL (eds): *Bedside Diagnostic Examination*, ed 3. New York, Macmillan Publishing Co, 1981, pp 636–770. *Physical examination of the musculoskeletal system.*

Gray H: *Anatomy of the Human Body*, ed 27. Philadelphia, Lea & Febiger, 1959. *Anatomical description of bursa and tendon.*

Hadler NM: *Medical Management of the Regional Musculoskeletal Diseases.* Orlando, Grune & Stratton, 1984, pp 105–122. *Diagnosis and treatment of shoulder pain.*

Justic EJ: Affections of muscles, tendons, and associate structures, in Edmondson AS, Crenshaw AH (eds): *Campbell's Operative Orthopaedics*, ed 6. St Louis, CV Mosby Co, 1980, pp 1379–1417. Surgical treatment of abnormalities of muscles, tendons, tendon sheath, fascia and bursa.

Kozin F: Painful shoulder and the reflex sympathetic dystrophy syndrome, in McCarty DJ (ed): *Arthritis and Allied Conditions*, ed 10. Philadelphia, Lea & Febiger, 1985, pp 1322–1355. Excellent discussion of the painful shoulder.

Pinals RS: Traumatic arthritis and allied conditions, in McCarty DJ (ed): *Arthritis and Allied Conditions*, ed 10. Philadelphia, Lea & Febiger, 1985, pp 1205–1222. *Textbook of rheumatology detailing clinical features of bursitis and tendinitis.*

INTERVERTEBRAL DISK DISEASE

Samuel E. Pitner, M.D.

Low-back pain and neck and arm pain are extremely common complaints of the patients of all physicians. These are commonly caused by lesions of the intervertebral disk that produce neurologic symptoms through compression of the nerve roots (radicles, hence the term *radiculopathy*) or spinal cord. The major mechanism of injury is by rupture of the nucleus pulposus through the annulus fibrosis with compression of a nerve root, the spinal cord, or both.

CLINICAL SIGNS AND SYMPTOMS

Most, but by no means all, intervertebral disk herniations are due to trauma. Severe trauma producing fractures of fracture-dislocations of the neck or spine also produces lesions of the intervertebral disks, but in these cases the disk lesions usually are the least significant part of the picture. Trauma is a more prominent part of the history in lumbar disk disease than in cervical disk disease.

In lumbar disk disease, a history of a twisting injury of the back, usually in lifting, is obtained in most cases. Initially, the patient may have episodes of neck or back pain without radiation along the course of a specific nerve root. In cervical disk disease, regardless of the exact level, intrascapular pain often is experienced. (At operation under local anesthesia, pinching the annulus fibrosis at any level with forceps produces intrascapular pain, so this pain in cervical disk disease usually is attributed to a beginning tear in the annulus prior to the actual extrusion of any disk material.) Eventually, in lesions in both areas, pain radiating along the course of a nerve root is present in addition to neck or low-back pain.

Nerve root (radicular) pain characteristically has a shooting or stabbing quality; in a fully developed case there also may be continuing paresthesia or weakness in the distribution of the involved root. In a typical case of a herniated lumbar disk, radicular pain is noted down the posterior (almost never anterior) thigh and into the leg to the ankle; good historians usually describe paresthesia or a different type of pain in the foot. Maneuvers that cause even slight movement of the compressed and irritated nerve root usually provoke radicular pain. Flexion of the neck or back frequently either exacerbates or brings out quiescent radicular pain. Changes in the pressure of the cerebrospinal fluid usually produce minute movements of the nerve root; therefore, such actions as coughing or sneezing or even an inadvertent Valsalva maneuver such as straining at stool will bring on radicular pain.

Rarely, one can see severe motor impairment such as a foot drop without local back pain. In cases where the spinal cord itself is compressed, progressive paraparesis with neurogenic bowel and bladder dysfunction often is the primary complaint rather than pain.

Findings on physical examination generally can be considered to be either nonspecific signs associated with nerve root irritation in general or specific neurologic localizing signs indicating compression of a given nerve root.

Because the posterior primary rami of the cervical and lumbar spinal nerve roots go directly to the large longitudinal paravertebral ("strap") muscles of the neck and back prior to entering the brachial or lumbosacral plexi, irritation of the nerve roots produces spasm and tenderness in these muscles. This in turn limits motion of the spine or neck, particularly flexion, and may produce some scoliosis in the case of a lumbar lesion. Paravertebral muscle spasm often can be detected by palpation. In the cervical region, pushing downward from the vertex of the skull and compressing the neck may cause increased bulging of the disk material and may induce radicular pain in the arm; manual traction upward may relieve such pain if present. In contrast to the circumstance with cervical lesions, where movements of the arms only rarely produce enough movement of nerve roots to precipitate pain, many maneuvers by the examiner of the legs of patients with lumbar lesions, particularly flexion of the extended leg at the hip ("straight-leg raising test"), put the sciatic nerve under tension and produce both back pain and radicular pain in the distribution of the involved nerve root. This is particularly diagnostic if this maneuver in the opposite and usually uninvolved leg produces pain down the other leg—a "crossed" response.

The preceding findings suggest an intervertebral disk lesion but cannot be considered as diagnostic without signs that indicate involvement of a specific nerve root. (Multiple nerve roots are involved in well under 5% of cases, and lesions of thoracic intervertebral disks account for only 1% of all disk lesions.) Table 149–1 lists the expected findings on neurologic examination by the most commonly involved nerve roots. The responsible disk lesion is usually at least one interspace higher than the involved nerve root. In many cases, clinical localization based on the neurologic examination is more accurate than either electrodiagnostic or special radiologic diagnostic studies.

A minority of patients will have a massive extrusion of disk material that will cause a permanent, usually painful, neurologic impairment unless it is removed surgically. A somewhat larger group has chronic and even progressive pain and impairment from the onset of symptoms. However, the majority of patients, for reasons that are not well understood, often will have continuing exacerbations and remissions of their symptoms. Medical treatment seems to help only the latter group.

PATHOPHYSIOLOGY

Many blame the prevalence of back pain on the predecessor of *Homo erectus* for having come down out of the trees, pointing out that the human spine, in spite of its need to bear a much greater amount of weight, really is not that different from the spines of quadrupeds. The central, semiliquid portion of the intervertebral disk, the nucleus pulposus, often has to bear weights of over 100 lb, depending on its location, even in a person standing upright without additional stress. The pressure in the intervertebral area is reduced markedly by the recumbent position. (An even more striking reduction is present with zero gravity—the heights of the astronauts are said to have increased so much when in space because of the increased vertical dimension of the intervertebral space that there were problems in fitting spacesuits!)

Beginning as early as age 25 years, there is some dessication of the contents of the intervertebral disk space, with progressive loss of its height on x-ray films of the patient in the upright position. This shortening gives rise to bulging of the annulus fibrosis, which is continuous with the periosteum of the adjacent vertebral body. The traction that ensues may elevate the periosteum and stimulate new bone growth in the area, eventually producing the radiographic picture of vertebral "lipping" and the growth of bone spurs, which themselves may extend into the spinal canal or the neural foramina and give rise to spinal cord or nerve root compression. This mechanism, which is secondary to disk disease, is a very common cause of radiculopathy in older patients.

A sudden increase in pressure in the intervertebral space may cause the nucleus pulposis itself to herniate, sometimes into the vertebral body itself (producing so-called Schmorl's nodules on x- ray films), but more commonly through a tear in the annulus fibrosis itself. This can occur anywhere around the periphery of the disk space, but produces neurologic symptoms only if it protrudes posteriorly ("central herniation") involving the spinal cord or posteriolaterally, involving the nerve root in the neural foramen. The posterior longitudinal ligament of the spine, although less dense than its anterior counterpart, provides a barrier to direct posterior herniation, so the vast majority of symptomatic herniations involve the nerve roots rather than the spinal cord. The consequences of this compression of the roots are the symptoms and signs described previously.

In the cervical area in particular, posterior lipping of the vertebral bodies and cartilaginous changes in the bulging annulus fibrosis can produce a posterior "bar" that intrudes posteriorly into the spinal canal, sometimes re-

TABLE 149–1.
Nerve Root Lesions with Herniated Cervical and Lumbar Intervertebral Disks*

SPINAL AREA	NERVE ROOT INVOLVED	USUAL DISK	MOTOR LOSS	SENSORY LOSS	REFLEX LOSS
CERVICAL					
	C6	C5–C6	Biceps Wrist extensors	Lateral forearm	Radial periosteal ("brachioradialis")
	C7	C6–C7	Triceps Wrist flexors Finger extensors	Middle finger	Triceps
	C5	C4–C5	Biceps Deltoid	Lateral arm	Biceps
	C8	C4–C5	Hand intrinsics Finger flexors	Medial forearm Little finger	None!
LUMBAR					
	S1	L5–S1	Peroneus longus and peroneus brevis	Lateral foot	Achilles ("ankle jerk")
	L5	L4–L5	Extensor hallucis longus	Lateral leg and dorsum of foot	None!
	L4	L3–L4	Tibialis anterior	Medial leg, medial foot occasionally	Patellar ("knee jerk")

* Modified from Hoppenfeld S.: *Orthopaedic Neurology: A Diagnostic Guide to Neurologic Levels.* Philadelphia, JB Lippincott Co, 1977.

Note: The nerve roots most commonly involved in both the cervical and lumbar areas by herniation of the nucleus pulposis are listed above in the order of relative frequency, not in anatomical order. In both the cervical and lumbar areas, the interspaces where the greatest movement on flexion and extension occurs are most frequently involved. Note that at five of these seven levels the neurologic examination gives objective evidence of involvement because the appropriate deep tendon reflex is diminished or absent.

ferred to as cervical spondylosis. Extension of the neck in even normal individuals decreases the anteroposterior diameter of the cervical spinal canal. If an individual who has a congenitally small diameter of the spinal canal in the cervical area develops cervical spondylosis, an extension injury to the neck can produce devastating trauma to the spinal cord without any fracture present. More commonly in such cases, repeated minimal stretching of the spinal cord, which is to an extent anchored in place by both the nerve roots and the dentate ligaments, is produced by extension within the physiologic range, with resultant progressive spastic paraparesis or quadriparesis. This condition, cervical spondylosis with myelopathy, is one of the more common causes of a usually painless and progressive spinal cord lesion producing quadriparesis or paraparesis in older patients. An analogous, but much less frequent, situation occurs in the lumbar spine, below the termination of the spinal cord opposite the body of the first lumbar vertebra. In this situation, all or part of the nerve roots making up the cauda equina are compressed. This sometimes is referred to as spinal stenosis. Often these patients have neurologic symptoms brought on by exercise of the legs and may have abnormal findings on neurologic examination only after exercise; this pattern sometimes has been referred

to as "intermittent claudication of the cauda equina."

CLINICAL–PATHOLOGIC CORRELATIONS

The major clinical–pathologic correlations are shown in Table 149–2.

DIFFERENTIAL DIAGNOSIS

The major disease processes that must be considered in the differential diagnosis of lesions of the intervertebral disk are listed in Table 149–3. Many of these entities can be excluded on the basis of the history and physical examination whereas others may require extensive laboratory or other studies beyond the scope of this discussion.

DIAGNOSIS

X-ray films of the cervical or lumbosacral spine should be obtained in all cases but are of limited diagnostic value. Lateral views may show loss of the normal lordotic curvature in both cervical and lumbar areas as a result of paraver-

---

TABLE 149–2.
Clinical–Pathologic Correlations for Intervertebral Disk Lesions

CLINICAL FINDINGS	PATHOLOGIC FINDINGS
Spinal osteoarthritis becomes apparent on x-rays but is not necessarily symptomatic; spurs in neural foramina can cause radiculopathy and simulate a herniated nucleus pulposus	Desiccation of disk with aging; bulging of annulus fibrosis with periosteal elevation; new bone formed
Cervical: if cervical spondylosis with myelopathy, progressive spastic paraparesis; quadriparesis	Above pathology combined with congenitally small AP diameter of spinal canal
Lumbar: spinal stenosis; possible "intermittent claudication of cauda equina"	
Neck pain and back pain, usually without definite neurologic localizing signs; cervical often also causes intrascapular pain	Incomplete tears of the annulus fibrosis; bulging of annulus without actual herniation of nucleus pulposus
Posterolateral herniation compresses nerve root and produces radicular pain and findings outlined in Table 149–1.	Herniation of all or part of nucleus pulposus through tear in annulus fibrosis with nerve root compression
Rarer, direct posterior (central) herniation compresses cervical spinal cord resulting in quadriparesis or paraparesis; in lumbar region, cauda equina can be involved with flaccid partial paraparesis	

tebral muscle spasm. Narrowing of a disk space, particularly if associated with early osteoarthritic changes, is of some value, particularly in the younger patient with only one level involved, but most people over 50 years of age show some spinal osteoarthritic changes, and it is very difficult to separate the symptomatic from the asymptomatic patients on the basis of x-ray findings alone. Oblique views, particularly in the cervical area, may show osteophytes projecting into the neural foramina. Only the later generations of computed tomography (CT) scanners have sufficient resolution to be helpful in the diagnosis of disk lesions, so spinal CT is in its infancy, at least as far as its use without associated myelography is concerned. Because it is much less affected by bone than CT, nuclear magnetic resonance (NMR) scanning holds even more promise for noninvasive imaging of the intervertebral disk and the spinal epidural space.

The electromyogram (EMG), particularly in combination with determination of nerve conduction velocities and other electrodiagnostic studies, is of great value in determining denervation in the muscles supplied by a given nerve root, as well as in excuding other conditions such as entrapment neuropathies or generalized peripheral neuropathies (see Chap 129, Neuromuscular Disorders). An EMG can correctly localize the involved root with 90% accuracy in most studies.

Except for actual surgical exploration, myelography traditionally has been regarded as the most accurate way to make the diagnosis of a herniated nucleus pulposus. This procedure, which requires hospitalization, consists of performing a lumbar or cisternal puncture and injecting a radiopaque contrast material into the spinal subarachnoid space. Formerly, iodized compounds in a heavy oil base were used, with the material being heavier than the spinal fluid and gravitating to the desired level as the patient is maneuvered under fluoroscopy on the radiographic table in order to visualize the suspected area. Now, metrizamide and other water-soluble agents are used, often in conjunction with the CT scan. Normally, the subarachnoid space extends for several millimeters down the nerve root sleeve along with the nerve root; failure of the nerve root to fill with contrast material usually indicates compression of the nerve root by a herniated nucleus

TABLE 149–3.
Differential Diagnosis of Intervertebral Disk Disease

ALL SPINAL AREAS
Osteoarthritis
Ankylosing spondylitis
Fibrositis syndrome
Postural pain
Disk space infection
Neoplasms
Metastatic to bone
Benign spinal cord or bone tumors
Primary malignant (rare)
Referred pain from disease of thoracic or abdominal viscera (e.g., aneurysm)

CERVICAL AREA
Brachial plexitis
Pulmonary apex malignancy (Pancoast's tumor)
Thoracic outlet syndromes
Adhesive capsulitis, acromial or biceps bursitis, and rotator cuff tears
Shoulder-hand syndrome
Ulnar compression neuropathy*
Carpal tunnel syndrome*

LUMBAR AREA
Chronic lumbosacral strain
Spondylolisthesis
Referred pain from hip disease
Lumbosacral plexus trauma*
Meralgia paresthetica*
(lateral femoral cutaneous nerve entrapment)
Sciatic nerve injury or common peroneal nerve compression palsy*

* These usually do not cause neck or back pain, but they mimic nerve root compression on the neurologic examination.

pulposus (Fig 149–1). Myelography is uncomfortable at best and has a very low but definite rate of complications, ranging from seizures of various types during the procedure itself to a delayed and devastating arachnoiditis producing paraplegia. It is not a procedure to be undertaken lightly, and usually is best reserved for precise localization of disk pathology in the patient who is going to require surgical therapy.

PRINCIPLES OF PREVENTION AND THERAPY

Proper lifting techniques can reduce the number of low-back injuries. Only time will tell if the legislatively mandated headrests for automobile seats will reduce the small number

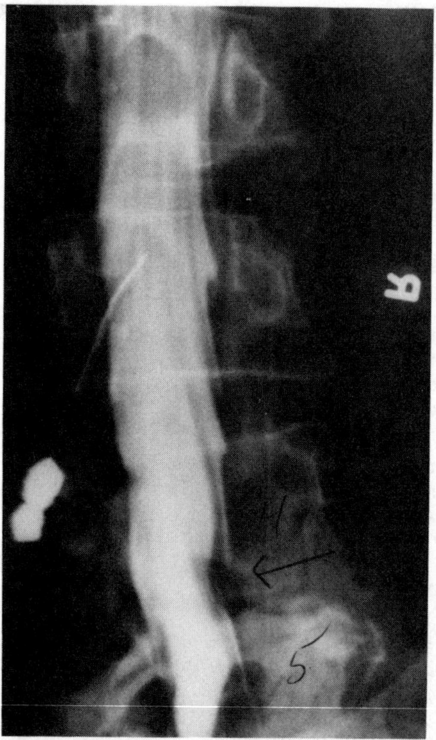

FIG 149–1.
Lumbar myelogram demonstrating protrusion of the L4–L5 intervertebral disk with compression of the fifth lumbar nerve root. The cerebrospinal fluid has been replaced by a radiopaque contrast medium, which outlines the inferior portion of the spinal subarachnoid space (white). The slight vertical filling defects are normal nerve roots. The arrow indicates the concave filling defect produced by the herniated nucleus pulposus. The nerve root sleeves fill on the left (white extensions downward at approximately a 45° angle), but the one in the area of the filling defect does not. (Courtesy Dr. Rich Carroll, Miami Valley Hospital Radiology Department.)

of cervical disk herniations produced by so-called whiplash injuries.

Rest is the mainstay of medical treatment of intervertebral disk lesions in the acute stage. In cases of lumbar lesions this is best accomplished by complete bedrest, usually with a bed board firming up the (usually) too soft mattress. Traction, either by a pelvic band attached to weights or Buck's extension with weights attached to the legs themselves is used by many in conjunction with bedrest; although critics point out that while the weights used usually don't open the disk space further, all agree that traction certainly enforces bedrest!

In cases of cervical disk lesions, the neck can be rested by using one of a variety of neck braces or soft cervical collars for several weeks. After the acute phase, cervical traction usually is helpful, particularly to those patients with radicular pain. Some advocate the use of neck bracing in the few patients who have cervical spondylosis with myelopathy.

Medication for pain usually is required; however, muscle relaxants have generally not been effective in the management of these acute cases of disk disease. In the case of low-back pain, after the acute symptoms have subsided, the use of exercises such as the Williams low-back exercises may be helpful. Transcutaneous electric nerve stimulation (TENS) units may be helpful in more chronic cases, as may be treatment regimens at "pain centers."

Significant focal muscle weakness from the onset, failure to improve or actual deterioration while undergoing medical treatment, and repeated episodes of discogenic pain and impairment are the three major indications for surgical treatment. Although myelography should be reserved for patients coming to surgical treatment, it is not necessary in all cases if there is firm clinical or electrodiagnostic evidence as to the specific nerve root involved. Chemonucleolysis, or lysis of the nucleus pulposus by the operative injection of chymopapain is a highly controversial treatment for lumbar disk disease, and the agent is not generally available for use in this country; many consider the risk of fatal anaphylactic shock associated with this agent to be unacceptable. Hemilaminectomy with surgical removal of all extruded disk material and as much of that remaining in the interspace as possible is the standard operative procedure. Proponents of techniques utilizing the operating microscope and of smaller incisions and lesser bone removal claim shorter postoperative morbidity. For cervical disk lesions some still favor the standard operation, and, in cases of cervical spondylosis with myelopathy, opening the dura mater and sectioning the dentate ligaments. More commonly, an anterior approach through the neck to the cervical spine is used, and fusion of one or more levels of the cervical spine after removing the offending disk ("anterior interbody fusion") is carried out, both in cases of typical "soft disks" and in patients with spondylosis and myelopathy.

Although all physicians and medical students encounter "the low-back loser," results of operative treatment of intervertebral disk disease are fairly good. Operative mortality is negligible, although in up to 4% of patients in some series, recovery is delayed by the occurrence of an inflammatory but apparently not infectious diskitis. Reports of long-term follow-up studies of patients give failure rates that range from a low of 2% to a high of 17%; the latter figure includes patients relieved of their radicular pain but with continuing back pain, as well as patients in whom disk disease occurs later at new levels. Many advocate spinal fusion in patients who are not relieved by the standard operation, but this approach is controversial. It is generally agreed that a point of diminishing returns soon comes into play in patients with repeated back operations. Complex issues of litigation and other compensation often become involved. Many studies point out the importance of depression and the premorbid personalities of many of these patients.

REFERENCES

Cailliet R: *Low Back Pain Syndrome*, ed 3. Philadelphia, FA Davis, 1981. *This short paperback by an experienced physiatrist contains a wealth of practical information on the diagnosis and medical management of all causes of low-back pain.*

Cailliet R: *Neck and Arm Pain*, ed 2. Philadelphia, FA Davis, 1981. *This companion volume to the one listed above presents a realistic and adequate discussion of the topic in the least space possible.*

Cyriax J: *Textbook of Orthopaedic Medicine, vol I, Diagnosis of Soft Tissue Lesions*, ed 8. London, Bailliere Tindall, 1982. *Never one to avoid controversy, this author incorporates the insights of osteopathy into his approach to low-back and neck pain.*

DePalma AF, Rothman RH: *The Intervertebral Disc.* Philadelphia, WB Saunders Co, 1970. *This book presents an in-depth view of disk disease from an American orthopedic standpoint.*

Hardy RW Jr (ed): *Lumbar Disc Disease.* New York, Raven Press, 1982 (editor of series, Seminars in Neurological Surgery). *This volume provides neurologic approach to this common problem that is much better than any other cited source in discussing problems such as myelopathy associated with disk disease.*

Hoppenfeld S: *Orthopaedic Neurology: A Diagnostic Guide to Neurologic Levels.* Philadelphia, JB Lippencott Co, 1977. *The essentials of localization of nerve root and spinal cord lesions are spelled out so that students, interns, residents, and even professors of medicine and neurology can understand them!*

Spurling RG: *Lesions of the Lumbar Intervertebral Disc.* Springfield, Ill, Charles C Thomas, 1953. *This book describes how lumbar intervertebral disk disease looked to an experienced neurosurgeon at a point in time halfway between its first description and the time of this writing. No description of the physical findings in patients with lumbar intervertebral disk disease has ever surpassed this one, not even those with CT scans or findings using other modern techniques.*

INDEX

Abdominal abscesses, 18
Abdominal carcinomatosis, 75
Abdominal distention, 70
Abdominal guarding, 78, 395
Abdominal perforation, 402
Abdominal trauma, 77–81
Abducens palsies, 682
Abortion
    diagnosis and differential
        diagnosis of, 628–629
    mid-trimester, 629
    pathophysiology of, 628
    signs and symptoms of, 628
    therapy for, 629
Abrasions, 101–102
Abruptio placentae, 630, 631
Acetaminophen, 268
Acetylcholine, 54, 295
Acetylcholine receptor, 760
Acetylcholinesterase, 762
Acetylcholinesterase
        antagonists, 762
Achilles peritendonitis, 871
Achilles tendonitis, 871
Acid-base balance, 529
Acid-base disorders, 8–10, 538,
        540
    therapy for, 14–15
    types of, 9t, 10–14
Acidemia, 8
Acid-fast bacilli, 334
Acidosis, 8, 532
Acoustic schwannomas, 729,
        731
Acquired immunodeficiency
        syndrome. See AIDS
Acral cyanosis, 285
Acromegaly, 732
ACTH. See
        Adrenocorticotrophic
        hormone
Actinomycetes infection, 279
Acute viral syndrome, 319
Acyclovir, 312
Addison's disease, 526
Adenocanthomas, 639
Adenocarcinomas
    colorecal, 411
    of prostate, 601
Adenoids, 658
Adenomas, colorectal, 412
Adenomyosis, 619
Adenosine arabinoside, 691

Adenosine deaminase
        deficiency, 322
ADH. See Antidiuretic hormone
Adrenal crisis, 505
    diagnosis and differential
        diagnosis of, 507–509
    pathophysiology of, 506–507
    prevention of and therapy for,
        509
    signs and symptoms of, 506
Adrenal insufficiency, 505, 506
Adrenocortical insufficiency,
        506, 507
    treatment of, 509
Adrenocorticosteroids, 244
Adrenocorticotrophic hormone,
        505–509
Adriamycin, 134
Adult diarrheal illness. See
        Diarrhea
Adult respiratory distress
        syndrome
    clinical–pathologic
        correlations of, 237
    diagnosis and differential
        diagnosis of, 237–239
    pathophysiology of, 236–237
    prevention of and therapy for,
        239–240
    sequential phases of, 235
    signs and symptoms of, 235
Aeroallergens, 231
Affective disorders, 774, 777.
        See also specific
        disorders
Agoraphobia, 771–772
AIDS, 20, 303
    asymptomatic infection with,
        319
    clinical–pathologic
        correlations of, 321
    dementia and, 56
    diagnosis and differential
        diagnosis of, 322
    epidemiology of, 317–318
    etiology of, 317
    high-risk groups for, 317
    pathophysiology of, 321
    prevention of and therapy for,
        322–323
    signs and symptoms of,
        318–321
AIDS-related complex, 319–320

AION. See Anterior idiopathic
        ischemic optic
        neuropathy
Air hunger, 231
Airflow obstruction, chronic
    diagnosis and differential
        diagnosis of, 202–203
    pathophysiology of, 200–202
    prevention of and therapy for,
        203
    signs and symptoms of,
        199–200
Airway obstruction, 97
Albumin levels, 369, 371
Alcohol
    gallbladder disease and, 377
    liver disease and, 369–370,
        434
    megaloblastic anemia and,
        440–444
Alcohol withdrawal, 786
Alcoholic cardiomyopathy, 134
Alcoholic cirrhosis, 493
    clinical–pathologic
        correlations of, 370
    differential diagnosis and
        diagnosis of, 370–371
    pathophysiology, 369–370
    signs and symptoms, 368–369
    treatment of, 371–372
Alcoholic neuropathies, 762
Alcoholism, 553, 758–787
Aldosterone, 31, 505–508, 572,
        578
Aldosteronism, 12, 34, 131
Alginic acid, 348
Alkalemia, 8–9
Alkalosis, 8, 532. See also
        Metabolic alkalosis;
        Respiratory alkalosis
Allergens, 229
Allergic conjunctivitis, 689
Allergic granulomatosis, 242,
        809
Allergic rhinitis, 268, 279
Allergy, to insect venom, 82–84
Allogeneic bone marrow
        transplantation, 455
Allopurinol, 566, 841
Alopecia, patchy, 313
Alpha-adrenergic blockers, 819
Alpha$_1$-antitrypsin, 200–201
    deficiency, 254

Alpha₁ globulin, 375
Alpha-fetoprotein, 375–376
ALS. *See* Amyotrophic lateral
    sclerosis
Aluminum hydroxide, 595
Aluminum levels in brain, 54
Alveolar collapse, 97
Alveolar edema, 237
Alveolar-arterial oxygen
    difference, 242
Alzheimer's disease, 50,
    51–52
  diagnosis of, 52
  etiology of, 54
  pathology of, 52–54
  treatment of, 54–55
Amantadine, 276, 748
Amaurosis fugax, 669, 695
Amblyopia, 679, 680
Amebiasis, 381, 383
Amebic liver abscesses, 383
Amenorrhea, 620
  compartment I disorders of,
      624
  compartment II disorders of,
      624–625
  compartment III disorders of,
      625–626
  compartment IV disorders of,
      626
  evaluation of, 621–624
  exercise and, 627
  hormone replacement therapy
      for, 627
American Rheumatism
    Association
  criteria, 796
Ametropia, 675–677
Amiloride, 591
Aminophylline, 234
Ammonium chloride, 15
Amphetamines, 788
Amphotericin, 737
Amphotericin B, 307, 341, 849,
    855
Ampicillin, 279, 294, 737
Ampulla of Vater, 70
Amputation, 186, 299
Amylase levels, 377, 379
Amyloid, 52
Amyloidosis, 474, 597, 794
Amyotrophic lateral sclerosis,
    758
Amyotrophies, 757
ANA test. *See* Antinuclear
    antibody test
Anaerobic bacteria, 224, 226,
    278–279
Anaerobic glycolysis, 111
Anaerobic necrotizing
    pneumonitis, 224
Anaerobic osteomyelitis,
    855
Anal canal, 406
Anal eroticism, 410

Anal hygiene, 407–408
Anal itch, 409–410
Anal lymphatic plexus, 406
Anal tumors, 410–411
Analgesic-sedative effects, 787
Anaphylactic reaction, 82
Anaplastic carcinomas, 464
Androgen-insensitivity
    syndrome, 624
Anemia, 450. *See also* Iron
    deficiency anemia
  clinical–pathologic
      correlations of, 437
  hemolytic, 803
    diagnosis and differential
        diagnosis of, 437–438
    pathophysiology, 434–437
    prevention of and therapy
        for, 438–439
    signs and symptoms of,
        433–434
  in inflammatory bowel
      disease, 389–390
  megaloblastic
    diagnosis and differential
        diagnosis of, 442–443
    pathophysiology of,
        441–442
    signs and symptoms of,
        440–441
  prevention of and therapy for,
      443–444
  with starvation, 88
Aneurysmal subarachnoid
    hemorrhage, 717
Aneurysms
  abdominal aortic, 181, 186
  aortic, 180
  false, 119
  intracranial, 41
  localization of, 812
  peripheral arteria, 181
  popliteal, 186
  poststenotic, 183
  ventricular, 134
Angel dust, 789
Angiitis, 242
Angina decubitus, 109
Angina pectoris, 117
  clinical–pathologic
      correlations of, 111–113
  diagnosis and differential
      diagnosis of, 113
  pathophysiology of, 111
  postinfarction, 119
  signs and symptoms of,
      109–111
  therapy for, 113–116
Angiodysplasia, 67, 404
Angiography, 184
Angiotensin-converting enzyme,
    249
  inhibitors, 36
Angiotrophic embolization, 69
Angor animi, 109

Anion gap, 10
Anisakis removal, 330
Ankle fracture-dislocations, 859
Ankle-systolic index, 183
Ankylosing spondylitis, 846,
    872
Ankylosis, 846
Anorectal abscess, 408–409
Anorectal examination, 407
Anorexia, 626
Anoscopy, 415
Anserine bursitis, 871
Antacids, 348
Anterior horn cell diseases, 760
Anterior idiopathic ischemic
    optic neuropathy, 670
Anthracycline derivative
    toxicity, 134
Antianxiety drugs, 774
Antibiotics
  for bacteremia, 288
  for bowel obstruction, 76
  for brain abscess, 743
  for burns, 100
  with catheterization, 589
  colitis and, 300
  for conjunctivitis, 672
  for corneal abrasion, 671
  for cystic fibrosis, 253
  for diarrhea, 387
  for endocarditis prevention,
      293
  for fever of unknown origin,
      20
  for gallbladder disease, 360
  immunocompromise from,
      305
  for immunocompromised
      host, 308
  for magnesium ammonium
      phosphate stones, 566
  for meningitis, 738–739
  for osteomyelitis, 856–857
  for otitis media, 660
  for progressive system
      sclerosis, 823
  for pseudomembranous
      colitis, 301
  for syphilis, 314
  for urinary tract infections,
      283
Anticholinergic drugs, 748
Anticholinesterase drugs, 750,
    752
Anticoagulants, 194
Anticoagulation, 194
Anticonvulsant therapy, 722,
    744
Antidepressants, 773–774, 776,
    778
  tricyclic, 777, 778
Antidiarrheal agents, 387
Antidiuresis mechanism, 525
Antidiuretic hormone, 481, 483,
    578

for diabetes insipidus, 486
nullification of, 528
syndrome of inappropriate,
    525, 527, 528t
Antiepileptic drugs, 722
Antifungal therapy, 307
Anti-glomerular basement
    membrane nephritis, 567,
    569, 574, 576
Antihistamines
    for allergy, 84, 689
    for otitis media, 660
    in sinus infections, 279
Antihypertensive drugs, 35
    with pregnancy-induced
        hypertension, 633
Anti-inflammatory drugs,
        nonsteroidal
    for fever of unknown origin,
        22
    for gout, 841
    for osteoarthritis, 836
    for rheumatoid arthritis, 798
    with systemic lupus
        erythematosus, 806
Antimalarial drugs, 245, 806
Antimicrobial therapy for brain
        abscess, 743
Antinuclear antibodies, 822
    in systemic lupus
        erythematosus, 799,
        801–803
Antinuclear antibody test, 3,
        797, 804, 812, 822, 826
Antinuclear double-stranded
        DNA test, 4
Anti-parietal cell antibodies,
        442
Antiplatelet antibodies, 803
Antipsychotic drugs, 783, 784
Antithrombin III, 194
Antithrombolytic agents, 717
Antithyroglobulin antibodies,
        501
Antitoxin, 297, 750
Antituberculous drugs, 855
Antivenom IgE antibodies, 82
Anxiety disorders, 771–774
Aortic coarctations, 289
Aortic regurgitation
    clinical–pathologic
        correlations of, 171
    diagnosis and differential
        diagnosis of, 171–174
    pathophysiology of, 171
    signs and symptoms of,
        170–171
    treatment of, 174
Aortic stenosis, 109
    aortic regurgitation and, 174
    clinical–pathologic
        correlations of, 168–169
    diagnosis and differential
        diagnosis of, 169–170
    pathophysiology of, 166–167

signs and symptoms of,
    165–166
    therapy for, 170
Aortic valve calcification, 169
Aortic valve disease, 165–174
Aortography, 813
Aortoiliac insufficiency, 181
Aortoiliac occlusive disease,
    181
Aphakia, 676
Apnea, 58
Appendectomy, 399
Appendiceal abscess, 396
Appendicitis, 74, 391
    acute
        diagnosis of, 397–399
        differential diagnosis of,
            396
        signs and symptoms of,
            394–396
        therapy for, 399
    retrocecal, 395
Appendicolith, 394
ARC. See AIDS-related complex
ARDS. See Adult respiratory
        distress syndrome
Argon-laser trabeculoplasty, 685
Arrhythmias, 118. See also
        specific types of
    cardiomyopathy and, 134
Arterial insufficiency, 180
Arteriovenous malformations,
        67
Arthritis. See also Rheumatoid
        arthritis
    gout and, 838
    septic, 844–849
Asbestos exposure, 208
Ascites, 371, 373
Ascorbic acid. See Vitamin C
Aseptic meningitis, 733, 736
Asherman's syndrome, 624
Aspartate transcarbamyolase, 5
Aspergillus fumigatus infection,
        251, 252
Aspergillus infection, 243, 279,
        306
Aspiration
    as main route to lung, 224
    risk of, 223, 226
Aspiration lung abscess, 225,
        226
Aspiration pneumonia, 217, 224
Aspirin, 618
    for common cold, 268
    for deep vein thrombosis, 194
    sensitivity to, 231
Asplenia and infections, 303
AST. See Asparate
        transcarbamyolase
Asthma, 199, 203
    assessing severity of, 228t,
        229
    clinical–pathologic
        correlations of, 230

diagnosis/differential
        diagnosis of, 230–231
    diurnal cycle of, 231
    pathophysiology of, 229
    prevention of and therapy for,
        231–234
    severity scale of, 227
    signs and symptoms of,
        227–229
    untreated, 229
Astigmatism, 42, 67
Astrocytoma, 730, 732
Astrocytosis, reactive, 754
Asymmetric septal hypertrophy,
        134
Atheromas, 182
Atherosclerosis, 182
Atherosclerotic plaques, 113,
        119
Athetosis, 764
Atonic seizures, 721
ATP deficiency, 554–555
Atrial arrhythmias, 152–158
Atrial dilation, acute, 117
Atrial fibrillation, 125, 157–158,
        162
    in mitral valve disease, 163
Atrial flutter, 157
Atrial infarction, 117
"Atrial" natriuretic peptide, 33
Atrial premature contractions,
        153–154
Atrial septal defect, 163
Atrial tachycardia, 154–155
Atrial thrombi, 160
Atrioventricular block, 118, 157
Atrophic vaginitis, 634
Atropine, 298
Atypical angina pectoris, 109
Atypical pneumonia
    diagnosis of, 221–222
    differential diagnosis of, 221
    prevention of and therapy for,
        222
    signs and symptoms of,
        218–220
Audiologic evaluation, 660, 661
Audiometry, 654
Austin Flint murmur, 171
Autoantibodies, 456, 801, 803
Autodigestion, 378
Autoimmune cytopenias, 460
Autoimmune disease, 762
Autoimmune inner ear disease,
        656
Autoimmune process, 749
Autoimmune thyroiditis, 501
Automaticity, 152
AV block. See Atrioventricular
        block
Axillary metastases, 612
Azidothymidine, 323
Azotemia, 495, 590
    prerenal, 583, 584
Azothioprine, 245, 752, 798, 806

Back bracing, for scoliosis,
862–863
Back injuries, 877–878
Back pain
in children, 866
psychologic factors in,
878–879
scoliosis and, 861–862
Bacteremia
with catheterization, 305
clinical–pathologic
correlations of, 286–287
diagnosis/differential
diagnosis of, 287–288
with mitral valve disease, 161
pathophysiology of, 285–286
prevention of and therapy for,
288
with pseudomembranous
colitis, 301
signs and symptoms of,
284–285
surgical procedures associated
with, 293
Bacteria opsonization, 303
Bacterial endocarditis. See
Endocarditis, infective
Bacterial infections, 251
Bacterial pneumonias, 217
Bacteroides species, 226
Baker's cysts, 183, 192, 871
Balloon angioplasty, 184
Balloon counterpulsation,
intra-aortic, 123
Balloon tamponade, 69
Barbiturates
with pregnancy-induced
hypertension, 633
for tetanus, 297
Barium enema, 392
for colorectal carcinoma, 415
for peptic ulcers, 352
in unprepared colon, 398
Barkan's membrane, 686
Baroreceptor activation, 578
Barrett's esophagus, 345, 346
Bartter's syndrome, 533
Basic energy expenditure, 97
Basophilia, 447
Bayes' theorem, 4
Belladonna, 298
Bell's palsy, 656
Bence Jones proteinuria, 474,
597
Benzodiazepine abuse, 787
Berger's disease, 567, 569,
574–575, 576
Beta-adrenergic agonists, 234
Beta-adrenergic blockers
for cardiomyopathy, 143
for glaucoma, 684
for hyperthyroidism, 494
for myocardial infarction, 125
for tachyarrhythmias, 497
Beta-blockers, 116, 163

Beta-human chorionic
gonadotropin test,
628–629
Beta-lactam antibiotics, 660
Bicarbonate, 8, 10, 13–15
Bicarbonaturia, 547
Bicuspid aortic valves,
calcification of, 165
Bifocals, 680
Bigeminy, 144
Bile duct injuries, 77
Biliary colic, 358
Biliary imaging techniques, 359
Biliary obstruction, 24
Bilirubin, 23, 369
glucuronidation of, 24
neurotoxicity of, 768
Biofeedback techniques
with dyspnea, 60
for tinnitus, 656
Birth control pills
breast cancer and, 610
with dysmenorrhea, 619
migraine and, 38
with systemic lupus
erythematosus, 805
Bladder, neurogenic, 282
Bladder diverticulae, 282
Bladder infection, 280
Blaisdell ligation treatment, 407
Bland diet, 353
Bleeding. See also Hemorrhage
normal, 423
into respiratory tract, 62
Blepharitis, marginal, 688
Blindness, 672
Blisters (burns), 96
Blood clotting, 423
Blood factor replacement, 428
Blood flow studies, 819
Blood glucose level, 34, 515
Blood pressure, 28. See also
Hypertension
determination of, 31
Blood transfusions, 69, 428, 476
Blood viscosity studies, 817
Blood-brain barrier breakdown,
708
Blunt trauma to abdomen,
77–78
Bohr effect, 10
Bone deformities, 438
Bone healing, 858
Bone loss, 832
Bone marrow
aspiration, 474
infiltration of with plasma
cells, 473
plasmacytosis, 473
transplantation, 455, 460
Bone necrosis, 853
Bone redistribution, 593
Bony spurs, 872, 874
Botulism, 297–299, 750
Bouchard's nodes, 834

Boutonniere deformities, 793
Bowel carcinoma, 403
Bowel fistula formation,
402–404
Bowel obstruction
clinical–pathologic
correlations of, 71t
diagnosis of, 74–75
differential diagnosis of,
73–74
mechanical causes of, 73
mortality rate of, 76
pathophysiology of, 72–73
signs and symptoms of, 70–72
therapy of, 75–76
Bowel perforations, 381
Bowel strangulation, 71, 73, 76
Bradycardia, 120
Bradykinesia, 745, 747
Bradykinin, 111, 378
Brain abscess, 278
diagnosis and differential
diagnosis of, 742–743
metastatic, 742
pathophysiology of, 741–742
prevention of and therapy for,
743–744
ruptured, 744
signs and symptoms of,
740–741
Brain death, 48–49
Brain injury, 766
Brain stem auditory evoked
potentials, 769
Brain tissue herniation, 727
Brain tumor, 729–732, 742
headache and, 42
metastatic, 725
primary, 725
Brainstem lesions, 44–45, 47
Branch retinal artery occlusion,
694–695
Branch retinal vein occlusion,
693–694
Breast abscess drainage, 609
Breast biopsy, 607, 609
Breast cancer
clinical–pathologic
correlations, 613
diagnosis and differential
diagnosis of, 613–615
inflammatory, 611, 615
pathophysiology of, 611–612
prevention of and therapy for,
615–616
signs and symptoms of,
610–611
Breast disease, benign
diagnosis and differential
diagnosis of, 607–608
pathophysiology of, 606–607
signs and symptoms of, 606
treatment of, 609
Breast needle aspiration, 614
Breast self-examination, 614

Brodie's abscess, 852
Bromocriptine, 748
Bronchial adenoma, 63
Bronchial breath sounds, 258
Bronchial tree obstruction, 215
Bronchiectasis, 62, 250, 251, 666
Bronchiolitis, 242
Bronchitis, 199
    as cause of hemoptysis, 63
    chronic, 202, 203, 250, 666
Bronchoalveolar lavage, 244, 248
Bronchodilator, 203, 242
    for cystic fibrosis, 253
Bronchogenic carcinoma, 63, 204
Bronchopneumonia, 210
Bronchoscopy, 226, 306
Bronchospasm, 201, 230
    reversal of, 229, 234
Brucellosis, 16–18
Brudzinski's maneuver, 733
Bruits, carotid, 708
Buck's extension, 878
Buffers, 8, 15
Bullous emphysema, 254
Bundle branch block, complete
    left, 121
Burkitt's lymphoma, 270, 462
Burn injuries
    associated injuries of, 97
    classification of, 95, 99, 101–102
    clinical–pathologic
        correlations of, 97–99
    healing of, 102
    psychosocial effects of, 99
    severity of, 96
    signs and symptoms of, 95–96
    stress-related changes with, 99
    therapy for, 99–100
Bursitis
    pathophysiology and
        diagnosis of, 867–872
    of shoulder, 868–870
    therapy for, 872
Butterfly rash, 799

Cachexia, 412
Cadmium exposure, 596
Calcaneal bursitis, 871
Calcaneal spur, 872
Calcific drusen, 696
Calcific periarthritis, 594
Calcific tendonitis, 869
Calcification, 546, 594
Calcitonin
    in calcium level control, 546, 547
    osteoporosis and, 830, 832
    production of, 637

Calcium
    concentrations of, 546. See
        also Hypercalcemia;
        Hypocalcemia
    deficiency of in menopause, 638
    hypertension and, 33
    negative balance of, 637
    osteoporosis and, 830, 832
    supplements, 550
Calcium alginate swabs, 314
Calcium carbonate, 595
Calcium channel-blocking
    agents, 36
Calcium gluconate, 551
Calcium lactate, 566
Calcium oxalate stones, 839
Calcium pyrophosphate
    deposition disease
    (CPDD). See Pseudogout
Calcium stones, 562, 566
Calcium-channel blockers
    for angina pectoris, 116
    for cardiomyopathy, 143
Calculi, 282
Campyobacter infection, 381–382
Candida albicans, 311
Candida endophthalmitis, 302, 307
Candida infections, 291, 311
    meningitis, 737
Candidiasis, 311
Cannabinoids, 788–789
Capillaries, leaky, 237
Captopril, 143, 823
Carbidopa, 748
Carbon dioxide retention, 15
Carbonic acid/bicarbonate, 8
Carbonic anhydrase inhibitors, 685
Carcino embryonic antigen, 414
Carcinoma. See also specific
        sites of
    lobular, 612
    of stomach, 354–357
Carcinomatous meningitis, 735
Cardiac arrest, 529, 546
Cardiac arrhythmias
    in magnesium deficiency, 541
    mechanisms of, 152–153
    treatment of, 122
Cardiac catheterization, 125, 132
Cardiac dysrhythmias, 181–182
Cardiac massage, external, 118
Cardiac output, 31, 128
Cardiac tamponade, 176, 179
Cardiac transplantation, 143
Cardiac trauma
    mortality from, 175
    penetrating, 176
        diagnosis of, 177–179
Cardiogenic shock, 118, 125
Cardiomegaly, 128

Cardiomyopathy
    clinical–pathologic
        correlations of, 138–140
    diagnosis of, 141, 163
    differential diagnosis of, 140–141
    pathophysiology of, 138
    prevention of and therapy for, 141–143
    signs and symptoms of, 134–138
Cardiopulmonary disease, 273
Cardiopulmonary resuscitation, 151
Cardioversion, 122, 150
    for atrial fibrillation, 158
    for atrial flutter, 157
Carmustine, 476
Carotid artery circulation, 707
Caseous necrosis, 332
Cataracts, 685, 699
Catecholamine depletors, 819
Catecholamines
    cellular effects of, 491
    increased, 554
    potassium levels and, 532
    release of, 119, 517
    supersensitivity to, 138
Catheterization
    infection associated with, 303, 305
    osteomyelitis and, 850, 854
    risks of, 288
Cat-scratch disease, 17
Cavalryman's disease, 871
Cavernous sinus thrombus, 278
Cecal wall perforation, 71
Cecum, dilation of, 71
Cefaclor, 279
Cefoperazone, 738
Cefotaxime, 738
Ceftazidime, 738
Ceftriaxone, 738
Cefuroxime, 738
Celiac sprue, 383
Cellular casts, 585
Cellular damage
    from burn, 96
    from noxious gas, 97
Cellulitis
    with deep vein thrombosis, 192
    with sinusitis, 278
    with venous insufficiency, 187, 189
Central nervous system. See
        also specific diseases of
    chronic infections of, 56
    progressive disorders of, 768
    tumors of, 732. See also
        Intracranial tumors
Central retinal artery occlusion, 695
Central retinal vein occlusion, 694

Cephalic tetanus, 295
Cephalosporin
    for lung abscess, 226
    for septic arthritis, 849
    for urinary tract infections,
        283
Cerebellar astrocytomas, 729
Cerebellar hemorrhage, 714
Cerebellopontine angle tumor,
    652
Cerebral angiography, 711
Cerebral blood flow, 707
Cerebral edema, 727
Cerebral embolism, 712
Cerebral gangliosides, 297
Cerebral hemorrhage, 714, 715
Cerebral infarction, 711
Cerebral ischemia, 707
Cerebral palsy, 764
    clinical–pathologic
        correlations of, 766–768
    diagnosis and differential
        diagnosis of, 768–769
    estropia with, 679
    signs and symptoms of,
        765–766
    therapy for, 769–770
Cerebral stroke, 669
Cerebral vascular accidents, 31
Cerebral vascular disease,
        707–713
Cerebritis, 741
Cerebrospinal fluid
        examination, 737, 738
Cerebrovasospasm, 788
Cervical cancer, 641–643
Cervical disk herniations, 878
Cervical dysplasia, 643
Cervical spondylosis, 876
Cervical sympathectomy, 819
Cervicovaginal cytologic smears,
    646
Cesarean delivery, 631
    with pregnancy-induced
        hypertension, 633
Chagas' disease, 325
Chalazion, 689
Chancres, 313
Chemical meningitis, 735
Chemonucleolysis, 878
Chemotherapeutic agents, 207
    immunocompromise from,
        304–305
Chemotherapy
    for acute nonlymphocytic
        leukemia, 454
    for breast cancer, 616
    for chronic lymphocytic
        leukemia, 460
    for gastric carcinoma, 357
    for hepatocellular carcinoma,
        376
    for Hodgkin's disease,
        470–471
    for hypernephroma, 599
    for lung cancer, 208, 209

    with multiple myeloma, 476
    for non-Hodgkin's lymphoma,
        465
    for osteomyelitis, 855
    for ovarian carcinoma,
        646–647
    for prostate cancer, 605
    for retinoblastomas, 699
    for tuberculosis, 336
Chest pain
    episodic, 113, 114–115t
    with mitral valve prolapse,
        162
Chest pain syndrome, 109. See
        also Angina pectoris
Chest trauma, 64
Cheyne-Stokes respiration
    with coma, 45
    with congestive heart failure,
        126
    in dyspnea, 58
CHF. See Congestive heart
        failure
Chlamydia psittaci, 218, 222
Chlamydia trachomatis, 309,
        314–315
    blindness due to, 672
Chlorambucil, 245, 460
Chloramphenicol
    for abortion treatment, 629
    in atypical pneumonia
        treatment, 222
    for brain abscess, 743
Chloride ion loss, 12
Chlorine gas exposure, 244
Chloroquine, 806
Cholangitis, 378
Cholecalciferol-binding
        globulin, 579
Cholecystectomy, 360
Cholecystitis, 359–360
Cholecystography, oral, 359
Cholecystokinin, 359–360
Cholelithiasis, 378
Cholestasis, 27
Cholesteatoma, 651, 656, 657
Cholesterol levels, 34, 360
Cholestyramine, 387
Choline, 54
Choline esterase inhibitors, 54
Cholinergic crisis, 762
Cholinergic drugs, 749
Cholinergic neuronal system
        damage, 54
Cholinesterase inhibitors, 749
Chorea, 51, 55
Choreoathetoid movements, 748
Chorioretinitis, 246, 339
Choroid, melanoma of, 701–702
Choroid tubercles, 302
Chronic airflow obstruction. See
        Airflow obstruction,
        chronic
Chronic renal failure, 31
Churg-Strauss syndrome, 242,
        809

Chymopapain, 878
Cigarette smoking
    atherosclerosis and, 182
    cessation of, 116, 203
    changes in lung with, 201
    chronic airflow obstruction
        with, 199
    inflammatory reaction to,
        200
    laryngeal infections and, 663
    lung cancer and, 204, 208
Cilial dysfunction, 278
Ciliary body, melanoma of, 701
Ciliary clearance, 213
Ciliary spasm, 684
Cimetidine, 69, 253, 380, 823
Circle of Willis, 710
Cirrhosis, 24
    alcoholic. See Alcoholic
        cirrhosis
    biliary, 493
    clinical–pathologic
        correlations of, 370
    diagnosis and differential
        diagnosis of, 370–371
    liver transplantation for, 28
    macronodular, 370
    micronodular, 27, 369
    pathophysiology of, 369–370
    signs and symptoms of,
        368–369
    treatment of, 370–371
Cisplatin, 552
Classic migraine, 38
Claudication, 181
Clavicle fractures, 859
Cleft palate, 657
Clergyman's knee, 871
Climacteric, 633
    clinical–pathologic
        correlations of, 635
    diagnosis of, 635–637
    pathophysiology of, 637
    signs and symptoms of,
        634–635
    therapy for, 638
Clindamycin, 226
Cloacogenic carcinoma, 411
Clonidine, 387
Clortrimazole, 311
Closed loop bowel obstruction,
        73
Clostridial infections, 295–301
Clostridium botulinum, 297,
        750
Clostridium difficile, 300–301
Clostridium perfringens, 299,
        383
Clostridium tetani infection,
        295
Clotting factor activation, 427
Cluster headache, 38
CMV. See Cytomegalovirus
Coagulation, 454
Coagulation cascade, 286
Coagulation disorders

pathophysiology of, 425–426
signs and symptoms of,
    423–424
therapy for, 426–428
Coagulation factors, 286
    defects of, 425
Coagulopathies, 585
    in abruptio placentae, 631
    bacteremia and, 287
    therapy for, 367
Coarse granular casts, 585
Cobb measurement method,
    861
Codeine, 393
Cognitive dysfunction, 50. See
    also Dementia
Cognitive therapy, 780
Cogwheel rigidity, 745–746
Cold agglutinins, 221
Cold challenge, 819
Colectomy, 404, 415
Colitis, 382
    acute, 300
    ischemic, 392
    radiation-induced, 306, 392
    ulcerative, 387, 389
        treatment of, 393
Collagen synthesis, 369–370
Collagen vascular disease, 826
Collagenases, 795
Colles' fracture, 634, 859
Colocutaneous fistula, 404
Colon
    cancer, 396
    hemorrhage of, 66, 404–405
    obstruction of, 71, 396
    perforation of, 78
    polyps, 412
    trauma to, 78
Colon-cutoff sign, 380
Colorectal carcinoma
    clinical–pathologic
        correlations of, 412
    diagnosis for, 414–415
    differential diagnosis for,
        413–414
    signs and symptoms of,
        411–412
    therapy for, 415
Colostomy, 405
Colposcopy, 642
Coma
    brain death and, 48–49
    with calcium level
        disturbances, 546
    course and prognosis of, 48
    differential diagnosis of, 48
    with hypernatremia, 522
    pathophysiology and
        classification of, 45–47
    pupillary responses in, 45
    respiratory patterns in, 45
    signs and symptoms of, 44–45
Comedo carcinomas, 615
Commissurotomy, 170
Common cold

diagnosis and differential
    diagnosis of, 268
pathophysiology of, 267
signs and symptoms of,
    266–267
treatment of, 268
Complement-fixing antibodies,
    221
Compound wounds
    healing stages of, 102–104
    treatment of, 104–105
Computed tomography, 722,
    741–742, 744
Condolomata, 642
Condyloma acuminatum, 309
Condyloma lata, 313
Congenital heart disease, 141
Congestive heart failure, 259
    with atrial fibrillation, 158
    cardiomyopathy and, 134
    clinical–pathologic
        correlations of, 129
    control of, 174
    diagnosis of, 131–132
    differential diagnosis of,
        129–131
    in glomerulonephritis, 572
    pathophysiology of, 128–129
    prevention of and therapy for,
        132–133
    signs and symptoms of,
        126–128
Conjunctiva, 689–691
    disease of, 688–691
    melanoma of, 700
    papillary hypertrophy of, 689
Conjunctivitis, 670, 672, 689
    allergic, 689
Connective tissue disease, 817
Consciousness, diminished,
    44–45. See also Coma
Constrictive pericarditis, 141
Contraception
    with cystic fibrosis, 253
    oral. See Birth control pills
Conversion aphonia, 666
Convulsions, 546. See also
    Seizures
Coombs' test, 221, 800, 803
Cor pulmonale, 243, 247
Corneal abrasion, 671
Corneal irregularity, 677
Corneal opacity, 679
Corneal surface disease,
    671–672
Corneal ulcer, 671–672, 690
Coronary angiography, 119
Coronary arteritis, 119
Coronary artery disease, 140
    atrial tachycardia and, 155
    with untreated hypertension,
        31
Coronary atherosclerosis, 125
Coronary bypass surgery, 116,
    497
Coronary spasm, 111, 113

Coronary vasodilation, 116
Coronary vasospasm, 119
Corticosteroids
    adrenal, 505
    in ARDS, 240
    for autoimmune cytopenias,
        460
    for cardiomyopathy, 143
    concentration of, 508
    with cranial inflammation, 42
    for fever of unknown origin,
        20
    for giant cell arteritis, 827
    for herpes simplex keratitis,
        691
    for immune hemolysis, 439
    for inflammatory bowel
        disease, 393
    for insect venom allergy, 84
    with multiple myeloma, 476
    for myasthenia gravis, 750, 752
    for myocardial infarction, 123
    in nephrotic syndrome, 582
    in neuromuscular disorders,
        762
    for polymyalgia rheumatica,
        827
    for progressive system
        sclerosis, 823
    for rheumatoid arthritis, 798
    for systemic vasculitis, 815
    for ulcerative colitis, 389
    for uveitis, 673
Cortisol, 31, 505–507
Corynebacterium infections, 303
Counterimmunoelectrophoresis,
    848
Cranial inflammation, 42
Creatine phosphokinase levels,
    762
Crescendo angina, 109
CREST syndrome, 819, 821
Creutzfeldt-Jakob disease, 54, 56
Crigler-Najjar Type II syndrome,
    28
Crohn's disease, 18, 387,
    389–390, 413
    treatment of, 393
Crohn's Disease Activity Index,
    389
Crohn's granulomatous colitis,
    403
Crohn's proctitis, 410
Crush fractures, 859
Cryoglobulinemia syndrome,
    809
Cryoglobulins, 575, 797
Cryopexy, 697
Cryotherapy, 410
Cryptococcus neoformans
    infection, 305, 737
Cryptosporidium, 320
Cullen's sign, 77, 377
Curare-like drugs, 297
Curling's ulcers, 99
Cushing's syndrome, 12, 732

Cyclic adenosine
monophosphate, 542, 547
Cyclooxygenase blockers, 240
Cyclophosphamide
for chronic lymphocytic
leukemia, 460
for interstitial lung disease,
245
with multiple myeloma, 476
with systemic lupus
erythematosus, 806
for systemic vasculitis, 815
Cysosarcoma phylloides, 615
Cystic fibrosis, 254
clinical–pathologic
correlations of, 252
complications of, 251
diagnosis/differential
diagnosis of, 252–253
pathophysiology of, 251–252
prevention of and therapy for,
253
signs and symptoms of,
250–251
Cystine stones, 563, 566
Cystinuria, 563
Cystitis, 280
Cystosarcoma phylloides, 606,
607, 609
Cytomegalovirus, 18, 269, 272
in AIDS, 320
Cytotoxic drugs, 798
Cytotoxic edema, 727
Cytoxan, 699

DC countershock, 151
Debridement, 102, 299
Decompressive laminectomy,
732
Decongestants, 268
for otitis media, 660
in sinus infections, 279
Decubitus ulcers, 754
Defibrillation, 118, 151
Dehydration, 70, 521
testing, 483
Delirium, 51
Delirium tremens, 787
Delta virus, 362
Demence precoce, 781
Dementia. See also Alzheimer's
disease; Huntington's
disease; Parkinsonism;
Wilson's disease
clinical–pathologic
correlations of, 51–56
diagnosis of, 51
signs and symptoms of, 50–51
Dementia praecox. See
Schizophrenia
Demyelination, 668, 754, 755
Dental abscess, 279
Dental infections, 660
Depressant abuse, 786–787
Depression, 774–775

back pain and, 879
and dementia, 51
diagnosis of, 777–778
pathophysiology of, 776–777
signs and symptoms of, 776
therapy for, 778–780
Deprivation amblyopia, 679
deQuervain's disease, 870. See
also Thyroiditis, subacute
Dermatomyositis, 762
Desensitization therapy, 773
Desipramine, 777
Dexamethasone, 509
Dexamethasone-suppression
test, 777
Dextran, 194
Diabetes
with hypertension, 29
osteomyelitis and, 850, 853
Diabetes insipidus
central, 483–486
differential diagnosis of, 483
with hypernatremia, 523
hypernatremia with, 521–522
nephrogenic, 486
pathophysiology of, 482–483
signs and symptoms of,
481–482
therapy for, 483–486
Diabetes mellitus, 510
blood glucose testing for, 34
with cardiomyopathy, 134
clinical–pathologic
correlations of, 512–513
differential diagnosis of,
513–514
gestational, 511
natural history of, 511–512
pathophysiology of, 512
prevention of and therapy for,
514–515
signs and symptoms of, 511
types I and II, 510
urinary tract infection and,
282
Diabetic ketoacidosis, 15, 511
Diabetic retinopathy, 512,
691–692
Diagnosis, 3–4
Diagnostic tests, 3–5
false-positive results, 5, 6
invasive vs. noninvasive, 6–7
Dialysis, 538, 545
peritoneal, 589
Diaphragmatic irritation, 77
Diarrhea
clinical–pathologic
correlations for, 385
diagnosis and differential
diagnosis of, 385
due to infective causes, 390
with inflammatory bowel
disease, 387
nocturnal, 381
pathophysiology of, 383–385

secretory, 384
signs and symptoms of,
381–383
small-volume, 381
therapy for, 386–387
Diastolic dysfunction, 138
Diastolic murmur, 160
Diastolic rumble, 161, 171
Diazepam, 60, 297, 633
Digitalis, 143
Digitalis intoxication, 155
Digoxin, 316
Dilatation and curettage, 619,
641
Dilated cardiomyopathy, 134,
136, 138
Diphenoxylate, 393
Diphosphonates, 552
Diphtheria, 266
Diphtheroids, 291
Diplopia, 679, 681
Disciform degeneration, 696
Discoid lupus erythematosus,
799
Disease, probability of, 4–5
Diuresis, 483
Diuretics
for congestive heart failure,
132
in fibrocystic disease, 609
for hypercalciuria, 566
hyponatremia and, 526
with mitral valve stenosis,
163
non–potassium-sparing, 12
osmoic, 712
potassium-sparing, 538
with pregnancy-induced
hypertension, 633
for vertigo, 656
Diverticular bleeding, 66
Diverticulitis, 74, 392, 413
Diverticulosis coli, 400–401
complications of, 402–405
signs and symptoms of,
401–402
therapy for, 405
Dizziness. See Vertigo
DNA strands, 362
DNA synthesis, impaired, 442
DNA test, antinuclear double-
stranded, 4
DNAases, 266
Dobutamine, 123, 143
Dohle's inclusion bodies, 316
Dopamine, 123
imbalance of, 746–748
Dopamine hydrochloride, 316
Dopamine-acetyl-choline
balance, 746
Dopaminergic agonists, 748
Dowager's hump, 634
Down's syndrome, 54, 451, 657
Doxorubicin, 357
Doxycycline, 325

Dressler's syndrome, 176
Drug abuse, 785–790, 850
  screening for, 790
Drug fever, 16
Drug flashbacks, 789
Drug tolerance, 785
Drusen, 696
Dsypareunia, 634
Duodenal ulcers, 349–351, 353
Duodenum, 70
Dysesthesia, 758
Dyskinesis, 748
Dysmenorrhea
  differential diagnosis of,
    618–619
  pathophysiology of, 617–618
  signs and symptoms, 617
  therapy of, 619
Dysphagia, 302, 356, 821
Dysphonia, 666
Dyspnea
  with chronic airflow
    obstruction, 199
  with congestive heart failure,
    126
  as indicator of heart disease, 4
  nonpulmonary conditions
    and, 59
  pathophysiology of, 58–60
  with pneumothorax, 254
  pulmonary conditions and, 59
  signs and symptoms of, 57–58
  treatment of, 60

Ear physiology, 652–653
Eaton-Lambert syndrome, 750
EBV. *See* Epstein-Barr virus
Echinococcus infestation, 325
Echovirus type 9 meningitis,
    736
Ecthyma gangrenosum, 284, 302
Ectopic hormone production,
    373
Ectopic impulse generation, 754
Ectopic pregnancy, 628, 629
Ectropion, 689
Edema
  from burns, 96
  with venous insufficiency,
    187, 189
Edrophonium, 299, 749, 760
EEG abnormalities in migraine,
    40
Egophony, 258
Elbow fractures, 859
Electrocoagulation, 410, 415
Electroconvulsive therapy, 776,
    779
Electroencephalography, 722
Electrolyte abnormalities, 134,
    543
Electrolyte balance, 386
Electromyography, 762
Electronystagmography, 654
ELISA tests, 322, 330

Embolic strokes, 710
Embolism, 160, 711
Emmetropia, 675
Emphysema, 199, 254
  subcutaneous, 256, 257
Empty sella syndrome, 625–626
Empyema, 217, 262
Encephalopathy, 367, 372, 768
Endarteritis, 180
Endocarditis, 18, 174
  bacterial, 161, 174
  infective
    clinical–pathologic
      correlations of, 291–292
    diagnosis of, 292–293
    differential diagnosis of,
      292
    pathophysiology of,
      290–291
    prevention of and therapy
      for, 293–294
    signs and symptoms of,
      289–290
Endocrine disease, 29
Endocrine insufficiency, 378
Endogenous pyrogen, 285
Endometrial cancer, 639, 641
Endometrial edenocarcinomas,
    639
Endometrial polyps, 619
Endometriosis, 617
Endoscopy, 69
Endotoxic shock. *See* Septic
    shock
Endotoxin, 285–286, 426
Entamoeba histolytica infection,
    383
Entercolic fistula, 404
Enteritis, 74, 384
Enterobacteriaceae infections,
    303
Enterofistulas, 387
Entrapment neuropathy, 794
Entropion, 688
Envenomation, 83
Enzyme deficiencies, 435
Eosinophilic granuloma, 254
Eosinophilic pneumonia, 243
Ependymoma, 732
Epicardial coronary artery
    damage, 176
Epidermal wounds, 101–102
Epididymitis, 418
Epidural abscess, 735
Epidural hemorrhage, 718
Epidural metastatic cancer, 732
Epigastric hernia, 417
Epilepsy, 719. *See also* Seizures
Epinephrine, 83–84
Epistaxis, 302, 423
Epitaxy, 562
Epithelial ovarian tumors, 644
Epithelization, 102
Epstein-Barr nuclear antigen,
    272

Epstein-Barr pharyngitis, 266
Epstein-Barr virus, 269–270, 462
Ergot, 41
Ergotrate, 41
Erythema nodosum, 247, 809
Erythrocyte sedimentation rate,
    20, 824, 826
Erythrocytosis, 374
Erythromycin, 222, 325
Erythromycin-sulfonamide, 660
Escherichia coli, 283
  toxigenic, 383
Esodeviations, 678–681
Esophageal function tests, 113
Esophageal pH, 347
Esophageal reflux
  clinical–pathologic
    correlations of, 346
  diagnosis of, 347
  differential diagnosis of,
    346–347
  pathophysiology of, 346
  signs and symptoms of,
    345–346
  therapy for, 347–348
Esophageal ulcers, 345
Esophageal varices, bleeding,
    371
Esophagitis, 302, 345, 346, 352,
    392
Esotropia, 677
Estradiol, 637, 640
Estrogen, 609, 633
  beyond menopause, 637
  deficiency, 832
Estrogen receptors in breast
    tumor, 614–616
Estrogen replacement therapy,
    638, 805, 832
Estrogen-progestin therapy, 638
  risks of, 832
Estrone, 637
Estropia, 679–681
Ethambutal, 849
Ethanol, 747
Ethmoid sinusitis, 674
Ethosuximide, 722
Eustachian tube function,
    abnormal, 658
Euthyroid sick syndrome, 495
Evoked compound muscle
    action potential, 750–751
Evoked potentials testing, 756
Exercise
  amenorrhea and, 627
  stress tests, 113
Exocrine insufficiency, 378
Exodeviation, 678
Exotoxins, 426
Expiratory volume, 1-second
    forced. *See* FEV$_1$
Extrapyramidal syndromes, 745.
    See also Parkinson's
    disease
Eye trauma, 674, 681

Eyeglasses, 680
Eyelid diseases, 688–691
Eyes, refractive errors of,
    675–678

Facial nerve decompression,
    656
Facial nerve lesion, 654
Facial paralysis, 652, 656
Factitious fever, 16
Familial Mediterranean fever,
    18
Fanconi's syndrome, 553, 580
Fasciitis, 853
Fasciolopsis infestation, 325
Fecal occult blood testing, 414
Fecalith, 394
Femoral hernia, 71, 417
Femoral shaft fractures, 859
Ferritin, 431, 432
Ferrous gluconate, 432
Ferrous sulfate, 432
Fetal monitoring, 632
FEV_1, 227, 229, 233
Fever of unknown origin
    comparative causes of, 19t
    diagnosis of, 18–22
    pathophysiology of, 17
    signs and symptoms of, 16–17
Fibrin, 236
Fibrinogen scanning, 193
Fibrinolysis, 191, 424, 428
Fibrinolytic therapy, 194
Fibroadenoma, 606, 608, 609
Fibroblast tissue, 97
Fibroblasts, 104
Fibrocystic disease, 606,
    608–609
Fibroplasia, 103–104
Fibrosarcoma, 597
Fibrosis, 244–245
    pulmonary, 249
Finger fractures, 859
Fischl index, 233–234
Fissure in ano, 408
Fistual in ano, 409
Floppy baby syndrome, 298
Floppy valve syndrome, 161
Fluid management, 239, 288
Fluorescein angiography, 693
Fluorescent antibody staining,
    222
Fluorescent treponemal
    antibody absorption test,
    314
5-Fluorocytosine, 849
5-Fluorouracil, 357
Focal defects, 735
Folate deficiency, 390, 440–441
Folate levels, 443
Foley catheterization risks, 288
Folic acid, 440
    deficiency, 87
    recommended daily
        allowance for, 443–444

Folliculogenesis, 621, 623
Food allergies, 231
Food poisoning, 383
Foramen ovale opening, 120
Forearm fractures, 859
Foreign body aspiration, 64
Fracture
    common, 858–859
    complications of, 859
    compression, 828, 831
    open, 853
Friedreich's ataxia, 134
Frontal lobe "release" signs,
    50–51
FTA-ABS test. See Fluorescent
    treponemal antibody
    absorption test
Functional falsetto, 667
Functional residual capacity,
    237
Fungal infection, 251, 293
    in acute sinusitis, 279
    meningitis, 736–737
Furosemide, 552
Fusion beats, 149

Gait apraxia, 747
Gait ataxia, 753
Galactorrhea, 623, 625, 732
Gallbladder disease
    alcohol and, 377
    clinical–pathologic
        correlations of, 360
    diagnosis of, 359
    differential diagnosis of,
        358–359
    malignancy, 26
    pathophysiology of, 359–360
    signs and symptoms of, 358
    therapy for, 360
Gallbladder injuries, 77
Gallbladder obstruction, 360
Gallium lung scans, 245
Gallium scanning for
        hepatocellular carcinoma,
        375
Gallop rhythm, 131
Gallstones, 26, 359
    reformation of, 360
    surgery for, 380
Gametogenesis, defective, 623
Gammapathy, monoclonal,
    473–475
Gangrene, 181, 299–300
Gardnerella vaginalis, 311
Gas exchange alterations, 237
Gas gangrene, 299–300
Gastrectomy, 381, 551
Gastric carcinoma
    clinical–pathologic
        correlations of, 356
    diagnosis of, 357
    differential diagnosis of, 356
    pathophysiology, 355

    signs and symptoms, 354–355
    therapy for, 357
Gastric lavage, 69
Gastric pH, 353
Gastric polyps, 356
Gastric ulcers, 349–352, 354,
    356
Gastrin, 384
Gastrinoma, 352
Gastritis, 351
Gastroenteritis, 382
Gastroesophageal dysphagia,
    345
Gastroesophageal reflux,
    345–347. See also
        Esophageal reflux
Gastrointestinal bleeding, 389.
        See also Hemorrhage
    clinical–pathologic
        correlations of, 67
    diagnosis of, 68
    differential diagnosis of, 67
    pathophysiology of, 66–67
    with peptic ulcer disease,
        350–351
    with renal failure, 589
    signs and symptoms of, 65–66
    therapy of, 68–69
Gastrointestinal hormones, 384
Gastrointestinal perforation, 69
Genetic diseases, 85–87
Genitourinary tract
        instrumentation, 282
Gentamicin, 294
Gentian violet, 311
Gerota's fascia, 597
Giant cell arteritis, 670, 810, 824
    diagnosis and differential
        diagnosis of, 826
    pathophysiology of, 826–827
    signs and symptoms of,
        825–826
    therapy for, 827
Giardia infestation, 325, 383
Gigantism, 732
Gilbert's disease, 28
Gingivitis, 302–303
Glasgow Coma Scale, 48
Glass microsphere injection, 717
Glaucoma, 673, 683, 697
    angle-closure, 685–686, 692
    congenital, 686–688
    neovascular, 692
    open-angle, 676, 684–685
    secondary, 688
    surgery for, 685
Glaucomatous cupping, 684
Glioblastoma multiforme,
    729–730
Glioblastomas, 727–728
Gliomas, 725, 727
Globin abnormalities, 436
Globin synthesis, abnormal, 436
Glomerular disease, 570. See
        also Nephrotic syndrome

Glomerular filtration rate, 572, 576, 590, 594, 595
  impairment of, 570
Glomerular hyperfiltration, 577
Glomerulonephritis
  chronic, 568, 572
  diagnosis and differential diagnosis of, 573–575
  diffuse proliferative, 799
  idiopathic, 576
  membranoproliferative, 569–570, 575, 576, 582
  membranous, 582, 803
  mesangial, 582, 803
  minimal change, 580
  pathophysiology of, 570–573
  postinfectious, 567, 569
  poststreptococcal, 568, 574, 576
  prevention of and therapy for, 575–577
  rapidly progressive, 567, 569
  signs and symptoms of, 567–570
  with streptococcal pharyngitis, 265
Glomerulonephritis syndromes, 572
Glucagon, 512, 516, 520
Glucocorticoids, 234, 551
  supplementary, 509
Gluconate, 566
Gluconeogenesis, 88
Glucose
  for hepatitis, 367
  intolerance, 510–511, 513–514
  production, 516
Glucose oxidase, 515
Glucose tolerance test, 514
Glucose-6-phosphatase dehydrogenase deficiency, 433–435, 438
Glucose-6-phosphate dehydrogenase, 446
Glucuronyl transferase, 28
Glycogen depletion, 516
Glycogenolysis, 520
Glycohemoglobin, 514
Goiter
  in Graves' disease, 3
  toxic, 493, 502
Gonad disorders, 624–625
Gonadal agenesis, 625
Gonadal dysgenesis, 625
Gonadotropin levels, 623
Gonioscopic evaluation, 686
Gonococcal arthritis, 845
Gonococcal infection, 844
  of eye, 672
Gonococcal proctitis, 410
Gonorrhea, 309, 312–313
  prostate cancer and, 604
Goodpasture's syndrome, 63, 241, 569, 585

Goodsalls' rule, 409
Gorlin formula, 161
Gout
  clinical–pathologic correlations of, 839
  diagnosis and differential diagnosis of, 839–841
  pathophysiology of, 838–839
  prevention of and therapy for, 841
  signs and symptoms of, 838
Gouty arthritis, 838, 839
Gower's sign, 760
Graft-versus-host disease, 470
Granulocytopenia, 303
Granulomas, 246, 340, 473, 728, 796
  caseating, 334
  hypercalcemia and, 549
  noncaseating, 248, 470
Granulomatous angiitis, 825
Granulomatous colitis, 404
Granulomatous enteritis, 74
Granulomatous hepatitis, 18
Granulomatous ileitis, 387
Graves' disease, 3, 442, 502
Grey Turner's sign, 377
Groin muscle injury, 418
Ground substance, 104
Guanidine, 750
Guillain-Barre syndrome, 274, 299, 758
  treatment of, 762
Gynecologic screening techniques, 646

H₂-receptor blockers, 353
Hageman factor activation, 286
Hallucinations, 51
Hallucinogens, 789
Halsted's operation. *See* Radical mastectomy
Ham test, 437
Handwashing practice, 288
Hangover headache, 41
Haptoglobin, 437
Hartmann procedure, 405
Harvard brain-death criteria, 48–49
Hashimoto's thyroiditis, 442, 499, 501
Hashish, 788–789
Hashitoxicosis, 487
HbSC disease, 434
HBV vaccine, 376
Headache, *See also* Migraine
  causes of, 38t
  chronic recurrent, 37
  diagnosis of, 42
  features of, 39t
  hypertension and, 42
  posttraumatic, 42
  of psychogenic origin, 41
  with subarachnoid hemorrhage, 716

  treatment for, 42, 43t
  types of, 37–42
Hearing loss, 651–652, 653
  with otitis media, 657
  treatment of, 654–656
Heart block
  complete, 117–118
  with hypercalcemia, 546
  sudden death with, 249
Heart disease
  indicators of, 4
  traumatic, 175–179
Heart failure, 126
Hebephrenia, 781
Heberden's nodes, 834
Helmithic worms, 329
Hemangiomas, 67, 664
Hemarthroses, 424
Hematemesis, 61, 65
Hematochezia, 65, 66
Hematomas, 423
Hematopoietic system, 17
Hematoxylin bodies, 803
Hematuria, 568, 596, 598
  with abdominal trauma, 78
  gross, 569
Hemihypesthesia, 714
Hemiparesis, 714, 764
Hemochromatosis, 27
Hemodialysis, 545
  hypernatremia with, 521
  osteomyelitis and, 850
Hemodynamic disturbances, 122–123
Hemoglobin, 432
Hemoglobin C, 433
Hemoglobin fraction, 515
Hemoglobinopathies, 438
Hemoglobinuria, 437, 584
  paroxysmal nocturnal, 434
Hemolysis, mechanical, 436
Hemolytic anemia. *See* Anemia, hemolytic
Hemolytic uremic syndrome, 574
Hemophilia, 423, 428
Hemophilus infections
  of throat, 663
  influenzae, 736
  in sinus infections, 278, 279
Hemoptysis
  diagnosis of, 64
  differential diagnosis of, 63–64
  pathophysiology of, 62–63
  signs and symptoms of, 61–62
  therapy for, 64
Hemorrhage. *See also specific sites of*
  chronic, 433
  from colon, 404–405
  epidural, 718
  intracerebral, 522–523, 714–716
  intracranial, 714–718, 768

Hemorrhage. *(cont.)*
  occult, 432
  with septic shock, 286
  splinter, 290
  subarachnoid, 716–717
  subdural, 717–718
Hemorrhagic infarct, 710–711
Hemorrhoidal arteries, 406
Hemorrhoidal veins, 406
Hemorrhoidectomy, 407
Hemorrhoids, 66, 407–408
Henderson-Hasselbach
    equation, 8
Henoch-Schonlein purpura,
    569–570, 574, 807–809
Heparin
  for acute myocadial
      infarction, 122
  for deep vein thrombosis,
      193–194
Hepatectomy, partial, 375
Hepatic transplantation, 376
Hepatitis, 24, 432. *See also* Viral
    hepatitis
  acute, 361
  alcoholic, 370
  chronic active, 27, 364, 366
  chronic persistent, 364
  lupoid chronic active, 367
Hepatitis A, 26
Hepatitis B, 26, 362, 364
  prevention of, 813
Hepatitis B antigen, 811
Hepatitis B virus surface
    antigen. *See* HGsAg
Hepatocellular carcinoma
  diagnosis of, 374–375
  pathophysiology of, 374
  signs and symptoms of,
      373–374
  therapy of, 375–376
Hepatojugular reflux, 128
Hepatomegaly, 270
Hepatorenal syndrome, 372
Hernias, 416
  differential diagnosis of, 418
  incarcerated or strangulated, 417
  pathophysiology of, 417–418
  signs and symptoms of, 417
  therapy for, 418–419
Herniography, 418
Heroin addiction, 787
  endocarditis in, 289, 291
Herpes, 309, 311–312
Herpes simplex infections, 736
Herpes simplex keratitis,
    690–691
  of cornea, 671
Herpes simplex
    keratoconjunctivitis, 690
Herpes zoster, 456
Heterografts, 291
Heterophorias, 42
Heterotropias, 42
HGsAg, 374

Hip fractures, 828, 859
  postmenopausal, 634
Hip-joint pain, 833
Histamine headache, 40
Histoplasma capsulatum
    infection, 338
Histoplasmin skin test, 339
Histoplasmosis
  clinical–pathologic
      correlations of, 341
  diagnosis of, 339
  differential diagnosis of,
      339–340
  disseminated, 339
  with fever, 17
  pathophysiology of, 340
  signs and symptoms, 338–339
  therapy for, 341
HIV. *See* Human
    immunodeficiency virus
Hives, 82
HLA type DR4 gene, 795
HLA-B27, 382
Hoarseness, 661
  intermittent, 667
  with organic pathological
      disorders, 662–665
  with vocal function disorders,
      665–667
Hodgkin's disease, 18
  diagnosis of, 468–469
  immunocompromise with,
      305
  pathophysiology and clinical
      correlations of, 469–470
  signs and symtoms of,
      466–467
  staging for, 466–467, 468
  therapy for, 470–471
Holter monitoring, 146
Homans' sign, 190
Hookworm infestation, 325
Hoover's sign, 200
Hordeolum, 689
Hormone replacement therapy,
    672. *See also* Estrogen
    replacement therapy
Homones
  abnormal levels of with fever,
      17
  deficiency, 516
  disease of affecting larynx,
      663
  manipulation of, 616
Horner syndrome, 708
Hot flashes, 634, 638
Housemaid's knee, 871
HTLV-III, 317
HTLV-III antibody, 322
Human immunodeficiency
    virus, 317
Human immunovirus antibody
    seroconversion, 319
Human T-cell leukemia virus-
    III. *See* HTLV-III

Humeral neck fractures, 859
Huntington's disease, 55–56
Hyaline drusen, 696
Hyaluronidase, 123
Hydatidiform mole, 628, 629
Hydralazine, 143
Hydrocele, 418
Hydrocephalus, 727
  communicating, 748
  estropia with, 679
  normal pressure, 55
  obstructive, 729
Hydrochloric acid, 15
Hydrocortisone, 509
Hydronephrosis, 594
Hydroxychloroquine, 806
25-Hydroxycholecalciferol, 579
Hymenoptera insect venom, 82
Hyperalimentation, 855
Hyperamylasemia, 379
Hyperapnea, 58
Hyperbaric oxygen therapy, 300,
    857
Hypercalcemia, 248, 374, 476,
    508
  clinical–pathologic
      correlations of, 549
  diagnosis and differential
      diagnosis of, 549–551
  pathophysiology of, 546–549
  prevention of and therapy for,
      551–552
  signs and symptoms of, 546
  in squamous cell neoplasms,
      208
  treatment of, 476
Hypercalciuria, 248, 562, 566
Hypercholesterolemia, 26, 182,
    374
Hypercoagulability, 191, 580
Hyperdeviation, 679
Hyperglycemia, 15, 374
  with diabetes, 510, 511, 513
Hyperinsulinism, endogenous,
    520
Hyperkalemia, 131, 182, 507,
    508, 588
  differential diagnosis of, 534t
  drug-induced, 591
  prevention and therapy for,
      533–538
  signs and symptoms of,
      529–530
Hyperkeratosis, 663–664
Hyperlipidemia, 374, 526
Hyperlipoproteinemia, 593
Hypermagnesemia, 589
  clinical–pathologic
      correlations of, 543
  diagnosis and differential
      diagnosis of, 543–544
  pathophysiology of, 542–543
  signs and symptoms of,
      541–542
  therapy for, 544–545

Hypermetabolism, 90, 487
Hypernatremia
  clinical–pathologic
      correlations of, 523
  differential diagnosis of, 522
  pathophysiology of, 522–523
  signs and symptoms of,
      521–522
  therapy for, 523
Hypernephroma
  clinical–pathologic
      correlations of, 598
  diagnosis and differential
      diagnosis of, 598–599
  pathophysiology of, 597
  prevention of and therapy for,
      599
  signs and symptoms of,
      596–597
Hyperopia, 676–677
Hyperoxaluria, 562–563, 566
Hyperparathyroidism, 550–551,
      595
  with nephrotic syndrome, 579
  primary, 562
  secondary, 593
Hyperphosphatemia, 588, 593
Hyperpigmentation, 506, 508
Hyperpituitarism, 663
Hyperreactive airways, 199
Hyperreflexia, 766
Hypersensitivity, delayed, 332
Hypersensitivity response, 229
Hypersensitivity vasculitis,
      807–809
  treatment of, 813
Hypersplenism, 434, 437–438
Hypertension, 28–29, 182,
      692–693
  with cardiomyopathy, 134
  clinical–pathologic
      correlations for, 33, 34t
  detection and prevention of,
      133
  diagnosis of, 34–35
  differential diagnosis of,
      33–34
  features of diseases causing,
      32t
  headache with, 42
  heart disease with, 141
  with intracerebral
      hemorrhage, 715
  pathophysiology of, 31–33
  pregnancy-induced, 631–633
  prevention of and therapy for,
      35–36
  screening tests for, 34–35
  signs and symptoms of, 29–31
  types of, 30t
  untreated, 31
  with volume expansion, 591
Hypertensive cardiovascular
      disease, 141
Hyperthyroidism, 383, 499

clinical–pathologic
      correlations of, 491
  diagnosis and differential
      diagnosis of, 491–493
  pathophysiology of, 489–491
  signs and symptoms of,
      487–489
  therapy for, 493–494
Hypertrophic cardiomyopathy,
      109, 134, 136, 138
Hypertrophic scars, 104
Hyperuricemia, 589, 838
  treatment of, 841
Hyperuricemic nephropathy,
      584
Hyperuricosuria, 563
Hyperventilation, 9, 129
Hypervitaminosis D, 549
Hypervolemia, 523, 595
Hypesthesia, 38
Hyphema, 673
Hypnotic-sedative drugs, abuse
      of, 786–787
Hypoalbuminemia, 87, 88, 300,
      551
Hypoaldosteronism, 591
Hypocalcemia, 588–589, 593
  clinical–pathologic
      correlations of, 549
  diagnosis and differential
      diagnosis of, 549–551
  with magnesium deficiency,
      544
  pathophysiology of, 546–549
  prevention of and therapy for,
      551–552
  signs and symptoms of, 546
Hypochloremia, 131
Hypogammaglobulinemia, 456,
      473, 474
Hypoglycemia, 374, 497, 508,
      520
  fasting
      clinical–pathologic
          correlations of, 516–517
      diagnosis and differential
          diagnosis of, 517–520
      pathophysiology of, 516
      prevention of and therapy
          for, 520
      signs and symptoms of, 516
  insulin-induced, 509
  reactive, 516
  refractory, 514
Hypoglycorrhachia, 520
Hypokalemia, 12, 131
  chronic, 527
  diagnosis of, 533
  differential diagnosis of, 535t
  with magnesium deficiency,
      544
  signs and symptoms of, 529,
      530–531
Hypomagnesemia, 548
  diagnosis and differential

diagnosis of, 543–544
  pathophysiology of, 542–543
  signs and symptoms of, 541
  therapy for, 544–545
Hyponatremia, 131, 497, 507
  clinical–pathologic
      correlations of, 526
  diagnosis of, 526–527
  pathophysiology of, 525
  signs and symptoms of,
      524–525
  spurious, 526
  therapy for, 528
Hypophosphatemia
  clinical–pathologic
      correlations of, 554–555,
      557t
  diagnosis and differential
      diagnosis of, 555, 558t
  pathophysiology of, 554
  prevention of and therapy for,
      556
  signs and symptoms of, 553
Hypoproliferative anemia, 800
Hypotension postural, 521
Hypothalamic tumors, 522
Hypothalamic-pituitary-thyroid
      negative feedback system,
      489
Hypothalamus disorders, 626
Hypothyroidism, 499, 663
  diagnosis and differential
      diagnosis of, 495–497
  pathophysiology of, 495
  signs and symptoms of,
      494–495
  therapy for, 497
  transient, 496
Hypotonia, 765, 768
Hypoventilation, 15
Hypovolemia, 118
  with hypernatremia, 521
  with hyponatremia, 524,
      527–528
  prevention of, 595
Hypovolemic shock, 72
Hypoxemia, 202, 203, 243
Hypoxia, 768
Hypoxic-ischemic
      encephalopathy, 768
Hysterectomy
  for cervial cancer, 643
  hoarseness with, 663
  for ovarian carcinoma, 646
Hysteria, 753
Hysteroscopy, 619

Ibuprofen, 123, 618
IDT$_8$ antigen, 321
IgG-IgA nephritis. See Berger's
      disease
Ileocecal valve incompetence,
      71
Ileocolitis, 387. See also Crohn's
      disease

Ileus, 377
Iliocolonic intussusception, 74
Iliopectineal bursitis, 871
Imipramine, 777
Immotile cilia syndrome, 252
Immune-complex vasculitis, 291
Immune complexes, 801, 803
Immune globulin, 366
Immune hemolysis, 436, 439
Immunocompromised host
    infections
    diagnosis of, 306
    differential diagnosis of,
        305–306
    histoplasmosis in, 339
    osteomyelitis in, 855
    pathophysiology of, 303–305
    prevention of and therapy for,
        306–308
    signs and symptoms of,
        302–303
Immunodeficiencies, 322
Immunoglobulin, monoclonal,
    472–473
Immunologic tests, 751
Immunosuppression, 287, 302
Immunosuppressive drugs
    for interstitial lung disease,
        245
    for myasthenia gravis, 750
    septic arthritis and, 848
    with systemic lupus
        erythematosus, 806
Immunotherapy, 83–84, 599
Impaired cell-mediated
    immunity, 305
Impedance plethysmography,
    192
Indomethacin
    for dysmenorrhea, 618
    for gout, 841
    for hypercalcemia, 552
    for myocardial infarction, 123
Infantile marasmus, 87
Infantile progressive spinal
    muscular atrophy, 758
Infections
    as cause of hemoptysis, 63
    of CNS, 56
    with relapsing fever, 16
    starvation with, 88
Inflammatory bowel disease,
    381, 383, 846
Influenza, 268
    clinical–pathologic
        correlations of, 274–276
    diagnosis and differential
        diagnosis of, 276
    pathophysiology of, 274
    prevention of and therapy for,
        276
    signs and symptoms of,
        273–274
Influenza A virus, 273–274, 276
Influenza B virus, 273, 274, 276

Influenza C virus, 273
Influenza vaccines, 203, 245,
    253, 276
Infrapatella bursitis, 871
Inguinal hernia, 416–417
Inguinal herniorrhaphy, 419
Inhalation burns, 97
Inotrophic agents, 143
Insect venom allergy, 82–84
Insulin, 512
    for diabetes, 514
    for hypoglycemia, 520
    for ketoacidosis, 15
    potassium levels and, 532
Insulin antibodies, 520
Insulin receptors, 512
Interleukin-1, 285, 796
Interstitial lung disease
    clinical–pathologic
        correlations of, 243–244
    diagnosis of, 243
    differential diagnosis of, 243
    pathophysiology of, 242–243
    prevention of and therapy for,
        244–245
    signs and symptoms of,
        241–242
Interstitial nephritis, 584–585,
    589, 591
Intervertebral disk disease
    clinical–pathologic
        correlations of, 876
    diagnosis and differential
        diagnosis of, 876–877
    pathophysiology of, 874–876
    prevention of and therapy for,
        877–879
    signs and symptoms of,
        873–874
Intestinal motility. See also
    Diarrhea altered, 384
Intracerebral hemorrhage,
    714–716
Intracranial hemorrhage,
    714–718, 768
Intracranial mass lesions, 44
Intracranial pressure, increased,
    726–727
Intracranial tumors
    classification and biology of,
        725–726
    clinical–pathologic
        correlations of, 727–728
    CNS metastasis of, 732
    common brain tumors,
        729–732
    diagnosis of, 728–729
    pathophysiology of, 726–727
    spinal neoplasms, 732
    therapy for, 729
Intracranial vasculitis, 742
Intramural thrombus, 119
Intranuclear inclusions, 311
Intraocular pressure, 683
Intravenous fluids

    with bowel obstruction, 76
    for gastrointestinal
        hemorrhage, 68–69
Intraventricular conduction
    disturbances, 118
Intussusception, 74
Invasive test, 6–7
Involucrum, 852
Iodine therapy, 487, 489,
    493–494
Iododeoxyuridine, 691
Iridectomy, 686
Iris melanoma, 700–701
Iris cysts, 685
Iritis, 671
Iron deficiency anemia
    clinical–pathologic
        correlations of, 430–431
    diagnosis of, 432
    differential diagnosis of, 431
    pathophysiology of, 430
    prevention of and therapy for,
        432–433
    signs and symptoms of,
        429–430
    stomach carcinoma and,
        356–357
Iron overload, 25
Irritable bowel syndrome, 391
Ischemic bowel, 75
Ischemic cardiomyopathy, 134
Ischiogluteal bursitis, 870–871
Ischiorectal abscess, 408
Isoamylase assay, 379
Isoniazid, 245, 337, 849
Isoniazid hepatitis, 337
Isospora infestation, 325

Jaundice
    clinical–pathologic
        correlations of, 24–26
    diagnosis of, 26–27
    differential diagnosis of, 26
    fluctuating, 26
    with hepatitis, 361, 364
    hepatocellular, 27
    in Hodgkin's disease, 470
    pathophysiologic mechanisms
        of, 25t
    pathophysiology, 24
    prevention of and therapy for,
        28
    signs and symptoms of, 23–24
Jejunum, 70
Jimson weed poisoning, 298
Joint destruction, 845–846, 849
Jugular vein distention, 178

Kala-azar, 325, 329
Kaliuretic diuretics, 131
Kallikrein, 111
Kaposi's sarcoma, 320
Kartagener's syndrome, 252
Karyotypes, 451
Kawasaki disease, 809, 813, 815

Keloid scars, 104
Keratitis sicca, 672
Keratoconjunctivitis, 689
  herpes simplex, 690
Kernicterus, 764, 768
Kernig's maneuver, 733
Ketoconazole, 341
Kidney stones, 561, *See also*
    Nephrolithiasis
  diagnosis of, 563
  dissolving of, 565
  gout and, 838–839
  surgical removal of, 565–566
Kidneys
  asymmetric, 587
  damage to with burn injuries,
    99
  polycystic, 591, 596
  scarring of, 282
Kinins, 111
Kelebsiella infections, 283
Klebsiella pneumoniae
    infection, 215
Korotkoff sounds, 179
Kuru, 54
Kussmaul's sign, 178
Kveim test, 248
Kwashiorkor, 87, 90
Kyphosis, 634, 864

Labetalol, 297
Laboratory tests, 7
Labyrinthitis, purulent, 657
Lactate, 111, 848
Lactate dehydrogenase, 597
Lactation history, 610
Lactic acid, 15
  overproduction of, 285
Lactic acidosis, 15, 521
Lactose intolerance, 383
Lactulose, 367
Lagophthalmos, 689
Laminar air flow, 307
Laminectomy, 476
Laparoscopy, 375, 619
Laparotomy, second-look, 647
Laryngeal papilloma, 665
Laryngeal paralysis, 664–665
Laryngeal web, 662
Laryngitis, chronic, 666
Laryngomalacia, 662
Larynx
  carcinoma of, 664
  disease of, 661–667
  organic pathology of
    congenital, 662
    hormonal, 663
    infections, 662–663
    neoplastic, 663–664
    paralytic, 664–665
Laser iridotomy, 686
Laser photocoagulation, 693
Lateral humeral epicondylitis,
    870
Latex agglutination test, 306

LAV. *See* Lymphadenopathy-
    associated virus
Learned pain syndrome, 121
Lecithin, 54
Legionella infections, 215, 218,
    306
Legionella pneumonia, 219–220,
    222
Leiomyoma, 356
Leishmaniasis, 325
Leptomeningeal carcinomatosis,
    732
Leriche's syndrome, 181
Leukemia, 18
  acute lymphoblastic, 457–458
  acute nonlymphocytic
    clinical–pathologic
      correlations of, 452
    diagnosis and differential
      diagnosis of, 452–454
    pathophysiology of,
      451–452
    signs and symptoms of,
      450–451
    therapy for, 454–455
  chronic lymphocytic
    diagnosis, of, 459
    differential diagnosis of,
      457–459
    pathologic mechanisms of,
      456–457
    signs and symptoms of,
      455–456
    treatment of, 459–460
  hairy cell, 458
  nonlymphocytic, 434
  prolymphocytic, 458
  T-cell chronic lymphocytic,
    458
Leukocoria, 698
Leukocyte alkaline phosphatase,
    449
Leukocyte pyrogen, 17
Leukocytoclastic vasculitis, 803,
    813
Leukocytosis, 359, 447
Leukopenia, 215
Leukoplakia, 663
Leukotrienes, 229
Levodopa, 748
Levothyroxine, 503
Lewy body formation, 747
Lhermitte's phenomenon, 753
Libman-Sacks endocarditis, 800
Lidocaine, 122, 146
Lifting techniques, 877–878
Ligament of Treitz, 78
Ligandin, 23
Limb-salvage reconstruction,
    184
Lingula biopsy, 243
Lipase, 379
Lipiduria, 577
Lipogenesis, 512
Lipoid nephrosis, 580

Lipolysis inhibition, 512
Lipoprotein electrophoresis, 526
Listeria monocytogenes fever,
    305
Listeria monocytogenes
    infection, 736
Lithogenic bile, 359
Lithotripsy, percutaneous, 566
Little's disease, 764
Livedo reticularis, 748, 809
Liver
  damage to, 25–26. *See also*
    Jaundice
  injury, end-stage, 369
  laceration, 77
  size of, 24
  transplantation, 28, 372
  tumors, 373
Liver disease, 370, 432. *See also*
    Cirrhosis
  alcoholic, 434
  with gastrointestinal bleeding,
    66
Liver transaminase, 597
Loa loa infestation, 325
  surgical removal of, 330
Lobular carcinoma, 612, 615
Lockjaw. *See* Tetanus
Loperamide, 387
Lord procedure, 408
Lordosis, 864
Lower esophageal sphincter
    pressure, 346, 348
LSD, 789
Lumbar disk disease, 873, 878
Lumbar puncture, 738, 739
Lumpectomy, 615
Lung abscess, 63
  clinical–pathologic
    correlations of, 225
  diagnosis of, 225–226
  differential diagnosis of, 225
  pathophysiology of, 224–225
  prevention of and therapy for,
    226
  signs and symptoms of,
    223–224
Lung biopsy, open, 306
Lung cancer, 549
  clinical–pathologic
    correlations of, 206
  diagnosis of, 207–208
  differential diagnosis of,
    206–207
  pathophysiology of, 206
  prevention of and therapy for,
    208–209
  signs and symptoms of,
    204–206
  staging of, 207–208
Lung disease. *See also* Lung
    abscess; Lung cancer
  anaerobic infections, 217
  chronic, 60, 131
  interstitial, 241–245

Lung parenchyma destruction, 223
Lung pseudotumors, 260
Lungs
  airflow resistance in, 201
  elastic recoil of, 201
  mechanics of, changes in, 237
Lupoid chronic active hepatitis, 367
Luteinizing hormone releasing hormone, 605
Lymph nodes
  enlargement of, 459, 470
  as source of fever, 17
Lymphadenectomy, 599
Lymphadenitis, suppurative cervical, 265
Lymphadenopathy, 247, 463, 469
Lymphadenopathy-associated virus, 317
Lymphocytes, 244
Lymphocytosis, 458–460
Lymphokines, 242, 248
Lymphoma, 356, 457
  malignant, 462
  non-Hodgkin's, 469
    clinical–pathologic correlations of, 463
    diagnosis of, 464–465
    differential diagnosis, of, 463–464
    pathophysiology of, 462–463
    signs and symptoms of, 461–462
    therapy for, 465
  staging criteria for, 464–465
Lymphoproliferation, 461–462
Lymphoproliferative disorders, 436
Lymphoreticular system, 17
Lymphosarcoma cell leukemia, 457

M hemoglobins, 434
M protein, 265
Machado test, 329
Macrophages, 244
Macular degeneration, senile, 695–696
Macular edema, 693
Magnesium, 541. See also Hypermagnesemia; Hypomagnesemia
  excretion of, 542
  renal reabsorption of, 547
Magnesium ammonium phosphate stones, 561, 563
  treatment of, 566
Magnesium salts, 383

Magnetic resonance imaging, 599
Malabsorption diseases, 26, 252
Malabsorption screen tests, 385
Malaria, 18, 325, 330
Malaria parasites, 329
Maldevelopmental tumors, 728
Malignant mesothelioma, 208
Malignant melanoma, 700–702
Mallory-Weiss tear, 65–66
Malnutrition
  anemia and, 444
  clinical–pathologic correlations, 90
  coagulation disorders and, 425
  in Crohn's disease, 389
  diagnosis, 91–94
  differential diagnosis, 90
  for gastric carcinoma, 357
  nosocomial, 88
  pathophysiology, 88–90
  signs and symptoms of, 87–88
  stomach carcinoma and, 356
  therapy for and prevention of, 94
Mammary duct estasia, 606
Mammography, 610
Manganese intoxication, 747
MAOIs. See Monoamine oxidase inhibitors
Marfan's syndrome, 85, 183
Marijuana, 788–789
Mast cells, 229
Mastectomy, 615
Mastoid disease, 656
Mastoiditis, 657
McBurney's point, 395
Meconium ileus, 252
Mediastinal fibrosis, 339
Medroxyprogesterone, 599
Medullary carcinoma, 608
Medullary cystic disease, 591
Medulloblastoma, 731
Megaloblastic anemia, 443
Megaloblastic madness, 441
Meibomian squamous carcinoma, 689
Melena, 65, 66
Membranoproliferative glomerulonephritis, 567
Memory loss, 54
MEN. See Multiple endocrine neoplastic syndromes
Meniere's disease, 653
Meningeal irritation, 717
Meningiomas, 727–728, 729, 731, 732
Meningitis, 278, 305
  clinical–pathologic correlations of, 735
  dementia and, 56
  diagnosis and differential diagnosis of, 735–738

  headache with, 42
  pathophysiology of, 734–735
  signs and symptoms, 733–734
  treatment of, 738–739
Menopause, 633
  clinical–pathologic correlations of, 635
  diagnosis of, 635–637
  pathophysiology of, 637
  premature, 623
  signs and symptoms of, 634–635
  therapy for, 638
Menotoxin, 617
Menstrual history, 610, 620
Menstruation
  missing periods in, 628
  normal, 620–621
  problems with. See Amenorrhea; Dysmenorrhea
Mental retardation, 769
6-Mercaptopurine, 752
Mesenteric infarction, 396
Metabolic acidosis, 9t, 10–12, 75, 588, 590
  bacteremia and, 287
  cause of, 9
  in septicemia, 285
Metabolic alkalosis, 9–15
Metallic foreign body, 857
Metaphysis, 850, 852
Metastatic infections, 210
Metastatic ocular tumors, 702
Methadone maintenance, 788
Methenamine, 283
Methicillin, 316
Methotrexate, 245
Methylmalonic acid, 442
Methylxanthines, 609
Metoclopramide, 348
Metronidazole, 301, 311, 743
Microadenomas, 732
Middle ear, disease of. See Otitis media
Middle ear effusion, 658, 659
Migraines, 37–40
Miliary tuberculosis, 17, 333
Milk, phosphate in, 556
Mineralocorticoid steroid excess, 15
Mineralocorticoids, 532
Minithoractomy, 262
Mitomycin C, 357
Mitral insufficiency, 160, 162, 164
Mitral regurgitation, 118, 159, 166
Mitral valve disease
  clinical–pathologic correlations of, 161
  diagnosis of, 162–163
  differential diagnosis of, 161–162

pathophysiology of, 161
prevention of and therapy for, 163–165
signs and symptoms of, 159–161
Mitral valve prolapse, 109, 160–162, 292
with chest pain, 162
diagnosis of, 163
with panic disorder, 773
treatment of, 164
Mitral valve stenosis, 159, 161–163
Mondor's disease, 606, 608
Mono spot test, 272
Monoamine oxidase inhibitors, 778–779
Monodeiodination, 493
Mononeuritis multiplex, 809
Mononeuropathy, 757
Mononucleosis, infectious
diagnosis and differential diagnosis of, 272
pathophysiology of, 270–272
signs and symptoms of, 269–270
Morphine, 121, 297
Mosaicism, 625
Movement disorders, 769
Moxolactam, 738
Mucociliary apparatus dysfunction, 213
Mucocutaneous junction, 407
Mucocutaneous lymph node syndrome, 809
Mucomycosis, 279
Müllerian anomalies, 624
Multifocal atrial tachycardia, 156–157
Multiple endocrine neoplastic syndrome, 33
Multiple infarct dementia, 55
Multiple sclerosis
clinical–pathologic correlations of, 755
diagnosis of, 756
genetic factors in, 755
pathophysiology of, 754–755
signs and symptoms of, 753–754
therapy for, 756–757
Muscle contraction headache, 40
Muscle necrosis, 530
Muscle tone evaluation, 766
Muscle weakness, 529
Muscular dystrophies, 758, 762
Duchenne type, 134, 762, 864
Myasthenia gravis, 299, 757–758
clinical–pathologic correlations of, 750
diagnosis and differential diagnosis of, 750–752
pathophysiology of, 750

signs and symptoms of, 749–750
therapy for, 752
treatment of, 762
Mycobacteria, 335
Mycobacterium avium-intracellulare, 320
Mycobacterium tuberculosis, 331, 333, 335
Mycoplasma pneumoniae, 218–219, 266
diagnosis of, 221–222
Mycostatin, 410
Myelin basic protein, 756
Myelin formation, 754
Myelodysplasia, 450, 452
Myelofibrosis, 445
with myeloid metaplasia, 445, 446, 449
Myelogenous leukemia, chronic, 445, 446, 447–449
Myelography, 877
Myeloid metaplasia, myelofibrosis with, 445
Myeloma, multiple
diagnosis of, 474–476
differential diagnosis of, 473–474
pathophysiology of, 473
signs and symptoms of, 472–473
therapy for, 476
Myelopathy, 878
Myeloproliferative diseases
diagnosis of, 449
differential diagnosis of, 447–449
pathophysiology of, 446–447
signs and symptoms of, 445–446
therapy for, 449
Myocardial abscesses, 291
Myocardial contusion, 175
clinical–pathologic correlations of, 176
pathophysiology of, 176
Myocardial infarction
acute
diagnosis of, 121
differential diagnosis of, 120 121
pathophysiology and correlations of, 119–120
prevention of and therapy for, 121–125
prognosis of, 124–125
signs and symptoms of, 117–119
interventional therapy for, 123
nonfatal, 111
premature ventricular complexes in, 145
silent, 121

Myocardial ischemia, 109, 111
Myocardial laceration, 176
Myocardial rupture, 176
Myocarditis, 800
Myoclonic seizures, 721
Myoclonus, 51
Myoglobin casts, 585
Myoglobinuria, 181, 437, 553, 584
Myopathy, 758
Myopia, 675–676
enlarged scleral canals with, 685
headache with, 42
uncorrected, 677
Myotonic dystrophy, 85, 134
Myxedema coma, 497
Myxoma, 18

Nafcillin, 294, 316
Nail-fold biopsies, 817
Nail-fold capillary abnormalities, 816
Naloxone, 288
Naproxen, 306, 618
Narcotic abuse, 787–788
Narcotics, 121
Nasal polyps, 250
Nasal vasomotor reaction headache, 40
Nasopharyngeal carcinoma, 270
Nasopharyngeal secretions, 658
Nasopharyngeal tumors, 658
Nearsightedness. See Myopia
Necrotizing pneumonia, 224
Neisseria gonorrhea, 266
Neisseria meningitidis meningitis, 736
Neomycin, 367
Neonatal bleeding, 423
Neonatal meningitis, 736
Neonatal osteomyelitis, 853, 854
Neoplasms
with fever, 17
hemoptysis and, 63
infections from, 303–304
rectal, 381
squamous cell, 208
Neoplastic fever, 306
Neovascularization, 692, 693, 697
Nephritic edema, 572
Nephritic glomerular injury, 567
Nephritic syndromes, 567, 568, 570
Nephritis, salt-losing, 591
Nephrolithiasis
clinical–pathologic correlations of, 563
diagnosis and differential diagnosis of, 563–565
pathophysiology of, 561–563

Nephrolithiasis *(cont.)*
  prevention of and therapy for,
    565–566
  signs and symptoms of, 561
Nephrosclerosis, 591
Nephrotic syndrome, 131
  clinical–pathologic
    correlations of, 579–580
  diagnosis and differential
    diagnosis of, 580–582
  pathophysiology of, 578–579
  signs and symptoms of,
    577–578
  therapy for, 582
Nephrotoxic antibiotics, 588,
    589
Nerve conduction velocity
    studies, 762
Nerve root pain, 873
Nerve sheath tumors, 731
Nesidioblastosis, 520
Neurofibrillary tangles, 52
Neurofibromas, 731
Neurofibromatosis, 85
Neurohormonal control
    mechanism defect, 777
Neuroleptic agents, 745
Neurologic dysfunction, diffuse,
    717
Neuromuscular blockade,
    prolonged, 685
Neuromuscular disorders, 757,
    763
  diagnosis of, 762
  pathophysiology of, 760–762
  prevention of and therapy for,
    762
  signs and symptoms of,
    758–760
Neuromuscular irritability, 543
Neuromuscular junction
    disorder, 760
Neuromuscular scoliosis, 864
Neuro-otologic surgery, 656
Neurotransmitters, 777
  balance of, 745–746
Neurotropism, 691
Neurovascular compression
    syndromes, 820
Neutron activation analysis, 832
Neutropenia, 303, 450
Neutrophils, 244
Nicotinic acid deficiency, 87
Nifedipine, 121
Night sweats, 470
Nipple discharge, bloody, 608
Nipple trauma, 607
Nitrates, 116, 143
Nitrofurantoin, 283
Nitroprusside, 143
Nitrosamines, 355
Nocardia infection, 305–306
Non-A, non-B hepatitis, 361,
    362, 364, 366

Non-Hodgkin's lymphoma, 18
Noninvasive tests, 6–7
Nonmigrainous vascular
    headaches, 41
Non-Q infarct, 120
Nontransmural infarct, 120
Norepinephrine, 31, 777
Nose drops, 268
Nosocomial organisms, 288
Noxious gas–induced injuries,
    97
Nuclear magnetic resonance,
    743
Nutrition
  with ARDS, 240
  burns and, 97–99, 100
  for cystic fibrosis, 253
  deficiencies with
    cardiomyopathy, 134
  in depression, 778
Nutrition profile, 91
Nutritional assessment
    checklist, 94
Nystagmus, 652

Oat cell cancer of lung, 750
Obsessive-compulsive
    disorders, 773
Obstipation, 72
Obstructive arterial disease, 180
Obtundation, 44
Obturator hernia, 71
Occlusive cerebral vascular
    disease, 707–713
Ocular deviations in adults,
    681–682
Ocular disorders
  acute painless monocular
    visual loss, 668–670
  orbital disease, 673–674
  red eye, 670–673
  uveitis, 673
Ocular malignancy
  diagnosis of, 698–699
  signs and symptoms of, 698
  therapy for, 699–700
Ocular trauma, 670, 672–673
Ocular tumors, metastatic, 702
Oculocephalic responses, 45
Oculomotor palsies, 681
Oculovestibular responses, 45
Odynophagia, 302
Olecranon bursitis, 870
Oligoclonal banding, 756
Oligodendroglioma, 728,
    730–731
Omentectomy, 646
Onchocerca removal, 330
Oncogenes, 451–452
Onion skin lesions, 803
Oophorectomy, prophylactic,
    646
Ophthalmoplegia, 681
Ophthalmoscopy, 697

Opiate antagonists, 788
Opioid abuse, 787–788
Opisthotonos, 295
Optic disc atrophy, 683
Optic neuritis, 668–669
optic neuropathy, ischemic,
    669–670
Orbital cellulitis, 673–674
Orbital disease, 673–674
Orbital rhabdomyosarcoma,
    702
Orchiectomy, 605
Organomegaly, 768
Oropharynx, 215
Orthopedic surgery, 770
Orthophosphates, 566
Orthopnea, 57, 126
Osmoreceptors, integrity of, 482
Osmotic diarrhea, 383
Ossicular reconstruction, 656
Osteitis fibrosa cystica, 593
Osteoarthritis
  clinical–pathologic
    correlations of, 835
  diagnosis and differential
    diagnosis of, 835–836,
    837t
  pathophysiology of, 834–835
  signs and symptoms of,
    833–834
  therapy for, 836
Osteoblastic metasases, 612
Osteoclastic activating factor,
    548–549
Osteolytic lesions, 476
Osteomalacia, 553–554, 579,
    593
Osteomyelitis
  clinical–pathologic
    correlations of, 853
  diagnosis and differential
    diagnosis of, 853–856
  pathophysiology of, 850–853
  signs and symptoms of, 850
  therapy for, 856–857
Osteopenia, 637, 797, 828
Osteophytes, 833, 835
Osteoporosis, 476
  clinical–pathologic
    correlations of, 830
  diagnosis and differential
    diagnosis of, 830–832
  pathophysiology of, 828–830
  postmenopausal, 634
  prevention of and therapy for,
    832
  signs and symptoms of, 828
  suspicion of, 635
Osteosclerosis, 593
Otalgia, 651, 659, 660
Otitis media, 652
  chronic, 250
  clinical–pathologic
    correlations of, 659

diagnosis and differential
diagnosis of, 660
pathophysiology of, 658–659
prevention of and therapy for,
660–661
signs and symptoms of,
657–658
with streptococcal
pharyngitis, 265
Otologic disease
diagnosis and differential
diagnosis of, 653–654,
655t
pathophysiology of, 652–653
prevention of and therapy for,
654, 656
signs and symptoms of,
651–652
Otorrhea, 651, 659
Ototoxic drugs, 652
Ovarian carcinoma
diagnosis and differential
diagnosis of, 645–646
pathophysiology of, 644
prevention of and therapy for,
646–647
signs and symptoms of, 644
Ovarian failure, premature, 625
Ovarian function, 621, 633. See
also Menopause;
Menstruation
Oxacillin, 316
Oxygen delivery, 239
Oxygen therapy, 203
Oxygen toxicity, 239
Oxytetracycline, 222
Oxytocin stimulation, 629

Pacemakers, 143
Pacing stress studies, 113
PaCO₂. See Partial pressure of
carbon dioxide
Paget's disease, 411, 610, 613
Palindromic rheumatism, 793
Palliative nephrectomy, 599
Palliative therapy, 470–471
Pancoast's tumors, 204
Pancreatic abscesses, 378
Pancreatic enzyme deficiency,
250
Pancreatic injury, 77
Pancreatitis, 74, 351
chronic, 378
clinical–pathologic
correlations of, 378
diagnosis of, 379–380
differential diagnosis of,
378–379
pathophysiology of, 378
signs and symptoms of,
377–378
therapy for, 380
Pancytopenia, 434, 455, 460
complications of, 302

Panhypopituitarism, 732
Panic disorder, 772–773
Pannus, 796
Pap smear, 312, 641, 642
Papillary carcinomas, 615
Papillary muscle dysfunction,
118
Papillary necrosis, 585
Papilledema, 733, 735
Papillomas, intraductal, 606,
608–609
Paradoxic pulse, 177–179
Paralytic ileus, 74–75
Paranasal sinus infection,
277–280
Paranasal sinus neoplasms,
279
Paraneoplastic syndrome, 204,
205t, 208, 596
Parasitic diseases
diagnosis and differential
diagnosis of, 329–330
pathophysiology, 325–329
prevention of and therapy for,
330
signs and symptoms of,
324–325
Parathyroid hormone, 542
in calcium level control,
546–547
control of, 546
hypomagnesemia and, 549
osteoporosis and, 830
stimulation of, 593
Parathyroid insufficiency, 549
Parathyroidectomy, subtotal,
595
Paravertebral muscle spasm,
876–877
Parenteral alimentation, 88, 357
Parenteral iron, 433
Parkinson's disease, 56
clinical–pathologic
correlations of, 747
diagnosis and differential
diagnosis of, 747–748
pathophysiology of, 746–747
prevention of and therapy for,
748
signs and symptoms of,
745–746
Paroxysmal nocturnal dyspnea,
57, 126
Paroxysmal supraventricular
tachycardia, 152
clinical significance of,
154–155
diagnostic criteria for, 154
signs and symptoms of,
155–156
treatment of, 156
Parrot fever. See Psittacosis
Partial pressure of carbon
dioxide, 8–9

in mixed acid-base
disturbances, 14
Patent ductus arteriosus, 289
Paul-Bunnell heterophile
agglutination test, 272
PCP, 789
Peak expiratory flow rates, 227
Pectinate line, 407
PEEP. See Positive end-
expiratory pressure
PEFR. See Peak expiratory flow
rates
Pelvic abscess, 312
Pelvic fractures, 859
Pelvic inflammatory disease,
396, 617, 619
Penetrating injuries
of abdomen, 77, 78
to chest, 175–179
ocular, 672–673
Penicillamine
for cystine stone, 566
for progressive system
sclerosis, 823
for rheumatoid arthritis, 798
for Wilson's disease, 28, 366
Penicillin
for aortic regurgitation, 174
in atypical pneumonia
treatment, 222
for endocarditis, 294
for lung abscess, 226
for septic arthritis, 849
for staphylococcal infections,
316
for tetanus, 297
for urinary tract infections,
283
Peptic ulcers, 392
clinical–pathologic
correlations of, 351
diagnosis of, 352–353
differential diagnosis of,
351–352
pathophysiology of, 350
penetrating, 351
perforated, 354
signs and symptoms of,
349–350
treatment of, 353–354
Percutaneous transluminal
coronary angioplasty,
111, 116, 125
Perianal abscesses, 387
Perianal diseases, 406–411
Perianal hidradenitis
suppurativa, 409
Pericardial knock, 136
Pericardial tamponade, 77
Pericardiocentesis, 179
Pericarditis, 800
constrictive, 141
fibrinous, 118
nonspecific, 18

Pericolic abscess, gross, 402
Perineal ecchymosis, 78
Periorbital cellulitis, 673–674
Peripartum cardiomyopathy, 134
Peripheral artery disease, 180
  clinical–pathologic correlations of, 183
  diagnosis of, 183–184
  differential diagnosis of, 183
  pathophysiology of, 182–183
  signs and symptoms of, 181–182
  treatment of, 184–186
Peripheral iridectomy, 686
Peripheral neuropathies, 757, 760
Peripheral vascular insufficiency, 853
Peripheral vasoconstriction, 120
Peripheral visual field evaluation, 668
Perirectal abscess, 302
Peristalsis, visible, 71
Peritoneal dialysis, 380
Peritoneal dialysis catheter, 79
Peritoneal irritation, 71, 78
Peritoneal lavage, 79
Peritoneovenous shunting, 372, 419
Peritonsillar abscess, 265
Pernicious anemia, 440, 495
pH levels, 8, 9t
Ph1 chromosome, absence of, 449
Pharyngitis, exudative, 266, 269
Pharynx inflammation, 265–266
Phencyclidine, 789
Phenobarbital, 722
L-Phenylalanine, 476
Phenytoin, 722
Pheochromocytoma, 41, 119
Phleborrheography, 193
Phlebotomy, 28, 449
Phlegmon, 377
Phobias, 771–772
Phoria, 678, 681
Phosphate, 8, 552–553, 556. *See also* Hypophosphatemia
  depletion, 542
Phosphaturia, 547
Phosphorus, 830
Photon absorptiometry, 831
Photophobia, 38, 672, 689
Physical signs, 6
Physical therapy, 100, 798
Physostigmine, 762
Pi system, 200
Pica, 429
Picornavirus, 362
Pituitary adenoma, 487, 732
Pituitary apoplexy, 732
Pituitary function disorders, 625–626

Pituitary gonadotropin assay, 635
Pituitary insufficiency, 496
Pituitary tumors, 625
Placenta, retained, 629
Placenta previa, 630, 631
Plantar fasciitis, 872
Plaques of demyelination, 754
Plasma cell proliferation, 472–473
Plasmacytosis, 474
Plasmapheresis, 752, 820
Plasminogen activation, 286
Plasminogen activators, 124
Platelet disorders, 424, 426, 427t, 803
Platelet microemboli, 160
Pleural biopsy, 259
Pleural effusion
  diagnosis of, 260–262
  differential diagnosis of, 259–260
  pathophysiology and clinical–pathologic correlations of, 258–259
  signs and symptoms of, 258
  therapy for, 262
Pleural fluid evaluation, 217, 261t
Pleural friction rub, 258
Pleural plaques, 262
Pleuritis, 800
Pleurodesis, 262
Plication, 194
Plummer-Vinson syndrome, 429
Pluripotent bone marrow stem cells, 445
Pneumococcal meningitis, 736
Pneumococcal pneumonia, 217
Pneumococcal vaccine, 203, 217, 307
Pneumocystis carinii, 243, 305, 320
Pneumomediastinum, 255
Pneumonia, 210
  acute bacterial, 213–216
    prevention of and therapy for, 217
    signs and symptoms of, 210–212
  atypical, 218–222
  eosinophilic, 243
  with lung abscess, 224, 225
  from obstructing neoplasms, 304
Pneumonic influenza, 273
Pneumonitis, 224, 306
Pneumoperitoneum, 78
Pneumothorax
  clinical–pathologic correlations of, 255
  diagnosis of, 255–256
  pathophysiology of, 255
  signs and symptoms of, 254–255

tension, 77
  therapy for, 256–257
Podagra, 838
Poiseuille equation, 182
Polio, 299
Polyarteritis nodosa, 63, 573, 793, 809, 810, 811
Polyarthralgia, 844–845
Polyarticular synovitis, 793
Polycystic kidneys, 591, 596
Polycythemia, secondary, 243
Polycythemia vera, 445–446, 447
Polydipsia, 481–483, 522
Polydrug abusers, 789–790
Polymyalgia rheumatica, 796, 810, 813, 824–825
  diagnosis and differential diagnosis of, 826
  pathophysiology of, 826–827
  signs and symptoms of, 825–826
  therapy for, 827
Polymyositis, 469
Polyneuropathy, 757, 758, 760
Polypropylene mesh prosthesis, 419
Polyuria, 481, 482
Pontiac fever, 219
Pontine hemorrhage, 714
Popliteal cyst, 192, 793–794, 871
Porphyria, acute intermittent, 85
Porphyria cutanea tarda, 374
Positive end-expiratory pressure measurement of, 239
Postmenopausal bleeding, 634
Postphlebitic syndrome, 190
Postsynaptic acetylcholine, 761–762
Post-traumatic stress disorder, 773–774
Potassium, 6, 529, 531, 540
  in aldosteronism, 34
  depletion, 15, 75, 533
  excretion of, 532–533
  transcellular distribution of, 538
Potassium disorders. *See also* Hyperkalemia; Hypokalemia
  diagnosis and differential diagnosis of, 533
  pathophysiology of, 531–533
  prevention of and therapy for, 533–540
  signs and symptoms of, 529–531
Potassium restriction, 575–576
Potassium supplements, 538
Pott's puffy tumor, 278
PPD test. *See* Purified protein derivative skin test
Prednisone, 476
Preeclampsia-eclampsia, 631

Pregnancy complications, 628–633
  hypertension in, 36, 631–633
  urinary tract infections and, 282
Premature ventricular complexes, 144–146
Prepatellar bursitis, 871
Prerenal azotemia, 583, 584
Presbyopia, 42, 677
Primidone, 722
Prinzmetal's angina, 109
Procainamide, 150
Proctitis, 302, 306, 389, 410
Proctocolectomy, 393
Proctoscopy, 392
Proctosigmoidoscopy, 385
Progesterone, 609
Progesterone receptors, 614
Progestogen challenge test, 621
Proinsulin, 520
Prolactin, 496, 621, 732
Prolactin-secreting tumors, 625
Promethazine, 60
Propionibacterium acnei, 811
Propranolol, 503, 747
Prostaglandin F$_2$, 618
Prostaglandin synthetase inhibitors, 486, 552, 618
Prostaglandins, 549, 617, 619, 820
Prostate cancer
  clinical–pathologic correlations of, 602–603
  diagnosis and differential diagnosis of, 603–604
  metastases of, 602, 603
  pathophysiology of, 601–602
  prevention of and therapy for, 604–605
  signs and symptoms of, 600–601
  stages of, 601, 604
Prostate enlargement, 280
Prosthetic intravascular devices, 289
Prosthetic valve endocarditis, 290
Protein buffers, 8
Protein deficiency, 88, 90, 579. See also Kwashiorkor
Protein electrophoreses, 474
Protein malnutrition, 425
Protein restriction, 576
Protein synthesis, 25
Proteinuria, 572–573, 574. See also Bence Jones proteinuria
  in nephrotic syndrome, 578
  with pregnancy-induced hypertension, 632
Proteus infections, 283
Protozoal diseases, 243, 382
PRPP synthetase, 838
Pruritus ani, 325, 409–410

Pseudocysts, 377–378, 380
Pseudogout, 843
  diagnosis and differential diagnosis of, 842
  pathophysiology and clinical–pathologic correlations of, 842
  signs and symptoms of, 841–842
  therapy for, 842
Pseudohyperkalemia, 533
Pseudohypoparathyroidism, 551
Pseudomembrane formation, 300
Pseudomembranous colitis, 300–301, 387
Pseudomonas aeruginosa, 251, 253, 284, 305
Pseudomonas aeruginosa osteomyelitis, 854
Pseudomonas cepacia infection, 252
Pseudomonas endarteritis, 302
Pseudomonas infections, 283, 303
Pseudomonas vaccine, 307
Pseudomyasthenic syndrome, 750
Pseudo-osteoarthritis, 841
Pseudorheumatoid arthritis, 841
Psittacosis, 218–219, 221
Psoriasis, 846
Psychogenic seizures, 721
Psychologic therapies, 779–780
Psychosocial therapy, 784
  for burn victims, 100
Psychotherapy, 772, 774
  group, 779–780
PTCA. See Percutaneous transluminal coronary angioplasty
Pulmonary capillary pressure increases, 132
Pulmonary capillary wedge pressure, 238
Pulmonary edema, 64, 128, 131, 162
Pulmonary embolism, 119, 129, 190, 215
Pulmonary fibrosis, 241, 249
Pulmonary hemorrhage, 64
Pulmonary histoplasmosis, 338
Pulmonary hypertension, 128, 247
Pulmonary infarction, 63
Pulmonary infections, 218, 223
Pulmonary nodule, 206, 207
Pulmonary vasculature disturbances, 62–63
Pulse-volume recorder, 184
^{32}P-uptake test, 699
Purified protein derivative skin test, 331, 332, 335, 336t
Purine metabolism, 838
Purine nucleoside

phosphorylase deficiency, 322
Purine restriction, 841
Purulent sputum, 215, 216
Pyelography, infusion, 599
Pyelonephritis, 282, 396
Pyelophlebitis, 396
Pyloric dysfunction, 350
Pylorus, 70
Pyogenic meningitis, 733
Pyomyositis, 853
Pyridostigmine, 762
Pyridostigmine bromide, 752
Pyridoxine, 566
  deficiency, 87
Pyrogenic exotoxin C, 315
Pyruvate kinase deficiency, 435

Q fever, 218
Q infarct, 120
Quinidine, 158, 385

Radiation as cause of colitis, 392
Radiation enteritis, 384
Radiation therapy
  for cancer, 208, 615, 643
  for Hodgkin's disease, 470
  for hypernephroma, 599
  immunocompromise with, 304–306
  with multiple myeloma, 476
  for non-Hodgkin's lymphoma, 465
  for retinoblastomas, 699
Radical mastectomy, 615
Radiculopathy, 757
Radioactive iodine uptake, 501
Radioallergosorbent test, 83
Radiohumeral bursitis, 870
Radionuclide ventriculography, 113
Rai staging of leukemia, 459
RAIU. See Radioactive iodine uptake
Range of motion therapy, 770, 798
RAS. See Reticular activating system
Rashes, 17
RAST. See Radioallergosorbent test
Raynaud's disease, 816
Raynaud's phenomenon, 799
  diagnosis and differential diagnosis of, 819
  pathophysiology of, 817–819
  prevention of and therapy for, 819–820
  with progressive systemic sclerosis, 821
  signs and symptoms of, 816–817
Rebound tenderness, 78
Rectal bleeding, 381, 387, 413, 630

Rectal examination, 601
Rectal prolapse, 250–251
Rectovaginal fistula, 409
Rectum injury, 78
Red cell casts, 585
Red cell membrane
      abnormalities, 434
Red eye, 670–673
Reentry, 148, 152
Reflex eye movement, 45
Reflex testing, 766
Reflexes, deep tendon, 760, 766
Reflux esophagitis, 113
Refractive errors, 675–677
Rehabilitative surgery, 798
Rehydration, 552
Reiter's syndrome, 314, 382,
      846, 847, 872
Relapsing fever, 16
Renal arteriography, 599
Renal biopsy, 582
   risks of, 7
Renal cell carcinoma. See
      Hypernephroma
Renal colic, 561
Renal disease, 29, 567, See also
      specific disorders
   end-stage, 281, 570
Renal failure, 538
   acute
      diagnosis and differential
         diagnosis of, 585–588
      pathophysiology of,
         583–585
      prevention of and therapy
         for, 588–589
      signs and symptoms of, 583
   chronic
      diagnosis and differential
         diagnosis of, 594–595
      signs and symptoms of,
         590–594
   with influenza, 274
   progressive, 281
   therapy for, 595
Renal injury, 282
Renal insufficiency, 839
Renal osteodystrophy, 593, 595
Renal parenchymal diseases,
      585
Renal stones, 838
Renal tubular acidosis, 10–11
Renal tubular disorders, 553
Renal vein thrombosis, 578
Renin, 578, 597
Respiratory acidosis, 9t, 12–13
   in ARDS, 235
   treatment of, 15
Respiratory alkalosis, 9t, 12–14
   in ARDS, 235
   treatment of, 15
Respiratory failure, 200, 247
   progressive, 229
   treatment of, 15
Respiratory infections

short-term upper, 662
upper, 265–268
Respiratory insufficiency,
      progressive, 235
Respiratory secretion
      evaluation, 215–216
Respiratory syncytial virus, 268
Rest angina, 109
Restrictive cardiomyopathy,
      134, 136, 138
Reticular activating system,
      45–47
Reticuloendothelial system
      malignancies, 469
Retinal artery occlusion,
      694–695
Retinal detachment, 685, 697
   tractional, 692
Retinal disease, 691–692,
      695–697
   hypertensive, 692–693
   retinal artery occlusion,
      694–695
   retinal vein occlusion,
      693–694
Retinal vein occlusion, 693–694
Retinal venules, nicking of, 693
Retinoblastoma, 725
   diagnosis of, 698–699
   signs and symptoms of, 698
   therapy for, 699–700
Retinopathy
   diabetic, 512
   with hypertension, 29
   microvascular, 511
   of prematurity, 697
Retrocalcaneal bursitis, 871
Retropharyngeal abscess, 265
Retrovirus infection, 317
Revascularization, 121
Reverse isolation, 307
Reverse transcriptase, 317
Reye's syndrome, 274, 276
Rh immune globulin, 629
Rh incompatibility, 765, 768
Rhabdomyolysis, 530, 553
Rhabdomyosarcoma, 702
Rhegmatogenous detachment,
      697
Rheumatic endocarditis, 174
Rheumatic fever, 18, 159–160,
      265
Rheumatic heart disease, 141,
      165
Rheumatoid arthritis, 469, 841,
      847
   clinical–pathologic
      correlations of, 796
   diagnosis and differential
      diagnosis of, 796–798
   pathophysiology of, 795–796
   prevention of and therapy for,
      798
   signs and symptoms of,
      793–795

Rheumatoid factor, 794, 795
Rheumatoid factor test, 826
Riboflavin deficiency, 87
Ribonuclear protein antibodies,
      822
Rickets, 553–554
Riedel's struma, 503
Rifampin, 337, 849
Rinne test, 651
Risus sradonicus, 295
RNA viruses, 451
Root canal disease, 279
Roth's spots, 290
RSV. See Respiratory syncytial
      virus
Rugger jersey spine, 593

S_3 ventricular gallop, 4
Saccular aneurysms, 810
Salicylates, 798, 815
Salmonella colitis, 382
Salmonella gastroenteritis, 381
Sarcoidosis, 17–18, 56, 138, 241,
      246–247, 549
   management of, 249
   pathophysiology of, 248–249
Sarcomas, 464
Sarcomatous tumors of orbit,
      700
Scars, 101–102, 104
Schaumann's bodies, 248
Scheuermann's disease, 864
Schilling test, 443
Schistosoma, 325, 330
Schizophrenia, 780–783
   psychopharmacologic
      investigations of, 782–783
   psychosocial factors of, 782
   therapy for, 783–784
Schmorl's nodes, 830, 874
Schwannomas, 731–732
Scintillating scotoma, 38
Scirrhous carcinoma, 615
Scirrhous desmoplastic
      reaction, 611
Scleral buckling surgery, 697
Sclerodactyly, 821
Scleroderma, 816, 821. See also
      Sclerosis, progressive
      systemic
Sclerosing adenosis, 607, 608
Sclerosis, 819
Sclerosis, progressive systemic
   diagnosis and differential
      diagnosis of, 822
   pathophysiology of, 822–823
   signs and symptoms of,
      821–822
   therapy for, 823
Sclerotic bone, 835
Scoliosis, 860–861
   back pain and, 861–862
   infantile and juvenile,
      863–864
   treatment for, 862–864

Scotoma, central, 668
Scrotal hematoma, 78
Scurvy, 424, 425
Seat belt injury, 77
Segmental mastectomy, 615
Seizures, 522, 722
  diagnosis and differential
      diagnosis of, 721–722
  generalized, 719–720, 721
  partial, 720, 721
  pathophysiology and
      classification of, 719–720
  with pregnancy-induced
      hypertension, 633
  signs and symptoms of,
      720–721
  therapy for, 722–724
  with tetanus, 297
Sella turcica, 624
Sengstaken-Balkemore tube, 69
Senile macular degeneration,
    695–696
Senile plaques, 52
Sensorineural hearing loss, 656
Sentinal loop, 380
Sentinel pile, 408
Sepsis, 284
Septic arthritis, 839
  clinical–pathologic
      correlations of, 846
  diagnosis and differential
      diagnosis of, 846–849
  pathophysiology of, 846
  prevention of and therapy for,
      849
  signs and symptoms of,
      844–846
Septic shock, 286–287
  with abortions, 629
  with bacteremia, 284–288
  treatment of, 288
Septicemia, 284–285, 305
Serologic testing, 222
Serotonin, 777
Serratia infections, 283
Serum protein electrophoresis,
    526
Serum sickness, 809
Sexually transmitted diseases,
    309–316. See also specific
    diseases
Shigella enteritis, 382
Shigellosis, 381
Shock, 82, 177, 507–508
Shunt nephritis, 568, 576
SIADH. See Antidiuretic
    hormone, syndrome of
    inappropriate
Sickle cell crises, 438
Sickle cell disease, 433–434,
    850
Sickle cell trait, 673
SIDS. See Sudden infant death
    syndrome
Sigmoidoscopy, 415

Silhouette sign, 260
Silicosis, 241, 244, 331
Sinus bradycardia, 117
Sinus drainage, 280
Sinus pain, 277
Sinusitis, 250, 265
  acute
    diagnosis of, 279
    differential diagnosis of,
      279
    pathophysiology of,
      278–279
    signs and symptoms of,
      277–278
    therapy for, 279–280
  chronic, 40, 277–280
Sipple's syndrome, 33
Sippy diet, 353
Skin, 95
  burn injuries to, 95–100
  loss of function of, 97
Skin grafting, 100
Skin testing
  for insect venom allergy, 83
  for anergy, 20
Skin-fold thickness index, 94
Skull erosion, 729
SLE. See Systemic lupus
    erythematosis
Sleep abnormalities, 777–778
Small-bowel obstruction, 75
Smoke inhalation, 200, 213
Smoking, elimination of, 599.
    See also Cigarette
    smoking
Sociotherapies, 783
Sodium, 31–33
Sodium bicarbonate excess, 521
Sodium fluoride, 832
Sodium restriction, 35, 163, 575
Sodium-potassium ATPase
    enzyme system, 532
Somatosensory evoked
    potentials, 769
South American
    trypanosomiasis, 325
Spastic cerebral palsy, 764
Spastic dysphonia, 664–665
Spectinomycin, 313
Speech discrimination, 653
Spherocylindrid lenses, 677
Spinal deformities, 860–866
Spinal injuries, 859, 865
Spinal neoplasms, 732
Spinal stenosis, 876
Spinal tap, 726
Spirometry, 231
Spironolactone, 591
Spleen enlargement, 459
Splenectomy, 434, 438, 439
Splenic rupture, 77
Splenomegaly, 247, 270, 445
Splinting, 798
Spondylarthropathies, 796
Spondylolisthesis, 865–866

Spondylolysis, 865
Spondylosis, 878
Sputum, purulent, 215
Sputum tests, 216
Squamous cell epithelioma, 410
Squamous cell neoplasms, 208
Stable angina pectoris, 109
Stannosis, 241
Stanozolol, 819
Staphylococcal enterotoxin F,
    315
Staphylococcal infections, 226,
    383
  of brain, 743
  treatment of, 316
  in urinary tract, 283
Staphylococcus aureus
    infection, 251, 252,
    290–291
Staphylococcus aureus
    pneumonia, 215, 254
Staphylococcus epidermidis,
    291, 305
Staphylococcus osteomyelitis,
    854–855
Starvation, 88. See also
    Malnutrition
Status asthmaticus, 809
Status epilepticus, 724
Steering wheel syndrome, 175
Stenosis, critical, 182
Steroid therapy, 203, 842
Steroidogensis, 637
Still's disease, 18, 793
Stimulant abuse, 788
Stinging insects, 82
Stomach lymphoma, 356
Strabismus, 678–679, 697
Strep throat, 269
Streptococcal pharyngitis,
    265–266
  clinical–pathologic
      correlations of, 266
  pathophysiology of, 265–266
  signs and symptoms of, 265
Streptococcus infection, 736
  of throat, 663
Streptococcus osteomyelitis,
    854
Streptococcus pneumonia,
    278–279
Streptococcus pyogenes
    infection, 265
Streptokinase, 123, 194
Streptolysins, 265–266
Streptomycin, 294
Stress disorder, post-traumatic,
    773–774
Stress tests, 4
Stress ulcers, 99
Stress-management techniques,
    231
Stroke, 716
  clinical–pathologic
      correlations of, 709t, 710

Stroke, (cont.)
diagnosis and differential
diagnosis of, 710–711
pathophysiology of, 708–710
signs and symptoms of,
707–708
therapy for, 712–713
Stroke-in-evolution, 707, 712
Strongyloides infestation, 325
Struvite. *See* Magnesium
ammonium phosphate
stones
Stupor, 44
Subacromial bursitis, 869
Subarachnoid leakage, 718
Subarchnoid hemorrhage,
716–717
Subcutaneous nodules, 793
Subdural empyema, 735, 742
Subdural hematomas, 718
Subdural hemorrhage, 717–718
Subendocardial hemorrhage,
176
Subepicardial hemorrhage, 176
Subfacial herniation, 727
Sublingual nitroglycerin, 116
Suboccipital headache, 42
Substance abuse, 785–790
Sucralfate, 348
Sudden death, 714
Sudden infant death syndrome,
298
Sulfa preparations, 283
Sulfasalazine, 393
Sulfonylurea, 520
Sulfonylurea hypoglycemia
agents, 514
Sulphasalzine therapy, 390
Support groups, 773
Suppressor/cytotoxic function,
321
Suppurative sinusitis, 277
Supralevator abscess, 408
Supraventricular arrhythmias,
152
Supraventricular
tachyarrhythmias, 149
Swan-Ganz catheter, 122, 125
Swan-neck deformities, 793
Swayback deformity, 864
Sweat test, 252–253
Sympathetic stimulation, 128
Synovial biopsy, 797, 848
Synovial fluid examination, 848
Synovitis, 835
Syphilis, 309, 313–314
dementia and, 56
Systemic lupus erythematosus,
3, 18, 63, 469, 596, 796,
836, 847–848
diagnosis and differential
diagnosis of, 803–805
pathophysiology of, 801–803
signs and symptoms of,
799–801
therapy for, 805–806

Systemic vasculitis
clinical–pathologic
correlations of, 812
diagnosis and differential
diagnosis of, 812–813
pathophysiology of, 810–811
prevention of and therapy for,
813–815
signs and symptoms of,
807–810
Systolic click, 160
Systolic function impairment,
128–129, 141
Systolic thrill, 166

Tachypnea, 199, 241
Taenia infestation, 329
Takayasu's arteritis, 810, 813,
815
Tamm-Horsfall protein
secretion, 572
Tamoxifen, 609, 616
Tapeworms, 325
Tardive dyskinesia, 746, 784
Telangiectases, 67, 821
Temporal arteritis, 42, 670
Temporal artery biopsy, 813
Temporomandibular joint
disease, 42
Temporomandibular joint
neuralgia, 651
Tendonitis
pathophysiology and
diagnosis of, 867–872
of shoulder, 868–870
therapy for, 872
Tennis elbow, 870
Tenosynovitis, 867, 871
Tenovaginitis, 870
TENS. *See* Transcutaneous
electric nerve stimulation
Tensilon test, 760
Tension pneumothorax, 257
Test panel, 5–6
Testicular torsion, 418
Tetanospasmin, 295
Tetanus, 99, 295–297
Tetanus immune globulin, 297
Tetanus toxoid boosters, 297
Tetany, 543, 546
Tetracycline, 222, 315
Thalamic hemorrhage, 715
Thalassemia major, 438
Thalassemia syndromes, 436
Thalassemia trait, 431
Thallium 201 myocardial
perfusion imaging, 113
Thermal injuries. *See* Burn
injuries
Thiamine deficiency, 87
Thiazides, 549, 566
Thioamide, 493
Third-trimester bleeding,
630–631
Thoracentesis, 262
Thoracolumbar injuries, 865

Thoractomy, 179
Throat clearing, compulsive,
665, 666
Thrombectomy, 194
Thrombi, 236
Thrombocythemia, essential,
445, 446, 449
Thrombocytopenia, 286, 424,
426, 428, 450, 459, 803
Thrombocytosis, 432, 447, 449
Thromboembolism, 158
Thrombolytic therapy, 121,
123–125
Thrombophlebitis, 119, 129,
189, 606
Thrombosed hemorrhoids, 408
Thrombosis, 711
acute occlusion from, 182
deep vein
clinical–pathologic
correlations of, 192
diagnosis of, 192–193
differential diagnosis of,
192
pathophysiology of,
190–192
prevention of and therapy
for, 193–194
signs and symptoms of, 190
microvascular, 795
with myocardial infarction,
125
Thrombotic thrombocytopenia
purpura, 574
Thromboxane, 426, 820
Thymectomy, 762
Thyroid blocking antibodies,
496
Thyroid function tests, 502
Thyroid gland autonomy, 491
Thyroid hormone, 489, 609
Thyroid replacement, 497
discontinuation of, 496–497
Thyroid storm, 487
Thyroid surgery, 493–494
Thyroid-binding globulin, 493
Thyroidectomy, 494
Thyroid-hormone resistance
syndromes, 493
Thyroiditis
acute nonsuppurative, 487,
494
acute suppurative, 499
chronic lymphocytic, 501
clinical–pathologic
correlations of, 502
diagnosis and differential
diagnosis of, 502–503,
504*t*
pathophysiology of, 501
signs and symptoms of,
499–501
subacute, 496, 499, 501
toxic chronic lymphocytic,
494
treatment of, 503

Thyroid-stimulating hormone, 486–497, 501
Thyrotoxicosis, 750
Thyrotropin-releasing hormone stimulation test, 491, 495
Thyroxin-binding globulin, 491
Thyroxine deficiency, 494
TIAs. *See* Transient ischemic attacks
Tibial fractures, 859
Tick paralysis, 299
Tinnitus, 652, 656, 659, 731
T-lymphocytes, 321
  in demyelination process, 754–755
  immunoregulatory, 801
Tonic contraction, 295
Tonic-clonic seizures, 720, 721, 724
Tonsillar herniation, 727
Tonsils
  enlargement of, 269
  inflammation of, 265–266
Torsade-de-pointes, 150
Total parenteral hyperalimentation, 392
Toxemia, 631
Toxic adenoma, 487
Toxic lesions, 44, 45, 47
Toxic megacolon, 300, 301, 381
Toxic shock syndrome, 315–316
Toxic-metabolic dementias, 56
Toxoplasma gondii, 269, 272
Trabeculae thinning, 828, 830
Tracheobronchial tree injuries, 97
Tracheostomy, 297
Traction, 878
Traction headache, 41–42
Transbronchial biopsy, 306
Transcortin levels, 578
Transcutaneous electric nerve stimulation, 878
Transferrin, 430, 431, 578
Transient cerebral ischemia, 708
Transient ischemic attacks, 707, 710–711, 713–714
Transluminal angioplasty, 121
Transmural infarct, 120
Transudates, 259, 260
Trauma, abdominal, 77–81
Traumatic heart disease
  clinical–pathologic correlations of, 176–177
  diagnosis of, 177–179
  pathophysiology of, 176
  prevention of and therapy for, 179
  signs and symptoms of, 175–176
Traumatic tattoo, 102
Travelers' diarrhea, 382–383
Tremors, 747
Trendelenburg's test, 187
Trental, 184
Treponema pallidum, 313

Triamterene, 591
Trichinella spiralis infestation, 329
Trichomonas infection, 309
Tricyclics. *See* Antidepressants, tricyclic
Trigeminal schwannomas, 731
Trigeminy, 144
Triidothyronine deficiency, 494
Triiodothyronin, 497
Trimethoprim-sulfamethoxazole, 279, 307
Trismus, 295
Trisomy 21. *See* Down's syndrome
Trochanteric bursitis, 870
Trochlear palsies, 681–682
Trophic ulcers, 853
Tropia, 678, 681
Trypsin, 378
Trypsinogen, 379
Tubal pregnancy, 398
Tube thoracostomy, 262
Tube-dilution susceptibility testing, 293
Tuberculosis, 18, 243, 392, 506, 663
  clinical–pathologic correlations of, 334
  diagnosis of, 335–336
  differential diagnosis of, 334–335
  pathophysiology of, 332–333
  prevention of and therapy for, 336–337
  signs and symptoms of, 331–332
Tuberculous infections, 844
Tuberculous meningitis, 736, 737
Tuberculous osteomyelitis, 855
Tuberculous sclerosis, 725
Tubular necrosis, acute, 583
Tumors, 355t
  gastrointestinal bleeding and, 66–67
  of posterior fossa, 42
  of stomach, 354
Turner's sign, 77
Turner's syndrome, 624–625
Tylectomy, 615
Tympanic membrane, 658
  mobility of, 660
  perforation of, 659
Tympanocentesis, 660
Tympanometry, 653, 660
Typhoid fever, 18

Ulceration, 189
Ulcerative colitis, 387
Ultrasonography, 184, 193, 359, 375
Umbilical hernia, 419
Uncal herniation, 718, 727

Unstable angina pectoris, 109, 117
Uranium mining, 208
Urate levels, 838
Uremic neuropathy, 594
Uremic pericarditis, 591–593
Uremic syndrome, 602
Ureter injury, 78
Ureteral obstruction, 418
Ureteral stricture, 282
Urethra infection, 280
Urethral injuries, 78
Urethral obstruction, 280
Urethritis, 280, 283, 314
Uric acid, 34, 838
Uric acid stones, 563, 566
Uric acid-calcium oxalate, 839
Uricosuric drugs, 841
Urinary obstruction, 282, 602
Urinary sodium level, 585
Urinary tract hypertonicity, 282
Urinary tract infection, 280
  diagnosis of, 283
  pathophysiology of, 282–283
  prevention of and therapy for, 283
  signs and symptoms of, 281
Urine volume, 282
Urobilinogen, 23
Uterine carcinoma
  of uterine cervix, 641–643
  of uterine corpus, 639–641
Uterine hyperplasia, 640
Uterine leiomyoma, 619
Uterine target organ disorders, 624
Uveitis, 246, 670, 673

Vaginal bleeding, 630, 640
  premenopausal, 639, 640–641
Vaginal discharge, 309–310
Vaginal strawberry spots, 311
Vaginitis, 309–311, 634
Vagotomy, 381
Valvular disease, 292
Valvular incompetency, 187, 189
Valvuloplasty, 170
Vancomycin, 294, 301, 849
Varicose veins, 187, 188
Vascular claudication, 800
Vascular disease, 585
  of brain, 707–713
Vascular headache, 37–40
Vascular lesions, 67
Vascular tissue-phase defects, 425
Vasculitis, 807–815, 827
Vasoactive intestinal polypeptide, 384
Vasoconstriction, 693
Vasoconstrictors, 689
Vasodilator therapy, 36, 132–133, 143, 656
Vasogenic edema, 727
Vasomotor nephropathy, 583

Vasomotor rhinitis, 40, 268, 279
Vasopressin, 69, 481, 483–486
Vasopressin analogue, 483–486
Vasospasm, 180
VDRL tests, 221
Vegetations, 290, 293
Vein stripping, 189
Vein transplant, 189
Venacaval ligation, 194
Venacavography, 599
Venereal disease, 604
Venom immunotherapy, 83, 84
Venous insufficiency, 131
    clinical–pathologic
        correlations of, 188
    diagnosis of, 189
    differential diagnosis of,
        188–189
    pathophysiology of, 187–188
    signs and symptoms of, 187
    therapy for, 189
Venous occlusions, 189
Venous stasis, 191, 194
Ventilation, 15
Ventral hernia, 417
Ventricle, 118
Ventricular arrhythmias, 529
    diagnosis of, 149
    differential diagnosis of,
        149–150
    pathophysiology of, 147–149
    precipitating factors of, 146t
    signs and symptoms of,
        144–146
    treatment of, 146, 150–151
Ventricular fibrillation, 117,
    144, 151
Ventricular flutter, 151
Ventricular hypertrophy, 34
Ventricular infarction, right, 117
Ventricular premature beats,
    149
    grading system, 147t, 148
Ventricular tachycardia, 117,
    125
    diagnosis of, 149
    differential diagnosis of,
        149–150
    pathophysiology of, 147–149
    signs and symptoms of,
        146–147
    treatment of, 150–151
Ventriculography, 132
Verrucous endocarditis, 800
Vertebral artery circulation, 707
Vertebral column fractures,
    864–865

Vertebral osteomyelitis, 855
Vertigo, 652, 653, 656
Vesicoureteral reflux, 280, 282
Vincent's angina, 266
Vincristine, 245, 476, 699
Viral encephalitides, 56, 742
Viral hepatitis
    clinical–pathologic
        correlations of, 364–366
    diagnosis of, 366
    differential diagnosis of, 366
    pathophysiology of, 362–364
    prevention of and therapy for,
        366–367
    signs and symptoms of,
        361–362
Viral infections, 251
    cardiomyopathy and, 134
    of CNS, 755
    upper respiratory, 213
Viral meningitis, 736
Viral pneumonia, 131
Virchow's triad, 191, 192t, 193
Viridans streptococci, 291
Visual accommodation, 676, 677
Visual acuity, best-corrected,
    679
Visual acuity testing, 677–678
Visual evoked potentials, 769
Visual field examination, 685
Visual loss. See also Blindness
    acute painless monocular,
        668–670
    central, 696
    from macular edema, 693
    with uveitis, 673
Vitamin A
    deficiency, 87
    excessive, 550
    malabsorption, 26
Vitamin B_{12}, 440
    deficiency, 440, 441–443
Vitamin C, 355
    deficiency, 87
Vitamin D
    in calcium level control, 546,
        547
    deficiency of, 26, 549,
        553–554, 579
    excessive, 550
    intoxication, 551
    for osteoporosis, 832
    supplementation, 551, 579
Vitamin deficiency, 87, 90
Vitamin E, 609, 697
Vitamin K deficiency, 26, 423,
    425, 428

Vitrectomy, 697
Vitreous hemorrhage, 692, 697
Vocal cords, 663
    failure of, 661–667
Vocal function disorders
    abusive, 665–666
    functional, 666–667
Vocal nodules, 665
Vocal polyps, 665–666
Voice abuse, 664
Voice therapy, 667
Volume depletion, 12, 372
Volvulus, 72, 74
von Hippel-Lindau disease, 596,
    725
Von Recklinghausen's disease,
    725, 731
von Willebrand's disease, 423
von Willebrand's factor, 425
Vulvar irritation, 311

Waldenstrom's
    macroglobulinemia, 458,
    474
Warfarin, 194
"Watch tick" test, 651
Water loss, systemic, 482, 483
Water restriction, 575
Water-drinking, compulsive,
    522, 523
Wegener's granulomatosis, 63,
    574, 810, 813, 815
Weight reduction, 35, 116
Werdnig-Hoffmann disease, 758
Wet gangrene, 181
Wheezing, 230
Whipple's disease, 17, 56
Whipple's triad, 519, 520
Wilson's disease, 28, 56, 366
Withdrawal bleeding, 621
Wolff-Parkinson-White
    syndrome, 121, 149, 158
Wound healing, 101–105
Wound infection, 105
Wound inspection, 101

Xanthine oxidase inhibitors
    for gout, 841

Yersinia infection, 382

Zero-decibel loss, 653
Zollinger-Ellison syndrome, 352
Zoster immune globulin, 307